# Sleep Disorders Medicine

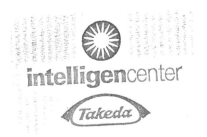

# Sleep Disorders Medicine:
## Basic Science, Technical Considerations, and Clinical Aspects

SECOND EDITION

Edited by

## Sudhansu Chokroverty, M.D., F.R.C.P., F.A.C.P.

Professor of Neurology, New York Medical College, Valhalla; Clinical Professor of Neurology, University of Medicine and Dentistry of New Jersey–Robert Wood Johnson Medical School, New Brunswick; Associate Chairman of Neurology, Chairman, Division of Neurophysiology, and Director, Center of Sleep Medicine, Saint Vincent's Hospital and Medical Center of New York

Foreword by

## Robert B. Daroff, M.D.

Professor of Neurology and Associate Dean, Case Western Reserve University School of Medicine, Cleveland; Chief of Staff and Senior Vice President for Academic Affairs, University Hospitals of Cleveland

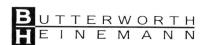

Boston   Oxford   Johannesburg   Melbourne   New Delhi   Singapore

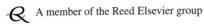

**Library of Congress Cataloging-in-Publication Data**

Sleep disorders medicine: basic science, technical considerations,
    and clinical aspects / [edited by] Sudhansu Chokroverty. -- 2nd ed.
        p.   cm.
    Includes bibliographical references and index.
    ISBN 0-7506-9954-X
    1. Sleep disorders.   I. Chokroverty, Sudhansu.
    [DNLM: 1. Sleep Disorders. 2. Sleep--physiology.   WM 188 S6323
1999]
    RC547.S534  1999
    616.8'498--dc21
    DNLM/DLC
    for Library of Congress                                                98-4115
                                                                              CIP


**British Library Cataloguing-in-Publication Data**
A catalogue record for this book is available from the British Library.

The publisher offers special discounts on bulk orders of this book.
For information, please contact:

Manager of Special Sales
Butterworth–Heinemann
225 Wildwood Avenue
Woburn, MA 01801-2041
Tel: 781-904-2500
Fax: 781-904-2620

For information on all Butterworth–Heinemann medical publications available,
contact our World Wide Web home page at: http://www.bh.com

10 9 8 7 6 5

Printed in the United States of America

*To my wife, Manisha Chokroverty, M.D.; my daughters, Linda Chokroverty, M.D.,
and Keka Chokroverty, B.A.; and my parents, Debendranath Chokroverty, M.A., LLB, FCA,
and Ashalata Chokroverty*

# Contents

# Contributing Authors

**Michael W. Anderson, Ph.D.**
Director, The Sleep Disorders Center, Overland Park Regional Medical Center, Overland Park, Kansas

**Richard P. Allen, Ph.D.**
Assistant Professor of Neurology, Johns Hopkins University School of Medicine, Baltimore; Co-Director of Sleep Disorders, Department of Neurology, Johns Hopkins Bayview Medical Center, Baltimore

**Barbara G. Bigby, M.A.**
Associate Director, Medical Research Center of Scripps Clinic, La Jolla, California

**Roger J. Broughton, M.D.**
Professor of Neurology and Cellular and Molecular Medicine (with cross appointment, School of Psychology), University of Ottawa, Ottawa, Ontario; Medical Director, Sleep Medicine Center, Ottawa Hospital (General Site), Ottawa

**Daniel J. Buysse**
Associate Professor of Psychiatry, Sleep and Chronobiology Center, University of Pittsburgh Medical Center, Pittsburgh

**Rafael de Jesus Cabeza, Ph.D.**
Assistant Professor of Biological Sciences, The University of Texas at El Paso

**Rosalind D. Cartwright, Ph.D.**
Professor and Chairman of Psychology, Rush Medical College of Rush University, Chicago; Director, Sleep Disorder Service and Research Center, Rush-Presbyterian-St. Luke's Medical Center, Chicago

**Sudhansu Chokroverty, M.D., F.R.C.P., F.A.C.P.**
Professor of Neurology, New York Medical College, Valhalla; Clinical Professor of Neurology, University of Medicine and Dentistry of New Jersey–Robert Wood Johnson Medical School, New Brunswick; Associate Chairman of Neurology, Chairman, Division of Neurophysiology, and Director, Center of Sleep Medicine, Saint Vincent's Hospital and Medical Center of New York

**William C. Dement, M.D., Ph.D.**
Lowell W. and Josephine Q. Berry Professor of Psychiatry and Behavioral Sciences, Stanford University School of Medicine, Stanford, California; Director, UCSF Stanford Health Care Sleep Disorders Clinic and Laboratory, Palo Alto, California

**Karl Doghramji, M.D.**
Associate Professor of Psychiatry and Human Behavior, Jefferson Medical College of Thomas Jefferson University, Philadelphia; Director, Sleep Disorders Center, Thomas Jefferson University Hospital, Philadelphia

**Milton G. Ettinger, M.D.**
Professor of Neurology, University of Minnesota Medical School—Minneapolis; Retired Chief of Neurology, Hennepin County Medical Center, Minneapolis

**Richard Ferber, M.D.**
Associate Professor of Clinical Neurology, Harvard Medical School, Boston; Director, Center for Pediatric Sleep Disorders, Department of Neurology, Children's Hospital, Boston

**J. Christian Gillin, M.D.**
Professor of Psychiatry and Director of Mental Health Clinical Research Center, University of California, San Diego, School of Medicine; Staff Psychiatrist, VA San Diego Healthcare System, San Diego

**Christian Guilleminault, M.D.**
Professor, Center for Excellence in Research, Diagnosis, and Treatment of Sleep Disorders, Stanford University School of Medicine, Stanford, California

**Wayne A. Hening, M.D., Ph.D.**
Clinical Assistant Professor of Neurology, University of Medicine and Dentistry of New Jersey–Robert Wood Johnson Medical School, New Brunswick

**Max Hirshkowitz, Ph.D.**
Associate Professor of Psychiatry, Baylor College of Medicine, Houston; Director, Sleep Research Center, Psychiatry Services, Veterans Affairs Medical Center, Houston

**Sharon A. Keenan, Ph.D.**
Director of The School of Sleep Medicine, Palo Alto, California

**Thomas S. Kilduff, Ph.D.**
Senior Research Scientist, Center for Sleep and Circadian Neurobiology, Departments of Biological Sciences and Department of Psychiatry and Behavioral Sciences, Stanford University School of Medicine, Stanford, California

**John B. Kostis, M.D.**
Professor and Chairman of Medicine, John G. Detwiler Professor of Cardiology, and Professor of Pharmacology, University of Medicine and Dentistry of New Jersey–Robert Wood Johnson Medical School, New Brunswick; Chief of Medical Service, Robert Wood Johnson University Hospital, New Brunswick

**Clete A. Kushida, M.D., Ph.D.**
Director, Stanford University Center for Human Sleep Research; Staff Physician and Clinical Instructor, Stanford University Sleep Disorders Clinic, Stanford University School of Medicine, Stanford, California

**Mark W. Mahowald, M.D.**
Professor of Neurology, University of Minnesota Medical School—Minneapolis; Director, Minnesota Regional Sleep Disorders Center, Hennepin County Medical Center, Minneapolis

**Robert W. McCarley, M.D.**
Professor of Psychiatry, Harvard Medical School, Boston; Deputy Chief of Staff, Mental Health Services, Department of Psychiatry, Brockton/West Roxbury Veterans Administration Medical Center, Brockton, Massachusetts

**Emmanuel Mignot, M.D., Ph.D.**
Associate Professor of Psychiatry and Director of the Center for Narcolepsy Research, Stanford University School of Medicine, Stanford, California

**Merrill M. Mitler, Ph.D.**
Professor of Neuropharmacology, The Scripps Research Institute, La Jolla, California; Psychologist, The Scripps Clinic, La Jolla

**Constance A. Moore, M.D,**
Director, Veterans Affairs Medical Center and Baylor Sleep Disorders Center, Baylor College of Medicine, Houston

**Maurice M. Ohayon, M.D., D.Sc., Ph.D.**
Director, Centre de Reserche Philippe Pinel de Montréal, Montréal, Quebec

**Richard A. Parisi, M.D.**
Associate Professor of Medicine, University of Medicine and Dentistry of New Jersey–Robert Wood Johnson Medical School, New Brunswick; Robert Wood Johnson University Hospital

**J. Steven Poceta, M.D.**
Consultant in Neurology and Sleep Disorders, Division of Neurology, The Scripps Clinic, La Jolla, California

**Christine M. Quinto, M.D.**
Research Fellow in Clinical Neurophysiology, St. Vincent's Hospital and Medical Center of New York and New York Medical College, Valhalla

**Anstella Robinson, M.D.**
Stanford University Sleep Disorders Clinic, Stanford University School of Medicine, Stanford, California

**Timothy A. Roehrs, Ph.D.**
Adjunct Professor of Psychiatry and Behavioral Neurosciences, Wayne State University School of Medicine, Detroit; Director of Research, Sleep Disorders and Research Center, Henry Ford Hospital, Detroit

**Leon Rosenthal, M.D.**
Adjunct Associate Professor, Wayne State University School of Medicine, Detroit; Medical Director, Sleep Disorders and Research Center, Henry Ford Hospital, Detroit

**Thomas Roth, Ph.D.**
Chief, Division of Sleep Medicine, Henry Ford Hospital, Detroit, Michigan

**Mark H. Sanders, M.D.**
Professor of Medicine and Anesthesiology, Division of Pulmonary, Allergy, and Critical Care Medicine, University of Pittsburgh School of Medicine; Chief of Pulmonary Sleep Disorders Program, University of Pittsburgh Medical Center; Assistant Chief, Pulmonary Service, Veterans Affairs Medical Center, Pittsburgh

**Carlos H. Schenck, M.D.**
Associate Professor of Psychiatry, University of Minnesota Medical School—Minneapolis; Staff Psychiatrist, Minnesota Regional Sleep Disorders Center, Hennepin County Medical Center, Minneapolis

**Daniel M. Shindler, M.D.**
Associate Clinical Professor of Medicine, University of Medicine and Dentistry of New Jersey–Robert Wood Johnson Medical School, New Brunswick; Director, Echocardiography Laboratory, Robert Wood Johnson University Hospital, New Brunswick

**Arthur J. Spielman, Ph.D.**
Professor of Psychology and Director, Sleep Disorders Center, City College of the City of New York; Director, Westchester Division of The Sleep Disorders Center of Columbia-Presbyterian Medical Center, New York

**Mircea Steriade, M.D., D.Sc.**
Professor of Physiology, Laval University School of Medicine, Quebec

**Ronald A. Stiller, Ph.D., M.D.**
Clinical Assistant Professor of Medicine, University of Pittsburgh School of Medicine; Director, Sleep Laboratory, University of Pittsburgh Medical Center–Shadyside Hospital, Pittsburgh

**Patrick J. Strollo, Jr., M.D.**
Associate Professor of Medicine and Anesthesiology, Division of Pulmonary, Allergy, and Critical Care Medicine, University of Pittsburgh School of Medicine

**Michael J. Thorpy, M.D.**
Associate Professor of Neurology, Albert Einstein College of Medicine of Yeshiva University, Bronx, New York; Director, Sleep Disorders Center, Montefiore Medical Center, Bronx

**Thaddeus Walczak, M.D., F.A.C.P.**
Assistant Professor of Neurology and Director, Epilepsy Monitoring Unit, Columbia University College of Physicians and Surgeons, New York; Attending Neurologist, Columbia-Presbyterian Medical Center, New York

**Arthur S. Walters, M.D.**
Associate Professor of Neurology, University of Medicine and Dentistry of New Jersey–Robert Wood Johnson Medical School, New Brunswick; Staff Physician, Neurology Service, Lyons Veterans Affairs Medical Center, Lyons, New Jersey

**Virgil D. Wooten, M.D.**
Director, Sleep Disorders Center of Greater Cincinnati, TriHealth, Bethesda Oak Hospital, Cincinnati; Volunteer Professor of Psychiatry, University of Cincinnati College of Medicine

**Rebecca K. Zoltoski, Ph.D.**
Assistant Professor of Basic Health and Sciences, Illinois College of Optometry, Chicago

# Foreword

In the foreword to the first edition of *Sleep Disorders Medicine*, published in 1995, Norman H. Edelman cited the *1993 Report of the National Commission on Sleep Disorders Research* indicating that 40 million Americans suffered from sleep disorders, often unrecognized. He commented on the multidisciplinary approach necessary for the diagnosis and management of sleep disorders and noted that the contributors to the text reflected the relevant diverse disciplines. The popularity and success of the first edition prompted this important second edition, which will be welcomed by both sleep experts and their novice trainees.

In Chapter 2, Dr. Chokroverty reviews the societal and medical concepts of sleep from biblical times to the present. The advances in our understanding of sleep over the past several decades are remarkable. Although Aserinsky and Kleitman described rapid eye movement (REM) sleep in 1953, I never heard it mentioned while a medical student in the late 1950s, nor as a neurology resident in the early 1960s. My personal introduction to REM sleep came in a 1964 chapter written by William C. Dement (who wrote Chapter 1 of this text) in a book on eye movements emanating from a National Institutes of Health–sponsored symposium in 1961. Dement's chapter contained 113 references reflecting research largely undertaken in the 8 years after the discovery of REM—research not then translated into clinical or bedside relevance for a neurology trainee. Fortunately, the basic and clinical sciences of sleep are now being incorporated into many medical school curricula and are essential aspects of training for neurologists, pulmonologists, and psychiatrists—both adult and pediatric.

This second edition contains eight new chapters: Neurophysiologic Mechanisms of Non–Rapid Eye Movement Sleep (Chapter 4), Dreaming in Sleep Disordered Patients (Chapter 7), Circadian Regulation of Sleep (Chapter 8), Maintenance of Wakefulness Test (Chapter 14), Computerized and Portable Sleep Recording (Chapter 15), Epidemiology of Sleep Disorders (Chapter 20), Human and Animal Genetics of Sleep and Sleep Disorders (Chapter 21), and Sleep-Related Violence and Forensic Medicine Issues (Chapter 35). These are welcome additions to an already superb text.

I have always regarded Dr. Chokroverty as one of our best neurologic scholars, educators, and critical thinkers. His interests are catholic and his acumen acute—a man for all neurologic seasons. He and his contributors deserve our grateful kudos for this new edition.

*Robert B. Daroff*

# Preface to the Second Edition

Sleep and its mysteries are continuing to unravel. Electrifying progress has been made in the field of sleep medicine in this century. The discovery of electroencephalography in 1929, rapid eye movement (REM) sleep in 1953, existence of human pacemaker (circadian clock) in the suprachiasmatic nuclei in 1972, location of the site of dysfunction in obstructive sleep apnea syndrome in 1965, noninvasive treatment using continuous positive airway pressure in upper airway obstructive sleep apnea syndrome in 1981, and the clock gene in the fruit fly *Drosophila* in the 1990s are examples of some of these advances. Despite this tremendous progress, we keep asking the basic questions without arriving at satisfactory answers: What is sleep? and Why do we sleep?

It is, however, gratifying to see that sleep medicine is gradually taking its rightful place as society is becoming increasingly aware of the growing importance of sleep and its disorders. This awareness is reflected in the frequent publication of sleep-related articles in the lay press (television, radio, and print media). The medical profession and the allied health profession are also taking increasing interest in the field. This bodes well for the science and art of sleep medicine and is a tremendous boost to those who have a sleep disorder—approximately one-third of the population.

The medical profession is coming to terms with a fact aptly summarized by Eugene Robin about 40 years ago (cited by Richard Martin in the preface of the second edition of *Cardiorespiratory Disorders During Sleep*): "The sleeping patient is still a patient. His disease not only goes on while he sleeps, but indeed may progress in an entirely different fashion from its progression during the waking state." Sleep medicine is now taking its place as an important medical discipline. A sleep center has now been established—the National Center for Sleep Disorders Research (NCSDR)—within the National Institutes of Health. Thanks to the efforts of the NCSDR, American Sleep Disorders Association, American Thoracic Society, National Sleep Foundation, and the Sleep Section of the American Academy of Neurology, the medical profession and the public alike are aware of the fact that sleep disorders are a serious health hazard.

Since the publication of the first edition of this book in 1995, an exponential growth in the science of sleep has taken place. Remarkable progress has been made in our understanding of the molecular biological and the basic science aspects of sleep, including new information about the role of sleep factors (e.g., adenosine) in the homeostatic regulation of sleep (Chapter 3); circadian rhythm, chronophysiology, chronopharmacology and chronotherapy (Chapters 8 and 30); the immune system and sleep (Chapter 2); and the impact of genetics (Chapter 21) on sleep medicine.

In this edition, eight new chapters have been added. In the first edition, no chapter covering dreams was included. Rosalind D. Cartwright has written such a chapter for this edition (Chapter 7). A new chapter dealing extensively with the mechanism of non-REM sleep has been written by Mircea Steriade (Chapter 4). Thomas S. Kilduff's and Clete A. Kushida's chapter on the basic science aspect of circadian regulation is new to this edition (Chapter 8). A chapter on the maintenance of wakefulness test by Karl Doghramji (Chapter 14) complements the Multiple Sleep Latency Test chapter (Chapter 13). To reflect the increasing application of computers in medicine, Max Hirshkowitz and Constance A. Moore have contributed a chapter on computer and portable sleep recording (Chapter 15). Chapter 20, on the epidemiology of sleep disorders, by Maurice M. Ohayon and Christian Guilleminault, and Chapter 21, on genetics in sleep medicine, by Emmanuel Mignot, both serve to increase our understanding of the importance of neurobiology and epidemiology of sleep disorders. The insomnia chapter of the first edition, written by Dr. Walsh, has been replaced by Arthur J. Spielman's chapter, which provides a structured interview and a thorough discussion of treatment planning (Chapter 24). Finally, as societies throughout the world witness increased violence, the chapter on sleep-related violence and forensic medicine issues by Mark W. Mahowald and Carlos H. Schenck is timely (Chapter 35). The other existing chapters have been largely revised and updated with recent references and some new illustrations. The chapter on ambulatory cassette recording that appeared in the first edition has been deleted.

The purpose of the second edition remains the same as that of the first edition, namely, to provide a comprehensive understanding of the clinical sleep disorders with adequate emphasis on the underlying basic science foundation for the clinicians and scientists with an interest in sleep disorders. The format also remains the same: Initial descriptions of the basic aspects of sleep are followed by discussions of sleep technology and finally comprehensive descriptions of clinical sleep disorders.

*Sudhansu Chokroverty*

# Preface to the First Edition

Sleep, that gentle tyrant,[1] has aroused the interest of mankind since time immemorial, as reflected in the writings of the Eastern and Western religions and civilizations (e.g., Upanishad,[2] circa 1000 BC wrote about "the dreaming" and "a deep dreamless sleep"; see Chapter 2). Even though there are many poetic, philosophical, and religious references to the phenomenon, and to the mystical nature of sleep, the science of sleep has been very slow to evolve. In the last 40 years, however, an explosive growth took place in the basic and clinical aspects of sleep research. Recent major discoveries and advances include the discovery of REM sleep and the cyclic pattern of non-REM–REM sleep stages throughout a human being's night sleep; the standardized sleep-scoring technique; the discovery of the mechanism of sleep apnea and better management of this disorder; better understanding of the nature of narcolepsy; an awareness of the parasomnias, their treatment, and their differentiation from epilepsy; phototherapy for circadian rhythm and other sleep disorders; pharmacotherapy for insomnias; and better understanding of the treatment of sleep apnea and hypoventilation related to neuromuscular disorders. Other significant recent developments include the formation of the Association of Sleep Disorders Centers, growing numbers of sleep disorders centers, formal certification for accreditation of such centers, formation of the American Board of Sleep Medicine to test practitioners' competency in sleep disorders medicine, publication of the scientific journal *Sleep*, and incorporation of the subject of sleep in other subspecialty board examinations (e.g., American Board of Clinical Neurophysiology: Added Qualifications in Clinical Neurophysiology). Growing awareness in the medical profession of the importance of sleep is reflected in the development of training programs in sleep disorders medicine, approval by the American Academy of Neurology for a section on sleep, and the formation of the National Commission on Sleep Disorders Research (NCSDR). The latter is significant because experts in the sleep field are now voicing their concerns in the political arena. The study of sleep has come a long way, and in this Decade of the Brain it is hoped that sleep medicine will find its rightful place as an independent specialty in the broad field of medicine.

---

[1]Webb WB. Sleep: The Gentle Tyrant. Bolton, MA: Anker Publishing, 1992.
[2]Wolpert S. A New History of India. New York: Oxford University Press, 1982;48.

Dement[3] defined sleep disorders medicine as the branch of medicine that deals with the sleeping brain and all manifestations and pathologies deriving therefrom. Sleep disturbances affect as many as one-third of all American adults, and about 40 million Americans suffer from chronic disorders of sleep and wakefulness. The majority of those affected remain undiagnosed and untreated (executive summary and findings NCSDR).[4] Therefore, education in sleep disorders medicine is urgently needed. This book aims to provide clinicians in many disciplines who have an interest in sleep and sleep disorders with a comprehensive scientific basis for understanding sleep, as well as to present information on the diagnosis and treatment of a wide variety of sleep disorders, which are, increasingly, being recognized. The purpose, therefore, is to produce a comprehensive treatise on sleep disorders medicine, not only for beginners but also for those who are already engaged in the art and science of sleep medicine. Thus, it is meant to be a practical exposition of the subject that also provides an appropriate foundation in the basic science. With these objectives in mind the monograph is divided into three sections: basic aspects of sleep, sleep technology, and the clinical science of sleep. The monograph is directed to all who are interested in sleep disorders medicine and should, therefore, be useful to neurologists, internists (particularly those subspecializing in pulmonary, cardiovascular, or gastrointestinal medicine), psychiatrists, psychologists, pediatricians, otolaryngologists, neurosurgeons, general practitioners dealing with many apparently undiagnosed sleep disorders patients, and neuroscientists with an interest in sleep research.

*Sudhansu Chokroverty*

---

[3]Dement WC. A personal history of sleep disorders medicine. J Clin Neurophysiol 1990;7:17.
[4]National Commission on Sleep Disorders Research. Report of the National Commission on Sleep Disorders Research. DHHS Pub. No. 92-XXXX. Washington, DC: U.S. Government Printing Office, 1992.

# Acknowledgments

I am indebted to all the contributors for their scholarly contributions. I am especially grateful to Robert B. Daroff, one of the finest clinicians, neuroscientists, and educators, for his kind and thoughtful foreword to the second edition. I wish to thank all the authors, editors, and publishers who granted us permission to reproduce illustrations that were published in other books and journals, as well as the American Sleep Disorders Association for giving me permission to reproduce the glossary of terms that appeared in the *International Classification of Sleep Disorders* and the graph showing the rapid growth of the sleep disorders centers.

It is my pleasure to acknowledge the efforts of my assistant, Erika Thompson, for typing and retyping several chapters in addition to her other duties.

Special thanks are due to Susan Pioli, Director of Medical Publishing at Butterworth–Heinemann, for her professionalism, helpful suggestions, pleasant discourse, and patience. I must also acknowledge with great appreciation, the splendid support of Jana Friedman, Associate Editor, and the staff at Butterworth–Heinemann for the production of the book.

Last but not the least, I wish to express my utmost appreciation to my wife, Manisha Chokroverty, M.D., for patience, tolerance, support, and encouragement throughout the long period, including the precious weekends, during production of this book.

*Sudhansu Chokroverty*

# Sleep Disorders Medicine

# Part I
# Basic Aspects of Sleep

# Chapter 1
# Introduction

William C. Dement

Sleep disorders medicine is based primarily on the understanding that human beings have two fully functioning brains—the brain in wakefulness and the brain in sleep. Cerebral activity has contrasting consequences in the state of wakefulness versus the state of sleep. In addition, the brain's two major functional states influence each other. Problems during wakefulness affect sleep, and disordered sleep or disordered sleep mechanisms impair the functions of wakefulness. Perhaps the most common complaint addressed in sleep disorders medicine is impaired daytime alertness (i.e., excessive sleepiness).

Critical to sleep disorders medicine is the fact that some function (e.g., breathing) may be normal during the state of wakefulness but pathologic during sleep. Moreover, a host of nonsleep disorders are, or may be, modified by sleep. It should no longer be necessary to argue that an understanding of a patient's health includes equal consideration of the state of the patient asleep and awake. The knowledge that patient care is a 24-hour commitment is fundamental to one aspect of sleep medicine: circadian regulation of sleep and wakefulness. It is worth suggesting that of all industries operating on a 24-hour schedule, it is the medical profession that should lead the way in developing techniques for resetting the biological clock to promote full alertness and optimal performance in those who must work at night.

## WHAT IS SLEEP DISORDERS MEDICINE?

"Sleep disorders medicine is a clinical specialty which deals with the diagnosis and treatment of patients who complain about disturbed nocturnal sleep, excessive daytime sleepiness, or some other sleep-related problem."[1] The spectrum of disorders and problems in this area is extremely broad, ranging from the minor such as a day or two of mild jet lag, to the catastrophic such as sudden infant death syndrome, fatal familial insomnia, or an automobile accident caused by a patient with sleep apnea who falls asleep at the wheel. The dysfunctions may be primary, involving the basic neural mechanisms of sleep and arousal, or secondary, in association with other physical, psychiatric, or neurologic illnesses. Where the associations with disturbed sleep are very strong, such as in endogenous depression and immune disorders, it has not yet been established that sleep mechanisms play a causal role. However, progress is being made in this area.

In sleep disorders medicine it is critical to examine the sleeping patient and to evaluate the impact of sleep on waking functions. Physicians in the field have an enormous responsibility to address the societal implications of sleep disorders and problems, particularly impaired alertness. This responsibility is heightened by the fact that the transfer of sleep medicine's knowledge base to the mainstream education system is far from complete, and effective public and professional awareness has not been accomplished. All physicians should be sensitive to the level of alertness in their patients and the potential consequences of falling asleep in the workplace, at the wheel, or elsewhere.

## A BRIEF HISTORY

Well into the nineteenth century the phenomenon of sleep escaped systematic observation, despite the fact that sleep occupies one-third of a human lifetime. All other things being equal, we may assume that there were a variety of reasons not to study sleep, one of which was the unpleasant necessity of staying awake at night.[2]

Although there is some evidence of sleep disorder research in the 1960s, including a fee-for-service narcolepsy clinic at Stanford University and research on illnesses related to inadequate sleep such as asthma and hypothyroidism at the University of California, Los Angeles,[3,4] sleep disorders medicine can be identified as having begun in earnest at Stanford University in 1970. The researchers at Stanford routinely used respiration and cardiac sensors together with electroencephalography, electro-oculography, and electromyography in all-night, polygraphic recordings. Continuous all-night recording using this array of data-gathering techniques was finally named polysomnography by Holland and colleagues,[5] and patients at Stanford paid for the tests as part of a clinical fee-for-service arrangement.

The Stanford model included responsibility for medical management and care of patients beyond mere interpretation of the test results and an assessment of daytime sleepiness. After several false starts, the latter effort culminated in the development of the Multiple Sleep Latency Test,[6,7] and the framework for the development of the discipline of sleep medicine was complete.

The comprehensive evaluation of sleep in patients who complained about their daytime alertness rapidly led to a series of discoveries, including the high prevalence of obstructive sleep apnea in patients complaining of sleepiness, the role of periodic limb movement in insomnia, the sleep misperception syndrome first called *pseudoinsomnia*, and so on. As with the beginning of any medical practice, the case-

series approach, wherein patients are evaluated and carefully tabulated, was very important.[8]

## THE PRESENT

Nasal continuous positive airway pressure and uvulopalatopharyngoplasty replaced tracheostomy as treatment for obstructive sleep apnea in 1981.[9,10] At that time, the field of sleep medicine entered a period of significant growth that has not abated. The number of accredited sleep disorders centers and laboratories has increased almost exponentially since 1977 (Figure 1-1). In 1990, a congressionally mandated national commission began its study of sleep deprivation and sleep disorders in American society with the goal of resolving some of the problems impeding access to treatment for millions of patients. The last decade of the twentieth century, however, will be recognized as a time when federal growth began to slow to a stop. Consequently, the growth of sleep medicine as a specialty practice has also slowed, although it is far from stopping. Nevertheless, the increasing competition for limited federal funds means that there is a great need for sleep disorders medicine to enter the mainstream of the health care system and for the knowledge obtained in this field to be disseminated throughout our education system.

With the incorporation of the American Board of Sleep Medicine, the creation of the National Center on Sleep Disorders Research, the continuing strength of patient and professional sleep societies, and recognized textbooks, a healthy foundation of sleep medicine is certainly in place. The population prevalence of obstructive sleep apnea has been established—this one illness afflicts 30 million people.[11] Gallup Polls suggest that one-half of all Americans have a sleep disorder. Given the grossly inadequate public and professional awareness of sleep disorders and problems, one must conclude that most of the millions of individuals afflicted with sleep disorders, some of which can lead to death, do not recognize their disorder and therefore do not obtain the benefits available to them.

There is a continuing need for effective presentation of the organized body of knowledge of sleep disorders medicine, and this book responds to that need. Every individual involved in this field must work toward the goal of improving education on sleep disorders, work that is not only critical for

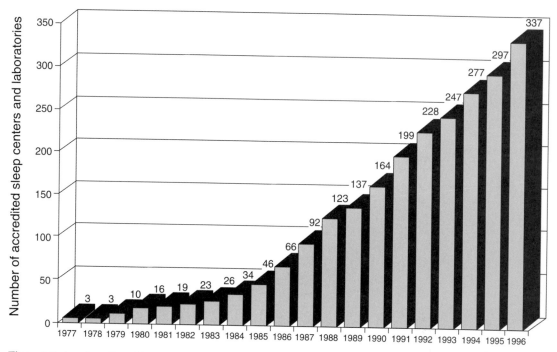

**Figure 1-1.** American Sleep Disorders Association (ASDA)–accredited sleep centers and laboratories shown graphically. (Reprinted with permission from ASDA.)

medical school students, but important for all other levels of scholarship as well.

## REFERENCES

1. Walsh J. Sleep Disorders Medicine. Rochester, MN: Association of Professional Sleep Societies, 1986.
2. Dement W. A personal history of sleep disorders medicine. Clin Neurophysiol 1990;7:17.
3. Kales A, Beall GN, Bajor GF, et al. Sleep studies in asthmatic adults: relationship of attacks to sleep stage and time of night. J Allergy Clin Immunol 1968;41:164.
4. Kales A, Heuser G, Jacobsen A, et al. All night sleep studies in hypothyroid patients, before and after treatment. J Clin Endocrinol Metab 1967;27:1593.
5. Holland V, Dement W, Raynal D. Polysomnography responding to a need for improved communication. Presented at annual meeting of Sleep Research Society, Jackson Hole, Wyoming, 1974.
6. Carskadon M, Dement W. Sleep tendency: an objective measure of sleep loss. Sleep Res 1977;6:200.
7. Richardson G, Carskadon M, Flagg W, et al. Excessive daytime sleepiness in man: multiple sleep latency measurement in narcoleptic and control subjects. Electroencephalogr Clin Neurophysiol 1978;45:621.
8. Dement W, Guilleminault C, Zarcone V. The Pathologies of Sleep: A Case Series Approach. In: D Tower (ed), The Nervous System (Vol 2). The Clinical Neurosciences. New York: Raven, 1975;501.
9. Fujita S, Conway W, Zorick F, et al. Surgical correction of anatomic abnormalities in obstructive sleep apnea syndrome: uvulopalatopharyngoplasty. Otolaryngol Head Neck Surg 1981;89:923.
10. Sullivan CE, Issa FG, Berthon-Jones M, Eves L. Reversal of obstructive sleep apnea by continuous positive airway pressure applied through the nares. Lancet 1981;1:862.
11. Young T, Palta M, Dempsey J, et al. The occurrence of sleep-disordered breathing among middle-aged adults. N Engl J Med 1993;328:1230.

# Chapter 2
# An Overview of Sleep

Sudhansu Chokroverty

## HISTORICAL PERSPECTIVE

Since the dawn of civilization, the mysteries of sleep have intrigued poets, artists, philosophers, and mythologists. The fascination with sleep is reflected in literature, folklore, religion, and medicine. *Upanishad*[1,2] (circa 1000 BC), the ancient Indian textbook of philosophy, sought to divide human existence into four states: the waking, the dreaming, the deep dreamless sleep, and the superconscious ("the very self"). One finds the description of pathologic sleepiness (possibly a case of Kleine-Levin syndrome) in the mythologic character Kumbhakarna in the great Indian epic *Ramayana*[3,4] (circa 1000 BC). Kumbhakarna would sleep for months at a time, then get up to eat and drink voraciously before falling asleep again.

The definition of sleep and a description of its functions have always baffled scientists. Moruzzi,[5] while describing the historical development of the deafferentation hypothesis of sleep, quoted the concept Lucretius articulated 2,000 years ago—that sleep is the *absence of wakefulness.* A variation of the same concept was expressed by Hartley[6] in 1749, and again in 1830 by Macnish.[7] Macnish defined sleep as *suspension of sensorial power,* in which the voluntary functions are in abeyance, but the involuntary powers, such as circulation or respiration, remain intact. The modern sleep scientist defines sleep on the basis of both behavioral and physiologic criteria.[8,9] The behavioral criteria include (1) lack of mobility or slight mobility, (2) closed eyes, (3) reduced response to external stim-

ulation (i.e., increased arousal threshold), (4) characteristic sleeping posture, and (5) reversibly unconscious state.[8] The physiologic criteria (see Sleep Architecture and Sleep Profile) are based on the findings from electroencephalography (EEG), electro-oculography (EOG), and electromyography (EMG).

Throughout literature, a close relationship between sleep and death has been perceived, but the rapid reversibility of sleep episodes differentiates sleep from coma and death. There are myriad references to sleep, death, and dream in poetic and religious writings, including the following quotations: "The deepest sleep resembles death" (*The Bible*, I Samuel 26:12); "sleep and death are similar . . . sleep is one-sixtieth [i.e., one piece] of death" (*The Talmud*, Berachoth 576); "There she [Aphrodite] met sleep, the brother of death" (Homer's *Iliad*, circa 700 BC); "To sleep perchance to dream. . . . For in that sleep of death what dreams may come?" (Shakespeare's *Hamlet*); "How wonderful is death; Death and his brother sleep" (Shelly's "Queen Mab").

Sleep and wakefulness, the two basic processes of life, are like two different worlds, with independent controls and functions. The reader should consult Borbely's monograph *Secrets of Sleep*[2] for an interesting historical introduction to sleep.

What is the origin of sleep? The words *sleep* and *somnolence* are derived from the Latin word *somnus;* the German words *sleps, slaf,* or *schlaf;* and the Greek word *hypnos.* Hippocrates, the father of medicine, postulated a humoral mechanism for sleep and asserted that sleep was caused by the retreat of blood and warmth into the inner regions of the body, whereas the Greek philosopher Aristotle thought sleep was related to food, which generates heat and causes sleepiness. Paracelsus, a sixteenth-century physician, wrote that "natural" sleep lasted 6 hours, eliminating tiredness and refreshing the sleeper. He also suggested that people not sleep too much or too little, but awake when the sun rises and go to bed at sunset. This advice from Paracelsus is strikingly similar to modern thinking about sleep. Views about sleep in the seventeenth and eighteenth centuries were expressed by Alexander Stuart, the British physician and physiologist, and by the Swiss physician, Albrecht von Haller. According to Stuart, sleep was due to a deficit of the "animal spirits"; von Haller wrote that the flow of the "spirits" to the nerves was cut off by the thickened blood in the heart, resulting in sleep. Nineteenth-century scientists used principles of physiology and chemistry to explain sleep. Both Humboldt and Pfluger thought that sleep resulted from a reduction or lack of oxygen in the brain.[2]

Ideas about sleep were not based on solid scientific experiments until the twentieth century. Ishimori,[10] in 1909, and Legendre and Pieron,[11] in 1913, observed sleep-promoting substances in the cerebrospinal fluid of animals during prolonged wakefulness. The discovery of the EEG waves in dogs by the English physician Caton[12] in 1875 and of the alpha waves from the surface of the human brain by the German physician Hans Berger[13] in 1929 provided the framework for contemporary sleep research. It is interesting to note that Kohlschutter, a nineteenth-century German physiologist, thought sleep was deepest in the first few hours and became lighter as time went on.[2] Modern sleep laboratory studies have generally confirmed these observations.

The golden age of sleep research began in 1937 with the discovery by American physiologist Loomis and colleagues[14] of different stages of sleep reflected in EEG changes. Aserinsky and Kleitman's[15] discovery of rapid eye movement (REM) sleep in the 1950s at the University of Chicago electrified the scientific community and propelled sleep research to the forefront. This was followed by Rechtschaffen and Kales'[16] technique of sleep scoring based on results of the EEG, EMG, and EOG, which has become the gold standard for sleep scoring throughout the world. The other significant milestone in the history of sleep medicine was the discovery in 1965 (independently) by Gastaut and

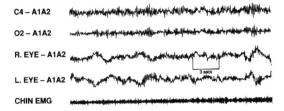

**Figure 2-1.** Polysomnographic recording shows wakefulness. Note 9–10 Hz alpha activity in the EEG (C4-A1A2; O2-A1A2: International nomenclature) mixed with some low-amplitude beta activity. Chin EMG (electromyography) shows much tonic activity. Waking eye movements are seen in the electro-oculographies (right and left eyes are referred to linked ear—A1A2). Paper speed: 10 mm/sec. Timer: 3 secs. Calibration: 50 μV for EEG and eye channels; 20 μV for EMG channel.

colleagues[17] in France and Jung and Kuhlo[18] in Germany of upper airway obstruction during sleep in patients with sleep apnea syndrome.

## SLEEP ARCHITECTURE AND SLEEP PROFILE

Sleep is not a homogeneous state. It has two separate and distinct states based on behavioral and physiologic characteristics: non–rapid eye movement (NREM) and REM sleep.[16,19–21]

### Non–Rapid Eye Movement Sleep

NREM sleep accounts for 75–80% of sleep time in an adult human. NREM sleep is further divided into four stages, primarily on the basis of EEG criteria: stage I, comprising approximately 3–8% of sleep time; stage II, occupying approximately 45–55% of total sleep time; and stages III and IV, making up approximately 15–20% of sleep time. Stages III and IV NREM sleep are together described as *slow-wave sleep* (SWS).

The beginning of stage I NREM sleep in adults is heralded by the diminution of the alpha waves of wakefulness in the EEG (Figure 2-1) to fewer than 50% in an epoch (Figure 2-2). The alpha waves are replaced by theta (and some beta) waves, accompanied by slow, rolling eye movements represented in the EOG recordings. Muscle tone decreases slightly, detected by the EMG.

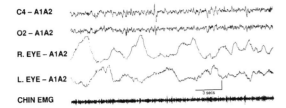

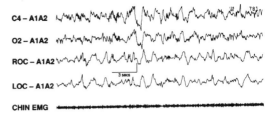

**Figure 2-2.** Polysomnographic recording shows stage I NREM sleep. EEGs (top two channels) show a decrease of alpha activity to less than 50% and low-amplitude, mixed-frequency activities in the range of 3–7 Hz. Note vertex sharp waves in the midportion of the EEGs. Electro-oculo-graphies (right and left eyes) show slow, rolling eye movements. Tonic electromyography (EMG) persists. Paper speed, timer, and calibration are as in Figure 2-1.

**Figure 2-4.** Polysomnographic recording shows stage III NREM sleep. EEG (top two channels) shows 20–50% of the epoch occupied by waves of 2 Hz or less with amplitudes greater than 75 μV from peak to peak. Paper speed, timer, and calibration are as in Figure 2-1.

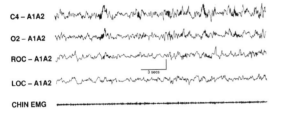

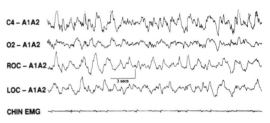

**Figure 2-3.** Polysomnographic recording shows stage II NREM sleep. Note 14-Hz sleep spindles in the EEG channels. No eye movements are seen. Tonic electromyography (EMG) persists, although EMG activity is less than in wakefulness and stage I. Paper speed, timer, and calibration are as in Figure 2-1. (ROC, LOC = electro-oculography of right and left eye, respectively.)

**Figure 2-5.** Polysomnographic recording shows stage IV NREM sleep. More than 50% of the epoch in the EEG (top two channels) now consists of waves of 2 Hz or less with amplitudes greater than 75 μV. Electro-oculographies (third and fourth channels from top) are contaminated with EEG waves. Paper speed, timer, and calibration are as in Figure 2-1.

Within a few minutes, the hypnogram shows bursts of 12- to 16-Hz sleep spindles intermixed with K complexes. Vertex sharp waves are noted toward the end of stage I and are also present in stage II NREM sleep (Figure 2-3), which is dominated by the spindles. The EOG does not register eye movements in stage II, and tone as measured by the EMG is less than in wakefulness or stage I sleep. The EEG shows theta and delta waves (fewer than 20%) in stage II sleep, which lasts approximately 30–60 minutes. Sleep next progresses to the stages of SWS, characterized by delta waves on the EEG. The delta waves constitute 20–50% of the EEG in stage III (Figure 2-4) and more than 50% in stage IV (Figure 2-5). Toward the end of the SWS, or deep sleep, body movements are registered as artifacts in the polysomnographic recordings. Stages III and IV NREM sleep are briefly interrupted by stage II NREM sleep, which is followed by the first REM sleep approximately 60–90 minutes after sleep onset.

### Rapid Eye Movement Sleep

REM sleep accounts for 20–25% of total sleep time. Based on EEG, EMG, and EOG criteria, REM sleep can be divided into two stages: tonic and phasic. A desynchronized EEG, hypotonia or atonia of the major muscle groups, and depression of monosynaptic and polysynaptic reflexes are characteristics of the tonic stage. The phasic stage is discontinuous and superimposed on the tonic stage. The phasic events are marked by bursts of REM, myoclonic twitchings of the facial and limb muscles, irregularities of heart rate and respiration with variable blood pressure, spontaneous activity of the middle ear muscles, and tongue movements.[21,22] The EEG during REM sleep (Figure 2-6) is characterized by a

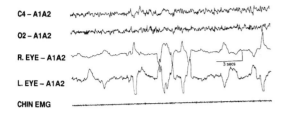

C4 – A1A2

O2 – A1A2

R. EYE – A1A2

3 secs

L. EYE – A1A2

CHIN EMG

**Figure 2-6.** REM sleep stage is shown in the polysomno-graphic recording. EEG (top two channels) shows low-amplitude, mixed-frequency theta, including some alpha activity without any sleep spindles or K complexes. REMs are seen in the electro-oculographies (third and fourth channels from above, right and left eyes). EMG (electromyography) shows marked reduction or absence of tonic activities. Paper speed, timer, and calibration are as in Figure 2-1.

low-voltage fast pattern mixed with a small amount of theta rhythm, and, often, "sawtooth" waves that may herald the onset of REM sleep.

The first REM period lasts only a few minutes; progression to stage II is next, followed by stage III and IV NREM sleep before the second REM sleep begins. A full sleep cycle consists of a sequence of NREM and REM, and each cycle lasts approximately 90–110 minutes. Generally, four to six full sleep cycles are observed during a night's sleep. The first two cycles are dominated by SWS (stages III and IV NREM sleep). These stages are noted only briefly in the later cycles, sometimes not at all. In contrast, the REM sleep cycle increases in duration from the first to the last full sleep cycle, and the longest REM cycle, occurring

toward the end of the night, may last as long as 1 hour. Thus, the SWS is dominant in the first third of the night and REM sleep is dominant in the last third. This characteristic sleep cycling is noted in both humans and animals. Table 2-1 lists the behavioral and physiologic characteristics of states of awareness.

## ONTOGENY OF SLEEP

Newborns have a polyphasic sleep pattern and spend about two-thirds of their first few days of life sleeping. On falling asleep, a newborn baby goes immediately into REM sleep, or active sleep, which is accompanied by restless movements of the arms and legs and the facial muscles. In premature babies it is often difficult to differentiate REM from wakefulness. This multiphasic sleep pattern gradually changes into the monophasic adult pattern.[20,23–25] By the age of about 3 months, the usual NREM-REM cyclic pattern is evident. Polyphasic sleep changes to biphasic sleep in preschool children, and finally to monophasic sleep in adults. Sleep reverts to biphasic or multiphasic in the elderly.

During the first few months of an infant's life REM sleep decreases. The EEG begins to show an adult sleep pattern with the appearance of spindles at approximately 3 months,[26] and K complexes at 6 months.[27] Although an NREM-REM cycle is noted in children, it is shorter lived than in adults. At age 1 year the cycle may last 45–50 minutes, whereas at age 5–10 years it increases to 60–70 minutes. At

**Table 2-1.** Behavioral and Physiologic Criteria for States of Awareness

| Criteria | Awake | NREM Sleep | REM Sleep |
|---|---|---|---|
| **Behavioral** | | | |
| Posture | Erect, sitting, or recumbent | Recumbent | Recumbent |
| Mobility | ++ | + | ± or − |
| Response to stimulation | ++ | + or ± | ± or − |
| Level of alertness | Alert | Reversibly unconscious | Reversibly unconscious |
| Eye movements | Waking eye movements | Slow eye movements | Rapid eye movements |
| **Physiologic** | | | |
| EEG | Alpha waves or desynchronized | Synchronized; spindles, V waves, K complexes, slow waves | Desynchronized; theta waves; "sawtooth" waves |
| Muscle tone (electro-myography) | ++ | + | ± or − |
| Electro-oculography | Waking eye movements | Slow eye movements | Rapid eye movements |

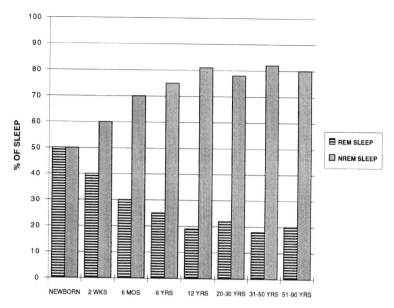

**Figure 2-7.** Graphic representation of percentages of REM and NREM sleep at different ages. Note the dramatic changes in REM sleep in the early years. (Adapted from HP Roffwarg, JN Muzzio, WC Dement. Ontogenic development of the human sleep-dream cycle. Science 1966;152:604–619.)

approximately age 10, adult REM sleep cycles (90–110 minutes) and REM percentages (20–25%) are observed. In older people, delta waves are less pronounced but the percentage of REM sleep remains relatively constant. Older adults have difficulty sleeping and often awaken frequently during the early morning. Elderly people often complain about increasingly poor sleep. The evolution of sleep stage distribution in newborns, infants, children, adults, and elders is shown schematically in Figure 2-7. Figure 2-8 shows night sleep histograms of a child, a young adult, and an elderly person.

## SLEEP HABITS

Sleep specialists sometimes divide people into two groups, "evening types" and "morning types."[2] The morning types wake up early feeling rested and refreshed, and work efficiently in the morning. These people get tired and go to bed early in the evening. In contrast, evening types have difficulty getting up early and they feel tired in the morning; they feel fresh and energetic toward the end of the day. These people perform best in the evening. They go to sleep late at night and wake up late in the morning. The body temperature rhythm takes on different curves in these two types of people.[2] The body temperature reaches the evening peak an hour

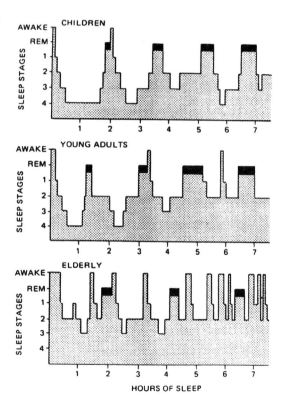

**Figure 2-8.** Night sleep histogram from a child, a young adult, and an elderly person. Note significant reduction of stage IV NREM sleep as one grows older. (Reproduced with permission from A Kales, JD Kales. Sleep disorders: recent findings in the diagnosis and treatment of disturbed sleep. N Engl J Med 1974;290:487.)

earlier in morning types than in evening types. What determines a morning or evening type is not known, but heredity may play a role.

## NEED FOR SLEEP

The average adult's sleep requirement is approximately 7½–8 hours, regardless of environmental or cultural differences.[25,28–30] Webb and Friel[31] observed that approximately 1.1% of college students sleep fewer than 5.5 hours and 3.2% sleep 9.5 hours.

The most important epidemiologic study to determine a relationship between the duration of sleep and the health of the individual was conducted by Kripke and colleagues.[32] They found that the chances of death from coronary artery disease, cancer, or stroke are greater for those who sleep fewer than 4 hours or more than 9 hours than for those who sleep an average of 7–8 hours. No personality trait or other psychological factor has been found that might differentiate "long" or "short" sleepers from average sleepers.

Taub and Berger[33] have clearly shown that our efficiency decreases if we sleep too much. These authors have also drawn attention to the fact that sometimes exhaustion and irritability may follow excessive sleep, which they refer to as the *Rip Van Winkle effect*.[34] The study by Benoit and colleagues[35] showed that long sleepers spend more time asleep but have less stage III and stage IV and more stage II sleep than short sleepers.

## DREAM AND SLEEP

Humankind has been fascinated by dreams since time immemorial. Since the discovery of REM sleep by Aserinsky and Kleitman,[15] dream research has taken a new direction. It is now believed that most dreams occur on awakening from REM sleep, but dreams also occur on awakening from NREM sleep.[2,25,36] However, there are some differences in the dreams experienced in the two kinds of sleep. REM sleep dreams appear to be more emotionally charged, complex, and bizarre, whereas NREM dreams are more realistic and rational. It should be remembered that people awakening from REM sleep are generally oriented, but are somewhat disoriented and confused on awakening from NREM sleep.

What is the significance of dreams? The most important contemporary dream research has been conducted by Hobson and McCarley,[37] who suggest that dreams result from activation of the neural networks in the brain. According to Koukkou and Lehmann,[38] dreams result from restructuring and reinterpretation of data stored in memory. This resembles Jouvet's[39] hypothesis of REM sleep relating to recently acquired information. According to molecular biologists Crick and Mitchison,[40] the function of dreaming is to unlearn, that is, to remove unnecessary and useless information from the brain. The biological significance of dreams at present remains unknown.

## PHYLOGENY OF SLEEP

Studies have been conducted to find out if, like humans, other mammals have sleep stages.[2,41–44] The EEG recordings of mammals show similarities to those of humans. Both REM and NREM sleep stages can be differentiated by EEG, EMG, and EOG in animals. Although dolphins and Australian spiny anteaters (the monotremes, or egg-laying mammals, *echidna*) show no REM sleep on recordings,[2,45,46] some recent evidence suggests that these egg-laying mammals do have REM sleep.[47,48] Siegel and colleagues[48] suggest that the echidna combines REM and NREM aspects of sleep in a single sleep state. These authors further suggest that REM and NREM sleep evolved from a single, phylogenetically older sleep state.

Like humans, mammals can be short or long sleepers. There are considerable similarities between sleep length and length of sleep cycles in small and large animals. Small animals with a high metabolic rate have a shorter life span and sleep longer than larger animals with lower metabolic rates.[49] Smaller animals also have a shorter REM-NREM cycle than larger animals.

A striking finding in dolphins is that during sleep half the brain shows the characteristic EEG features of sleep while the other half shows the EEG features of waking.[50] Each sleep episode lasts approximately 30–60 minutes; then the roles of the two halves of the brain reverse. Similar unihemispheric sleep episodes are known to occur in the pilot whale and porpoise.[8]

Both vertebrates and invertebrates display sleep and wakefulness.[51] Most animals show the basic rest-activity rhythms during a 24-hour period.

There is behavioral and EEG evidence of sleep in birds but the avian REM-NREM cycles are very short.[52] Although birds are thought to have evolved from reptiles, the question of the existence of REM sleep in reptiles remains somewhat controversial.[51] Another controversy centers on the question of whether REM and NREM sleep evolved independently in birds and mammals. Sleep has also been noted in invertebrates, such as insects, scorpions, and worms, based on behavioral criteria.[53]

In conclusion, the purpose of studying the phylogeny of sleep is to understand the neurophysiologic and neuroanatomic correlates of sleep as one ascends the ladder of phylogeny from inframammalian to mammalian species. Tobler[8] concluded that sleep is homeostatically regulated, in a strikingly similar manner, in a broad range of mammalian species. These similarities in sleep and its regulation among mammals suggest common underlying mechanisms that have been preserved in the evolutionary process.

## CIRCADIAN SLEEP-WAKE RHYTHM

The existence of circadian rhythms has been recognized since the eighteenth century, when the French astronomer de Mairan[54] noted a diurnal rhythm in heliotrope plants. The plants closed their leaves at sunset and opened them at sunrise, even when they were kept in darkness, shielded from direct sunlight. The discovery of 24-hour rhythm in the movements of plant leaves suggested to de Mairan an "internal clock" in the plant. Experiments by chronobiologists Pittendrigh[55] and Aschoff[56] clearly proved the existence of 24-hour rhythms in animals.

The term *circadian rhythm*, coined by chronobiologist Halberg,[57] is derived from the Latin *circa*, which means *about*, and *dian*, which means *day*. Experimental isolation from all environmental time cues (German *Zeitgebers*), has clearly demonstrated the existence of a circadian rhythm in humans independent of environmental stimuli.[58,59] The circadian cycle lasts approximately 25 hours (ranging from 24.7 to 25.2 hours) instead of the 24 hours of a day-night cycle.[2,60,61] Ordinarily, environmental cues of light and darkness synchronize or entrain the rhythms to the night-day cycle; however, the existence of environment-independent, autonomous rhythm suggests that the human body also has an internal biological clock.[2,58-61]

The experiments in rats in 1972 by Stephan and Zucker[62] and Moore and Eichler[63] clearly identified the site of the biological clock, located in the suprachiasmatic nucleus in the hypothalamus, above the optic chiasma. Experimental stimulation, ablation, and lesion of these nuclei altered circadian rhythms. The existence of the suprachiasmatic nucleus (SCN) in humans was confirmed by Lydic and colleagues.[64] There has been clear demonstration of the neuroanatomic connection between the retina and the suprachiasmatic nuclei—the retinohypothalamic pathway[65]—that sends the environmental cues of light to the SCN. The SCN serves as a pacemaker, and the neurons in the SCN are responsible for generating the circadian rhythms.[59,66-68] Several neurotransmitters have been located within terminals of the SCN afferents and interneurons, including serotonin, neuropeptide Y, vasopressin, vasoactive intestinal peptide, and γ-aminobutyric acid.[59,68,69]

Daily rhythms are noted in several other human physiologic processes. Body temperature rhythm is sinusoidal, and cortisol and growth hormone secretion rhythms are pulsatile. It is well-known that plasma levels of prolactin, growth hormone, and testosterone are all increased during sleep at night[25] (see Chapter 6). Melatonin, the hormone synthesized by the pineal gland (see Chapter 6), is secreted maximally during night and may be an important modulator of human circadian rhythm entrainment by the light-dark cycle. Sleep decreases body temperature, whereas activity and wakefulness increase it. It should be noted that internal desynchronization occurs during free-running experiments, and the rhythm of body temperature dissociates from the sleep rhythm as a result of that desynchronization.[2,25,59-61] This raises the question of whether there is more than one circadian (or internal) clock or circadian oscillator.[2] The existence of two oscillators was postulated by Kronauer and colleagues.[70] They suggested that a 25-hour rhythm exists for temperature, cortisol, and REM sleep, and that the second oscillator is somewhat labile and consists of the sleep-wake rhythm. Other authors,[71] however, have suggested that one oscillator could explain both phenomena. It is important to be aware of circadian rhythms, because several sleep disturbances are related to alterations in them, such as those associated with shift work and jet lag.

## CHRONOBIOLOGY, CHRONOPHARMACOLOGY, AND CHRONOTHERAPY

Sleep specialists are becoming aware of the importance of chronobiology, chronopharmacology, and chronotherapy.[72] *Chronobiology* refers to the study of the body's biological responses to time-related events. All biological functions of the cells, organs, and the entire body have circadian (approximately 24 hours), ultradian (<24 hours), or infradian (>24 hours) rhythms. It is important, therefore, to understand how the body responds to treatment at different times throughout the circadian cycle,[72] and that circadian timing may alter the pathophysiologic responses in various disease states (e.g., resulting exacerbation of bronchial asthma at night and a high incidence of stroke late at night and myocardial infarction early in the morning; see Chapter 29).

Biological responses to medications may also depend on the circadian timing of administration of the drugs. Potential differences of responses of antibiotics to bacteria, or of cancer cells to chemotherapy or radiotherapy, depending on the time of administration, illustrate the importance of chronopharmacology.[72]

Circadian rhythms can be manipulated to treat certain disorders, a technique called *chronotherapy.* Examples of this are phase advance or phase delay of sleep rhythms and application of bright light at certain periods of the evening and morning.

## SLEEP DEPRIVATION AND SLEEPINESS

Many Americans (e.g., doctors, nurses, firefighters, interstate truck drivers, police officers, overnight train engineers) work irregular sleep-wake schedules and alternating shifts, making them chronically sleep deprived.[73,74] A survey study[73] found that, compared with the population at the turn of the century (1910–1911), Americans are sleeping 1.5 hours less per 24-hour period. This does not mean we need less sleep today but that people are sleep deprived. It should be noted, however, that there may be a sampling error in these surveys (i.e., approximately 2,000 people were surveyed in 1910–1911, vs. 311 in the later survey). Factors that have been suggested to be responsible for this reduction of total sleep include environmental and cultural changes, such as increased environmental light; increased industrialization; growing numbers of people doing shift work; and the advent of television and radio. A review of the epidemiologic study by Partinen[75] estimated a prevalence of excessive sleepiness in Westerners at 5–36% of the total population. In contrast, Harrison and Horne[76] argued that most people are not chronically sleep deprived but simply choose not to sleep as much as they could.

What are the consequences of sleep deprivation? This question has been explored in studies of total, partial, and selective sleep deprivation (e.g., REM sleep or SWS deprivation). These studies have conclusively proved that sleep deprivation causes sleepiness; decrement of performance, vigilance, attention, and concentration; and increased reaction time. The performance decrement resulting from sleep deprivation may be related to periods of microsleep. *Microsleep* is defined as transient physiologic sleep (i.e., 3- to 14-second EEG patterns change from those of wakefulness to those of stage I NREM sleep) with or without rolling eye movements and behavioral sleep (e.g., drooping or heaviness of the eyelids, slight sagging and nodding of the head). Sleep deprivation does not cause permanent memory loss or other central nervous system (CNS) changes.

The most common cause of excessive daytime sleepiness (EDS) today is sleep deprivation. In the survey by Partinen,[75] up to one-third of young adults have EDS secondary to chronic partial sleep deprivation, and approximately 7% of middle-aged individuals have EDS secondary to sleep disorders and 2% secondary to shift work. Sleep deprivation poses danger to the individuals experiencing it as well as to others, making people prone to accidents in the work place, particularly in industrial and transportation work. The incidence of automobile crashes increases with driver fatigue and sleepiness. Fatigue resulting from sleep deprivation may have been responsible for many major national and international catastrophes (e.g., the Exxon Valdez oil spill, Bhopal chemical explosion in India, Three Mile Island nuclear accident, Challenger explosion, and Chernobyl nuclear plant disaster in the former USSR).[77]

There are two types of sleepiness: physiologic and subjective.[78] *Physiologic sleepiness* indicates the body's need for sleep. *Subjective sleepiness* is the individual's perception of sleepiness, which depends on external factors such as being in a stimulating environment, ingestion of coffee or other caffeinated beverages, and so on. Human beings are particularly vulnerable to sleepiness during two periods: (1) from 2:00 to 6:00 AM, particularly 3:00–5:00 AM, and (2) from 2:00 to 6:00 PM, especially 3:00–5:00 PM. Catastrophes have occurred most frequently during these two periods.[79] Physiological sleepiness depends on sleep factor and circadian phase. *Sleep factor* refers to a prior period of wakefulness and sleep debt. After a prolonged period of wakefulness, there is an increasing tendency to sleep. The recovery from sleep debt is aided by an additional amount of sleep. This additional sleep does not equal the exact number of hours of sleep debt, however; a sleep-deprived individual needs additional SWS to restore the body. The circadian factor determines the body's level of sleepiness from 3:00 to 5:00 AM and from 3:00 to 5:00 PM (sleepiness will be less intense in the second period). Scheduled naps of 20–30 minutes may help sleep-deprived patients overcome their sleepiness. Prophylactic naps before planned deprivation may improve performance.[78]

### Sleep-Deprivation Experiments

Although neither humans nor animals can do without sleep, the amount of sleep necessary to individual people or species varies widely. We know that a lack of sleep leads to sleepiness, but we do not know the exact functions of sleep. Sleep-deprivation experiments in animals have clearly shown that sleep is necessary for survival. The experiments of Rechtschaffen and colleagues[80] with rats using the carousel device have provided evidence for the necessity of sleep. All rats deprived of sleep for 10–30 days died after having lost weight, despite increases in their food intake. The rats also lost temperature control. Rats deprived only of REM sleep lived longer. Complete sleep-deprivation experiments for prolonged periods (weeks to months) cannot be conducted in humans for obvious ethical reasons.

### Total Sleep Deprivation

One of the early sleep-deprivation experiments in humans was conducted in 1896 by Patrick and Gilbert,[81] who studied the effects of a 90-hour period of sleep deprivation on three healthy young men. One reported sensory illusions, which disappeared completely when, at the end of the experiment, he was allowed to sleep for 10 hours. All subjects had difficulty staying awake, but felt totally fresh and rested after they were allowed to sleep.

A spectacular experiment in this century was conducted in 1965. A 17-year-old California college student named Randy Gardner tried to set a new world record for staying awake. Dement and colleagues[82] observed him during the later part of the experiment. Gardner stayed awake for 264 hours and 12 minutes, then slept for 14 hours and 40 minutes. He was recovered fully when he awoke. The conclusion drawn from the experiment is that it is possible to deprive people of sleep for a prolonged period without causing serious mental impairment. An important observation is the loss of performance with long sleep deprivation, which is due to loss of motivation and the frequent occurrence of microsleep.

In another experiment, Johnson and MacLeod[83] showed that it is possible to intentionally reduce total sleeping time by 1–2 hours without suffering any adverse effect. The experiments by Carskadon and Dement[84,85] showed that sleep deprivation increases the tendency to sleep during the day. This has been conclusively proved using the multiple sleep latency test with subjects.[85,86]

During the recovery sleep period after sleep deprivation, the percentage of SWS (stages III and IV NREM) increases considerably. Similarly, after a long period of sleep deprivation, the REM sleep percentage increases during recovery sleep. (This increase has not been demonstrated after a short period of sleep deprivation, that is, up to 4 days.) These experiments suggest that different mechanisms regulate NREM and REM sleep.[2]

### Partial Sleep Deprivation

Measurements of mood and performance after partial sleep deprivation (e.g., restricting sleep to 4.5–5.5 hours for 2–3 months) showed only minimal deficits in performance, which may have been related to decreased motivation. Thus, both total and partial sleep deprivation produce minimal deleterious effects in humans.[25,87,88]

### Selective REM Sleep Deprivation

Dement[89] performed REM-deprivation experiments (by awakening the subject for 5 minutes at the moment the polysomnographic [PSG] recording demonstrated onset of REM sleep). PSG results showed increased REM pressure (i.e., earlier and more frequent onset of REM sleep during successive nights) and REM rebound (i.e., quantitative increase of REM percentage during recovery nights). These findings were subsequently replicated by Borbely[2] and others,[90, 91] but Dement's third observation— a psychotic reaction following REM deprivation—could not be replicated in subsequent investigations.[90]

### Stage IV Sleep Deprivation

Agnew and colleagues[92] reported that, after stage IV NREM sleep deprivation for two consecutive nights, there was an increase in stage IV sleep during the recovery night. Two important points were raised by this group's later experiments: (1) REM rebound was more significant than stage IV rebound during recovery nights, and (2) it was more difficult to deprive a person of stage IV sleep than of REM sleep.[91]

The effects of total sleep deprivation, as well as of REM sleep deprivation, are similar in animals and humans, suggesting that the sleep stages and the fundamental regulatory mechanisms for controlling sleep are the same in all mammals.

## SLEEP, IMMUNE SYSTEM, AND SLEEP FACTORS

Cytokines are proteins that play an important role in immune regulation; they include interleukin (IL), tumor necrosis factor (TNF), and interferons (IFNs). A number of cytokines have been shown to promote sleep in animals, including IL-1, IFN-$\alpha$, and TNF.[93–95] Other sleep-promoting substances called *sleep factors* are increased in concentration during prolonged wakefulness or during infection.[96,97] The other endogenous compounds that

enhance sleep include delta sleep–inducing peptides, muramyl peptides, cholecystokinin, arginine vasotocin, vasoactive intestinal peptide, growth hormone–releasing factor, and somatostatin.[93,97] It has been shown that adenosine may fulfill the major criteria for neural sleep factor, that is, mediating the somnogenic effects of prolonged wakefulness.[98]

The cytokines play a role in the cellular and immune changes noted during sleep deprivation.[99] The precise nature of the immune response after sleep deprivation has, however, remained controversial, and the results of studies on the subject have been inconsistent.[100] These inconsistencies may reflect different stress reactions of subjects and different circadian factors (e.g., timing of drawing of blood for estimation of plasma levels).[100]

Infection (bacterial, viral, and fungal) enhances NREM sleep but suppresses REM sleep. It has been postulated that sleep acts as a host defense against infection and facilitates the healing process.[99,100] It is also believed that sleep deprivation may increase vulnerability to infection. The results of experiments with animals suggest that sleep deprivation alters immune function.[100,101] The relationship between sleep deprivation and immune system disturbances in humans, however, remains controversial.[100]

## THEORIES OF THE FUNCTION OF SLEEP

Despite considerable progress in understanding the mechanisms of NREM and REM sleep and the neurobiology of sleep, we still do not know the exact function of sleep. Several theories of the function of sleep that have been proposed are described briefly in the following sections. Summaries of sleep theories can be found in Hobson[102] and Horne.[103]

### Restorative Theory

Proponents of the restorative theory ascribe body tissue restoration to NREM sleep and brain tissue restoration to REM sleep.[104–107] The findings of increased secretion of anabolic hormones[108–110] (e.g., growth hormone, prolactin, testosterone, luteinizing hormone) and decreased levels of catabolic hormones[111] (e.g., cortisol) during sleep, along with the subjective feeling of being refreshed after sleep, may support such a contention.[25] Increased SWS after sleep deprivation[2] further supports the role of NREM sleep as restorative. The critical role of REM sleep for the development of the CNS of young organisms, and increased protein synthesis in the brain during REM sleep, are cited as evidence of restoration of brain functions by REM sleep.[112] Several studies of brain basal metabolism suggest an enhanced synthesis of macromolecules such as nucleic acids and proteins in the brain during sleep,[113] but the data remain scarce and controversial. Confirmation of such cerebral anabolic processes would provide an outstanding argument in favor of the restorative theory of sleep.

### Energy Conservation Theory

Zepelin and Rechtschaffen[49] found that animals with a high metabolic rate sleep longer than those with a slower metabolism, suggesting that energy is conserved during sleep. During NREM sleep, brain energy metabolism and cerebral blood flow decrease, whereas during REM sleep, the level of metabolism is similar to that of wakefulness and the cerebral blood flow increases. Although these findings might suggest that NREM sleep helps conserve energy, the fact that only 120 calories are conserved in 8 hours of sleep makes the energy conservation theory less than satisfactory. Considering that humans spend one-third of their lives sleeping,[114] one would expect far more calories to be conserved during an 8-hour period if energy conservation was the function of sleep.

### Adaptive Theory

In both animals and humans, sleep is an adaptive behavior that allows the creature to survive under a variety of environmental conditions.[115,116]

### Instinctive Theory

The instinctive theory views sleep as an instinct,[104,117] which relates to the theory of adaptation and energy conservation.

### Memory Reinforcement and Consolidation Theory

The theory of memory reinforcement and consolidation applies particularly to REM sleep, which is thought to facilitate memory and learning. In fact, McGaugh and colleagues[118] suggested that sleep-

and waking-related fluctuations of hormones and neurotransmitters may modulate memory processes. Crick and Mitchison[40] suggested that REM sleep removes undesirable data from the memory. They also suggested that the facts that REM deprivation produces a large rebound and that REM sleep occurs in almost all mammals make it probable that REM sleep has some important biological function.[119]

The theory that memory reinforcement and consolidation take place during REM sleep has been strengthened by scientific data provided by Karni and colleagues.[120] These authors conducted selective REM and SWS deprivation in six young adults. They found that perceptual learning during REM deprivation was significantly less compared with perceptual learning during SWS deprivation. In addition, SWS deprivation had a significant detrimental effect on a task that was already learned. These data suggest that REM deprivation affected the consolidation of the recent perceptual experience, thus supporting the theory of long-term consolidation during REM sleep.

### Synaptic and Neuronal Network Integrity Theory

There is a new theory emerging that suggests the primary function of sleep is the maintenance of synaptic and neuronal network integrity.[114,121–123] According to this theory, sleep is important for the maintenance of synapses that have been insufficiently stimulated during wakefulness. Intermittent stimulation of the neural network is necessary to preserve CNS function. This theory further suggests that NREM and REM sleep serve the same function of synaptic reorganization.[121] This emerging concept of the "dynamic stabilization" (i.e., repetitive activations of brain synapses and neural circuitry) theory of sleep suggests that REM sleep maintains motor circuits, whereas NREM sleep maintains nonmotor activities.[121–123]

### Thermoregulatory Function Theory

According to the theory of thermoregulatory function, sleep maintains thermoregulatory homeostasis.[114] Severe thermoregulatory abnormalities after total sleep deprivation and the influence of the preoptic and anterior hypothalamic thermosensitive neurons on sleep and arousal can be cited as evidence of the thermoregulatory function of sleep.

## REFERENCES

1. Wolpert S. A New History of India. New York: Oxford University Press, 1982;48.
2. Borbely A. Secrets of Sleep. New York: Basic Books, 1984.
3. Mazumda S. Ramayana. Calcutta: Deva Shahittya Kutir, 1979.
4. Parkes JD. Sleep and Its Disorders. Philadelphia: Saunders, 1985;314.
5. Moruzzi G. The historical development of the deafferentation hypothesis of sleep. Proc Am Philosoph Soc 1964;108:19.
6. Hartley D. Observations on Man, His Frame, His Duty, and His Expectations. London: Leake and Frederick, 1749.
7. Macnish R. The Philosophy of Sleep. Glasgow: E. M'Phun, 1830.
8. Tobler I. Is sleep fundamentally different between mammalian species? Behav Brain Res 1995;69:35.
9. Mahowald MW, Schenck CH. Status dissociatus: a perspective on states of being. Sleep 1991;14:69.
10. Ishimori K. True causes of sleep—a hypnogenic substance as evidenced in the brain of sleep-deprived animals. Igakkai Zasshi (Tokyo) 1909;23:429.
11. Legendre R, Pieron H. Recherches sur le besoin de sommeil consecutif a une veille prolongée. Z Allerg Physiol 1913;14:235.
12. Caton R. The electric currents of the brain. BMJ 1875;2:278.
13 Berger H. Uber das Elektroenkephalogramm des Menschen. Arch Psychiatr Nervenber 1929;87:527.
14. Loomis AL, Harvey EN, Hobart GA. Cerebral states during sleep, as studied by human brain potentials. J Exp Physiol 1937;21:127.
15. Aserinsky E, Kleitman N. Regularly occurring periods of eye motility and concomitant phenomena during sleep. Science 1953;118:273.
16. Rechtschaffen A, Kales A. A Manual of Standardized Terminology, Techniques and Scoring Systems for Sleep Stages of Human Subjects. Los Angeles: UCLA Brain Information Service/Brain Research Institute, 1968.
17. Gastaut H, Tassinari C, Duron B. Étude polygraphique des manifestations épisodiques (hypniques et respiratoires) du syndrome de Pickwick. Rev Neurol 1965;112:568.
18. Jung R, Kuhlo W. Neurophysiological studies of abnormal night sleep and the Pickwickian syndrome. Prog Brain Res 1965;18:140.
19. William RL, Agnew HW Jr, Webb WB. Sleep patterns in young adults: an EEG study. Electroencephalogr Clin Neurophysiol 1964;17:376.
20. Williams RL, Karacan I, Hursch CJ. Electroencephalography (EEG) of Human Sleep: Clinical Applications. New York: Wiley, 1974.
21. Chokroverty S. Sleep and Breathing in Neurological Disorders. In NH Edelman, TV Santiago (eds), Breathing Disorders of Sleep. New York: Churchill Livingstone, 1986;225.
22. Chokroverty S. Phasic tongue movements in human rapid-eye movement in sleep. Neurology 1980;30:665.
23. Roffwarg HP, Muzzio JN, Dement WC. Ontogenetic development of the human sleep-dream cycle. Science 1966;152:604.
24. Anders TF. Maturation of Sleep Patterns in the Newborn Infant. In ED Weitzman (ed), Advances in Sleep Research. New York: Spectrum, 1975;43.
25. Anch AM, Browman CP, Mitler MM, et al. Sleep: A Scientific Perspective. Englewood Cliffs, NJ: Prentice Hall, 1988.
26. Metcalf DR. The effects of extrauterine experience on the ontogenesis of EEG sleep spindles. Psychosom Med 1969;31:393.
27. Metcalf DR, Mondale J, Burler FK. Ontogenesis of spontaneous K complexes. Psychophysiology 1971;8:340.
28. Kleitman N. Sleep and Wakefulness (rev ed). Chicago: University of Chicago Press, 1963.
29. White RM Jr. The Lengths of Sleep. Washington, DC: America Psychological Association, 1975.
30. Browman CP, Gordon GC, Tepas DI, et al. Reported sleep and drug use of workers: a preliminary report. Sleep Res 1977;6:111.
31. Webb WB, Friel J. Sleep stages and personalities characteristics of "natural" long and short sleepers. Science 1971;171:587.
32. Kripke DF, Simons RN, Garfinkel L, et al. Short and long sleep and sleeping pills: is increased mortality associated? Arch Gen Psychiatry 1979;36:103.
33. Taub JM, Berger RJ. Effects of acute sleep pattern alteration depend upon sleep duration. Physiol Psychol 1976;4:412.
34. Taub JM, Berger RJ. Extended sleep and performance: the Rip Van Winkle effect. Psychonom Sci 1969;16:204.
35. Benoit O, Foret J, Bouard G. The time course of slow-wave sleep and REM sleep in habitual long and short sleepers: effect of prior wakefulness. Hum Neurobiol 1983;2:91.
36. Foulkes D. Dream research: 1953–1993. Sleep 1996; 19:609.
37. Hobson JA, McCarley RW. The brain as a dream state generator: an activation synthesis hypothesis of the dream process. Am J Psychiatry 1977;134:1335.
38. Koukkou M, Lehmann D. Psychophysiologie des Traumens und der Neurosentherapie: das Zustands-Wechsel-Modell, eine Synopsis. Fortschr Neurol Psychiatr 1980;48:324.
39. Jouvet M. Le sommeil paradoxal, est-il responsable d'une programmation genetique de cerveau? Soc Seances Soc Biol Fil 1978;172:9.
40. Crick F, Mitchison G. The function of dream sleep. Nature 1983;304:111.
41. Zepelin H. Mammalian Sleep. In MH Kryger, T Roth, WC Dement (eds), Principles and Practice of Sleep Medicine. Philadelphia: Saunders, 1994;69.

42. Tauber ES. Phylogeny of Sleep. In ED Weitzman (ed), Advances in Sleep Research (Vol I). Flushing, NY: Spectrum, 1974;133.

43. Tobler I, Horne J. Phylogenetic Approaches to the Functions of Sleep. In WP Koella (ed), Sleep 1982. Basel: S Karger, 1983;126.

44. Tobler I. Evolution of the Sleep Process: A Phylogenetic Approach. In AA Borbely, JL Valatx (eds), Sleep Mechanisms: Experimental Brain Research. Heidelberg: Springer, 1984;8(Suppl):227.

45. Allison T, Van Twyver H, Goff WR. Electrophysiological studies of the echidna, *Tachyglossus aculeatus*. I. Waking and sleep. Arch Ital Biol 1972;110:145.

46. Mukhametov LM. Sleep in marine mammals. Exp Brain Res 1984;8:S227.

47. Berger RJ, Nicol SC, Andersen NA, Phillips NH. Paradoxical sleep in the echidna. Sleep Res 1995;24A:199.

48. Siegel JM, Manger PR, Nienhuis R, et al. The echidna *Tachyglossus aculeatus* combines REM and NREM aspects in a single sleep state: implications for the evolution of sleep. J Neurosci 1996;16:3500.

49. Zepelin H, Rechtschaffen A. Mammalian sleep, longevity and energy metabolism. Brain Behav Evol 1974;10:425.

50. Mukhametov LM, Supin AY, Poliakova IG. Interhemispheric asymmetry of the electroencephalographic sleep patterns in dolphins. Brain Res 1977;124:581.

51. Hartse KM. Sleep in Insects and Nonmammalian Vertebrates. In MH Kryger, T Roth, WC Dement (eds), Principles and Practice of Sleep Medicine (2nd ed). Philadelphia: Saunders, 1994;95.

52. Amlaner CJ Jr, Ball NJ. Avian Sleep. In MH Kryger, T Roth, WC Dement (eds), Principles and Practice of Sleep Medicine (2nd ed). Philadelphia: Saunders, 1994;81.

53. Flannigan WF Jr. Behavioral States and Electroencephalogram of Reptiles. In MH Chase (ed), The Sleeping Brain: Perspectives in Brain Sciences. Los Angeles: UCLA Brain Information Service/Brain Research Institute, 1972;14.

54. de Mairan JJ. Observation Botanique. Histoire de l' Academie Royale des Sciences. Paris: Imprimerie Royale, 1731;35.

55. Pittendrigh CS. Circadian rhythms and the circadian organization of living systems. Cold Spring Harb Symp Quant Biol 1960;25:159.

56. Aschoff J. Exogenous and endogenous components in circadian rhythms. Cold Spring Harb Symp Quant Biol 1960;25:11.

57. Halberg F. Physiologic 24-hour periodicity: general and procedural considerations with reference to the adrenal cycle. Z Vit Morm Fermentforschung 1959;10:225.

58. Aschoff J. Circadian rhythms in man. Science 1965; 148:1427.

59. Miller JD, Morin LP, Schwartz WJ, Moore RY. New insights into the mammalian circadian clock. Sleep 1996;19:641.

60. Moore-Ede M, Sulzman FM, Fuller CA. The Clocks that Time Us. Cambridge, MA: Harvard University Press, 1982.

61. Wever RA. The Circadian System of Man: Results of Experiments Under Temporal Isolation. New York: Springer, 1979.

62. Stephan FK, Zucker I. Circadian rhythms in drinking behavior and locomotor activity of rats are eliminated by hypothalamic lesions. Proc Natl Acad Sci U S A 1972;69:1583.

63. Moore RY, Eichler VB. Loss of a circadian adrenal corticosterone rhythm following suprachiasmatic lesion in the rat. Brain Res 1972;42:201.

64. Lydic R, Schoene WC, Czeisler CA, et al. Suprachiasmatic region of the human hypothalamus: homolog to the primate circadian pacemaker? Sleep 1980; 2:355.

65. Moore RY, Lenn NJ. A retinohypothalamic projection in the rat. J Comp Neurol 1972;146:1.

66. Schwartz WJ. Understanding circadian clocks: from c-Fos to fly balls. Ann Neurol 1997;41:289.

67. Ralph MR, Joyner AL, Lehman MN. Culture and transplantation of the mammalian circadian pacemaker. J Biol Rhythms 1993;8:S83.

68. Murphy PJ, Campbell SS. Physiology of the circadian system in animals and humans. J Clin Neurophysiol 1996;13:2.

69. Inouye ST, Shibata S. Neurochemical organization of circadian rhythm in the suprachiasmatic nucleus. Neurosci Res 1994;20:109.

70. Kronauer RE, Czeisler CA, Pilato SF, et al. Mathematical model of the human circadian system with two interacting oscillators. Am J Physiol 1982; 242:R3.

71. Daan S, Beersma DGM, Borbely AA. The timing of human sleep: recovery process gated by a circadian pacemaker. Am J Physiol 1984;246:R161.

72. Kraft M, Martin RJ. Chronobiology and chronotherapy in medicine. Dis Mon 1995;41:501.

73. Webb WB, Agnew HW. Are we chronically sleep-deprived? Bull Psychonomic Soc 1975;6:47.

74. Bonnet MH, Arand DL. We are chronically sleep-deprived. Sleep 1995;18:908.

75. Partinen M. Epidemiology of Sleep Disorders. In MH Kryger, T Roth, WC Dement (eds), Principles and Practice of Sleep Medicine (2nd ed). Philadelphia: Saunders, 1994;437.

76. Harrison Y, Horne JA. Should we be taking more sleep? Sleep 1995;18:901.

77. National Commission on Sleep Disorders. Wake up America. Washington, DC: US Government Printing Office, 1993.

78. Dinges DF, Broughton RJ. Sleep and Alertness: Chronobiological, Behavioral and Medical Aspects of Napping. New York: Raven, 1989.

79. Mitler NM, Carskadon MA, Czeisler CA, et al. Catastrophes, sleep and public policy. Sleep 1988;11:100.

80. Rechtschaffen A, Gilliland MA, Bergmann BM, et al. Physiological correlates of prolonged sleep deprivation in rats. Science 1983;221:182.

81. Patrick GT, Gilbert JA. On the effects of loss of sleep. Psychol Rev 1896;3:469.

82. Dement WC. Some Must Watch While Some Must Sleep. San Francisco: WH Freeman, 1974.

83. Johnson LC, MacLeod WL. Sleep and awake behavior during gradual sleep reduction. Percept Mot Skills 1973;36:87.

84. Carskadon MA, Dement WC. Effects of total sleep loss on sleep tendency. Percept Mot Skills 1979;48:495.

85. Carskadon MA, Dement WC. Cumulative effects of sleep restriction on daytime sleepiness. Psychophysiology 1981;18:107.

86. Dement WC, Carskadon MA. An Essay on Sleepiness. In M Baldy-Moulinier (ed), Actualites en Médecine Experimentale, en Hommage au Professeur P Passouant. Montpellier: Euromed, 1981;47.

87. Webb WB, Agnew HR Jr. The effects of a chronic limitation of sleep length. Psychophysiology 1974;11:265.

88. Friedmann JK, Globus G, Huntley A, et al. Performance and mood during and after gradual sleep reduction. Psychophysiology 1977;14:245.

89. Dement W. The effect of dream deprivation. Science 1960;131:1705.

90. Kales A, Hoedemaker FS, Jacobson A, et al. Dream deprivation: an experimental reappraisal. Nature 1964; 204:1337.

91. Agnew HW Jr, Webb WB, Williams RL. Comparison of stage 4 and 1-REM sleep deprivation. Percept Mot Skills 1967;24:851.

92. Agnew HW Jr, Webb WB, Williams RL. The effects of stage 4 sleep deprivation. Electroencephalogr Clin Neurophysiol 1964;17:68.

93. Krueger JM. Somnogenic activity of immune response modifiers. Trends Pharmacol Sci 1990;11:122.

94. DeSarro GB, Masuda Y, Ascioti C, et al. Behavioral and ECog spectrum changes induced by intracerebral infusion of interferons and interleukin-2 in rats are antagonized by naloxone. Neuropharmacology 1990;29:167.

95. Schoham S, Davenne D, Cady AB, et al. Recombinant tumor necrosis factor and interleukin-1 enhance slow wave sleep. Am J Physiol 1987;253:R142.

96. Borbely AA, Tobler I. Endogenous sleep-promoting substances and sleep regulation. Physiol Rev 1989;69:605.

97. Inoue S. Biology of Sleep Substances. Orlando: CRC, 1989.

98. Porkka-Heiskanen T, Strecker E, Thakkar M, et al. Adenosine: a mediator of the sleep-inducing effects of prolonged wakefulness. Science 1997;276:1265.

99. Moldofsky H. Sleep and the immune system. Int J Immunopharmacol 1995;17:649.

100. Dinges DF, Douglas SD, Hamarman S, et al. Sleep deprivation and human immune function. Adv Neuroimmunol 1995;5:97.

101. Toth LA. Sleep, sleep deprivation and infectious diseases: studies in animals. Adv Neuroimmunol 1995;5:79.

102. Hobson JA. Sleep. New York: Scientific American Library, 1989;189.

103. Horne J. Why We Sleep. New York: Oxford University Press, 1988.

104. Moruzzi G. The sleep-waking cycle. Ergeb Physiol 1972;64:1.

105. Hartmann E. The Functions of Sleep. New Haven: Yale University Press, 1973.

106. Oswald I. Sleep. Middlesex, UK: Penguin, 1974.

107. Adam K, Oswald I. Sleep is for tissue restoration. J R Coll Phys 1977;11:376.

108. Takahashi Y, Kipnis D, Daughaday W. Growth hormone secretion during sleep. J Clin Invest 1968;47:2079.

109. Sassin JF, Frantz AG, Kapen S, et al. The nocturnal rise of human prolactin is dependent on sleep. J Clin Endocrinol Metab 1973;37:436.

110. Boyar RM, Rosenfeld RS, Kapen S, et al. Human puberty: simultaneous augmented secretion of luteinizing hormone and testosterone during sleep. J Clin Invest 1974;54:609.

111. Weitzman ED, Hellman L. Temporal Organization of the 24-Hour Pattern of the Hypothalamic-Pituitary Axis. In M Ferin, F Halberg, RM Richart, et al. (eds), Biorhythms and Human Reproduction. New York: Wiley, 1974;371.

112. Drucker-Colin R. Protein Molecules and the Regulation of REM Sleep: Possible Implications for Function. In R Drucker-Colin, M Shkurovich, MD Sterman (eds), The Functions of Sleep. New York: Academic, 1979;99.

113. Maquet P. Sleep function (S and cerebral metabolism). Behav Brain Res 1995;69:75.

114. Mahowald MW, Chokroverty S, Kader G, Schenck CH. Sleep Disorders. Continuum (Vol 3, No. 4). A progra, of the American Academy of Neurology. Baltimore: Williams and Wilkins, 1997.

115. Meddis R. The Sleep Instinct. London: Routledge, 1977.

116. Webb WB. Sleep: The Gentle Tyrant. Bolton, MA: Anker, 1992.

117. McGinty DJ, Harper TM, Fairbanks MK. Neuronal Unit Activity and the Control of Sleep States. In E Weitzman (ed), Advances in Sleep Research (Vol I). New York: Spectrum, 1974;173.

118. McGaugh JL, Gold PE, Van Buskirk RB, et al. Modulating Influences of Hormones and Catecholamines on Memory Storage Processes. In GH Gispen, TB van Wimersma-Gridanus, B Bohus, et al. (eds), Hormones, Homeostasis and the Brain. Amsterdam: Elsevier, 1975;151.

119. Crick F, Mitchison G. REM sleep and neural nets. Behav Brain Res 1995;69:147.

120. Karni A, Tanne D, Rubenstein BS, et al. Dependence on REM sleep of overnight improvement of a perceptual skill. Science 1994;265:679.

121. Krueger JM, Obal F Jr, Kapas L, Fang J. Brain organization and sleep function. Behav Brain Res 1995;69:177.

122. Kavanau JL. Memory, sleep and the evolution of mechanisms of synaptic efficacy maintenance. Neuroscience 1997;79:7.

123. Kavanau JL. Origin and evolution of sleep: roles of vision and endothermy. Brain Res Bull 1997;42:245.

# Chapter 3

# Sleep Neurophysiology: Basic Mechanisms Underlying Control of Wakefulness and Sleep

Robert W. McCarley

This chapter presents an overview of the current knowledge of the neurophysiology and cellular pharmacology of sleep mechanisms. It is written from the belief that this field is entering a "golden age" of development of knowledge about sleep mechanisms due to the capability of current cellular neurophysiologic, pharmacologic, and molecular techniques to provide focused, detailed, and replicable studies. These studies will enrich the knowledge of sleep phenomenology and pathology derived from electroencephalography (EEG) analysis. This chapter has a cellular neurophysiologic and neuropharmacologic focus, with most of the emphasis on mechanisms relevant to rapid eye movement (REM) sleep. The cellular pharmacology and physiology of non-REM (NREM) sleep is treated in Chapter 4. The present chapter discusses evidence that adenosine (AD) is a sleep factor mediating the sleep-inducing effects of prolonged wakefulness. Molecular biological and anatomic evidence pointing to a set of NREM sleep–active neurons in the ventrolateral preoptic areas as important for NREM sleep is also considered. A detailed historical introduction to the topics of this chapter is available in Steriade and McCarley.[1] For the reader interested in an update on the terminology and techniques of cellular physiology, one of the standard neurobiology texts should be consulted (e.g., Kandel and colleagues[2]). Overviews of REM sleep physiology are also available[3,4]; the present chapter draws on these accounts and presents more recent developments. Although the present chapter touches on the literature on humoral factors in sleep, for more detail the reader is referred to recent reviews (e.g., Hayaishi and Inoue,[5] and the chapter by Kueger and Fang in this volume).

This chapter begins with brief and elementary overviews of sleep architecture and phylogeny/ontogeny, providing a basis for the later mechanistic discussions. The subject of REM sleep and the relevant anatomy and physiology are then discussed, followed by a consideration of AD as a sleep factor and present molecular biological research.

## SLEEP ARCHITECTURE

Sleep may be divided into two phases: (1) REM sleep is most often associated with vivid dreaming and a high level of brain activity. (2) The other phase of sleep, called *NREM sleep,* is usually associated with reduced neuronal activity; thought content during this state in humans is, unlike dreams, typically nonvisual and consisting of ruminative thoughts.

As shown in Figure 3-1, as one goes to sleep, the low-voltage fast (LVF) EEG of waking gradually gives way to a slowing of frequency. As sleep moves toward the deepest stages, there is an abundance of *delta waves,* EEG waves with high amplitude and a frequency ranging from 0.5 to less than 0.4 Hz. The first REM period usually occurs approximately 70 minutes after the onset of sleep. REM sleep in

This chapter was supported by awards from the National Institutes of Mental Health (MH R37 39, 683) and the Department of Veterans Affairs.

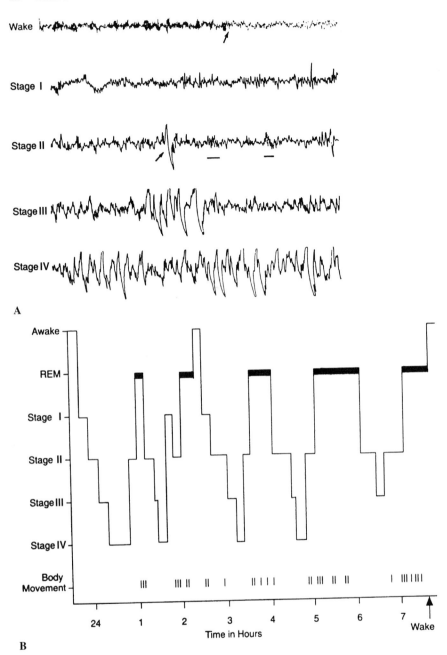

**Figure 3-1.** EEG patterns associated with wakefulness and the stages of sleep (**A**) and the time course of sleep stages over a night's sleep (**B**) in a healthy young man. During wakefulness there is a low-voltage fast (LVF) EEG pattern, often with alpha waves, as shown here. There is a transition to stage I sleep (*arrow*), with loss of the alpha rhythm, and the presence of a low voltage fast EEG. As sleep deepens, the EEG frequency slows more and more. Stage II is characterized by the presence of K complexes (*arrow*) and sleep spindles (*underlined*). During stage III, delta waves (0.5–0.3 Hz) appear, and they are present more than 50% of the time in stage IV. During REM sleep (*black bars*) the EEG pattern returns to an LVF pattern. The percentage of time spent in REM sleep increases with successive sleep cycles, whereas the percentage of time spent in stages III and IV decreases. (In waking, EEG segments recorded from occipital electrodes; all other segments recorded from central electrodes.) (Adapted from RW McCarley. Sleep, Dreams and States of Consciousness. In PM Conn [ed], Neuroscience in Medicine. Philadelphia: Lippincott, 1995;537.)

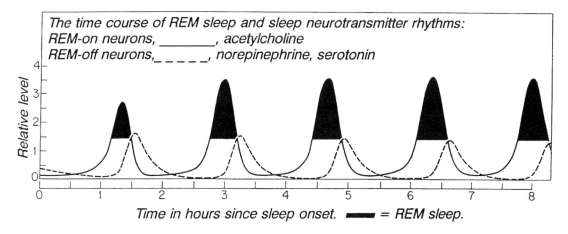

**Figure 3-2.** Schematic of a night's course of REM sleep in human beings showing the occurrence and intensity of REM sleep as dependent on the activity of populations of REM-on, REM sleep–promoting neurons (*solid line*). As the REM sleep–promoting neuronal activity reaches a certain threshold, the full set of REM sleep signs occurs (black areas under curve indicate REM sleep). Note, however, that, unlike the steplike EEG diagnosis of stages in Figure 3-1, the underlying neuronal activity is a continuous function. The shorter, less intense first REM episode occurs because of circadian modulation of the REM sleep oscillator. The neurotransmitter acetylcholine is important in REM production, acting to excite populations of brain stem reticular formation neurons to produce the set of REM signs. Other neuronal populations using the monoamine neurotransmitters serotonin and norepinephrine are REM sleep–suppressive; the time course of their activity is sketched by the dotted line. These curves were generated by the limit cycle reciprocal interaction model,[54,61] which accurately models the time course and percentage of REM sleep.

humans is defined by the presence of LVF EEG activity, suppression of muscle tone (typically measured in the chin muscles), and the presence of REMs. The first REM sleep episode in humans is short. After the first REM sleep episode, the stages of the sleep cycle are repeated, and NREM sleep occurs. Approximately 90 minutes after the start of the first REM period, another REM sleep episode takes place. This rhythmic cycling persists throughout the night. A sleep cycle is approximately 90 minutes in humans, and the duration of each REM sleep episode after the first is approximately 30 minutes. Figure 3-2 includes a schematic of the time course of REM sleep and a representation of the intensity of REM-related neuronal activity. Over the course of the night, delta-wave activity tends to diminish and NREM sleep has waves of higher frequencies and lower amplitude.

## SLEEP ONTOGENY AND PHYLOGENY

Periods of immobility and rest have been observed in many lower animals, including insects and lizards. Because of the absence of a cortical brain structure like that of humans, it is difficult to say whether the absence of slow waves in these animals means they do not have the equivalent of human SWS or whether SWS is expressed in a form not detectable with EEG recordings. REM sleep is present in all non–egg-laying mammals, and data suggest it is also present in egg-laying mammals, such as the spiny anteater and the duckbill platypus. Birds have very brief bouts of REM sleep. REM sleep cycles vary in duration according to the size of the animal, with elephants having the longest cycle and smaller animals having shorter cycles. For example, the cat has a sleep cycle of approximately 22 minutes, whereas the rat cycle is approximately 12 minutes.

In utero, mammals spend a large percentage of time in REM sleep, ranging from 50% to 80% of a 24-hour day. Animals born with immature nervous systems have a much higher percentage of REM sleep than do the adults of the same species. For example, sleep occupies two-thirds of the human newborn's time, with REM sleep occupying one-half of the total sleep time, or approximately one-third of the entire 24-hour period. The percentage of REM sleep declines rapidly in early childhood, so that by approximately age 10 the adult percentage of REM sleep is reached—20% of total sleep time. The predominance of REM sleep in the young suggests an important function in promoting nervous system growth and development.

Delta sleep is minimally present in the newborn but increases over the first years of life, reaching a maximum at approximately age 10 and declining thereafter. Feinberg and coworkers[7] have noted that the first three decades of the time course of this delta activity can be matched to a gamma probability distribution, and that approximately the same time course is present for synaptic density and positron emission tomography measurements of metabolic rate in the human frontal cortex. They speculate that the reduction in these three variables (delta sleep, synaptic density, and matabolic rate) may reflect a pruning of redundant cortical synapses that is a key factor in cognitive maturation, allowing greater specialization and sustained problem solving.

## REM SLEEP PHYSIOLOGY AND RELEVANT BRAIN ANATOMY: REM-PROMOTING SYSTEMS

### *Transection Studies*

Lesion studies performed by Jouvet and coworkers in France demonstrated that the brain stem contains the neural machinery of the REM sleep rhythm (reviewed in Steriade and McCarley[1]). As illustrated in Figure 3-3, a transection made just above the junction of the pons and midbrain produced a state in which periodic occurrence of REM sleep was found in recordings made in the isolated brain stem. Recordings in the isolated forebrain, however, showed no signs of REM sleep. Thus, although forebrain mechanisms (including those related to circadian rhythms) modulate REM sleep, the fundamental rhythm-generating machinery is in the brain stem, and it is here that anatomic and physiologic studies have focused. Figure 3-3 also shows the cell groups important in REM sleep—the cholinergic neurons, which act as promoters of REM phenomena, and the monoaminergic neurons, which may act to suppress most components of REM sleep. Note that Figure 3-3 shows that the Jouvet transection spared these essential brain stem zones.

### *Effector Neurons for Different Components of REM Sleep*

Effector neurons are those neurons directly in the neural pathways leading to the production of different REM sleep components, such as REM. A series of physiologic investigations over the past three decades has shown that what has been called the *behavioral state* of REM sleep in nonhuman mammals is dissociable into different components under control of different mechanisms and with different anatomic loci. The reader familiar with the pathology of human REM sleep will find this concept easy to understand, given that much pathology consists of inappropriate expression or suppression of individual components of REM sleep. As in humans, the cardinal signs of REM sleep in nonhuman mammals are muscle atonia, EEG activation (LVF pattern, sometimes termed *desynchronization*), and REM.

*PGO waves* are another important component of REM sleep found in recordings from deep brain structures in many animals (they are visible in the cat recording in Figure 3-4). PGO waves are spiky EEG waves that arise in the *P*ons and are transmitted to the thalamic lateral *G*eniculate nucleus (a visual system nucleus) and to the visual *O*ccipital cortex, hence the name *PGO* waves. There is suggestive evidence that PGO waves are present in humans but the depth recordings necessary to establish their existence have not been done. PGO waves are EEG signs of neural activation; they index an important mode of brain stem activation of the forebrain during REM sleep. It is worth noting that they are also present in nonvisual thalamic nuclei, although their timing is linked to eye movements, with the first wave of the usual burst of three to five waves occurring just before an eye movement.

Most of the physiologic events of REM sleep have effector neurons located in the brain stem reticular formation, with important neurons especially concentrated in the *pontine reticular formation* (PRF) (see Figure 3-3 for location). Thus, PRF neuronal recordings are of special interest for understanding the mechanisms of production of the events of REM sleep. Intracellular recordings of PTF neurons (see Figure 3-4) show that these effector neurons have relatively hyperpolarized membrane potentials and generate almost no action potentials during NREM sleep. As illustrated in Figure 3-4, PRF neurons begin to depolarize even before the occurrence of the first

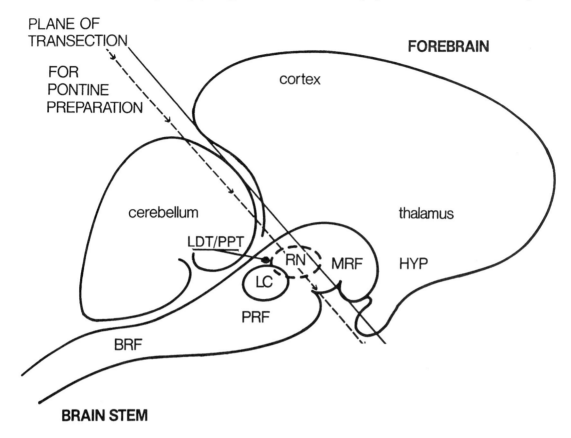

**Figure 3-3.** Schematic of a sagittal section of a mammalian brain (cat) showing the plane of transection that preserves REM sleep signs caudal to the transection, but abolishes them rostral to the transection. Laterodorsal and pedunculopontine tegmental nuclei (LDT/PPT) make up the principal site of cholinergic (acetylcholine-containing) neurons important for REM sleep and EEG desynchronization (as shown in Figure 3-6, these nuclei are more extensive than indicated on this sketch). Locus coeruleus (LC) is where most norepinephrine-containing neurons are located. The dorsal raphe nucleus (RN) is the site of serotonin-containing neurons. (BRF = bulbar reticular formation; PRF = pontine reticular formation; MRF = mesencephalic reticular formation; HYP = hypothalamus.) (Adapted from RW McCarley. Sleep, Dreams and States of Consciousness. In PM Conn [ed], Neuroscience in Medicine. Philadelphia: Lippincott, 1995.)

EEG sign of the approach of REM sleep—the PGO waves that occur 30–60 seconds before the onset of the rest of the EEG signs of REM sleep. As PRF neuronal depolarization proceeds and the threshold for action potential production is reached, these neurons begin to discharge (i.e., generate action potentials). Their discharge rate increases as REM sleep is approached and the high level of discharge is maintained throughout REM sleep due to the maintenance of this membrane depolarization.

Throughout the entire REM sleep episode almost the entire population of PRF neurons remains depolarized. The resultant increased action potential activity leads to the production of those REM sleep components that have their phys-

iologic bases in activity of PRF neurons. Figure 3-5 provides a schematic overview of REM sleep arising from increases in activity of the various populations of reticular formation neurons that are important effectors of REM sleep phenomena. PRF neurons are important for REMs (the generator for saccades is in the PRF) and PGO waves, and a group of dorsolateral PRF neurons controls the muscle atonia of REM sleep (these neurons become active just before the onset of muscle atonia). Neurons in the *midbrain reticular formation,* (see location in Figure 3-3), are especially important for EEG activation, the LVF EEG pattern. These neurons were originally described as making up the *ascending reticular activating system*

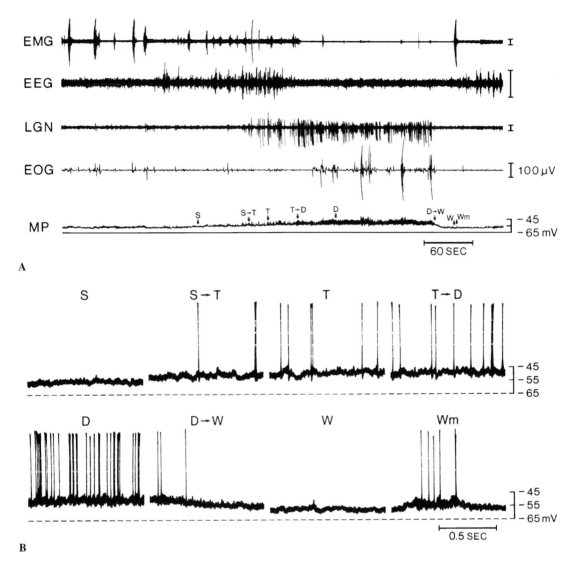

**Figure 3-4.** Changes in action-potential frequency and membrane potential of an intracellularly recorded medial pontine reticular formation neuron in a cat over a sleep-wake cycle. The inkwriter record of the defining state and the record of the membrane potential (MP) with action potentials filtered out (**A**) and cathode ray oscilloscope photographs taken at the indicated points in the inkwriter record (**B**) are shown. The record begins in waking (W): Note that there is eye movement activity in the electrooculogram (EOG) record and low-voltage fast EEG activity. The transient bursts of high-amplitude activity in the nuchal electromyogram (EMG) record indicate somatic movement. In W the membrane potential was approximately –60 mV, and remained at approximately the same level with the onset of sleep (S) (note EEG slow-wave activity). Postsynaptic potential (PSP) activity in S was low. Even before the onset of the first PGO wave in the LGN record, the MP showed a gradual onset of MP depolarization. By the time of the first LGN PGO wave (S → T) the PSP activity increased and there was one action potential. With the advent of more PGO waves (*segment T*, transition period) and the onset of REM sleep (D, for desynchronized sleep, another name for REM sleep) there was further MP depolarization and an accompanying increase in action potentials and PSPs (**B**, T and T → D); the increase in PSPs is visible as the thickening of the inkwriter MP trace. With the onset of D and during runs of the phasic activity of PGO waves and REMs, there were storms of depolarizing PSP activity and corresponding action potentials (*segment D*). The MP remained tonically depolarized at approximately –50 mV throughout D, with further phasic depolarizations. With the end of D and the onset of W (D → W) there was a membrane repolarization to approximately the same tonic –57-mV level seen in the initial W episode. At walking with movement (Wm), a somatic movement was accompanied by increased PSPs, a transient (phasic) membrane depolarization, and a burst of action potentials, before the MP returned to its baseline W polarization level. (EEG = sensorimotor cortex EEG; LGN = EEG record from lateral geniculate nucleus.) (Data from Ito and McCarley. Adapted from M Steriade, RW McCarley. Brainstem Control of Wakefulness and Sleep. New York: Plenum, 1990.)

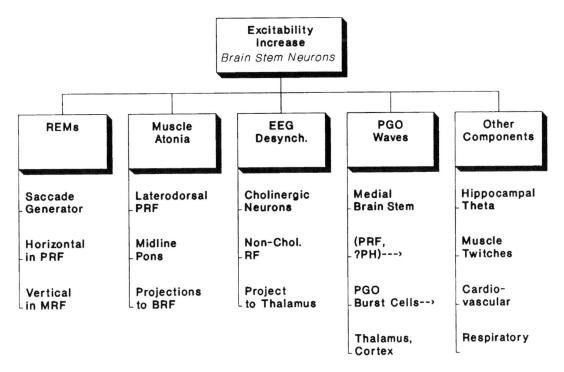

**Figure 3-5.** Schematic of REM sleep control. Increasing the excitability (activity) of brain stem neuronal pools subserving each of the major components of the state causes the occurrence of this component. For example, the neuronal pool important for REM is suggested to be the brain stem's saccade-generating system, whose main machinery is in the paramedian pontine reticular formation. Although vertical saccades are fewer in REM sleep, their presence suggests similar involvement of the mesencephalic reticular formation. Information under the other system components sketches the major features of the anatomy and projections of neuronal pools important for muscle atonia, EEG desynchronization, and PGO waves. The last part of the diagram lists other components of REM sleep.

(ARAS), the set of neurons responsible for EEG activation. Subsequent work has enlarged this original ARAS concept to include cholinergic neurons, with contributions to EEG activation also coming from monoaminergic systems (neurons using serotonin and norepinephrine [NE] as neurotransmitters).

### Cholinergic Mechanisms and the Initiation and Coordination of REM Sleep

Work during the last few years has led to an appreciation of the importance of the neurotransmitter acetylcholine (ACh) for REM sleep and of the nature of the anatomy and physiology of the cholinergic influences on REM sleep. Current data suggest cholinergic influences act by increasing the excitability of brain stem reticular neurons that

are important as effectors in REM sleep and that cholinergic neurons may directly mediate PGO wave transmission from brain stem to forebrain. There is now rather widespread agreement among physiologists on the importance of cholinergic mechanisms, and the essential data supporting this conclusion are outlined in the following sections.

### Production of a REM Sleep–Like State by Injection of Acetylcholine Agonists

It has been known since the mid-1960s that cholinergic agonist injection into the PRF produces a state that very closely mimics natural REM sleep (for a review and detailed literature citations for this section, see Steriade and McCarley[1]). The latencies to onset and duration are dose-dependent; within the PRF, most workers have found the shortest latencies to come from injections in dorsoros-

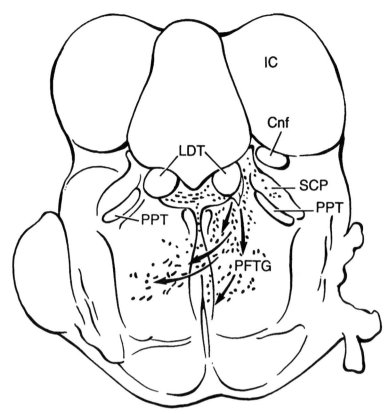

**Figure 3-6.** This schematic of frontal section of the brain stem at the pons-midbrain junction shows the location of the acetylcholine-containing neurons most important for REM sleep—the laterodorsal tegmental nucleus and the pedunculopontine tegmental nucleus (LDT and PPT)—and a schematic of projections of the LDT (on one side) to the pontine reticular formation. (IC = inferior colliculus; Cnf = cuneiform nucleus; SCP = superior cerebellar peduncle; PFTG = abbreviation of one component of PRF.) (Adapted from A Mitani, K Ito, AH Hallanger, et al. Cholinergic projections from the laterodorsal and pedunculopontine tegmental nuclei to the pontine gigantocellular tegmental field in the cat. Brain Res 1988;451:397.)

tral pontine reticular sites, although some work suggests a ventral site to be equally, or even more, effective.[8] Muscarinic cholinergic receptors appear to be of major importance, with nicotinic receptors playing a lesser role. Thus, this series of studies suggests that cholinergic pharmacologic manipulations can produce REM sleep. The obvious follow-up question is whether cholinergic mechanisms are important in natural REM sleep. Current anatomic, lesion, and physiologic data strongly suggest that the answer is "yes," and the next sections summarize this evidence.

*Cholinergic Projections to Reticular Formation Neurons*

Cholinergic projections in brain stem and to brain stem sites arise from two nuclei at the pons-midbrain junction that contain cholinergic neurons, the *laterodorsal tegmental nucleus* (LDT) and the *pedunculopontine tegmental nucleus* (PPT). A sagittal schematic of their location is marked in Figure 3-3,

and Figure 3-6, a coronal view, shows their projections to critical PRF zones (as first shown by Mitani and coworkers[9] and repeatedly confirmed). One study has found extensive LDT and PPT innervation of both pontine and bulbar reticular formation, as well as cranial nerve nuclei, by projections that are often bilateral. This finding indicates the relatively global nature of the projections of LDT and PPT, such as one would expect for pathways important in behavioral state control.[9] A similar series of studies has documented the extensive rostral projections of cholinergic neurons to the thalamus and basal forebrain (BF), where their actions are important for EEG activation—a topic discussed in the following section.

*Direct Excitation of Pontine Reticular Formation Neurons by Cholinergic Agonists*

In vivo injections of cholinergic agonists have several intrinsic limitations in testing hypotheses about cholinergic effects. Fortunately, these can be overcome by use of the in vitro pontine brain stem slice

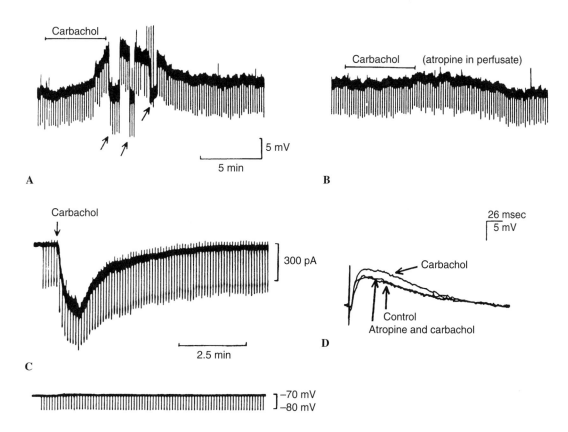

**Figure 3-7.** The cholinergic agonist carbachol depolarizes and increases the postsynaptic potential (PSP) responsiveness of medial pontine reticular formation (mPRF) neurons recorded in vitro. (**A**) Chart record of a typical depolarizing response of an mPRF neuron to bath application of 0.5 μmol/liter carbachol. Downward deflections are due to intracellular current pulses (pA = picoamperes) applied to assess input resistance. Membrane potential was returned to the baseline potential (*arrows*); the increased amplitude of voltage deflections indicates increased input resistance. (**B**) Atropine (0.5 μmol/liter) blocks the depolarizing response to carbachol (same neuron as in **A**). (**C**) Decreased membrane conductance during micropipette pressure application of carbachol (1 mmol/liter) for 1 second at 3 psi (*arrow*) is indicated by the decreased amplitude of downward deflections in the upper current record in response to 10-mV, 400-msec membrane potential shift commands (*lower record*) in a neuron under voltage-clamp control. (**D**) Three superimposed oscilloscope traces from an mPRF neuron of a PSP elicited by stimulation of the contralateral medial PRF (stimulation artifact is the first biphasic positive-negative deflection). Topmost trace is during bath perfusion with carbachol (0.5 μmol/liter), and bottom traces are during the control condition and during bath perfusion with both carbachol and atropine (0.5 μmol/liter). Note the 20% increase of PSP amplitude in the presence of carbachol compared to control and carbachol-atropine conditions. (Adapted from RW Greene, U Gerber, RW McCarley. Cholinergic activation of medial pontine reticular formation neurons in vitro. Brain Res 1989;476:154.)

preparation. This preparation offers the ability to apply agonists and antagonists in physiologic concentrations, which are usually in the low micromolar range. Effective in vivo injections use concentrations that are a thousandfold greater, in the millimolar range, and thus raise the possibility of mediation of effects by nonphysiologic mechanisms. That cholinergic excitation is via physiologic mechanisms is implied by in vitro experiments, in which applications of micromolar amounts of cholinergic agonists in vitro produce an excitation of a majority (80%) of reticular formation neurons (Figure 3-7).[10] Another advantage of the in vitro preparation is the ability to use a sodium-dependent action potential blocker, tetrodotoxin. These experiments show that the excitatory effects of cholinergic agonists on PRF neurons are direct (see review in Greene and McCarley[12]). Furthermore, the depolarizing, excitatory effects of cholinergic agonists (see Figure 3-7) mimic the changes seen in PRF neurons during natural REM sleep (see Figure 3-4).

*Laterodorsal and Pedunculopontine Tegmental Nuclei: Lesion and Stimulation Effects*

Extensive destruction of the cell bodies of LDT and PPT neurons by local injections of excitatory amino acids leads to a marked reduction of REM sleep.[13] Low-level (10 µA) electrical stimulation of LDT increases REM sleep.[14]

*Discharge Activity of Laterodorsal and Pedunculopontine Tegmental Nuclei Neurons Across the REM Cycle*

A subset of LDT and PPT neurons has been shown to discharge selectively during REM sleep, with the onset of increased discharges occurring before the onset of REM sleep[15–17] (see Figure 3-2). This LDT and PPT discharge pattern and the presence of excitatory projections to the PRF suggest that LDT and PPT cholinergic neurons may be important in producing the depolarization of reticular effector neurons, leading to production of the events characterizing REM sleep. The LDT, PPT, and reticular formation neurons that become active in REM sleep are often referred to as *REM-on neurons*. Subgroups of PRF neurons may show discharges during waking motoric activity, either somatic or oculomotor, but a sustained depolarization (see Figure 3-4) throughout almost all of the population occurs only during REM sleep.

*Production of the Low-Voltage Fast EEG Pattern of REM Sleep and Waking*

Rostral projections of another subgroup of LDT and PPT neurons are important for the EEG activation of both REM sleep and waking. This topic is discussed in NREM Sleep Mechanisms.

**Neurotransmitters and Pontine Reticular Formation Neurons**

At this point it is useful to present a summary of the neurotransmitters affecting PRF neurons, which we have characterized as the "effector neurons" for REM phenomena. It is important to emphasize that these data come primarily from studies on medial PRF neurons and that other reticular neurons may have different response profiles, although there is no reason now to suspect that populations in other areas will be strikingly different. It is also important to note that the list of neurotransmitters, receptor types, and ionic mechanisms is incomplete.

Knowledge of neurotransmitter effects is useful not only from a basic science point of view, but also in terms of predicting the kinds of effects produced by pharmacologic agents. Figure 3-8 summarizes effects in terms of excitation and inhibition, and describes the various ionic currents that mediate neurotransmitter effects. An important consideration in interpreting Figure 3-8 is that different neurons may have different sets of receptors and be involved in different behavioral systems. For example, the set of neurons with excitatory responses to serotonin apparently includes a class that may mediate rapid reticulospinal excitatory responses, such as those in startle, and that are not very important for sleep. For the neurons that are important to REM sleep, it is reasonable to predict that pharmacologic agents that excite will promote REM sleep phenomena, whereas those that inhibit will have the opposite effect. This is most likely with cholinergic compounds, which have excitatory actions on approximately 80% of PRF neurons—including those important in REM sleep. This figure is based on work, too extensive to cite here, of members of the Harvard-Brockton group, including Greene, Stevens, Gerber, Haas, Luebke, Birnstiel, and the present author. (Papers by Stevens and coworkers[18,19] and Gerber and coworkers,[20] as well as the Steriade and McCarley book,[1] provide references to the literature.)

The reader should be aware of the many peptides that are colocalized with the neurotransmitter ACh in LDT and PPT neurons; this colocalization likely also means they have synaptic corelease with ACh. The peptide substance P is found in approximately 40% of LDT and PPT neurons and, overall, more than 15 different colocalized peptides have been described. The role of these peptides in modulating ACh activity relevant to wakefulness and sleep is not entirely clear, but it should be emphasized that the colocalized vasoactive intestinal peptide has been reported by several investigators as an enhancer of REM sleep when injected intraventricularly.[4]

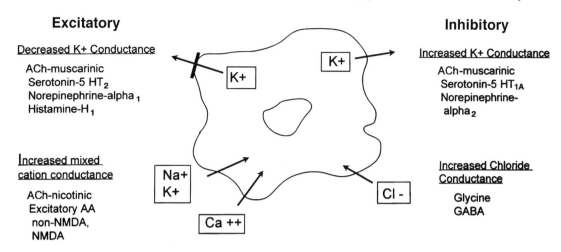

**Figure 3-8.** Neurotransmitter actions on medial pontine reticular formation (mPRF) neurons in vitro. Classes or receptor-mediated excitatory and inhibitory postsynaptic effects on mPRF neurons and the ionic currents mediating these effects are shown here. It is important to note that different mPRF neurons may have different sets of receptors and be involved in different behavioral systems. For example, the set of neurons with excitatory responses to serotonin apparently includes a class that may mediate rapid reticulospinal excitatory responses, such as those in startle, and that are not so important for sleep. For neurons that are important in REM sleep, it is reasonable to predict that pharmacologic agents that excite will promote REM sleep phenomena, whereas those that inhibit will have the opposite effect. This is clearest with cholinergic compounds, which have excitatory actions on approximately 80% of mPRF neurons. This figure is based on in vitro work by the author and other workers in their laboratory, as described in the text. (GABA = γ-aminobutyric acid; AA = amino acids; NMDA = N-methyl-D-aspartate; ACh = acetylcholine.)

### Muscle Atonia

Muscle atonia is an important REM feature from a clinical standpoint because disorders of muscle atonia are present in many patients who present to sleep disorders clinicians. Three important zones for atonia are listed below, according to their projections:

pontine reticular formation
→ bulbar reticular formation
→ motoneurons

### Motoneurons

The target of the muscle inhibition system is the alpha motoneuron. REM sleep effects on motoneurons have been principally investigated at the cellular level by Morales and Chase[21,22] and Chase and coworkers,[23] both in trigeminal motoneurons and spinal alpha motoneurons. Figure 3-9 illustrates the phenomenon of membrane hyperpolarization of motoneurons that accompanies REM sleep. Morales and Chase[21,22] recorded antidromically identified lumbar motoneurons in naturally sleeping cats, using the chronic intra-

cellular recording techniques they pioneered. Mean resting potential in wakefulness (W) was –65 mV, and there was a slight hyperpolarization from active W to SWS. During the passage from SWS to REM sleep, there was a marked membrane hyperpolarization, averaging 6.7 mV with a range of 4–10 mV; this hyperpolarization was temporally coincident with the loss of nuchal EMG activity. On transition to W, the level of polarization decreased. Chase and colleagues[22] found that the microiontophoretic application of strychnine (but not picrotoxin or bicuculline) onto lumbar motoneurons was effective in abolishing the large-amplitude, spontaneous inhibitory postsynaptic potentials of REM sleep, suggesting that glycine is the principal neurotransmitter mediating these potentials in lumbar motoneurons. Other data[1] suggest that the projections providing this inhibitory input ultimately arise from the bulbar reticular formation, perhaps with an intermediate synapse in the spinal cord.

### Pontine and Bulbar Reticular Formation

Jouvet[24] and Sastre and Jouvet[25] in Lyon, France, reported that bilateral lesions of the pontine reticular

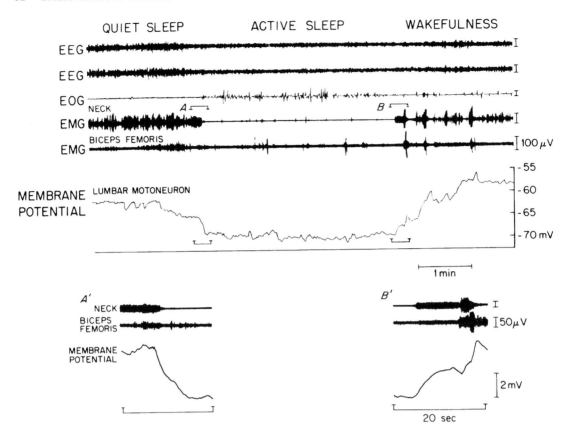

**Figure 3-9.** Intracellular record from a lumbar motoneuron during sleep and wakefulness with correlation of membrane potential and behavioral state. This figure highlights the membrane hyperpolarization that accompanies active sleep (REM sleep). Hyperpolarization commenced before the cessation of muscle tone, which was accompanied by a further and rather sharp increase in membrane polarization (*A*; shown oscilloscopically at higher gain and expanded time base in *A'*). At the termination of active sleep, the membrane depolarized coincident with the resumption of muscle tone and behavioral awakening (*B, B'*). Note the brief periods of depolarization during active sleep and wakefulness, which were accompanied by phasic increases in muscle activity (i.e., muscular twitches during active sleep and leg movements during wakefulness). Spike potentials often occurred during these periods of depolarization but are not evident in this high frequency–filtered record. The first and second polygraph traces are those of EEG activity recorded from the left and right frontal-parietal cortex, respectively. (Adapted from FR Morales, MH Chase. Intracellular recording of lumbar motoneuron membrane potential during sleep and wakefulness. Exp Neurol 1978;62:821.)

region just ventral to the locus coeruleus (LC), termed by this group the *peri-LC alpha*, and its descending pathway to the bulbar reticular formation abolished the muscle atonia of REM sleep (Figure 3-10). It should be emphasized that this zone is a reticular zone, not one containing noradrenergic neurons like the LC proper, and that the name refers only to proximity to the LC. The Lyon group also reported that not only was the nuchal muscle atonia of REM suppressed, but that cats with such lesions exhibited oneiric behavior, including locomotion, attack behavior, and behavior with head raised and with horizontal and vertical movements "as

if watching something." Hendricks and collaborators[26] confirmed the basic finding of REM without atonia with bilateral pontine tegmental lesions but reported that lesions extending beyond the LC alpha region and its efferent pathway to bulb were necessary for more than a minimal release of muscle tone and to produce the elaborate oneiric behaviors. They found particular lesion locations were associated with particular sets of behaviors: For example, attack behavior was associated with lesions that extended into midbrain and interrupted amygdalar pathways; locomotion with lesions near the brain stem locomotor region; and orienting

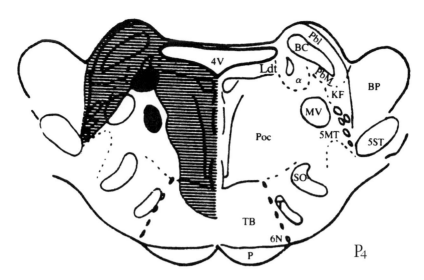

**Figure 3-10.** Frontal section of the pons of the cat. The solid areas indicate the localization of the lesions, which suppress postural atonia during REM sleep according to Jouvet. These lesions coincide with the reticular formation zone, termed *locus coeruleus alpha*, or its descending pathway. The horizontal hatching corresponds to lesions that do not suppress postural atonia. (Pbl = nucleus parabrachialis lateralis; Ldt = nucleus lateralis tegmenti dorsalis; PbM = nucleus parabrachialis medialis; KF = nucleus Kolliker-Fuse; Poc = nucleus pontis caudalis; BP = brachium pontis; MV and 5MT = motor nucleus and mesencephalic tract of trigeminal nerve; 5ST = sensory nucleus of trigeminal nerve; BC = brachium conjunctivum; 4V = fourth ventricle; TB = trapezoid body; SO = superior olivary nucleus; 6N = sixth nucleus; P = pyramidal tract.) (Adapted from M Jouvet. What does a cat dream about? Trends Neurosci 1979;2:15.)

behavior with small, symmetric dorsolateral pontine lesions. Finally, the presence of attack and locomotion behaviors in REM sleep without atonia was reported to be associated with an increased incidence of these behaviors in waking, leading to the interpretation that the lesions may have done more than simply counteract a behaviorally nonspecific muscle inhibition during REM sleep—they may have released the particular behaviors appearing in both REM and waking. Still another zone of neurons and pathways associated with muscle suppression has been reported by Mori[27] in the midline. The exact location and number of inhibitory pathways is still a matter of some controversy, with all investigators agreeing on the important, if not exclusive, role of the peri-LC alpha (or, as it is often termed, the *dorsolateral reticular small cell group*).

An overview of reticular areas important in muscle atonia, and evidence about important neurotransmitters is provided in Figure 3-11, adapted from Lai and Siegel,[28] and in Siegel.[29] Figure 3-11 shows sites in which, in decerebrate cats, injection of glutamate or cholinergic agonists induced atonia. The strong data implicating ACh in REM phenomena have been described under cholinergic mechanisms and the ini-

tiation and coordination of REM sleep. Precise in vitro evidence for glutamatergic reticular formation neurotransmission has been obtained by the Brockton group.[30] Lai and Siegel[31] have obtained evidence that the glutamate-effective sites show muscle atonia to non–$N$-methyl-$D$-aspartate (NMDA) agonists, whereas NMDA agonists produced increased muscle tone and locomotion, suggesting that REM sleep–related activation and inhibition of muscular activity might be mediated by different receptors responding to glutamate.

## REM SLEEP–SUPPRESSING SYSTEMS: INHIBITION OF CHOLINERGIC NEURONS

*REM-on neurons* are defined as those neurons that become active in REM sleep compared with SWS and waking and that presumably have a protagonist role in production of REM sleep phenomena. Neurons with a reciprocal discharge time course that becomes inactive as REM sleep is approached and entered are called *REM-off neurons* (see schematic of discharge time course in Figure 3-2). REM-off

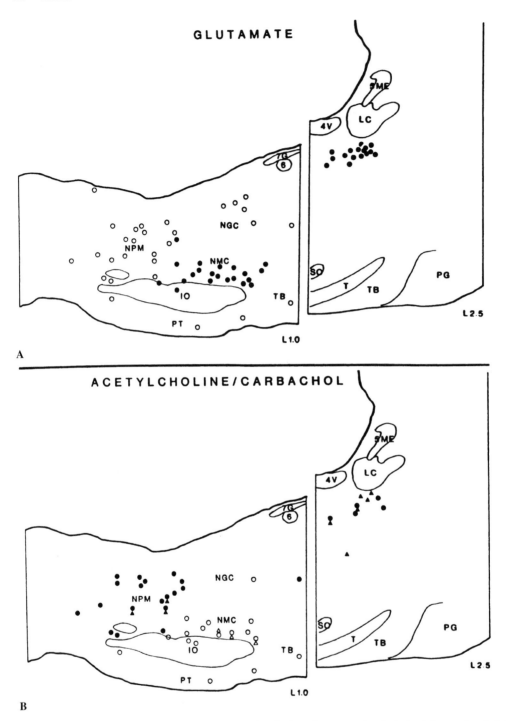

**Figure 3-11.** Pontobulbar inhibitory areas on sagittal section. In decerebrate cats, electrical stimulation produced atonia at all indicated points. Filled symbols indicate where muscle atonia was produced by injections of glutamate (0.2 mol/liter) (**A**) or cholinergic agonists (1.1 mol/liter acetylcholine [**B**, *circles*] or 0.01 mol/liter carbachol [**B**, *triangles*]). Open symbols indicate no effect. (IO = inferior olive; LC = locus coeruleus; 7G and 6 = genu of seventh nerve and sixth nucleus; NGC = bulbar nucleus gigantocellularis; NMC = nucleus magnocellularis; NPM = nucleus paramedianus; PG = pontine gray; PT = pyramidal tract; SO = superior olivary nucleus; TB = trapezoid body; T = trapezoid fibers; 4V = fourth ventricle.) (Adapted from YY Lai and JM Siegel. Medullary regions mediating atonia. J Neurosci 1988;8:4790.)

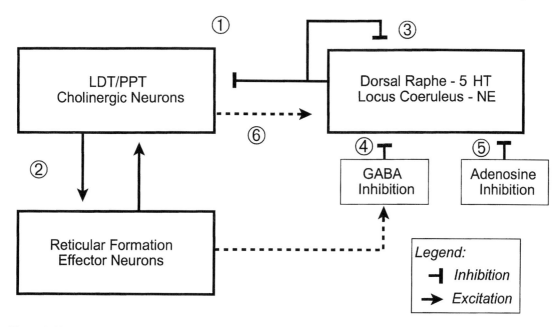

**Figure 3-12.** Reciprocal interaction model of REM sleep control. Cholinergic neurons activate reticular formation neurons in a positive feedback interaction to produce the onset of REM sleep. REM sleep is terminated by the inhibitory activity of REM-off aminergic neurons 3, which become active at the end of a REM sleep period due to their recruitment by REM-on activity. REM-off neuronal activity decreases in slow-wave sleep and becomes minimal at the onset of REM sleep due to self-inhibitory feedback and adenosinergic inhibition. GABA-ergic input is important for maintaining inhibition during REM sleep. This decreased REM-off activity disinhibits REM-on neurons and allows the onset of a REM sleep episode. The cycle then repeats itself. (GABA = γ-aminobutyric acid; LDT/PPT = laterodorsal tegmental/pedunculopontine tegmental nucleus; 5 HT = serotonin; NE = norepinephrine.)

neurons are most active in waking, have discharge activity that declines in SWS, and are virtually silent in REM sleep until they resume discharge toward the later portion of the REM sleep episode. Electrophysiologic data suggest REM-off neurons include the following three classes of aminergic neurons (see Figure 3-3 for anatomy): (1) *NE-containing neurons* are principally located in the LC, called the "blue spot" because of its appearance in the unstained brain (first demonstrated to be REM-off by Hobson and associates[32]). (2) *Serotonin-containing neurons* are located in the *raphe system* of the brain stem, the midline collection of neurons that extends from the bulb to the midbrain, with higher concentrations of serotonin-containing neurons among the more rostral neurons (REM-off neurons in the dorsal raphe, the midbrain nucleus, were first recorded by McGinty and Harper[33]). (3) *Histamine-containing neurons* are located in the posterior hypothalamus, and recording experiments suggest they are REM-off (see English summary in Lin and colleagues[34]). This system has

been conceptualized as one of the wakefulness-promoting systems, in agreement with drowsiness as a common side effect of antihistaminics, and is a projection target for the sleep-active neurons discussed in the final section of this chapter. Transection studies indicate, however, that the histaminergic neurons are not essential for the REM sleep oscillation.[35]

A strikingly inverse time course over the REM sleep cycle between PGO wave activity and the discharge activity of dorsal raphe neurons (presumptively serotonergic) has been demonstrated by Lydic and colleagues.[36] A similar inverse pattern of activity of REM-off neurons in the LC with REM-on neurons led a structural and mathematical model of REM sleep by McCarley and Hobson[37] (reciprocal interaction model), that had as one of its postulates that the REM-off neurons inhibited the REM-promoting, REM-on neurons. For many years this was regarded as a highly controversial postulate. In vitro work since the early 1990s, however, has supported this hypothesis. Figure 3-12 sketches the

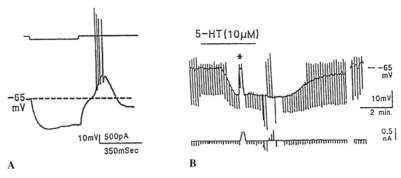

**Figure 3-13.** Serotonin (5-HT) inhibits cholinergic low-threshold burst neurons in the laterodorsal tegmental nucleus. Intracellular recordings from a rat in vitro preparation. **(A)** With the membrane potential held at –65 mV, a hyperpolarizing current step results in a rebound low-threshold burst, the likely mechanism for the production of bursts seen in extracellular in vivo recordings of PGO burst neurons. **(B)** Application of 10 μmol/liter 5-HT to a cholinergic bursting neuron results in a hyperpolarization of the membrane potential (*top trace*), a response that other experiments showed persisted in the presence of tetrodotoxin, indicating the inhibition was a direct serotonergic effect. The voltage deflections in the top trace are responses to constant current pulses used to measure input resistance; repolarization of the membrane to resting levels (*asterisk*) demonstrated that there was a decrease in input resistance that was independent of the change in membrane potential and thus due to a direct drug action. The same current that was effective in producing a burst in **A** did not result in a burst during the application of 5-HT (not shown in this figure); other experiments indicated that a 5-HT$_{1A}$ receptor mediated these effects. (Modified from JI Luebke, RW Greene, K Semba, et al. Serotonin hyperpolarizes cholinergic low threshold burst neurons in the rat laterodorsal tegmental nucleus in vitro. Proc Natl Acad Sci U S A 1992;89:743.)

structural model, which may be helpful to the reader in following the discussion in the following paragraph. Portions of the model that have empirical support and those that remain conjectural are differentiated in the discussion. Step 1 in the model, the postulated inhibitory effect of serotonin and NE on LDT and PPT cholinergic neurons, is treated first.

There is anatomic evidence indicating that the dorsal raphe sends serotonergic projections and that the LC sends norepinephrinergic projections to both LDT and PPT (see reviews[38–40]). In vitro experiments in a number of laboratories have now shown that serotonin inhibits cholinergic neurons of the LDT and PPT.[41–43] For example, Luebke and coworkers[42] showed that approximately two-thirds of histologically identified cholinergic neurons recorded in the rat in vitro preparation responded to the application of serotonin with a membrane hyperpolarization and decrease in input resistance (Figure 3-13). Whole-cell patch clamp recordings revealed that the hyperpolarizing response was mediated by an inwardly rectifying potassium current. Pharmacologic studies have shown that the serotonin (5-hydroxytryptamine [5-HT]) effect was mimicked by application of the selective 5-HT$_{1A}$ receptor agonist 8-hydroxy-2-(di-n-propylamino)

tetralin (8-OH-DPAT), implying mediation of the 5-HT$_{1A}$ receptor. The same results were obtained with tetrodotoxin present in the bathing medium (blocking sodium-dependent action potentials), indicating that the serotonin effects were direct. Williams and Reiner[44] obtained very similar inhibitory results with NE. Ninety-two percent of histologically identified cholinergic LDT neurons in the rat in vitro preparation were hyperpolarized in response to NE, whereas noncholinergic neurons exhibited mixed responses. Interestingly, the NE response in the cholinergic LDT neurons was mediated by an inwardly rectifying potassium current, similar to that activated by serotonin.

The in vitro data were quite clear about the strong inhibitory effect of serotonin on cholinergic LDT neurons. However, the systems neurophysiology question remained as to the strength of this input. As mentioned before, dorsal raphe neurons (presumably serotonergic) slow and virtually cease discharge with the approach and onset of REM sleep. Whether this withdrawal of inhibitory input could be sufficiently strong to disinhibit the cholinergic neurons and permit the occurrence of a REM sleep episode (see Figure 3-12, action labeled 1) was still unclear. The capability to use microdialysis techniques in the

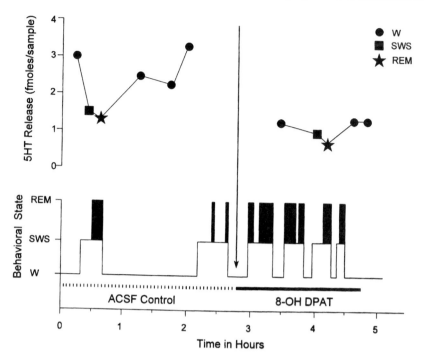

**Figure 3-14.** Effects of microdialysis delivery of 8-OH-DPAT to the dorsal raphe nucleus (DRN) on serotonin (5-HT) release and REM sleep. Time course of 5-HT levels (*top*) and behavioral state (*bottom*) before and during DRN 8-OH-DPAT perfusion in a typical experiment are shown. Note that, in the control perfusion of artificial cerebrospinal fluid (ACSF), waking DRN 5-HT levels (*circles*) are higher than those in slow-wave sleep (SWS) (*squares*) and REM sleep (*stars*). Each 5-HT value is expressed as fmol/7.5-μl sample and was obtained during an uninterrupted 5-minute sequence of the behavioral state. With the onset of 10 μmol/liter 8-OH-DPAT perfusion (*arrow; filled horizontal bar* indicates duration), the 5-HT level dropped quickly to levels as low as those normally present in SWS or REM. Behaviorally, 8-OH-DPAT administration increased REM sleep (*black bars*) more than 300%. (Adapted from CM Portas, M Thakkar, D Rainnie, RW McCarley. Microdialysis perfusion of 8-OH-DPAT in the dorsal raphe nucleus decreases serotonin release and increases REM sleep in the freely moving cat. J Neurosci 1996;16:2820.)

dorsal raphe nucleus (DRN) of freely moving cats offered what appeared to be a happy opportunity for a direct test of the hypothesis of serotonergic inhibition of REM sleep. Portas and McCarley[45] inserted microdialysis probes into the DRN; using high-performance liquid chromatography (HPLC) and electrochemical detection techniques they were able to detect changes of a few femtomoles in serotonin concentrations. In samples collected over spontaneously occurring sleep cycles, the serotonin concentrations in the DRN had the same ordering as did presumably serotonergic unit discharge rates: Waking > NREM sleep (= SWS) > REM sleep. This presumably reflected the detection of serotonin released by DRN recurrent collaterals, and this state-related ordering of concentrations matched that

found in distant, forebrain DRN projection sites, as reported in cats[46] and in rats.[47,48]

Portas and colleagues[49] reasoned that, if one were able to inhibit DRN serotonergic activity, the degree of subsequent enhancement of REM sleep would provide an index of the strength of DRN inhibitory control. For inhibition of the DRN the specific 5-HT$_{1A}$ agonist 8-OH-DPAT was selected, because it was known to exert powerful inhibitory effects via somatodendritic 5-HT$_{1A}$ receptors.[50] As illustrated in Figure 3-14, the experimental protocol was to measure behavioral state percentages and serotonin concentrations during a control period, and then to add 8-OH-DPAT (10 μmol/liter concentration) to the artificial cerebrospinal fluid (ACSF) flowing into the dialysis probe. The effects during the period of perfusion with 8-OH-DPAT were clear: (1) There was a strong reduction of 5-HT extracellular concentration, indicating inhibition of DRN activity, and (2) there was a 300% increase in the percentage of REM sleep, presumably reflecting the disinhibition of brain stem LDT and PPT cholinergic neurons.

The finding that 8-OH-DPAT delivery through a probe in the aqueduct did not increase REM sleep, but tended to increase waking and decrease SWS, suggested DRN specificity of effects. These data on REM sleep provided the first biochemically validated and direct evidence that suppression of DRN serotonergic activity increases REM sleep, and furnished a key complement to the previously cited in vitro data indicating that mesopontine cholinergic neurons, a target of DRN projections, are inhibited by 5-HT.[42] The 8-OH-DPAT–induced reduction of DRN 5-HT is consistent with the hypothesis that the concomitant REM sleep disinhibition is mediated by DRN serotonergic projections to the LDT and PPT cholinergic neurons implicated in REM sleep production.

### Inhibition of REM-On Versus Wake/REM-On Neurons

This section describes a direct test of the postulate that REM-on neurons are inhibited by monoaminergic neurons and provides an answer to the question of why some neurons in the LDT and PPT cholinergic zone are REM-on whereas others are selectively active in both wakefulness and REM sleep (wake/REM-on neurons).

Our laboratory has tested the hypothesis that REM-on neurons are not active in waking because they are inhibited at $5\text{-HT}_{1A}$ receptors by projections from waking-active 5-HT DRN neurons, whereas wake/REM-on neurons are not inhibited. We have developed techniques for simultaneous unit recording from microwire bundles implanted adjacent to microdialysis probes used to perfuse pharmacologic agents or collect samples for neurotransmitter analysis. Using this technique, we have examined the effect of microdialysis perfusion of the $5\text{-HT}_{1A}$ agonist 8-OH-DPAT on the discharge activity of neurons within the REM-on (and presumptively cholinergic) zone. Our prediction was that 8-OH-DPAT would suppress discharge of REM-on but not wake/REM-on neurons. This experiment first involved recording an LDT or PPT neuron to determine if it was a REM-on neuron (operationally defined as having a discharge rate in REM sleep with PGOs or eye movements, termed *REM+*, that was twice that in other states) or a wake/REM-on neuron (operationally defined as having discharge rates in active wake (movement present) and REM sleep higher than in NREM, but with REM+ rates less than twice those in active wake.

Our preliminary data[51] indicate that all REM-on neurons thus far recorded ($N = 7$) were markedly inhibited by 10 µmol/liter 8-OH-DPAT in the perfusate (mean 89% reduction in discharge rate), whereas, in contrast, none of the wake/REM-on ($N = 20$) neurons was markedly inhibited. These differences in responsiveness were highly statistically significant, and of further note is that suppression began within 2 minutes after the 8-OH-DPAT reached the brain. The data thus far acquired suggest that $5\text{-HT}_{1A}$ agonist responsiveness has an either-or, present-or-absent nature. Neurons with intermediate responsiveness, however, may be encountered as we acquire more data. The absence of responsiveness could result from absence of innervation of the $5\text{-HT}_{1A}$ receptor or a lesser sensitivity to 5-HT. Future immunohistochemical studies can, of course, determine the percentage of neurons with $5\text{-HT}_{1A}$ receptors.

### REM-On Cholinergic Neurons

The following discussion treats the subject of increased activity of REM-on cholinergic neurons after disinhibition from decreased activity of serotonin- and NE-containing neurons. Positive feedback mechanisms are also addressed.

Evidence for disinhibition of LDT and PPT neurons by the gradual reduction in firing that occurs in LC and dorsal raphe neurons during the NREM portion of the cycle preceding REM sleep onset has been discussed and illustrated (see Figure 3-12, label 1). Extensive evidence that discharge of LDT and PPT neurons excites reticular formation neurons, which, in turn, generate the occurrence of REM sleep events such as REMs and muscle atonia, has also been presented (see Figure 3-12, label 2). Note that in the model, the recruitment of discharge activity in the populations of LDT, PPT, and reticular formation neurons is facilitated by the presence of excitatory projections of PRF neurons back onto the LDT and PPT population. The original reciprocal interaction model[37] postulated a positive feedback in the REM sleep–generating population; in the model, this positive feedback was required for the coordination and recruitment of activity and was compatible with the exponential recruitment curve of reticular neurons in experimental data. With respect to recurrent projections, there is anatomic evidence for projection from one cholinergic zone to another, such as LDT-LDT projections from one side to the other, as well as between LDT and PPT.[9,39,52] At the electron microscopic level, chlorine acetyltransferase (ChAT+) axon terminals form somatodendritic synaptic contacts with ChAT+ neurons,[53] further consistent with recurrent collateral innervation. Obviously, whether this recurrent cholinergic innervation is excitatory or inhibitory is important from the point of view of regulation of the cholinergic system. Contrary to the original simple postulate of direct positive feedback, we now know that this recurrent cholinergic innervation is inhibitory.[41,54]

Based on experimental data, it is suggested that the positive feedback comes through another, indirect connection, via the PRF.[55] The data can be summarized as follows: (1) There are anatomically documented reciprocal LDT and PPT–reticular connections. (2) Cholinergic projections to reticular formation are primarily excitatory.[11] (3) Data indicate excitatory amino acid (EAA) synaptic input to cholinergic LDT neurons.[56] (4) There is evidence that many PRF neurons use EAA neurotransmission.[19]

### Why Do REM-Off Neurons Turn Off?

The following causal events for REM sleep production have been presented (the numbers refer to Figure 3-12):

1. REM-off neurons turn off → disinhibition of REM-on cholinergic neurons in LDT and PPT
2. REM-on cholinergic neuronal activity → excitation of reticular effector neurons → REM sleep events, and positive feedback on LDT and PPT cholinergic neurons

What initiates this chain is a topic of intense current investigation. The currently postulated mecha-

nisms and evidence bearing on them are presented in the following discussion, which is confined to DRN neurons. Although many parallel points are valid for LC neurons, the overall empirical evidence is less abundant. There appear to be four main possible answers to why REM-off neurons turn off; these are not mutually exclusive, nor exhaustive of all possible mechanisms.

The first suggestion, offered by McCarley and Hobson,[37] is that recurrent inhibitory feedback of serotonergic and adrenergic collaterals might diminish activity. There might not only be immediate ion channel effects of recurrent collaterals but also long-lasting second messenger mechanisms. The recurrent inhibition (see Figure 3-12, label 3) is well-documented, although second-messenger effects have not been demonstrated. With respect to possible second-messenger mechanisms, the DRN somatodendritic $5\text{-}HT_{1A}$ receptor is coupled through a G protein ($G_{i/o}$) family effector to a reduction in cyclic adenosine monophosphate (cAMP), as well as to changes in ion channel permeabilities, to $K^+$? and $Ca^{2+}$; changes in cAMP and $Ca^{2+}$ might induce effects more long-lasting than simple ionic flux changes, such as receptor phosphorylation (see summary review in Peroutka[57] and Watson and Girdlestone[58]). An alternative possibility is recurrent feedback effects on the serotonin transporter. Although such effects remain a possibility, they have not been empirically demonstrated.

A second possibility, raised by the studies of Nitz and Siegel,[58] is that γ-aminobutyric acid (GABA) input silences the discharge of DRN serotonergic neurons (see Figure 3-12, label 4). Nitz and Siegel have provided microdialysis evidence that DRN GABA levels are increased during REM sleep, and Peyron and coworkers[60] have documented GABAergic projections to the dorsal raphe from several sites, including the brain stem reticular formation. Figure 3-12 suggests this increased GABAergic input may be activated as part of the increased reticular formation activity during REM sleep. This input would then diminish DRN activity in the period just before and during REM sleep (as illustrated in Figure 3-12, this is the period during which REM-on neurons become active). However, this would not explain the initial decrease in REM-off activity, which precedes any REM-on activity (see Figure 3-12). Although this increased GABAergic input could come from other sites, Nitz and Siegel did not find evidence of increased DRN GABA levels during NREM sleep, the time when DRN neurons are beginning to decrease rates. These considerations suggest that GABA may not be the initiator of the decrease in REM-off neuronal discharge rates, although it may contribute to the virtual silence of activity during REM sleep.

A third possibility raised by our studies on adenosine (AD) is that serotonergic neuronal discharge, slowing after prolonged wakefulness, might be due to a buildup of AD, which acts, directly or indirectly, to inhibit discharge (see Figure 3-12, label 5). An extensive discussion of AD is given under Adenosine and REM Sleep: Influences on DRN REM-off Neurons. A fourth possibility, raised by our in vitro preliminary data, is that the discharge slowing is due to a dysfacilitation of nicotinic cholinergic presynaptic enhancement of adrenergic ($\alpha_1$) excitatory input to DRN, occurring because both wake/REM-on cholinergic and adrenergic neurons slow discharge rate with transition to SWS.[61]

### Termination of REM Sleep Episodes and REM-Off Neurons

There is some question as to what terminates REM sleep episodes and why REM-off neurons turn on the end of REM sleep. The original reciprocal interaction model postulated was that REM-on cholinergic neurons slowly excite the REM-off, REM-suppressive neurons in the dorsal raphe and LC (see Figure 3-12, label 6). As the REM-off neurons become active at the end of a REM sleep period due to their recruitment by REM-on activity, they terminate REM sleep because of their inhibition of REM-on neurons. With respect to excitation of REM-off neurons by REM-on neurons, there is anatomic evidence (reviewed in Steriade and McCarley[1] and Jones[39]) for cholinergic projections to both LC and DRN. In vivo data indicate excitatory effects of ACh on LC neurons, and, thus, this mechanism seems plausible for NE LC neurons. As has been mentioned, however, new data from the author's laboratory do not indicate such clear excitatory effects on dorsal raphe,[61] although the resumption of adrenergic input would tend to activate DRN neurons.

In summary, the basic structure of the reciprocal interaction model, as described in 1986,[62] still appears reasonable. The major empirical advances since the early 1990s have been the recognition of the importance of ACh and the very recent documentation of serotonergic inhibition of cholinergic neurons. Several important areas for future physiologic investigation include the mechanisms of coupling between circadian and REM sleep control systems and the mechanisms of REM sleep rebound.

## NREM SLEEP MECHANISMS

### Importance of Cholinergic Activity in Suppression of EEG Synchronization and Slow-Wave Activity

One of the major recent advances has been the growing understanding of the importance of a cholinergic activating system in EEG activation. This is often termed *EEG desynchronization*, but EEG activation is preferable, because this is the EEG pattern accompanying cortical activity and because higher frequency rhythmic activity (gamma activity, approximately 40 Hz) may be present, although the amplitude is low. The cholinergic system is likely a major component of the *ascending reticular activating system*, a concept that arose before methods were available for labeling neurons using specific neurotransmitters. We now know that a subset of the cholinergic LDT and PPT neurons has high discharge rates in waking and REM sleep, and low discharge rates in SWS; this group is anatomically interspersed with the physiologically distinct REM-selective cholinergic neurons (see previous section on Inhibition of REM-On versus Wake/REM-On Neurons). There is also extensive anatomic evidence that these cholinergic neurons project to thalamic nuclei important in EEG activation and synchronization. In vitro and in vivo neurophysiologic studies have both indicated that the target neurons in the thalamus respond to cholinergic agonists in a way consistent with EEG activation, as is discussed in Chapter 4. Cholinergic systems are not the only substrate of EEG desynchronization; brain stem reticular formation projections to the thalamus (using EAA) may also play an important role, and NE projections from the LC may be relevant during waking (LC neurons are silent in REM sleep).

In addition to brain stem cholinergic systems, cholinergic input to the cortex from the BF cholinergic nucleus basalis of Meynert is also important for

EEG activation. Many neurons in this zone are active in both waking and REM sleep and both lesion and pharmacologic data suggest their importance in REM sleep (see review by Szymusiak[63]). This BF cholinergic zone is discussed in the next section.

### Adenosine and the Sleep-Inducing Effects of Prolonged Wakefulness

The way in which a population of mesopontine and BF cholinergic neurons selectively discharges during both REM sleep and waking has been discussed, as well as the possibility that these neurons contribute to the production of EEG arousal. Such EEG arousal diminishes as a function of the duration of prior wakefulness or of brain hyperthermia. How these cholinergic neurons might be modulated by factors that diminish EEG arousal has been an open question (see discussion in Rainnie and colleagues[64]). Using an in vitro rat brain stem slice preparation, our laboratory demonstrated that both mesopontine and BF cholinergic neurons are under the tonic inhibitory control of endogenous AD, a neuromodulator. Other data suggested that the extracellular concentration of AD was proportional to brain metabolic rate (see citations in Rainnie and colleagues[64]). Whole-cell and extracellular recordings of identified cholinergic neurons showed an AD inhibitory tone that was mediated postsynaptically by an inwardly rectifying potassium conductance and by an inhibition of the hyperpolarization-activated current $I_H$. These data provided a potential coupling mechanism linking neuronal control of EEG arousal with the effects of prior wakefulness and brain hyperthermia (states of increased metabolism relative to SWS), as well as the ubiquitous use of the AD-receptor blockers caffeine and theophylline to promote alertness.

It was essential to demonstrate that AD fulfilled the following additional major in vivo criteria for a sleep factor mediating the somnogenic effects of prolonged wakefulness: (1) AD increases with prolonged wakefulness and decreases during recovery sleep, and (2) an increase in extracellular AD concentration leads to a decrease in wakefulness. The first series of studies[65] examined the in vivo effect, on electrographically defined behavioral states, of microdialysis perfusion of AD into the cholinergic zones of the substantia innominata of BF and the

brain stem LDT nucleus of freely moving cats. Unilateral, localized perfusion of 300 µmol/liter AD into either the cholinergic BF or the cholinergic LDT caused a marked alteration in sleep-wake architecture, with a dramatic decrease in waking to approximately 50% of the control level. Perfusion into the BF also resulted in a significant increase in REM sleep, whereas SWS, although increased, was not statistically different from control values. In contrast, AD perfusion into the LDT produced statistically significant increases in both SWS and REM sleep, the magnitude of which were proportional to decreases in waking. EEG power spectral analysis showed that AD perfusion into the BF increased the relative power in the delta-frequency band, whereas higher frequency bands (theta, alpha, beta, and gamma) showed decreases. These data supported the hypothesis that AD might play a key role as an endogenous modulator of wakefulness and sleep. Although the effects of perfused AD were clear, the possibility remained that AD fluctuations might not occur under physiologic circumstances.

We evaluated the extracellular concentration of AD during spontaneously occurring behavioral states and during prolonged wakefulness and recovery. We also evaluated the effects on sleep and wakefulness of pharmacologically increasing AD concentration.[66] The results of this study are compatible with AD's being an endogenous sleep factor, mediating the sleep-inducing effects of prolonged wakefulness. Microdialysate samples were collected from male cats prepared for chronic sleep studies with EEG, EOG, EMG, and PGO electrodes, as well as microdialysis probes.

The microdialysis probes were placed in the BF cholinergic region, termed the *substantia innominata* in the cat and, as a control, in the relay thalamic zone of the ventroanterior and ventrolateral nucleus (VA/VL). Using ultraviolet detection, the microbore HPLC system could detect levels as low as 50 fmol. Mean AD concentration in samples collected during spontaneous wakefulness was significantly higher than those collected during NREM sleep for both the BF and VA/VL of thalamus. Absolute values were approximately 41 nmol/liter in waking and 33 nmol/liter in NREM sleep, a reduction of approximately 25%. This finding is in line with our expectation that AD levels may be globally increased throughout the brain during waking. (In these experiments, it was diffi-

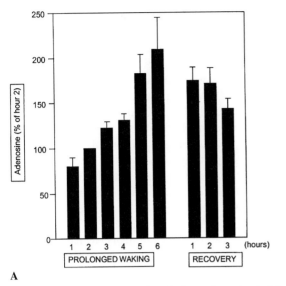
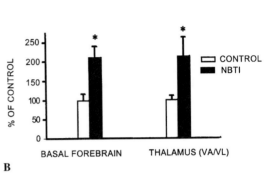

**Figure 3-15.** (A) Adenosine values during prolonged wakefulness and recovery sleep. The graph shows mean basal fore-brain extracellular adenosine values (+ SEM) by hour during 6 hours of prolonged wakefulness (9:00 AM to 3:00 PM) and in the subsequent 3 hours of spontaneous recovery sleep (N = 6). Values are normalized relative to the second hour of deprivation (due to technical problems, values for the three first hours were missing). Repeated measures analysis of variance (ANOVA): between subjects, df = 5, NS; between treatments df = 8, F = 7.0, P <.0001; paired t-test between the second and the last hour of wakefulness, t(5) = 3.14, P <.05. (B) Effects of local perfusion of the adenosine-transport inhibitor NBTI (1 μmol/liter). Microdialysis perfusion of NBTI increases adenosine levels in both the basal forebrain (paired t-test, t[5] = 4.79, P <.01) and in the thalamus (paired t-test, t[4] = 3.92, P <.05) approximately twofold (comparison of the means of last three samples before and the means of the first three samples after onset of NBTI perfusion).

cult to get sufficiently long, pure REM sleep samples to determine AD values during this state.) The next step was to determine if AD levels increased during sleep deprivation, as would be expected if AD were a somnogenic factor. As illustrated in Figure 3-15A, mean AD concentrations increased steadily in the BF during 6 hours of continuous, EEG-verified wakefulness produced by gentle handling or playing (9 AM to 3 PM), and declined slowly during a 3-hour recovery period.

We then evaluated whether microdialysis application of the AD transport inhibitor S-(4-nitrobenzyl)-6-thioinosine (NBTI) could be used to produce a local increase in AD that would affect sleep. Perfusion of 1 μmol/liter NBTI increased extracellular AD in both cholinergic BF and thalamus approximately twofold (Figure 3-15B). We then evaluated the behavioral effects of the NBTI-induced AD increases in cholinergic BF and thalamus to determine if there was any evidence for site specificity of the behavioral effects of increasing extracellular AD. Cholinergic neurons have widespread and strategic efferent targets in the thalamic and corti-

cal systems important for the control of EEG arousal, and thus may constitute a relatively selective site of AD action. There was a significant decrease in wakefulness when 1 μmol/liter NBTI was (unilaterally) perfused in the BF, but not when perfused in the thalamus, despite the fact that both treatments yielded similar increases in local AD concentrations (Figure 3-15C). These data are consistent with a selective AD effect on behavioral state in the BF cholinergic zone, as contrasted with the noncholinergic thalamus. Finally, the state distributions in the period after the approximately twofold elevation of BF AD after prolonged wakefulness were closely mimicked by the approximately twofold elevation of BF AD with unilateral NBTI perfusion (Figure 3-15D). These data support a causal role for AD in increasing NREM sleep.

These data are the first to show changes in AD during spontaneously occurring behavioral states. They are compatible with the data of Huston and associates[67] showing AD increases in the striatum and hippocampus during the circadian phase of activity in the rat as contrasted with the circadian

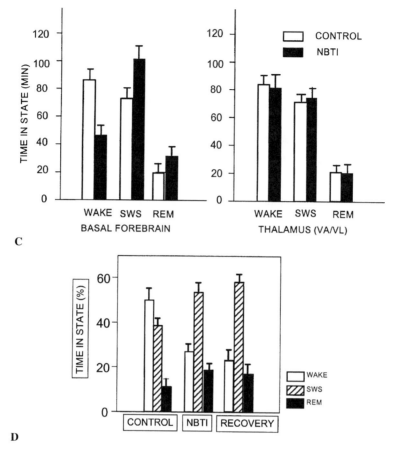

**Figure 3-15.** *continued.* **(C)** NBTI administration causes sleep-wake changes in the basal forebrain (*left*) but not in the ventroanterior and ventrolateral nucleus (VA/VL) thalamus (*right*). Basal forebrain: paired *t*-test, $t(5) = 3.47$, $P < .05$ for waking, $t(5) = 3.78$, $P < .05$ for slow-wave sleep (SWS), and $t(5) = 2.76$, $P < .05$ for REM sleep. Thalamus: $P = NS$ for all states. Ordinate: minutes in each state during the 3-hour recording period. **(D)** Comparison of the effects of prolonged wakefulness and NBTI perfusion in basal forebrain on the percentage of time spent in each behavioral state. Both during NBTI treatment and recovery sleep, SWS was increased as compared to control sleep (40% and 50%, respectively; repeated measures ANOVA, between subjects ($N = 5$) NS, between treatments df = 2, F = 5.92, $P < .05$; post hoc Neuman-Keul $P < .05$, no difference between NBTI-treated and recovery sleep groups). During NBTI treatment and recovery sleep, wakefulness was decreased (45% and 50%, respectively; repeated measures ANOVA, between subjects [$n = 5$] NS, between treatments df = 2, F = 9.41, $P < .01$; post hoc Neuman-Keul $P < .05$; no difference between NBTI-treated and recovery sleep groups). REM sleep in the NBTI-treated and recovery sleep groups had similar percentage increases (65% and 50%, respectively) and did not statistically differ. (Adapted from T Porkka Heiskanen, RE Strecker, M Thakkar, et al. Adenosine: a mediator of the sleep-inducing effects of prolonged wakefulness. Science 1997;276:1265.)

phase of inactivity (no EEG recordings were done). The data bear an intriguing relationship to the work of Hayaishi,[68] given the fact that recent data[69] suggest that somnogenic effects of prostaglandin $D_2$ may be mediated by AD.

This series of experiments has shown that (1) extracellular AD concentrations changed according to behavioral state, being higher during wakefulness than in sleep; (2) during prolonged wakefulness there was a progressive increase in extracellular AD concentrations; (3) NBTI-induced elevations of extracellular AD concentrations did not decrease wakefulness and increase sleep similarly in all brain areas, but did so in the vicinity of the cholinergic neurons of the BF; and (4) induction of a similar level of elevation of extracellular AD concentrations in the BF by two methods (prolonged wakefulness and NBTI infusion) induced similar decreases in wakefulness and increases in SWS.

The nature of the mechanism of the observed changes in extracellular concentrations of AD that occur in association with sleep-wakefulness changes remains an open question. Mechanisms that influence extracellular AD levels include modulation of AD anabolic and catabolic enzyme activity and AD transport rate constants or activities.[70–72] Increases in metabolic activity during wakefulness could increase intracellular AD concentrations and, by altering the transmembrane AD gradient, reduce or even reverse the direction of the inward diffusion of AD via its facilitated nucleoside transporters; this possibility has been reviewed by Brundege and Dunwiddie,[73] who also provide direct evidence for an increase in intracellular AD's leading to an increase in extracellular AD's actions on receptors. Similar AD increases may occur in other central nervous system regions, and indeed, diurnal variations of AD levels in the frontal cortex and hippocampus have been reported, although these studies did not measure behavioral state–related changes.[67,74] We suggest that AD's powerful state-altering effects in the cholinergic BF region occur primarily because of the cholinergic neurons' widespread and strategic efferent targets in the thalamic and cortical systems important for the control of EEG arousal.[1,39] Increased AD concentrations in the cholinergic BF zone would thus decrease EEG arousal, increase drowsiness, and promote EEG delta-wave activity during subsequent sleep. We suggest that extracellular AD levels decrease in SWS because of the reduced metabolic activity of sleep, especially delta-wave sleep, a time when cholinergic neurons are relatively quiescent. This postulate is congruent with the observed declining exponential time course of delta-wave activity over a night's sleep.[75]

Taken together, these results suggest that AD is a physiologic sleep factor that mediates somnogenic effects of prior wakefulness. The duration and depth of sleep after wakefulness appear to be profoundly modulated by the elevated concentrations of AD. Krueger and Fang[6] have reviewed putative sleep factors affecting SWS. The four putative factors (other than AD) meeting their criteria for promising candidates have a time course and spectrum of effects quite different from AD. Fever may be induced by the cytokine interleukin-1α, and both it and the cytokine tumor necrosis factor–α are intimately linked with host defense mechanisms, although both may separately influence SWS. These two cytokines and growth hormone–releasing hormone, another putative sleep factor,[76,77] have not been demonstrated to show spontaneous variation in the time epochs associated with individual bouts of wakefulness and SWS, but rather to show diurnal variation. Prostaglandin $D_2$, whose synthesis has been localized to the pia-arachnoid membranes, also has not been demonstrated to show spontaneous variation during bouts of wakefulness and SWS.[68]

## Adenosine and REM Sleep: Influences on DRN REM-Off Neurons

After considering the effects of AD on NREM sleep, effects strongly mediated by cholinergic neurons, one might wonder if AD has any effect on REM sleep. This is a reasonable question, because the DRN serotonin and the LC NE systems that are important in suppressing the cholinergic REM-on neurons also have a role in promotion of wakefulness. We selected the DRN as an initial site for evaluation of the behavioral state effect of NBTI perfusion. We reasoned that increased AD buildup in wakefulness might act to promote the slowing of discharge of serotonergic neurons that begins with the onset of SWS and becomes maximal in REM sleep. AD suppression of 5-HT neuronal activity might occur as the result of either direct (postsynaptic) or indirect effects, including actions on nonserotonergic neurons or presynaptic actions on inputs to serotonergic neurons. The effects on slowing of DRN serotonergic activity might be expected to produce a decrease in wakefulness and an increase in REM sleep.

In comparison with ACSF control perfusion, perfusion of 1 μmol/liter NBTI led to a clear-cut increase in REM sleep (approximately twofold), with a concomitant 20% decrease in wakefulness. In the preliminary data obtained from six experiments, the REM sleep data are statistically significant but, because of more variability, the waking data are not. SWS was virtually unchanged. Thus, although application of NBTI to the cholinergic BF appears to act significantly on wakefulness and

NREM sleep, and on REM sleep to a lesser degree, the main effect of DRN perfusion of NBTI appears to be an increase in REM sleep. BF effects are most easily interpreted as the inhibition of cholinergic neurons.[64] The actions on the DRN may be the direct result of inhibition of 5-HT neurons; this would disinhibit cholinergic REM-on neurons (see section Why Do REM-Off Neurons Turn Off?) and produce REM sleep. It should be noted that NBTI's effects on the DRN (increased REM sleep) are like those seen with 8-OH-DPAT inhibition of DRN 5-HT neurons.[49] Further experiments are under way, including efforts to determine DRN 5-HT levels and unit activity in the course of NBTI perfusion. We think the AD actions may represent physiologic as well as pharmacologic effects, because a significant reduction of extracellular AD is found in spontaneous NREM sleep compared with waking.

The results of our studies are intriguing in terms of a hypothesis about AD control of multiple EEG arousal systems. Our data suggest, for the first time, that 5-HT neuronal activity is under adenosinergic modulation. Functionally, this would be compatible with the role of AD as a sleep factor mediating the effects of prolonged wakefulness. Cholinergic neurons are important in maintaining EEG arousal, but 5-HT neurons also play a role.[78] Thus AD inhibition might act on 5-HT as well as cholinergic components of the arousal system. The state-alerting effects of AD appear to be more selective for neuronal systems highly involved in state regulation, such as the cholinergic and serotonergic systems. Although control sites other than the VA/VL of the thalamus need to be tested, the data thus far suggest that AD effects on behavioral state are not global but relatively selective, in contrast with the hypothesis of Bennington and Heller.[79]

The AD effects on DRN are most interesting in providing yet another potential mechanism for regulating the discharge of 5-HT neurons and, in particular, the progressive slowing of the discharge that begins at the onset of SWS and progresses to a virtual silence with the onset of REM sleep. The data strongly suggest that AD acts to suppress DRN discharge activity and 5-HT release, based on the association of decreased 5-HT neuronal discharge with a decrease in waking and an increase in REM sleep (see Figure 3-12 for a sketch of this possibility). Experiments in progress are designed to provide more direct evidence. Increased AD concentrations appear to be a particularly attractive candidate for the mechanism leading to a slowing of DRN activity after periods of prolonged wakefulness, a time when maximal AD concentrations would be present.

## FUNCTIONAL QUESTIONS ABOUT SLEEP AND THE USE OF IMMEDIATE EARLY GENES AS MARKERS OF ACTIVATION

Perhaps the major unsolved problem in sleep research is the function(s) of sleep. There are many plausible theories about REM sleep. Its prominence in the developing animal implies a possible functional role promoting development. A reasonable extension postulates that REM sleep "exercises" neural circuits in the adult, keeping functionally fit the many neural pathways not used on a regular basis in heavily encephalized higher animals. Without the development of knowledge about the deeper consequences of REM sleep for neuronal biology, however, such theories will remain speculative. The consequences of REM sleep–like states for cellular biology are beginning to be explored, and the effect of these states on immediate early genes is now a topic of considerable interest. The following paragraphs are a brief introduction to the topic.

Neurotransmitters may activate mechanisms regulating the transcription of DNA. The induction of the *immediate early genes* (IEG) such as c-*fos* and *jun* is one example of this mechanism. The term *fos* was first used to describe the oncogene (cancer gene) encoded by the *F*inkel-Biskis-Jenkins murine *o*steogenic *s*arcoma virus. The normal *cel*lular sequences from which the viral oncogene v-*fos* was derived are referred to as the *fos proto-oncogene* or c-*fos*. In normal cells, the level of the protein product of the c-*fos* gene, Fos, is highly regulated; many stimuli, some associated with cellular differentiation and some linked with neuronal excitation, lead to a transient induction of c-*fos* messenger RNA (mRNA). The name for the immediate early gene *jun* was derived in similar fashion from the oncogene carried by the avian sarcoma virus (ASV)-17; "*ju-n*ana" is the Japanese word for the number 17. An extensive discussion of stimulus-transcription coupling can be found in Morgan and Curran.[80]

In the following schematic, arrows are used to indicate successive steps in the cascade involving c-*fos*.

Neurotransmitter/receptor binding

→ change in second messenger levels

→ induction of transcription of the genes c-*fos* and *jun*

→ c-*fos* and *jun* mRNAs present in cytoplasm for approximately 1–2 hours

→ translation of Fos and Jun proteins

→ possible alterations in post-translational modification (e.g., phosphorylation) of Fos by stimuli

→ translocation to nucleus and formation of a Fos/Jun dimer (Fos has a half-life of approximately 2 hours)

→ Fos/Jun dimer complex binds to DNA regulatory element (AP-1 site)

→ increase in transcription of DNA

→ increase in production of a particular protein

The area of stimulus-transcription coupling is one of intense current work and hence of great flux in defining both (1) which neurotransmitters and stimuli lead to IEG production and (2) which proteins are regulated by this transcriptional control, a much more difficult question.

Neurotransmitters and receptors reported to modulate c-*fos* expression include excitatory amino acids (especially NMDA, but also kainate), dopamine, opioids, cholecystokinin, progesterone, interleukin-1, and nicotine. Stimuli and conditions known to activate c-*fos* include heat shock, dehydration, electrical stimulation, seizures (especially in the hippocampus), manipulation of internal calcium concentration, treadmill locomotion, and stimulation with light (for further information, see the list of published studies furnished by Morgan and Curran[80]). Although this list is long, it should not be assumed that all cellular activation leads to c-*fos* production, nor that c-*fos* production is nonspecific.

There appears to be a relatively specific production of c-*fos* in the hypothalamic suprachiasmatic nucleus (SCN). The SCN contains the basic mechanisms of the circadian clock, which regulates the circadian oscillations of many body systems, including temperature and sleep. This clock may be reset to an earlier time (this kind of reset is called *phase advancing*) in response to a light stimulus occurring just before the expected onset of light in the environment. Several groups of investigators have found that light stimuli applied at this time—but not at other circadian times that do not induce the same phase reset—have the capability

of inducing c-*fos*. Although it has been hypothesized that the transcriptional regulation of DNA is important in resetting the circadian clock, this has not yet been proved.

The induction of immediate early genes may be very important for REM sleep function, because this process may mediate long-term alterations of neuronal connectivity and activity. Initial studies[81–83] have used cholinergic induction of a REM sleep–like state as a model. Compared with vehicle control, induction of a REM sleep–like state by carbachol microinjections in the medial PRF led to a marked increase in Fos-like immunoreactivity in cells in several brain stem areas thought to be important in REM sleep. Longer REM sleep–like episodes were associated with more Fos-like immunoreactivity cells than the shorter-duration ones. Fos-like immunoreactivity increases were found in the LDT and PPT nuclei, where some Fos-like immunoreactive cells were immunohistochemically identified as cholinergic; the LC, where some of the Fos-like immunoreactivity cells were identified to be catecholaminergic; the dorsal raphe; and the PRF. These findings suggest that immediate early gene activation is associated with the carbachol-induced REM sleep–like state. Future studies are needed to explore the presence of IEG induction in natural REM sleep. This line of investigation, although in its infancy, offers the potential for answers about the functional consequences of REM sleep.

Sherin and associates[84] have used Fos immunohistochemistry to identify groups of cells in the ventrolateral preoptic area of the hypothalamus that may form an important component of NREM sleep induction. This brain area had been implicated in sleep control by clinical neurologic data and experimental lesions; however, the precise localization of any selectively sleep-active neurons had been difficult to establish physiologically. The reasoning was that heightened Fos immunoreactivity might show the locus of sleep-active neurons in this zone. As shown in Figure 3-16, the extent of Fos immunoreactivity was directly proportional to the duration of time the experimental animals slept, regardless of circadian phase. Double labeling with the retrograde tracer cholera toxin B showed that these neurons projected to the tuberomammillary nucleus. This nucleus is the locus of the histamine neurons that are selectively active in arousal and may comprise an important element of arousal systems. Further work by Sherin since this publication (personal communication, 1997) sug-

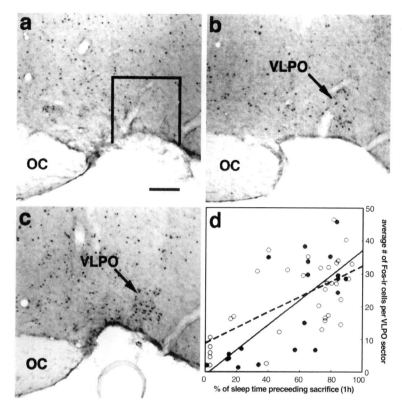

**Figure 3-16. (A–C)** Photomicrographs of *fos*-immunostained (*fos*-ir) coronal sections through the preoptic hypothalamus of spontaneously behaving rats that slept 15% (**A**) and 63% (**B**), and a sleep-deprived rat that slept 83% (**C**), of the hour before they were killed; *fos*-ir cells (black nuclei) are apparent in the ventrolateral preoptic area (VLPO) of animals that slept most of the hour before they were killed (**B** and **C**; *arrows*). (**D**) Correlation between the number of *fos*-ir cells counted in each preoptic sector containing the VLPO (shown in **A**) and percent of total sleep time for spontaneously behaving rats (*closed circles*; solid regression line: Pearson's correlation coefficient r = 0.743, *P* <.0001) and sleep-deprived rats (*open circles*, dashed regression line; R = 0.704, *P* <.0001). Scale bar = 150 μmol/liter. (OC = optic chiasm.) (Adapted from JE Sherin, PJ Shiromani, RW McCarley, CB Saper. Activation of ventrolateral preoptic neurons during sleep. Science 1996;271:216.)

gests that these neurons are GABAergic and that they send projections to the brain stem LDT, PPT, LC, and DRN nuclei, which are important in behavioral state regulation, as well as to the LC and the DRN.

## REFERENCES

1. Steriade M, McCarley RW. Brainstem Control of Wakefulness and Sleep. New York: Plenum, 1990.
2. Kandel E, Schwarz JH, Jessell TM (eds). Principles of Neural Science. New York: Elsevier, 1991.
3. McCarley RW. Sleep, Dreams and States of Consciousness. In PM Conn (ed), Neuroscience in Medicine. Philadelphia: Lippincott, 1995.
4. McCarley RW, Greene RW, Rainnie D, Portas CM. Brain stem neuromodulation and REM sleep. Semin Neurosci 1995;7:341.
5. Hayaishi O, Inoue S (eds). Sleep and Sleep Disorders: From Molecule to Behavior. Tokyo: Academic/Harcourt Brace Japan, 1997.
6. Krueger JM, Fang J. Cytokines in sleep regulation. In O Hayaishi, S Inoue (eds), Sleep and Sleep Disorders: From Molecule to Behavior. Tokyo: Academic/Harcourt Brace Japan, 1997:261–280.
7. Feinberg I, Thode HC, Chugani HT, March JD. Gamma function describes maturational curves for delta wave amplitude, cortical metabolic rate and synaptic density. J Theor Biol 1990;142:149.
8. Reinoso-Suárez F, Rodrigo-Angulo ML, Rodríguez-Veiga E, DeAndres I. Thalamic Connections of the Oral Pontine Tegmentum Sites whose Cholinergic Stimulation Produces Enhancement of Paradoxical Sleep Signs. In M Mancia, G Marini (eds), The Diencephalon and Sleep. New York: Raven, 1990.
9. Mitani A, Ito K, Hallanger AH, et al. Cholinergic projections from the laterodorsal and pedunculopontine tegmental nuclei to the pontine gigantocellular tegmental field in the cat. Brain Res 1988;451:397.
10. Yanagihara M, Ito K, Dauphin L, et al. Multiple brainstem projection targets of laterodorsal tegmental (LDT) and pedunculopontine tegmental (PPT) nucleus cholinergic neurons in the rat. Soc Neurosci Abstr 1991;17:1163.
11. Greene RW, Gerber U, McCarley RW. Cholinergic activation of medial pontine reticular formation neurons in vitro. Brain Res 1989;476:154.

12. Greene RW, McCarley RW. Cholinergic Neurotransmission in the Brainstem: Implications for Behavioral State Control. In M Steriade, D Biesold (eds), Brain Cholinergic Systems. New York: Oxford University Press, 1990.

13. Webster HH, Jones BE. Neurotoxic lesions of the dorsolateral pontomesencephalic tegmentum-cholinergic area in the cat. II. Effects upon sleep-waking states. Brain Res 1988;458:285.

14. Thakkar M, Portas CM, McCarley RW. Chronic low amplitude electrical stimulation of the laterodorsal tegmental nucleus of freely moving cats increases REM sleep. Brain Res 1996;723:223.

15. El Mansari M, Sakai K, Jouvet M. Responses of presumed cholinergic mesopontine tegmental neurons to carbachol microinjections in freely moving cats. Exp Brain Res 1990;83:115.

16. Kayama Y, Ohta M, Jodo E. Firing of 'possibly' cholinergic neurons in the rat laterodorsal tegmental nucleus during sleep and wakefulness. Brain Res 1992;569:210.

17. Steriade M, Datta S, Pare D, et al. Neuronal activities in brain-stem cholinergic nuclei related to tonic activation processes in thalamocortical systems. J Neurosci 1990;10:2541.

18. Stevens DR, McCarley RW, Greene RW. 5HT$_1$ and 5HT$_2$ receptors hyperpolarize and depolarize separate populations of medial pontine reticular neurons in vitro. Neuroscience 1992;47:545.

19. Stevens DR, McCarley RW, Greene RW. Excitatory amino acid-mediated responses and synaptic potentials in medial pontine reticular formation neurons of the rat in vitro. J Neurosci 1992;12:4188.

20. Gerber U, Stevens DS, McCarley RW, Greene RW. A muscarinic-gated conductance increase in medial pontine reticular neurons of the rat in vitro. J Neurosci 1991;11:3861.

21. Morales FR, Chase MH. Intracellular recording of lumbar motoneuron membrane potential during sleep and wakefulness. Exp Neurol 1978;62:821.

22. Morales FR, Chase MH. Postsynaptic control of lumbar motoneuron excitability during active sleep in the chronic cat. Brain Res 1981;225:279.

23. Chase MH, Soja PJ, Morales FR. Evidence that glycine mediates the postsynaptic potentials that inhibit lumbar motorneuron during the atonia of active sleep. J Neurosci 1989;9:743.

24. Jouvet M. What does a cat dream about? Trends Neurosci 1979;2:15.

25. Sastre JP, Jouvet M. Le comportement onirique du chat. Physiol Behav 1979;22:979.

26. Hendricks JC, Morrison AR, Mann GL. Different behaviors during paradoxical sleep without atonia depend on pontine lesion site. Brain Res 1982;239:81.

27. Mori S. Integration of posture and locomotion in acute decerebrate cats and in awake, freely moving cats. Prog Neurobiol 1987;28:161.

28. Lai YY, Siegel JM. Medullary regions mediating atonia. J Neurosci 1988;8:4790.

29. Siegel JM. Brainstem Mechanisms Generating REM Sleep. In MK Kryger, T Roth, WC Dement (eds), Principle and Practice of Sleep Medicine (2nd ed). New York: Saunders, 1994.

30. Stevens DR, Greene RW, McCarley RW. Pontine Reticular Formation Neurons: Excitatory Amino Acid Receptor-Mediated Responses. In J Horne (ed), Sleep 90. Bochum, Germany: Pontenagel, 1990.

31. Lai YY, Siegel JM. Pontomedullary glutamate receptors mediating locomotion and muscle tone suppression. J Neurosci 1991;11:2931.

32. Hobson JA, McCarley RW, Wyzinski PW. Sleep cycle oscillation: reciprocal discharge by two brain stem neuronal groups. Science 1975;189:55.

33. McGinty DJ, Harper RM. Dorsal raphe neurons: depression of firing during sleep in cats. Brain Res 1976;101:569.

34. Lin JS, Sakai K, Vanni-Mercier G, et al. Involvement of histaminergic neurons in arousal mechanisms demonstrated with H3-receptor ligands in the cat. Brain Res 1990;523:325.

35. Jouvet M. Recherches sur les structures nerveuses et les mécanismes responsables des différentes phases du sommeil physiologique. Arch Ital Biol 1962; 100:125.

36. Lydic R, McCarley RW, Hobson JA. Serotonin neurons and sleep: I. Long term recordings of dorsal raphe discharge frequency and PGO waves. Arch Ital Biol 1987;125:317.

37. McCarley RW, Hobson JA. Neuronal excitability modulation over the sleep cycle: a structural and mathematical model. Science 1975;189:58.

38. Honda T, Semba K. Serotonergic synaptic input to cholinergic neurons in the rat mesopontine tegmentum. Brain Res 1994;647:299.

39. Jones BE. Paradoxical sleep and its chemical/structural substrates in the brain. Neuroscience 1991;40:637.

40. Steininger TL, Wainer BH, Blakely RD, Rye DB. Serotonergic dorsal raphe nucleus projections to the cholinergic and noncholinergic neurons of the pedunculopontine tegmental region: a light and electron microscope anterograde tracing and immunohistochemical study. J Comp Neurol 1997;382:302.

41. Leonard CS, Llinás RR. Serotonergic and cholinergic inhibition of mesopontine cholinergic neurons controlling REM sleep: an in vitro electrophysiological study. Neuroscience 1994;59:309.

42. Luebke JI, Greene RW, Semba K, et al. Serotonin hyperpolarizes cholinergic low threshold burst neurons in the rat laterodorsal tegmental nucleus in vitro. Proc Natl Acad Sci U S A 1992;89:743.

43. Mühlethaler M, Khateb A, Serafin M. Effects of Monoamines and Opiates on Pedunculopontine Neurons. In M Mancia, G Marini (eds), The Diencephalon and Sleep. New York: Raven, 1990.

44. Williams JA, Reiner PB. Noradrenaline hyperpolarizes identified rat mesopontine cholinergic neurons in vitro. J Neurosci 1993;13:3878.
45. Portas CM, McCarley RW. Behavioral state-related changes of extracellular serotonin concentration in the dorsal raphe nucleus: a microdialysis study in the freely moving cat. Brain Res 1994;648:306.
46. Wilkinson LO, Auerbach SB, Jacobs BL. Extracellular serotonin levels change with behavioral state but not with pyrogen-induced hyperthermia. J Neurosci 1991;11:2732.
47. Auerbach SB, Minzenberg MJ, Wilkinson LO. Extracellular serotonin and 5-hydroxyindolacetic acid in hypothalamus of the unanesthetized rat measured by in vivo dialysis coupled to high performance liquid chromatography with electrochemical detection: dialysate serotonin reflects neuronal release. Brain Res 1989;499:281.
48. Imeri L, De Simoni MG, Giglio R, et al. Changes in the serotoninergic system during the sleep-wake cycle: simultaneous polygraphic and voltammetric recordings in hypothalamus using a telemetry system. Neuroscience 1994;58:353.
49. Portas CM, Thakkar M, Rainnie D, McCarley RW. Microdialysis perfusion of 8-OH-DPAT in the dorsal raphe nucleus decreases serotonin release and increases REM sleep in the freely moving cat. J Neurosci 1996;16:2820.
50. Sprouse JS, Aghajanian GK. Electrophysiological responses of serotonergic dorsal raphe neurons to 5-$HT_{1A}$ and 5-$HT_{1B}$ agonists. Synapse 1987;1:3.
51. Thakkar M, Strecker R, McCarley RW. The 5-$HT_{1A}$ agonist 8-OH-DPAT inhibits REM-on neurons but has no effect on W/R-on neurons: a combined microdialysis and unit recording study. Sleep Res 1997; 26:52
52. Semba K, Fibiger HC. Afferent connections of the laterodorsal and the pedunculopontine tegmental nuclei in the rat: a retro- and antero-grade transport and immunohistochemical study. J Comp Neurol 1992;323:387.
53. Honda T, Semba K. An ultrastructural study of cholinergic and non-cholinergic neurons in the laterodorsal and pedunculopontine tegmental nuclei in rat. Neuroscience 1995;68:837.
54. Luebke JI, McCarley RW, Greene RW. Inhibitory action of muscarinic agonists on neurons in the rat laterodorsal tegmental nucleus in vitro. J Neurophysiol 1993;70:2128.
55. McCarley RW, Massaquoi SG. The limit cycle reciprocal interaction model of REM cycle control: new neurobiological structure. J Sleep Res 1992;1:132.
56. Sanchez R, Leonard CS. NMDA receptor–mediated synaptic input to nitric oxide synthase-containing neurons of the guinea pig mesopontine tegmentum in vitro. Neurosci Lett 1994;179:141.
57. Peroutka SJ. 5-HT receptors: past, present and future. Trends Neurosci 1995;18:68.
58. Alexander SPH, Peters JA. TIPS receptor and ion channel nomenclature supplement. Trends Pharmacol Sci 1997;7:46.
59. Nitz D, Siegel JM. GABA release in the cat locus coeruleus as a function of the sleep/wake cycle. Neuroscience 1997;78:795.
60. Peyron C, Rampon C, Jouvet M, Luppi P-H. Identification of neurons which could be responsible for the cessation of activity of serotonergic cells of the dorsal raphe nucleus during sleep. Sleep Res 1997;26:92.
61. Li X, Rainnie DG, McCarley RW, Greene RW. Nicotinic pre- and post-synaptic effects in dorsal raphe nucleus. Soc Neurosci Abstr 1996;22:1740.
62. McCarley RW, Massaquoi SG. A limit cycle mathematical model of the REM sleep oscillator system. Am J Physiol 1986;251:R1011.
63. Szymusiak R. Magnocellular nuclei of the basal forebrain: substrates of sleep and arousal regulation. Sleep 1995;18:478.
64. Rainnie DG, Grunze HCR, McCarley RW, Greene RW. Adenosine inhibits mesopontine cholinergic neurons: implications for EEG arousal. Science 1994;263:689.
65. Portas CM, Thakkar M, Rainnie DG, et al. Role of adenosine in behavioral state modulation: a microdialysis study in the freely moving cat. Neuroscience 1997;79:225.
66. Porkka-Heiskanen T, Strecker RE, Thakkar M, et al. Adenosine: a mediator of the sleep-inducing effects of prolonged wakefulness. Science 1997;276:1265.
67. Huston JP, Haas HL, Boix F, et al. Extracellular adenosine levels in neostriatum and hippocampus during rest and activity periods of rats. Neuroscience 1996;73:99.
68. Hayaishi O. Sleep-wake regulation by prostaglandins $D_2$ and $E_2$. J Biol Chem 1988;263:14593.
69. Hayaishi O. Prostaglandin $D_2$ and Sleep. In O Hayaishi, S Inoue (eds), Sleep and Sleep Disorders: From Molecule to Behavior. Tokyo: Academic/Harcourt Brace Japan, 1997;3–10.
70. Gu JG, Geiger JD. Transport and metabolism of D-[3H]adenosine and L-[3H]adenosine in rat cerebral cortical synaptoneurosomes. J Neurochem 1992;58:1699.
71. Padua R, Geiger JD, Dambock S, Nagy JI. 2'-Deoxycoformycin inhibition of adenosine deaminase in rat brain: in vivo and in vitro analysis of specificity, potency, and enzyme recovery. J Neurochem 1990;54:1169.
72. Wu PH, Barraco RA, Phillis JW. Further studies on the inhibition of adenosine uptake into rat brain synaptosomes by adenosine derivatives and methylaxanthines. Gen Pharmacol 1984;15:251.
73. Brundege JM, Dunwiddie TV. Modulation of excitatory synaptic transmission by adenosine released from single hippocampal pyramidal neurons. J Neurosci 1996;16:5603.
74. Chagoya de Sanchez V, Hernandez Munoz R, Suarez J, et al. Day-night variations of adenosine and its metabolizing enzymes in the brain cortex of the rat—possible physiological significance for the energetic homeostasis and the sleep-wake cycle. Brain Res 1993; 612:115.
75. Borbely AA. A two process model of sleep regulation. Hum Neurobiol 1982;1:195.

76. Obal F Jr, Alfoldi P, Cady AB, et al. Growth hormone-releasing factor enhances sleep in rats and rabbits. Am J Physiol 1988;255:R310.

77. Toppila J, Asikainen M, Alanko L, et al. The effect of REM sleep deprivation on somatostatin and growth hormone-releasing hormone gene expression in the rat hypothalamus. J Sleep Res 1996;5:115.

78. McCormick DA, Pape H-C. Noradrenergic and serotonergic modulation of a hyperpolarization-activated cation current in thalamic relay neurons. J Physiol 1990;431:319.

79. Bennington JH, Heller HC. Restoration of brain energy metabolism as the function of sleep. Prog Neurobiol 1995;45:347.

80. Morgan TJ, Curran T. Stimulus-Transcription Coupling in the Nervous System: Involvement of the Inducible Proto-Oncogenes *fos* and *jun*. In WM Cowan, EM Shooter, CF Stevens, RF Thompson (eds), Annual Review of Neuroscience. Palo Alto, CA: Annual Reviews, 1991;421.

81. Shiromani PJ, Kilduff TS, Bloom FE, McCarley RW. Cholinergically-induced REM sleep triggers Fos-like immunoreactivity in dorsolateral pontine regions associated with REM sleep. Brain Res 1992;580:351.

82. Shiromani PS, Malik M, Winston S, McCarley RW. Time course of Fos-like immunoreactivity associated with cholinergically-induced REM sleep. J Neurosci 1995;15:3500.

83. Shiromani PJ, Winston S, McCarley RW. Pontine cholinergic neurons show Fos-like immunoreactivity associated with cholinergically-induced REM sleep. Mol Brain Res 1996;38:77.

84. Sherin JE, Shiromani PJ, McCarley RW, Saper CB. Activation of ventrolateral preoptic neurons during sleep. Science 1996;271:216.

# Chapter 4

# Neurophysiologic Mechanisms of Non–Rapid Eye Movement (Resting) Sleep

## Mircea Steriade

The behavioral state of sleep consists of two basic stages, as distinct as night and day. *Resting* sleep, also termed *quiet* and characterized by the large-scale synchronization of brain electrical activity recorded by the electroencephalogram (EEG), is associated with the suspension of conscious processes and is antinomic to the wake state. The *active* stage of sleep, usually termed *REM sleep* because of the rapid eye movements that characterize it, is accompanied by dreaming episodes and tempestuous activity of the brain, similar to or even exceeding the level of alertness seen during the state of wakefulness.

The dual nature of sleep is reflected by very dissimilar brain oscillations during the two sleep stages. During resting sleep, EEG displays low-frequency (<15-Hz) thalamic and cortical rhythms that are synchronized among large neuronal populations and whose basic components are prolonged inhibitions. One of the functional roles played by these inhibitory processes is to disconnect the brain from the outside world. Both thalamic and cortical cells continue to discharge at surprisingly high rates for a presumably inactive state, however, thus suggesting that some important brain operations take place during this stage of sleep. During dreaming sleep, the low-frequency EEG rhythms are suppressed and fast oscillations (20–40 Hz) appear. Contrary to low-frequency rhythms, the synchronization of fast rhythms is confined to more restricted territories.

This chapter deals with (1) the notion of *sleep centers* as opposed to distributed systems, in relation to the concepts of the passive or active nature

of sleep; (2) the physiologic and behavioral evidence for brain deafferentation during sleep and the brain level at which the disconnection from signals arising in the outside world takes place; (3) the various types of low-frequency oscillations that appear in different non-REM (NREM) sleep stages; and (4) the cellular substrates and possible functions of these rhythms. A more detailed treatment of these topics may be found in monographs on the thalamocortical (TC) systems,[1,2] which play a major role in the generation of NREM oscillations, and the modulation of these systems by ascending brain stem reticular projections that contribute to the shift from NREM sleep to waking and REM sleep.[3]

## DISTRIBUTED SYSTEMS GENERATING THE STATE OF RESTING SLEEP

The hypotheses postulating that sleep is a passive phenomenon due to the closure of cerebral gates (brain deafferentation) or, alternatively, an active phenomenon promoted by inhibitory mechanisms arising in some hypnogenic cerebral areas, have long been considered as opposing views. The passive and active mechanisms are probably successive steps within a chain of events, however, and they may be complementary rather than opposing.

The concept of *sleep centers* that has prevailed in the literature implies that circumscribed brain territories may generate different behavioral states of vigilance. Since the early clinical-anatomic studies

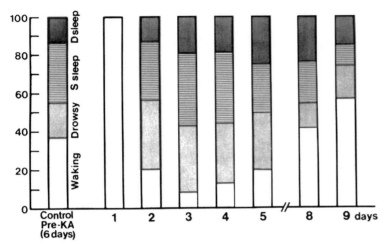

**Figure 4-1.** Evolution of wake-sleep cycle after kainate (KA) injection in the mesencephalic reticular formation in chronically implanted cat. Control was taken from average of 6 days before injection. S sleep indicates NREM sleep. D sleep indicates REM sleep. Note permanent arousal during 1 day (corresponding to the period of KA-induced excitation of midbrain reticular perikarya), diminution in waking duration for the next 4 days, and recovery, even above control value, after 8–9 days. See histology and electrographic patterns in Steriade.[12]

of the 1920s, it has been thought that waking and sleep are generated within the posterior and anterior parts of the hypothalamus, respectively. Sleeping sickness followed lesions of the posterior hypothalamus, whereas postencephalitic insomnia was associated with prominent damage in the preoptic area of the anterior hypothalamus (reviewed in Moruzzi[4]). The clinical-anatomic observations have been followed by experimental studies suggesting the antagonistic nature of the anterior (hypnogenic) and posterior (awakening) areas of the hypothalamus[5] and proposing that an inhibitory circuit links the anterior hypothalamus to posterior arousing areas.[6] This hypothesis found support in experiments reporting long-term insomnia produced by electrolytic lesions of the preoptic area.[7] The descending circuit is now substantiated by the identification of inhibitory pathways from the anterior to the posterior hypothalamus,[8] and physiologically by the specific activation of some ventrolateral preoptic neurons during NREM sleep.[9] Recordings of neuronal activity within and around the anterior hypothalamic area, however, which includes heterogenous neuronal types using different neurotransmitters and having different projection fields, show great variability in relation to behavioral states of vigilance, with most neurons displaying an increased rate of discharge during wakefulness.[10]

That insomnia is produced by anterior hypothalamic lesions does not imply that the anterior hypothalamic area is *necessary* for sleep. After insomnia resulting from the lesion of preoptic neurons,

reversible inactivation of posterior hypothalamic neurons produces recovery of sleep.[11] Thus, sleep can be restored by the removal of activating actions exerted by posterior hypothalamic histaminergic neurons, and there is no need to consider the "active inhibitory hypnogenic" properties of preoptic neurons as indispensable for NREM sleep.

Rather than being generated in discrete brain centers, waking and sleep states are produced by complex chains of interconnected systems. Most experimental data favor this contention. It follows that a lesion of one sector of interconnected neuronal groups will *not* be followed by a permanent disturbance in a given state of vigilance, but by compensatory phenomena due to the presence of remaining circuits, consisting of neurons with properties similar to those of lesioned neurons. After large chemical lesions of activating mesencephalic tegmental neurons, the state of NREM sleep increases in duration, at the expense of wakefulness, over the course of 3–4 days; however, this is followed by a period in which waking recovers and even exceeds control values, possibly due to denervation hypersensitivity in target neurons of the thalamus and nucleus basalis[12] (Figure 4-1).

There is a redundancy of brain stem and supramesencephalic neurons that possess activating properties. Some neurotransmitters exert actions on postsynaptic targets that are very similar to those of neurotransmitters released by parallel projection pathways. For example, mesopontine cholinergic cells project to the thalamus[13,14] and exert activating effects during both waking and REM sleep.[15] However, many other brain stem reticular cells, probably using glutamate as a neurotransmitter, also project to the thalamus and similarly display increased firing rates reliably preceding brain-active states, waking and REM sleep.[16] Acetylcholine (ACh) exerts activating effects on TC neurons partly due to the blockage of a "leak" $K^+$ conductance, similar to the glutamatergic action mediated by metabotropic glutamate receptors on the same neurons.[17] It is no surprise, then, that after extensive lesions of mesopontine cholinergic nuclei, TC systems continue to display signs of activation. This is due to the fact that many other brain stem–projecting (among them glutamatergic) systems remain intact. Although there is a large body of cellular studies, mainly from in vitro experiments, concerning the actions of different neurotransmitters, the synergistic or competitive effects of chemical substances released in concert on natural awakening from sleep are still unknown. To give only one example, ACh inhibits thalamic reticular (RE) GABAergic neurons, whereas norepinephrine and serotonin, which are simultaneously released on arousal, exert depolarizing actions on the same inhibitory neurons.[18] The study of these competitive actions remains a tantalizing task for the future.

One of the major factors accounting for sleep-inducing effects of prolonged wakefulness is adenosine (AD). Both mesopontine and basal forebrain cholinergic neurons are under the tonic inhibitory control of endogenous AD, and the extracellular concentration of AD is proportional to brain metabolic rate. AD exerts an inhibitory tone on mesopontine cholinergic neurons by an inwardly rectifying potassium conductance and by an inhibition of a hyperpolarization-activated current ($I_H$).[19] That AD mediates the hypnogenic effects of prolonged wakefulness was demonstrated by microdialysis studies showing that an increase in extracellular AD concentration leads to a decrease in wakefulness (see details in Chapter 3). The conclusion of these experiments is that AD is a physiologic sleep factor that mediates somnogenic effects of prior wakefulness.

To summarize, the idea of *sleep centers* should be abandoned because none of the previously hypothesized centers has proved necessary and sufficient for the induction and maintenance of NREM sleep. On the basis of cellular studies indicating that some neurons display signs of increased activity preceding the electrographic signs defining various behavioral states of vigilance, the notion of *prime-mover* cells was introduced. This concept is sterile because whenever such presumptive cells are detected, the question arises: What is behind this neuronal change? The search is only transferred one synapse before, climbing a hypothetical hierarchic line.

In fact, NREM sleep is generated by a series of phenomena generated in interconnected structures, including inhibition of activating cellular aggregates, thus finally resulting in disfacilitation of target structures, as postulated by the passive theory of sleep. At this time, the best candidate for a neuronal circuit implicated in the process of falling asleep is the inhibitory GABAergic projection from the preoptic area in the anterior hypothalamus to the activating histaminergic area in the tuberoinfundibular region of the posterior hypothalamus. The rostral projections of the latter are the thalamus and cerebral cortex. Thus, the inhibition of histaminergic neurons results in disfacilitation of the thalamus and cerebral cortex. In addition to rostral targets in the diencephalon and telencephalon, the histaminergic neurons of the posterior hypothalamus also project downward to the reticular core of the upper brain stem and excite mesopontine cholinergic neurons.[20] Thus, the inhibition exerted on these posterior hypothalamic neurons by the GABAergic anterior hypothalamic cells also results in disfacilitation of mesopontine cholinergic neurons, with obvious deafferentation consequences in TC systems. All the above represent an avalanche of disfacilitatory processes[15,16] (Figure 4-2).

## BRAIN DISCONNECTION FROM THE EXTERNAL WORLD DURING NREM SLEEP

The idea that sleep is essentially caused by the diminution or cessation of sensory signals assailing the brain during wakefulness is two millennia old and was substantiated more recently by transection experiments. When the brain stem is transected at the bulbospinal level, the encephalon displays fluctuations between waking and sleep, whereas a transection at the upper brain stem is followed by ocular and EEG signs resembling those of deep barbiturate narcosis.[21] The conclusion of Bremer's experiments[21] was that the cerebral tonus is maintained by a steady flow of sensory input reaching the brain

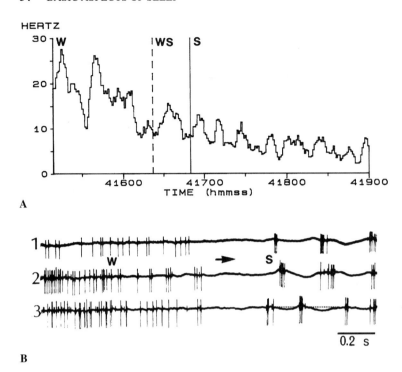

**Figure 4-2.** Neuronal activities during transition from wake (W) to sleep (S) suggests that an avalanche of disfacilitory processes underlies the process of falling asleep. **(A)** Thalamic-projecting neuron from the pedunculopontine tegmental cholinergic nucleus decreases firing rate (ordinate) from W to S (WS indicates the transitional period marked by the first EEG signs). Abscissa (~4 minutes) indicates time (hours, minutes, seconds). **(B)** Corticothalamic neuron stops firing for 0.3–0.4 seconds during transition from W to S. (Adapted from M Steriade, S Datta, D Paré, et al. Neuronal activities in brainstem cholinergic nuclei related to tonic activation processes in thalamocortical systems. J Neurosci 1990;10:2541; and M Steriade. Cortical long-axoned cells and putative interneurons during the sleep-waking cycle. Behav Brain Sci 1978;3:465.)

stem between the medulla and midbrain, and that sleep results from the withdrawal of sensory bombardment. Subsequently, the EEG activation exerted by the ascending brain stem reticular neurons has been demonstrated.[4]

Animal experiments and clinical studies have corroborated Bremer's pioneering observations. Gross impairments of the state of vigilance, leading to hypersomnia, result from lesions of the mesopontine reticular neurons or bilateral lesions of thalamic intralaminar nuclei, which represent the rostral continuation of the brain stem reticular formation.[22] Thalamic intralaminar neurons are directly excited from the mesopontine reticular core, and they project to widespread cortical areas where they exert excitatory actions.[23] Studies of patients with prolonged lethargy led to the conclusion that the brain stem–thalamocortical circuit effectively contributes to the maintenance of alertness in higher mammals, especially in primates. The role of thalamic intralaminar nuclei in regulating arousal is also suggested by the fact that their activity increases during a task requiring alertness and attention in humans.[24] Parallel extrathalamic pathways, through which brain stem reticular neurons influence the cerebral cortex, are relayed by histaminergic projections of posterior

hypothalamic (tuberoinfundibular) neurons and by cholinergic projections of the nucleus basalis.[25]

The basic mechanism of falling asleep is the transformation of a brain responsive to external signals into a closed brain. In humans, the onset of sleep is associated with functional blindness.[26] The obliteration of messages from the outside world at sleep onset is due to inhibitory processes that are reflected in peculiar EEG rhythms generated in the thalamus and cerebral cortex, as well as to the decreased excitability of both thalamic and cortical neurons.

That the transmission of afferent signals is reduced at the thalamic level from the very onset of natural sleep was first shown by recording field potentials in dorsal thalamic nuclei.[27] It was demonstrated that the thalamic responses to stimuli applied to prethalamic axon bundles are diminished from the drowsy state and that the postsynaptic waves are completely obliterated during further deepening of sleep, despite no measurable change in the presynaptic component that monitors the magnitude of prethalamic input[28] (Figure 4-3). Indeed, simultaneous recordings from the thalamus and different relay stations in the brain stem or the retinogeniculate axons showed that, during the period of falling asleep, the diminished postsynaptic responses in dorsal thalamic nuclei are not paralleled

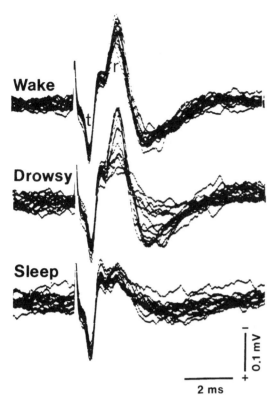

**Wake**

**Drowsy**

**Sleep**

0.1 mV

2 ms

**Figure 4-3.** Blockade of synaptic transmission in thalamus at sleep onset in behaving cat with implanted electrodes. Field potentials evoked in the ventral lateral (motor) thalamic nucleus by stimulation of axons in the cerebellothalamic pathway. Evoked responses consist of a presynaptic (tract, t) component and a monosynaptically relayed (r) wave. Note progressively diminished amplitude of r wave during drowsiness, up to its complete obliteration during slow-wave sleep, despite lack of changes in afferent volley monitored by t component. (Adapted from M Steriade. Alertness, Quiet Sleep, Dreaming. In A Peters, EG Jones [eds], Cerebral Cortex [Vol. 9]. Normal and Altered States of Function. New York: Plenum, 1991;279.)

by alterations in afferent pathways. *This demonstrates that the thalamus is the first relay station at which reduction of afferent signals takes place when falling asleep.* Intracellular recordings have shown that the diminution or suppression of the monosynaptic response of TC neurons to afferent volleys occurs during the inhibitory postsynaptic potentials (IPSPs) related to sleep spindles.[29] Thalamic gating deprives the cerebral cortex of the input required to elaborate a response and is responsible for the decreased transfer of information at the cortical level. These processes

constitute a necessary deafferentation prelude for deepening the state of sleep.

Instead of high-security, short-latency (1–2 msec), single-spike responses to prethalamic stimuli during waking, the same TC neuron fails to discharge or respond during EEG-synchronized sleep, with occasional spike-bursts at a high frequency (200–400 Hz), occurring at longer latencies (5–12 msec). This fact, described in earlier extracellular studies,[30] was explained by low-threshold burst responses[31] that are uncovered by the hyperpolarization of TC neurons during resting sleep.[1,2]

The thalamic blockade of afferent signals from the very onset of sleep is associated with a diminished cortical reactivity to afferent stimuli. Field potential recordings in animals and humans reached similar conclusions concerning the decreased cortical responsiveness at sleep onset and during later stages of NREM sleep. With testing stimuli applied to prethalamic pathways, the earliest component of the cortical-evoked response is dramatically reduced with transition from wakefulness to drowsiness, with the consequence that the cortically elaborated postsynaptic component is also greatly diminished.[27] The decreased transfer of information through cortical circuits is not merely due to the decreased input from the thalamus, however; it also depends on intrinsic cortical events. In monkeys, the cortical field response evoked by a somatosensory stimulus consists of an abrupt surface-positive component (P1) peaking at approximately 12 msec, and a surface-negativity wave (N1) at approximately 50 msec after the stimulus. P1 persists in anesthetized monkeys, whereas N1 does not.[32] It seems that P1 amplitude is a simple function of stimulus intensity, whereas N1 amplitude depends on behavioral discrimination. In humans, the most sensitive components of cortical-evoked potentials during shifts in states of vigilance are fast frequency wavelets (FFWs) superimposed on the major waves at frontal and parietal scalp electrodes. The FFWs are attenuated or totally disappear with transition from wakefulness to the early stages of NREM sleep.[33]

## GROUPING OF SLEEP RHYTHMS BY THE SLOW CORTICAL OSCILLATION

Much more is known about the cellular mechanisms underlying different oscillations that characterize NREM sleep than about the functions of these oscillations or the neural and humoral processes responsible for sleep. The principal neurons involved in sleep oscillations are cortical pyramidal cells, GABAergic RE thalamic cells, and TC cells. Cortical cells project to the thalamus and excite both RE and TC cells, TC cells project to the cortex and give off collaterals to RE cells, and RE cells do not project to the cortex but project back to TC cells, thus forming an intrathalamic, recurrent inhibitory circuit (Figure 4-4). The local-circuit GABAergic neurons, intrinsic to virtually every thalamic nucleus of felines and primates, play an important role in inhibitory processes that assist discriminatory functions but have only an ancillary role in sleep oscillations.

Three major sleep oscillations are generated in the thalamus and cerebral cortex: sleep spindles, delta oscillations, and slow cortical oscillations. Each of these can be generated in different structures, even after their complete disconnection.

### Sleep Spindles

Sleep spindles (7–14 Hz) occur during early stages of sleep and are generated in the thalamus, even after complete decortication. Spindles are due to the pacemaking role of RE neurons that impose rhythmic IPSPs on target TC cells (see Figure 4-4). The crucial role played by the GABAergic RE cells was demonstrated by the absence of spindles after disruption of the connection arising in the RE nucleus.[34] Moreover, spindles have been recorded in the deafferented rostral pole of the thalamic RE nucleus.[35]

### Delta Oscillations

Delta oscillations (1–4 Hz) appear during later stages of NREM sleep and consist of two components. One of them is generated in the neocortex, demonstrated by the fact that it survives extensive thalamectomy. The other component is thalamic and can thus be recorded in vivo after decortication[36] as well as in thalamic slices.[37,38] The stereotyped thalamic delta oscillation results from the interplay between two voltage-gated currents of TC cells.[37,38] This interplay is dependent on the hyperpolarization of TC cells, which occurs during NREM sleep

because of the withdrawal of brain stem–ascending, activating impulses.[3] Although the thalamic delta oscillation is generated in single TC cells, it can be expressed at the global EEG level, because TC cells can be synchronized by corticothalamic volleys, engaging RE and TC neurons.[39]

### Slow Cortical Oscillation

The slow cortical oscillation (<1 Hz, typically 0.6–0.9 Hz) was discovered in intracellular recordings from cortical neurons in anesthetized animals.[40] It consists of prolonged depolarizations and hyperpolarizations (Figure 4-5). The same oscillatory type was also investigated during natural NREM sleep of behaving cats[41,42] as well as during natural NREM sleep in humans.[43,44] The slow oscillation is generated within cortical networks; because it survives extensive thalamic lesions,[45] it does not appear in the thalamus after decortication,[46] and its synchronization is disrupted after disconnection of cortical synaptic linkages.[47] After preliminary data showing the presence of slow oscillation during natural sleep in humans,[40] the human slow oscillation (<1 Hz) was reported in parallel studies from two laboratories.[43,44] The different aspects of the human slow sleep oscillation are as follows: During stage II of NREM sleep, scalp recordings show a prevalent peak (0.8 Hz) within the frequency range of the slow oscillation as well as a minor mode around 15 Hz reflecting spindle waves. The depth-negative components of the slow oscillation, followed or not by spindles, represent the K complexes. The frequency of K complexes (peaks at 0.5 Hz in stage II, at 0.7 Hz in stages III and IV) is very similar, up to identity, to the frequency of the slow oscillation during natural sleep. The power spectrum reveals a major peak around 1 Hz that becomes evident from stage II and continues throughout resting sleep. The slow oscillation is particularly abundant in frontoparietal leads.

Does the slow oscillation belong to the same category of brain rhythms as sleep delta waves? Is the slow oscillation similar to the so-called cyclic alternating pattern during sleep? The reasons why the answers to the above two questions are clearly negative are outlined in the remainder of this section.

Although the delta rhythm is commonly viewed as a cortical oscillation, at least two types of rhythms

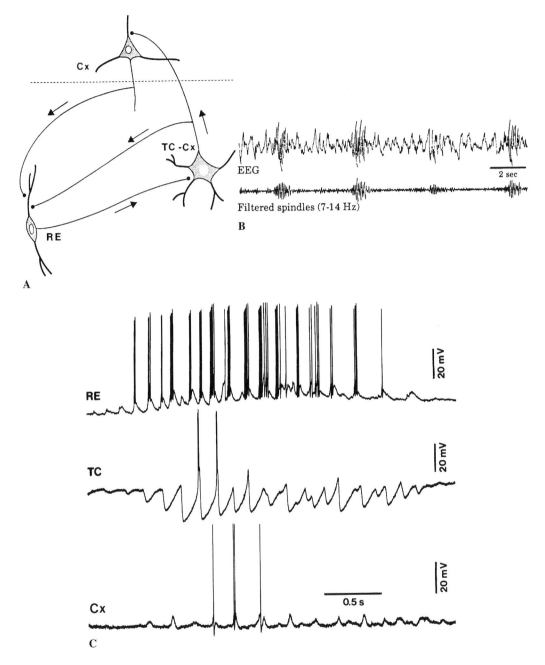

**Figure 4-4.** Generation of sleep spindles in the recurrent inhibitory circuit formed by thalamic reticular (RE) and thalamocortical (TC) neurons, and their reflection in cortical (Cx) neurons and EEG. (**A**) Network of RE, TC, and Cx neurons. (**B**) Four spindle sequences recurring rhythmically. (**C**) Intracellular recordings of RE, TC, and Cx cells during one spindle sequence. Note rhythmic spike-bursts with a depolarizing envelope in GABAergic RE cell, rhythmic inhibitory postsynaptic potentials occasionally leading to rebound spike-bursts in TC cell, and rhythmic excitatory postsynaptic potentials in target Cx cell. (Modified from M Steriade, M Deschênes. Intrathalamic and Brainstem-Thalamic Networks Involved in Resting and Alert States. In M Bentivoglio, R Spreafico [eds], Cellular Thalamic Mechanisms. Amsterdam: Elsevier, 1988;37.)

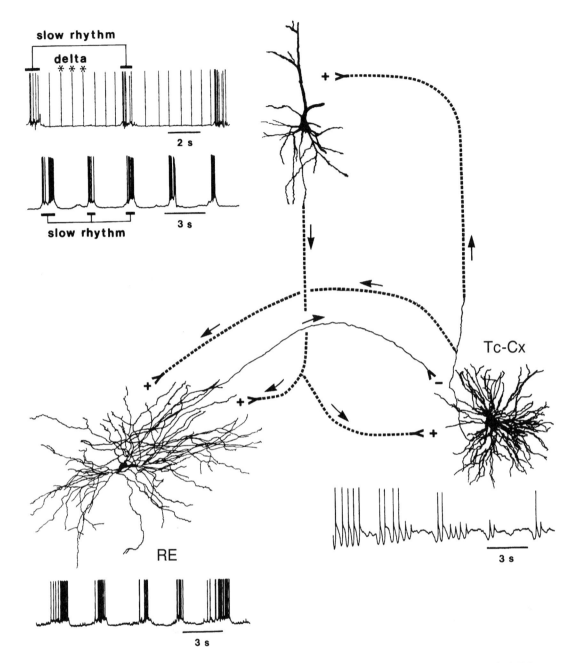

**Figure 4-5.** Slow (<1 Hz) cortical (Cx) oscillation and its effects on thalamic reticular (RE) and thalamocortical (TC) neurons. Neurons are intracellularly stained. Direction of axons is indicated by arrows and excitatory or inhibitory signs are indicated by + or −. Note similar slow oscillation in Cx (*second trace*) and RE neurons, combined slow rhythm and clocklike (thalamically generated) rhythm in Cx cell (*first trace*), and rhythmic disruption of clocklike delta rhythm in TC cell due to increased membrane conductance produced by slow oscillation in corticothalamic cells. (Modified from M Steriade, A Nuñez, F Amzica. A novel slow [<1 Hz] oscillation of neocortical neurons in vivo: depolarizing and hyperpolarizing components. J Neurosci 1993;13:3266; and M Steriade, D Contreras, R Curró Dossi, A Nuñez. The slow [<1 Hz] oscillation in reticular thalamic and thalamocortical neurons: scenario of sleep rhythms generation in interacting thalamic and neocortical networks. J Neurosci 1993;13:3284.)

are within the frequency range of 1–4 Hz, one originating in the thalamus, the other in the neocortex (as discussed earlier). We have demonstrated that cortical delta waves, associated with discharges of regular-spiking and intrinsically bursting cells, are grouped by the slow oscillation.[45] These data point to the distinctiveness of the two (slow and delta) oscillations. The other, stereotyped (clocklike), delta oscillation is generated in the thalamus. Intracellular recordings of cortical neurons showed that clocklike delta potentials of thalamic origin occur simultaneously with, but distinctly from, the slow oscillation during a progressive increase in EEG synchronization[45] (see Figure 4-5). Again, this indicates that the two (delta and slow) oscillations are different types of brain rhythmic activities. With the benefit of hindsight, one can see, in previous EEG recordings, cyclic groups of delta waves at 3–4 Hz recurring with a slow rhythm of 0.3–0.4 Hz in animals and during light sleep in humans.

As to the "cyclic alternating pattern" of EEG waves grouped in sequences recurring at intervals of 20 or more seconds,[48] it is basically different from the slow oscillation because it is associated with the enhancement of muscle tone and heart rate and was described by the term of *arousal-related phasic events*. In contrast, the slow oscillation is blocked during cholinergic- and noradrenergic-mediated arousal in acute experiments[49] and during natural waking in behaving animals.[42]

The distinction of NREM sleep oscillations into three types is useful for analytic purposes. In the intact brain, however, the thalamus and cortex are interacting and their rhythms are combined in complex wave sequences. Thus, although spindles may be generated through the network and intrinsic properties of thalamic RE neurons, the mechanisms for the generation of spindles in the intact brain require reciprocal interactions between thalamic and cortical neurons. Indeed, spindles are evoked by corticothalamic projections[50,51] and they are grouped within periodic sequences that display a similar rhythm (0.2–0.5 Hz)[1,2] to that of the slow cortical oscillation. Although the origin of the slow rhythm of spindle sequences is still a mystery and may partially depend on intrinsic properties of thalamic neurons, each synchronous corticothalamic excitatory volley is effective in driving thalamic RE cells and in synchronizing them within the frequency range of spindles. Moreover, the spectacular

synchronization and near-simultaneity of spindles in the thalamus and over the cortex is produced by corticothalamic projections, because spindles are more disorganized in decorticated animals.[52,53] Thus, although spindles appear after decortication and can even be recorded in thalamic slices,[54–56] the widespread synchronization of this thalamically generated oscillation, as seen during natural sleep in animals and humans, depends on feedback projections from the neocortex. The interaction between the cortex and the thalamus is also evident when analyzing the relation between the thalamic delta oscillation and the cortical slow oscillation. The intrinsic delta oscillation of TC neurons is periodically interrupted by excitatory impulses of cortical origin within the frequency of slow oscillation (see Figure 4-5, lower right trace) because depolarizing input brings TC cells out of the voltage range where the stereotyped delta rhythm is generated.

The data presented in this section emphasize the necessity of investigating brains with intact circuitry when exploring the cellular mechanisms of NREM sleep rhythms.

## POSSIBLE FUNCTIONS OF SLEEP OSCILLATIONS

Despite the diversity of NREM sleep rhythms, their functional outcome may be similar. As the major components of these oscillations are hyperpolarizations in thalamic and cortical neurons,[1,2] their obvious role is brain disconnection from the outside world. The reduction in neuronal responsiveness might be considered evidence for the hypothesis that the function of resting sleep is the restoration of brain energy metabolism through the replenishment of cerebral glycogen stores that are depleted during waking.[57]

The deafferentation process that occurs from the very onset of sleep and is a prerequisite to falling deeply asleep may be just the tip of the iceberg. The high-frequency spike-bursts, repeated rhythmically during both thalamic-generated spindles and delta oscillations, may prevent the metabolic inertia that would result from complete absence of discharges in TC cells, if the hyperpolarization were to persist, uninterrupted, for tens of minutes or for hours during sleep. Counteraction of this metabolic inertia would favor a quick passage from quiet sleep to either wakefulness or REM sleep.[58] Thus, the rhythmic bursts of thalamic cells may keep themselves, as well as cortical neurons, in a state of biochemical readiness for a rapid transition to an active state. In addition, the flux of ions, particularly that of $Ca^{2+}$, across the membrane will maintain biochemical processes in the cell that are sensitive to intracellular ion concentrations.[59] Indeed, the massive fluxes of $Ca^{2+}$ associated with the generation of rhythmic spike-bursts during NREM sleep may modulate the $Ca^{2+}$-dependent gene expression and $Ca^{2+}$-dependent second messengers. Thus, the possibility exists that sleep rhythms reorchestrate the intracellular processes of neurons to perform tasks best done during quiet sleep.

Sleep oscillations may also assist the brain in complex operations, including plasticity and memory. Contrary to previous assumptions that the whole sleeping system lies dormant for the most part and that sleep is characterized by mental blankness, many cells recorded from neocortical areas of animals have been found to be firing as actively in NREM sleep as in waking, although the firing patterns change from one state to the other.[60,61] One of the mysteries of sleep is the question of why cortical cells are so active when the brain is supposed to rest. Various hypotheses propose that dreaming sleep, a behavioral state known for its association with a highly activated brain, maintains brain hardwiring[62] and consolidates the circuitry encoding memory traces.[63] It is now proposed that in resting sleep, a state that is usually viewed as being associated with the obliteration of all forms of consciousness, the cyclic spike-trains or spike-bursts may reorganize and specify the circuitry and stimulate the dendrites of neocortical neurons to grow more spines, thereby leading to consolidation of memory traces acquired during wakefulness.[64] This hypothesis rests on the suggestion that the rich neuronal activity during the depolarizing components of sleep oscillations prevailingly affects certain cellular groups for which plasticity is important, as is the case for neurons from association areas.

# REFERENCES

1. Steriade M, Jones EG, Llinás RR. Thalamic Oscillations and Signaling. New York: Wiley-Interscience, 1990.
2. Steriade M, Jones EG, McCormick DA. Thalamus. Oxford: Elsevier, 1997.
3. Steriade M, McCarley RW. Brainstem Control of Wakefulness and Sleep. New York: Plenum, 1990.
4. Moruzzi G. The sleep-waking cycle. Ergeb Physiol 1972;64:1.
5. Nauta WJH. Hypothalamic regulation of sleep in rats. Experimental study. J Neurophysiol 1946;9:285.
6. Bremer F. Preoptic hypnogenic focus and mesencephalic reticular formation. Brain Res 1970;21:132.
7. McGinty DJ, Sterman MB. Sleep suppression after basal forebrain lesions in the cat. Science 1968;60:1253.
8. Gritti I, Mainville L, Jones BE. Projections of GABAergic and cholinergic basal forebrain and GABAergic preoptic-anterior hypothalamic neurons to the posterior lateral hypothalamus of the rat. J Comp Neurol 1994;339:251.
9. Sherin JE, Shiromani PJ, McCarley RW, Saper CB. Activation of ventrolateral preoptic neurons during sleep. Science 1996;271:216.
10. Szymusiak R, McGinty D. Sleep-waking discharge of basal forebrain projection neurons in cats. Brain Res Bull 1989;22:423.
11. Sallanon M, Denoyer M, Kitahama K, et al. Long-lasting insomnia induced by preoptic neurons lesions and its transient reversal by muscimol injection into the posterior hypothalamus in the cat. Neuroscience 1989;32:669.
12. Steriade M. Cellular Mechanisms of Wakefulness and Sleep. In A Mayes (ed), Sleep Mechanisms and Functions in Humans and Animals. Wokingham, UK: Van Rostrand Reinhold, 1983;161.
13. Steriade M, Paré D, Parent A, Smith Y. Projections of cholinergic and non-cholinergic neurons of the brainstem core to relay and associational thalamic nuclei in the cat and macaque monkey. Neuroscience 1988;25:47.
14. Paré D, Smith Y, Parent A, Steriade M. Projections of brainstem core cholinergic and non-cholinergic neurons of cat to intralaminar and reticular thalamic nuclei. Neuroscience 1988;25:69.
15. Steriade M, Datta S, Paré D, et al. Neuronal activities in brainstem cholinergic nuclei related to tonic activation processes in thalamocortical systems. J Neurosci 1990;10:2541.
16. Steriade M, Oakson G, Ropert N. Firing rates and patterns of midbrain reticular neurons during steady and transitional states of the sleep-waking cycle. Exp Brain Res 1982;46:37.
17. McCormick DA, von Krosigk M. Corticothalamic activation modulates thalamic firing through activation of glutamate metabotropic receptors. Proc Natl Acad Sci U S A 1992;89:2774.
18. McCormick DA. Neurotransmitter actions in the thalamus and cerebral cortex and their role in modulation of thalamocortical activity. Prog Neurobiol 1992;39:337.
19. Rainnie DG, Grunze HCR, McCarley RW, Greene RW. Adenosine inhibition of mesopontine cholinergic neurons. Science 1994;263:689.
20. Lin JS, Hou Y, Sakai K, Jouvet M. Histaminergic descending inputs to the mesopontine tegmentum and

their role in the control of cortical activation and wakefulness in the cat. J Neurosci 1996;16:1523.

21. Bremer F. Cerveau "isolé" et physiologie du sommeil. C R Séances Soc Biol Fil 1935;118:1235.

22. Façon E, Steriade M, Wertheim N. Hypersomnie prolongée engendrée par des lésions bilatérales du système activateur médial: le syndrome thrombotique de la bifurcation du tronc basilaire. Rev Neurol (Paris) 1958;98:117.

23. Steriade M, Glenn LL. Neocortical and caudate projections of intralaminar thalamic neurons and their synaptic excitation from the midbrain reticular core. J Neurophysiol 1982;48:352.

24. Kinomura S, Larsson J, Gulyás B, Roland P. Activation by attention of the human reticular formation and thalamic intralaminar nuclei. Science 1996;271:512.

25. Steriade M, Buzsáki G. Parallel Activation of Thalamic and Cortical Neurons by Brainstem and Basal Forebrain Cholinergic Systems. In M Steriade, D Biesold (eds), Brain Cholinergic Systems. Oxford: Oxford University Press, 1990;3.

26. Rechtschaffen A, Foulkes D. Effects of visual stimuli on dream content. Percept Mot Skills 1965;19:1149.

27. Steriade M, Iosif G, Apostol V. Responsiveness of thalamic and cortical motor relays during arousal and various stages of sleep. J Neurophysiol 1969;32:384.

28. Steriade M. Alertness, Quiet Sleep, Dreaming. In A Peters, EG Jones (eds), Cerebral Cortex (Vol 9), Normal and Altered States of Function. New York: Plenum, 1991;279.

29. Timofeev I, Contreras D, Steriade M. Synaptic responsiveness of cortical and thalamic neurones during various phases of slow sleep oscillation in cat. J Physiol (Lond) 1996;494:265.

30. Steriade M, Apostol V, Oakson G. Control of unitary activities in cerebellothalamic pathway during wakefulness and synchronized sleep. J Neurophysiol 1971;34:384.

31. Llinás RR. The intrinsic electrophysiological properties of mammalian neurons and CNS function. Science 1988;242:1654.

32. Arezzo JC, Vaughn HG Jr, Legatt AD. Topography and intracranial sources of somatosensory evoked potentials in the monkey. II. Cortical components. Electroencephalogr Clin Neurophysiol 1981;28:1.

33. Yamada T, Kameyama S, Fuchigami Y, et al. Changes of short latency somatosensory evoked potential in sleep. Electroencephalogr Clin Neurophysiol 1988;70:126.

34. Steriade M, Deschênes M, Domich L, Mulle C. Abolition of spindle oscillations in thalamic neurons disconnected from nucleus reticularis thalami. J Neurophysiol 1985;54:1473.

35. Steriade M, Domich L, Oakson G, Deschênes M. The deafferented reticularis thalami nucleus generates spindle rhythmicity. J Neurophysiol 1987;57:260.

36. Curró Dossi R, Nuñez A, Steriade M. Electrophysiology of a slow (0.5–4 Hz) intrinsic oscillation of cat thalamocortical neurones in vivo. J Physiol (Lond) 1992;447:215.

37. McCormick DA, Pape HC. Properties of a hyperpolarization-activated cation current and its role in rhythmic oscillation in thalamic relay neurones. J Physiol (Lond) 1990;431:291.

38. Leresche N, Lightowler S, Soltesz I, et al. Low-frequency oscillatory activities intrinsic to rat and cat thalamocortical cells. J Physiol (Lond) 1991;441:155.

39. Steriade M, Curró Dossi R, Nuñez A. Network modulation of a slow intrinsic oscillation of cat thalamocortical neurons implicated in sleep delta waves: cortical potentiation and brainstem cholinergic suppression. J Neurosci 1991;11:3200.

40. Steriade M, Nuñez A, Amzica F. A novel slow (<1 Hz) oscillation of neocortical neurons in vivo: depolarizing and hyperpolarizing components. J Neurosci 1993; 13:3266.

41. Steriade M, Amzica F, Contreras D. Synchronization of fast (30–40 Hz) spontaneous cortical rhythms during brain activation. J Neurosci 1996;16:392.

42. Steriade M, Contreras D, Amzica F, Timofeev I. Synchronization of fast (30–40 Hz) spontaneous oscillations in intrathalamic and thalamocortical networks. J Neurosci 1996;16:2788.

43. Achermann P, Borbély A. Low-frequency (<1 Hz) oscillation in the human sleep electroencephalogram. Neuroscience 1997;81:213.

44. Amzica F, Steriade M. The K-complex: its slow (<1 Hz) rhythmicity and relation to delta waves. Neurology 1997;49:952.

45. Steriade M, Nuñez A, Amzica F. Intracellular analysis of relations between the slow (<1 Hz) neocortical oscillation and other sleep rhythms of the electroencephalogram. J Neurosci 1993;13:3266.

46. Timofeev I, Steriade M. Low-frequency rhythms in the thalamus of intact and decorticated cats. J Neurophysiol 1996;76:4152.

47. Amzica F, Steriade M. Disconnection of intracortical synaptic linkages disrupts synchronization of a slow oscillation. J Neurosci 1995;15:4658.

48. Terzano MG, Parrino L. Clinical applications of cyclic alternating pattern. Physiol Behav 1993;54:807.

49. Steriade M, Amzica F, Nuñez A. Cholinergic and noradrenergic modulation of the slow (~0.3 Hz) oscillation in neocortical cells. J Neurophysiol 1993; 70:1384.

50. Steriade M, Wyzinski P, Apostol V. Corticofugal Projections Governing Rhythmic Thalamic Activity. In TL Frigyesi, E Rinvik, MD Yahr (eds), Corticothalamic Projections and Sensorimotor Activities. New York: Raven, 1972;221.

51. Contreras D, Steriade M. Spindle oscillation: the role of corticothalamic feedback in a thalamically generated rhythm. J Physiol (Lond) 1996;490:159.

52. Contreras D, Destexhe A, Sejnowski TJ, Steriade M. Control of spatiotemporal coherence of a thalamic oscillation by corticothalamic feedback. Science 1996; 274:771.

53. Contreras D, Destexhe A, Sejnowski TJ, Steriade M. Spatiotemporal patterns of spindle oscillations in cortex and thalamus. J Neurosci 1997;17:1179.

54. Von Krosigk M, Bal T, McCormick DA. Cellular mechanisms of a synchronized oscillation in the thalamus. Science 1993;261:361.

55. Bal T, von Krosigk M, McCormick DA. Synaptic and membrane mechanisms underlying synchronized oscillations in the ferret LGNd in vitro. J Physiol (Lond) 1995;483:641.

56. Bal T, von Krosigk M, McCormick DA. Role of the ferret perigeniculate nucleus in the generation of synchronized oscillations in vitro. J Physiol (Lond) 1995; 483:665.

57. Benington J, Heller HC. Restoration of brain energy metabolism as the function of sleep. Prog Neurobiol 1995;45:347.

58. Steriade M. Brain Electrical Activity and Sensory Processing During Waking and Sleep States. In MM Kryger, T Roth, WC Dement (eds), Principles and Practice of Sleep Medicine. Philadelphia: Saunders, 1989;86.

59. Steriade M, McCormick DA, Sejnowski TJ. Thalamocortical oscillations in the sleeping and aroused brain. Science 1993;262:679.

60. Evarts EV. Temporal patterns of discharge of pyramidal tract neurons during sleep and waking in the monkey. J Neurophysiol 1964;27:152.

61. Steriade M, Deschênes M, Oakson G. Inhibitory processes and interneuronal apparatus in motor cortex during sleep and waking. I. Background firing and responsiveness of pyramidal tract neurons and interneurons. J Neurophysiol 1974;37:1065.

62. Roffwarg HP, Muzio JN, Dement WC. Ontogenetic development of the human sleep-dream cycle. Science 1966;152:604.

63. Steriade M. Cortical long-axoned cells and putative interneurons during the sleep-waking cycle. Behav Brain Sci 1978;3:465.

64. Steriade M, Contreras D, Curró Dossi R, Nuñez A. The slow (<1 Hz) oscillation in reticular thalamic and thalamocortical neurons: scenario of sleep rhythms generation in interacting thalamic and neocortical networks. J Neurosci 1993;13:3284.

# Chapter 5
# Biochemical Pharmacology of Sleep

Rebecca K. Zoltoski, Rafael de Jesus Cabeza,
and J. Christian Gillin

What is sleep and what purpose does it serve? These questions have been the topic of philosophic, psychological, and physiologic inquiry for centuries. It was only in this century, however, with the advent of the polygraph and the discovery of electroencephalography (EEG), that the basic architecture of sleep was characterized.[1,2] Speculation about the function of sleep has been and remains based on the ideas of circadian rhythms and homeostasis. The first idea emphasizes the daily cycles of rest and activity, with the implication that the survival of the species is facilitated by the appropriate timing of sleep and wakefulness over the 24-hour day. The second idea regards sleep as important for necessary repair or the maintenance of homeostasis; that is, after wakefulness and activity, sleep has some sort of restorative purpose. Unfortunately for these hypotheses, no specific physiologic repair or homeostatic process has yet been identified during sleep. Although we have a better idea of how sleep and wakefulness are structured and generated, the functions of sleep remain an enigma.

Various theoretical models have been proposed to account for the regulation of sleep and wakefulness. One model, which takes into account both circadian and homeostatic considerations, is the two-process model developed by Borbely and associates.[3] The two processes it postulates are process S and process C. Process S is a homeostatic process: The longer the organism is awake, the greater the propensity to sleep and to have a more "intense" sleep, specifically measured as the power density in the delta frequency (0.25–<4.00 Hz) EEG band during non–rapid eye movement (NREM) sleep. Because a positive correlation exists between the length of time spent awake and the propensity for sleep, the model hypothesizes the existence of an endogenous sleep factor that is synthesized or accumulated exponentially during waking and is catabolized or dissipated exponentially during sleep. The decline of delta EEG power (0.25–<4.00 Hz) across the sleep period may be an indirect measure of this restorative function of sleep; evidence suggests that protein synthesis during sleep is significantly correlated with the amount of delta sleep.[4,5] Process C, the second component of the two-process model, reflects an oscillatory process that determines the threshold of sensitivity to the homeostatic factor and thus affects the propensity for sleep and waking. Process C is hypothesized to entrain or be entrained with other oscillators responsible for biological rhythms, such as temperature, cortisol secretion, and REM sleep.

The two-process model of sleep regulation has important implications for clinicians as well as basic scientists. In evaluating and treating patients with sleep-wake disorders, the clinician must evaluate not only how much the patient sleeps, but the history,

This chapter is supported in part by a grant from the National Institute of Mental Health (NIMH), #2-P30-MH30914, NIMH #5-RO1-MH57134, and a Veterans Administration Merit Review grant.

timing, and duration of sleep-wake episodes as well. Normal sleep architecture and duration are generally promoted when sleep is preceded by a long period of wakefulness and when it occurs at the appropriate phase of the circadian sleep-wake cycle. Two peaks of normal sleep propensity—presumably reflecting process C—have been identified in humans entrained to the customary sleep-wake schedule. These peaks occur at night and at midafternoon.[6]

Two behavioral states exist in most mammals and birds: wakefulness and sleep. (A possible exception is the common shrew, which apparently failed to have polygraphically defined sleep during a 2-week study in the laboratory.[7]) Thus, animals can be awake and conscious of their environment, or they can be asleep, and only responsive to strong stimuli. In most animals, sleep itself is composed of two very different states: (1) NREM sleep, a state characterized by a global lowering of brain metabolism, and (2) REM sleep, characterized by a level of brain metabolism comparable to waking.[8–10] NREM sleep is normally divided into stages dependent on the EEG pattern. REM sleep can be subdivided into *tonic* and *phasic* REM sleep. Tonic events include a desynchronized EEG (high-frequency, low-amplitude waves), a persistent atonia of antigravity muscles, and hippocampal theta activity. Phasic events include REM, periodic twitches of skeletal muscles, variability of autonomic function (e.g., heart rate and respiration), and the presence of pontine-geniculate-occipital (PGO) spikes. In human studies, the "intensity" of REM sleep is often measured by the amount of ocular activity per minute of REM sleep, sometimes referred to as *REM density*. Under normal entrained conditions, NREM sleep always precedes REM sleep. These two sleep states alternate in an ultradian (more than one cycle per 24 hours) cycle, which in humans is approximately 90 minutes.

Most species entrain their wake-sleep cycle to the daily light-dark periods. In the case of homeotherms, the entrainment of the circadian wake-sleep cycle to the daily light-dark period requires a small group of oscillatory cells located within the floor of the third ventricle directly above the optic chiasm, the suprachiasmatic nucleus (SCN). The SCN receives information about environmental lighting conditions via pathways leading from the retina (the retinal-hypothalamic pathway) and from the intrageniculate leaflet.[11–13] The light-dark cycle provides the major *Zeitgeber*, or time giver, which entrains the phase

position of the SCN endogenous oscillations to the environment. One important output eventually reaches the pineal gland, via the superior cervical ganglia, and times the circadian release of melatonin, which occurs only during the dark period. Ablation of this nucleus disrupts both the entrainment of the sleep-wake cycle to the light-dark cycle and the circadian organization of sleep and wakefulness, as well as the circadian changes in body temperature, cortisol secretion, and REM sleep.[11,14] Animals whose SCN have been lesioned show a succession of short bouts of sleep and activity distributed randomly over the 24-hour day without a circadian predominance of one over the other. Nevertheless, SCN-lesioned animals show a rebound compensation in sleep after sleep deprivation, suggesting that the physiologic mechanisms regulating the homeostasis of sleep and wakefulness can be physiologically isolated from those responsible for the circadian organization of sleep and wakefulness.[15] These observations also suggest that basic mechanisms generating sleep and wakefulness do not reside within the SCN. The SCN, however, may well be the anatomic site for process C. A major function is to provide temporal organization over the 24-hour day to a variety of circadian processes, including sleep and wakefulness.

An implication of the two-process model is that duration of wakefulness is positively correlated with the increased sleep propensity, perhaps due to an endogenous sleep-promoting compound.[3] An interesting further implication is that many so-called hypnotic agents may promote sleep by unmasking a prior *sleep debt* in addition to or instead of inherent sleep-inducing/wakefulness-suppressing properties. For example, alcohol's sleep-promoting properties probably depend on a prior sleep debt.[16] Likewise, Edgar et al.[17] have reported that triazolam, a benzodiazepine hypnotic, does not induce sleep in the SCN-lesioned rat; because the rat sleeps in short bursts occurring frequently around the clock, it is assumed that it does not develop a sleep debt that could be unmasked by triazolam.

Because the circadian clock plays such an important role in the timing and character of sleep, considerable research has been conducted in recent years to determine ways to regulate the clock. Under normal circumstances, information about ambient light is conveyed from the retina directly and indirectly to the SCN and synchronizes the phase position of the clock with the outside world. The gradually increasing light intensity that comes with dawn probably plays a particularly important role in this process. Properly administered bright light, however, can be used not only to synchronize the clock but to shift the phase position of the clock in the desired direction. A pulse of bright light (e.g., 1,500 lux for 30 minutes) at the onset of the normal rest period will delay the phase position of the clock, especially if the subject is in the dark at the end of the rest period. Alternatively, the clock can be phase-advanced by exposure to darkness at the beginning of the rest period and to light at the end of the rest period. These findings have important implications for the clinical management of jet lag, sleep-wake problems associated with shift work, and circadian rhythm disorders.[18]

The scientific understanding of the molecular mechanisms responsible for the regulation of the SCN or "biological clock" has grown dramatically in recent years and has significant implications for understanding the regulation of the sleep-wake cycle. Much of the most exciting research has been conducted in the eye of the fruit fly (*Drosophila melanogaster*), where a self-regulating feedback system, involving the rise and fall of two proteins (per and tim) have been shown to control the circadian rest-activity cycle. So-called clock genes have also been detected in mice.[19] In addition, as is reviewed later in this chapter, administration of melatonin may also shift the biological clock. As knowledge increases about the regulation of the circadian system, new avenues will emerge that promise better management of sleep-wake problems.

Although the two-process model has been useful in the search for factors or processes that affect the sleep-wake cycle, it does not address the regulation of NREM versus REM sleep with the same rigor. The length of the NREM-REM cycle is species-dependent and in humans has a period of approximately 90 minutes. According to the reciprocal interaction model of REM sleep, the ultradian cycle of REM and NREM sleep results from the reciprocal interactions between cholinergic, REM facilitatory neurons (REM-on cells) and REM inhibitory neurons (REM-off cells), possible noradrenergic and serotonergic cells.[20,21]

It is important at this juncture to mention two points that should be kept in mind throughout the reading of this chapter. The models we have described, the two-process model and the reciprocal interaction model, have predictive and heuristic value but are not yet firmly supported by anatomic, physiologic, and neurochemical evidence. Furthermore, the models were developed in an effort to describe sleep; the physiologic mechanisms of wakefulness, therefore, are not considered in depth. Thus, it is hoped that the following discussion of the pharmacology of all three states, wakefulness, REM sleep, and NREM sleep, is helpful in gaining a better understanding and appreciation of the pharmacology of sleep.

## PHARMACOLOGY OF WAKEFULNESS AND SLEEP

As proposed by Koella,[22] the sleep organizing and regulation apparatus (SORA) may comprise a coordinating center with two programs, one sustaining wakefulness and the other sleep. The output of these processes is controlled by the various neurotransmitters, such as acetylcholine (ACh), dopamine (DA), norepinephrine (NE), and serotonin (5-HT for 5-hydroxytryptamine) with the assistance of inhibitory neurotransmitters, in the coordination with the excitatory and inhibitory flow as processed through the SORA. The overall net output of this apparatus determines which of the three different states, waking and NREM and REM sleep, is predominant. There are situations, however, in which the appearance of any given state is incomplete. One example of this is narcolepsy, in which it appears that there is an inappropriate intrusion of components of REM sleep into wakefulness, resulting in cataplexy, sleep paralysis, and hypnagogic hallucinations.[23] Pharmacologic studies in human narcoleptics, as well as the canine model, have aided in our understanding of the pharmacology of these three states.

### Wakefulness

Wakefulness is maintained by the tonic activity of neurons distributed throughout the brain stem reticular formation that project to the thalamus, the hypothalamus, and the basal forebrain (BF).[2] The major neurotransmitter systems that appear to regulate wakefulness are the dopaminergic and noradrenergic neurons of the pontomesencephalic tegmentum, the posterior hypothalamic histaminergic neurons, and the cholinergic neurons of the BF. These regions all project diffusely to and through the forebrain to subcortical and cortical areas.

*Dopamine*

The effects of amphetamines[24] and cocaine[25] on sleep suggest a role for DA and other amines in promoting wakefulness. Stimulants increase wakefulness and decrease REM sleep. Withdrawal from stimulants in chronic users increases both total sleep and REM sleep.[26] The effect of amphetamine on sleep can largely be blocked by pretreatment with pimozide, a dopaminergic receptor antagonist.[27]

Evidence from studies using intracranial injections of DA[28,29]; treatment with the precursor L-dopa[30]; and lesions of the ventral tegmentum and substantia nigra, which are dopaminergic,[31,32] suggests that DA is important in the maintenance of waking. Biochemical and electrophysiologic studies also suggest that DA activity is associated with waking rather than sleep. DA content is high during waking,[33] and its turnover decreases during the transition from waking to sleep.[34] Thus pharmacologic, biochemical, and electrophysiologic studies on DA suggest that it maintains behavioral waking.

In rats and dogs, moderate to high doses of apomorphine, a DA agonist, increase wakefulness at the expense of sleep, with REM sleep being more sensitive to its effects than NREM sleep[35,36]; administration of pimozide, a DA antagonist, has the opposite effect.[37] In humans, after intravenous (IV) infusion of apomorphine at moderate to high doses, a complete abolition of REM sleep, a severe reduction in stage II, and a marked increase in stage IV were noticed.[38]

Five DA receptor subtypes have been identified.[39] Drugs that selectively stimulate $D_1$ and $D_2$ have been used to assess their relative role in wakefulness. The $D_1$ agonist A68930 increased waking time and reduced the amount of REM sleep in the rat. SCH 23390, also a $D_1$ antagonist, blocked these effects.[40] Studies assessing the role of the $D_2$ receptor have been less clear. Early reports using the DA antagonists haloperidol and sulpiride suggested that the dopaminergic effect of increasing waking and decreasing REM sleep were mediated via the $D_2$ receptor.[41] However, a new $D_2$ antagonist, remoxipride, had no sedative effect.[42] These conflicting results may be due to drug selectivity problems.

In narcoleptics, both human and canine, a decrease in DA activity or turnover has been reported,[43–45] as well as an upregulation of $D_1$ and $D_2$ receptors.[46] Drugs that alter the synaptic availability of DA have little effect in humans or canine narcoleptic symptoms, however, with the exception of cataplexy.[45,47,48] Therefore, the mechanisms for these observations are still unclear.

In summary, drugs that increase availability of DA also increase wakefulness and decrease sleep, which appears to be mediated through the $D_1$ and possibly the $D_2$ receptors. Despite these observations implicating DA in the regulation of sleep and wakefulness, its role remains unclear. Single-cell recordings of dopaminergic neurons in the substantia nigra, for example, show only minor changes across the sleep-wake cycle.[49] Therefore, it is possible that DA plays a role in maintaining wakefulness in narcolepsy or other hypersomnolent states, or under the influence of powerful stimulants, but it is not involved in the normal sleep-wake cycle.

*Norepinephrine*

Recordings of unit activity of noradrenergic neurons in the locus ceruleus (LC) have shown that the firing rate of these cells is state dependent, so that most cells exhibit a high firing rate during wakefulness that then decreases over NREM sleep until they are virtually silent during REM sleep.[50]

Pharmacologic studies have shown that there is an important interaction of α- and β-adrenergic receptors in the maintenance and components of the sleep-wake cycle. The noradrenergic receptor family has been further extended to include at least two types of α and three types of β receptors.[39] Peripheral administration of the $α_1$-adrenoceptor antagonist phenoxybenzamine increases wakefulness and reduces REM sleep.[51] Peripheral administration of clonidine, an $α_2$-adrenoceptor agonist, increases drowsiness and decreases sleep in rats, cats, and humans.[52–54] In addition, local administration of clonidine into the LC increases wakefulness and suppresses REM sleep.[54] Finally, localized microinjection of clonidine into the medial preoptic area increased sleep, whereas yohimbine, an $α_2$-adrenoceptor antagonist, inhibited this effect.[55] Single-cell recordings in the medial preoptic area after administration of NA suggests that it promotes wakefulness by inhibiting sleep-active neurons and exciting waking-active neurons.[56]

In rats, systemic administration of the adrenergic receptor antagonist propranolol, which may decrease noradrenergic activity, increases wakefulness and inhibits REM sleep,[54] whereas in cats, localized administration of propranolol into the medial pontine reticular formation (mPRF) had no effect on wakefulness, but increased REM sleep.[57] In rats, however, localized administration of the adrenoceptor agonist isoproterenol into the medial septal region of the BF increases waking time while suppressing REM sleep.[58]

In narcolepsy, increased noradrenergic turnover and $\alpha_2$-adrenoceptor density has been reported in humans.[46,59] In addition, pharmacologic studies using the canine narcolepsy model have shown that increasing noradrenergic transmission reduces cataplexy.[47] Therefore, abnormal noradrenergic function has been implicated in cataplexy associated with narcolepsy.

In general, the noradrenergic system promotes wakefulness; however, the action of peripherally administered drugs must be assessed by the availability of the drugs to the various brain regions. Further studies are needed to fully assess the relative importance of various noradrenergic brain regions and receptor subtypes in stimulating wakefulness.

*Histamine*

The proposal that histamine (HA) plays a neuroregulatory role in sleep and waking derives mainly from pharmacologic studies in which the arousing effect of HA and the sedative and sleep-inducing effects of some antihistamines were described.[60–62] In humans, $H_1$-receptor antagonists impair vigilance and shorten latency to drowsy sleep, but have little or no effect on nocturnal sleep. $H_2$-receptor antagonists, however, do not appear to impair vigilance,[63] but cause an increase in the amount of slow-wave sleep (SWS) and number of movements in and out of NREM sleep.[61] It should be noted, however, that antihistamines may significantly improve sleep in individuals with stuffy noses that interfere with breathing during sleep.

An ascending histaminergic pathway from the posterior hypothalamus innervates the cortex, striatum, hippocampus, and amygdala of the forebrain with cell bodies originating in the posterior hypothalamus and midbrain regions.[64,65] In particular, studies suggest that neurons in the ventrolateral preoptic area (VLPO) of the anterior hypothalamus are involved in the generation of NREM sleep.[66] Projections from the VLPO may inhibit the histaminergic tuberomamillary neurons in the caudal hypothalamus, thereby promoting NREM sleep. In addition, a descending histaminergic pathway extends from the posterior hypothalamus to the mesopontine tegmentum,[64,67] where many of these fibers intermingle with the cholinergic, adrenergic, and other neuronal populations that play a key role in the generation of wakefulness and REM sleep.[30,68]

In the rat, a circadian rhythm of HA concentration has its peak in the light phase. The enzymes that synthesize histamine (histidine decarboxylase) and destroy it (histamine-$N$-methyl-transferase) also show a circadian pattern, with their activity highest during the dark phase.[69] This seems to indicate that the peak turnover rate occurs during their active phase. In monkeys, an increased release of HA in the posterior hypothalamus occurs on awakening and is maintained during each waking episode.[70] Administration of substances that impair HA transmission or synthesis increase NREM, whereas enhancement of HA transmission increases quiet wakefulness.[71–73] More specifically, the administration of centrally penetrating $H_1$-receptor antagonists induces sedation and NREM sleep.[71,73] Additionally, microinjection of the $H_1$-receptor agonist 2-thiazolylethylamine into the mesopontine tegmentum of cats causes an increase in quiet wakefulness, which could be blocked with mepyramine, an $H_1$-receptor antagonist.[68]

It would appear that histamine antagonism has a more obvious effect during wakefulness than during sleep, and it is therefore suggested that the histaminergic system may be more concerned with vigilance than the underlying state of sleep and wakefulness. The tendency to decrease wakefulness and increase NREM sleep suggests a complementary role of the $H_1$ and $H_2$ systems in the control of sleep, and it is tentatively suggested that they may modulate the balance between wakefulness and NREM sleep.[74]

In summary, experiments in humans support the role of histaminergic mechanisms in the control of the sleep-wakefulness continuum, although their limited effect during nocturnal sleep and their more obvious effect during wakefulness suggest that the histaminergic system may be more concerned with maintaining vigilance during the wakeful state than the underlying state of wakefulness itself. Histaminergic mechanisms may also have a subtle role in maintaining the balance between the cortical desynchronization of wakefulness and synchronization of slow-wave activity during nocturnal sleep. One postulated mechanism of this phenomenon is that histaminergic descending pathways into the mesopontine tegmentum would promote waking via activation of $H_1$ receptors located on cholinergic neurons.[68]

### Acetylcholine

Cholinergic mechanisms clearly play a role in maintaining arousal at both cortical[75,76] and subcortical sites.[77,78] For example, ACh is released from the cerebral cortex and hippocampus during activation,[79,80] including REM sleep.[81] In addition, IV administration of physostigmine during NREM sleep in humans induces REM sleep at low doses and wakefulness at high doses; furthermore, consistent with the concept that the first NREM period is "deeper" than the second, a dose that induces REM during the first NREM period induces wakefulness during the second NREM period.[82] On the other hand, diminished cortical cholinergic activity is associated with a synchronized EEG (delta waves or high-amplitude, slow-frequency waves), whether achieved by lesions of the nucleus basalis (the origin of cholinergic projections to the cortex) or the administration of muscarinic antagonists.[76]

These BF regions are recognized as important sites for regulation of neocortical and limbic system arousal, to modulate sensory and cognitive processing.[83] Loss of BF cholinergic neurons is a critical feature of the neuropathology of Alzheimer's disease.[84] This loss appears to lead to cognitive attention deficits, as patterned by excitotoxin-induced lesions of cholinergic regions of the BF in animals.[85] It has been further hypothesized that the cholinergic BF neurons interact with neurons that use γ-aminobutyric acid (GABA) to regulate behavioral states.[58]

### Non–Rapid Eye Movement Sleep

Lesion and recording studies have identified cells that are most active during NREM sleep in the lower brain stem,[2] the anterior hypothalamus–preoptic area, and the BF area. These cells may be necessary to NREM sleep.[83,86,87] These sleep-on cells located in the anterior hypothalamus–preoptic area are intermingled with cells involved in heat loss. Many anatomic and chemical substrates that produce increases in temperature and result in heat loss may also induce NREM sleep. This suggests that sleep-generating and temperature-regulating mechanisms are closely linked anatomically or chemically. However, the causal and functional relationship of this link is speculative at this time.

The initiation of NREM sleep involves the dampening of the activity of those systems involved in wakefulness. This process, by nature of the anatomic connections of the neurons, involves an antagonistic, inhibitory action by other neuronal populations that are discussed in the next section.

### Serotonin

A role for 5-HT in sleep has been suggested by the observation that L-tryptophan, a precursor of 5-HT, is a *natural hypnotic* that increases NREM sleep time and decreases sleep latency.[88,89] It should be noted, however, that tryptophan is not currently used clinically, because it was implicated in the eosinophilic myalgia syndrome.

The mechanism responsible for the role of 5-HT in sleep is not clear. Jouvet's original monoamine theory of sleep[30,90] first recognized the importance of 5-HT in initiating and maintaining sleep. Briefly, lesions of the dorsal raphe nucleus (DRN) as well as pharmacologic depletion of brain 5-HT by *para*-chlorophenylalanine (PCPA), a tryptophan-hydroxylase inhibitor, produced insomnia lasting 3–4 days in cats.[91,92] This insomnia could be reversed by treatment with 5-hydroxytryptophan, the 5-HT precursor that bypassed synthesis inhibition. Later studies, however, have refuted the original hypothesis that 5-HT was the "sleep" neurotransmitter. In cats given daily PCPA treatment, NREM sleep returned to 70% of normal in 1 week, although brain 5-HT levels were still depleted by 90–95%.[93] Other methods of depleting brain 5-HT, such as the neurotoxin 5,7-dihydroxytryptamine, did not effect sleep despite a 78% forebrain depletion of 5-HT.[94] Furthermore, in vivo voltammetric studies demonstrated that the intracerebral release of 5-HT did not increase with sleep onset.[95]

The profound but temporary insomnia induced by 5-HT depletion, by either PCPA or lesions of the DRN, may have resulted from the rapidity with which brain levels fell rather than the absolute levels of 5-HT. This interpretation is consistent with the hyperexcitable state, including convulsions, associated with abrupt discontinuation of high 5-hydroxytryptophan doses in schizophrenic patients.[96]

Not only the level of 5-HT but also the number of specific 5-HT–binding sites exhibit a 24-hour rhythm.[97] Unlike the 5-HT levels that are increased in the forebrain during recovery after sleep deprivation,[98] however, the receptor levels are unchanged by sleep deprivation.[99] Attempts to measure 5-HT levels in various brain regions during the different stages have yielded interesting results. Using microdialysis in the DRN of freely moving cats, an increased level of 5-HT was noted during waking as compared to NREM and REM sleep.[100] Also, using in vivo voltammetry in the posterior hypothalamus, an increased level of 5-HT metabolites were observed during wakefulness as compared to both NREM and REM sleep.[101]

Numerous distinct binding sites for 5-HT have been identified.[39] The 5-HT$_1$ agonist eltoprazine has been reported to increase NREM sleep at the expense of REM sleep in cats.[102] In humans, REM sleep may be inhibited by either ipsapirone, a direct 5-HT$_{1A}$–receptor agonist,[103] or indirectly by pindolol, a 5-HT$_{1A}$–receptor antagonist that disinhibits DRN neurons.[104] The role of the 5-HT$_2$ receptor in sleep has been implicated by studies using ritanserin, a specific antagonist at this receptor. Administration of ritanserin (5–10 mg) increased stage III and IV sleep in humans with a tendency toward decreased waking and REM sleep.[105–107] Ritanserin administration in cats, however, has been shown to decrease NREM sleep and increase wakefulness.[108] Therefore, it may be that serotonergic projections from the DRN to 5-HT$_{1A}$ receptors on the cholinergic brain stem inhibit REM sleep.[109]

In summary, the overwhelming evidence indicates that 5-HT is probably not involved in NREM sleep itself, but may be involved in the regulation of the stages of sleep. Jouvet and his colleagues have formulated a new conception of the role of 5-HT in sleep mechanisms: 5-HT, released by axonal nerve endings in the basal hypothalamus as a neurotransmitter during waking, might act as a neurohormone and induce the synthesis or liberation of hypnogenic factor(s) that would be secondarily responsible for NREM and REM sleep.[110]

*Circulating Factors*

Legendre and Pieron[111,112] and Ishimori[113] introduced the idea of a sleep-inducing factor called *hypnotoxin*. Sleep was induced in a naive recipient after intraventricular injection of a cerebrospinal fluid (CSF) sample obtained from a sleep-deprived dog.[111–113] Pieron's hypnotoxin theory was confirmed with the use of better quantitative measurements and properly controlled experiments by Schnedorf and Ivy.[114] Many substances capable of affecting sleep fit into the hypnotoxin category. Initial studies describing the effects of these substances administered separately are helpful in understanding their possible role, but subsequent studies analyzing sequential administration of several substances have provided more insight.[115,116] Because the role of these multiple substances in regulating sleep-wake states is not completely understood, however, these substances are discussed individually in the following sections.

**Delta Sleep–Inducing Peptide.** The intracerebroventricular (ICV) infusion of extracorporeal dialysates from the blood of donor rabbits in a state of electrically induced sleep has been reported to induce NREM sleep in recipient rabbits.[117] A nonpeptide (delta sleep–inducing peptide [DSIP]) that has been isolated from these dialysates appears to be responsible for this effect.[118,119] Further experiments have shown that this effect is repeatable in rats and cats even when the drug is administered IV or subcutaneously, in addition to intraventricularly (for review, see Inoue[120]). In humans, IV infusions of DSIP in the morning or at night increased total sleep time.[121–124] In rats and in humans, plasma DSIP exhibited a circadian rhythm, with a peak in the late afternoon and a trough in the early morning,[125,126] with no correlation between levels and sleep stages.[125] Finally, DSIP decreases at the initiation of sleep at different circadian times, suggesting that the initiation of sleep influences the levels of DSIP.[127] Constant exposure to light abolishes this circadian rhythm.[126]

In addition to its effects on sleep, DSIP has many extra-sleep effects. It increases body temperature with no apparent effect on brain temperature.[128] In addition, DSIP-induced decreases in blood pressure,[129] anxiousness,[130] and locomotor activity[131–133] have been reported.

In humans, beneficial applications of DSIP have been reported for insomniacs,[122,134–136] a narcoleptic,[137] opiate addicts and alcoholics,[130] as well as patients with chronic, pronounced pain episodes.[138] Reports regarding chronic psychophysiologic insomniacs have claimed a complete elimination of insomnia, including improvements in sleep, daytime mood state, circadian rhythmicity of sleep, and cognitive and psychomotor performance after 6 days of DSIP treatment.[139–142] Monti et al.[143] have not been able to repeat these findings. Therefore, its clinical usefulness still needs to be determined.

It has been observed that DSIP not only affects sleep, but also modulates a variety of physiologic activities in humans and animals. Graf and colleagues[144] have proposed that DSIP, in addition to facilitating sleep, may exert a chronopharmacologic action as a natural programming substance by inducing changes in cerebral neurotransmitters and plasma proteins. In support of this idea, Tobler and Borbely[132] noted a delayed effect of DSIP on rat locomotor activity. Inoue[145,146] observed circadian rest-activity, rhythm-dependent, sleep-modulatory effects of DSIP on rats. From these observations, it has been suggested that DSIP might be the first peptide representative of a possibly large group of *psychophysiologic programming substances* within a yet-unknown hierarchic, multidimensional network of priming molecular mechanisms.[147] Therefore, optimal functioning of an individual in a complex situation can occur with DSIP possibly involved in a high-level control of sleep and waking.

**Sleep-Promoting Substances: Uridine and SPS-B.**
Sleep-promoting substance (SPS) extracted from the water dialysates of brain stems of rats deprived of sleep for 24 hours contains a number of active components. In addition to uridine, which was first identified in 1983,[148,149] there are at least four other partially purified fractions.[150] Of these, SPS-B has been shown to cause an excess of sleep. ICV infusion of the most recently purified form of SPS-B has been shown to elicit a profound sleep-enhancing effect in freely behaving rats at the beginning of their nocturnal period.[120] This effect was caused by the more frequent occurrence of NREM and REM sleep episodes with normal sleep-waking behavior. However, further purification as well as identification of this substance is necessary before its definitive role in sleep modulation can be assessed.

Uridine, after a nocturnal ICV infusion, caused more frequent occurrence of NREM and REM sleep episodes without affecting the duration of the episodes. Diurnal infusion had no effect on sleep patterns.[115] Extra-sleep effects of uridine include a reduction of spontaneous locomotor activity[151,152] with no change in temperature.[150,153,154] These data support the conclusion that uridine may be involved in the feedback mechanisms that regulate the sleep pressure at a dependent normal level, which is preprogrammed in accordance with the phase of the circadian rest activity rhythm.[150,153,155]

**Muramyl Peptides.**    In 1984, Martin et al.[156] and Krueger et al.[157] reported that factor S, which was obtained from the CSF of sleep-deprived goats, bovine and rabbit cerebral tissue, and human urine, was identified as a muramyl tetrapeptide. In addition, a muramyl tripeptide from humans was identified as an active somnogen. It has been proposed that muramyl peptides (MPs) can induce sleep, which in turn enhances immunoreaction, serving a recuperative function in the mammalian body.[158–161] MPs are known as components of peptidoglycans, which form the backbone of bacterial cell walls and exert profound pyrogenic and immunostimulatory activities in the mammalian body.[162–164] The pyrogenic effects can be dissociated from the sleep-inducing effects.[165–168] Although MPs cannot be biosynthesized in the mammalian body,[163] a chemically unidentified sleep-enhancing substance was produced during the digestion of bacteria by macrophages,[169] suggesting that mammals can process bacterial cell walls to produce biologically active MPs. It appears that the somnogenic activity of MPs, which are concerned mainly with the induction of excess NREM sleep, is mediated through the monokine, interleukin-1 (IL-1). The somnogenic effect can be elicited sooner by IL-1 than by MPs in rabbits.[158,163,166–168,170]

**Interleukin-1.**    Krueger et al.[159] have proposed that sleep has a reciprocal relationship with the immune system. That is, sleep itself may enhance certain aspects of immune regulation and may, in turn be enhanced by certain immune modulators. In support of this, Moldofsky et al.[171] reported that serum IL-1 and other immune modulators were elevated during sleep in humans. IL-1 belongs to a family of polypeptides that mediate a variety of host-defense functions and possess pyrogenic activity. IL-1 is liberated by macrophages to activate T lymphocytes and induce fever by acting on hypothalamic cells.

IL-1 purified from human or rabbit mononuclear cells enhanced NREM sleep in a dose-dependent fashion immediately after intraventricular or IV infusion into rabbits or rats.[172–175] In addition, IL-1 elicited hyperthermia. In rabbits, this hyperthermic response, but not the typical temperature changes that occur at transition time, could be prevented by simultaneous ICV infusion of anisomycin without abolishing the somnogenic effect.[172,176] Furthermore, in the rat the increase of slow-wave activity was not correlated with the enhanced body temperature.[173] These results indicate that the effect of IL-1 on sleep is not a secondary effect of hyperthermia. In humans, a peak in the plasma IL-1 level occurs during SWS shortly after sleep onset.[171]

The central nervous system and the immune system play a role in host defense mechanisms. Many regulatory substances, such as IL-1, MPs, and vasoactive intestinal peptide/growth hormone–releasing factor (VIP/GRF)–like peptides are shared by both systems and have profound effects on both sleep and specific aspects of the immune response. Krueger and coworkers[159] have found close relationships between immune reactions and NREM sleep occurrence. Further mammalian macrophages process bacterial cell walls, which contain polymers of MPs and release somnogenic substances. Both glia and macrophages possess binding sites for MPs and both produce several somnogenic immunoactive substances, such as IL-1, prostaglandins (PGs), and interferon-α. Furthermore, studies suggest that the gene responsible for canine narcolepsy is homologous to the human immunoglobulin μ-switch gene, thereby supporting a possible relationship between immune function and control of sleep.[177] Irwin et al.[178] reported that natural killer cell activity, a measure of immune response, was positively and significantly correlated with various aspects of NREM sleep in both normal controls and depressed patients. Furthermore, sleep deprivation actually reduces natural killer cell activity in normal controls.[179] Together, these findings strongly suggest an interaction between sleep and the immune response and suggest a role for sleep in recuperative processes.

**Arginine Vasotocin.** Arginine vasotocin (AVT), a naturally occurring peptide isolated from the pineal gland, inhibits gonadotropin release, modifies conditioned behavior, and possibly enhances NREM sleep. Intraventricular administration of AVT in cats and rabbits induces NREM and decreases REM sleep.[180,181] In rats, however, only a decrease in REM latency was observed.[132,182] In addition, in humans, subcutaneous administration of AVT increased REM sleep. The conclusion from these ambiguous results is that the somnogenic properties of AVT appear to be mediated through indirect effects and await further confirmation.

**Adenosine.** Adenosine (AD) is a naturally occurring purine nucleoside that causes sedation and inhibits neuronal firing activity. Caffeine decreases sleep, particularly NREM sleep, and shortens REM latency, presumably because it blocks the AD receptors.[183]

Many studies indicate that AD enhances deep NREM and REM sleep. Briefly, in rats and dogs, intraventricular or intraperitoneal administration of AD or an AD $A_1$–receptor agonist increases NREM sleep.[184–186] In addition, deoxycoformycin, an AD deaminase inhibitor, enhanced REM sleep, and, at higher doses, NREM sleep.[186,187] Finally, the AD precursor S-adenosylhomocysteine enhanced NREM and REM sleep in rats, cats, and rabbits.[188]

AD $A_1$ receptors, which are more responsive to the doses of AD used in the previously mentioned study,[185] have been studied after REM sleep deprivation. After a 48- or 96-hour deprivation, the AD receptor number was elevated; however, after the 48-hour deprivation, AD levels were unchanged.[189]

The exact role of AD on alertness remains to be determined. It is hypothesized that AD is an endogenous mediator of sleep need. Using power spectral analysis, stimulation of $A_1$ receptors with $N_6$-cyclopentyladenosine produced an EEG pattern similar to the one produced after sleep deprivation.[190,191] Therefore, AD may be involved in the homeostatic feedback control of sleep expression. A particularly interesting hypothesis has been proposed regarding the role of AD in the induction, maintenance, and function of sleep. Bennington and Heller[192] proposed that high-energy, phosphorylated compounds (such as adenosine triphosphate and adenosine 5' triphosphate) in the brain are dephosphorylated during wakefulness, with a resultant increase in AD concentrations. In their theory, not only does AD promote sleep, but sleep provides a time to rephosphorylate AD and restore the level of high-energy compounds in the brain. Consistent with this theory, Porkka-Heiskanen et al.[193] have reported that extracellular concentrations of AD increase progressively with duration of wakefulness in the BF. AD inhibits BF cholinergic neurons that promote cortical arousal. Finally, the concentration of extracellular AD decreases with sleep. In summary, these results suggest that the duration and depth of sleep are increased by elevated concentrations of AD after wakefulness.

**Prostaglandins.** Ueno et al.[194,195] and Matsumura et al.[196] have developed the PG-dependent humoral theory of sleep regulation. Two different PGs, $PGD_2$ and $PGE_2$, have been shown to interact reciprocally to affect sleep. Whereas $PGD_2$ increases, $PGE_2$ decreases sleep time in a dose-dependent manner. $PGD_2$, when injected into the preoptic area or infused ICV in femtomolar quantities, induces both NREM and REM sleep in rats and monkeys.[197–201] In addition, the PGD synthetase activity exhibits a circadian fluctuation that parallels the sleep-wake cycle, so that there is more activity during the quiescent phases of the animal's activity cycle. Finally, infusion of the inhibitors of PG synthesis, diclofenac sodium and inorganic selenium compounds, into rats inhibits sleep.[202,203] After termination of the infusion, a rebound in sleep was reported. These results are consistent with the notion that $PGD_2$ is involved in physiologic induction of sleep in rats. It was further shown that $PGE_2$ increases wakefulness. When AH6809, a $PGE_2$ antagonist, was infused centrally in both monkeys and rats, a dose-dependent increase in sleep was reported.[196,204] Therefore, reciprocal activities of $PGD_2$ and $PGE_2$ in or near the preoptic area and posterior hypothalamus may regulate the state of vigilance.[205]

**Melatonin.** Melatonin is a major hormone of the mammalian pineal gland. Its synthesis and release into the general circulation is timed by one or more biological clocks but occurs only in humans in darkness. In studies examining individuals in near-dark conditions, the onset and offset of melatonin secretion have been used to determine the phase position of the circadian oscillator or oscillators. The general physiologic function of melatonin in humans remains unknown, although in some other mammals it appears to regulate seasonal breeding behavior.

Abnormalities of melatonin secretion have been described in three psychiatric syndromes: (1) seasonal affective disorder with winter depression, (2) major depressive disorders, and (3) premenstrual disorder. Seasonal affective disorder is associated with hypersomniac, hyperphagic depressions

each winter in northerly climates.[206] It can be treated with the extension of the daily photoperiod with bright lights. It has been suggested that the seasonal affective disorder in humans is associated closely with a phase delay of the circadian rhythm of melatonin secretion. In contrast, most but not all studies in patients with major depression report low total amount of nocturnal melatonin.[207] In women with premenstrual depression, total melatonin secretion is low at all phases of the menstrual cycle, possibly because of early offset of melatonin secretion.[208]

Melatonin secretion at night generally declines with normal and pathologic aging, such as that which occurs with Alzheimer's disease. Whether endogenous nocturnal melatonin secretion is etiologically associated with poor sleep is uncertain, despite claims by some that administration of exogenous melatonin "restores natural sleep." In any case, many unanswered questions remain about the efficacy, safety, dosage, or timing of the administration of exogenous melatonin. Because melatonin is regulated as a food supplement rather than a drug, the U.S. Food and Drug Administration does not require rigorous data supporting clinical efficacy, safety, or composition of products labeled and sold as melatonin.

Melatonin has been reported to enhance sleep in cats, rats, young chickens, and humans.[209–213] In humans, for example, an IV bedtime dose of 50 mg reduced sleep latency,[212] whereas three oral daytime doses of 80 mg enhanced sleepiness.[214] On the other hand, no effect was reported after a 1- or 5-mg oral dose administered at bedtime, except a prolongation of REM sleep latency after the large dose.[215] In other studies, sleep propensity was increased in normal subjects given much lower doses (0.1, 0.3, or 1.0 mg), either in the daytime[216] or in the evening.[217] The daily administration of 2 mg melatonin in the late afternoon induced unusual tiredness in the early evening after 4–5 days and an increase in plasma levels that exceeded endogenous nighttime levels by a factor of 10–100.[218,219]

Although it appears unlikely that melatonin is directly involved in sleep regulation, due to the pharmacologically high doses needed to alter sleep, it does appear that it may affect sleep indirectly by altering the phase of the circadian pacemaker.[220] If this preliminary finding is confirmed by further studies, it will be important from both a clinical and pre-clinical point of view. Clinically, it might provide the first pharmacologic means of shifting the phase position of the circadian rhythm. Preclinically, it will be the first demonstration that a pharmacologic agent affects the human circadian rhythm in a manner consistent with a traditional phase-response curve.

### γ-Aminobutyric Acid

Evidence for a role of GABA in the induction of sleep was supplied by the benzodiazepine hypnotics, which enhance GABAergic inhibitory transmission.[221] The benzodiazepines also have nonspecific effects, however, such as anxiolysis and muscle relaxation. It has been reported that classic benzodiazepines do not alter the effect of GABA agonist–stimulated sleep.[222] Nevertheless, lowering of the level of behavioral vigilance and induction as well as maintenance of sleep are among the more prominent effects. After administration of L-cycloserine, an inhibitor of the GABA-degrading enzyme GABA-transaminase, to rats, rabbits, and cats, similar results to that obtained with benzodiazepines, with the exception of no increased agitation at high doses, was noticed.[223] For example, at low doses, an augmentation of REM sleep with no change in NREM sleep was reported, whereas at high doses, REM sleep was inhibited. In addition, a prolonged transition phase between NREM and REM sleep was noticed.[223]

Microdialysis techniques have been used to assess changes in GABA levels across states. In the posterior hypothalamus, an area involved in cortical desynchronization, a selective increase in GABA release was reported.[224] When muscimol, a GABA agonist, was injected into this area, NREM sleep increased.

As proposed by Koella,[22] the SORA may comprise a coordinating center with two programs, one sustaining wakefulness and the other sleep. The output of these different channels is controlled by the various neurotransmitters; however, GABA, which is an inhibitory neurotransmitter, may play a local transmission-modulation role in the coordination of the excitatory and inhibitory flow as processed through the SORA.

### Rapid Eye Movement Sleep

REM sleep has been called *paradoxical sleep* because the brain is metabolically, physiologically,

and psychologically active, unlike during NREM sleep. During REM sleep the brain neither depends on external stimuli for its increased activity nor expresses a motor output in response to activation of the central motor systems. Because of this cyclic central activation, some have suggested that REM sleep is important to brain metabolic processes.

In any mammalian or avian species, the amount of REM sleep increases as body and brain size increase. The time between any two REM sleep episodes decreases as the basal metabolic rate of a given homeothermic species increases,[2] a finding consistent with the hypothesis that REM sleep is important to some brain metabolic process.

The anatomic substrates responsible for the generation of REM sleep are apparently located within the pons. By using complete transections of the brain at specific points, Jouvet[30] demonstrated the cyclic appearance of REM sleep–like phenomena such as REM and atonia. More specific intrapontine lesions indicated that different pathways were involved in tonic and phasic events. Lesions of the dorsolateral pontomesencephalic tegmentum, which send projections to the thalamus, caused phasic events such as PGO spikes to disappear, but not tonic events (muscle atonia and cortical activation).[225] In fact, microdialysis probes placed in the thalamus of rats show a sodium- and calcium-dependent increase in ACh release during REM sleep,[226] supporting the notion that the cholinergic projections from the pons are responsible for the PGO spikes seen during REM sleep. Anatomic studies in the rat suggest that cortical activation depends on cholinergic projections from the pons to the thalamus, hypothalamus, and BF,[77,227,228] and thus offer a possible explanation as to why these lesions, which disrupted the connections to the thalamus but may not have altered those connections to either the hypothalamus or the BF, did not affect cortical activation during REM sleep. The tonic atonia that accompanies REM sleep is generated at the level of the pons but involves a critical relay at the medulla. As early as 1946 it was shown that electrical stimulation of the ventromedial medulla induces muscle atonia not unlike that seen in REM sleep.[229] Muscle atonia may be mediated by several centers, as is suggested by the work of Nishino and coworkers,[230] who demonstrated that cholinergic stimulation of the BF by high amounts of carbachol, a cholinergic agonist, could induce atonia. Another tonic phenomenon of REM sleep that can be cholinergically induced is hippocampal theta activity. Injection of carbachol into either the pedunculopontine tegmental nucleus (PPT) or the pontis oralis nucleus (PO) caused the appearance of hippocampal theta activity with the PO site having a latency approximately one-third of the PPT (approximately 1.7 minutes) suggesting that the PO may be a relay site between the PPT and the generation of the theta activity of the hippocampus.[231]

The prime candidates for the cholinergic cells that facilitate REM sleep are located in the lateral dorsal tegmental nucleus (LDT) and the PPT group.[232-235] These cells display increased firing rates before and during REM sleep, especially in association with PGO spikes. Nonselective lesions of the dorsolateral tegmentum with kainic acid or electricity markedly attenuate REM sleep. The LDT and PPT send projections to the thalamus, where they may inhibit the mechanisms responsible for sleep spindles and delta EEG waves; to the mPRF, where application of cholinomimetic agents trigger REM sleep; and to the medulla, where they facilitate the atonia of REM sleep. The NE and 5-HT neurons in the LC and dorsal raphe, respectively, lie close to the cholinergic neurons in the LDT and PPT and apparently can inhibit them, either directly or indirectly, via GABA interneurons.

The ability of several types of pharmacologic agents to affect REM sleep can be understood within the conceptual framework provided by the reciprocal interaction model. Some cholinomimetic agents and some aminergic antagonists augment REM sleep, whereas anticholinergic agents and aminergic agonists often attenuate or block it. Although this model is of heuristic value, it is undoubtedly simplistic, as other endogenous substances affect REM sleep and not all pharmacologic predictions of the model have been confirmed in actual experiments. For example, lesions of the LC and dorsal raphe do not increase total REM sleep.[2]

*Cholinergic Agents*

The importance of cholinergic mechanisms in the control of REM sleep is firmly established. An interesting historical footnote relays that a dream inspired Otto Loewi to conduct the experiment that established ACh as a neurotransmitter.[236] Thus, we may surmise that ACh triggered the dream that led to the discovery of one of its roles in the brain.

By placing ACh crystals directly on the pons and BF of a cat, Hernandez-Peon was the first to

observe that cholinergic agonists induce REM sleep.[237-239] Although this technique was crude and fraught with interpretation problems, the observation of REM sleep induction by cholinomimetic agents has been repeatedly confirmed using a variety of agents such as carbachol (a nonhydrolyzable analogue of ACh), bethanechol (a muscarinic agonist), and neostigmine (an acetylcholinesterase inhibitor). Baghdoyan and coworkers[240] have shown that stimulation with carbachol of either the BF or the pons of cats can increase REM sleep but that simultaneous injections into both sites is less effective than the injection into the pons alone, suggesting that a regulatory interaction may exist between these two cholinoceptive sites. The effects on REM sleep of physostigmine, an acetylcholinesterase inhibitor, were variable in animals, sometimes increasing REM sleep and at other times having no effect. Injections of cholinergic agonists into the mPRF effectively induce REM sleep or its components but may result in longer latency than is seen with injections into the dorsal or medial pontine tegmentum. In contrast, injections of carbachol into the rostral midbrain or the medullary reticular formation induced waking and decreased REM sleep.[241-244] Similar results have been observed in the rat.[245,246] Systemic administration of two different acetylcholinesterase inhibitors in humans, at doses producing few side effects, caused a shortening of the REM sleep latency and, in the case of galanthamine, also increased the REM sleep density.[247,248] It is important to note that sites that can be stimulated by carbachol to induce REM sleep can also increase wakefulness. Injection of 1–10 ng carbachol into the posterior oral pontine reticular nucleus of the rat increased REM sleep, but injection of 500 ng carbachol into this same site increased wakefulness with no effect on REM sleep.[246] Although this finding might imply involvement of two different receptor systems in the generation of the two states, it is more likely that high concentration of carbachol may diffuse sufficiently far to trigger cholinoceptive centers involved in wakefulness.

A particularly striking observation is that a single injection of carbachol into the peribrachial region of cats increases REM sleep threefold, with a latency of approximately 1 day, and that the increased REM sleep lasts at least 2 weeks, decaying in what appears to be a monotonic fashion.[249,250]

This region of the brain stem is involved in the generation of PGO spikes. The first effect of carbachol infusion is an ipsilateral increase in PGO spiking, followed by bilateral increases in PGO spiking along with the increased REM sleep. The increased PGO spike activity even intrudes into SWS (a phenomenon seen briefly only during the transition between SWS and REM sleep).[249,251] These findings suggest that prolonged periods of PGO spikes prime REM sleep and may be involved in its temporal regulation via the activity of the peribrachial nucleus; however, studies using agents that affect serotonergic activity suggest that PGO spikes are not sufficient in themselves (see Serotonergic Compounds, later).[250,251]

Other pharmacologic evidence in support of a role for ACh in the generation of REM sleep is that hemicholinium-3, an inhibitor of the high-affinity choline uptake system and thus of ACh synthesis, completely blocked the appearance of REM sleep and decreased waking time when given to cats ICV.[252] In a related finding, administration of vesamicol, a drug that inhibits vesicular transport of ACh and thus its release, into the left lateral ventricle of rats caused a dose-dependent inhibition of REM sleep with a marked REM rebound after withdrawal from a 2-day dosing with the drug.[253] An increase in the release of ACh from the feline pons during REM sleep as compared with either SWS or waking has been reported,[254,255] further strengthening the evidence for a role for endogenous ACh in REM sleep. The release of ACh to trigger REM sleep appears to be regulated by several factors, including nitric oxide and morphine-like endogenous substances. When an inhibitor of nitric oxide synthase is used, there is a decrease in the endogenously released ACh from the mPRF of cats across all three states (wakefulness, NREM sleep, and REM sleep), suggesting that this neurotransmitter may play an important role in the normal control of ACh release from this REM sleep regulatory site.[255] Injections of morphine into this same site, or given systemically, inhibited REM sleep and decreased stimulated ACh release at the gigantocellular tegmental field of the mPRF.[256,257] As might be expected, not only does the release of ACh by these cholinergic terminals appear to be regulated, but the response of the cholinoceptive areas involved in the generation of REM sleep can be regulated. In an interesting report, Prospéro-García and colleagues[258] have noted that pretreatment with systemic chlor-amphenicol, an antibiotic, can prevent the induction of REM sleep by carbachol injected into the mPRF.

**Acetylcholine Receptor Subsystems.** The actions of ACh on cholinoceptive cells are determined by the receptor system that is activated by ACh. Two major cholinergic receptor types are known, the nicotinic and the muscarinic. These two receptor types are phylogenetically unrelated to each other, with the nicotinic receptor type functioning as an ion channel and the muscarinic type transducing the signal intracellularly (both excitatory as well as inhibitory) by acting on various G proteins. The nicotinic receptors of the central nervous system have a wide range of subunit composition variability but all that have been studied electrophysiologically so far cause membrane depolarization and thus cellular excitation. This is not the case for the muscarinic receptors that have been separated into five types ($M_1$, $M_2$, $M_3$, $M_4$, and $M_5$) based on their protein sequences as determined by studying messenger RNA (mRNA). These five types of receptors can easily be separated into two classes based on whether their activation leads to inhibition ($M_2$ and $M_4$) or excitation ($M_1$, $M_3$, and $M_5$). The $M_2$ and $M_4$ receptor types inhibit cellular excitation by either inhibiting the enzyme adenylyl cyclase or by turning on a $K^+$ current. The $M_1$, $M_3$, and $M_5$ types increase cellular excitation by stimulation of the enzyme phospholipase C, which in turn, through its second messengers, increases the level of free cytoplasmic $Ca^{+2}$.[259]

Attempts to map the cholinergic receptor densities at various sites in the brain stem areas important to REM sleep regulation have yielded interesting results. Nicotinic receptors have been studied using the binding of [$^3$H]-nicotine and [$^{125}$I] α-bungarotoxin to identify various classes of nicotinic receptors.[260] In the developing human brain, there is a high density of nicotinic receptors in the tegmental nuclei (PPT, dorsal raphe, LC, etc.), which decline by 60–70% by birth.[261] In rats, as in humans, the density of nicotinic receptors in REM sleep–regulating sites is relatively low. The presence of muscarinic receptors has been studied using a variety of techniques including [$^3$H]-3-quinuclidinyl benzilate binding and the detection of mRNA for several muscarinic receptors. These studies have found that $M_1$, $M_2$, and $M_3$ receptors are located throughout the brain stem of the cat but that most are concentrated in the raphe nuclei and LC, with fewer of the receptors existing in the PRF.[262–264] In total sleep–deprived rats, no changes were seen in the number of nicotinic receptors, and a change in the muscarinic receptors was observed in the septal area only.[265] In a similar study looking at the expression in REM sleep–deprived rats of mRNAs for the $M_1$, $M_2$, and $M_3$ receptors, the level of $M_3$ mRNA was increased in the pontine nuclei but the $M_2$ mRNA levels were decreased in these same nuclei.[266]

Much work has been done in an attempt to elucidate which receptor systems may be involved in the overall generation of REM sleep and its components. The largest volume of work and the earliest implications of a receptor system playing a role in REM sleep generation are devoted to the muscarinic family, although subsequent work indicates that nicotinic receptors also play an important role. The following sections begin with a discussion of the evidence for involvement of a muscarinic receptor system in REM sleep.

**Muscarinic Receptors.** Administration of scopolamine, a muscarinic antagonist, has been shown to inhibit REM sleep in both rats and humans. Tolerance to the REM sleep suppression develops over a period of several days.[267] REM sleep rebound occurred in rats when scopolamine was abruptly discontinued and accompanied by a significant increase in the density of muscarinic receptors in the caudate but not in the brain stem.[268] This suggests that the REM sleep rebound experienced on discontinuation of the scopolamine is not the result of an upregulation of muscarinic receptors in the centers thought to generate REM sleep. These results and the receptor studies mentioned in the previous section do not make it possible to discern which, if any, of the cholinergic receptor systems might play a role in the REM sleep rebound seen with total or REM sleep deprivation.

Administration of cholinomimetic agonists to humans also induces REM sleep, depending on the timing and dose of the drug. For example, physostigmine can induce either REM sleep in small doses or wakefulness in large doses when infused during the first or second NREM periods; the latency to REM sleep induction was longer when physostigmine was infused just after sleep onset than when it was infused 35 minutes after sleep onset. Furthermore, the dose of physostigmine (0.5 mg) that induced

REM sleep when infused 35 minutes into the first NREM period induced wakefulness when infused midway through the second NREM period.[82] These differential effects of physostigmine may reflect the dynamic relationships between REM inhibitory and facilitatory processes that evolve with the sleep cycle and have been partially modeled according to the mathematical implications of the reciprocal interaction model.[269] Pretreatment with scopolamine (but not methylscopolamine, which fails to cross the blood-brain barrier) blocked the REM-inducing effects of arecoline in humans, further suggesting that arecoline-induced REM sleep is mediated by muscarinic receptors. Other cholinergic agonists reported to facilitate REM sleep in humans include RS 86, pilocarpine, and SDZ 210-086.[270–272] It is of great clinical interest that both arecoline and RS 86 shorten REM sleep latency more in patients with depression than in control volunteers.[270,271,273] This finding has now been replicated in more than nine separate studies, including one group of patients who had never received antidepressants before or who had been off antidepressants for at least 4 months. In some but not all studies, the arecoline-induced REM sleep was significantly correlated with REM sleep latency. Because REM sleep latency is typically short in patients who meet formal criteria for depression, this finding suggests that short REM sleep latency might be related to upregulated muscarinic neurotransmission or diminished aminergic neurotransmission. It is important to note that when REM latency shortenings are studied in depressed versus control subjects, using arecoline or RS 86, age-matched controls are critical because the timing and induction of REM sleep is significantly affected by age.[261] These observations are consistent with the cholinergic-aminergic imbalance hypothesis of depression, which suggests that depression results from an increased ratio of cholinergic to aminergic neurotransmission.[274] Although this hypothesis has proved to be of great value in understanding many aspects of the therapeutics used in depression, it cannot explain all pharmacologic effects seen, even on REM sleep–latency shortening, and therefore needs expansion and further consideration.[275,276] Riemann and colleagues[277] have reported faster REM sleep induction with RS 86 in schizophrenic patients than in controls, with a greater effect seen in depressives versus schizophrenics.[278,279] Although they did not specifically assess their patients with this hypothesis in mind, this observation may be consistent with the suggestion that the so-called negative symptoms of schizophrenia (e.g., anhedonia, apathy, dysphoria) reflect muscarinic, cholinergic-receptor supersensitivity.[279,280]

To determine the cholinergic receptor specificity in the generation of REM sleep, Velazquez-Moctezuma and coworkers[281–283] administered equimolar amounts of the $M_2$-receptor agonists cis-dioxolane and oxotremorine-M into the mPRF of cats. They reported rapid induction and increased percentage of REM sleep over a 5-hour recording period.[281–283] The same molar dose of the $M_1$ agonist McN-A-343 had no effect on REM sleep compared to saline. Although these results suggest that in the cat an $M_2$ receptor in the mPRF mediates REM sleep, the study does not exclude the possible role of other muscarinic receptor subtypes. $M_2$-receptor subtypes are located predominantly in the mPRF, whereas $M_1$-receptor subtypes are located in areas of the forebrain. Consistent with the hypothesis that $M_1$-receptor subtypes are involved in REM sleep, systemic administration of biperiden and other relatively selective antagonists of $M_1$ receptors has been reported to reduce REM sleep. In humans and cats, acute administration of biperiden (2–8 mg in humans, 0.1 mg/kg in cats) increased the latency to REM sleep and decreased REM sleep time.[284–286] Furthermore, Salin-Pascual and colleagues[285] found that biperiden blocked the increase in REM sleep induced by auditory stimulation during REM sleep in humans. In addition, Zoltoski and colleagues[287] have reported that systemic administration of scopolamine, trihexyphenidyl (a relatively selective $M_1$ antagonist), and biperiden exerted a dose-dependent inhibition of REM sleep in rats.

Of interest are the observations that the REM sleep rebound is different after the repeated administration of biperiden (over four nights)[285] and scopolamine (over three nights)[284] to humans. Although REM sleep latency was shortened in both instances, REM sleep time was increased compared to baseline after the abrupt discontinuation of scopolamine but not biperiden. This finding suggests that both receptor subtypes mediate induction of REM sleep but that only $M_2$ receptors increase total REM sleep time.

The role of muscarinic receptors was further suggested by a study of the Flinders sensitive line (FSL) of rats. These rats have been selectively bred by Overstreet and coworkers[288,289] for more than 20 generations for their sensitivity to the hypothermic effects of cholinergic agonists. The rats display an increased density of muscarinic cholinergic receptors as assessed by the binding of quinuclidinyl benzilate (QNB). The data showed a short REM latency and significantly increased REM sleep percentage (resulting from shorter REM sleep–cycle lengths rather than longer duration of each REM sleep period[290]). Also of interest, the FSL strain has been proposed as a rodent model of depression.[289,291] The exact mechanisms of the sleep and behavior changes in the FSL remain to be determined.

In human narcolepsy, as well as in the canine model of narcolepsy, REM sleep latency is very short. Although the neural mechanisms responsible are unknown, an increased density of muscarinic receptors (assessed by QNB binding) has been found in the brain stem of narcoleptic versus nonnarcoleptic dogs.[292] In addition, other data suggest decreased turnover of dopamine.[44]

**Nicotinic Receptors.** Soldatos and associates[293] reported that smokers had a significantly longer sleep latency than nonsmokers and that their sleep improved immediately after discontinuing smoking. Subsequent studies suggest that the sleep of smokers who have just started to abstain from cigarettes is more fragmented, with more awakenings occurring during the night, and that replacement of nicotine by patches helps to alleviate these symptoms of withdrawal.[294,295] In studies in which the nicotine patch (7.0–17.5 mg nicotine) has been used in nonsmoking volunteers, treatment has been reported to decrease REM sleep time and REM percentage (i.e., REM density) with a rebound of REM sleep occurring in one study on the recovery night.[296–298] Although few side effects were reported in these studies, it is likely that nicotine has a strong stimulating effect in nicotine-naive subjects and may account for the reduction in REM sleep and sleep time. It is well-established that chronic nicotine treatment (>1 week) causes a change in the number of nicotinic receptors in the brain and that responses to nicotine are altered by such treatment.[260] Thus, it is difficult to compare the effects of the nicotine patch on sleep architecture between smokers and nonsmokers. Interestingly, one study looked at depressed patients as well as controls (both groups nonsmoking) and found that the depressed patients actually had an increase in REM sleep—unlike the controls, who showed the decrease in REM sleep previously mentioned.[298]

It has been difficult to assess the function of nicotinic receptors in the regulation and generation of REM sleep from human studies because it is difficult to separate general effects on several sites from specific effects at only one site. Animal studies in which microinfusion of nicotinic agents into specific brain regions has been carried out have been more enlightening. Hu and colleagues[299] have reported that both mecamylamine and hexamethonium, antagonists of neuronal nicotinic receptors, blocked the generation of PGO spikes in reserpinized cats. Velazquez-Moctezuma and colleagues[300] reached similar conclusions, suggesting that PGO spike–generation is partially mediated by a nicotinic mechanism, that cortical activation as measured by a desynchronized EEG contains an $M_1$ component, and that the muscle atonia seen during REM sleep is mediated by an $M_2$-receptor system. Velazquez-Moctezuma's group[301] also reported that administration of nicotine into the mPRF induced REM sleep in cats. One study has looked at the ability of nicotine to depolarize neurons of the mPRF and thus stimulate these neurons.[302] As might be expected, the stimulatory effect of nicotine was not blocked by atropine; surprisingly, however, neither could the effect be blocked by neuronal nicotinic antagonists such as mecamylamine and hexamethonium. The stimulatory effect of nicotine on these mPRF neurons could be blocked, however, by the neuromuscular nicotinic receptor antagonist tubocurare.

Much work remains to be done if the role of nicotinic receptors in REM sleep is to be understood. As more selective agonists and antagonists are developed for the various nicotinic receptor forms it will be necessary to evaluate these drugs with respect to their effects on sleep architecture.

*Noradrenergic Compounds*

Many cells of the LC cease firing during the transition from NREM to REM sleep (or during REM sleep) and become active again as soon as REM sleep is terminated. This, along with evidence provided here, suggests not only that REM sleep needs cholinergic action to be generated but that the effects of NE are directly inhibitory. Williams and Reiner[303] have found that NE can directly hyperpolarize cholinergic cells of the mesopontine tegmentum of the rat and that this effect cannot be due to indirect actions via another substance. Consistent with the reciprocal interaction model, which predicts that affecting the adrenergic system will affect REM sleep and vice versa, it was observed that 96 hours of REM sleep deprivation in rats led to an increase in NE concentrations in the neocortex, hippocampus, and hypothalamus, along with an increase in the tyrosine hydroxylase mRNA levels in the LC.[304] In fact, Siegel and Rogawski[305] proposed that REM sleep resensitizes or upregulates noradrenergic receptors again, an idea consistent with a reciprocal interaction between the LC and the REM sleep regulatory centers of the pons. Also supporting these notions are observations made in the canine model of narcolepsy. Drugs that mainly affect the adrenergic systems were the most powerful at preventing cataplexy in narcoleptic dogs.[47] In general, compounds that decrease the content or release of NE increase the amount of REM sleep and compounds that increase NE activity decrease REM sleep.

Amphetamine releases NE (as well as other amines) from nerve terminals, inhibits its reuptake, and can have other adrenergic effects. As mentioned earlier, D-amphetamine decreases both the percentage of REM and total sleep. Long-term (but not short-term) treatment with this stimulant leads to a large REM sleep rebound.[306] In addition, addicts demonstrate hypersomnia, short REM sleep latencies, and increased amounts and percentage of REM sleep during the first several weeks after withdrawal from cocaine and amphetamine.[26] Although amphetamine and other stimulants do release NE, they have numerous other neuropharmacologic effects that complicate interpretation. For example, pretreatment with a dopamine antagonist, pimozide, blocked the REM sleep–inhibiting and alerting effects of amphetamine in humans.[27]

The compound α-methyl-*p*-tyrosine (AMPT) is an inhibitor of the catecholamine-synthesizing enzyme tyrosine hydroxylase and depletes the neurotransmitter stores of NE and DA at the nerve terminal. Cats treated with this compound show an increase in the amount of REM sleep, although little happens to NREM sleep.[307] The same basic observation was made when healthy volunteers were given AMPT, except that there was an increase in NREM sleep as well.[308,309] In addition, profound insomnia for 1–2 days resulted from the discontinuation of the AMPT that had been administered for 3 days previously. Reserpine, a drug that depletes tissue of NE, DA, and 5-HT by preventing their reentry into the vesicles from which they are released, can also increase the amount of REM sleep and shorten the latency to REM sleep in both cats and humans.[310] These findings are consistent with the view that aminergic neurotransmitters inhibit REM sleep. Work with more selective adrenergic agonists and antagonists further supports the idea of an inhibitory role for NE in REM sleep.

**Adrenergic Receptor Subtypes.** Adrenergic receptors are subdivided into two major types, $\alpha$- and $\beta$-adrenergic receptors, based on their ability to interact differentially with a family of adrenergic pharmacologic agents. Like cholinergic receptors, these major classifications of receptors are further subdivided based on similar pharmacologic criteria of differential compound effects into the $\alpha_{1A}$, $\alpha_{1B}$, $\alpha_{1D}$, $\alpha_{2A}$, $\alpha_{2B}$, $\alpha_{2C}$, $\alpha_{2D}$, $\beta_1$, $\beta_2$, and $\beta_3$ receptors. The $\alpha_1$ receptors work by increasing the turnover of inositol triphosphates and increasing diacylglycerol, both of which increase the free cytoplasmic $Ca^{+2}$ levels and thus excitability. The $\alpha_2$ receptors work by inhibiting the enzyme adenylyl cyclase, thereby decreasing the levels of cyclic adenosine monophosphate (cAMP), and are thus inhibitory. Finally, all of the $\beta$ receptors work by increasing the levels of cAMP.[311]

As predicted by the reciprocal interaction hypothesis, the compound methoxamine, an $\alpha_1$-receptor agonist, decreases REM sleep in rats, whereas the $\alpha_1$-receptor antagonist prazosin increases REM sleep.[312] IV administration of thymozamine, an $\alpha_1$-receptor antagonist, also increases REM sleep in humans.[313] Cirelli and colleagues[314] confirmed the effects of methoxamine in cats and found that this effect was blockable by prazosin pretreatment. They did not get consistent results, however, when prazosin was used alone.[314] These findings suggest that NE is capable of inhibiting the development of REM sleep by an $\alpha_1$-receptor system, but it is not yet possible to determine how important the $\alpha_1$-receptor system is to the regulation of REM sleep by the normal, endogenous release of NE. Activation of $\alpha_1$ receptors leads to increased wakefulness and a decrease in both NREM and REM sleep.

Studies conducted using the $\alpha_2$-receptor agonist clonidine reported modest decreases in REM sleep in both humans and cats.[315,316] One study found that clonidine's effect on REM sleep was less marked in patients with affective disorders than in controls.[317] Yohimbine, an $\alpha_2$-receptor antagonist, does decrease REM sleep in rats, supposedly by increasing the release of NE.[312] However, injections of idazoxan, a different $\alpha_2$-receptor antagonist, into the mPRF of cats greatly increased REM sleep.[318] Further work is needed with $\alpha_2$ receptor–specific drugs to clarify what role this receptor system plays in REM sleep regulation. As part of the reciprocal interaction hypothesis, it has been postulated that NE systems are inhibitory to the generation of PGO spikes.[319] Clonidine reduced PGO spike activity, whereas idazoxan antagonized this effect.[320] As stated earlier, many noradrenergic cells in the LC cease firing in association with PGO spikes.

The narcolepsy syndrome is characterized by excessive daytime sleepiness, cataplexy, sleep paralysis, and hypnagogic hallucinations. The noradrenergic and serotonergic systems appear to be involved, because antidepressants, which mainly potentiate both systems by reuptake blockade, are effective in treating the various symptoms of narcolepsy, both human and canine.[47,321,322] Moreover, in both narcoleptic patients and dogs, prazosin, an $\alpha_1$-adrenergic blocker, precipitates cataplexy, whereas clonidine, an $\alpha_2$-adrenergic agonist, decreases cataplectic attacks.[321] In general, it appears that NE acts to suppress cataplexy,[323] although its exact mechanism and role in the narcoleptic tetrad still need to be determined.

The results of studies using $\alpha$ receptor–specific agents indicate that both types of receptors may play a role in the LC control of the pontine cholinergic cells important to the generation of REM sleep. How each receptor subtype works in the normal control or what percentage of the overall effect is due to each subtype of receptor remains to be determined. Because the $\alpha_1$- and $\alpha_2$-receptor systems tend to have opposite effects on cellular activity, it will be important to determine exactly how each subsystem acts and whether the receptors are found presynaptic or postsynaptic to the NE terminal.

The use of $\beta$-selective drugs such as propranolol has produced inconsistent or no effects on REM sleep. The role played by the $\beta$ receptors in mediating NE's actions in the pons is therefore unclear.[312]

*Serotonergic Compounds*

The second major group of cells that are relatively quiescent during REM sleep are located within the raphe nucleus. For this reason, 5-HT has also been proposed as an inhibitor of REM sleep. Consistent with this hypothesis, in vivo microdialysis measures of extracellular 5-HT from the mPRF of a cat showed the highest levels during waking and the lowest levels during REM sleep.[324] The levels of 5-HT present during REM sleep were approximately half of those during waking, with approximately 90% of the waking levels being released during NREM sleep. Also predicted by the reciprocal interaction hypothesis is that levels of 5-HT in the dorsal raphe should be lower during REM sleep than in other behavioral states. Portas and McCarley[100] have reported that this is indeed the case. By placing microdialysis probes in the dorsal raphe of cats, they showed that 5-HT levels were highest during waking, approximately 50% of waking levels during NREM sleep, and approximately 38% of waking during REM sleep. Furthermore, 5-HT levels fluctuated during changes in behavioral state in the hypoglossal nucleus, an area known to be affected by REM sleep. As in other studies, there was a decrease in the 5-HT levels of the hypoglossal nucleus after induction of REM sleep by carbachol injections into the mPRF of the cat.[325] Together, the results of these studies suggest that the activity of 5-HT–containing terminals is lowest during the REM sleep period in a variety of places predicted by the reciprocal interaction hypothesis. Extensive electrophysiologic data concerning the serotonergic cells of the dorsal raphe are consistent with the neurochemical studies just outlined.

Pharmacologic attempts to investigate the importance of 5-HT have used the 5-HT–depleting drug PCPA and various agents that block the reuptake of 5-HT. With these pharmacologic approaches, one can see what decreasing or increasing activity of the serotonergic system does to REM sleep. PCPA can initially prevent sleep when given in large enough doses to animals. Even with continued treatment, however, sleep returns to normal with time, although the 5-HT level remains low.[93] PGO spikes continued to appear appear during wakefulness and NREM sleep, suggesting that serotonergic cells inhibit PGO spike activity. It is interesting that this increased PGO spike activity is not accompanied by an increase in REM sleep, suggesting that the increased PGO spike activity is not sufficient for priming REM sleep (see Cholinergic Agents, earlier). When given to humans, smaller doses of the drug (approximately one-tenth of that used in animals) decreased REM sleep but had little effect on NREM sleep. The decrease in REM sleep could be sustained for several weeks. When some of these patients were given the 5-HT precursor 5-hydroxytryptophan, which can circumvent the PCPA block, REM sleep returned to normal with no rebound.[308] Likewise, when PCPA treatment was discontinued, normal REM sleep returned within a few days in both humans and animals. Rats injected with zimeldine (20 mg/kg), a 5-HT reuptake inhibitor that increases the concentration of 5-HT found in the synaptic cleft, showed a decrease or abolition of REM sleep for 6–8 hours after treatment.[326,327] Surprisingly, high doses of the general 5-HT receptor antagonist methiothepin (2 mg/kg) did not reverse the effects of zimeldine on REM sleep, but reduced REM sleep as well.[327] Hamsters treated with fluoxetine (5–40 mg/kg), another 5-HT reuptake blocker, showed a dose-dependent decrease in REM sleep and brain temperature with an increase in NREM sleep.[328] At the highest doses, fluoxetine also increased wakefulness. With chronic treatment, however, REM sleep returned to normal, suggesting that some feedback control exists at the level of the serotonergic cell's activity or at the level of serotonergic receptor number or sensitivity. When healthy human volunteers were given fluoxetine (20 mg/day) for six days, they showed a decrease in REM sleep with small increases in stage II and III NREM sleep.[329] Similarly, when a group of patients suffering from major depression were given paroxetine, also a 5-HT reuptake blocker, they responded with a decrease in REM sleep.[330] Lysergic acid diethylamide tends to increase REM sleep in humans,[331,332] possibly because it shuts down serotonergic neurons (as it does in the DRN of the rat[333]). Furthermore, 5-HT potentiators such as fenfluramine, which releases 5-HT, and fluoxetine decrease both total and REM sleep.[308]

**Serotonergic Receptor Subtypes.** Serotonergic receptors come in a large family of subtypes. The 5-HT$_1$ subtype is further divided into five subtypes (A–F), but all decrease cAMP for their signal transduction mechanism. Therefore, 5-HT$_1$ receptors primarily inhibit cell activity. The 5-HT$_2$ subtype exists in three pharmacologically distinct forms (A–C), but all increase inositol triphosphate and diacylglycerol as their signal transduction mechanism and are thus mainly cell-activity stimulators. The remaining subtypes are 5-HT$_3$, 5-HT$_4$, 5-HT$_5$, 5-HT$_6$, and 5-HT$_7$. The 5-HT$_3$ receptor activates a cation channel that leads to a direct depolarization of the neuronal membrane and thus excitation. Most of the remaining receptor subtypes mentioned above activate adenylyl cyclase and therefore increase the cytoplasmic levels of cAMP. Only three receptor subtypes have been widely studied with respect to sleep: 5-HT$_1$, 5-HT$_2$, and 5-HT$_3$.

In general, systemic administration of 5-HT$_1$ agonists has an inhibitory effect on REM sleep, and this effect is not blockable by 5-HT$_1$ antagonists. Rats injected with the 5-HT$_{1A}$ receptor agonist 8-hydroxy-2-(n-dipropylamino) tetralin (8-OH-DPAT) (0.010–0.375 mg/kg) showed a suppression of REM sleep regardless of dose, increased NREM sleep at the low dose, and increasing wakefulness at the high dose.[334] In rats depleted of 5-HT by ICV administration of 5,7-dihydroxytryptamine, however, only the highest dose of 8-OH-DPAT produced the previous effects on REM sleep. When other 5-HT$_1$ receptor agonists were studied (buspirone, ipsapirone, and gepirone) similar effects were obtained, but pretreatment with the 5-HT$_{1A}$ antagonist (-)-pindolol was unable to reverse the REM sleep depressant effect of the agonists.[335] Other work on rats using a variety of 5-HT$_1$ agonists has shown the same inhibitory effect on REM sleep and an inability to block this effect using several 5-HT$_1$ antagonists.[336] In one study in which both the 5-HT$_{1A}$ antagonist NAN-190 and the 5-HT reuptake blocker citalopram were used, it was found that both, alone or together, caused a decrease in REM sleep.[337] When given together, citalopram augmented NAN-190's REM sleep inhibitory effect. Similar results have been obtained with cats in which intraperitoneal treatment with eltoprazine, another 5-HT$_1$ agonist, caused a marked decrease in REM sleep.[338] After treatment with eltoprazine for 5–7 days, there was a twofold REM sleep rebound, as compared to pretreatment, which could be attenuated by the anticholinergic agent scopolamine.[339,340] As in one of the rat studies, eltoprazine caused a NREM sleep increase.[338,339] Although the results are consistent,

it is hard to interpret this body of data, given that the agonist effects are not blockable by antagonists of the supposedly same receptor class. One possible explanation is that the agonists and antagonists are working on separate 5-HT$_1$–subtype receptors. In addition, systemic administration makes interpreting the site of action impossible. Sanford and colleagues[341] microinfused 8-OH-DPAT into the peribrachial region of the feline PPT and found a REM sleep–suppressing effect. This effect was found to be due to a decrease in REM sleep–bout frequency, not to changes in REM sleep–bout duration, suggesting that a 5-HT$_{1A}$–receptor system is involved in the initiation but not the maintenance of REM sleep.[341] When Portas and coworkers[342] perfused 8-OH-DPAT into the DRN of cats, they found that the release of 5-HT was halved and REM sleep was augmented. These last two results strongly suggest that 5-HT$_1$ agonists and antagonists need to be studied by discrete microinfusions into specific brain regions if the role of these receptors in REM sleep regulation is to be understood.

There has been less investigation of the role of 5-HT$_2$ and 5-HT$_3$ receptors in REM sleep. Sommerfelt and Ursin[108] orally administered the 5-HT$_{2A}$ antagonist ritanserin to cats and found that there was a decrease in REM sleep and an increase in REM sleep latency. Because 5-HT$_2$ receptors are generally stimulatory, these results indicate that some subset of 5-HT receptors plays a role in stimulating REM sleep and that not all 5-HT effects need be inhibitory to this behavioral state. Given the results using reuptake inhibitors, however, this also suggests that the overwhelming effect of 5-HT is to inhibit REM sleep. Ponzoni and colleagues[343] studied the 5-HT$_3$ receptor agonist m-chlorophenylbiguanide by injecting it ICV into rats and found that waking was increased at the expense of both REM and NREM sleep. This effect was blockable by the 5-HT$_3$ antagonist MDL 72222. In a separate study, they found that injection of m-chlorophenylbiguanide into the nucleus accumbens of rats had no effect on REM sleep but still had the previously noted effect on waking and NREM sleep.[344]

Although difficult to interpret, most work on 5-HT receptor subtypes suggests that the main effect of 5-HT is to inhibit REM sleep, as proposed by the reciprocal interaction model of REM sleep. Further work is needed to make a reasonable hypothesis about the role that the plethora of 5-HT receptors may play in REM sleep. As can be gleaned from these results, more selective agonist-antagonist pairs must be used in discrete brain regions before this important area of REM sleep control can be better understood.

*Neuropeptides and Other Possible Modulators*

Knowledge of the biology of central nervous system neuropeptides and neuromodulators is growing quickly, but is not yet as detailed as knowledge of the classic neurotransmitters. Thus, the location and function of many of these compounds is not clearly understood, and this precludes their integration into any present model of REM sleep induction and maintenance. Furthermore, because many of these substances might not cross the blood-brain barrier, studies carried out in humans may point to systemic effects and not to a central function. Whether some of the effects noted in animals represent pharmacologic rather than physiologic effects also remains to be determined.

AVT can totally block REM sleep and greatly increase NREM sleep for at least 5 hours in cats that receive as little as $10^{-18}$ mol ICV. The same effect can be obtained by a 100-fold larger dose of the peptide given intraperitoneally.[180] When anti-AVT antiserum is given ICV to cats, not only is there an increase in the amount of REM sleep, but there is the intrusion of REM sleep episodes occurring at sleep onset, a condition not seen in normal animals.[181] If the DRN is lesioned, no effect of ICV AVT is observed in cats for 5 days after the lesion.[345] This suggests that the inhibition of REM sleep by AVT in the cat is dependent on the actions of 5-HT, an area of investigation that requires more work. The fact that antiserum raised against AVT can augment REM sleep, however, supports the notion of an endogenous role for AVT in regulating REM sleep.

A large body of literature suggests that vasoactive intestinal polypeptide (VIP) increases REM sleep in animals. ICV administration of 30 pmol VIP to rats at the beginning of the light or rest phase enhanced REM sleep within 1 hour after injection. A tenfold larger dose produced the same effect but with a 24-hour delay, suggesting a complicated modulatory role of REM sleep by VIP.[346] Cats treated with 30 pmol ICV gave similar results to those obtained in the rats, but with a 5-hour delay of the effects.[347] To better estimate whether VIP

normally plays a role in modulating REM sleep, an anti-VIP antiserum was administered to rats ICV, resulting in an increase in waking and a decrease in REM sleep that was not associated with a decrease in NREM sleep.[346] In fact, some work suggests that VIP may be responsible for the REM sleep rebound seen after sleep deprivation. When cats were sleep deprived, it was found that the level of VIP in the CSF was increased.[348] Furthermore, removal of CSF from these animals attenuated the REM sleep rebound. As noted earlier, PCPA treatment leads to a large decrease in the concentration of 5-HT and to a long-lasting insomnia. When PCPA-treated cats were given either ICV VIP (200 ng) or intramuscular atropine (0.5 mg/kg) it was found that each substance alone or in combination was able to augment the decrease in REM sleep seen with PCPA treatment.[349] Similar results were obtained in PCPA-treated rats when the VIP was directly injected into the DRN.[350] When VIP is given systemically to rats, it also enhances REM sleep and treatment is correlated with an increased amount of prolactin in the blood.[351] The REM sleep enhancement can be blocked by the coadministration of an antiprolactin antisera and VIP. Thus, there is reasonable support for the theory that both VIP and AVT play a normal role in modulating the REM sleep–generating or sustaining system of the brain (or both systems), and that in the case of VIP this effect may be mediated by the release of prolactin.

A third peptide with interesting effects on REM sleep is somatostatin (SS). When rats were infused ICV with SS over 2 days, REM sleep increased and no effect on NREM sleep was observed. When SS administration was discontinued, sleep state percentages returned to pretreatment levels.[352,353] Furthermore, if cysteamine (a drug that depletes SS stores) is given ICV (40 or 90 µg per day), there is a dose-dependent decrease in the amount of REM sleep, again with no statistically significant change in NREM sleep. If SS can increase REM sleep, depriving animals of REM sleep might increase the expression of SS mRNA. This was found to be the case in rats that were REM sleep deprived for 24–72 hours. The number of cells in the arcuate nucleus expressing SS increased with 24 hours of REM sleep deprivation, but not with 72 hours of deprivation. The number of cells in the periventricular nucleus expressing SS increased after 72 hours of deprivation, but not after 24 hours.[354] When SS was given systemically to male volunteers, however, no changes were seen in REM or NREM sleep, although one study found a trend toward increased REM density.[355,356] Analogues of SS have similar effects on REM sleep. SS has also been reported to overcome the REM sleep–suppressing effect of scopolamine.[357,358] In addition, increased REM sleep induced by carbachol treatment may be dependent on SS, because pretreatment with an anti-SS antiserum was reported to block the carbachol stimulatory effect.[359] A new endogenous, somatostatin-like peptide named *cortistatin* has been discovered. This peptide counters some of the effects of ACh, however, and can inhibit REM sleep when given ICV to rats.[360]

## CONCLUSIONS

Sleep researchers have made significant progress in recent years in identifying the neurochemical and neurophysiologic mechanisms responsible for sleep and, especially, REM sleep. Indeed, we now probably know as much about the physiologic control of REM sleep as we know about any higher basic behavioral state, such as eating, sexual behavior, or memory. Clearly, the current widely accepted paradigm is that REM sleep is promoted by cholinergic neurons originating within the brain stem, most probably in the LDT nucleus and PPT group, and inhibited by noradrenergic and serotonergic neurons located within the LC and dorsal raphe, respectively. Cholinergic neurons play a widespread and crucial role in the orchestration of REM sleep through their projections to the mPRF, medulla, and forebrain areas in the thalamus and BF.

Although many interesting clues to the neurochemical and neurophysiologic mechanisms involved in the control of NREM sleep have been discovered, much remains to be firmly established. Clearly, the role of the thalamus and BF have been established in specific EEG manifestations of NREM sleep. Still, the specific mechanisms involved in the induction and maintenance of NREM sleep appear to be varied and complicated—not yet readily put into a simple framework.

Considerable interest is currently directed toward hypothetical endogenous "sleep hormones," immunologic modulatory factors that might promote sleep,

and thermoregulatory processes involved in the induction and possible functions of sleep.

A broader view of sleep is also emerging, one that includes wakefulness and a relationship to underlying circadian processes. Moreover, as we learn more about the manipulation of underlying circadian processes and thermoregulation, we can anticipate new approaches to the management of sleep-wake disorders.

## REFERENCES

1. Rechtschaffen A, Kales AA. A Manual of Standardized Terminology, Techniques, and Scoring System for Sleep Stages of Human Subjects. Washington, DC: Public Health Service, 1968.
2. Jones BE. Paradoxical sleep and its chemical/structural substrates in the brain. Neuroscience 1991;40:637.
3. Daan S, Beersma DGM, Borbely AA. Timing of human sleep: recovery process gated by a circadian pacemaker. Am J Physiol 1984;246:R161.
4. Nakanishi H, Sun Y, Nakamura RK, et al. Positive correlations between cerebral protein synthesis rates and deep sleep in macaca mulatta. Eur J Neurosci 1997;9:271.
5. Ramm P, Smith CT. Rates of cerebral protein synthesis are linked to slow wave sleep in the rat. Physiol Behav 1990;48:749.
6. Dijk D-J, Czeisler CA. Paradoxical timing of the circadian rhythm of sleep propensity serves to consolidate sleep and wakefulness in humans. Neurosci Lett 1994;166:63.
7. Tobler I. Evolution and Comparative Physiology of Sleep in Animals. In R Lydic, JF Biebuyck (eds), Clinical Physiology of Sleep. Bethesda, MD: American Physiological Society, 1988;21.
8. Buchsbaum MS, Gillin JC, Wu J, et al. Regional cerebral glucose metabolic rate in human sleep assessed by positron emission tomography. Life Sci 1989;45:1349.
9. Kennedy C, Gillin JC, Mendelson WB, et al. Local cerebral glucose utilization in non–rapid eye movement sleep. Nature 1982;297:325.
10. Nakamura R, Kennedy C, Gillin JC, et al. Hypnogenic center theory of sleep: no support from metabolic mapping in monkeys. Brain Res 1983;268:372.
11. Moore RY, Eichler VB. Loss of a circadian adrenal corticosterone rhythm following suprachiasmatic lesions in the rat. Brain Res 1972;42:201.
12. Moore RY, Lenn NJ. A retinohypothalamic projection in the rat. J Comp Neurol 1972;142:1.
13. Smale L, Blanchard J, Moore RY, et al. Immunocytochemical characterization of the suprachiasmatic nucleus and the intergeniculate leaflet in the diurnal ground squirrel, *Spermophilus lateralis*. Brain Res 1991;563:77.

14. Eastman CI, Mistlberger RE, Rechtschaffen A. Suprachiasmatic nuclei lesions eliminate circadian temperature and sleep rhythms in the rat. Physiol Behav 1983;32:357.
15. Mistlberger RE, Bergmann BM, Waldenar W, et al. Recovery sleep following sleep deprivation in intact and suprachiasmatic nuclei lesioned rats. Sleep 1983;6:217.
16. Zwyghuizen-Doorenbos A, Roehrs T, Lamphere J, et al. Increased daytime sleepiness enhances ethanol's sedative effects. Neuropsychopharmacology 1988;1:279.
17. Edgar DM, Seidel WF, Martin CE, et al. Triazolam fails to induce sleep in suprachiasmatic nucleus-lesioned rats. Neurosci Lett 1991;125:125.
18. Terman M, Lewy AJ, Dijk D-J, et al. Light treatment for sleep disorders: consensus report. IV. Sleep phase and duration disturbances. J Biol Rhythms 1995;10:135.
19. Hotz Vitaterna M, King DP, Chang AM, et al. Mutagenesis and mapping of a mouse gene clock, essential for circadian behavior. Science 1994;264:629.
20. McCarley RW, Hobson JA. Neuronal excitability modulation over the sleep cycle: a structural and mathematical model. Science 1975;189:58.
21. Hobson JA, McCarley RW, Wyzinski PW. Sleep cycle oscillation: reciprocal discharge by two brainstem neuronal groups. Science 1975;189:55.
22. Koella WP. The organization and regulation of sleep. A review of the experimental evidence and a novel integrated model of the organizing and regulating apparatus. Experientia 1984;40:309.
23. Mahowald MW, Schenck CH. Dissociated states of wakefulness and sleep. Neurology 1992;42:44.
24. Gillin JC, van Kammen DP, Graves J, et al. Differential effects of D- and L-amphetamine on the sleep of depressed patients. Life Sci 1975;17:1233.
25. Post RM, Gillin JC, Goodwin FK, et al. The effect of orally administered cocaine on sleep of depressed patients. Psychopharmacology 1974;37:59.
26. Watson R, Hartmann E, Schildkraut JJ. Amphetamine withdrawal: affective state sleep patterns, and MHPG excretion. Am J Psychiatry 1972;129:39.
27. Gillin JC, van Kammen D, Bunney WE Jr. Pimozide attenuates effects of D-amphetamine in EEG sleep patterns in psychiatric patients. Life Sci 1978;22:1805.
28. Benkert O, Kohler B. Intrahypothalamic and intrastriatal dopamine and norepinephrine injection in relation to motor hyperactivity in the rat. Psychopharmacology 1972;24:318.
29. Fog R. Stereotyped and non-stereotyped behavior in rats induced by various stimulant drugs. Psychopharmacology 1969;14:299.
30. Jouvet M. The role of monoamines and acetylcholine-containing neurons in the regulation of the sleep-waking cycle. Ergeb Physiol 1972;64:166.
31. Jones BE, Bobillier P, Jouvet M. Effets de la destruction des neurones contenant des catecholamines du mesencephale sur le cycle veille sommeils du chat. C R Seances Soc Biol Fill 1969;163:176.
32. Jones BE, Bobillier P, Pin C, et al. The effects of lesions of catecholamine-containing neurons on monoamine content of the brain and EEG and behavioral waking in the cat. Brain Res 1973;58:157.
33. Scheving LE, Harrison WH, Gordon P, et al. Daily fluctuation (circadian and ultradian) in biogenic amines of the rat brain. Am J Physiol 1968;214:166.
34. Kovacevic R, Radulovacki M. Monoamine changes in the brain of cats during slow wave sleep. Science 1976;193:1025.
35. Kafi S, Gaillard JM. Brain dopamine receptors and sleep in the rat: effects of stimulant blockade. Eur J Pharmacol 1976;38:357.
36. Wauquier A, Van den Broeck WAE, Niemegeers CJE. On the Antagonistic Effects of Pimozide and Clompenidine on Apomorphine-Disturbed Sleepwakefulness in Dogs. In WP Koella (ed), Sleep 1980. Basel: Karger, 1981;279.
37. Wauquier A, Van den Broeck WAE, Janssen PAJ. Biphasic effects of pimozide on sleep-wakefulness in dogs. Life Sci 1980;27:1469.
38. Cianchetti C, Masala C, Corsini GU, et al. Effect of apomorphine on human sleep. Life Sci 1978;23:403.
39. Stone TW. Neuropharmacology. Oxford: Freeman, 1995.
40. Trampus M, Ferri N, Adami M, et al. The dopamine $D_1$ receptor agonists, A68930 and SKF 38393, induce arousal and suppress REM sleep in the rat. Eur J Pharmacol 1993;235:83.
41. Cianchetti C. Dopamine Agonists and Sleep in Man. In A Wauquier, JM Gaillard, JM Monti, et al. (eds), Sleep: Neurotransmitters and Neuromodulators. New York: Raven, 1985;121.
42. Ongini E, Bo P, Dionisotti S, et al. Effects of remoxipride, a dopamine D-2 antagonist antipsychotic, on sleep-waking patterns and EEG activity in rats and rabbits. Psychopharmacology (Berl) 1992;107:236.
43. Montplaisir J, de Champlain J, Young SN, et al. Narcolepsy and idiopathic hyperinsomnia: biogenic amines and related compounds in CSF. Neurology 1982;32:1299.
44. Faull KF, Zeller-DeAmicis LC, Radde L, et al. Biogenic amine concentrations in the brains of normal and narcoleptic canines: current status. Sleep 1986;9:107.
45. Parkes JD, Fenton G, Struthers G, et al. Narcolepsy and cataplexy. Clinical features, treament, and cerebrospinal fluid findings. Q J Med 1974;43:525.
46. Kish SJ, Mamelak M, Slimovitch C, et al. Brain neurotransmitter changes in human narcolepsy. Neurology 1992;42:229.
47. Mignot E, Renaud A, Nishino S, et al. Canine cataplexy is preferentially controlled by adrenergic mechanisms: evidence using monoamine selective uptake inhibitors and release enhancers. Psychopharmacology (Berl) 1993;113:76.
48. Reid MS, Tafti M, Nishino S, et al. Local administration of dopaminergic drugs into the ventral tegmental area modulates cataplexy in the narcoleptic canine. Brain Res 1996;733:83.

49. Miller JD, Farber J, Gatz P, et al. Activity of mesencephalic dopamine and non-dopamine neurons across stages of sleep and walking in the rat. Brain Res 1983;273:133.

50. Aston-Jones G, Bloom FE. Norepinephrine-containing locus coeruleus neurons in behaving rats exhibit pronounced responses to non-noxious environmental stimuli. J Neurosci 1981;1:887.

51. Skarby T, Andersson K-E, Edvinsson L. Characterization of the postsynaptic alpha-adrenoceptor in isolated feline cerebral arteries. Acta Physiol Scand 1981;112:105.

52. Kleinlogel H, Scholtysik G, Sayers AC. Effects of clonidine and BS 100-141 on the EEG sleep pattern in rats. Eur J Pharmacol 1975;33:159.

53. Autret A, Beillevaire T, Cathala H-P, et al. The effect of clonidine on sleep patterns in man. Eur J Clin Pharmacol 1977;12:319.

54. Putkonen PTS, Leppavuori A, Stenberg D. Paradoxical sleep inhibition by central alpha-adrenoceptor stimulant clonidine antagonized by alpha-receptor blocker yohimbine. Life Sci 1977;21:1059.

55. Ramesh V, Kumar VM, John J, et al. Medial preoptic alpha-2 adrenoceptors in the regulation of sleep-wakefulness. Physiol Behav 1995;57:171.

56. Osaka T, Matsumura H. Noradrenaline inhibits preoptic sleep-active neurons through alpha 2-receptors in the rat. Neurosci Res 1995;21:323.

57. Tononi G, Pompeiano M, Pompeiano O. Modulation of desynchronized sleep through microinjection of B-adrenergic agonists and antagonists in the dorsal pontine tegmentum of the cat. Eur J Physiol 1989;415:142.

58. Berridge CW, Foote SL. Enhancement of behavioral and electroencephalographic indices of waking following stimulation of noradrenergic β-receptors within the medial septal region of the basal forebrain. J Neurosci 1996;16:6999.

59. Aldrich MS, Hollingsworth Z, Penney JB. Adrenergic receptor autoradiography of human narcoleptic brain. Sleep Res 1991;20A:280.

60. Monnier M, Sauer R, Hatt AM. The activating effects of histamine on the central nervous system. Int Rev Neurobiol 1970;12:265.

61. Nicholson AN, Pascoe PA, Stone BM. Histaminergic systems and sleep: studies in man with histamine $H_1$ and $H_2$ receptor antagonists. Neuropharmacology 1985;24:245.

62. Monti JM. Involvement of histamine in the control of the waking state. Life Sci 1993;53:1331.

63. Nicholson AN, Stone BM. The $H_2$ antagonists cimetidine and ranitidine: studies on performance. Eur J Clin Pharmacol 1984;26:579.

64. Inagaki N, Yamatodani A, Ando-Yamamoto M, et al. Organization of histaminergic fibers in the rat brain. J Comp Neurol 1988;273:283.

65. Lin JS, Luppi PH, Salvert D, et al. Histamine-containing neurons in the cat hypothalamus. C R Acad Sci 1986;303:371.

66. Sherin JE, Shiromani PJ, McCarley RW, et al. Activation of ventrolateral preoptic neurons during sleep. Science 1996;271:216.

67. Lin JS, Kitahama K, Fort P, et al. Histaminergic system in the cat hypothalamus with reference to type B monoamine oxidase. J Comp Neurol 1993;330:405.

68. Lin JS, Hou Y, Sakai K, et al. Histaminergic descending inputs to the mesopontine tegmentum and their role in the control of cortical activation and wakefulness in the cat. J Neurosci 1996;16:1523.

69. Orr E, Quay WB. Hypothalamic 24-hour rhythms in histamine, histidine decarboxylase, and histamine-$N$-methyltransferase. Endocrinology 1975;96:941.

70. Onoé H, Yamatodani A, Watanabe Y, et al. Prostaglandin E2 and histamine in the posterior hypothalamus. J Sleep Res 1992;1:S166.

71. Lin JS, Sakai K, Jouvet M. Evidence for histaminergic arousal mechanisms in the hypothalamus of cats. Neuropharmacology 1988;27:111.

72. Lin JS, Sakai K, Vanni-Mercier G, et al. Involvement of histaminergic neurons in arousal mechanisms demonstrated with $H_3$-receptor ligands in the cat. Brain Res 1990;523:325.

73. Monti JM, Jantos H, Boussard M, et al. Effects of selective activation or blockade of the histamine $H_3$ receptor on sleep and wakefulness. Eur J Pharmacol 1991;205:283.

74. Nicholson AN. Histaminergic Systems: Daytime Alertness and Nocturnal Sleep. In A Wauquier, JM Gaillard, JM Monti, et al. (eds), Sleep: Neurotransmitters and Neuromodulators. New York: Raven, 1985;211.

75. Vanderwolf CH, Robinson TE. Reticulo-cortical activity and behavior: a critique of the arousal theory and new synthesis. Behav Brain Sci 1981;4:459.

76. Buzsaki G, Bickford RG, Ponomareff G, et al. Nucleus basalis and thalamic control of neocortical activity in the freely moving rat. J Neurosci 1988;8:4007.

77. Steriade M, Datla S, Pare D, et al. Neuronal activities in brainstem cholinergic nuclei related to tonic activation patterns in thalamocortical systems. J Neurosci 1990;10:2541.

78. Steriade M, Dossi RC, Nunez A. Network modulation of a slow intrinsic oscillation of cat thalamocortical neurons implicated in sleep delta waves: cortically induced synchronization and brainstem cholinergic suppression. J Neurosci 1991;11:3200.

79. Celesia GG, Jasper HH. Acetylcholine released from cerebral cortex in relation to state of activation. Neurology 1966;16:1053.

80. Marrosu F, Portas C, Mascia MS, et al. Microdialysis measurement of cortical and hippocampal acetylcholine release during sleep-waking cycle in freely moving cats. Brain Res 1995;671:329.

81. Jasper H, Tessier J. Acetylcholine liberation from cerebral cortex during paradoxical (REM) sleep. Science 1971;172:601.

82. Sitaram N, Gillin JC. Development and use of pharmacological probes of the CNS in man: evidence of cholinergic abnormality in primary affective illness. Biol Psychiatry 1980;15:925.

83. Szymusiak R. Magnocellular nuclei of the basal fore-brain: substrates of sleep and arousal regulation. Sleep 1995;18:478.

84. Bartus RT, Dean RL, Beer B, et al. The cholinergic hypothesis of geriatric memory dysfunction. Science 1982;217:408.

85. Dekker AJAM, Connor DJ, Thal LJ. The role of cholinergic projections from the nucleus basalis in memory. Neurosci Biobehav Rev 1991;15:299.

86. McGinty DJ, Sterman MB. Sleep suppression after basal forebrain lesions in the cat. Science 1968;160:1253.

87. McGinty D. Hypothalamic Thermoregulatory Control of Slow Wave Sleep. In M Mancia, G Marini (eds), The Diencephalon and Sleep. New York: Raven, 1990;97.

88. Wyatt RJ, Kupfer DJ, Sjoersma A, et al. Effects of L-tryptophan (a natural sedative) on human sleep. Lancet 1970;2:842.

89. Hartmann E. L-Tryptophan as an hypnotic agent: a review. Waking Sleeping 1977;1:155.

90. Jouvet M. Neuropharmacology of the sleep-waking cycle. Handbook Psychopharmacol 1977;8:233.

91. Koella WP, Feldstein A, Czicman JS. The effect of *para*-chlorophenylalanine on the sleep of cats. Electroencephalogr Clin Neurophysiol 1968;25:481.

92. Weitzman E, Rapport MM, McGregor P, et al. Sleep patterns of the monkey and brain serotonin concentration: effect of *p*-chlorophenylalanine. Science 1968;160:1361.

93. Dement W, Mitler M, Henriksen S. Sleep changes during chronic administration of parachlorophenylalanine. Rev Can Biol (Suppl) 1972;31:239.

94. Ross CA, Trulson ME, Jacobs BL. Depletion of brain serotonin following intraventricular 5,7-dihydroxytryptamine fails to disrupt sleep in the rat. Brain Res 1976;114:517.

95. Cespuglio R, Saika N, Gharib A, et al. Voltammetric detection of the release of 5-hydroxyindole compounds through the sleep-waking cycle of the rat. Exp Brain Res 1990;80:121.

96. Wyatt RJ, Gillin JC. Development of Tolerance to and Dependence of Endogenous Neurotransmitters. In AJ Mandell (ed), Neurobiological Mechanisms of Adaptation and Behavior. New York: Raven, 1975;47.

97. Wesemann W, Rotsch M, Schulz E, et al. Circadian rhythm of serotonin binding in rat brain I. Effect of the light-dark cycle. Chronobiol Int 1986;3:135.

98. Borbely AA, Steigrad P, Tobler I. Effect of sleep deprivation on brain serotonin in the rat. Behav Brain Res 1980;1:205.

99. Wesemann W, Rotsch M, Schulz E, et al. Circadian rhythm of serotonin binding in rat brain. II. Influence of sleep deprivation and imipramine. Chronobiol Int 1986;3:141.

100. Portas CM, McCarley RW. Behavioral state-related changes of extracellular serotonin concentration in the dorsal raphe nucleus: a microdialysis study in the freely moving cat. Brain Res 1994;648:306.

101. Imeri L, De Simoni MG, Giglio R, et al. Changes in the serotonergic system during the sleep-wake cycle: simultaneous polygraphic and voltammetric recordings in hypothalamus using a telemetry system. Neuroscience 1994;58:353.

102. Quattrochi JJ, Mamelak AN, Binder D, et al. Dose-related suppression of REM sleep and PGO waves by the serotonin-1 agonist eltoprazine. Neuropsychopharmacology 1993;8:7.

103. Gillin JC, Sohn SM, Lardon M, et al. Ipsapirone, a 5-$HT_{1A}$ agonist, suppresses REM sleep equally in unmedicated depressed patients and normal controls. Neuropsychopharmacology 1996;15:109.

104. Seifritz E, Stahl SM, Gillin JC. Human sleep EEG following the 5-$HT_{1A}$ antagonist pindolol: possible disinhibition of raphe neuron activity. Brain Res 1997;759:84.

105. Declerck AC, Wauquier A, Van der Ham-Veltman PHM, et al. Increase in slow wave sleep in humans with serotonin-$S_2$ antagonist ritanserin. Curr Ther Res Clin Exp 1987;41:427.

106. Idzikowski C, Cowen PJ, Nutt D, et al. The effects of chronic ritanserin treatment on sleep and the neuroendocrine response to L-tryptophan. Psychopharmacology 1987;93:416.

107. Idzikowski C, Mills FJ, Glennard R. 5-Hydroxytryptamine-2 antagonist increases human slow wave sleep. Brain Res 1986;378:164.

108. Sommerfelt L, Ursin R. The 5-$HT_2$ antagonist ritanserin decreases sleep in cats. Sleep 1993;16:15.

109. Luebke JI, Greene RW, Semba K, et al. Serotonin hyperpolarizes cholinergic low-threshold burst neurons in the rat laterodorsal tegmental nucleus in vitro. Proc Natl Acad Sci U S A 1992;89:743.

110. Jouvet M, Buda C, Cespuglio R, et al. Hypnogenic Effects of Some Hypothalamo-Pituitary Peptides. In WE Bunney Jr, E Costa, SG Potkin (eds), Clinical Neuropharmacology (Vol 9, Suppl 4). New York: Raven, 1986;465.

111. Legendre R, Pieron H. Le probleme des facteurs du sommeil. Resultats d'injections vasculaires et intracerebrales de liquides insomniques. C R Seances Soc Biol Fil 1910;62:1077.

112. Legendre R, Pieron H. Recherches sur le besoin de sommeil consecutif a une veille prolongee. Z Allerg Physiol 1913;14:235.

113. Ishimoro K. True cause of sleep—a hypnogenic substance as evidenced in the brain of sleep-deprived animals. Igakkai Zasshi (Tokyo) 1909;23:429.

114. Schnedorf JG, Ivy AC. An examination of the hypnotoxin theory of sleep. Am J Physiol 1939;125:491.

115. Inoue S. Sleep-promoting substance (SPS) and physiological sleep regulation. Zoolog Sci 1993;10:557.

116. Kimura-Takeuchi M, Inoue S. Differential sleep modulation by sequentially administered muramyl dipeptide and uridine. Brain Res Bull 1993;31:33.

117. Monnier M, Hosli L. Dialysis of sleep and waking factors in blood of rabbit. Science 1964;146:796.

118. Schoenenberger GA, Monnier M. Characterization of a delta-electroencephalogram (sleep)-inducing peptide. Proc Natl Acad Sci U S A 1977;74:1282.

119. Schoenenberger GA, Maier PF, Tober HJ, et al. The delta EEG (sleep)–inducing peptide (DSIP). XI. Amino-acid analysis, sequence, synthesis and activity of the nonapeptide. Pflugers Arch 1978;376:119.

120. Inoue S. Biology of Sleep Substances. Boca Raton, FL: CRC, 1989.

121. Schneider-Helmert D, Gniess F, Monnier M, et al. Acute and delayed effects of DSIP (delta sleep–inducing peptide) on human sleep behavior. Int J Clin Pharmacol Ther Toxicol 1981;19:341.

122. Schneider-Helmert D, Schoenenberger GA. Effects of DSIP in man. Multifunctional psychophysiological properties besides induction of natural sleep. Neuropsychobiology 1983;9:197.

123. Blois R, Monnier M, Tissot R, et al. Effect of DSIP on Diurnal and Nocturnal Sleep in Man. In WP Koella (ed), Sleep 1980. Basel: Karger, 1981;301.

124. Schneider-Helmert D, Gniess F, Schoenenberger GA. Effect of DSIP Applications in Healthy and Insomniac Adults. In WP Koella (ed), Sleep 1980. Basel: Karger, 1981;417.

125. Kato N, Nagaki S, Takahashi Y, et al. DSIP-Like Material in Rat Brain, Human Cerebrospinal Fluid, and Plasma as Determined by Enzyme Immunoassay. In S Inoue, AA Borbely (eds), Endogenous Sleep Substances and Sleep Regulation. Tokyo: Japanese Scientific Society Press, 1985;141.

126. Fischman AJ, Kastin AJ, Graf M. Circadian variation of DSIP-like material in rat plasma. Life Sci 1984;35:2079.

127. Seifritz E, Muller MJ, Schonenberger GA, et al. Human plasma DSIP decreases at the initiation of sleep at different circadian times. Peptides 1995;16:1475.

128. Obal F Jr, Torok A, Alfoldi P, et al. Effects of intracerebroventricular injection of delta sleep–inducing peptide (DSIP) and an analogue on sleep and brain temperature in rats at night. Pharmacol Biochem Behav 1985;23:953.

129. Graf MV, Kastin AJ, Schoenenberger GA. Delta sleep–inducing peptide in spontaneously hyperactive rats. Pharmacol Biochem Behav 1986;24:1797.

130. Dick P, Costa C, Fayolle K, et al. DSIP in the treatment of withdrawal syndromes from alcohol and opiates. Eur Neurol 1984;23:364.

131. Monnier M, Hatt AM, Cueni LB, et al. Humoral transmission of sleep. VI. Purification and assessment of a hypnogenic fraction of "sleep dialysate" (factor delta). Pflugers Arch 1972;331:257.

132. Tobler I, Borbely AA. Effect of delta sleep inducing peptide (DSIP) and arginine vasotocin (AVT) on sleep and locomotor activity in the rat. Waking Sleeping 1980;4:139.

133. Schoenenberger GA, Graf M. Effects of DSIP and DSIP-P on Different Biorhythmic Parameters. In A Wauquier, JM Gaillard, JM Monti, et al. (eds), Sleep: Neurotransmitters and Neuromodulators. New York: Raven, 1985;265.

134. Schneider-Helmert D. Influences of DSIP on Sleep and Waking Behavior in Man. In WP Koella (ed), Sleep 1982. Basel: Karger, 1983;117.

135. Schneider-Helmert D. DSIP in insomnia. Eur Neurol 1984;23:358.

136. Kaeser HE. A clinical trial with DSIP. Eur Neurol 1984;23:386.

137. Schneider-Helmert D. Effects of DSIP on narcolepsy. Eur Neurol 1984;23:353.

138. Larbig W, Gerber WD, Kluck M, et al. Therapeutic effects of delta-sleep–inducing peptide (DSIP) in patients with chronic, pronounced pain episodes. A clinical pilot study. Eur Neurol 1984;23:372.

139. Hermann E, Ernst A, Schneider-Helmert D. Effects of DSIP on daytime mood states of insomniacs. Sleep Res Abstr 1987;16:222.

140. Hofman WF, Schneider-Helmert D. The influence of DSIP on the rhythm of spontaneous sleep tendency in insomniacs and normal subjects. Sleep Res Abstr 1987;16:615.

141. Schneider-Helmert D, Hermann E, Schoenenberger GA. Efficacy of DSIP for withdrawal treatment of low-dose benzodiazepine dependent insomniacs. Sleep Res Abstr 1987;16:133.

142. Schneider-Helmert D, Schoenenberger GA, Hermann E. Advancing delayed sleep phase by treatment with DSIP. Sleep Res Abstr 1987;16:222.

143. Monti JM, Debellis J, Alterwain P, et al. Study of delta sleep-inducing peptide efficacy in improving sleep on short-term administration of chronic insomniacs. Int J Clin Pharmacol Res 1987;7:105.

144. Graf MV, Christen H, Schoenenberger GA. DSIP/DSIP-P and circadian motor activity of rats under continuous light. Peptides 1982;3:623.

145. Inoue S, Honda K, Komoda Y, et al. Little sleep-promoting effects of three sleep substances diurnally infused in unrestrained rats. Neurosci Lett 1984;49:207.

146. Inoue S, Honda K, Komoda Y, et al. Differential sleep-promoting effects of five sleep substances nocturnally infused in unrestrained rats. Proc Natl Acad Sci U S A 1984;81:6240.

147. Schneider-Helmert D. DSIP: Clinical Application of the Programming Effect. In S Inoue, D Schneider-Helmert (eds), Sleep Peptides: Basic and Clinical Approaches. Berlin: Springer, 1988;175.

148. Komoda Y, Ishikawa M, Nagasaki H, et al. Uridine, a sleep-promoting substance from brainstems of sleep-deprived rats. Biomed Res 1983;4:S223.

149. Komoda Y, Ishikawa M, Nagasaki H, et al. Purification, isolation, and identification of sleep-promoting substances (SPS) from brainstems of sleep-deprived rats. Folia Psychiatr Neurol (Japan) 1985;39:210.

150. Inoue S, Honda K, Komoda Y. Sleep-Promoting Substances. In A Wauquier, JM Gaillard, JM Monti, et al. (eds), Sleep: Neurotransmitters and Neuromodulators. New York: Raven, 1985;305.

151. Krooth RS, Hsaio WL, Lam GFM. Effects of natural pyrimidines and of certain related compounds on the

spontaneous activity in the mouse. J Pharmacol Exp Ther 1978;207:504.

152. Yamamoto I, Kimura T, Tateoka Y, et al. Central depressant activities of $N_3$-allyluridine and $N_3$-allylthymidine. Res Commun Chem Pathol Pharmacol 1986;52:321.

153. Honda K, Komoda Y, Inoue S. Effects of Sleep-Promoting Substances on the Rat Circadian Sleep-Waking Cycles. In S Inoue, AA Borbely (eds), Endogenous Sleep Substances and Sleep Regulation. Tokyo: Japanese Scientific Society Press, 1985;203.

154. Honda K, Komoda Y, Nishida S, et al. Uridine as an active component of sleep-promoting substance: its effects on the nocturnal sleep in rats. Neurosci Res 1984;1:243.

155. Inoue S. Sleep Substances: Their Roles and Evolution. In S Inoue, AA Borbely (eds), Endogenous Sleep Substances and Sleep Regulation. Tokyo: Japanese Scientific Society Press, 1985;3.

156. Martin SA, Karnovsky ML, Krueger JM, et al. Peptideglycans as promoters of slow-wave sleep. I. Structure of the sleep-promoting factor isolated from human urine. J Biol Chem 1984;259:12652.

157. Krueger JM, Karnovsky ML, Martin SA, et al. Peptideglycans as promotors of slow wave sleep. II. Somnogenic and pyrogenic activities of some naturally occurring muramyl peptides; correlations with mass spectrometric structure determination. J Biol Chem 1984;259:12659.

158. Krueger JM. Muramyl peptide enhancement of slow-wave sleep. Methods Find Exp Clin Pharmacol 1986;8:105.

159. Krueger JM, Walter J, Levin C. Factor S and Related Somnogens: An Immune Theory for Slow Wave Sleep. In DJ McGinty, R Drucker-Colin, A Morrison, et al. (eds), Brain Mechanisms of Sleep. New York: Raven, 1987;253.

160. Krueger JM, Toth LA, Cady AB, et al. Immunomodulation and Sleep. In S Inoue, D Schneider-Helmert (eds), Sleep Peptides: Basic and Clinical Approaches. Berlin: Springer, 1988;95.

161. Krueger JM, Karnovsky ML. Sleep and immune response. Ann N Y Acad Sci 1987;496:510.

162. Adam A, Lederer E. Muramyl peptides: immunomodulators, sleep factors, and vitamins. Med Res Rev 1984;4:111.

163. Karnovsky ML. Muramyl peptides in mammalian tissues and their effects at the cellular level. Fed Proc 1986;45:2556.

164. Werner GH, Floch F, Migliore-Samour D, et al. Immunomodulating peptides. Experientia 1986;42:521.

165. Krueger JM. Muramyl Peptides and Interleukin-1 as Promoters of Slow Wave Sleep. In S Inoue, AA Borbely (eds), Endogenous Sleep Substances and Sleep Regulation. Tokyo: Japanese Scientific Society Press, 1985;181.

166. Krueger JM, Pappenheimer JR, Karnovsky ML. Sleep-promoting effects of muramyl peptides. Proc Natl Acad Sci U S A 1982;79:6102.

167. Krueger JM, Walter J, Karnovsky ML, et al. Muramyl peptides. Variation of somnogenic activity with structure. J Exp Med 1984;159:68.

168. Krueger JM. Endogenous Sleep Factors. In A Wauquier, JM Gaillard, JM Monti, et al. (eds), Sleep: Neurotransmitters and Neuromodulators. New York: Raven, 1985;319.

169. Johanssen L, Wecke J, Krueger JM. Macrophages produce a sleep-enhancing substance(s) during the digestion of bacteria. Int Symp Current Trends Slow Wave Sleep Res Abstr 1987;42.

170. Imeri L, Opp MR, Krueger JM. An IL-1 receptor and an IL-1 receptor antagonist attenuate muramyl dipeptide- and IL-1–induced sleep and fever. Am J Physiol 1993;265:R907.

171. Moldofsky H, Lue FA, Eisen J, et al. The relationship of interleukin-1 and immune functions to sleep in humans. Psychosom Med 1986;48:309.

172. Walter J, Davenne D, Shoham S, et al. Brain temperature changes coupled to sleep states persist during interleukin-1–enhanced sleep. Am J Physiol 1986;250:R96.

173. Tobler I, Borbely AA, Schwyzer M, et al. Interleukin-1 derived from astrocytes enhances slow wave activity in sleep EEG of the rat. Eur J Pharmacol 1984;104:191.

174. Shoham S, Davenne D, Cady AB, et al. Recombinant tumor necrosis factor and interleukin-1 enhance slow-wave sleep in rabbits. Am J Physiol 1987;253:R142.

175. Krueger JM, Walter J, Dinarello CA, et al. Sleep-promoting effects of endogenous pyrogen (interleukin-1). Am J Physiol 1984;246:R994.

176. Krueger JM, Karaszewski JH, Davenne D, et al. Somnogenic muramyl peptides. Fed Proc 1986;45:2552.

177. Mignot E, Wang C, Rattazzi C, et al. Genetic linkage of autosomal recessive canine narcolepsy with a μ immunoglobulin heavy-chain switch-like segment. Proc Natl Acad Sci U S A 1991;88:3475.

178. Irwin M, Smith TL, Gillin JC. Electroencephalographic sleep and natural killer activity in depressed patients and controls. Psychosom Med 1992;54:10.

179. Irwin M, McClintick J, Costlow C, et al. Partial night sleep deprivation reduces natural killer and cellular immune responses in humans. FASEB J 1996;10:643.

180. Pavel S, Psatta D, Goldstein R. Slow wave sleep induced in cats by extremely small amounts of synthetic and pineal vasotocin injected into the third ventricle of the brain. Brain Res Bull 1977;2:251.

181. Goldstein R, Psatta D. Sleep in the cat: raphe dorsalis and vasotocin. Sleep 1984;7:373.

182. Mendelson WB, Gillin JC, Pisner G, et al. Arginine vasotocin and sleep in the rat. Brain Res 1980;182:246.

183. Karacan I, Thornby JI, Anch AM. Dose-related sleep disturbances induced by coffee and caffeine. Clin Pharmacol Ther 1976;20:682.

184. Radulovacki M, Miletich RS, Green RD. $N_6$(L-phenylisopropyl)adenosine (L-PIA) increases slow wave sleep (S2) and decreases wakefulness in rats. Brain Res 1982;246:178.

185. Radulovacki M, Virus RM, Djuricic-Nedelson M, et al. Adenosine analogs and sleep in rats. J Pharmacol Exp Ther 1984;228:268.
186. Radulovacki M, Virus RM, Rapoza D, et al. A comparison of the dose response effects of pyrimidine ribonucleosides and adenosine on sleep in rats. Psychopharmacology 1985;87:136.
187. Radulovacki M, Virus RM, Djuricic-Nedelson M, et al. Hypnotic effects of deoxycorformycin in rats. Brain Res 1983;271:392.
188. Sarda N, Dubois M, Gharib A, et al. Increase of paradoxical sleep induced by S-adenosyl-L-homocysteine. Neurosci Lett 1982;30:69.
189. Yanik G, Radulovacki M. REM sleep deprivation upregulates adenosine $A_1$ receptors. Brain Res 1987;402:362.
190. Benington JH, Kodali SK, Heller HC. Stimulation of $A_1$ adenosine receptors mimics the electroencephalographic effects of sleep deprivation. Brain Res 1995;692:79.
191. Schwierin B, Borbely AA, Tobler I. Effects of $N_6$-cyclopentyladenosine and caffeine on sleep regulation in the rat. Eur J Pharmacol 1996;300:163.
192. Benington JH, Heller HC. Restoration of brain energy metabolism as the function of sleep. Prog Neurobiol 1995;45:347.
193. Porkka-Heiskanen T, Strecker RE, Thakkar M, et al. Adenosine: a mediator of the sleep-inducing effects of prolonged wakefulness. Science 1997;276:1268.
194. Ueno R, Hayaishi O, Osama H, et al. Prostaglandin $D_2$ Regulates Physiological Sleep. In S Inoue, AA Borbely (eds), Endogenous Sleep Substances and Sleep Regulation. Tokyo: Japanese Scientific Society Press, 1985;193.
195. Ueno R, Honda K, Inoue S, et al. Prostaglandin $D_2$, a cerebral sleep-inducing substance in rats. Proc Natl Acad Sci U S A 1983;80:1735.
196. Matsumura H, Honda K, Goh Y, et al. Awaking effect of prostaglandin $E_2$ in freely moving rats. Brain Res 1989;481:242.
197. Ueno R, Ishikawa Y, Nakayama T, et al. Prostaglandin $D_2$ induces sleep when microinjected into the preoptic area of conscious rats. Biochem Biophys Res Commun 1982;109:576.
198. Hayaishi O, Ueno R, Onoe H, et al. Prostaglandin $D_2$ induces sleep when infused into the cerebral ventricle of conscious monkeys. Adv Prostaglandin Thromboxane Leukot Res 1987;17B:946.
199. Hayaishi O. Prostaglandin $D_2$ and sleep. Adv Prostaglandin Thromboxane Leukot Res 1989;19:26.
200. Onoe H, Ueno R, Fujita I, et al. Prostaglandin $D_2$, a cerebral sleep-inducing substance in monkeys. Proc Natl Acad Sci U S A 1988;85:4082.
201. Koyama Y, Hayaishi O. Modulation by prostaglandins of activity of sleep-related neurons in the preoptic/anterior hypothalamic areas in rats. Brain Res Bull 1994;33:367.
202. Naito K, Osama H, Ueno R, et al. Suppression of sleep by prostaglandin synthesis inhibitors in unrestrained rats. Brain Res 1988;71(3A):A298.
203. Takahata R, Matsumura H, Kantha SS, et al. Intravenous administration of inorganic selenium compounds, inhibitors of prostaglandin D synthase, inhibits sleep in freely moving rats. Brain Res 1993;623:65.
204. Matsumura H, Goh Y, Ueno R, et al. Awaking effect of $PGE_2$ microinjected into the preoptic area of rats. Brain Res 1988;444:265.
205. Hayaishi O. Molecular mechanisms of sleep-wake regulation: roles of prostaglandins $D_2$ and $E_2$. FASEB J 1991;5:2575.
206. Rosenthal NE, Sack DA, Gillin JC, et al. Seasonal affective disorder. Arch Gen Psychiatry 1984;41:72.
207. Wetterberg L, Beck-Friis J, Kjellman BF. Melatonin as a Marker for a Subgroup of Depression in Adults. In M Shafii, SL Shafii (eds), Biological Rhythms, Mood Disorders, Light Therapy, and the Pineal Gland. Washington, D.C.: American Psychiatric Press, 1990;69.
208. Parry BL, Berga S, Kripke D, et al. Altered waveform of plasma nocturnal melatonin secretion in premenstrual depression. Arch Gen Psychiatry 1990;47:1139.
209. Marczynski TJ, Yamaguchi N, Ling GM, et al. Sleep induced by the administration of melatonin (5-methoxy-N-acetyltryptamine) to the hypothalamus in unrestrained cats. Experientia 1964;20:435.
210. Hishikawa Y, Cramer H, Kuhlo W. Natural and melatonin-induced sleep in young chickens—a behavioral and electrographic study. Exp Brain Res 1969;7:84.
211. Anton-Tay F, Diaz JL, Fernandez-Guardiola A. On the effect of melatonin on human brain. Its possible therapeutic implications. Life Sci 1971;10:841.
212. Cramer H, Rudolph J, Consbruch U, et al. On the effects of melatonin on sleep and behavior in man. Adv Biochem Psychopharmacol 1974;11:187.
213. Holmes SW, Sugden D. Effects of melatonin on sleep and neurochemistry in the rat. Br J Pharmacol 1982;76:95.
214. Lieberman HR, Waldhauser F, Garfield G, et al. Effects of melatonin on human mood and performance. Brain Res 1984;323:201.
215. James SP, Mendelson WB, Sack DA, et al. The effect of melatonin on normal sleep. Neuropsychopharmacology 1987;1:41.
216. Dollins AB, Zhdanova IV, Wurtman RJ, et al. Effect of inducing nocturnal serum melatonin concentration in daytime on sleep, mood, body temperature, and performance. Proc Natl Acad Sci U S A 1994;91:1824.
217. Zhdanova IV, Wurtman RJ, Lynch HJ, et al. Sleep-inducing effects of low doses of melatonin ingested in the evening. Clin Pharmacol Ther 1995;57:552.
218. Arendt J, Borbely AA, Franey C, et al. Effects of chronic, small doses of melatonin given in the late afternoon on fatigue in man: a preliminary study. Neurosci Lett 1984;45:317.
219. Arendt J, Bojkowski C, Folkard S, et al. Photoperiodism, Melatonin and the Pineal. In D Evered, S Clark (eds), Ciba Foundation Symposium, 117. London: Pitman, 1985.

220. Lewy AJ, Ahmed S, Sack RL. Phase shifting the human circadian clock using melatonin. Behav Brain Res 1995;73:131.

221. Mendelson WB, Canin M, Cook JM, et al. A benzodiazepine receptor antagonist decreases sleep and reverses the hypnotic actions of flurazepam. Science 1983;219:414.

222. Mendelson WB, Monti D. Do benzodiazepines induce sleep by a GABAergic mechanism? Life Sci 1993; 53:PL81.

223. Scherschlicht R. Role for GABA in the Control of the Sleep-Wakefulness Cycle. In A Wauquier, J Gaillard, JM Monti, et al. (eds), Sleep: Neurotransmitters and Neuromodulators. New York: Raven, 1985;237.

224. Nitz D, Siegel JM. GABA release in posterior hypothalamus across sleep-wake cycle. Am J Physiol 1996;271:1707.

225. Henley K, Morrison AD. A re-evaluation of the effects of lesions of the pontine tegmentum and locus coeruleus on phenomena of paradoxical sleep in the cat. Acta Neurobiol Exp 1974;34:215.

226. Williams JA, Comisarow J, Day J, et al. State-dependent release of acetylcholine in rat thalamus measured by in vivo microdialysis. J Neurosci 1994;14:5236.

227. Jones BE, Tian-Zhu Y. The efferent projections from the reticular formation and the locus coeruleus by anterograde and retrograde axonal transport in the rat. J Comp Neurol 1985;242:56.

228. Steriade M, McCarley RW. Brainstem Control of Wakefulness and Sleep. New York: Plenum, 1990.

229. Magoun HW, Rhines R. An inhibitory mechanism in the bulbar reticular formation. J Neurophysiol 1946;9:165.

230. Nishino S, Tafti M, Reid MS, et al. Muscle atonia is triggered by cholinergic stimulation of the basal forebrain: implication for the pathophysiology of canine narcolepsy. J Neurosci 1995;15:4806.

231. Vertes RP, Colon LV, Fortin WJ, et al. Brainstem sites for the carbachol elicitation of the hippocampal theta rhythm in the rat. Exp Brain Res 1993;96:419.

232. Friedman L, Jones BE. Computer graphic analysis of sleep-wakefulness state changes after pontine lesions. Brain Res Bull 1984;13:53.

233. Friedman L, Jones BE. Study of sleep-wakefulness states by computer graphics and cluster analysis before and after lesions of pontine tegmentum in the cat. Electroencephalogr Clin Neurophysiol 1984;57:43.

234. Mitani A, Ito K, Hallanger AE, et al. Cholinergic projections from the laterodorsal and pedunculopontine tegmental nuclei to the pontine giganticellular tegmental field in the cat. Brain Res 1988;451:397.

235. Shiromani PJ, Armstrong DM, Gillin JC. Cholinergic neurons from the dorsolateral pons project to the medial pons: a WGA-HRP and choline acetyltransferase immunohistochemical study. Neurosci Lett 1988;95:19.

236. Friedman AK. Circumstances influencing Otto Loewi's discovery of chemical transmission in the nervous system. Pflugers Arch 1971;325:85.

237. Mazzuchelli-O'Flaherty AL, O'Flaherty JJ, Hernandez-Peon R. Sleep and other behavioral responses induced by acetylcholinergic stimulation of frontal and mesial cortex. Brain Res 1967;4:268.

238. Hernandez-Peon R, Chavez-Ibarra G, Morgane PJ, et al. Limbic cholinergic pathways involved in sleep and emotional behavior. Exp Neurol 1963;8:93.

239. Hernandez-Peon R, O'Flaherty JJ, Mazzuchelli-O'Flaherty AL. Sleep and other behavioral effects induced by acetylcholinergic stimulation of basal temporal cortex and striate structures. Brain Res 1967;4:243.

240. Baghdoyan HA, Spotts JL, Snyder SG. Simultaneous pontine and basal forebrain microinjections of carbachol suppress REM sleep. J Neurosci 1993;13:229.

241. Baghdoyan HA, Rodrigo-Angula ML, McCarley RW, et al. Site-specific enhancement and suppression of desynchronized sleep signs following cholinergic stimulation of three brainstem sites. Brain Res 1984;306:39.

242. Baghdoyan HA, Lydic R, Clifton CW, et al. The carbachol-induced enhancement of desynchronized sleep signs is dose dependent and antagonized by centrally administered atropine. Neuropsychopharmacology 1989;2:67.

243. Vanni-Mercier G, Sakai K, Lin DS, et al. Mapping of cholinoreceptive brainstem structures responsible for the generation of paradoxical sleep in the cat. Arch Ital Biol 1989;127:133.

244. Baghdoyan HA, Rodrigo-Angulo ML, McCarley RW, et al. A neuroanatomical gradient in the pontine tegmentum for the cholinoceptive induction of desynchronized sleep signs. Brain Res 1987;414:245.

245. Gnadt JW, Pegram GV. Cholinergic brainstem mechanisms of REM sleep in the rat. Brain Res 1986;384:29.

246. Bourgin P, Escourrou P, Gaultier C, et al. Induction of rapid eye movement by carbachol infusion into the pontine reticular formation in the rat. Neuroreport 1995;6:532.

247. Riemann D, Gann H, Dressing H, et al. Influence of the cholinesterase inhibitor galanthamine hydrobromide on normal sleep. Psychiatry Res 1994;51:253.

248. Riemann D, Lis S, Fritsch-Montero R, et al. Effect of tetrahydroaminoacridine on sleep in healthy subjects. Biol Psychiatry 1996;39:796.

249. Datta S, Calvo JM, Quattrochi JJ, et al. Long-term enhancement of REM sleep following cholinergic stimulation. Neuroreport 1991;2:619.

250. Calvo JM, Datta S, Quattrochi J, et al. Cholinergic microstimulation of the peribrachial nucleus in the cat. II. Delayed and prolonged increases in REM sleep. Arch Ital Biol 1992;130:285.

251. Datta S, Calvo JM, Quattrochi J, et al. Cholinergic microstimulation of the peribrachial nucleus in the cat. I. Immediate and prolonged increases in ponto-geniculo-occipital waves. Arch Ital Biol 1992;130:263.

252. Hazra J. Effect of hemicholinium 3 on slow wave and paradoxical sleep of cat. Eur J Pharmacol 1970;11:395.

253. Salin-Pascual RJ, Jimenez-Anguiano A. Vesamicol, an acetylcholine uptake blocker in presynaptic vesicles,

suppresses rapid eye movement (REM) sleep in the rat. Psychopharmacology 1995;121:485.

254. Kodama T, Takahashi Y, Honda Y. Enhancement of ACh release during paradoxical sleep in the dorsal tegmental field of the cat brain stem. Neurosci Lett 1990;114:277.

255. Leonard TO, Lydic R. Nitric oxide synthase inhibition decreases pontine acetylcholine release. Neuroreport 1995;6:1525.

256. Keifer JC, Baghdoyan HA, Lydic R. Sleep disruption and increased apneas after pontine microinjection of morphine. Anesthesiology 1992;77:973.

257. Lydic R, Keifer JC, Baghdoyan HA, et al. Microdialysis of the pontine reticular formation reveals inhibition of acetylcholine release by morphine. Anesthesiology 1993;79:1003.

258. Prospéro-García O, Jiménez-Anguiano A, Drucker-Colín R. Chloramphenicol prevents carbachol-induced REM sleep in cats. Neurosci Lett 1993;154:168.

259. Taylor P, Heller-Brown J. Acetylcholine. In GJ Siegel, BW Agranoff, RW Albers, et al. (eds), Basic Neurochemistry (5th ed). New York: Raven, 1994;231.

260. el-Bizri H, Clarke PBS. Regulation of nicotinic receptors in rat brain follow quasi-irreversible nicotinic blockade by chlorisondamine and chronic treatment with nicotine. Br J Pharmacol 1994;113:917.

261. Riemann D, Hohagen F, Bahro M, et al. Sleep in depression: the influence of age, gender, and diagnostic subtype on baseline sleep and the cholinergic REM induction test with RS 86. Eur Arch Psychiatry Clin Neurosci 1994;243:279.

262. Baghdoyan HA, Carlson BX, Roth MT. Pharmacological characterization of muscarinic cholinergic receptors in cat pons and cortex. Preliminary study. Pharmacology 1994;48:77.

263. Baghdoyan HA, Mallios VJ, Duckrow RB, et al. Localization of muscarinic receptor subtypes in brain stem areas regulating sleep. Neuroreport 1994;5:1631.

264. Gillin JC, Salin-Pascual RJ, Velazquez-Moctezuma J, et al. Cholinergic Receptor Subtypes and REM Sleep in Animals and Normal Controls. In Progress in Brain Research (Vol 98). Amsterdam: Elsevier, 1993;379.

265. Tsai LL, Bergmann BM, Perry BD, et al. Effects of chronic sleep deprivation on central cholinergic receptors in rat brain. Brain Res 1994;642:95.

266. Kushida CA, Zoltoski RK, Gillin JC. The expression of $m_1$-$m_3$ muscarinic receptor mRNAs in rat brain following REM sleep deprivation. Neuroreport 1995;6:1705.

267. Gillin JC, Sutton L, Ruiz C, et al. The effects of scopolamine on sleep and mood in depressed patients with a history of alcoholism and a normal comparison group. Biol Psychiatry 1991;30:157.

268. Sutin EL, Shiromani PJ, Kelsoe JR, et al. Rapid-eye movement sleep and muscarinic receptor binding in rats are augmented during withdrawal from chronic scopolamine treatment. Life Sci 1986;39:2419.

269. McCarley RW, Massaquoi SG. A limit cycle mathematical model of the REM sleep oscillatory system. Am J Physiol 1986;251:R1011.

270. Berger M, Riemann D, Hoechli D, et al. The cholinergic REM sleep induction test with RS86: state or trait-marker of depression? Arch Gen Psychiatry 1989;46:421.

271. Berkowitz A, Janowsky D, Gillin JC. Pilocarpine, an orally active, muscarinic, cholinergic agonist, induces REM sleep and reduces delta sleep in normal volunteers. Psychiatry Res 1990;33:113-119.

272. Hohagen F, Riemann D, Spiegel R, et al. Influence of the cholinergic agonist SDZ 210-086 on sleep in healthy subjects. Neuropsychopharmacology 1993;9:225-232.

273. Dahl RE, Ryan ND, Perel J, et al. Cholinergic REM induction test with arecoline in depressed children. Psychiatry Res 1994;51:269.

274. Janowsky DS, El-Yousef MK, Davis JM. A cholinergic-adrenergic hypothesis of mania and depression. Lancet 1972;2:632.

275. LeBon O. Is REM latency a dying concept? Acta Psychiatr Belg 1992;92:131.

276. Fritze J. The adrenergic-cholinergic imbalance hypothesis of depression: a review and a perspective. Rev Neurosci 1993;4:63.

277. Riemann D, Gann H, Fleckenstein P, et al. Effect of RS 86 on REM latency in schizophrenia. Psychiatry Res 1991;38:89.

278. Riemann D, Hohagen F, Bahro M, et al. Cholinergic neurotransmission, REM sleep, and depression. J Psychosom Res 1994;38:S15.

279. Riemann D, Hohagen F, Krieger S, et al. Cholinergic REM induction test: muscarinic supersensitivity underlies polysomnographic findings in both depression and schizophrenia. J Psychiatr Res 1994;28:195.

280. Tandon R, Greden JF. Cholinergic hyperactivity and negative schizophrenic symptoms. Arch Gen Psychiatry 1989;46:747.

281. Velazquez-Moctezuma J, Shalauta MD, Gillin JC, et al. Cholinergic antagonists and REM sleep generation. Brain Res 1991;543:175.

282. Velazquez-Moctezuma J, Gillin JC, Shiromani PJ. Effect of specific $M_1$, $M_2$ muscarinic receptor agonists on REM sleep generation. Brain Res 1989;503:128.

283. Velazquez-Moctezuma J, Shiromani PJ, Gillin JC. Acetylcholine and Acetylcholine Receptor Subtypes in REM Sleep Generation. In Progress in Brain Research (84th ed). Amsterdam: Elsevier, 1990;407.

284. Gillin JC, Sutton L, Ruiz C, et al. Dose dependent inhibition of REM sleep in normal volunteers by biperiden, a muscarinic antagonist. Biol Psychiatry 1991;30:151.

285. Salin-Pascual RJ, Granados-Fuentes D, Galacia-Polo L, et al. Biperiden administration in normal sleep and after REM sleep deprivation in healthy volunteers. Neuropsychopharmacology 1991;5:97.

286. Salin-Pascual RJ, Jimenez-Anguiano A, Granados-Fuentes D, et al. Effects of biperiden on sleep at base-

line and after 72 h of REM sleep deprivation in the cat. Psychopharmacology (Berlin) 1992;106:540.

287. Zoltoski RK, Velazquez-Moctezuma J, Shalauta M, et al. Effects of muscarinic antagonists on sleep. Soc Neurosci Abstr 1990;16:1254.

288. Overstreet DH, Russell RW, Helps SC, et al. Selective breeding for sensitivity to the anticholinesterase DFP. Psychopharmacology 1979;65:15.

289. Overstreet DH. The Flinders sensitive line rats: a genetic animal model of depression. Neurosci Biobehav Rev 1993;17:51.

290. Shiromani PJ, Overstreet D, Levy D, et al. Increased REM sleep in rats genetically bred for cholinergic hyperactivity. Neuropsychopharmacology 1988;1:127.

291. Overstreet DH. Selective breeding for increased cholinergic function: development of a new animal model of depression. Biol Psychiatry 1986;21:49.

292. Kilduff TS, Bowersox S, Kaitin K, et al. Muscarinic cholinergic receptors and the canine model of narcolepsy. Sleep 1986;9:102.

293. Soldatos CR, Kales JD, Scharf MB. Cigarette smoking associated with sleep difficulty. Science 1980;207:551.

294. Prosise GL, Bonnet MH, Berry RB, et al. Effects of abstinence from smoking on sleep and daytime sleepiness. Chest 1994;105:1136.

295. Wetter DW, Fiore MC, Baker TB, et al. Tobacco withdrawal and nicotine replacement influence objective measures of sleep. J Consult Clin Psychol 1995;636:658.

296. Gillin JC, Lardon M, Ruiz C, et al. Dose-dependent effects of transdermal nicotine on early morning awakening and rapid eye movement sleep time in nonsmoking normal volunteers. J Clin Psychopharmacol 1994;14:264.

297. Davila DG, Hurt RD, Offord KP, et al. Acute effects of transdermal nicotine on sleep architecture, snoring, and sleep-disordered breathing in nonsmokers. Am J Respir Crit Care Med 1994;150:469.

298. Salin-Pascual RJ, De La Fuente JR, Galicia-Polo L, et al. Effects of transdermal nicotine on mood and sleep in nonsmoking major depressed patients. Psychopharmacology 1995;121:476.

299. Hu B, Bouhassira D, Steriade M, et al. The blockage of PGO waves in the cat LGN by nicotinic antagonists. Brain Res 1988;473:394.

300. Velazquez-Moctezuma J, Shalauta MD, Gillin JC, et al. Differential effects of cholinergic antagonists on REM sleep components. Psychopharmacol Bull 1990;26:349.

301. Velazquez-Moctezuma J, Shalauta MD, Gillin JC, et al. Microinjections of nicotine in the medial pontine reticular formation elicits REM sleep. Neurosci Lett 1990;115:265.

302. Stevens DR, Birnstiel S, Gerber U, et al. Nicotinic depolarization of rat medial pontine reticular formation neurons studied in vitro. Neuroscience 1993;57:419.

303. Williams JA, Reiner PB. Noradrenaline hyperpolarizes identified rat mesopontine cholinergic neurons in vitro. J Neurosci 1993;13:3878.

304. Porkka-Heiskanen T, Smith SE, Taira T, et al. Noradrenergic activity in rat brain during rapid eye movement sleep deprivation and rebound sleep. Am J Physiol 1995;268:R1456.

305. Siegel JM, Rogawski MA. A function for REM sleep: regulation of noradrenergic receptor sensitivity. Brain Res Rev 1988;13:213.

306. Rechtschaffen A, Maron L. The effect of amphetamine on the sleep cycle. Electroencephalogr Clin Neurophysiol 1964;16:438.

307. Stern WC, Morgane PJ. Theoretical view of REM sleep function: maintenance of catecholamine systems in the central nervous system. Behav Biol 1974;11:1.

308. Wyatt RJ. The serotonin-catecholamine dream bicycle: a clinical study. Biol Psychiatry 1972;5:33.

309. Sitaram N, Gillin JC, Bunney WE Jr. Cholinergic and Catecholaminergic Receptor Sensitivity Illness: Strategy and Theory. In RM Post, JC Ballenger (eds), Neurobiology of Mood Disorders. Baltimore: Williams & Wilkins, 1984;629.

310. Coulter JD, Lester BK. Reserpine and sleep. Psychopharmacology 1971;19:134.

311. Weiner N, Molinoff PB. Catecholamines. In GJ Siegel, BW Agranoff, RW Albers, et al. (eds), Basic Neurochemistry (5th ed). New York: Raven, 1994;261.

312. Hilakivi I, Leppavouri A. Effects of methoxamine, an alpha-1 adrenoceptor agonist, and prazosin, an alpha-1 antagonist, on the stages of the sleep-wake cycle in the rat. Acta Physiol Scand 1984;120:363.

313. Oswald I, Adam K, Allen S, et al. Alpha adrenergic blocker, thymoxamine and mesoridazine both increase human REM sleep duration. Sleep Res Abstr 1974;3:62.

314. Cirelli C, Tononi G, Pompeiano M, et al. Modulation of desynchronized sleep through microinjection of $\alpha_1$-adrenergic agonists and antagonists in the dorsal pontine tegmentum of the cat. Pflugers Arch-Eur J Physiol 1992;422:273.

315. Nicholson AN, Pascoe PA. Presynaptic alpha$_2$-adrenoceptor function and sleep in man: Studies with clonidine and idazoxan. Neuropharmacology 1991;30:367.

316. Hilakivi I. The role of beta- and alpha-adrenoreceptors in the regulation of the stages of the sleep-waking cycle in the cat. Brain Res 1983;277:109.

317. Schittecatte M, Charles G, Machowski R, et al. Reduced clonidine rapid eye movement sleep suppression in patients with primary major affective illness. Arch Gen Psychiatry 1992;49:637.

318. Bier MJ, McCarley RW. REM-enhancing effects of the adrenergic antagonist idazoxan infused into the medial pontine reticular formation of the freely moving cat. Brain Res 1994;634:333.

319. Ruch-Monachon MA, Jalfre M, Haefely W. Drugs and PGO waves in the lateral geniculate body of the curarized cat. I. PGO wave activity induced by Ro4-1284 and by p-chlorophenylalanine (PCPA) as a basis for neuropharmacologic studies. Arch Int Pharmacodyn Ther 1976;219:251.

320. Depoorte H. Adrenergic Agonists and Antagonists and Sleep-Wakefulness Stages. In A Wauquier, JM Gaillard, JM Monti, et al. (eds), Sleep: Neurotransmitters and Neuromodulators. New York: Raven, 1985;79.

321. Mignot E, Guilleminault C, Bowersox S, et al. Role of central alpha-1 adrenoceptors in canine narcolepsy. J Clin Invest 1988;82:885.

322. Guilleminault C. Narcolepsy Syndrome. In MH Kryger, T Roth, WC Dement (eds), Principles and Practices of Sleep Medicine. New York: Saunders, 1989;338.

323. Aldrich MS, Rogers AE. Exacerbation of human cataplexy by prazosin. Sleep 1989;12:254.

324. Iwakiri H, Matsuyama K, Mori S. Extracellular levels of serotonin in the medial pontine reticular formation in relation to sleep-wake cycle in cats: a microdialysis study. Neurosci Res 1993;18:157.

325. Kubin L, Reignier C, Tojima H, et al. Changes in serotonin level in the hypoglossal nucleus region during carbachol-induced atonia. Brain Res 1994;645:291.

326. Olsen OE, Neckelmann D, Ursin R. Diurnal differences in L-tryptophan sleep and temperature effects in the rat. Behav Brain Res 1994;65:195.

327. Bjorvatn B, Bjorkum AA, Neckelmann D, et al. Sleep/waking and EEG power spectrum effects of a non-selective serotonin (5-HT) antagonist and a selective 5-HT reuptake inhibitor given alone and in combination. Sleep 1995;18:451.

328. Gao B, Duncan WC Jr, Wehr TA. Fluoxetine decreases brain temperature and REM sleep in Syrian hamsters. Psychopharmacology (Berlin) 1992;106:321.

329. Vasar V, Appelberg B, Rimon R. The effect of fluoxetine on sleep: a longitudinal, double-blind polysomnographic study of healthy volunteers. J Sleep Res 1992: 59.

330. Staner L, Kerkhofs M, Detroux D, et al. Acute, subchronic, and withdrawal sleep EEG changes during treatment with paroxetine and amitriptyline: a double-blind randomized trial in major depression. Sleep 1995;18:470.

331. Muzio JN, Roffwarg HP, Kaufman E. Alterations in the nocturnal sleep cycle resulting from LSD. Electroencephalogr Clin Neurophysiol 1966;21:313.

332. Torda C. Contribution to the serotonin theory of dreaming (LSD infusion). N Y J Med 1968;68:1135.

333. Haigler HJ, Aghajanian GK. Lysergic acid diethylamide and serotonin: a comparison of effects on serotonergic neurons and neurons receiving a serotonergic input. J Pharmacol Exp Ther 1974;188:688.

334. Monti JM, Jantos H, Silveira R, et al. Depletion of brain serotonin by 5,7-DHT: effects on the 8-OH-DPAT–induced changes of sleep and waking in the rat. Psychopharmacology 1992;106:321.

335. Monti JM, Jantos H, Silveira R, et al. Sleep and waking in 5,7-DHT-lesioned or (-)-pindolol-pretreated rats after administration of buspirone, ipsapirone, or gepirone. Pharmacol Biochem Behav 1995;52:305.

336. Dzoljic MR, Ukponmwan OE, Saxena PR. 5-HT$_1$-like receptor agonists enhance wakefulness. Neuropharmacology 1992;31:623.

337. Neckelmann D, Bjorkum AA, Bjorvatn B, et al. Sleep and EEG power spectrum effects of the 5-HT$_{1A}$ antagonist NAN-190 alone and in combination with citalopram. Behav Brain Res 1996;75:159.

338. Quattrochi JJ, Mamelak A, Binder D, et al. Dose-related suppression of REM sleep and PGO waves by the serotonin-1 agonist eltoprazine. Neuropsychopharmacology 1993;8:7.

339. Quattrochi JJ, Mamelak A, Binder D, et al. Dynamic suppression of REM sleep by parenteral administration of the serotonin-1 agonist eltoprazine. Sleep 1992;15:125.

340. Stickgold R, Williams J, Datta S, et al. Suppression of eltoprazine-induced REM sleep rebound by scopolamine. Neuropharmacology 1993;32:447.

341. Sanford LD, Ross RJ, Seggos AE, et al. Central administration of two 5-HT receptor agonists: effect on REM sleep initiation and PGO waves. Pharmacol Biochem Behav 1994;49:93.

342. Portas CM, Thakkar M, Rainnie DG, et al. Microdialysis perfusion of 8-hydroxy-2-(di-n-propylamino)tetralin (8-OH-DPAT) in the dorsal raphe nucleus decreases serotonin release and increases rapid eye movement sleep in the freely moving cat. J Neurosci 1996;16:2820.

343. Ponzoni A, Monti JM, Jantos H. The effects of selective activation of the 5-HT$_3$ receptor with m-chlorophenylbiguanide on sleep and wakefulness in the rat. Eur J Pharmacol 1993;249:259.

344. Ponzoni A, Monti JM, Jantos H, et al. Increased waking after intra-accumbens injection of m-chlorophenylbiguanide: prevention with serotonin or dopamine receptor antagonists. Eur J Pharmacol 1995;278:111.

345. Pavel S. Pineal vasotocin and sleep: involvement of serotonin containing neurons. Brain Res Bull 1979;4:731.

346. Riou F, Cespuglio R, Jouvet M. Endogenous peptides and sleep in the rat. III. The hypnogenic properties of vasoactive intestinal peptide. Neuropeptides 1982;2:265.

347. Prospero-Garcia O, Morales M, Arankowsky-Sandoval G, et al. Vasoactive intestinal polypeptide (VIP) and cerebrospinal fluid (CSF) of sleep-deprived cats restores REM sleep in insomniac recipients. Brain Res 1986;385:169.

348. Jimenez-Anguiano A, Baez-Saldana A, Drucker-Colin R. Cerebrospinal fluid (CSF) extracted immediately after REM sleep deprivation prevents REM rebound and contains vasoactive intestinal peptide (VIP). Brain Res 1993;631:345.

349. Prospero-Garcia O, Jimenez-Anguiano A, Drucker-Colin R. The combination of VIP and atropine induces REM sleep in cats rendered insomniac by PCPA. Neuropsychopharmacology 1993;8:387.

350. el Kafi B, Leger L, Seguin S, et al. Sleep permissive components with the dorsal raphe nucleus in the rat. Brain Res 1995;686:150.

351. Obal F, Payne L, Kacsoh B, et al. Involvement of prolactin in the REM sleep-promoting activity of systemic vasoactive intestinal peptide (VIP). Brain Res 1994;645:143.

352. Danguir J, De Saint-Hilaire-Kafi S. Reversal of desipramine-induced suppression of paradoxical sleep

by a long-acting somatostatin analogue (octreotide) in rats. Neurosci Lett 1989;98:154.

353. Danguir J. Intracerebroventricular infusion of somatostatin selectively increases paradoxical sleep in rats. Brain Res 1986;367:26.

354. Toppila J, Asikainen M, Alanko L, et al. The effect of REM sleep deprivation on somatostatin and growth hormone-releasing hormone gene expression in the rat hypothalamus. J Sleep Res 1996;5:115.

355. Kupfer DJ, Jarrett DB, Ehlers CL. The effect of SRIF on the EEG sleep of normal men. Psychoneuroendocrinology 1992;17:37.

356. Steiger A, Guldner J, Hemmeter U, et al. Effects of growth hormone-releasing hormone and somatostatin on sleep EEG and nocturnal hormone secre-

tion in male controls. Neuroendocrinology 1992; 56:566.

357. Danguir J. The somatostatin analogue SMS 201-995 promotes paradoxical sleep in aged rats. Neurobiol Aging 1989;93:349.

358. Danguir J, De Saint-Hilaire-Kafi S. Scopolamine-induced suppression of paradoxical sleep is reversed by the somatostatin analogue SMS 201-995 in rats. Pharmacol Biochem Behav 1988;30:295.

359. Danguir J, De Saint-Hilaire-Kafi S. Somatostatin antiserum blocks carbachol-induced increase in paradoxical sleep in the rat. Brain Res Bull 1988;20:9.

360. de Lecea L, Criado JR, Prospéro-García O, et al. A cortical neuropeptide with neuronal depressant and sleep-modulating properties. Nature 1996;381:242.

# Chapter 6
# Physiologic Changes in Sleep

## Sudhansu Chokroverty

Awareness about the importance of sleep and its effect on the human organism is growing. Adult humans spend approximately one-third of their lives sleeping, yet we do not have a clear understanding of the functions of sleep. We do know that a vast number of physiologic changes take place during sleep in humans and other mammals. Almost every system in the body undergoes change during sleep—most in the form of reduced activity, although some systems show increased activity. The physiology of wakefulness has been studied intensively, but comparatively little has been written about physiologic changes during sleep. It is important to be aware of these changes in different body systems to understand how they may affect various sleep disorders. A striking example is sleep apnea syndrome, which causes dramatic changes in respiratory control and the upper airway muscles during sleep that direct our attention to a very important pathophysiologic mechanism and a therapeutic intervention for this disorder. Similarly, physiologic changes in several other body systems are important to understanding the pathophysiology of many medical disorders, including disturbances of sleep.

Physiologic changes are known to occur in both the somatic nervous system and the autonomic nervous system (ANS) during sleep. Important changes in the endocrine system and temperature regulation are also associated with sleep. All of these factors have effects that are important for understanding clinical disorders. This chapter provides a review of the physiologic changes in the ANS; the respiratory,

cardiovascular, and neuromuscular systems; and the gastrointestinal tract during sleep. Some attention is also given to thermal and endocrine regulation. For a more detailed discussion, readers are referred to excellent reviews by Orem and Barnes[1] and Lydic and Biebuyck.[2]

## AUTONOMIC NERVOUS SYSTEM AND SLEEP

### Central Autonomic Network

The existence of a central autonomic network in the brain stem with ascending and descending projections that are often reciprocally connected has been clearly shown by work done over the past 20 years (Figures 6-1 and 6-2).[3–8] The nucleus tractus solitarius (NTS) may be considered a central station in the central autonomic network. The NTS, which is located in the dorsal region of the medulla ventral to the dorsal vagal nucleus, is the single most important structure of the autonomic network and is influenced by higher brain stem, diencephalon, forebrain, and neocortical regions (Figure 6-3; see also Figures 6-1 and 6-2). The NTS receives afferent fibers— from the cardiovascular system and the respiratory and gastrointestinal tracts—important for influencing autonomic control of cardiac rhythm and rate, circulation, respiration, and gastrointestinal motility and secretion (Figure 6-4). Efferent projections arise from the NTS and are sent to the supramedullary

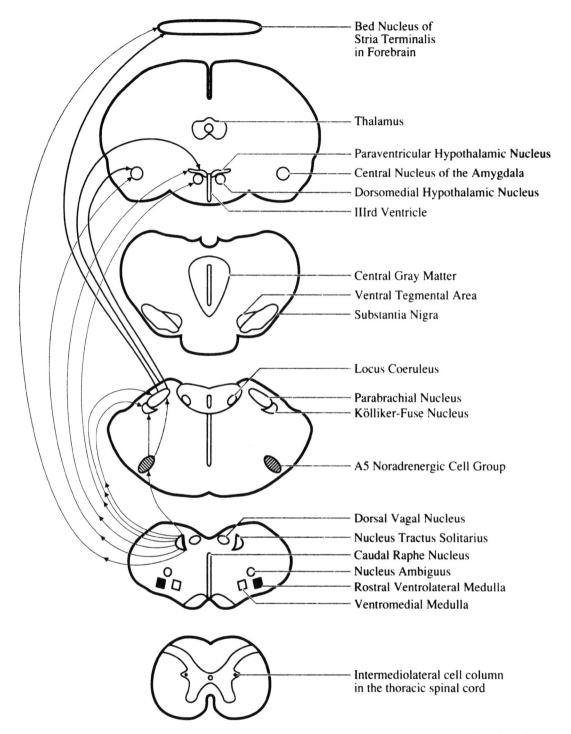

**Figure 6-1.** The ascending projections from the central autonomic network. (Reprinted with permission from S Chokroverty. Functional anatomy of the autonomic nervous system correlated with symptomatology of neurologic disease. In American Academy of Neurology Course No. 246. San Diego: American Academy of Neurology, 1992;49.)

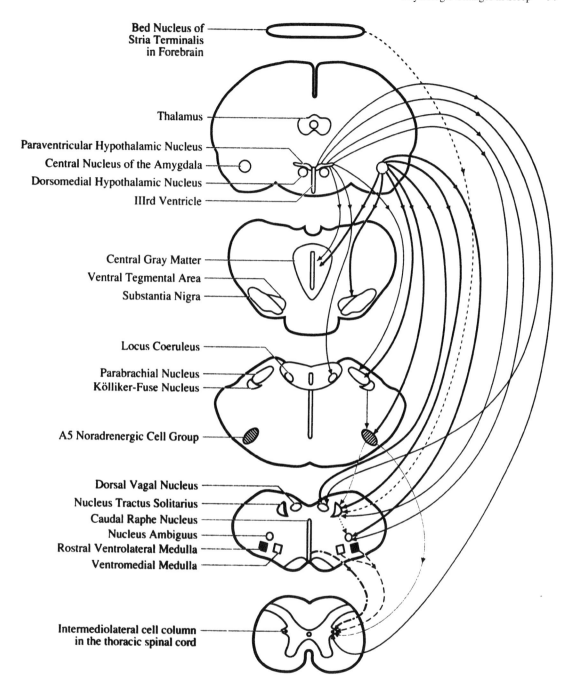

**Figure 6-2.** The descending projections from the central autonomic network. (Reprinted with permission from S Chokroverty. Functional anatomy of the autonomic nervous system correlated with symptomatology of neurologic disease. In American Academy of Neurology Course No. 246. San Diego: American Academy of Neurology, 1992;49.)

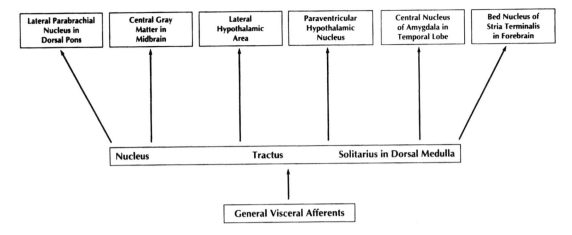

**Figure 6-3.** Schematic diagram of central autonomic network: ascending projections from nucleus tractus solitarius. (Reproduced with permission from S Chokroverty. Functional anatomy of the autonomic nervous system: autonomic dysfunction and disorders of the CNS. In American Academy of Neurology Course No. 144. Boston: American Academy of Neurology, 1991;77.)

structures, including hypothalamic and limbic regions, and to the ventral medulla, which exerts significant control over cardiovascular regulation.[4,9,10] The ventral medulla sends efferent projections to the intermediolateral neurons of the spinal cord (see Figures 6-1 and 6-2). The final common pathways from the NTS are the vagus nerve and sympathetic fibers, which send projections to the intermediolateral neurons of the spinal cord to orchestrate the central autonomic network for integrating various autonomic functions that maintain internal homeostasis. The NTS also contains the lower brain stem hypnogenic and central respiratory neurons. Dysfunction of the ANS, therefore, may have a serious impact on human sleep and respiration.

The cardiovascular system and respiration play significant roles in the maintenance of the internal homeostasis in human beings.[9,10] Cardiovascular control in humans is maintained reflexively, involving peripheral receptors in the heart and blood vessels with afferents to the central nervous system (CNS) and efferents to the heart and blood vessels. Sympathetic preganglionic neurons regulating the cardiovascular system are located predominantly (90%) in the intermediolateral neurons of the thoracic spinal cord, with a small number (10%) in the adjacent spinal structures. Parasympathetic preganglionic neurons controlling the heart and circulation are located in the nucleus ambiguus as well as in

the dorsal motor nucleus of the vagus in the medulla. Sympathetic preganglionic neurons in the intermediolateral column of the spinal cord as well as parasympathetic preganglionic neurons in the nucleus ambiguus and dorsal motor nucleus of the vagus are the central determinants of cardiovascular regulation. Both the sympathetic and parasympathetic preganglionic neurons have extensive connections to the central autonomic network, which in turn is influenced by peripheral afferents (Figure 6-5; see also Figures 6-1 through 6-4). There is direct projection from the hypothalamic paraventricular nucleus to sympathetic preganglionic neurons in the spinal cord (see Figures 6-2 and 6-5).

### Autonomic Changes During Sleep

During sleep in normal individuals, there are profound changes in the functions of the ANS.[3,4,6,11] Most of the autonomic changes that occur during sleep involve the heart, circulation, respiration, and thermal regulation. There are also pupillary changes. Pupilloconstriction occurs during non–rapid eye movement (NREM) sleep and is maintained during REM sleep due to tonic parasympathetic drive. Phasic dilation during phasic REM sleep results from central inhibition of parasympathetic outflow to the iris.

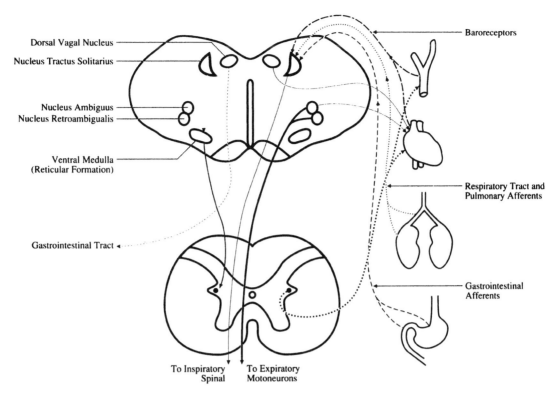

**Figure 6-4.** The visceral afferents to and efferents from the nucleus tractus solitarius. (Reprinted with permission from S Chokroverty. Functional anatomy of the autonomic nervous system correlated with symptomatology of neurologic disease. In American Academy of Neurology Course No. 246, San Diego: American Academy of Neurology, 1992;49.)

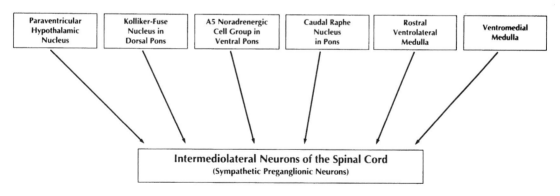

**Figure 6-5.** Schematic diagram to show descending hypothalamic and brain stem inputs to intermediolateral neurons in the spinal cord. (Reprinted with permission from S Chokroverty. Functional anatomy of the autonomic nervous system correlated with symptomatology of neurologic disease. In American Academy of Neurology Course No. 246, San Diego: American Academy of Neurology, 1992;49.)

Autonomic functions during wakefulness must be compared to those during sleep to understand ANS changes in sleep.[6,11] The basic ANS changes during sleep include increased parasympathetic tone and decreased sympathetic activity during NREM sleep. During REM sleep, there is further increase of parasympathetic tone and further decrease of sympathetic activity; intermittently, however, there

Awake

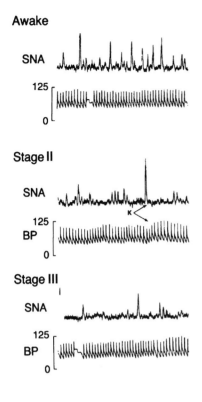

Stage IV

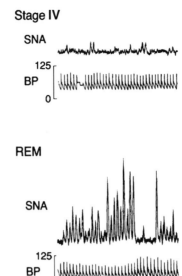

**Figure 6-6.** Sympathetic nerve activity (SNA) and mean blood pressure (BP) recordings in a normal subject while awake and during NREM stages II, III, and IV and during REM sleep. Note gradual decrement of SNA during NREM stages II–IV but profound increase of SNA during REM sleep. Arousal stimuli during stage II NREM sleep elicited K complexes in the EEG (not shown) accompanied by increased SNA. (Reproduced with permission VK Somers, ME Dyken, AL Mark, FM Abboud. Sympathetic nerve activity during sleep in normal subjects. N Engl J Med 1993;328:303.)

is an increase of sympathetic activity during phasic REM sleep.

There is also a profound change of sympathetic activity in muscle and skin blood vessels. Microneurographic technique measures peripheral sympathetic nerve activity in the muscle and skin vascular beds. The technique permits direct intraneural recording of efferent sympathetic nerve activity involving the muscle and skin blood vessels by using tungsten microelectrodes.[12–16]

Muscle sympathetic nerve activity is reduced by more than half from wakefulness to stage IV NREM sleep but increases to levels above waking values during REM sleep.[15] Although sympathetic nerve activity increases in the skeletal muscle vessels (vasoconstriction) during REM sleep, the sympathetic drive decreases in the splanchnic and renal circulation (vasodilation).[15] Sympathetic nerve activity is lower during NREM sleep than during wakefulness but increases above the waking level during REM sleep, particularly during phasic REM sleep (Figures 6-6 and 6-7). During the arousal and appearance of K complexes in NREM sleep, the bursts of sympathetic activity transiently increase (see Figure 6-7).[15]

The implications of changes in the ANS during sleep in humans are profound. Disorders of the ANS in humans, such as multiple system atrophy, familial dysautonomia, and secondary autonomic failure (see Chapter 27), adversely affect respiratory and cardiovascular functions during sleep. A number of human primary sleep disorders may affect autonomic functions (e.g., obstructive sleep apnea [OSA] syndrome, cluster headache, sleep terrors, REM sleep–related sinus arrest and painful penile erections, and sleep-related abnormal swallowing syndrome).

## RESPIRATION AND SLEEP

### Functional Neuroanatomy of Respiration

Legallois[17] discovered in 1812 that breathing depends on a circumscribed region of the medulla. After an intensive period of research on the respiratory centers in the nineteenth century, Lumsden,[18,19] and later Pitts and coworkers,[20] laid the foundation (in the twentieth century) for modern concepts of the central respiratory neuronal networks. Based on sectioning at different

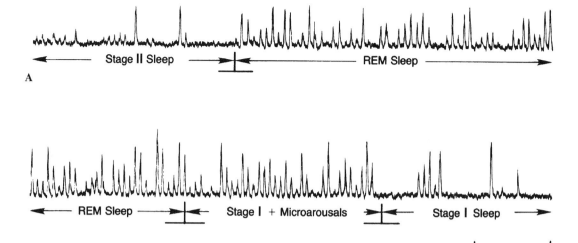

**Figure 6-7.** Changes in sympathetic nerve activity during the transition from NREM sleep stage II to REM sleep (**A**) and the transition from REM sleep to NREM sleep stage I with microarousals, and then to regular NREM sleep stage I (**B**). (Reproduced with permission. Somers VK, Dyken ME, Mark AL, Abboud FM. Sympathetic nerve activity during sleep in normal subjects. N Engl J Med 1993;328:303.)

levels of the brain stem of cats, Lumsden[18,19] proposed pneumotaxic and apneustic centers in the pons and expiratory and gasping centers in the medulla. Later, Pitts' group[20] concluded from experiments with cats that the inspiratory and expiratory centers were located in the medullary reticular formation.

There is a close interrelationship between the respiratory,[21–23] central autonomic,[5,24] and lower brain stem hypnogenic neurons[25–32] in the pontomedullary region. The hypothalamic and the lower brain stem hypnogenic neurons are also connected.[33] Reciprocal connections exist between the hypothalamus, central nucleus of amygdala, parabrachial and Kolliker-Fuse nuclei, and NTS of the medulla (see Figures 6-1 and 6-2).[8,24,34–36] In addition, the NTS connects with the nucleus ambiguus and retroambigualis (see Figure 6-2).[8,34–36] Thus, their anatomic relationships suggest close functional interdependence among the central autonomic network and respiratory and hypnogenic neurons. In addition, peripheral respiratory receptors (arising from the pulmonary and tracheobronchial tree) and chemoreceptors (peripheral and central) interact with the central autonomic network in the region of the NTS.[21–23,37,38]

Breathing is controlled during wakefulness and sleep by two separate and independent systems[22,23,39–42]: the metabolic or automatic,[22,23] and the voluntary or behavioral.[42] Both metabolic and voluntary systems operate during wakefulness, but breathing during sleep is entirely dependent on the inherent rhythmicity of the autonomic (automatic) respiratory control system located in the medulla.[39–41] Voluntary control is mediated through the behavioral system that influences ventilation during wakefulness as well as nonrespiratory functions[43,44] such as phonation and speech. In addition, the wakefulness stimulus, which is probably derived from the ascending reticular activating system,[45,46] represents a tonic stimulus to ventilation during wakefulness. McNicholas and coworkers[47] reported that the reticular arousal system, which is probably the same as the wakefulness stimulus,[45,46,48] exerts a tonic influence on the brain stem respiratory neurons.

Upper brain stem respiratory neurons are located in the rostral pons, in the region of the parabrachial and Kolliker-Fuse nuclei (pneumotaxic center), and in the dorsolateral region of the lower pons (apneustic center).[38] These two centers influence the automatic medullary respiratory neurons, which comprise two principal groups.[21–23,37–41,49,50] The dorsal respiratory group located in the NTS is responsible principally, but not exclusively, for inspi-

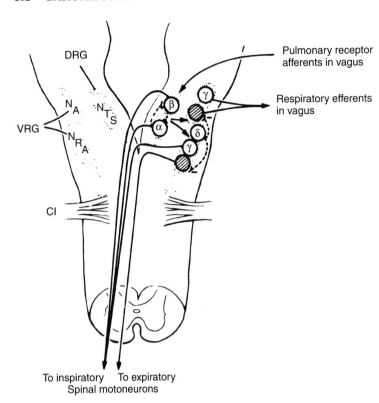

**Figure 6-8.** Schematic diagram of medullary respiratory neurons, cell types, and their interconnections. (DRG = dorsal respiratory group; VRG = ventral respiratory group; NTS = nucleus tractus solitarius; NA = nucleus ambiguus; NRA = nucleus retroambigualis; CI = first cervical root; α, β, γ, δ = designations for inspiratory cell subtypes; open circles = inspiratory cells; hatched circles = expiratory cells.) (Reproduced with permission from AJ Berger, RA Mitchell, JW Severinghaus. Regulation of respiration. N Engl J Med 1977;297:92, 138, 194.)

ration, and the ventral respiratory group located in the region of the nucleus ambiguus and retroambigualis is responsible for both inspiration and expiration (Figure 6-8). These respiratory premotor neurons send axons that decussate below the obex and descend in the reticulospinal tracts in the ventrolateral cervical spinal cord to form synapses with the spinal respiratory motor neurons innervating the various respiratory muscles (see Figures 6-8 and 6-4). Respiratory rhythmogenesis depends on tonic input from the peripheral and central structures converging on the medullary neurons.[18,37,51,52] The parasympathetic vagal afferents from the peripheral respiratory tracts, the carotid and aortic body peripheral chemoreceptors, the central chemoreceptors located on the ventrolateral surface of the medulla lateral to the pyramids, the supramedullary (forebrain, midbrain, and pontine regions), and the reticular activating systems all influence the medullary respiratory neurons to regulate the rate, rhythm, and amplitude of breathing and internal homeostasis.[5,37,38,52] Figure 6-9 shows the effects of various brain stem and vagal transections on ventilatory patterns.

The voluntary control system for breathing originating in the cerebral cortex (forebrain and limbic system) controls respiration during wakefulness and has some nonrespiratory functions.[37,42,52] This system descends with the corticobulbar and corticospinal tracts partly to the automatic medullary controlling system and to some degree both terminates and integrates there, but it primarily descends with the corticospinal tract to the spinal respiratory motor neurons, where the fibers finally integrate with the reticulospinal fibers originating from the automatic medullary respiratory neurons.[22,23,35,41,53]

### Control of Ventilation During Wakefulness

The function of ventilation is to maintain arterial homeostasis (i.e., normal partial pressure of oxygen [$Po_2$] and carbon dioxide [$Pco_2$]).[54] To maintain optimal $Po_2$ and $Pco_2$ levels, the metabolic or autonomic respiratory system uses primarily the peripheral and central chemoreceptors but also to some extent the body's metabolism and the intrapulmonary recep-

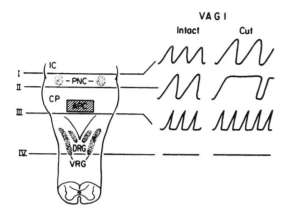

**VAG I**

Intact    Cut

**Figure 6-9.** Effects of various brain stem and vagal (VAG) transections on the ventilatory pattern of the anesthetized animal. On the left is a schematic representation of the dorsal surface of the lower brain stem, and on the right a representation of tidal volume with inspiration upward. Transection I, just rostral to the pneumotaxic center (PNC), causes slow, deep breathing in combination with vagotomy but does not affect normal breathing. Transection II, below PNC but above the apneustic center (APC), causes slow, deep breathing with intact vagi but apneusis (sustained inspiration) or apneustic breathing (increased inspiratory time) when the vagi are cut. Transection III, at the pontomedullary junction, generally causes regular gasping breathing which is not affected by vagotomy. Transection IV, at the medullospinal junction, causes respiratory arrest. (IC = inferior colliculus; CP = cerebellar peduncle; DRG = dorsal respiratory group; VRG = ventral respiratory group.) (Reproduced with permission from AJ Berger, RA Mitchell, JW Severinghaus. Regulation of respiration. N Engl J Med 1977;297:92, 138, 194.)

tors.[54] It is well-known that hypoxia and hypercapnia stimulate breathing.[55,56] Hypoxic ventilatory response is mediated through the carotid body chemoreceptors.[57,58] Normally, this response represents a hyperbolic curve that shows a sudden increase in ventilation when $P_{O_2}$ falls below 60 mm Hg[54,55] (Figure 6-10). On the other hand, hypercapnic[54,56] ventilatory response is linear (see Figure 6-10). This is mediated mainly through the medullary chemoreceptors[59] but also to some extent through the carotid body peripheral chemoreceptors.[57] When $P_{CO_2}$ falls below a certain minimum level, resting ventilation is inhibited.[54] The metabolic rate (e.g., carbon dioxide production [$\dot{V}_{CO_2}$] or oxygen consumption [$\dot{V}_{O_2}$], particularly $\dot{V}_{CO_2}$), affects ventilation in part.[54] During sleep, metabolism slows. The intrapulmonary receptors do not seem to play a major role in normal human ventilation.[54] The Hering-Breuer reflex,

important to respiration, depends on pulmonary stretch receptors. Vagal afferent stimulation by increasing lung inflation terminates inspiration.

### Control of Ventilation During Sleep

In normal persons, during both REM and NREM sleep, clear alterations are noted in tidal volume, alveolar ventilation, blood gases, and respiratory rate and rhythm.[39–42,52,60–65]

### Changes in Ventilation

During NREM sleep, minute ventilation falls by approximately 0.5–1.5 liters per minute,[54,61,63,66–69] and this is secondary to reduction in the tidal volume. REM sleep shows a similar reduction of minute ventilation, up to approximately 1.6 liters per minute.[54,63,67,69–71] Although there is a discrepancy in the literature regarding REM sleep–related ventilation in humans, it is generally accepted that most reduction occurs during phasic REM sleep.

The following factors, in combination, may be responsible for alveolar hypoventilation during sleep[54]: reduction of $\dot{V}_{CO_2}$ and $\dot{V}_{O_2}$ during sleep, absence of the tonic influence of the brain stem reticular formation (i.e., absence of the wakefulness stimulus), reduced chemosensitivity (see Chemosensitivity and Sleep), and increased upper airway resistance to airflow resulting from reduced activity of the pharyngeal dilator muscles during sleep.[67,72,73]

### Changes in Blood Gases

As a result of the fall of alveolar ventilation, the $P_{CO_2}$ rises by 2–8 mm Hg, $P_{O_2}$ decreases by 3–10 mm Hg, and oxygen saturation ($S_{aO_2}$) decreases by less than 2% during sleep.[61,63,64,74,75] These changes occur despite reductions of $\dot{V}_{O_2}$ and $\dot{V}_{CO_2}$ during sleep.[76]

### Respiratory Rate and Rhythm

In NREM sleep the respiratory rate primarily shows a decrement, whereas in REM sleep the respiration becomes irregular, especially during phasic REM.[54] There is also waxing and waning of

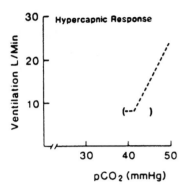

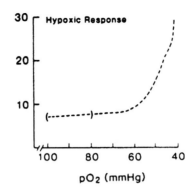

**Figure 6-10.** Schematic representation of normal hypercapnic and hypoxic ventilatory response. Normal ranges are indicated by parentheses. ($PCO_2$ = partial pressure of carbon dioxide; $PO_2$ = partial pressure of oxygen.) (Reproduced with permission from DP White. Central sleep apnea. Clin Chest Med 1985;6:626.)

the tidal volume during sleep onset resembling Cheyne-Stokes breathing,[61,64,77–80] which is related to several factors[54]: sudden loss of wakefulness stimulus, reduced chemosensitivity at sleep onset (see Chemosensitivity and Sleep), and transient arousal. During the deepening stage of NREM sleep, respiration becomes stable and rhythmic and depends entirely on the metabolic controlling system.[39–41,52,54,63]

### Chemosensitivity and Sleep

Hypoxic ventilatory response in humans is decreased in NREM sleep and further decreases during REM sleep (Figure 6-11).[81–84] This reduction could result from two factors: (1) increased upper airway resistance to airflow during all stages of sleep[67,72,73] and (2) decreased chemosensitivity.

Hypercapnic ventilatory response also decreases by approximately 20–50% during NREM sleep[61,64,68,85,86] and further during REM sleep (Figure 6-12).[85,86] This results from a combination of two factors[25]: (1) decreased number of functional medullary respiratory neurons during sleep and (2) increased upper airway resistance.[67,72,73] During sleep, the carbon dioxide response curve shifts to the right so that increasing amounts of $PCO_2$ are needed to stimulate ventilation.[75,79] These findings suggest decreased sensitivity of the central chemoreceptors subserving medullary respiratory neurons during sleep.[5]

### Metabolism and Ventilation During Sleep

There is a definite decrease in $\dot{V}CO_2$ and $\dot{V}O_2$ during sleep.[76,87,88] Metabolism slows suddenly at sleep

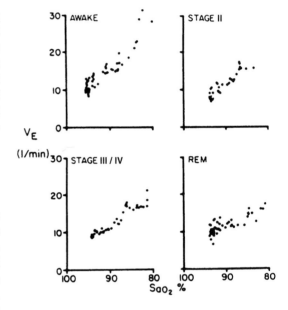

**Figure 6-11.** Hypoxic ventilatory response data show decreased responses during different stages of sleep. ($Sao_2$% = percentage of arterial oxygen saturation; VE = expired ventilation [liter/min]). (Reproduced with permission from NJ Douglas, DP White, JV Weil, et al. Hypoxic ventilatory response decreases during sleep in normal men. Am Rev Respir Dis 1982;125:286.)

onset and accelerates slowly in the early morning at approximately 5:00 AM.[76] During sleep, ventilation falls parallel to metabolism. The rise of $PCO_2$ during sleep, however, is due to alveolar hypoventilation and is not related to reduced metabolism.[54] The role of the intrapulmonary receptors during normal sleep in humans is unknown.[54]

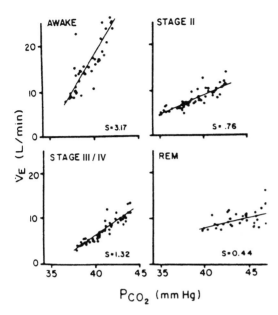

**Figure 6-12.** Hypercapnic ventilatory response data show decreased responses in sleep, the most marked ones in REM sleep. (Reproduced with permission from NJ Douglas, DP White, JV Weil, et al. Hypercapnic ventilatory response in sleeping adults. Am Rev Respir Dis 1982;126:758.)

### Changes in the Upper Airway and in Intercostal Muscle and Diaphragm Tone

Upper airway resistance increases during sleep as a result of hypotonia of the upper airway–dilating muscle[65,67,72,73,89,90] (see Physiologic Changes in the Neuromuscular System, later). There is also hypotonia of the intercostal muscles and atonia during REM sleep. The phasic activities in the diaphragm are maintained, but the tonic activity is reduced during REM sleep.[41] As a result of the supine position and hypotonia of intercostal muscles, the functional residual capacity decreases.[91,92] In most normal individuals, there are circadian changes in airway patency with mild bronchoconstriction during sleep at night.[93,94]

### Arousal Responses During Sleep

Hypercapnia is a stronger arousal stimulus than hypoxemia during sleep. An increase of $P_{CO_2}$ of 6–15 mm Hg causes consistent arousal during

sleep,[83] whereas $Sao_2$ would have to decrease to 75% before arousing a normal person.[81,95]

Laryngeal stimulation normally causes cough reflex response, but this is decreased during both states of sleep and is more markedly decreased during REM than NREM sleep.[96] Thus, clearance of aspirated gastric contents is impaired during sleep. In infants, laryngeal stimulation causes OSA, and this has been postulated as one mechanism for sudden infant death syndrome (SIDS).[97]

### Summary and Conclusions

During wakefulness both metabolic and voluntary control systems are active. In NREM sleep the voluntary system is inactive and respiration is entirely dependent on the metabolic controller—behavioral influences and wakefulness stimuli are not controlling respiration. The nature of ventilatory control during REM sleep has not been determined definitively, but most likely the behavioral mechanism is responsible for controlling breathing in REM sleep. Ventilation is unstable during sleep, and apneas may occur, particularly at sleep onset and during REM sleep. Respiratory homeostasis is thus relatively unprotected during sleep.

The major cause of hypoventilation and reduced ventilatory response to chemical stimuli during sleep is increased airway resistance.[67,72,73,98] The increased resistance results from reduced activity of the pharyngeal dilator muscles as well as decreased output from the sleep-related medullary respiratory neurons.[99] The reduction of the medullary respiratory neuronal activity in sleep causes a loss of the tonic and phasic motor output to the upper airway muscles resulting in an increase in airway resistance. Other factors that contribute to sleep-related hypoventilation include the following[39–41,52,54,100]: reduction of metabolic rate by approximately 10–15%; absence of wakefulness stimuli; reduced chemosensitivity; increased blood flow to the brain during REM sleep, which may depress central chemoreceptor activity; and functional alterations in the CNS during sleep (e.g., cerebral cortical suppression due to reticular inhibition and physiologic cortical deafferentation [presynaptic and postsynaptic inhibition of the afferent neurons[101]] as well as postsynaptic inhibition of motor neurons during REM sleep [see Physiologic Changes in the Neuromuscular System, later]).

Sleep-related changes in breathing may have profound implications in human sleep disorders. Increased upper airway resistance, which is noted during sleep in normal individuals, may predispose to upper airway occlusion and OSA in susceptible individuals.[65] Similarly, the circadian changes of mild brochoconstriction during sleep in normal individuals may be accentuated in patients with asthma, causing a marked decrease in peak flow rate, which may in turn cause severe broncho-spasm.[65,94] As a result of the complex effects of sleep on respiration, there is an overall reduction in ventilation during sleep compared to wakefulness.[65] This may not significantly affect a normal person, but may cause life-threatening hypoxemia and abnormal breathing patterns during sleep in patients with neuromuscular disorders, chronic obstructive pulmonary disease, and bronchial asthma, especially in those with daytime hypoxemia.[65]

## PHYSIOLOGIC CHANGES IN THE HEART AND CIRCULATION DURING SLEEP

Physiologic changes in the heart during sleep include alterations in heart rate and cardiac output. Changes in circulation during sleep include changes in blood pressure (BP), peripheral vascular resistance, and blood flow to various systems and regions.

### Heart Rate

The heart rate decreases during NREM sleep and shows frequent upward and downward swings during REM sleep.[6,11,102–110] Bradycardia during NREM sleep results from a tonic increase in parasympathetic activity (sympathectomy has little effect).[6,102–105] Bradycardia persists during REM sleep and becomes intense owing to tonically reduced sympathetic discharge. Phasic heart rate changes (bradytachycardia) during REM sleep are due to transient changes in both the cardiac sympathetic and parasympathetic activities.[6,102–105] Thus, parasympathetic activity predominates during sleep and an additional decrease of sympathetic activity is observed during REM sleep.

In several studies, the heart rate variability during sleep stages has been documented after spectral analysis.[106–109] The documentation of the high-frequency component of the electrocardiogram clearly indicates the prevalence of parasympathetic activity during both NREM and REM sleep. These studies also show intermittent increases of low-frequency components in the electrocardiogram, indicating intermittent sympathetic nervous system activation during REM sleep. Studies also show that the heart rate acceleration occurs at least 10 beats before the electroencephalogram (EEG) arousal.[106] In another study,[110] a global declining trend was present over successive NREM sleep episodes and over successive REM sleep episodes. A rapid increase of heart rate at the NREM-REM sleep transition was followed by a slow decline starting within the REM episodes. Heart rate variability was higher in REM than in NREM sleep. It was concluded that the global trends and ultradian variations of heart rate may represent sleep state–dependent modulations and circadian variations of the autonomic nervous system.[110]

### Cardiac Output

Cardiac output falls progressively during sleep, the greatest decrement occurring during the last sleep cycle, particularly during the last REM sleep cycle early in the morning.[102,111] This may help explain why normal individuals and patients with cardiopulmonary disease are most likely to die during the hours of early morning.[112] Maximal oxygen desaturation and periodic breathing are also noted at this time.

### Systemic Arterial Blood Pressure

BP falls by approximately 5–14% during NREM sleep and fluctuates during REM sleep.[102,103,113] These changes are related to alterations in the ANS.[6,11] Coote[114] concluded that the fall in BP during NREM sleep was secondary to a reduction in cardiac output, whereas the BP changes during REM sleep resulted from alterations in cardiac output and peripheral vascular resistance.

### Pulmonary Arterial Pressure

Pulmonary arterial pressure rises slightly during sleep. During wakefulness, the mean value is 18/8 mm Hg; during sleep, 23/12 mm Hg.[115]

*Peripheral Vascular Resistance*

During NREM sleep peripheral resistance (PR) remains unchanged or may fall slightly, whereas in REM sleep there is a decrease in PR due to vasodilation.[102,116,117]

*Blood Flow*

Cutaneous, muscular, and mesenteric vascular blood flow shows little change during NREM sleep, but during REM sleep, there is profound vasodilation resulting in increased blood flow in the mesenteric and renal vascular beds.[13–16,102,117,118] However, there is vasoconstriction causing decreased blood flow in the skeletal muscular and cutaneous vascular beds during REM sleep.[13–16,117] Mullen and coworkers[119] reported a decrease of plasma renin activity in humans during REM sleep, which indirectly suggests increased renal blood flow.

Cerebral blood flow (CBF) and cerebral metabolic rate for glucose and oxygen decrease by 5–23% during NREM stages I–IV,[120–127] whereas these values increase to 10% below up to 41% above the waking levels during REM sleep.[121-128] These data indirectly suggest[121] that NREM sleep is the state of resting brain with reduced neuronal activity, decreased synaptic transmission, and depressed cerebral metabolism. In contrast, these data are consistent with the assumption that REM sleep represents active brain state with increased neuronal activity and increased brain metabolism. The largest increases during REM sleep are noted in the hypothalamus and the brain stem structures, and the smallest increases are in the cerebral cortex and white matter. Maquet et al.[129] used positron emission tomography (PET) and statistical parametric mapping to study the brain state associated with REM sleep in seven subjects. They found that regional CBF is positively correlated with REM sleep in the pontine tegmentum, left thalamus, both amygdaloid complexes, the anterior cingulate cortex and the right parietal operculum. They found a negative correlation between regional blood flow and REM sleep in the dorsolateral prefrontal cortex, the parietal cortex (supramarginal gyrus), and the posterior cingulate cortex and precuneus. They concluded that the pattern of activation in the amygdala and the cortical areas provides a biological basis for

the processing of some types of memory during REM sleep. Braun et al.[130] measured CBF with $H_2(15)O$ and PET in 37 normal men during wakefulness, slow-wave sleep (SWS), and REM sleep, while monitoring the subjects polysomnographically throughout the course of a single night. They found profound deactivation during SWS in the centrencephalic regions, including the brain stem, thalamus, and basal forebrain, whereas REM sleep showed marked reactivation in the same areas. They also found similar state-dependent changes in the activity of the limbic and paralimbic areas, including the insula, cingulate, and mesial temporal cortices, during SWS and REM sleep. SWS was associated with selective deactivation of the association areas whereas activity in primary and secondary sensory cortices was preserved. They noted that deactivation of the association areas was common to both SWS and REM sleep states. Regional CBF studies during wakefulness and SWS with PET using the $H_2(15)O$ in human subjects by Hofle et al.[131] noted that delta activity covaried negatively with regional CBF most markedly in the thalamus and also in the brain stem reticular formation, cerebellum, and anterior cingulate and orbitofrontal cortex. They found a positive correlation between delta activity and regional CBF in the visual and auditory cortex, however, which possibly reflected processes of dreamlike mentation thought to occur during SWS.

In summary, these hemodynamic changes in the cardiovascular system result from alterations in the ANS.[6,11,105,114] In general, parasympathetic activity predominates during both NREM and REM sleep and is most predominant during REM sleep. In addition, there is sympathetic inhibition during REM sleep. The sympathetic activity during REM sleep is decreased in cardiac, renal, and splanchnic vessels, but increased in skeletal muscles, owing to an alteration in the brain stem sympathetic controlling mechanism. Furthermore, during phasic REM sleep, BP and heart rate are unstable owing to phasic vagal inhibition and sympathetic activation resulting from changes in brain stem neural activity. Heart rate and BP, therefore, fluctuate during REM sleep. Because of these hemodynamic and sympathetic alterations during REM sleep, which is prominent during the last third of total sleep in the early hours of the morning, the increased platelet aggregability, plaque rupture, and coronary arterial spasm could be initiated, possibly triggering thrombotic events causing myocardial infarction, ventricular arrhythmias, or even sudden cardiac death (see Chapter 29).

## PHYSIOLOGIC CHANGES IN THE NEUROMUSCULAR SYSTEM

Physiologic changes have been noted during sleep in both the somatic nervous system and the ANS that in turn produce changes in the somatic and smooth muscles of the body. This section presents a discussion of the physiologic changes noted during sleep in the somatic muscles, including cranial, limb, and respiratory muscles.

### Changes in Limb and Cranial Muscles

Alterations of limb and cranial muscle tone are noted during sleep. Muscle tone is maximal during wakefulness, slightly decreased in NREM sleep, and markedly decreased or absent in REM sleep. Electromyography (EMG), particularly of the submental muscle, is necessary to identify REM sleep and is thus important for scoring technique. In addition, transient myoclonic bursts are noted during REM sleep. An important EMG characteristic is documentation of periodic limb movements of sleep, which are noted in the majority of patients with restless legs syndrome; patients with a variety of sleep disorders; and normal individuals, most commonly elderly ones.

### Mechanism of Muscle Atonia or Hypotonia in REM Sleep

The dorsal pontine tegmentum appears to be an important central region responsible for limb muscle atonia in REM sleep.[26,132] Axonal projections from this pontine area (peri–locus ceruleus region) containing neurons of the nucleus reticularis pontis oralis via a medial[133] and a lateral tegmentoreticular tract[134] terminate on the medullary reticular formation (gigantocellular and magnocellular regions). Long, descending axons from this area (ventrolateral reticulospinal tract), terminating in the spinal cord,[135,136] cause REM sleep–specific inhibitory postsynaptic potentials (IPSPs) to produce muscle atonia.[137] Lesions of the dorsal pontine tegmentum abolish muscle atonia of REM sleep.[138–140] Similar episodes of REM sleep without muscle atonia have been observed in cats, also with localized lesions in the ventromedial medulla.[141]

Postsynaptic inhibition of the motor neurons is responsible for the atonia of the somatic muscles, as evidenced by intracellular recordings of spinal motor neurons in chronic spinal preparation of cats.[142] There was lumbar motor neuron hyperpolarization of 2–10 mV during REM sleep, and intracellular recordings revealed increased number and appearance of REM sleep–specific IPSPs in the lumbar motor neurons of cats.[143,144] These potentials are derived from inhibitory interneurons, possibly located either in the spinal cord or in the brain stem, from which long axons project to the spinal motor neurons.[143,145] These REM sleep–specific IPSPs are responsible for muscle atonia in REM sleep.[146] The neurotransmitter for mediation of such IPSPs appears to be glycine, not γ-aminobutyric acid (GABA).[146] The glycine antagonist strychnine, administered by microiontophoresis near the motor neurons, antagonizes the IPSP; the GABA antagonists picrotoxin and bicuculline do not. The identity of the individual interneurons in the spinal cord remains unknown—they could be Ia-inhibitory neurons but they are not Renshaw cells.

The IPSPs in the cranial motor neurons are also most likely strychnine sensitive, and a neurotransmitter could be GABA-B.[146]

### Upper Airway Muscles and Sleep

Changes occur in the function of the upper airway muscles during sleep that have important clinical implications, particularly for patients with sleep apnea syndrome. Upper respiratory tract subserves both respiratory and nonrespiratory functions.[147] In experimental studies in cats, pharyngeal motor neurons in the vagus and glossopharyngeal nerves were located in the medulla, overlapping the medullary respiratory neurons.[148] The experimental study by Bianchi and colleagues[149] demonstrated that after changes induced by chemical stimuli (normocapnic hypoxia and normoxic hypercapnia), pharyngeal motor activities are more sensitive than phrenic nerve activation. The influence of sleep on respiratory muscle function has been reviewed by Gothe et al.[150] and Horner.[151]

## Genioglossus Muscle

Genioglossal EMG activities consist of phasic inspiratory bursts and variable tonic discharges, which are decreased during NREM sleep and further decreased during REM sleep.[152–155] Selective reduction of genioglossal or hypoglossal nerve activity (i.e., disproportionately more reduction than the diaphragmatic or phrenic activities) has been noted with alcohol, diazepam, and many anesthetic agents.[152] On the other hand, protriptyline and strychnine each selectively increases such activity.[152]

## Palatal Muscles

Levator veli palatini and palatoglossus muscles in humans show phasic inspiratory and tonic expiratory activities,[156,157] but tensor veli palatini muscle shows tonic activity during both inspiration and expiration in wakefulness and sleep.[158,159] During sleep in normal individuals, palatal muscles (palatoglossus, tensor veli palatini, and levator veli palatini) show decreased tone causing increased upper airway resistance and decreased airway space.[158]

## Masseter Muscle

Masseter contraction closes the jaw and elevates the mandible. In sleep apnea patients, masseter activation is present during eupneic episodes but decreased during apneic ones. Masseter EMG activity decreases immediately before the apnea, is absent during the early part of the episode, and increases at the end of the apneic period.[160] Based on experiments using chemical stimuli, Suratt and Hollowell[160] concluded that masseter activity can be increased by hyperoxic hypercapnia and inspiratory resistance loading. It appears that phasic EMG bursts start in the masseter at the same time as in the genioglossus and the diaphragm. Suratt and Hollowell[160] did not find phasic activity in masseter muscle in normal subjects during regular breathing, but noted such activity during inspiratory stimulation such as inspiratory resistance loading or hypercapnia. In sleep apnea patients, spontaneous phasic masseter activity was noted during regular breathing.

## Intrinsic Laryngeal Muscle Activity

Intrinsic laryngeal muscles, controlled by the brain stem neuronal mechanism, play an important role in the regulation of breathing.[161] In addition, the larynx participates in phonation, deglutition, and airway protection.[162] The posterior cricoarytenoid (PCA) muscle is the main vocal cord abductor. Laryngeal EMG can be performed by placing hooked wire electrodes percutaneously through the cricothyroid membrane.[163]

PCA demonstrates phasic inspiratory bursts in normal subjects during wakefulness and NREM sleep.[161] In addition, there is tonic expiratory activity in wakefulness that disappears with NREM sleep. In REM sleep, PCA EMG shows fragmented inspiratory bursts and variable expiratory activity. During isocapnic hypoxia and hyperoxic hypercapnia, normal subjects show increased phasic inspiratory PCA activity but minimal increase of tonic expiratory activity.[161]

## Hyoid Muscles

Suprahyoid muscles (those inserted superiorly on hyoid bone) include geniohyoid, mylohyoid, hyoglossus, stylohyoid, and digastric muscles.[164] Infrahyoid muscles (those that insert inferiorly) include sternohyoid, omohyoid, and sternothyroid muscles.[164] It should be noted that the size and shape of the upper airways can be altered by movements of the hyoid bone. Motor neurons supplying these muscles are located in the pons, the medulla, and the upper cervical spinal cord. The hyoid muscles show inspiratory bursts during wakefulness and NREM sleep that are increased by hypercapnia. According to van Lunteren,[164] the relative contribution of hyoid, genioglossus, and other tongue muscles in the maintenance of pharyngeal patency needs to be clarified.

## REM Sleep–Related Alterations in Respiratory Muscle Activity

During REM sleep, activity of upper airway muscle and the diaphragm is reduced. Three types of REM sleep–related alterations in the respiration muscles have been described[165]: (1) *Atonia* of EMG activity throughout the REM sleep period is found. Somatic muscles characteristically show this response, which is related to glycine-mediated post-synaptic inhibition of motor neurons.[146] (2) Rhythmic activity of the diaphragm persists in REM sleep, but certain diaphragmatic motor units cease firing. Kline and coworkers[166] recently described *intermittent decrement of diaphragmatic activity* during single breaths. Upper airway muscles also show similar changes. (3) *Fractionations of diaphragmatic activity* refer to pauses lasting 40–80 msec and occur in clusters correlated with PGO (pontine-geniculate-occipital) waves, which are phasic events of REM sleep.[167]

What is the mechanism of muscle atonia in the upper airway muscles during REM sleep? Based on animal experiments, it is clearly established that glycine-mediated postsynaptic inhibition of the lumbar motor neurons (causing hyperpolarization) gives rise to somatic muscle atonia. Similar, postsynpatic inhibition (glycine- or GABA-mediated) has been postulated for trigeminal[168,169] but not for hypoglossal[170] motor neurons. The mechanism of dysfacilitation has been postulated as playing a major role in hypoglossal motor neuron activities causing decrement of genioglossal muscle activity during carbachol-induced REM sleep in animals.[151,171–173] Caudal raphe serotonergic neurons[174–176] and locus coeruleus noradrenergic neurons,[177,178] or "REM-off" neurons, have strong excitatory input to the hypoglossal neurons. The REM-off neurons shut off the activity during REM sleep, causing dysfacilitation of the hypoglossal motor neurons. A role for GABA- or glycine-mediated postsynaptic inhibition cannot be completely excluded.

### Upper Airway Reflexes

The negative intrathoracic pressure at the onset of inspiration generates a reflex response (increased activity) to the upper airway dilator muscles. During sleep, such reflex responses are decreased, making the upper airway susceptible to suction collapse.[151] This probably results from a decrement in the excitability of the upper airway motor neurons. In this connection, the observations of McNicholas et al.[179] of increased frequency of obstructive apneas and hypopneas in normal sleeping subjects after upper airway anesthesia and increased apnea index after upper airway anesthesia in snorers[180] support the importance of the upper airway reflexes in controlling the upper airway resistance and space. However, there is no clear indication of the impairment of upper airway reflex in OSA. Patients with OSA, in contrast to snorers and normal sleepers, do not show an increase in apnea index after upper airway anesthesia.[181,182] Alcohol, benzodiazepines, and age[151,183] clearly cause a decrement in upper airway reflex response.

### Summary and Clinical Relevance

There is considerable reduction of the activity of the upper airway dilator muscles during NREM sleep, with further reduction in REM sleep, causing increased upper airway resistance and narrowing of the upper airway space. The site of the upper airway obstruction in OSA is usually at the level of the soft palate, but in approximately half the patients the obstruction extends caudally to the region of the tongue, with further caudal extension during REM sleep.[151,184–191] Therefore, decreased tone in the palatal, genioglossal, and other upper airway muscles causing increased upper airway resistance and decreased airway space plays an important role in contributing upper airway obstruction in OSA, particularly because many OSA patients have smaller upper airways than individuals without OSA.[151,192–194]

## GASTROINTESTINAL PHYSIOLOGY DURING SLEEP

A brief summary of the physiology of the gastrointestinal tract during sleep is given in this section. For a more detailed discussion, readers are referred to Orr.[195] Gastrointestinal changes include alterations in gastric acid secretion, gastric volume and motility, swallowing, and esophageal peristalsis and intestinal motility.

Studying the physiology of the gastrointestinal system has been difficult traditionally, because of the lack of adequate technique. Techniques as well as facilities for making simultaneous polysomnographic (PSG) recordings are now available, allowing study of the alterations in gastrointestinal physiology during different stages of sleep. Before the advent of these techniques, scattered reports generally showed decreased motor and secretory functions during sleep. Subsequent methods have produced better and more consistent results, although findings are still somewhat contradictory overall. There is a dearth of adequate studies using PSG and other modern techniques to understand the physiologic alterations of gastrointestinal motility and secretions during sleep.

### Gastric Acid Secretion

During wakefulness, gastric acid secretion depends on food ingestion, increased salivation, and the activity of the gastric vagus nerve. Moore and Englert[196] showed a clear circadian rhythm for gastric acid secretion in humans. These authors noted peak gastric acid secretion between 10:00 PM and 2:00 AM in patients with duodenal ulcer. Acid secretion increases considerably during the day and at night.[197,198] The importance of vagal stimulation for the control of circadian oscillation of gastric acid secretion has been demonstrated by the absence of circadian rhythm for gastric acid secretion following vagotomy.[199]

Several studies have attempted to understand gastric acid secretion during different stages of sleep, but the results have not been consistent because of methodologic flaws and cumbersome techniques.[200–202] An important study was made by Orr and colleagues,[203] who examined five duodenal ulcer patients for five consecutive nights using PSG technique and continuous aspiration of gastric contents. They found no relationship between acid secretion and different stages of sleep or REM versus NREM sleep. The most striking finding was failure of inhibition of acid secretion during the first 2 hours of sleep, a result that agrees with the previous study by Levin and associates.[197]

### Gastric Motility

Findings regarding gastric motility have been contradictory. Both inhibition and enhancement of gastric motility have been noted during sleep.[204–206] In 1922, Wada[207] described cyclic gastric contractions in normal subjects during wakefulness and sleep. Finch and coworkers[208] later showed that gastroduodenal motility during sleep was related to sleep-stage shifts and body movements. Orr[195] reported that, although no definite statement regarding gastric motility can be made, there seems to be overall inhibition of gastric motor function during sleep.

### Esophageal Function

Swallowing is suppressed during sleep, particularly in stages III and IV of NREM sleep,[209–211] resulting in prolonged mucosal contact with refluxed acid. Johnson and DeMeester[212] considered prolonged acid clearance an important factor in the pathogenesis of esophagitis caused by nocturnal gastroesophageal reflux (GER). Salivary flow, which is important for acid neutralization, also is decreased during sleep,[195] a phenomenon that contributes to prolonged acid clearance.[213] In normal subjects during wakefulness, reflux may occur in the upright position, mainly postprandially, and these episodes are terminated in less than 4 minutes.[212] Studies by Orr and colleagues[209,213] clearly show that the arousal response associated with swallowing during sleep prevents prolonged acid clearance and GER during sleep in normal subjects. In normal individuals who experience episodes of GER, there is generally a reduction in lower esophageal sphincter pressure.[214] The availability of the method to measure GER during sleep by esophageal pH monitoring[215] has advanced understanding of swallowing and esophageal function during sleep.

### Intestinal Motility

Although methods are now available to accurately measure intestinal motility, the results of motility studies during sleep are contradictory.[195] A special pattern of motor activity, called *migrating motor complex* (MMC), recurs every 90 minutes in the stomach and small intestine.[216] This periodicity of the gut motor activity is similar to the cyclic REM-NREM sleep. In fact, a circadian rhythm in the propagation of the MMC has been documented with the slowest velocity occurring during sleep.[216–220] There are no clear changes in the MMC distribution between REM and NREM sleep stages. Consistent abnormalities in the MMC in different bowel diseases have not been documented.

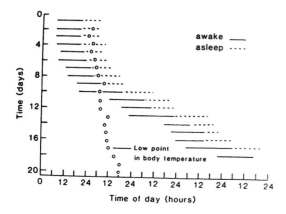

**Figure 6-13.** Synchronized (light-entrained) and desynchronized (free-running) rhythms in a person showing dissociation between body temperature and sleep-activity cycles. (Reproduced with permission from J Aschoff. Desynchronization and resynchronization of human circadian rhythms. Aerospace Med 1969;40:847.)

## THERMAL REGULATION IN SLEEP

### Changes in Body Temperature and Circadian Rhythm

That body temperature follows a circadian rhythm independent of the sleep-wake rhythm[221] has been demonstrated in experiments involving desynchronization and resynchronization of human circadian rhythms. It has been shown that when all environmental cues (*Zeitgebers*) are removed, the endogenous rhythms are freed from the influence of exogenous rhythms and a free-running rhythm ensues. During this time, it is clear that body temperature has a rhythm independent of the sleep-wake rhythm (Figure 6-13).[222] Nevertheless, body temperature has been linked intimately to the sleep-wake cycle.[223] Body temperature begins to fall with the onset of sleep, and the lowest temperature is noted during the third sleep cycle.[224,225]

### Role of REM Sleep in Thermal Regulation

During REM sleep, the thermoregulating mechanism appears to be inoperative.[223,226,227] Body temperature increases during REM sleep, and cyclic changes in the temperature occur throughout this period. Thermoregulatory responses such as sweating and panting are noted in NREM sleep, but are absent in REM sleep; in fact, animals display a state of poikilothermia during REM sleep. Brain temperature rises during REM sleep. Szymusiak and McGinty[228] speculated that REM sleep, by elevating brain temperature or by reversing the cooling trend in SWS, prepares the body for behavioral activation. It should be noted that the loss of thermoregulation in REM sleep is not related to inhibition of motor control but is determined by central integration or thermoafferent pathways, or may be due to both mechanisms.[223]

### Mechanism of Thermoregulation in Sleep

The function of sleep appears to be energy conservation, as evidenced by a reduction in body temperature and metabolism during sleep, especially NREM sleep.[224,225,229] Sleep onset in humans is associated with a reduction of body temperature of 1–2°C accompanied by heat loss due to vasodilation and increased sweating. These changes appear to be related to reduced thermal sensitivity of the preoptic nucleus of the hypothalamus.[229] MacFadyen and colleagues[230] observed increased SWS after 2–3 days of fasting in humans, suggesting that the length of hypometabolism helps conserve energy. Increased body temperature[231] and hypothalamic heating[232] are associated with increased SWS. If the body temperature is elevated during the waking periods, SWS increases.[233,234] SWS is accompanied by a drop in body and brain temperature. According to Aschoff,[221] the independent circadian rhythm of body temperature is unrelated to a reduction of motor activities at sleep onset. Exercise, a hot bath, and facial warming all increase SWS 4–5 hours later in response to heat loads.[235–238] Thus, sleep is controlled by thermoregulatory processes. The medial preoptic-anterior hypothalamic (POAH) neurons participate in both NREM sleep and thermoregulation.[235,239] McGinty and Szymusiak[235] cited the following evidence in support of this hypothesis: POAH warming will facilitate SWS, whereas lesions will suppress it; microinjection of putative sleep factors into POAH will promote SWS. Based on experiments in cats, Szymusiak and McGinty[228,240] hypothesized that the neuronal mechanisms in the POAH region are responsible for both thermal regulation and SWS generation and that SWS is essentially a thermoregulatory process. Although thermoregulation and sleep are clearly linked, they are also clearly separate.[241]

### Clinical Relevance

There are clinical implications for understanding thermoregulation in sleep. Jet lag and shift work may disrupt this linkage of thermoregulation and SWS generation and change the rhythms of sleep and body temperature, which may cause difficulty in initiating and maintaining sleep and disorganization of sleep architecture and daytime function.[223] Menopausal hot flashes are thought to be a disorder of thermoregulation initiating within the POAH. Woodward and Freedman[242] performed 24-hour ambulatory recordings of hot flashes and all night sleep characteristics on 12 postmenopausal women with hot flashes and seven without hot flashes to determine the effect of hot flashes on sleep patterns. They found that hot flashes were associated with increased stage IV sleep and that hot flashes occurring in the 2 hours before sleep onset were positively correlated with the amount of SWS. They concluded that the central thermoregulatory mechanism underlying hot flashes may affect hypnogenic pathways, inducing sleep and heat loss in the absence of a thermal load in these patients. It has been suggested that environmental temperature and hyperthermia play a role in SIDS.[243] However, multiple factors (e.g., sleep-related respiratory dysrhythmias and CNS disorders, particularly in the region of the arcuate nucleus in the medulla) are implicated in SIDS, and the primary cause of the syndrome remains unknown. Finally, it has been suggested that thermoregulatory dysfunction may cause sleep disturbance in patients with depression[244] but there is no compelling evidence to support this assumption.

## ENDOCRINE REGULATION IN SLEEP

Neuroendocrine secretion appears to be under circadian control—that is, it shows circadian rhythm in the plasma concentrations of the hormones. The characteristic pattern of endocrine gland secretion is episodic or pulsatile secretion every 1–2 hours, which suggests ultradian rhythmicity. Hormone secretion thus depends on the stages of sleep and time of day. Changes in the secretion of some major

hormones during sleep are described in the following paragraphs. Figure 6-14 shows a schematic of the patterns of neuroendocrine secretion during sleep in an adult human.

### Growth Hormone

Takahashi and colleagues[245] observed that the plasma concentration of growth hormone (GH) peaks 90 minutes after sleep onset in seven of eight normal subjects and lasts approximately 1.5–2.5 hours. The peak is related to SWS (stages III and IV of NREM sleep). Several subsequent reports showed nocturnal peaks of GH in association with SWS.[246–251] Although the major peak in plasma GH occurs during the early part of nocturnal sleep, it has been shown that in approximately one-fourth of young, healthy men, peaks in circulating GH occur before sleep onset.[251] Sleep deprivation causes suppression of GH secretion, which may be an age-dependent phenomenon that develops during early childhood. The sleep-related release of GH is absent before age 3 months and is reduced in old age.[250,252–254] It should be noted that GH secretion is regulated physiologically by opposite actions of GH-releasing hormone and somatostatin.[255] It has been suggested that somatostatin may induce sleep deterioration in the elderly.[255] Van Cauter and Plat[254] suggested that age-related decrements in GH secretion play a major role in the hyposomatotropism of senescence. The timing of the release of GH shifts if sleep is phase-advanced or -delayed, suggesting a close relationship between episodic GH secretion and sleep.[256] Sadamatsu et al.[257] measured 24-hour rhythms of plasma GH, prolactin, and thyroid-stimulating hormone (TSH) in nine normal adult men by means of serial blood sampling at 30-minute intervals. Their findings suggested two mechanisms regulating GH secretion: one that is sleep-independent and has an ultradian rhythm and another that is sleep-dependent.

There is some evidence of possible circadian influences on the regulation of GH secretion from a jet lag study by Goldstein and associates[258] and a study of GH secretory rate in night workers by Weibel et al.[259] Increased GH secretion has been noted after flights both eastward and westward.[258]

The tightly linked normal relationship between GH and SWS is disrupted during sleep disturbances. For example, in narcolepsy,[260] depression

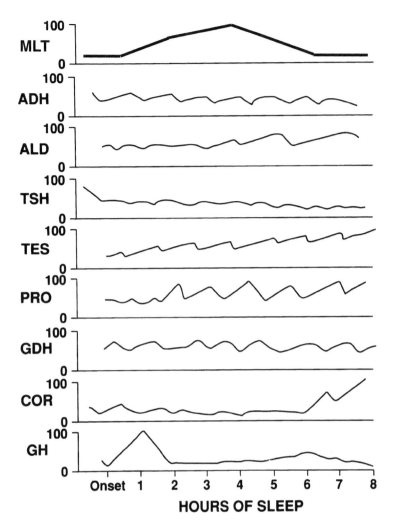

**Figure 6-14.** Schematic representation of the plasma levels of hormones in an adult during 8 hours of sleep. Zero indicates lowest secretory episode and 100 indicates peak. (MLT = melatonin; ADH = antidiuretic hormone; ALD = aldosterone; TSH = thyroid-stimulating hormone; TES = testosterone; PRO = prolactin; GDH = gonadotropic hormone; COR = cortisol; GH = growth hormone.) (Modified from R Rubin. Sleep endocrinology studies in man. Prog Brain Res 1975;42:73.)

HOURS OF SLEEP

of GH secretion is associated with sleep disturbance, and in some cases of insomnia,[261] there is a dissociation between SWS and GH secretion. Such dissociation also occurs in old age.[250,262,263] These findings suggest that there are independent mechanisms for controlling GH secretion and SWS. It is interesting to note that such a tight relationship is observed only in humans and baboons and not in rhesus monkeys and dogs,[264] a fact that may relate to the monophasic sleep patterns observed in baboons and humans.[265]

In acromegaly patients, GH secretion remains high throughout sleep and has no relationship to sleep onset or SWS.[266,267] Diminished, sleep-related secretion of GH is found in both sleep apnea and narcolepsy.[268] The pattern of GH secretion associated with clinical depression is contradictory: Both impairment and normal sleep-related GH secretion have been noted.[261,269,270] GH secretion is somewhat disturbed in alcoholics.[271] Schizophrenia, alcoholism, and depression in adults are associated with impaired sleep-related GH secretion.[270] Whether the impairment is related to an associated decrease in SWS or abnormalities of biogenic amine metabolism in these disorders cannot be stated with certainty. Cushing's syndrome is associated with decreased SWS and GH secretion. Nocturnal GH secretion was found to be higher than normal and SWS increased in two patients with thyrotoxicosis.[272] These abnormal findings normalized in response to antithyroid medication.

### Adrenocorticotropic Hormone and Cortisol Secretion

Adrenocorticotropic hormone (ACTH) stimulates cortisol secretion by the adrenal cortex. ACTH-cortisol secretion appears to be under circadian influence and is inhibited by sleep. The cortisol level is generally lowest in the early hours of sleep and highest in the early morning hours, from approximately 4:00 to 8:00 AM.[273–277] The inhibitory influence of early nocturnal sleep on pituitary-adrenal activity as evidenced by ACTH-cortisol levels is most marked during SWS.[275] Alford and coworkers[278] and Jacoby and colleagues,[279] however, documented both a circadian and an ultradian episodic pattern of secretion for cortisol and ACTH. It should be noted, however, that in contrast to nocturnal sleep, daytime sleep failed to significantly inhibit cortisol secretion, suggesting that sleep does not suppress cortisol release at any point of its circadian rhythm, but only within a limited range of entrainment.[280,281]

In general, the circadian rhythm of cortisol secretion remains undisturbed in disease states such as Cushing's syndrome and narcolepsy.[270] With depression, the earlier occurrence of the lowest point of cortisol levels is thought to indicate a circadian phase advance.[282] The failure of dexamethasone to suppress cortisol secretion in depressed persons is not necessarily positively correlated with reduced REM latencies noted in depression.[283] Sleep deprivation itself may be responsible for such failure, as is noted in normal individuals.[284]

### Prolactin Secretion

Plasma prolactin concentration has long been known to exhibit a sleep-dependent pattern, with the highest levels occurring during sleep and the lowest during waking.[270,285–287] The plasma prolactin level does not seem to have a definite circadian rhythm; it appears to be linked to sleep,[285,286] but is not related to specific sleep stages.[270] The prolactin level begins to rise approximately 60–90 minutes after sleep onset and peaks in the early morning hours from approximately 5:00 to 7:00 AM.[288] Studies by Mendelson

and coworkers,[270,289] Rubin et al.,[290] and Van Cauter and colleagues[291] clearly show no relationship between prolactin secretion and NREM-REM cycles. Subsequent studies, however, have clearly shown that prolactin secretion is also driven by a sleep-independent circadian pattern.[292,293] Waldstreicher et al.[292] studied 12 men and 10 women using a constant routine protocol, during which the subjects remained in semirecumbent wakefulness. The authors clearly documented a robust, sleep-independent, endogenous circadian rhythm of prolactin secretion in humans. The authors hypothesized that the endogenous components of the circadian rhythm of prolactin secretion, along with body temperature; urine production; and cortisol, TSH, and melatonin secretion, are driven by a central circadian pacemaker located in the suprachiasmatic nucleus of the hypothalamus.[292]

Prolactin secretion is suppressed by dopamine but stimulated by thyrotropin-releasing hormone.[270] Although prolactin secretion is related to sleep, the secretory pattern of prolactin does not decline with age like that of GH.[294]

### Gonadotropic Hormone (Gonadotropin)

The gonadotropin-releasing hormone (GnRH) produced by the hypothalamus stimulates the anterior pituitary gland to secrete leuteinizing hormone (LH) and follicle-stimulating hormone (FSH). In men, LH is the stimulus for the secretion of testosterone by the testes, and FSH stimulates spermatogenesis. In women, the ovarian hormones estrogen and progesterone are secreted by the ovaries in response to LH and FSH, which also are responsible for ovarian changes during the menstrual cycle. It has been difficult to study the relationship between FSH and LH plasma levels because of the limitations of assay sensitivity in measurements and the inaccuracies associated with pulsatile secretion of circulating gonadotropin. A clear relationship between FSH and LH plasma levels and the sleep-wake cycle or sleep stages in children or adults has not been found. In pubertal boys and girls, however, gonadotropin levels increase during sleep.[295–298] By using an ultrasensitive immunofluorometric assay to measure plasma LH and deconvolution analysis to depict LH secretory characteristics, it has been possible to show an increase in sleep-associated

GnRH and LH secretion during puberty and prepubertal stage.[299]

FSH and LH show pulsatile activities throughout the night without showing any relationship to testosterone secretion. During sleep early in puberty,[295] however, there is a marked rise of plasma LH concentration, in contrast to testosterone or prolactin. LH and FSH secretion show no distinct circadian rhythms. Plasma testosterone levels rise at sleep onset and continue to rise during sleep at night.[300] Based on the observation that LH and prolactin secretion precede testosterone secretion by 60–80 minutes, Rubin[265] suggested a relationship between these hormones.

### Thyroid-Stimulating Hormone

A distinct circadian rhythm has been established for the secretion of TSH in normal humans.[278,301,302] There is general agreement that TSH levels are low during the daytime, increase in the evening, peak shortly before sleep onset, and are inhibited by sleep.[250,270,302–304] However, TSH secretion does not depend on any specific sleep stage.[305] Exposure to bright light in the early evening can delay the TSH circadian rhythm, whereas exposure late at night or in the early morning can advance it.[250,304]

### Miscellaneous Hormones

Aldosterone shows a maximal rise just before a sleeper awakes.[306] Antidiuretic hormone shows episodic secretion without any relationship to sleep or sleep stages.[306] Plasma renin activity shows a marked drop during REM sleep.[119] Spectral analysis of the sleep EEG has shown that an increase in slow waves during sleep is associated with an increase in plasma renin activity, and a decrease in slow waves is associated with a decrease in plasma renin activity. This suggests a common mechanism controlling both slow-wave activity in EEG during sleep and renin released from the kidney.[307] Renin is a hormone secreted by the juxtaglomerular cells of the kidneys under the influence of the sympathetic nervous system, circulation, blood volume, and systemic BP.

In normal persons, nocturnal urine volume decreases owing to decreased glomerular filtration, alteration of renin release, and increased reabsorption of water.[308] Brandenberger and coworkers[309,310] demonstrated that 24-hour variations in plasma renin activity are not circadian in nature but are related to sleep processes and are dependent on the regularity and the length of the sleep cycles in an ultradian manner.

Kripke and associates[311] studied parathyroid hormone (PTH) in seven normal subjects for eight nights in the sleep laboratory. Plasma samples were obtained at 10- to 20-minute intervals for PTH and calcium determinations. PTH peaks tended to occur every 100 minutes, and PTH concentration was significantly related to cycles of stages III and IV NREM sleep. Total plasma calcium, however, was significantly related to cycles of REM and stage II NREM sleep.

### Melatonin

There has been a resurgence in the study of melatonin because of its possible role in circadian rhythm regulation, its generation by the suprachiasmatic nucleus (SCN), and its hypnotic effect. Melatonin is a hormone synthesized in the pineal gland, which lies in the center of the brain behind the third ventricle.[312–317] The hormone is not stored in the pineal gland but is released directly into the bloodstream or the cerebrospinal fluid. The precursor of melatonin is the circulating amino acid L-tryptophan. Tryptophan is converted to 5-hydroxytryptophan by the enzyme tryptophan hydroxylase and this is then decarboxylated to serotonin. The serotonin is catalyzed by acetyltransferase and hydroxyindole-o-methyltransferase, then converted into melatonin (N-acetyl-5-methoxytryptamine).[312–317] Melatonin is inactivated in the liver after conversion to 6-hydroxymelatonin, most of which is excreted in the urine and feces as a sulfate conjugate (6-sulfatoxymelatonin).[314,317] Evidence indicates that the environmental light-dark cycle and the SCN act in concert to produce the daily rhythm of melatonin production.[312–317] The neural pathway involved in this process includes the retinohypothalamic tract from the retinal ganglion cells to the SCN, efferent fibers from the SCN to the superior cervical ganglia through multiple synaptic connections, and the postganglionic efferent fibers from the superior cervical ganglia to the pineal gland.[312–317] This entire neural pathway is activated during the night, triggering melatonin production that is suppressed by exposure to bright light. A circadian rhythm generated by the rhythmic SCN output is responsible for the melatonin circadian rhythm.[314,315,317,318] The maximum nocturnal secretion of melatonin has been observed in young children aged 1–3 years; secretion begins to fall around puberty and decreases significantly in the elderly.[318–320] Melatonin begins to rise in the evening, attaining the maximum values between 3:00 and 5:00 AM, then decreasing to low levels during the day.[312–314,317]

Because of the important effect of melatonin on circadian rhythms and its possible hypnotic effect, there have been a few clinical applications of melatonin that appear promising. Placebo-controlled, double-blind studies using a large number of subjects need to be performed, however, before accepting melatonin as a treatment for various sleep disorders. Administration of melatonin has been shown to have some beneficial effects on the symptoms of jet lag[317,321] and on nighttime alertness and daytime sleep of shift workers.[317,322] Administration of melatonin has been found to be beneficial in some primary circadian rhythm sleep disorders such as delayed sleep phase syndrome[323,324] and non–24 hour sleep-wake[325,326] syndrome. In a subgroup of elderly subjects with reduced melatonin secretion at night, beneficial effects of melatonin on sleep disturbances in insomniac elderly subjects have been noted.[314,327] The hypnotic effect of melatonin has been noted in several reports.[314,328–330] Again, however, placebo-controlled, double-blind studies with large numbers of subjects are needed before considering the clinical applications of melatonin as a hypnotic agent. In conclusion, until further studies are conducted to determine the long-term effects of melatonin, its indiscriminate use (melatonin is available as a nutritional supplement without U.S. Food and Drug Administration control) should be discouraged. Furthermore, melatonin should only be administered to subjects with clearly documented melatonin deficiency.[314,315]

## REFERENCES

1. Orem J, Barnes CD. Physiology in Sleep. New York: Academic, 1980.
2. Lydic R, Biebuyck JF. Clinical Physiology of Sleep. Bethesda, MD: American Physiological Society, 1988.
3. Chokroverty S. Functional Anatomy of the Autonomic Nervous System: Autonomic Dysfunction and Disorders of the CNS. In American Academy of Neurology Course No. 144. Boston: American Academy of Neurology, 1991;77.
4. Lowey AD, Spyer KM. Central Regulation of Autonomic Functions. New York: Oxford University Press, 1990.
5. Chokroverty S. Sleep Apnea and Autonomic Failure. In PA Low (ed), Clinical Autonomic Disorders. Boston: Little, Brown, 1993;589.
6. Parmeggiani PL, Morrison AR. Alterations of Autonomic Functions During Sleep. In AD Lowey, KM Spyer (eds), Central Regulation of Autonomic Functions. New York: Oxford University Press, 1990;367.
7. Lowey AD. Central Autonomic Pathways. In PA Low (ed), Clinical Autonomic Disorders. Boston: Little, Brown, 1993;88.
8. Barron KD, Chokroverty S. Anatomy of the Autonomic Nervous System: Brain and Brainstem. In PA Low (ed), Clinical Autonomic Disorders. Boston: Little, Brown, 1993;3.
9. Spyer KM. The Central Nervous Organization of Reflex Circulatory Control. In AD Lowey, KM Spyer (eds), Central Regulation of Autonomic Functions. New York: Oxford University Press, 1990;168.
10. Guyenet PG. Role of the Ventral Medulla Oblongata in Blood Pressure Regulation. In AD Lowey, KM Spyer (eds), Central Regulation of Autonomic Functions. New York: Oxford University Press, 1990;145.
11. Parmeggiani PL. The Autonomic Nervous System in Sleep. In MH Kryger, T Roth, WC Dement (eds), Principles and Practice of Sleep Medicine (2nd ed). Philadelphia: Saunders, 1994;194.
12. Wallin G. Intraneural Recording and Autonomic Function in Man. In R Bannister (ed), Autonomic Failure: A Textbook of Clinical Disorders of the Autonomic Nervous System. Oxford, England: Oxford University Press, 1983;36.
13. Okada H, Iwase S, Manno T, et al. Changes in muscle sympathetic nerve activity during sleep in humans. Neurology 1991;46:1961.
14. Hornyak M, Cejnar M, Elam M, et al. Sympathetic muscle nerve activity during sleep in man. Brain 1991;114:1281.
15. Somers VK, Dyken ME, Mark AL, Abboud FM. Sympathetic nerve activity during sleep in normal subjects. N Engl J Med 1993;328:303.
16. Takeuchi S, Iwase S, Manno T, et al. Sleep-related changes in human muscle and skin sympathetic nerve activities. J Auton Nerv Syst 1994;47:121.
17. Legallois C. Experiences Sur le Principe de la Vie. Paris: d'Hautel, 1812.
18. Lumsden T. Observations on the respiratory centres in the cat. J Physiol (Lond) 1922–1923;57:153,354.
19. Lumsden T. The regulation of respiration. J Physiol (Lond) 1923–1924;58:81,111.
20. Pitts RF, Magoun HW, Ranson SW. Localization of the medullary respiratory centers in the cat. Am J Physiol 1939;126:673.

21. Mitchell RA, Berger AJ. Neural regulation of respiration. Am Rev Respir Dis 1975;111:206.

22. Berger AJ, Mitchell RA, Severinghaus JW. Regulation of respiration. N Engl J Med 1977;297:92,138,194.

23. Mitchell RA. Neural regulation of respiration. Clin Chest Med 1980;1:3.

24. Loewy AD, Spyer KM. Central Regulation of Autonomic Functions. New York: Oxford University Press, 1990.

25. Steriade M, McCarley RW. Brainstem Control of Wakefulness and Sleep. New York: Plenum, 1990.

26. Vertes RP. Brainstem control of the events of REM sleep. Prog Neurobiol 1984;22:241.

27. Moruzzi G. The sleep waking cycle. Ergeb Physiol 1972;64:1.

28. Hobson JA, Lydic R, Baghdoyan HA. Evolving concepts of sleep cycle generation: from brain centers to neuronal populations. Behav Brain Sci 1986;9:371.

29. Jouvet M. The role of monoamines and acteylcholine containing neurons in the regulation of the sleep-waking cycle. Ergeb Physiol 1972;64:166.

30. Batini C, Magni F, Palestini M, et al. Neural mechanisms underlying the enduring EEG and behavioral activation in the mid-pontine pretrigeminal preparation. Arch Ital Biol 1959;97:1.

31. Batini C, Moruzzi G, Palestini M, et al. Effect of complete pontine transections on the sleep-wakefulness rhythm: the mid-pontine pretrigeminal preparation. Arch Ital Biol 1959;97:1.

32. Bremer F. Cerebral hypnogenic centers. Ann Neurol 1977;2:1.

33. Ricardo JA, Koh ET. Anatomical evidence of direct projections from the nucleus of the solitary tract to the hypothalamus, amygdala, and other forebrain structures in the rat. Brain Res 1978;153:1.

34. Loewy AD. Central Autonomic Pathways. In PA Low (ed), Clinical Autonomic Disorders. Boston: Little, Brown, 1993;88.

35. Loewy AD. Anatomy of the Autonomic Nervous System: An Overview. In AD Loewy, KM Spyer (eds), Central Regulation of Autonomic Functions. New York: Oxford University Press, 1990;3.

36. Chokroverty S. Functional Anatomy of the Autonomic Nervous System Correlated with Symptomatology of Neurologic Disease. In American Academy of Neurology Course No. 246. San Diego: American Academy of Neurology, 1992;49.

37. Chokroverty S. The Spectrum of Ventilatory Disturbances in Movement Disorders. In S Chokroverty (ed), Movement Disorders. Costa Mesa, CA: PMA, 1990;365.

38. Cherniack NS, Longobardo GA. Abnormalities in Respiratory Rhythm. In AF Fishman, NS Cherniack, JG Widdicombe (eds), Handbook of Physiology, sec 3. The Respiratory System (Vol II, Part 2). Bethesda, MD: American Physiological Society, 1986;729.

39. Phillipson EA. Control of breathing during sleep. Am Rev Physiol 1978;18:909.

40. Phillipson EA. Respiratory adaptations in sleep. Ann Rev Physiol 1978;40:133.

41. Phillipson EA, Bowes G. Control of Breathing During Sleep. In AF Fishman, NS Cherniack, JG Widdicombe (eds), Handbook of Physiology, sec 3. The Respiratory System (Vol II, Part 2). Bethesda MD: American Physiological Society, 1986;649.

42. Plum F. Breathlessness in Neurological Disease: The Effects of Neurological Disease on the Act of Breathing. In JBL Howell, EJM Campbell (eds), Breathlessness. Oxford: Blackwell, 1966;203.

43. Sears TA, Newsom Davis J. The control of respiratory muscles during voluntary breathing. Ann N Y Acad Sci 1968;155:183.

44. Procter DF. Breathing Mechanics During Phonations and Singing. In B Wyke (ed), Ventilatory and Phonatory Control Systems. London: Oxford University Press, 1974;39.

45. Cohen MI, Hugelin A. Suprapontine reticular control of intrinsic respiratory mechanisms. Arch Ital Biol 1965;103:317.

46. Hugelin A, Cohen MI. The reticular activating system and respiratory regulation in the cat. Ann N Y Acad Sci 1963;109:586.

47. McNicholas WT, Rutherford R, Grossman R, et al. Abnormal respiratory pattern generation during sleep in patients with autonomic dysfunction. Am Rev Respir Dis 1983;128:429.

48. Fink BR. Influence of cerebral activity in wakefulness on regulation of breathing. J Appl Physiol 1961;16:15.

49. Merrill EG. The lateral respiratory neurons of the medulla: their associations with nucleus ambiguus, nucleus retroambigualis, the spinal accessory nucleus and the spinal cord. Brain Res 1970;24:11.

50. Nathan PW. The descending respiratory pathway in man. J Neurol Neurosurg Psychiatry 1963;26:487.

51. Wang SC, Ngai SH, Frumin MJ. Organization of central respiratory mechanisms in the brainstem of the cat: genesis of normal respiratory rhythmicity. Am J Physiol 1957;190:333.

52. Sullivan CE. Breathing in Sleep. In J Orem, CD Barnes (eds), Physiology in Sleep. New York: Academic, 1980;213.

53. Newsom Davis J. Control of Muscles in Breathing. In JG Widdicombe (ed), Respiratory Physiology: MTP International Review of Science (Vol 2). London: Butterworth, 1974;221.

54. White DP. Ventilation and the Control of Respiration During Sleep: Normal Mechanisms, Pathologic Nocturnal Hypoventilation, and Central Sleep Apnea. In RJ Martin (ed), Cardiorespiratory Disorders During Sleep. Mount Kisco, NY: Futura, 1990;53.

55. Weil J, Byrne-Quinn E, Sodal I, et al. Hypoxic ventilatory drive in normal man. J Clin Invest 1970;49:1061.

56. Read DJC. A clinical method for assessing the ventilatory response to carbon dioxide. Australas Ann Med 1967;16:20.

57. Whipp BJ, Wasserman K. Carotid bodies and ventilatory control dynamics in man. Fed Proc 1980;39:2668.

58. Hornbein TF. The Relationship Between Stimulus to Chemoreceptors and Their Response. In TW Torrance (ed), Arterial Chemoreceptors. Oxford, UK: Blackwell, 1968;65.

59. Loeschcke HH. Review lecture: central chemosensitivity and the reaction therapy. J Physiol (Lond) 1982;332:1.

60. Bulow K, Ingvar DH. Respiration and state of wakefulness in normals, studied by spirography, capnography and EEG. Acta Physiol Scand 1961;51:230.

61. Bulow K. Respiration and wakefulness in man. Acta Physiol Scand Suppl 1963;59:1.

62. Cherniack N. Respiratory dysrhythmias during sleep. N Engl J Med 1981;305:325.

63. Douglas J, White DP, Pickett CK, et al. Respiration during sleep in normal man. Thorax 1982;37:840.

64. Robin ED, Whaley RD, Crump CH, et al. Alveolar gas tensions, pulmonary ventilation, and blood pH during physiologic sleep in normal subjects. J Clin Invest 1958;37:981.

65. McNicholas WT. Impact of sleep in respiratory failure. Eur Respir J 1997;10:920.

66. Skatrud J, Dempsey J. Interaction of sleep state and chemical stimuli in sustaining rhythmic ventilation. J Appl Physiol 1983;55:813.

67. Hudgel DW, Martin RJ, Johnson B, et al. Mechanics of the respiratory system and breathing during sleep in normal humans. J Appl Physiol 1984;56:133.

68. Goethe B, Altose MD, Gotham MD, et al. Effect of quiet sleep on resting and $CO_2$-stimulated breathing in humans. J Appl Physiol 1981;50:724.

69. Tabachnik E, Muller NL, Bryant AC, et al. Changes in ventilation and chest wall mechanics during sleep in normal adolescents. J Appl Physiol 1981;51:557.

70. Krieger J, Turlot JC, Mangin P, et al. Breathing during sleep in normal young and elderly subjects: hypopneas, apneas, and correlated factors. Sleep 1983;6:108.

71. Lopes JM, Tabachnik E, Muller NL, et al. Total airway resistance and respiratory muscle activity during sleep. J Appl Physiol 1983;54:773.

72. Skatrud JB, Dempsey JA. Airway resistance and respiratory muscle function in snorers during NREM sleep. J Appl Physiol 1985;59:328.

73. Wiegand L, Zwillich CW, White DP. Collapsibility of the human upper airway during normal sleep. J Appl Physiol 1989;66:1800.

74. Birchfield RI, Sieker HO, Heyman A. Alterations in respiratory function during natural sleep. J Lab Clin Med 1959;54:216.

75. Reed DJ, Kellogg RH. Changes in respiratory response to $CO_2$ during natural sleep at sea level and at altitude. J Appl Physiol 1958;13:325.

76. White DP, Weil JV, Zwillich CW. Metabolic rate and breathing during sleep. J Appl Physiol 1985;59:384.

77. Block AJ, Boysen PG, Wynne JW, et al. Sleep apnea, hypopnea, and oxygen desaturation in normal subjects. N Engl J Med 1979;300:513.

78. Webb P. Periodic breathing during sleep. J Appl Physiol 1974;37:899.

79. Bellville JW, Howland WS, Seed JC, et al. The effect of sleep on the respiratory response to carbon dioxide. Anesthesiology 1959;20:628.

80. Gillam PMS. Patterns of respiration in human beings at rest and during sleep. Bull Eur Physiopathol Respir 1972;8:1059.

81. Berthon-Jones M, Sullivan CE. Ventilatory and arousal responses to hypoxia in sleeping humans. Am Rev Respir Dis 1982;125:632.

82. Douglas NJ, White DP, Weil JV, et al. Hypoxic ventilatory response decreases during sleep in normal men. Am Rev Respir Dis 1982;125:286.

83. Hedemark LL, Kronenberg RS. Ventilatory and heart rate responses to hypoxia and hypercapnia during sleep in adults. J Appl Physiol 1982;53:307.

84. White DP, Douglas NJ, Pickett CK, et al. Hypoxic ventilatory response during sleep in normal women. Am Rev Respir Dis 1982;126:530.

85. Douglas NJ, White DP, Weil JV, et al. Hypercapnic ventilatory response in sleeping adults. Am Rev Respir Dis 1982;126:758.

86. Berthon-Jones M, Sullivan CE. Ventilatory and arousal responses to hypercapnia in normal sleeping adults. J Appl Physiol 1984;57:59.

87. Brebbia DR, Altshuler KZ. Oxygen consumption rate and electroencephalographic stage of sleep. Science 1965;150:1621.

88. Buskirk ER, Thompson RH, Moore R, et al. Human energy expenditure studies in the National Institute of Arthritis and Metabolic Diseases metabolic chamber. Am J Clin Nutr 1960;8:602.

89. Anch AM, Remmers JE, Bunce H III. Supraglottic airway resistance in normal subjects and patients with occlusive sleep apnea. J Appl Physiol 1982;53:1158.

90. Skatrud JB, Dempsey JA, Badr S, et al. Effect of airway impedance on $CO_2$ retention and respiratory muscle activity during NREM sleep. J Appl Physiol 1988;65:1676.

91. Hudgel DW, Devadatta P. Decrease in functional residual capacity during sleep in normal humans. J Appl Physiol 1984;57:1319.

92. Tusiewicz K, Moldofsky H, Bryan AC, et al. Mechanics of the rib cage and diaphragm during sleep. J Appl Physiol 1977;43:600.

93. Kerr HD. Diurnal variation of respiratory function independent of air quality. Arch Environ Health 1973;26:144.

94. Hettzel MR, Clark TJH. Comparison of normal and asthmatic circadian rhythms in peak expiratory flow rate. Thorax 1980;35:732.

95. Gothe B, Goldman MD, Cherniack NS, et al. Effect of progressive hypoxia on breathing during sleep. Am Rev Respir Dis 1982;126:97.

96. Hara KS, Shepard JW Jr. Sleep and Critical Care Medicine. In RJ Martin (ed), Cardiorespiratory Disorders During Sleep. Mount Kisco, NY: Futura, 1990;323.

97. Thach BT, Davies AM, Koenig JS. Pathophysiology of Sudden Airway Obstruction in Sleeping Infants and its Relevance for SIDS. In PJ Schwartz, DP Southall, M Valdes-Dapena (eds), The Sudden Infant Death Syndrome: Cardiac and Respiratory Mechanisms and Interventions [Monogr]. Ann N Y Acad Sci 1988;533:314.

98. Dempsey JA, Henke KG, Skatrud JB. Regulation of Ventilation and Respiratory Muscle Function in NREM Sleep. In FG Issa, PM Suratt, JE Remmers (eds), Sleep and Respiration. New York: Wiley, 1990;145.

99. Orem J. The Nature of the Wakefulness Stimulus for Breathing. In FG Issa, PM Suratt, JE Remmers (eds), Sleep and Respiration. New York: Wiley, 1990;23.

100. Douglas NJ. Breathing During Sleep in Normal Subjects. In JH Peter, T Podszus, P Von Wichert (eds), Sleep-Related Disorders and Internal Diseases. Berlin: Springer, 1987;254.

101. Pompeiano O. Mechanism of sensorimotor integration during sleep. Prog Physiol Psychol 1973;3:1.

102. Khatri IM, Freis ED. Hemodynamic changes during sleep. J Appl Physiol 1967;22:867.

103. Snyder F, Hobson JA, Morrison DF, et al. Changes in respiration, heart rate, and systolic blood pressure in human sleep. J Appl Physiol 1964;19:417.

104. Burdick JA, Brinton G, Goldstein L, et al. Heart-rate variability in sleep and wakefulness. Cardiology 1970;55:79.

105. Baust W, Bohnert B. The regulation of heart rate during sleep. Exp Brain Res 1969;7:169.

106. Bonnett MH, Arand DL. Heart rate variability: sleep stage, time of night and arousal influences. Electroencephalogr Clin Neurophysiol 1997;102:390.

107. Toscani L, Gangemi PF, Pariji A, et al. Human heart rate variability and sleep stages. Ital J Neurol Sci 1996;17:437.

108. Finley JP, Nugent ST. Heart rate variability in infants, children and young adults. J Auton Nerv Syst 1995;51:103.

109. Vanoli E, Adamson PB, Ba-Lin, et al. Heart rate variability during specific sleep stages. A comparison of healthy subjects with patients after myocardial infarction. Circulation 1995;91:1918.

110. Cajochen C, Pischke J, Aeschbach D, Borboli AA. Heart rate dynamics during human sleep. Physiol Behav 1994;55:769.

111. Miller JC, Horvath SM. Cardiac output during human sleep. Aviat Space Environ Med 1976;47:1046.

112. Smolensky M, Halberg F, Sargent F II. Chronobiology of the Life Sequence. In S Itoh, K Ogata, H Yoshimura (eds), Advances in Climatic Physiology. New York: Springer, 1971.

113. Coccagna G, Mantovani M, Brignani F, et al. Arterial pressure changes during spontaneous sleep in man. Electroencephalogr Clin Neurophysiol 1971;31:277.

114. Coote JH. Respiratory and circulatory control during sleep. J Exp Biol 1982;100:223.

115. Lugaresi E, Coccagna G, Cirignotta F, et al. Breathing during sleep in man in normal and pathological conditions. Adv Exp Med Biol 1978;99:35.

116. Kumazawa T, Baccella G, Guazzi M, et al. Haemodynamic patterns during desynchronized sleep in intact cats and in cats with sino-aortic deafferentation. Circ Res 1969;24:923.

117. Mancia G, Baccella G, Adams DB, et al. Vasomotor regulation during sleep in the cat. Am J Physiol 1971;220:1086.

118. Watson WE. Distensibility of the capacitance blood vessels of the human hand during sleep. J Physiol 1962;161:392.

119. Mullen PE, James VHT, Lightman SL, et al. A relationship between plasma renin activity and the rapid eye movement phase of sleep in man. J Clin Endocrinol Metab 1980;50:466.

120. Greenberg JH. Sleep and the Cerebral Circulation. In J Orem, CD Barnes (eds), Physiology in Sleep. New York: Academic, 1980;57.

121. Hajak G, Klingelhofer J, Schulz-Varszegi M, et al. Relationship between cerebral blood flow verocities and cerebral electrical activity in sleep. Sleep 1994;17:11.

122. Buchsbaum MS, Gaillin JC, Wu J, et al. Regional cerebral glucose metabolic rate in human sleep assessed by positron emission tomography. Life Sci 1989;45:1349.

123. Heiss WD, Pawlik G, Herholz K. Regional cerebral glucose metabolism in man during wakefulness, sleep and dreaming. Brain Res 1985;327:362.

124. Madsen PL, Schmidt JF, Wildschiodtz G, et al. Cerebral oxygen metabolism and cerebral blood flow in humans during deep and rapid eye movement in sleep. J Appl Physiol 1991;70:2597.

125. Maquet P, Div D, Salmon E, et al. Cerebral glucose utilization during sleep-wake cycle in man determined by positron emission tomography and {18F} 2-fluoro-deoxy-D-glucose method. Brain Res 1997;513:136.

126. Meyer JS, Ishikawa Y, Hata T, Karacan I. Cerebral blood flow in normal and abnormal sleep and dreaming. Brain Cogn 1987;6:266.

127. Sacai F, Meyer JS, Karacan I, et al. Normal human sleep: regional cerebral hemodynamics. Ann Neurol 1980;7:471.

128. Madsen PL, Holm S, Vorstrup S, et al. Human regional cerebral blood flow during REM sleep. J Cereb Blood Flow Metab 1991;11:502.

129. Maquet P, Peters J, Aerts J, et al. Functional neuroanatomy of human rapid-eye-movement sleep and dreaming. Nature 1996;383:163.

130. Braun AR, Belkin TJ, Wesenten NJ, et al. Regional cerebral blood flow throughout the sleep-wake cycle. An $H_2(15)O$ PET study. Brain 1997;120:1173.

131. Hofle N, Paus T, Reutens D, et al. Regional cerebral blood flow changes as a function of delta and spindle activity during slow wave sleep in humans. J Neurosci 1997;17:4800.

132. Siegel JM. Brain Stem Mechanisms Generating REM Sleep. In MH Kryger, T Roth, WC Dement (eds), Principles and Practice of Sleep Medicine (2nd ed). Philadelphia: Saunders, 1994;125.

133. Ohta Y, Mori S, Kimura H. Neuronal structures of the brainstem participating in postural suppression in cats. Neurosci Res 1988;5:181.

134. Sakai K, Sastre JP, Salvert D, et al. Tegmentoreticular projections with special reference to the muscular atonia during paradoxical sleep in the cat. An HRP study. Brain Res 1979;176:233.

135. Bowker RM, Westlund KN, Sullivan MC, et al. Descending serotonergic, peptidergic and cholinergic pathways from the raphe nuclei: a multiple transmitter complex. Brain Res 1983;288:33.

136. Jones BE, Pare M, Beaudet A. Retrograde labeling of neurons in the brain stem following injections of [3H] choline into the rat spinal cord. Neuroscience 1986;18:901.

137. Chase MH, Morales FR, Boxer PA, et al. Effect of stimulation of the nucleus reticularis gigantocellularis on the membrane potential of cat lumbar motoneurons during sleep and wakefulness. Brain Res 1986;386:237.

138. Jouvet M. Locus coeruleus et sommeil paradoxal. C R Soc Biol 1965;159:895.

139. Henley K, Morrison AR. A re-evaluation of the effect of lesions on the pontine tegmentum and locus coeruleus on phenomena of paradoxical sleep in the cat. Acta Neurobiol Exp 1974;34:215.

140. Hendricks JC, Morrison AR, Mann GL. Different behaviors during paradoxical sleep without atonia depend on pontine lesion site. Brain Res 1982;239:81.

141. Schenkel E, Siegel JM. REM sleep without atonia after lesions of the medial medulla. Neurosci Lett 1989;98:159.

142. Chase MH. Synaptic mechanisms and circuitry involved in motoneuron control during sleep. Int Rev Neurobiol 1983;24:213.

143. Morales FR, Boxer PA, Chase MH. Behavioral state-specific inhibitory postsynaptic potentials impinge on cat lumbar motoneurons during active sleep. Exp Neurol 1987;98:418.

144. Morales FR, Chase MH. Repetitive synaptic potentials responsible for inhibition of spinal cord motoneurons during active sleep. Exp Neurol 1982;78:471.

145. Takakusaki K, Ohta Y, Mori S. Single medullary reticulospinal neurons exert postsynaptic inhibitory effects via inhibitory interneurons upon alphamotoneurons innervating cat hindlimb muscles. Exp Brain Res 1989;74:11.

146. Soja PJ, Morales FR, Chase MH. Postsynaptic Control of Lumbar Motoneurons During the Atonia of Active Sleep. In FG Issa, PM Suratt, JE Remmers (eds), Sleep and Respiration. New York: Wiley, 1990;9.

147. Iscoe S. Central Control of the Upper Airway. In OP Mathew, G Sant'Ambrogio (eds), Respiratory Function of the Upper Airway. New York: Marcel Dekker, 1988;125.

148. Kalia M. Anatomical organization of the central respiratory neurons. Ann Rev Physiol 1981;43:105.

149. Bianchi AL, Grelot L, Barillot JC. Motor Output to the Pharyngeal Muscles. In FG Issa, PM Suratt, JE Remmers (eds), Sleep and Respiration. New York: Wiley, 1990;89.

150. Gothe B, van Lunteren E, Dick TE. The Influence of Sleep and Respiratory Muscle Function. In NA Saunders, CE Sullivan (eds), Sleep and Breathing (2nd ed). New York: Marcel Dekker, 1994;239.

151. Horner RL. Motor control of the pharyngeal musculature and implications for the pathogenesis of obstructive sleep apnea. Sleep 1996;19:827.

152. Bartlett D Jr, Leiter JC, Knuth SL. Control and Actions of the Genioglossus Muscle. In FG Issa, PM Suratt, JE Remmers (eds), Sleep and Respiration. New York: Wiley, 1990;99.

153. Sauerland EK, Harper RM. The human tongue during sleep: electromyographic activity of the genioglossus muscle. Exp Neurol 1976;51:160.

154. Sauerland EK, Orr WC, Hairston LE. EMG patterns of oropharyngeal muscles during respiration in wakefulness and sleep. Electromyogr Clin Neurophysiol 1981;21:307.

155. Doble EA, Leiter JC, Knuth SL, et al. A noninvasive intraoral electromyographic electrode for genioglossus muscle. J Appl Physiol 1985;58:1378.

156. Mathur R, Mortimore IL, Jan MA, Douglas NJ. Effect of breathing, pressure and posture on palatoglossal and genioglossal tone. Clin Sci 1995;89:441.

157. Mortimore IL, Mathur R, Douglas NJ. Effect of posture, route of respiration, and negative pressure on palatal muscle activity in humans. J Appl Physiol 1995;79:448.

158. Tangel DJ, Mezzanotte WS, Sandberg EJ, White DP. Influences of sleep on tensor palatini EMG and upper airway resistance in normal men. J Appl Physiol 1991;70:2574.

159. Tangel DJ, Mezzanotte WS, Sandberg EJ, White DP. Influences of NREM sleep on the activity of tonic vs. inspiratory phasic muscles in normal men. J Appl Physiol 1992;73:1058.

160. Suratt PM, Hollowell DE. Inspiratory Activation of the Masseter. In FG Issa, PM Suratt, JE Remmers (eds), Sleep and Respiration. New York: Wiley, 1990;109.

161. Kuna SI, Insalaco G. Respiratory-Related Intrinsic Laryngeal Muscle Activity in Normal Adults. In FG Issa, PM Suratt, JE Remmers (eds), Sleep and Respiration. New York: Wiley, 1990;117.

162. Sant'Ambrogio G, Mathew OP. Laryngeal Function in Respiration. New York: Marcel Dekker, 1988.

163. Kuna ST, Smickley JS, Insalaco G. Posterior cricoarytenoid muscle activity during wakefulness and sleep in normal adults. Am Rev Respir Dis 1989;139:A446.

164. van Lunteren E. Role of Mammalian Hyoid Muscles in the Maintenance of Pharyngeal Patency. In FG Issa, PM Suratt, JE Remmers (eds), Sleep and Respiration. New York: Wiley, 1990;125.

165. Pack AI, Kline LR, Hendricks JC, et al. Neural Mechanisms in the Genesis of Sleep Apnea. In FG Issa, PM Suratt, JE Remmers (eds), Sleep and Respiration. New York: Wiley, 1990;177.

166. Kline LR, Hendricks JC, Davies RO, et al. Control of activity of the diaphragm in rapid eye movement sleep. J Appl Physiol 1986;61:1293.

167. Orem J. Neuronal mechanisms of respiration in REM sleep. Sleep 1980;3:251.

168. Soja PJ, Finch DM, Chase MH. Effect of inhibitory amino acid antagonists on masseteric reflex suppression during active sleep. Exp Neurol 1987;96:178.

169. Pedroarena C, Castillo P, Chase MH, Morales FR. The control of jaw-opener motoneurons during the active sleep. Brain Res 1994;653:31.

170. Kubin L, Kimura H, Tojima H, et al. Suppression of hypoglossal motoneurons during the carbachol-induced atonia of REM sleep is not caused by fast synaptic inhibition. Brain Res 1993;611:300.

171. Pack AI. Changes in Respiratory Motor Activity during Rapid Eye Movement Sleep. In JA Dempsey, AI Pack (eds), Regulation of Breathing. New York: Marcel Dekker, 1995;983.

172. Tojima H, Kubin L, Kimura H, Davies RO. Spontaneous ventilation and respiratory motor output during carachol-induced atonia of REM sleep in the decerebrate cat. Sleep 1992;15:404.

173. Horner RL, Kozar LF, Kimoff RJ, Phillipson EA. Effects of sleep on the tonic drive to respiratory muscle and the threshold for rhythm generation in the dog. J Physiol (Lond) 1994;474:525.

174. Manaker S, Tischler LJ, Morrison AR. Raphespinal and reticulospinal collaterals to the hypoglossal nucleus in the rat. J Comp Neurol 1992;322:68.

175. Manaker S, Tischler LJ. Origin of serotonergic afferents to the hypoglossal nucleus in the rat. J Comp Neurol 1993;334:466.

176. Li YQ, Takada M, Mizuno N. The sites of origin of serotonergic afferent fibers in the trigeminal motor, facial, and hypoglossal nuclei in the rat. Neurosci Res 1993;17:307.

177. Aldes LD. Topographically organized projections from the nucleus subcoeruleus to the hypoglossal nucleus in the rat: a light and electron microscopic study with complementary axonal transport techniques. J Comp Neurol 1990;302:643.

178. Aldes LD, Chapman ME, Chronister RB, Haycock JW. Sources of noradrenergic afferents to the hypoglossal nucleus in the rat. Brain Res Bull 1992;29:931.

179. McNicholas WT, Coffey M, McDonnell T, et al. Upper airway obstruction during sleep in normal subjects after selective topical oropharyngeal anesthesia. Am Rev Respir Dis 1987;135:1316.

180. Chadwick G, Crowley P, Fitzgerald MX, et al. Obstructive sleep apnea following topical oropharyngeal anesthesia in loud snorers. Am Rev Respir Dis 1991;143:810.

181. Deegan PC, Mulloy E, McNicholas WT. Topical oropharyngeal anesthesia in patients with obstructive sleep apnea. Am J Respir Crit Care Med 1995;151:1108.

182. Berry RB, Kouchi KG, Bower JL, Light RW. Effect of upper airway anesthesia on obstructive sleep apnea. Am J Respir Crit Care Med 1995;151:1857.

183. Pontoppidan H, Bleecher HK. Progressive loss of protective reflexes in the airway with the advance of age. JAMA 1960;174:2209.

184. Horner RL, Shea SA, McIvor J, Guz A. Pharyngeal size and shape during wakefulness and sleep in patients with obstructive sleep apnea. Q J Med 1989;72:719.

185. Guilleminault C, Hill MW, Simmons FB, Dement WC. Obstructive sleep apnea: electromyographic and fiberoptic studies. Exp Neurol 1978;62:48.

186. Weitzman ED, Pollak CP, Borowiecki B, et al. The Hypersomnia-Sleep Apnea Syndrome: Site and Mechanisms of Upper Airway Obstruction. In C Guilleminault, WC Dement (eds), Sleep Apnea Syndromes. New York: Liss, 1978;235.

187. Suratt PM, Dee P, Atkinson RL, et al. Fluoroscopic and computed tomographic features of the pharyngeal airway in obstructive sleep apnea. Am Rev Respir Dis 1983;127:487.

188. Stein GM, Gamsu G, de Geer G, et al. Cine CT in obstructive sleep apnea. Am J Radiol 1987;148:1069.

189. Hudgel DW. Variable site of airway narrowing among obstructive sleep apnea patients. J Appl Physiol 1986;61:1403.

190. Chaban R, Cole P, Hoffstein V. Site of upper airway obstruction in patients with idiopathic obstructive sleep apnea. Laryngoscope 1988;98:641.

191. Shepard JW Jr, Thawley SE. Localization of upper airway collapse during sleep in patients with obstructive sleep apnea. Am Rev Respir Dis 1990;141:1350.

192. Remmers JE, de Groot WJ, Sauerland EK, Anch AM. Pathogenesis of upper airway occlusion during sleep. J Appl Physiol 1978;44:931.

193. Sullivan CE, Issa FG, Berthon-Jones M, Saunders NA. Pathophysiology of Sleep Apnea. In NA Saunders, CE Sullivan (eds), Sleep and Breathing. New York: Marcel Dekker, 1984;299.

194. Orem J. Control of the Upper Airways During Sleep and the Hypersomnia-Sleep Apnea Syndrome. New York: Academic, 1980;273.

195. Orr WC. Gastrointestinal Physiology. In MH Kryger, T Roth, WC Dement (eds), Principles and Practice of Sleep Medicine. Philadelphia: Saunders, 1994;252.

196. Moore JG, Englert E. Circadian rhythm of gastric acid secretion in man. Nature 1970;226:1261.

197. Levin E, Kirsner JB, Palmer WL, et al. A comparison of the nocturnal gastric secretion in patients with duodenal ulcer in normal individuals. Gastroenterology 1948;10:952.

198. Feldman M, Richardson CT. Total 24-hour gastric acid secretion in patients with duodenal ulcer: comparison with normal subjects and effects of cimetidine and parietal cell vagotomy. Gastroenterology 1986;90:540.

199. McCloy RF, Girvan DP, Baron JH. Twenty-four-hour gastric acidity after vagotomy. Gut 1978;19:664.

200. Reichsman F, Cohen J, Colwill J, et al. Natural and histamine-induced gastric secretion during waking and sleeping states. Psychosomat Med 1960;1:14.

201. Armstrong RH, Burnap D, Jacobson A, et al. Dreams and acid secretions in duodenal ulcer patients. New Physician 1965;33:241.
202. Stacher G, Presslich B, Starker H. Gastric acid secretion and sleep stages during natural night sleep. Gastroenterology 1975;68:1449.
203. Orr WC, Hall WH, Stahl ML, et al. Sleep patterns and gastric acid secretion in duodenal ulcer disease. Arch Intern Med 1976;136:655.
204. Orr WC, Dubois A, Stahl ML, et al. Gastric function during sleep. Sleep Res 1978;7:72.
205. Bloom PB, Ross DL, Stunkard AJ, et al. Gastric and duodenal motility, food intake and hunger measured in man during a 24-hour period. Dig Dis Sci 1970;15:719.
206. Yaryura-Tobias HA, Hutcheson JS, White L. Relationship between stages of sleep and gastric motility. Behav Neuropsychiatry 1970;2:22.
207. Wada T. An experimental study of slumber in its relation to activity. Arch Psychol (Frankf) 1922;8:1.
208. Finch P, Ingram D, Henstridge J, et al. Relationship of fasting gastroduodenal motility to the sleep cycle. Gastroenterology 1982;83:605.
209. Orr W, Robinson M, Johnson L. Acid clearance during sleep in the pathogenesis of reflux esophagitis. Dig Dis Sci 1981;26:423.
210. Lear C, Flanagan J, Moorees C. The frequency of deglutition in man. Arch Oral Biol 1965;10:83.
211. Litcher J, Muir RC. The pattern of swallowing during sleep. Electroencephalogr Clin Neurophysiol 1975;38:427.
212. Johnson LF, DeMeester TR. Twenty-four-hour pH monitoring of the distal esophagus: a quantitative measure of gastroesophageal reflux. Am J Gastroenterol 1974;62:325.
213. Orr WC, Johnson LF, Robinson MG. The effect of sleep on swallowing, esophageal peristalsis, and acid clearance. Gastroenterology 1984;86:814.
214. Dent J, Dodds WJ, Friedman RH, et al. Mechanisms of gastroesophageal reflux in recumbent asymptomatic human subjects. J Clin Invest 1980;65:256.
215. Orr WC, Bollinger C, Stahl M. Measurement of Gastroesophageal Reflux During Sleep by Esophageal pH Monitoring. In C Guilleminault (ed), Sleeping and Waking Disorders: Indications and Techniques. Menlo Park, CA: Addison-Wesley, 1982;331.
216. Guyton AC, Hall JE. Textbook of Medical Physiology. Philadelphia: Saunders, 1996;810.
217. Kumar D, Wingate D, Ruckebusch Y. Circadian variation in the propagation velocity of the migrating motor complex. Gastroenterology 1986;91:926.
218. Kellow JE, Borody TJ, Phillips SF, et al. Human interdigestive motility: variations in patterns from esophagus to colon. Gastroenterology 1986;91:386.
219. Gorard DA, Vesselinova-Jenkins CK, Libby GW, Ferthing MJ. Migrating motor complex and sleep in health and irritable bowel syndrome. Dig Dis Sci 1995;40:2383.
220. David D, Mertz H, Fefer L, et al. Sleep and duodenal motor activity in patients with severe non-ulcer dyspepsia. Gut 1994;35:916.
221. Aschoff J. Circadian control of body temperature. J Therm Biol 1983;8:143.
222. Aschoff J. Desynchronization and resynchronization of human circadian rhythms. Aerospace Med 1969;40:847.
223. Heller HC, Glotzback S, Grahn D, et al. Sleep-Dependent Changes in the Thermoregulatory System. In R Lydic, JF Biebuyck (eds), Clinical Physiology of Sleep. Bethesda, MD: American Physiological Society, 1988;145.
224. Aschoff J. Circadian Rhythm of Activity and Body Temperature. In JD Hardy, AP Gagge, JAJ Stolwijk (eds), Physiological and Behavioral Temperature Regulation. Springfield, IL: Thomas, 1970;905.
225. Timbal J, Colin J, Boutelier C. Circadian variations in the sweating mechanism. J Appl Psychol 1975;39:226.
226. Parmeggiani PL. Temperature Regulation During Sleep: A Study in Homeostasis. In J Orem, CD Barnes (eds), Physiology in Sleep. New York: Academic, 1980;97.
227. Henane R, Buguet A, Roussel B, et al. Variations in evaporation and body temperatures during sleep in man. J Appl Physiol 1977;42:50.
228. Szymusiak R, McGinty D. Control of Slow Wave Sleep by Thermoregulatory Mechanisms. In FG Issa, PM Suratt, JE Remmers (eds), Sleep and Respiration. New York: Wiley, 1990;53.
229. Berger RJ, Phillips NH. Comparative Physiology of Sleep, Thermoregulation and Metabolism from the Perspective of Energy Metabolism. In FG Issa, PM Suratt, JE Remmers (eds), Sleep and Respiration. New York: Wiley, 1990;41.
230. MacFadyen H, Oswald I, Lewis SA. Starvation and human slow wave sleep. J Appl Physiol 1973;35:391.
231. Horne JA, Shackell BS. Slow wave sleep elevations after body heating: proximity to sleep and effects of aspirin. Sleep 1987;10:383.
232. Benedek GF, Obal F Jr, Lelkes Z, et al. Thermal and chemical stimulation of the hypothalamic heat detectors. The effects on the EEG. Acta Physiol Acad Sci Hungar 1982;60:27.
233. Bunnell DE, Agnew JA, Horvath SM, et al. Passive body heating and sleep: influence of proximity to sleep. Sleep 1988;11:210.
234. Horne JA, Reid AS. Night-time sleep EEG changes following body heating in a warm bath. Electroencephalogr Clin Neurophysiol 1985;60:154.
235. McGinty D, Szymusiak R. Neurobiology of Sleep. In NA Saunders, CE Sullivan (eds), Sleep and Breathing. New York: Marcel Dekker, 1994;1.
236. Jordon J, Montegomery I, Trinder J. The effect of afternoon body heating on body temperature and slow wave sleep. Psychophysiology 1990;27:560.
237. Horne JA, Moore VJ. Sleep EEG effects of exercise with and without additional body cooling. Electroencephalogr Clin Neurophysiol 1985;60:33.
238. Moriarty SR, Phillips NH, Berger RJ. Manipulation of tympanic temperature by facial heating or cooling influences SWS in humans. Sleep Res 1988;17:24.

239. Imeri L, Biancha S, Angeli P, Mancia M. Stimulation of cholinergic receptors in the medial preoptic area affect sleep and cortical temperature. Am J Physiol 1995;269:R294.

240. McGinty D, Szymusiak R. The Basal Forebrain and Slow Wave Sleep: Mechanistic and Functional Aspects. In A Wauquier (ed), Slow-Wave Sleep: Physiological, Pathophysiological and Functional Aspects. New York: Raven, 1989;61.

241. Krueger JM, Takahashi S. Thermoregulation and sleep. Closely linked but separable. Ann N Y Acad Sci 1997;813:281.

242. Woodward S, Freedman RR. The thermoregulatory effects of menopausal hot flashes on sleep. Sleep 1994;17:497.

243. Kinmonth AL. Review of the epidemiology of sudden infant death syndrome and its relationship to temperature regulation. Br J Gen Pract 1990;40:161.

244. Avery DH, Wildschiodtz G, Rafaelsen OJ. Nocturnal temperature in affective disorder. J Affect Disord 1982;4:61.

245. Takahashi Y, Kipnis D, Daughaday W. Growth hormone secretion during sleep. J Clin Invest 1968;47:2079.

246. Honda Y, Takahashi K, Takahashi S, et al. Growth hormone secretion during nocturnal sleep in normal subjects. J Clin Endocrinol Metab 1969;29:20.

247. Parker D, Sassin J, Mace J, et al. Human growth hormone release during sleep: electroencephalographic correlation. J Clin Endocrinol Metab 1969;29:871.

248. Sassin J, Parker D, Mace J, et al. Human growth hormone release: relation to slow-wave sleep and sleep-waking cycles. Science 1969;165:513.

249. Quabbe H. Chronobiology of growth hormone secretion. Chronobiologia 1977;4:217.

250. Van Kauter E, Turek FW. Endocrine and Other Biological Rhythms. In LJ DeGroot, M Besser, SG Burger, et al. (eds), Endocrinology (3rd ed). Philadelphia: Saunders, 1995;2487.

251. Gronfier C, Luthringer R, Follenius M. A quantitative evaluation of the relationship between growth hormone secretion and delta wave electroencephalographic activity during normal sleep and after enrichment in delta waves. Sleep 1996;19:817.

252. Mullington J, Hermann D, Holsbower F, Pollmacher T. Age-dependent suppression of nocturnal growth hormone levels during sleep deprivation. Neuroendocrinology 1996;64:233.

253. Veldhuis JD, Iranmanesh A. Physiological regulation of the human growth hormone (GH)-insulin-like growth factor type I (IGFI) axis: predominant impact of age, obesity, gonadal function and sleep. Sleep 1996;19:S221.

254. Van Cauter E, Plat L. Physiology of growth hormone secretion during sleep. J Pediatr 1996;128:S32.

255. Frieboes RM, Murck H, Schier T, et al. Somatostatin impairs sleep in elderly human subjects. Neuropsychopharmacology 1997;16:339.

256. Weitzman E, Boyar R, Kapen S, et al. The relationship of sleep and sleep stages to neuroendocrine secretion and biological rhythms in man. Recent Prog Horm Res 1975;31:401.

257. Sadamatsu M, Kato N, Iida H, et al. The 24-hour rhythms in plasma growth hormone, prolactin and thyroid stimulating hormone: effect of sleep deprivation. J Neuroendocrinol 1995;7:597.

258. Goldstein J, Cauter EV, DeSir D, et al. Effects of "jet lag" on hormonal patterns. IV. Time shifts increase growth hormone release. J Clin Endocrinol Metab 1983;56:433.

259. Weibel L, Follenius M, Spiegel K, et al. Growth hormone secretion in night workers. Chronobiol Int 1997;14:49.

260. Besset A, Bonardet A, Billiard M, et al. Circadian pattern of GH and cortisol in narcoleptic patients. Chronobiologia 1979;6:19.

261. Schilkrut R, Chandra O, Oswald N, et al. Growth hormone release during sleep and with thermal stimulation in depressed patients. Neuropsychobiology 1975;1:70.

262. Mendelson W. Studies of human growth hormone secretion in sleep and waking. Int Rev Neurobiol 1982;23:367.

263. Orr W, Vogel G, Stahl M, et al. Sleep patterns in growth hormone-deficient children and age-matched controls: developmental considerations. Neuroendocrinology 1977;24:347.

264. Takahashi Y. Growth Hormone Secretion During Sleep: A Review. In M Kawakami (ed), Biological Rhythms in Neuroendocrine Activity. Tokyo: Igaku-Shoin, 1974;316.

265. Rubin R. Sleep endocrinology studies in man. Prog Brain Res 1975;42:73.

266. Carlson HE, Gillin JC, Gorden P, et al. Absence of sleep related growth hormone peaks in aged normal subjects and in acromegaly. J Clin Endocrinol Metab 1972;34:1102.

267. Sassin J, Hellman L, Weitzman E. A circadian pattern of growth hormone secretion in acromegalics. Sleep Res 1972;1:189.

268. Clark RW, Schmidt HS, Malarkey WB. Disordered growth hormone and prolactin secretion in primary disorders of sleep. Neurology 1979;29:855.

269. Amsterdam JD, Schweitzer E, Winoker A. Multiple hormonal responses to insulin-induced hypoglycemia in depressed patients and normal volunteers. Am J Psychiatry 1987;144:170.

270. Mendelson WB. Human Sleep. New York: Plenum, 1987;129.

271. Othmer E, Goodwin D, Levine W, et al. Sleep-related growth hormone secretion in alcoholics. Clin Res 1972;20:726.

272. Dunleavy DL, Oswald I, Brown E, et al. Hyperthyroidism, sleep and growth hormone. Electroencephalogr Clin Neurophysiol 1974;36:259.

273. Weitzman ED, Fukushima D, Nogeri C, et al. Twenty-four hour pattern of the episodic secretion of cortisol in normal subjects. J Clin Endocrinol Metab 1971;33:14.

274. Hellman L, Nakada R, Curta J, et al. Cortisol is secreted episodically by normal man. J Clin Endocrinol Metab 1970;30:411.

275. Bierwolf C, Struve K, Marshall L, et al. Slow wave sleep drives inhibition of pituitary-adrenal secretion in humans. J Neuroendocrinol 1997;9:479.

276. Jarrett DB, Coble PA, Kupfer DJ. Reduced cortisol latency in depressive illness. Arch Gen Psychiatry 1983;40:506.

277. Kupfer D, Bulik C, Jarrett D. Nighttime plasma cortisol secretion and EEG sleep—are they associated? Psychiatr Res 1983;10:191.

278. Alford FP, Baker HW, Burger HG, et al. Temporal patterns of integrated plasma hormone levels during sleep and wakefulness. I. Thyroid-stimulating hormone, growth hormone and cortisol. J Clin Endocrinol Metab 1973;37:841.

279. Jacoby JH, Sassin JF, Greenstein M, et al. Patterns of spontaneous cortisol and growth hormone in rhesus monkeys during the sleep-wake cycle. Neuroendocrinology 1974;14:165.

280. Weibal L, Follenius M, Spiegel K, et al. Comparative effective of night and daytime sleep on the 24-hour cortisol secretory profile. Sleep 1995;18:549.

281. Pietrowsky R, Meyrer R, Kern W, et al. Effects of diurnal sleep on secretion of cortisol, luteinizing hormone and growth hormone in man. J Clin Endocrinol Metab 1994;78:683.

282. Fullerton DT, Wenzel FJ, Lohrenz FN, et al. Circadian rhythm of adrenal cortical activity in depression. Arch Gen Psychiatry 1968;19:674,682.

283. Rush AJ, Giles DE, Roffwarg HP, et al. Sleep EEG and dexamethasone suppression test findings in outpatients with unipolar major depressive disorders. Biol Psychiatry 1982;17:327.

284. Klein HE, Seibold B. DST in healthy volunteers and after sleep deprivation. Acta Psychiatr Scand 1985;72:16.

285. Sassin JF, Frantz AG, Kepen S, et al. The nocturnal rise of human prolactin is dependent on sleep. J Clin Endocrinol Metab 1973;37:436.

286. Parker D, Rossman L, Vanderhaan E. Sleep-related nyctohemeral and briefly episodic variation in human prolactin concentration. J Clin Endocrinol Metab 1973;36:1119.

287. Spiegel K, Luthringer R, Follenius M, et al. Temporal relationship between prolactin secretion and slow wave electroencephalic activity during sleep. Sleep 1995;18:543.

288. Sassin J, Frantz A, Weitzman E, et al. Human prolactin: 24 hour patterns with increased release during sleep. Science 1972;17:1205.

289. Mendelson W, Jacobs L, Reichman J, et al. Methysergide suppression of sleep-related prolactin secretion and enhancement of sleep-related growth hormone secretion. J Clin Invest 1975;56:690.

290. Rubin RT, Poland RE, Gouin PR, et al. Secretion of hormones influencing water and electrolyte balance (antidiuretic hormone, aldosterone, prolactin) during sleep in normal adult men. Psychosom Med 1978;40:44.

291. Van Cauter E, Desir D, Refetoff S, et al. The relationship between episodic variations of plasma prolactin and REM-non-REM cyclicity is an artifact. J Clin Endocrinol Metab 1982;54:70.

292. Waldstreicher J, Duffy JF, Brown EN, et al. Gender differences in the temporal organizations of prolactin (PRL) secretion: evidence for a sleep-independent circadian rhythm of circulating PRL levels—a clinical research center study. J Clin Endocrinol Metab 1996;81:1483.

293. Partsch CJ, Lerchl A, Sippel WG. Characteristics of pulsatile and circadian prolactin release and its variability in man. Exp Clin Endocrinol Diabetes 1995;103:33.

294. Parker DC, Rossman LG, Kripke TF, et al. Endocrine Rhythms Across Sleep-Wake Cycles in Normal Young Men under Basal State Conditions. In J Orem, CD Barnes (eds), Physiology in Sleep. New York: Academic, 1980;145.

295. Boyar R, Finkelstein J, Roffwarg H, et al. Synchronization of augmented luteinizing hormone secretion with sleep during puberty. N Engl J Med 1972;287:582.

296. Boyar RM, Rosenfeld RS, Kapen S, et al. Human puberty: simultaneous augmented secretion of luteinizing hormone and testosterone during sleep. J Clin Invest 1974;54:609.

297. Kapen S, Boyar RM, Finkelstein J, et al. Effect of sleep-wake cycle reversal on LH secretory pattern in puberty. J Clin Endocrinol Metab 1974;39:283.

298. Fevre M, Segel T, Marks JF, et al. LH and melatonin secretion patterns in pubertal boys. J Clin Endocrinol Metab 1978;47:1383.

299. Wu FC, Butler GE, Kelnar CJ, et al. Ontogeny of pulsatile gonadotropin releasing hormone secretion from mid-childhood, through puberty, to adulthood in the human male: a study using deconvolusion analysis and then the ultrasensitive immunofluorometric assay. J Clin Endocrinol Metab 1996;81:1798.

300. Evans JI, MacLean AM, Ismail AAA, et al. Concentration of plasma testosterone in normal men during sleep. Nature 1971;229:261.

301. Weeke J, Gundersen HJG. Circadian and 30 minute variations in serum TSH and thyroid hormones in normal subjects. Acta Endocrinol 1978;89:659.

302. Lucke C, Hehrmann R, von Mayersbach K, et al. Studies in circadian variations of plasma TSH, thyroxine and triiodothyronine in man. Acta Endocrinol 1976;86:81.

303. Parker D, Pekary A, Hershman J. Effect of normal and reversed sleep-wake cycles upon nyctohemeral rhythmicity of plasma thyrotropin: evidence suggestive of an inhibitory influence in sleep. J Clin Endocrinol Metab 1976;43:318.

304. Fisher DA. Physiological variations in thyroid hormones: physiological and pathophysiological considerations. Clin Chem 1996;42:135.

305. Peters J, Santa-Cruz F, Tower B, et al. Differential endocrine responses to thyrotropin-releasing hormone during the rapid eye movement and slow-wave sleep in man. J Clin Endocrinol Metab 1981;52:975.

306. Anch AM, Browman CP, Mitler MM, et al. Sleep: A Scientific Perspective. Engelwood Cliffs, NJ: Prentice Hall, 1988.

307. Luthringer R, Brandenberger G, Schaltenbrand N, et al. Slow wave electroencephalic activity parallels renin oscillations during sleep in humans. Electroencephalogr Clin Neurophysiol 1995;95:318.

308. Leaf A, Liddle GW. Summarization of the Effects of Hormones of Water and Electrolyde Metabolism. In RH Williams (ed), Textbook of Endocrinology. Philadelphia: Saunders, 1972;938.

309. Brandenberger G, Follenius M, Muzet A, et al. Ultradian oscillations in plasma renin activity: their relationships to meals and sleep stages. J Clin Endocrinol Metab 1985;61:280.

310. Brandenberger G, Follenius M, Goichot B, et al. Twenty-four-hour profiles of plasma renin activity in relation to the sleep-wake cycle. J Hypertens 1994;12:277.

311. Kripke DF, Lavie P, Parker D, et al. Plasma parathyroid hormone and calcium are related to sleep stage cycles. J Clin Endocrinol Metab 1978;47:1021.

312. Brzezinski A. Melatonin in humans. New Engl J Med 1997;336:186.

313. Penev PD, Zee PC. Melatonin: a clinical perspective. Ann Neurol 1997;42:545.

314. Zhdanova IV, Lynch HJ, Wurtman RJ. Melatonin: a sleep-promoting hormone. Sleep 1997;20:899.

315. Sack RL, Hughes RJ, Edgar DM, Lewy AJ. Sleep-promoting effects of melatonin: at what dose, under what conditions, and by what mechanisms? Sleep 1997;20:908.

316. Coon SL, Roseboom PH, Baler R, et al. Pineal serotonin N-acetyltransferase: expression cloning and molecular analysis. Science 1995;270:1681.

317. Arend TJ. Melatonin and the Mammalian Pineal Gland. London: Chapman & Hall, 1995.

318. Kennaway DJ, Goble FC, Stamp GE. Factors influencing the development of melatonin rhythmicity in humans. J Clin Endocrinol Metab 1996;81:1525.

319. Waldhauser F, Frisch H, Waldhauser M, et al. Fall in nocturnal serum melatonin during pre-puberty and pubescence. Lancet 1994;362.

320. Sack RL, Lewy AJ, Erb DL, et al. Human melatonin production decreases with age. J Pineal Res 1986;3:379.

321. Samel A, Wegmann H-M, Vijvoda M, et al. Influence of melatonin treatment on human circadian rhythmicity before and after a simulated 9-hr time shift. J Biol Rhythms 1991;6:235.

322. Dawson D, Encel N, Lushington K. Improving adaption to simulated night shift: timed exposure to bright light versus daytime melatonin administration. Sleep 1995;18:11.

323. Dahlitz M, Alvarez B, Vignau J, et al. Delayed sleep phase syndrome response to melatonin. Lancet 1991;337:1121.

324. Oldani A, Ferini-Strambi L, Zucconi M, et al. Melatonin and delayed sleep phase syndrome: ambulatory polygraphic evaluation. Neuroreport 1994;6:132.

325. Sack RL, Lewy AJ, Blood ML, et al. Melatonin administration to blind people: phase advances and entrainment. J Biol Rhythms 1991;6:249.

326. McArthur AJ, Lewy AJ, Sack RL. Non-24-hour sleep/wake syndrome in a sighted man: circadian rhythm studies and efficacy of melatonin treatment. Sleep 1995;19:544.

327. Haimov I, Laudon M, Zisapel L, et al. Sleep disorders and melatonin rhythms in elderly people. BMJ 1994;309:167.

328. Tzischinsky O, Lavie P. Melatonin possesses time-dependent hypnotic effects. Sleep 1994;17:638.

329. Tzischinsky O, Shlitner A, Lavie P. The association between nocturnal sleep gates and nocturnal onset of urinary aMT6s. J Biol Rhythms 1994;8:199.

330. Dawson D, Encel N. Melatonin and sleep in humans. J Pineal Res 1993;15:1.

# Chapter 7
# Dreaming in Sleep-Disordered Patients

Rosalind D. Cartwright

## A BRIEF HISTORICAL INTRODUCTION

The first edition of this book had no chapter on dreaming, and that, in itself, is a commentary on the perceived importance of this area to an understanding of sleep and its disorders. Research in dreaming has been at a low ebb. In fact, its demise was mourned in a review by Foulkes,[1] one of the pioneers of this work. But the reports of the death of interest in this area are greatly exaggerated. There was a period of reduced activity, roughly from the mid-1970s to the mid-1980s, which is remarkable in light of the fact that the field of sleep, with its dual emphasis on basic science and clinical studies, has been booming since the 1970s.

The increased activity in the field of sleep can be traced to the discovery of rapid eye movement (REM) sleep. At the time, the importance of this discovery was its close association to the psychological experience of dreaming. Once the objective, identifying characteristics of REM sleep were worked out, it was anticipated that these would provide the markers for exposing this highly private mental activity to systematic study, thus expanding our understanding of abnormal mental behavior. It seemed likely that we would soon be able to answer basic questions such as, "Is a dream equivalent to the hallucination of psychosis?" and if so, "Why is it that some people hallucinate and lose the ability to evaluate perceptions critically only when asleep, whereas others have these behaviors intrude into their waking life?" The idea that research on dreaming could provide

insights into mental disorders is now being realized due to a renewed interest in dreaming in sleep-disordered patients. This chapter explores the results of studies examining the REM sleep and dreams of subjects falling into three diagnoses: depression, posttraumatic stress disorder (PTSD), and sleep terrors.

The first decade or so (i.e., 1955–1965) of the laboratory work on dreaming involved studies that were, for the most part, descriptive—devoted to mapping the relation of dreams to REM sleep. These studies addressed questions such as the following: Does the dream fill the REM period or only occur in the brief seconds during the arousal? Are the various dreams of the night interconnected? What, if anything, is the nature of the mental activity occurring between the periods of REM sleep? This literature was built largely on studies with small subject pools made up of young, healthy, predominantly male, medical or undergraduate psychology students. Much of the core of knowledge gleaned from that early work about dreaming that we take on faith has never been replicated or has failed to be confirmed on replication. Only Snyder's analysis[2] of the content of the dreams, reported from 635 REM awakenings over 250 nights for 56 subjects, gives us a data base from a fairly homogeneous sample large enough for us to have some confidence in the reliability of the findings. His conclusion—that the typical dream is a "clear, coherent, and detailed account of a realistic situation involving the dreamer and other people caught up in very ordinary activities and preoccupations, and usually talking about them"—was not at all what was expected from reports of dreams as told during psychoanalytic sessions.[3] Snyder suggested that remembered dreams make up a highly selected sample, more memorable because they are more dramatic, vivid, and emotionally rich. Furthermore, he suggested, the dreams of people who are emotionally disturbed most likely reflect this disturbance, and therefore differ from the ordinary dreams of his normal subjects. Because much of the current literature is based on patients' reports to their therapists, it is important to keep in mind the distinction between recalled dreams and dreams collected in the laboratory.

Early studies revealed a number of pitfalls associated with studying dreaming under laboratory conditions. The first was the need to adapt subjects to the laboratory before a night of awakenings. Subjects typically do not sleep well the first night in the laboratory. Onset of the first REM sleep period is often delayed, or the period is aborted after only 1–2 minutes. Furthermore, dream content is likely to be influenced by the experimental setting.[4,5] As a result, laboratory dreams got the reputation of not being representative samples of home dreams. When subjects wrote descriptions of home dreams in daily diaries, the dreams were found to be more personal and emotional and included more sex and aggression than those reported when REM sleep was interrupted in laboratories. Like the problem of the atypical first night, the influence of laboratory conditions on the content of dreams can be overcome by ensuring the privacy of the subjects.[6,7]

Another problem that emerged from early studies was one of timing the awakening. Identifying REM is not all that is required to obtain good recall of the dream. If the experimenter waits to solicit a report until a REM period is clearly over and stage II sleep has returned, the percentage of awakenings yielding dream recall will drop markedly.[8] A standard protocol was developed for collecting dreams reliably in any laboratory, ensuring that reports can be compared with confidence that the method of collection is not responsible for any differences found.

The standard protocol calls for the following:

1. A minimum of one night of uninterrupted sleep before attempting to record dreams.

2. The subject should be given instructions before lights out that minimize the implicit demand that a dream be reported at each awakening: "I will be waking you periodically tonight and asking what is going through your mind at the time. You may be thinking, or dreaming or not experiencing anything at all. That's okay. I just want to know what your experience is at the time."

3. The awakening should be made during the ongoing REM after a standard number of minutes have elapsed. REM is identified by the absence of chin muscle tone and stage II signs (spindles and K complexes). A tape recorder is turned on at the appropriate time and the subject is called by name.

4. The amount of REM sleep permitted before the wake-up is lengthened progressively from one period of REM sleep to the next, to account for the increasing length of these successive periods. The most usual schedule followed for these awakenings is

> 5 minutes after the onset of REM I
> 10 minutes after the onset of REM II
> 15 minutes after the onset of REM III
> 20 minutes after the onset of REM IV

5. On each awakening the subject is asked, "What was going through your mind just before I called you?" If no recall is given immediately the subject is asked to "take a moment to see if anything comes back to you." If nothing is reported they are to be thanked and told to go back to sleep and that they will be called again later.

6. Experimenters must be careful not to lead the subjects' recall but to help them with nonspecific prompts such as, "Anything else?"

The early normative work on adults was extended to children to study how dreaming develops. Foulkes[9] concluded from his studies of children's dreams that their structure parallels the child's waking stages of cognitive development. This discovery, added to Snyder's[2] finding about the realistic nature of the content of the dreams of normal subjects, eroded some of the mystique of dreaming.

One of the clearest findings from 1970–1980 was the degree to which there are marked individual differences in dreaming behavior. Snyder[2] reported that some people always had interesting dreams, whereas dreams of others were consistently dull. Dement's[10] initial conclusion that we have a "need to dream" based on the rebound of REM sleep after its curtailment was modified by subsequent studies finding that some REM sleep–deprived subjects did not show later rebound. Those normals who did not experience a rebound accommodated to the deprivation of REM sleep by heightening their dreaming experience during stage II sleep.[11] Not only did REM sleep deprivation not always equal dream deprivation, it did not conform to the expected model of psychosis. After modest amounts of REM sleep deprivation, some subjects performed better rather than worse during the following day.

The idea that dreaming is exclusively related to REM sleep was also challenged by the finding that sleep onset mentation was almost equally imagistic,[12] although not as narratively coherent, as the dreams of REM sleep,[13] and that all of NREM sleep became more dreamlike when subjects were more anxious or unhappy.[14] All of this lead to a revised view of dreaming, not as an epiphenomenon of REM sleep, but as an independent psychological activity: a continuous stream of mental activity that surfaces in awareness when there is a state of high cerebral arousal in the absence of attention to external stimuli. These conditions are reliably present in REM but may also be present in NREM in particular persons and circumstances. This will be discussed under Clinical Sleep Disorders.

A contrasting explanation of dreaming was proposed in the activation-synthesis hypothesis,[15] which accounted for the central characteristics of dreams—the sensory images and their connecting narrative—as by-products of the phasic-tonic nature of REM sleep and its underlying neurophysiology. This hypothesis suggests that the sensory component of dreams is triggered by the phasic bursts of spikes arising from the pons before and during REM sleep, which stimulate the production of random images. When these reach the higher cortex, which is in a state of tonic excitation and motor inhibition, meaning is added to the images both singly and collectively. This explanation was attractive, as it was both parsimonious and parallel to how waking perception adds meaning to novel sensory stimuli. Awake or asleep, the interpretation of any ambiguous stimulus is strongly influenced by what we bring to it from past experience, present needs, and ongoing interests. This, the authors imply, gives the illusion that dreams have meaning, but the meaning is in the mind of the beholder.

The activation-synthesis hypothesis, which became extremely popular, discounted the idea that dreaming had any special function. This suggestion was supported by the fact that REM sleep is turned on and off regularly, whether we have more or less "need" of our dreams. Given that dreams were robbed of uniqueness of form,[9] content,[2] and meaning and function,[15] it is not surprising that the field of dream study went into decline.

## REVIVAL OF DREAM STUDY

Few studies of the dreams of psychiatric patients were attempted during the early years of laboratory dream work because medication effects were difficult to control, and diagnostically homogeneous samples were difficult to obtain.[16-19]

New sleep disorder centers moved the field forward, as well as the demand for help from patients who were experiencing sleep disruptions such as disturbing nightmares, repetitive dreams after trauma, and episodes of sleep terrors. It was through exposure to these sleep anomalies that sleep specialists were lured back to the investigation of dreaming and its relation to waking personality structure and to current and subsequent emotional states.

### *Dreaming and Affect*

What was missing in the reductionist explanations of dreaming was a serious consideration of what dreams had to do with the emotional life of the dreamer. Even in the dream reports of normal student samples, Snyder found that negative emotions predominated in the dreams. In his study, unpleasant emotions were twice as common as pleasant emotions, with fear and anxiety the most prominent and anger next.

Breger et al.[20] confirmed this emphasis on emotion in their study of the REM sleep–monitored dreams of patients before and after elective surgery. Breger concluded that dreaming is an emotional informational processing system and that dreams are the "output of particular memory systems operating under the guidance of programs that are peculiar to sleep." Some waking experience, thought, or fantasy activates an emotional reaction that potentiates an associated memory network to further internal activity. This does not stop at sleep onset. The systems that have been primed respond in REM sleep with output that is freer in its laws of association than waking logic permits. "Association may be by shape, color, common sound or function."[21] In other words, dream content is not the result of random stimulation to which interpretable meaning is added. It is associated in meaning with the waking emotional stimulus, however loosely, due to the persistent activity of a particular memory network already activated and held at the ready for further expression during the opportunity offered by REM sleep. Dreams function as "*attempts* at emotional problem solving."

Kramer[22,23] extended this psychological model to include the effect of dreams on the subsequent waking emotional state. His studies show that in normal samples, there is an overnight mood change, specifically from more to less unhappiness, which is related to the content of the intervening dreams. He sums up the function of dreaming as one of *selective* mood regulation.

Cartwright[24,25] subscribed to this interactive psychological proposal by adding that the degree and kind of presleep waking affect is important not only in determining the form of the dream, but also the functionality of that night's dreaming as a whole. If the presleep affect is negative and the level of the affect is high, the dreams might be repetitive in content, with poor quality dream work, and the morning mood will remain unchanged; if affect is moderate, the dreams might be sequential, showing progress across the night, and these will be followed by a reduction in negative morning mood; if affect is low, the dreams might be unrelated, as the affective networks have not been sufficiently perturbed to remain active, and the morning mood will be unaffected. Cartwright also suggested that the content stored in the emotional memory network, related to the presleep experience, determines what material is available for dream construction.

Hartmann[26] provided another structural variable: the nature of the subject's psychological "boundaries." The boundaries refer to the fluidity of associations between the realms of reality and fantasy and they are measured as "thick" or "thin" by a test developed by Hartmann. He concludes that the schizophrenic and the creative person both have thin boundaries between reality and fantasy, which result in flooding of negative affect during sleep and subsequent nightmares.

A psychological model provides a framework for studying the relationship of sleep symptoms to personality traits and to the presleep and postsleep affect states of disordered dreamers. The level of informa-

tion gathered about patients must be increased to include before- and after-sleep mood scales, such as the Profile of Mood States, and some standard psychological screening test for psychopathology, such as the Minnesota Multiphasic Personality Inventory. Patients most likely to require such a work-up include those with a mood disorder, PTSD, or adult parasomnias. Patients with these disorders may present at a sleep disorder service with the complaint of insomnia (secondary to depression), persistent nightmares (after a traumatic event), and nocturnal acting out of fight or flight behaviors, usually occurring early in sleep before the first period of REM sleep.

*Sleep and Dreaming in Depression*

Two groups of researchers are responsible for the interest in looking into the dreams of the depressed: (1) Kupfer et al.[27–29] showed that the depressed have abnormal REM parameters, including early onset and high eye movement density of the first REM sleep period. (2) Vogel et al.[30] demonstrated that REM sleep–deprivation improved waking mood due to a buildup of REM pressure. Depressed individuals clearly do not show successful overnight mood regulation and it is suspected that the emotional information processing that takes place during dreaming is dysfunctional and perhaps therefore best suppressed.

Cartwright and colleagues[31–34] examined the REM sleep and dreams of subjects who were and were not depressed while going through a divorce. Seventy unmedicated community volunteers, 40 of whom met Research Diagnostic Criteria for major depression, spent three successive nights in the laboratory on two occasions, 1 year apart. Dreams were collected on the third night. Dream masochism,[35] (the dreamer is deprived, attacked, excluded, or fails) was more characteristic of women than men. Depressed women were more masochistic in their dreams than depressed men, and, at follow-up, formerly depressed women had more masochistic dreams than those men who were formerly depressed. This supports an earlier study by Hauri,[36] who found that a remitted group of former, mostly female, depressed inpatients continued to have more negative dreams than a control group who were never depressed. Greenberg et al.[37] reported that negative dreams during depression indicate a poor prognosis. This was confirmed by Cartwright and Wood,[33] who found that depressed women classified as masochistic dreamers showed less improvement in their waking lives and more need for emotional support after 1 year than did depressed women who did not have masochistic dreams. They concluded that dream masochism may be a continuing cognitive-emotional sleep style that contributes to the vulnerability of women to major depression. A further analysis of their sample found that depressed mood as assessed by the Beck Depression Inventory (BDI),[38] both initially and at follow-up, was associated with the total number of laboratory-recorded dreams rated by the subjects as unpleasant. Early onset of REM sleep was also correlated with the number of unpleasant dreams. When partial correlations were controlled for sex and initial level of depression, the correlation of the number of unpleasant dreams and the degree of depressed mood 1 year later was still significant. A multiple regression equation that entered the initial BDI score, the number of unpleasant dreams, and the eye-movement density of the first period of REM sleep accounted for 54% of the variance in the depression level at the follow-up session.

A study by Thase et al.[39] showed a significant decrease in eye-movement density in a group of 45 depressed men treated with psychotherapy designed to reduce their waking negative cognitive patterns. A reduction in eye-movement density to normal levels occurred whether the treatment resulted in remission from depression or not. No dreams were collected in this study, and the therapy did not address problems revealed in the dreaming.

These findings suggest tentatively that a more positive waking cognitive style and a therapist's support may normalize one REM sleep parameter associated with depression, but that dysphoric mood will persist or recur if the dream content continues to be negative. Perhaps this is why Vogel's work[30] showed that suppressing REM sleep will improve mood in the depressed. The alternative strategy would be to address the unpleasant dream content directly in treatment with the intent to change it,[40] as has been found to be effective with nightmare patients.[41]

### Sleep and Dreaming in Post-Traumatic Stress Disorder

Repetitive dreams that replay trauma along with the accompanying emotions of rage, fear, or grief are one diagnostic symptom of post-traumatic stress disorder.[42] Lavie and Kaminer's[43,44] study of 23 survivors of the holocaust and 10 controls, more than 40 years after their traumatic experiences during World War II, supports Vogel's position that it is better emotionally to have no dreams than it is to have bad dreams.

Lavie divided the survivors into two groups on the basis of extensive testing. One was made up of those who had adapted well in waking life and the other those who did not. They were then studied for four nights in the laboratory, with dreams collected on nights 1, 3, and 4. In waking, the well-adjusted survivors had fewer PTSD symptoms, greater ego strength, less manifest anxiety, and their defensive style was repression. Their sleep included lower eye-movement density, and they experienced a lower percentage of dream recall, less complex dreams with lower salience, and less dream anxiety than those who were poorly adjusted. The authors interpret their results as demonstrating that repression of dreams and waking memories works to protect the mental health of the individual by sealing off the traumatic past to allow for a better life adjustment.

This calls into question Breger's emotional information processing model of dream function, in which waking emotional experience evokes a dream response that integrates the new experience with previous emotional experiences that have had successful resolutions in the past.[21] This model may not be applicable to long-lasting, highly stressful experiences that have no precedent in the life of the sleeper, and for which there is no solution. Under these circumstances, different personalities may respond differently. Those with thick boundaries, in Hartmann's terms,[26] can live with their unresolved, negative experiences because they can successfully suppress their memories and the dreams that evoke them. Those whose boundaries are "thin" may continue to have trouble adapting because they are less successful at suppressing their experiences and dreaming.

One difficulty in interpreting the results of Lavie's study and its implications for understanding dreaming is the remoteness of the time of testing from the initial traumatic experience. It is possible that adaptive dreaming can be successful in the case of extreme trauma, and that the well-adjusted survivors had long since accomplished their adaptive dreaming.

Vietnam veterans have been studied closer in time to their traumatic experiences. Even in this literature, however, there is confusion as to whether REM onset is lengthened[45] or shortened,[46] and whether the disturbed dreams occur only in REM sleep, only in NREM sleep, or in both.[47,48]

A review of the findings to date from studies of Vietnam veterans with traumatic dreams by Domhoff[49] points out the differences in characteristics between those combat veterans who do and do not develop PTSD with traumatic dreams. Those who developed this syndrome are younger, less well-educated, and more likely to have experienced the death of a friend than those who did not. The veterans who did not develop the syndrome resemble the description of Lavie's well-adjusted holocaust survivors: They "put up a wall between themselves and others while in Vietnam."

Over time, traumatic dreams become less like the original experience as they are merged with other memories. However, episodes that resemble the original trauma can occur when new stressors are experienced. Kramer et al.[48] reported that a later loss of a spouse to death or divorce in a veteran will trigger a resurgence of dreams of the original trauma. These traumatic dreams can occur in all stages of sleep and occur earlier in the night than do chronic nightmares, which tend to be late-night phenomena. Kramer et al. suggest that the emotion engendered by the traumatic event overwhelms the person's ability to assimilate the experience at the time and this allows the original trauma to re-emerge from the memory networks in dreams when a new traumatic event resembling the original occurs.

Laboratory studies of PTSD patients are difficult to carry out, given the frequency of dual diagnoses with depression and chronic alcoholism, the need to discontinue medication and the effects of withdrawal, and the difficulty of obtaining an example of the traumatic dream under the circumstance of the more emotionally secure environment of the laboratory. There is clearly a need for further work in this area, particularly longitudinal studies that reveal the course of changes in sleep and in dreaming over time. The data currently available support the emotional information processing model of dreaming. When strong negative affect is engendered in someone who is unprepared for it, who has no successful resolutions from previous experiences to rely on, and who must remain in the disturbing conditions over time, they are likely to have heightened arousal levels throughout all sleep. This makes it possible for dreams to occur in all sleep stages and for the dream content to appear more like the original event, rather than as material assimilated to other memories. Patients who present with recurrent nightmares may have been PTSD patients years ago and are now experiencing a relapse due to some new stress.

### Dreams in Sleep Terrors

Sleep terrors are defined as one of the parasomnias. These have been well-described by Broughton[50] as an arousal, usually from the first or second delta sleep cycle of the night, accompanied by a confusional state and the behavior and physiologic manifestations of terror. Sleep terrors are more common in children than adults. As they tend to happen during the transition from delta to REM sleep, they typically delay the appearance of the first period of REM sleep and may reduce the total amount of REM sleep on the nights they occur. The sleeper is usually inconsolable at the time and may engage in complex behaviors to rescue someone, escape, or fight an enemy. There is little or no recall once the episode is over and rarely any morning recall.

Several writers have noted that children who experience sleep terrors rarely have any associated psychopathology but that the adult patient is more likely to have some personality disturbance.[51] Minnesota Multiphasic Personality profiles of these patients seen in our laboratory show them to have elevated scores on the scale that measures impulses to act out with antisocial behaviors (the psychopathic deviant score). This desire to act out is being tightly controlled by the patient during waking.

There have been no formal laboratory studies reporting the REM dreams of these patients but reports of the mentation experienced at the time they are abruptly aroused from delta sleep in the laboratory are instructive. The mentation often includes a strong emotional issue.[52] One case example will illustrate this: The patient is a well-mannered, mild young man who suffered sleep terrors with an image of a bus about to run him over. He would jump out of bed to run out of the way of the bus. When asked in treatment to change the image to one with a more positive conclusion, he stated he would like to "turn around and shoot the son of a bitch." This alerted the therapist to the fact that the threat was from a man and came from behind. His sleep terrors had re-emerged after his marriage, which came after a period of quiescence beginning in his childhood.

The interpretation of these images is highly speculative and further work is needed to collect in the laboratory examples of the mentation behind sleep terrors. The available data do suggest, however, that the sleep terror patient has strong impulses that are unacceptable and are therefore carefully controlled by the patient during waking. In those individuals with a predisposition to delta arousals from childhood, the later exacerbation of these impulses may precipitate a resurgence of arousal before REM sleep to avoid their fuller expression in dreams. This is supported by preliminary data showing that these patients tend to have poor recall of any dreams until their terror episodes subside.

### Drugs and Dreams

Various medications have been associated with both increased and decreased experience of dreaming. For example, one of the claims of melatonin users is that melatonin results in an intensification of colorful dreams. Because both depression and PTSD are often treated with tricyclics, many of which have a REM sleep–supressing effect, it was speculated that part of their benefit for these disorders might stem from relieving the patient of bad dreams. This is bolstered by reports that reducing or eliminating these medications is often followed by increased intensity of nightmares. Erman[53] has reviewed the effects of antidepressants on nightmares. The logic that dream suppression is responsible for the effectiveness of the tricyclics is challenged by the observation that some of the newer serotonin-reuptake inhibitors are effective for mood improvement with little or no suppression of REM sleep.

There is a substantial history of usefulness and safety of clonazepam for the control of adult sleep terrors. This may be a result of its reputed effect of lightening the delta sleep in the first cycle, which allows the patient to move more smoothly into REM sleep. As yet there has been no study examining whether by eliminating the arousal that aborts the first period of REM sleep this medication also promotes more efficient "dream work" to take place.

## CONCLUSION

The two explanatory models of dreaming we have reviewed, the neurophysiologic activation-synthesis model and the psychological emotional information processing model, are not incompatible. It is possible that the state of arousal in REM sleep, although not determining dream content, does provide the conditions that allow the ongoing stream of thought to occupy awareness. Those in a state of hyperarousal due to unresolved negative affect may experience early onset of REM sleep (as in depression), develop the conditions for dreaming in NREM sleep (as in PTSD), or abort REM sleep (as in sleep terrors). All of these events are less efficient for mood regulation. Dreaming is a natural part of a 24-hour period of mental activity. The disturbance of dreaming in sleep-disordered patients provides an opportunity to understand more fully the nature and function of dreaming.

## REFERENCES

1. Foulkes D. Dream research 1953–1993. Sleep 1996; 19:609.
2. Snyder F. The Phenomenology of Dreaming. In L Madow, L Snow (eds), The Psychodynamic Implications of the Physiological Studies of Dreams. Springfield, IL: Thomas 1970;124.
3. Freud S. The Interpretation of Dreams. New York: Basic Books, 1955 (original date 1900).
4. Dement W, Kahn E, Roffwarg H. The influence of the laboratory situation on the dreams of the experimental subject. J Nerv Ment Dis 1965;140:119.
5. Domhoff W, Kamiya J. A comparison of home and laboratory dream reports. Arch Gen Psychiatry 1964;11:519.
6. Weisz R, Foulkes D. Home and laboratory dreams collected under uniform sampling conditions. Psychophysiology 1970;6:588.
7. Lloyd S, Cartwright R. The collection of home and laboratory dreams by means of an instrumental response technique. Dreaming 1995;63.
8. Dement W, Kleitman N. The relation of eye movements during sleep to dream: an objective method for the study of dreaming. J Exp Psychol 1957;53:339.
9. Foulkes D. Children's Dreams. New York: Wiley, 1982;275.
10. Dement W. The effect of dream deprivation. Science 1960;131:1705.
11. Cartwright R, Monroe L, Palmer C. Individual differences in response to REM deprivation. Arch Gen Psychiatry 1967;16:297.
12. Foulkes D, Vogel G. Mental activity at sleep onset. J Abnorm Psychol 1965;70:231.
13. Rechtschaffen A, Verdone P, Wheaton J. Reports of mental activity during sleep. Can Psychiatr Assoc J 1963;8:409.

14. Brown J, Cartwright R. Locating NREM dreaming through instrumental responses. Psychophysiology 1978;15:35.

15. Hobson A, McCarley R. The brain as a dream state generator: an activation synthesis hypothesis of the dream process. Am J Psychiatry 1977;134:1335.

16. Dement W. Dream recall and eye movements during sleep in schizophrenics and normals. J Nerv Ment Dis 1955;122:263.

17. Kramer M, Roth T. A comparison of dream content in dream reports of schizophrenic and depressed patient groups. Compr Psychiatry 1973;14:325.

18. Cartwright R. Sleep fantasy in normal and schizophrenic persons. J Abnorm Psychol 1972;80:275.

19. Freedman N, Grand S, Karacan I. An approach to the study of dreaming and changes in psychopathological states. J Nerv Ment Dis 1966;143:399.

20. Breger L, Hunter I, Lane R. The effect of stress on dreams. Psychol Issues Monogr 1971;7:No. 27.

21. Breger L. Dream Function: An Information Processing Model. In L Breger (ed), Clinical-Cognitive Psychology. Englewood Cliffs, NJ: Prentice-Hall, 1969;209.

22. Kramer M, Roth T. The Mood Regulating Function of Sleep. In W Koella, P Levin (eds), Sleep: Physiology, Biochemistry, Psychology, Pharmacology, Clinical Implications. Basel: Karger, 1973;563.

23. Kramer M. The Selective Mood Regulatory Function of Dreaming: An Update and Revision. In A Moffitt, M Kramer, R Hoffman (eds), The Functions of Dreaming. New York: New York University Press, 1993.

24. Cartwright R. The nature and function of repetitive dreams: a survey and speculation. Psychiatry 1979;42:131.

25. Cartwright R. Affect and dream work from an information processing point of view. Cogn Dream Res. 1986; 7:411.

26. Hartmann E. Boundaries of the Mind: A New Psychology of Personality. New York: Basic Books, 1991.

27. Kupfer D, Foster F. Interval between the onset of sleep and rapid eye movements as an indicator of depression. Lancet 1972;11:684.

28. Kupfer D. A psychobiological marker for primary depressive disease. Biol Psychiatry 1976;11:159.

29. Kupfer D, Foster F, Coble P, et al. The application of EEG sleep for the differential diagnosis of affective disorders. Am J Psychiatry 1978;37:247.

30. Vogel G, Thurmond A, Gibbons P, et al. REM sleep reduction effects on depression syndromes. Arch Gen Psychiatry 1975;32:765.

31. Cartwright R, Kravitz AH, Eastman C, et al. REM latency and recovery from depression: getting over divorce. Am J Psychiatry 1991;148:1530.

32. Cartwright R. "Masochism" in dreaming and its relation to depression. Dreaming 1992;2:79.

33. Cartwright R, Wood E. The contribution of dream masochism to the sex ratio difference in depression. Psychiatry Res 1993;46:165.

34. Cartwright R. REM dream characteristics related to the chronicity of depression. Sleep Res 1997;26:239.

35. Beck A. Depression. New York: Harper & Row, 1967;333.

36. Hauri P. Dreams in patients remitted from reactive depression. J Abnorm Psychol 1976;85:1.

37. Greenberg R, Pearlman C, Blacher R, et al. Depression: variability of intrapsychic and sleep parameters. J Am Acad Psychoanal 1990;18:233.

38. Beck A, Ward C, Mendelson W, et al. An inventory for measuring depression. Arch Gen Psychiatry 1961;4:561.

39. Thase M, Reynolds C, Frank E, et al. Polysomnographic studies of unmedicated depressed men before and after cognitive behavioral therapy. Am J Psychiatry 1994;151:1615.

40. Cartwright R, Lamberg L. Crisis Dreaming. New York: Harper Perennial, 1993.

41. Neidhardt E, Krakow B, Kellner R, et al. The beneficial effects of one treatment session and recording of nightmares on chronic nightmare sufferers. Sleep 1992;15:470.

42. Ross R, Ball W, Sullivan K, et al. Sleep disturbance as the hallmark of post traumatic stress disorder. Am J Psychiatry 1989;146:697.

43. Lavie P, Kaminer H. Dreams the poison sleep: dreaming in holocaust survivors. Dreaming 1991;1:11.

44. Lavie P, Kaminer H. Dreaming and Coping Style in Holocaust Survivors. In D Barrett (ed),Trauma and Dreams. Cambridge: Harvard University Press 1996;114.

45. Schlosberg A, Benjamin M. Sleep patterns in three combat fatigue cases. J Clin Psychiatry 1978;39:546.

46. Greenberg R, Pearlman C, Gampel D. War neuroses and the adaptive function of REM sleep. Br J Med Psychol 1972;45:27.

47. Hartmann E. The Nightmare: The Psychology and Biology of Terrifying Dreams. New York: Basic Books, 1984.

48. Kramer M, Schoen L, Kinney L. The Dream Experience in Dream-Disturbed Vietnam Veterans. In van der Kolk (ed), Post-Traumatic Stress Disorder: Psychological and Biological Sequelae. Washington: American Psychiatric Press, 1984.

49. Domhoff GW. The Repetition of Dreams and Dream Elements: A Possible Clue to a Function of Dreams. In A Moffitt, M Kramer, R Hoffman (eds), The Functions of Dreaming. Albany, NY: State University of New York Press 1993;293.

50. Broughton R. Parasomnias. In S Chokroverty (ed), Sleep Disorders Medicine: Basic Science, Technical Considerations, and Clinical Aspects (1st ed). Boston: Butterworth–Heinemann, 1994;381.

51. Kales A, Soldatos C, Caldwell A, et al. Somnambulism: clinical characteristics and personality patterns. Arch Gen Psychiatry 1980;37:1406.

52. Fisher C, Kahn E, Edwards S, et al. Psychophysiological study of nightmares and night terrors III mental content and recall of stage 4 night terrors. J Nerv Ment Dis 1974;15:174.

53. Erman M. Dream anxiety attacks (nightmares). Psychiatr Clin North Am 1987;10:667.

# Chapter 8
# Circadian Regulation of Sleep

## Thomas S. Kilduff and Clete A. Kushida

Sleep research since the 1970s has provided evidence that the occurrence of sleep is regulated by both homeostatic and circadian mechanisms. Although the homeostatic nature of sleep has probably been evident even to untrained observers for centuries, an appreciation of the role of the circadian system in gating the occurrence of sleep has been recognized only relatively recently. This chapter introduces the mammalian circadian system, discusses evidence suggesting roles of both homeostatic and circadian influences on sleep control, and presents three models for the interaction between these systems. The chapter concludes with a discussion of the impact of circadian rhythms on public health.

## THE MAMMALIAN CIRCADIAN SYSTEM

### Introduction to Circadian Terminology

One of the fundamental properties of living matter is an underlying rhythmicity. This property is so ubiquitous it has been suggested that it should be added to the list of the four characteristics of life—growth, reproduction, movement, and responsiveness (or irritability). Natural cycles vary in length from the firing of individual neurons at millisecond intervals to the 17-year growth-and-flight cycle of the periodic cicada. A more commonly observed periodicity is the cycle of activity and rest associated with the rhythmic geophysical fluctuations of light and darkness. Organisms that are active during the day and rest at night are called *diurnal*, whereas those active at night are *nocturnal*. Other animals, including many rodents and birds, that are active primarily at dawn and dusk are called *crepuscular*. In many cases, these cycles of activity and inactivity are not merely passive responses by the organism to changing environmental conditions; rather, they are endogenous and appear to be generated by an internal timing mechanism or pacemaker known as the *biological clock*.

The strongest test for the existence of an endogenous rhythm is its persistence when all exogenous periodic cues (e.g., cycles of light and dark, temperature and humidity fluctuations, social cues) have been removed from the organism's environment. If the observed variable remains periodic under such constant conditions, the rhythmicity is ascribed to an *endogenous pacemaker* or clock. The most commonly studied endogenous rhythms are *circadian*, those with periods approximately 24 hours in length (derived from Latin: *circa,* about; *diem,* day). Rhythms with periods shorter than a day are *ultradian* and those that approximate a year in length are *circannual*. Rhythms of these periodicities are not restricted to overtly observable behavior but include internal physiologic rhythms, such as the ultradian oscillations in heart rate, the circadian rhythm of melatonin release by the pineal gland, and circannual cycles of testicular regression and recrudescence in some rodent species.

Figure 8-1 illustrates some of the basic properties of circadian rhythms using the locomotor activity of

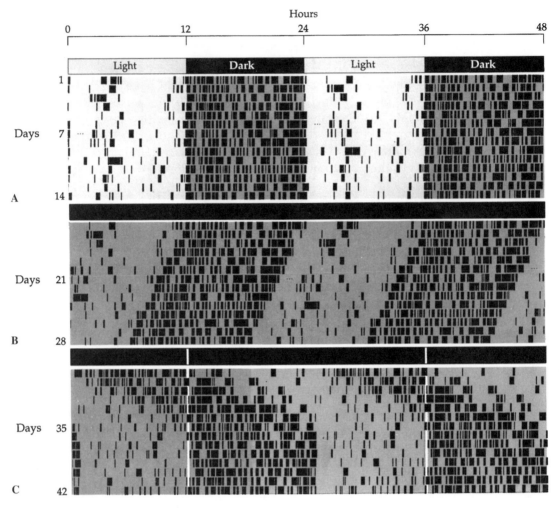

**Figure 8-1.** Wheel-running activity of a mouse recorded for 6 weeks in three experimental conditions. Vertical tick marks in each line indicate that running in the wheel has occurred during a particular 10-minute epoch; 48 hours of data are double-plotted in standard circadian fashion. **(A)** Animal is subjected to 12-hour light/12-hour dark photoperiod. Note that the major period of activity begins at light offset, as one would expect in a nocturnal animal. **(B)** Animal is subjected to continuous darkness for 14 days; note that the onset of activity drifts to an earlier time each successive day but that activity onset is fairly precise between days. **(C)** Animal is subjected to a single 10-minute light pulse every 24 hours for 2 weeks. Note that within 7 days, the mouse has synchronized its activity onset to the offset of the 10-minute light pulse. (Reprinted from WK Purves, GH Orians, HC Heller. Life: The Science of Biology [4th ed]. Sunderland, MA: Sinauer, 1995.)

the mouse as an example. In Figure 8-1A (days 1–14), wheel-running activity in this nocturnal species primarily occurs during the dark phase of a 12-hour light/12-hour dark (LD) cycle. On day 15 (Figure 8-1B), this periodic environmental cue is removed and the mouse's activity is recorded while in constant darkness (DD). Note that the mouse continues to run for a portion of each day during the period called its *subjective night* and is relatively inactive during its *subjective day*. The fact that the activity rhythm persists in DD indicates that the rhythm is truly endogenous and thus likely to be generated by an internal pacemaker. Note also that the animal begins its major activity period slightly earlier each day. If one were to fit a regression line to the onset of activity each day, the period of the activity rhythm generated by the endogenous pacemaker would be approximately 23.5 hours in DD. Thus, in retrospect, the LD cycle in days 1–14 must have synchronized the endogenous pacemaker, which had a period of 23.5 hours, to precisely 24 hours. Using the same terms physicists use to describe properties of harmonic oscillations, the environmental LD cycle *entrained* the internal pacemaker of the mouse. *Entrainment* is the process whereby the period of an external variable such as the LD cycle imposes itself on the organism's endogenous rhythm. Other commonly used terms in the discussion of rhythms are *amplitude*, referring to the magnitude of an observable rhythm, and *phase*, which refers to a particular point in the cycle.

Figure 8-1C illustrates another property of circadian rhythms regarding the entrainment process. In this case, the periodic environmental cue is a 10-minute pulse of light that recurs every 24 hours, rather than 12 hours of continuous light. Even this brief exposure to light is an effective stimulus, as the activity rhythm is clearly re-entrained by day 35 of the record. Note that entrainment occurs over the course of several cycles (days 29–35), while a stable phase relationship is gradually established between the periodic environmental stimulus and the endogenous rhythm. Environmental variables that are capable of entraining circadian rhythms are known as *entraining agents* or *Zeitgebers* (from the German: *Zeit,* time; *Geber,* giver). Although light is the most commonly studied entraining agent, temperature, food availability, and social interaction are also effective *Zeitgebers.*

Figure 8-2 demonstrates an important characteristic of circadian pacemakers: They can be reset to a new phase by a single presentation of an entraining agent. As in the case of many oscillators, resetting the pacemaker's underlying circadian rhythms is nonlinear—that is, the resultant phase after the perturbation is a function of the phase at which the perturbation occurred. Figure 8-2 presents an example in which a brief light pulse (approximately 15 minutes) is presented at five different circadian phases (A–E). The effect of the light pulse in resetting the circadian pacemaker is dependent on the phase at which the light pulse occurs. Whereas a light pulse at A during the subjective day is ineffective, light pulses at B and C during the early subjective night cause the onset of activity to occur later on subsequent days (a phase delay). Conversely, light pulses at D and E during the late subjective night cause advances of the activity rhythm on successive days. The sum of all these responses is presented in the lower half of Figure 8-2

as a *phase response curve*, which is a property of the underlying pacemaker.

At this point, it should be apparent that circadian biologists make inferences about the central pacemaker or clock based on measurements made on observable rhythms such as wheel-running activity. However, circadian experiments are guided by an explicit theoretical framework presented in Figure 8-3. Implicit in this model is the expectation that the inputs to the clock, the pacemaker itself, and the outputs from the pacemaker are anatomically localized. As described in the next section, this does appear to be the case for the circadian system of mammals.

## *Location of the Circadian Pacemaker*

The search for the pathway whereby light entrains circadian rhythms focused on the primary optic tract in the early 1970s. When the optic nerves were severed or the eyes removed, the circadian rhythms of laboratory mammals were found to free-run, even when the animals were kept under an LD cycle. If the optic tract was severed caudal to the decussation of the optic nerves in the optic chiasm, however, animals continued to entrain to an LD cycle. These results led to the conclusion that an area of the hypothalamus around the optic chiasm was important for the entrainment of circadian rhythms by light. Using sensitive autoradiographic techniques, a direct retinohypothalamic (RHT) projection was found to terminate in a small cluster of cells in the anterior hypothalamus known as the *suprachiasmatic nuclei* (SCN).[1,2] When the SCN were lesioned bilaterally, circadian rhythms were disrupted (Figure 8-4). This seminal observation made virtually simultaneously by two groups in 1972[3,4] led to a number of discoveries demonstrating that the circadian pacemaker (biological clock) of mammals is located in the SCN.

In addition to the behavioral and anatomic evidence presented earlier, both in vivo and in vitro physiologic experiments indicate that the SCN contain a light-entrainable circadian pacemaker. The SCN receive direct and indirect retinal projections necessary to entrain circadian rhythms to environmental cycles. The SCN make up the only area of the brain known to undergo a rhythm of glucose metabolism.[5,6] Surgical isolation of the SCN from other brain regions eliminates circadian rhythms of

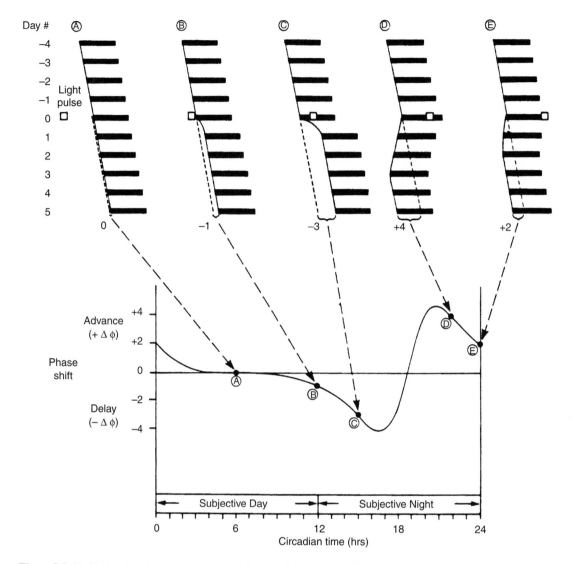

**Figure 8-2.** Derivation of a phase-response curve using resetting of the activity rhythm as an example. In each of the five experiments illustrated (A–E), a 15-minute light pulse is presented at a different circadian phase (relative to activity onset) to an animal being recorded in constant conditions. In contrast to Figure 8-1C, the 15-minute light pulse is presented on a single day rather than on multiple days. Note that the effect of the light pulse on the animal's activity on subsequent days depends on where the light pulse occurred in the animal's activity period: Light pulses early in the activity period (subjective night) delay activity onset on subsequent days whereas light pulses late during the activity period advance activity onset on succeeding days. (Reprinted with permission from MC Moore-Ede, FM Sulzman, CA Fuller. The Clocks That Time Us: Physiology of the Circadian Timing System. Cambridge, MA: Harvard University Press, 1982.)

electrical activity outside the surgically produced hypothalamic "island."[7] Tissue explants containing the SCN maintained in vitro continue to express circadian rhythms of single-unit activity,[8,9] glucose utilization,[10,11] and vasopressin release,[12,13] indicating that rhythm generation is intrinsic to the nucleus. In addition, circadian rhythmicity can be restored to arrhythmic, SCN-lesioned animals by implantation of fetal brain tissue containing SCN cells.[14,15] Most importantly, SCN transplants determine the *period* of circadian rhythms exhibited by the recipient animals.[16] Thus, the circadian clock in the SCN is a

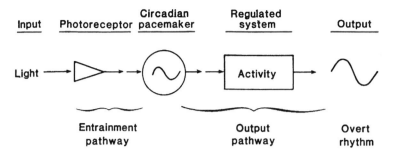

**Figure 8-3.** A schematic model of the elements of a circadian system. Research indicates that feedback to the central oscillator may occur from overt rhythms in many systems. (Reprinted with permission from A Eskin. Identification and physiology of circadian pacemakers. Introduction. Fed Proc 1979;38:2570.)

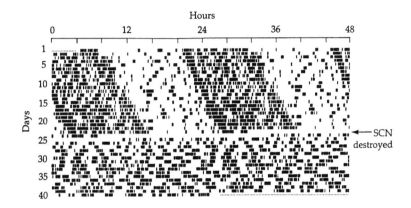

**Figure 8-4.** Activity of a mouse recorded in constant darkness for 40 days. Forty-eight hours of data are double-plotted in standard circadian fashion. Note that for the first 25 days, the onset of activity is slightly later each day (i.e., the period of the endogenous pacemaker is greater than 24 hours). On day 25, the mouse's suprachiasmatic nuclei (SCN) are lesioned bilaterally and the precise activity rhythm is permanently disrupted, indicating that the circadian pacemaker (or its output—see Figure 8-3) has been damaged. (Reprinted with permission from L Trachsel, DM Edgar, WF Seidel, et al. Sleep homeostasis in suprachiasmatic nuclei-lesioned rats: effects of sleep deprivation and triazolam administration. Brain Res 1992;589:253.)

self-sustaining oscillator that is a primary component of the mammalian circadian system.

### *Neurobiology of the Suprachiasmatic Nucleus*

The SCN are two small, paired nuclei, each containing approximately 8,000 neurons, which are located directly above the optic chiasm and to either side of the third ventricle. The SCN seem to be in the same general location but are more laterally placed in humans.

The SCN receive three major afferent projections. (1) As indicated earlier, photic information, which can entrain the circadian pacemaker to environmental LD cycles, is transmitted directly from the retina to the SCN via the RHT. The neurotransmitter released by these neurons is thought to be an excitatory amino acid or a dipeptide, (e.g., glutamate or *N*-acetylaspartylglutamate), but data on this point are not conclusive. The neuropeptide substance P has been suggested as a modulator of this projection.[17] (2) The SCN also receive an indirect retinal projection from the intergeniculate leaflet of the lateral geniculate nucleus via the geniculohypothalamic tract. The neurotransmitter of this projection is neuropeptide Y.[18] (3) Finally, the SCN receive a massive serotonergic input from the midbrain raphe nuclei[19] that is likely to mediate nonphotic input to the SCN. All three sets of afferents project to the ventrolateral portion of the SCN and may actually synapse on the same intrinsic neurons. These pathways and the concomitant neurotransmitter receptors represent potential sites at which

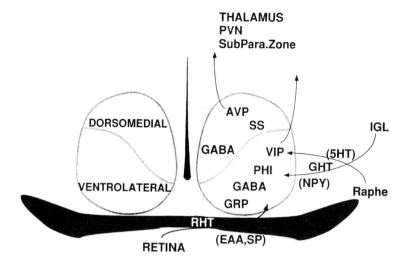

**Figure 8-5.** Schematic of the suprachiasmatic nuclei showing afferents, efferents and the distribution of neuropeptides and neurotransmitters within the dorsomedial and ventrolateral divisions. (PVN = paraventricular nuclei; AVP = arginine vasopressin; SS = somatostatin; GABA = γ-aminobutyric acid; VIP = vasoactive intestinal polypeptide; PHI = peptide histidine isoleucine; GRP = gastrin-releasing peptide; RHT = retinohypothalamic tract; EAA = excitatory amino acid; SP = substance P; IGL = intergeniculate leaflet; 5-HT = serotonin; GHT = geniculohypothalamic tract; NPY = neuropeptide Y.) (Reprinted with permission from S-IT Inouye, K Shinohara, K Tominaga, et al. Circadian Rhythms in Peptides and Their Precursor Messenger RNAs in the Suprachiasmatic Nucleus. In H Nakagawa, Y Oomura, K Nagai [eds], New Functional Aspects of the Suprachiasmatic Nucleus of the Hypothalamus. London: John Libbey, 1993;219.)

pharmacologic treatments can be directed to manipulate the biological clock.

Several neuropeptides are intrinsic to the SCN. Vasoactive intestinal polypeptide (VIP) cell bodies are found primarily in the ventrolateral SCN (the region receiving most of the afferent innervation and often called the *visual SCN*),[20] whereas arginine vasopressin–containing cell bodies are located primarily in the dorsomedial (nonvisual) SCN (Figure 8-5). Peptide histidine isoleucine and gastrin-releasing peptide are colocalized with VIP. γ-Aminobutyric acid (GABA)-ergic neurons are scattered throughout the SCN,[21] whereas somatostatin-containing cells are located between the ventrolateral and dorsomedial divisions of the SCN.[22] Although these are the most numerous cell types, several other neuroactive substances exist in the SCN.

Despite increasing knowledge about the efferent connections from the SCN to other brain regions, it is not well-understood how the SCN communicate time-of-day information to regulate behavioral states such as sleep and wakefulness or other regulated physiologic systems, with the exception of the pineal melatonin rhythm (see Melatonin and the Pineal Gland). The major efferent projections from the SCN are (1) dorsally to (a) the subparaventricular zone and paraventricular nuclei (PVN) of the hypothalamus and (b) to the thalamus, and (2) dorsocaudally to the dorsomedial hypothalamic nucleus.[23–25] Weaker projections to other hypothalamic nuclei also exist. Although these neural pathways represent the anatomic basis by which the SCN communicate with the rest of the central nervous system (CNS) to provide a circadian organization to behavior and internal synchronization of an organism's physiology, there is evidence suggesting that the SCN may also communicate via a humoral link to the rest of the brain.[26]

*Melatonin and the Pineal Gland*

The efferent pathway from the SCN to a regulated physiologic variable that is best understood is the pineal melatonin rhythm. This pathway involves an efferent from the SCN to the PVN of the hypothalamus, which projects directly to the intermediolateral (IML) horn of the spinal cord.[27–29] The IML in turn projects to the superior cervical ganglion, which provides sympathetic input to the pineal gland. Several of the neurotransmitters and receptors involved in this pathway have been determined. The net result is that basal levels of pineal (and plasma) melatonin occur throughout the day and peak melatonin concentrations occur at night, even if an organism is kept in constant conditions. High-affinity melatonin receptors exist in the SCN and relatively few other brain regions,[30,31] suggesting the possibility of a feedback loop between the SCN and pineal gland.

Melatonin (*N*-acetyl-5-methoxytryptamine) is synthesized in two steps from the neurotransmitter serotonin (5-hydroxytryptamine), with pineal *N*-acetyltransferase (NAT) being the rate-limiting step. NAT activity is under circadian control by the pathway described earlier and is very light-sensitive: Interruption of darkness by a brief pulse of light results in a rapid, dramatic decline of NAT activity and, consequently, pineal melatonin concentration. These properties suggest that melatonin serves as an internal humoral signal to communicate time-of-day information throughout the body, a suggestion that has made melatonin the subject of a great deal of interest. Furthermore, because melatonin can be detected in saliva as well as plasma, this hormone provides a useful marker of the circadian clock in clinical research. Indeed, in blind individuals, timed daily injections of melatonin can synchronize the internal melatonin rhythm, suggesting that this hormone can synchronize the biological clock in the SCN. In a study with rats, daily melatonin administration entrained activity rhythm and lesions of the SCN prevented the entraining effect.[32] The existence of high-affinity melatonin receptors in the rat SCN[30,31] lends further support to a physiologic role for melatonin in entrainment. These observations, as well as others, have spurred interest in melatonin as a potential "jet lag pill" that could hasten re-entrainment of the biological clock after intercontinental flights. At the present, however, large-scale, well-controlled studies have not been conducted to determine the efficacy and safety of this compound in humans.

### Gene Expression, the Phase-Shifting Response, and Entrainment

As indicated earlier, circadian rhythms are normally entrained to the external light-dark cycle, but persist under constant (free-running) environmental conditions. Figure 8-2 illustrates that a free-running activity rhythm can be phase-shifted by light pulses in a phase-dependent manner: Light pulses delivered early in the active period result in phase delays of the pacemaker, whereas pulses given late in the active period cause phase advances. This phase-dependent response to light is likely the basis of the photic entrainment process, especially in nocturnal species that only see light at dusk and dawn.

Inducing a phase-shift of the circadian system represents a long-term modification of the organism's behavior. Because other long-term changes in the CNS involve changes in gene expression, resetting the circadian clock might also be expected to involve a change in transcriptional processes. It is now understood that a specific class of genes known as *immediate early genes* (IEGs) are induced in the rodent SCN in response to photic stimulation, but only at circadian times when light pulses produce phase-shifts of the circadian system (i.e., the subjective night or active period in a nocturnal animal).[33–37] Furthermore, the luminance threshold for induction of IEGs is very similar to the threshold for photic-induced phase-shifts,[36] suggesting that IEG induction is a part of the pathway of the phase-shifting response. These observations are particularly significant because IEGs encode proteins that act as transcription factors to regulate the long-term response of cells to stimulation. Taken together, these data suggest that IEGs are a molecular component of the photic pathway for entrainment of mammalian circadian rhythms.

There is strong evidence for genetic regulation of the period of circadian pacemakers. In *Drosophila*, there are mutant strains at the *per* locus that are completely arrhythmic or have either a 19- or 29-hour rhythm instead of the 24-hour rhythm found in the wild type.[38] An elegant series of experiments has determined that the per protein interacts with the tim protein to regulate the circadian control of *per* transcription[39] and that the per protein itself may be a transcription factor. In mammals, the *tau* mutant hamster has a period of approximately 20 hours compared to 23.9–24.1 hours found in the wild type; heterozygotes show an intermediate period of 22 hours, indicating a single gene at this locus.[40] The identity of the gene and the protein it encodes is not known at the present time. The discovery of the clock mutation in mice[41] increases the likelihood that a molecular basis for the circadian oscillator within the mammalian SCN will be found in the not-too-distant future.

## HOMEOSTATIC AND CIRCADIAN INTERACTIONS IN SLEEP REGULATION

### *Evidence for Sleep Homeostasis*

Although the existence of compensatory sleep responses to sleep deprivation has probably been evident even to untrained observers for centuries, a rigorous quantification of the homeostatic response did not occur until spectral analysis was used to analyze electroencephalogram (EEG) signals. The occurrence of slow-wave sleep during the first third of the night, its decline across the rest period, and its recovery before rapid eye movement (REM) sleep after total sleep deprivation were noted by early sleep investigators. After spectral analysis was introduced, however, a number of studies suggested that the presence of EEG slow waves—activity in the 0.5- to <4.0-Hz (delta) range of the EEG during non-REM (NREM) sleep—was an important characteristic of sleep that may be related to the underlying homeostatic process. When EEG slow-wave activity (SWA) is subjected to Fourier analysis, the spectral power measured in the delta range during NREM sleep is high at the beginning of the rest period and then declines during sleep. Furthermore, this parameter of EEG delta power measured at sleep onset was found to increase in proportion to previous wake duration in humans and many other species.[42–45] Nap studies subsequently indicated buildup of SWA in proportion to the time elapsed since the previous night's sleep[46] and other studies have documented that sleep interruptions delay the peak in SWA.[47] EEG delta power has therefore been interpreted to represent the cortical manifestation of the recovery processes from previous waking activities occurring during sleep.[48,49] Thus, numerous studies of sleep deprivation in humans and animals support the idea that sleep is homeostatically regulated and that EEG delta power may be a useful physiologic index of sleep homeostasis.

### *Evidence for Circadian Involvement in Sleep Regulation*

The involvement of the circadian system in sleep regulation first became apparent in the late 1970s from both animal and human studies. In rats, ablation of the SCN resulted in arrhythmicity of the sleep-wake cycle.[50] In humans, a "90-minute day" study placed subjects on a schedule of 60 minutes of wakefulness and 30 minutes of sleep for five and one-third 24-hour periods, followed by two 24-hour recovery periods.[51,52] Circadian patterns of sleep-wake behavior persisted despite increasing sleep debt, thus providing evidence for a circadian process associated with sleep and alertness independent of the homeostatic sleep drive. Sleep studies of humans maintained in temporal isolation indicated that sleep onset was coupled with body temperature rhythm and that sleep duration was linked to the phase of temperature rhythm at sleep onset.[53] REM sleep in particular was found to be closely connected to the circadian pacemaker.[54] Forced desynchrony studies have demonstrated dramatic alerting effects of the circadian system across the circadian day, even after prolonged wakefulness.[55,56]

Given these observations of the involvement of the circadian system in sleep onset and duration, determining the role of the SCN in regulating the homeostatic response to sleep was the next step. This question was addressed by assessing the homeostatic response to sleep deprivation in animals in which the SCN was surgically ablated. Mistlberger et al.[57] assessed recovery sleep for 3–5 days after 24 hours of total sleep deprivation in normal rats and in rats lacking circadian rhythms of sleep because of lesioning of the SCN. All groups showed immediate rebounds of high-amplitude NREM sleep and para-doxical sleep, confined mostly to the first 12–18 hours of recovery, and decreases in moderate and low-amplitude NREM sleep during the first 6–12 hours of recovery. Total sleep rebound was distributed over a longer period in SCN-lesioned rats but total accumulated rebound sleep was similar in all groups. Thus, the SCN were proposed to modulate the timing but not the amount of accumulated total sleep rebound. Tobler et al.[58] also assessed the effects of 24-hour sleep deprivation on sleep in SCN-lesioned rats. As found in the Mistlberger et al.[57] study, sleep deprivation caused an increase in total sleep, REM sleep, and

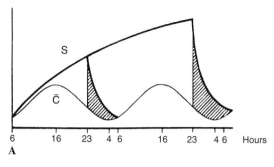

**Figure 8-6.** Three models incorporating homeostatic and circadian processes in sleep regulation. **(A)** The two-process model includes a sleep homeostatic process (S) and a circadian process (C). Sleep deprivation results in a sharp rise in sleep propensity as depicted in the second circadian cycle. (Reprinted with permission from AA Borbely. A two process model of sleep regulation. Hum Neurobiol 1982; 1:195.) **(B)** The opponent-process model proposes that the suprachiasmatic nuclei have an alerting function, opposing the sleep load that accumulates across the waking period. (Reprinted with permission from DM Edgar, WC Dement, CA Fuller, et al. Effect of SCN lesions on sleep in squirrel monkeys: evidence for opponent processes in sleep-wake regulation. J Neurosci 1993;13:1065.) **(C)** The three-process model includes a circadian process (C), a homeostatic process during waking (S), and a homeostatic process during sleep (S'), which are summed (S + C) to yield a scaled score of predicted alertness. (Reprinted with permission from T Akerstedt, S Folkard. Predicting duration of sleep from the three process model of regulation of alertness. Occup Environ Med 1996;53:136.)

the slow-wave sleep portion of NREM sleep. On the basis of these results, Tobler et al.[58] concluded that "the homeostatic component of sleep regulation is 'morphologically and functionally distinct' from the circadian component." In a study designed to assess the necessity of the SCN for the soporific effects of the benzodiazepine triazolam, Trachsel et al.[59] found that state-specific EEG power spectra profiles in SCN-lesioned rats were similar to those of intact animals, although EEG SWA in NREM sleep was markedly lower in SCN-lesioned rats. Because recovery from 6-hour sleep deprivation was characterized by a brief reduction of REM sleep and a long-lasting increase of NREM sleep time at the cost of wakefulness and because EEG SWA rebounded during the first 8 hours in recovery, the authors concluded that major EEG features of homeostatic sleep regulation

are present in SCN-lesioned rats. Thus, studies by three different laboratories support the concept that, although the circadian system is clearly involved in sleep expression, sleep homeostasis itself is not dependent on an intact circadian system.

### Models for the Interaction of Homeostatic and Circadian Factors in Sleep Regulation

Several models (Figure 8-6) have been proposed to conceptualize the interaction of circadian and homeostatic processes in sleep regulation. The elegant two-process model of sleep regulation,[48] which addresses the timing of sleep, was initially proposed by Borbely and colleagues[60] as a model of sleep regulation in the rat. In this model, a sleep homeostatic process that increases during waking and decreases during sleep (process S) is proposed to interact with input from the circadian system that is independent of sleep and waking (process C), to gate the occurrence of sleep and wakefulness. EEG SWA (i.e., EEG waveforms with frequencies of approximately 0.5–<4.0 Hz and amplitudes of at least 75 μV) was proposed as an indicator of the time course of process S. In later versions of the model, process S varies between upper and lower thresholds modulated by a single circadian process,[61] and the change, rather than the level, in process S corresponds to SWA.[62] In this model, once a threshold value of process S is reached, sleep will ensue only if process C is in the appropriate circadian phase. The two-process model, although seemingly simplistic, accounts remarkably well for the timing of sleep in humans and in several animal species.[42–45]

The opponent-process model[63] was proposed based on work showing that squirrel monkeys with SCN lesions were incapable of maintaining sustained wakefulness and exhibited ultradian sleep-wake patterns of approximately 4 hours. Thus, in contrast to intact squirrel monkeys that have consolidated sleep and waking periods, sleep and wakefulness was fragmented throughout the 24-hour period in lesioned monkeys. Furthermore, SCN-lesioned monkeys slept more than 3 hours longer per 24-hour period than their intact counterparts. These observations suggested that two opponent processes govern sleepiness and alertness: (1) a circadian pacemaker that actively promoted wakefulness and opposed accumulating diurnal sleep drive, and (2) a nocturnal sleep homeostatic process. This model provides a functional role for the SCN in sleep and wakefulness, particularly in the regulation of total sleep time.

The most recent three-process model of alertness regulation incorporates both circadian (C) and homeostatic (S) sleep loss components, which are summed to yield a scaled score of predicted alertness.[64,65] This computerized model can be used to predict sleep latency or duration of individuals with irregular sleep-wake patterns across a specified time span. Akerstedt and Folkard[64,65] suggested that this model may have practical applications in evaluating work and rest schedules to reduce risks of sleep loss.

These models provide building blocks for conceptualizing sleep homeostasis and circadian regulation of sleep-wake patterns and address issues of sleep propensity, the circadian timing of sleep, and

the presumed recovery processes that occur during sleep. These models do *not* address ultradian issues such as the NREM-REM sleep cycle, which has been addressed by others,[66,67] nor the consequences of longer-term sleep deprivation in rats, as investigated in detail by the Rechtschaffen laboratory.[68,69] Another significant model proposes that slow-wave sleep serves as a mechanism to cool the brain and implicates the preoptic anterior hypothalamic area as an important regulatory region for initiating sleep.[70] On the basis of extensive experimental evidence, prostaglandins $D_2$ and $E_2$ have been proposed as two biochemical regulators of sleep and wakefulness[71] and the leptomeninges have been described as the location of high concentrations of the synthetic enzyme prostaglandin D synthase.[72,73] Without denying the utility and validity of these models,[74,75] further exploration in this area is necessary. There are basic questions, such as the biochemical or molecular substrate of process S and the neurobiological pathway by which process C interacts with the sleep homeostatic mechanism, that must be addressed.

## FUNCTIONAL SIGNIFICANCE OF CIRCADIAN RHYTHMICITY

### *Circadian Rhythm Effects on Human Physiology and Metabolism*

Although most of the foregoing discussion of circadian rhythms has used activity rhythms as an example, virtually all physiologic and metabolic processes are characterized by rhythmicity, and there is good evidence for multiple autonomous oscillators in mammals. Therefore, it is most appropriate to describe the SCN as making up the central pacemaker coordinating the activities of these oscillators and providing synchronization of multiple internal rhythms. Coupled with these circadian rhythms of physiology and metabolism are circadian fluctuations in susceptibility to infection, drugs, and accidents. Cardiovascular disease (e.g., myocardial ischemia and infarction) worsens in the morning,[76,77] and exacerbation of pulmonary disorders are observed during sleep.[78,79] This cyclicity in metabolism, especially susceptibility to drugs, is becoming increasingly well-known and has led to the establishment of the discipline known as *chronopharmacology*. Among the more successful applications of the knowledge in this area to date have been the establishment of chemotherapeutic regimens that incorporate chronopharmacologic concepts. Knowledge of the circadian rhythmicity of specific diseases can enhance treatment through the determination of optimal times of drug administration.

### Impact of Circadian Rhythms on Public Health

Industrialization and technological advances have sped up the pace of daily life. Sleep is often considered a luxury, as overtime, shift work, and irregular sleep-wake schedules are increasingly more common. Automobile and industry-related accidents stemming from individual or corporate failure to consider sleep homeostasis and circadian rhythmicity result in tremendous private and public costs. Air and ground transportation workers are often subject to demanding schedules that are not optimized for circadian variations in sleepiness and alertness. This problem cannot be underestimated. A 1995 study showed that fatigue is a factor in 57% of accidents leading to the death of a truck driver and in 10% of fatal car accidents, and results in costs of up to $56 billion per year in America.[80] It is the responsibility of industrialized nations to recognize the adverse impact of sleep deprivation–related accidents on the health and welfare of its citizens. Health professionals and sleep specialists can help the governments of these nations enact legislation that would help reduce the potential of sleep deprivation–related accidents by limiting work schedules in the high-risk transportation industry.

## CONCLUSION AND FUTURE WORK

The relatively new field of chronobiology has already witnessed several important breakthroughs in our understanding of the circadian regulation of sleep. We know that the circadian pacemaker is located within the SCN of the hypothalamus. The afferent projections and at least some of the critical neurochemicals for the function of these nuclei have been identified. Unfortunately, how the SCN communicate temporal information to regulate physiologic and behavioral states, and their role in alertness is presently unknown. The efficacy of melatonin, genetic regulation of the circadian system, and the neurobiological substrates for sleep

homeostasis are areas of active investigation. Future work in the field of chronopharmacology will undoubtedly provide more effective treatments for common diseases. Finally, it cannot be overemphasized that continued ignorance of the effects of sleep homeostasis and circadian influences on sleep and wakefulness will result in both private tragedy and staggering societal costs.

*Acknowledgments*

This work was supported in part by grants from the National Institutes of Health (AG11084) and the Army Research Office (DAAH04-95-1-0616).

## REFERENCES

1. Moore RY, Lenn NJ. A retinohypothalamic projection in the rat. J Comp Neurol 1972;146:1.
2. Hendrickson AE, Wagoner N, Cowan WM. An autoradiographic and electron microscopic study of retino-hypothalamic connections. Z Zellforsch Mikroskop Anat 1972;135:1.
3. Moore RY, Eichler VB. Loss of circadian adrenal corticosterone rhythm following suprachiasmatic nucleus lesion in the rat. Brain Res 1972;42:201.
4. Stephan FK, Zucker I. Circadian rhythms in drinking behavior and locomotor activity are eliminated by suprachiasmatic lesions. Proc Natl Acad Sci U S A 1972;54:1521.
5. Schwartz WJ, Gainer H. Suprachiasmatic nucleus: use of $^{14}$C-labeled deoxyglucose uptake as a functional marker. Science 1977;197:1089.
6. Schwartz WJ, Davidsen L, Smith C. In vivo metabolic activity of a putative circadian oscillator, the suprachiasmatic nucleus. J Comp Neurol 1980;189:157.
7. Inouye S-IT, Kawamura H. Persistence of circadian rhythmicity in a hypothalamic 'island' containing the suprachiasmatic nucleus. Proc Natl Acad Sci U S A 1979;76:5962.
8. Green DJ, Gillette R. Circadian rhythm of firing rate recorded from single units in the rat suprachiasmatic brain slice. Brain Res 1982;245:198.
9. Gillette MU. The suprachiasmatic nuclei: circadian phase shifts induced at the time of hypothalamic slice preparation are preserved in vitro. Brain Res 1986; 379:176.
10. Newman GC, Hospod FE. Rhythm of suprachiasmatic nucleus 2-deoxyglucose uptake in vitro. Brain Res 1986;381:345.
11. Newman GC, Hospod FE, Patlak CS, Moore RY. Analysis of in vitro glucose utilization in a circadian pacemaker model. J Neurosci 1992;12:2015.

12. Gillette MU, Reppert SM. The hypothalamic suprachiasmatic nuclei: circadian patterns of vasopressin secretion and neuronal activity in vitro. Brain Res Bull 1987; 19:135.

13. Earnest DJ, Sladek CD. Circadian rhythms of vasopressin release from individual rat suprachiasmatic explants in vitro. Brain Res 1986;382:129.

14. Lehman MN, Silver R, Gladstone WR, et al. Circadian rhythmicity restored by neural transplant. Immunocytochemical characterization of the graft and its integration with the host brain. J Neurosci 1987;7:1626.

15. DeCoursey PJ, Buggy J. Circadian rhythmicity after neural transplant to hamster third ventricle: specificity of suprachiasmatic nuclei. Brain Res 1989;500:263.

16. Ralph MR, Foster RG, Davis FC, Menaker M. Transplanted suprachiasmatic nucleus determines circadian period. Science 1990;247:975.

17. Takatsuji K, Miguel-Hidalgo JJ, Tohyama M. Substance P–immunoreactive innervation from the retina to the suprachiasmatic nucleus in the rat. Brain Res 1991;568:223.

18. Card JP, Moore RY. Neuropeptide Y localization in the rat suprachiasmatic nucleus and periventricular hypothalamus. Neurosci Lett 1988;88:241.

19. Meyer-Bernstein EL, Morin LP. Differential serotonergic innervation of the suprachiasmatic nucleus and the intergeniculate leaflet and its role in circadian rhythm modulation. J Neurosci 1996;16:2097.

20. Card JP, Brecha N, Karten HJ, Moore RY. Immunocytochemical localization of vasoactive intestinal polypeptide-containing cells and processes in the suprachiasmatic nucleus of the rat: light and electron microscopic analysis. J Neurosci 1981;1:1289.

21. Moore RY, Speh JC. GABA is the principal neurotransmitter of the circadian system. Neurosci Lett 1993;150:112.

22. Card JP, Moore RY. The suprachiasmatic nucleus of the golden hamster: immunohistochemical analysis of cell and fiber distribution. Neuroscience 1984;13:415.

23. Watts AG, Swanson LW, Sanchez-Watts G. Efferent projections of the suprachiasmatic nucleus: I. Studies using anterograde transport of Phaseolus vulgaris leucoagglutinin in the rat. J Comp Neurol 1987;258:204.

24. Watts AG, Swanson LW. Efferent projections of the suprachiasmatic nucleus: II. Studies using retrograde transport of fluorescent dyes and simultaneous peptide immunohistochemistry in the rat. J Comp Neurol 1987;258:230.

25. Morin LP, Goodless-Sanchez N, Smale L, Moore RY. Projections of the suprachiasmatic nuclei, subparaventricular zone and retrochiasmatic area in the golden hamster. Neuroscience 1994;61:391.

26. Silver R, LeSauter J, Tresco P, Lehman M. A diffusible coupling signal from the transplanted suprachiasmatic nucleus controlling circadian locomotor rhythms. Nature 1996;382:810.

27. Pickard GE, Turek FW. The hypothalamic paraventricular nucleus mediates the photoperiodic control of reproduction but not the effects of light on the circadian rhythm of activity. Neurosci Lett 1983;43:67.

28. Klein DC, Smoot R, Weller JL, et al. Lesions of the paraventricular nucleus area of the hypothalamus disrupt the suprachiasmatic leads to spinal cord circuit in the melatonin rhythm generating system. Brain Res Bull 1983;10:647.

29. Lehman MN, Bittman EL, Newman SW. Role of the hypothalamic paraventricular nucleus in neuroendocrine responses to daylength in the golden hamster. Brain Res 1984;308:25.

30. Vanecek J, Pavlik A, Illnerova H. Hypothalamic melatonin receptor sites revealed by autoradiography. Brain Res 1987;435:359.

31. Weaver DR, Rivkees SA, Reppert SM. Localization and characterization of melatonin receptors in rodent brain by in vitro autoradiography. J Neurosci 1989;9:2581.

32. Cassone VM, Chesworth MJ, Armstrong SM. Entrainment of rat circadian rhythms by daily injection of melatonin depends upon the hypothalamic suprachiasmatic nuclei. Physiol Behav 1986;36:1111.

33. Aronin N, Sagar SM, Sharp FR, Schwartz WJ. Light regulates expression of a Fos-related protein in rat suprachiasmatic nuclei. 1990;87:5959.

34. Rea MA. Light increases Fos-related protein immunoreactivity in the rat suprachiasmatic nuclei. Brain Res Bull 1989;23:577.

35. Rusak B, Robertson HA, Wisden W, Hunt SP. Light pulses that shift rhythms induce gene expression in the suprachiasmatic nucleus. Science 1990;248:1237.

36. Kornhauser JM, Nelson DE, Mayo KE, Takahashi JS. Photic and circadian regulation of c-fos gene expression in the hamster suprachiasmatic nucleus. Neuron 1990;5:127.

37. Sutin EL, Kilduff TS. Circadian and light-induced expression of immediate early gene mRNAs in the rat suprachiasmatic nucleus. Brain Res Mol Brain Res 1992;15:281.

38. Konopka RJ, Benzer S. Clock mutants of Drosophila melanogaster. Proc Natl Acad Sci U S A 1971;68:2112.

39. Sehgal A, Price JL, Man B, Young MW. Loss of circadian behavioral rhythms and per RNA oscillations in the Drosophila mutant timeless. Science 1994;263:1603.

40. Ralph MR, Menaker M. A mutation of the circadian system in golden hamsters. Science 1988;241:1225.

41. Vitaterna MH, King DP, Chang A-M, et al. Mutagenesis and mapping of a mouse gene, clock, essential for circadian behavior. Science 1994;264:719.

42. Borbely AA, Baumann F, Brandeis D, et al. Sleep deprivation: effect on sleep stages and EEG power density in man. Electroencephalogr Clin Neurophysiol 1981;51:483.

43. Borbely AA, Tobler I, Hanagasioglu M. Effect of sleep deprivation on sleep and EEG power spectra in the rat. Behav Brain Res 1984;14:171.

44. Tobler I, Jaggi K. Sleep and EEG spectra in the Syrian hamster (Mesocricetus auratus) under baseline conditions and following sleep deprivation. J Comp Physiol [A] 1987;161:449.

45. Dijk DJ, Daan S. Sleep EEG spectral analysis in a diurnal rodent: *Eutamias sibiricus*. J Comp Physiol [A] 1989;165:205.

46. Dijk DJ, Beersma DG, Daan S. EEG power density during nap sleep: reflection of an hourglass measuring the duration of prior wakefulness. J Biol Rhythms 1987;2:207.

47. Dijk DJ, Beersma DG. Effects of SWS deprivation on subsequent EEG power density and spontaneous sleep duration. Electroencephalogr Clin Neurophysiol 1989;72:312.

48. Borbely AA. A two process model of sleep regulation. Hum Neurobiol 1982;1:195.

49. Borbely AA, Achermann P, Trachsel L, Tobler I. Sleep initiation and initial sleep intensity: interactions of homeostatic and circadian mechanisms. J Biol Rhythms 1989;4:149.

50. Ibuka N, Kawamura H. Loss of circadian sleep-wakefulness cycle in rats by suprachiasmatic nucleus lesion. Brain Res 1975;96:76.

51. Carskadon MA, Dement WC. Sleep studies on a 90-minute day. Electroencephalogr Clin Neurophysiol 1975;39:145.

52. Carskadon MA, Dement WC. Sleepiness and sleep state on a 90-min schedule. Psychophysiology 1977;14:127.

53. Czeisler C, Weitzman E, Moore-Ede M, et al. Human sleep: its duration and organization depend on its circadian phase. Science 1980;210:1264.

54. Czeisler C, Zimmerman J, Ronda J, et al. Timing of REM sleep is coupled to the circadian rhythm of body temperature in man. Sleep 1980;2:329.

55. Dijk DJ, Czeisler CA. Paradoxical timing of the circadian rhythm of sleep propensity serves to consolidate sleep and wakefulness in humans. Neurosci Lett 1994;166:63.

56. Dijk DJ, Czeisler CA. Contribution of the circadian pacemaker and the sleep homeostat to sleep propensity, sleep structure, electroencephalographic slow waves, and sleep spindle activity in humans. J Neurosci 1995;15(5 Pt 1):3526.

57. Mistlberger RE, Bergmann BM, Waldenar W, Rechtschaffen A. Recovery sleep following sleep deprivation in intact and suprachiasmatic nuclei-lesioned rats. Sleep 1983;6:217.

58. Tobler I, Borbely AA, Groos G. The effect of sleep deprivation on sleep in rats with suprachiasmatic lesions. Neurosci Lett 1983;42:49.

59. Trachsel L, Edgar DM, Seidel WF, et al. Sleep homeostasis in suprachiasmatic nuclei-lesioned rats: effects of sleep deprivation and triazolam administration. Brain Res 1992;589:253.

60. Borbely AA. Effects of light and circadian rhythm on the occurrence of REM sleep in the rat. Sleep 1980;2:289.

61. Daan S, Beersma DG, Borbely AA. Timing of human sleep: recovery process gated by a circadian pacemaker. Am J Physiol 1984;246(2 Pt 2):R161.

62. Achermann P, Dijk DJ, Brunner DP, Borbely AA. A model of human sleep homeostasis based on EEG slow-wave activity: quantitative comparison of data and simulations. Brain Res Bull 1993;31:97.

63. Edgar DM, Dement WC, Fuller CA. Effect of SCN lesions on sleep in squirrel monkeys: evidence for opponent processes in sleep-wake regulation. J Neurosci 1993;13:1065.

64. Akerstedt T, Folkard S. Predicting sleep latency from the three-process model of alertness regulation. Psychophysiology 1996;33:385.

65. Akerstedt T, Folkard S. Predicting duration of sleep from the three process model of regulation of alertness. Occup Environ Med 1996;53:136.

66. Hobson J, Lydic R, Baghdoyan H. Evolving concepts of sleep cycle generation: from brain centers to neuronal populations. Behav Brain Sci 1986;9:371.

67. Steriade M, McCarley R. Brainstem Control of Wakefulness and Sleep. New York: Plenum, 1990.

68. Rechtschaffen A, Bergmann BM, Everson CA, et al. Sleep deprivation in the rat: I. Conceptual issues. Sleep 1989;11:1.

69. Rechtschaffen A, Bergmann BM, Everson CA, et al. Sleep deprivation in the rat: X. Integration and discussion of the findings. Sleep 1989;12:68.

70. McGinty D, Szymusiak R. Keeping cool: a hypothesis about the mechanisms and functions of slow-wave sleep. Trends Neurosci 1990;13:480.

71. Hayaishi O. Molecular mechanisms of sleep-wake regulation: roles of prostaglandins $D_2$ and $E_2$. FASEB J 1991;5:2575.

72. Urade Y, Kitahama K, Ohishi H, et al. Dominant expression of mRNA for prostaglandin D synthase in leptomeninges, choroid plexus, and oligodendrocytes of the adult rat brain. Proc Natl Acad Sci U S A 1993;90:9070.

73. Blodorn B, Mader M, Urade Y, et al. Choroid plexus: the major site of mRNA expression for the beta-trace protein (prostaglandin D synthase) in human brain. Neurosci Lett 1996;209:117.

74. Krueger JM, Obal F Jr, Kapas L, Fang J. Brain organization and sleep function. Behav Brain Res 1995;69:177.

75. Benington JH, Heller HC. Restoration of brain energy metabolism as the function of sleep. Prog Neurobiol 1995;45:347.

76. Burkart F, Osswald S. Mechanisms of myocardial ischemia and circadian fluctuations of ischemic episodes. Schweiz Rundsch Med Prax 1992;81:171.

77. Herren T, Urban P, Rutishauser W. Consequences of circadian variability for the treatment of ischemic heart disease. Schweiz Rundsch Med Prax 1992; 81:176.

78. Petty T. Circadian variations in chronic asthma and chronic obstructive pulmonary disease. Am J Med 1988;85(Suppl B):21.

79. Zoratti E, Busse W. Nighttime asthma symptoms: no idle threat. Respir Dis 1990;11:137.

80. Bonnet M, Arand D. We are chronically sleep deprived. Sleep 1995;18:908.

# Part II
## Technical Considerations

# Chapter 9

# Polysomnographic Technique: An Overview

## Sharon A. Keenan

The term *polysomnography* (PSG) was proposed by Holland and colleagues[1] in 1974 to describe the recording, analysis, and interpretation of multiple, simultaneous physiologic parameters. PSG is an essential tool in the formulation of diagnoses for sleep disorders patients and in the enhancement of our understanding of both normal sleep and its disorders.[2–14] It is a complex procedure that should be performed by a trained technologist. Sleep laboratories continue to undergo technological evolution, particularly in terms of the increased reliance on computers and the collection of data outside of the traditional setting of the sleep laboratory. This evolution requires sophisticated knowledge of equipment and procedures.

This chapter is a review of the technical aspects of PSG, providing a step-by-step approach to classic in-laboratory PSG recording techniques. Problems likely to be encountered during a recording are examined, as are ways to alleviate them. Figures and actual tracings augment the text and help identify artifacts. A brief discussion of digital recording is included and comparisons between analog digital systems are made throughout the chapter. Elsewhere in this volume, specified protocols are discussed, physiologic recording techniques are reviewed, and an entire chapter is dedicated to the use of digital systems in the sleep laboratory. The reader is directed to other sources[15–27] for indications and standards of practice articles that have appeared in the literature since the first edition of this text.

## PATIENT CONTACT

A number of factors should be kept in mind when a PSG study is scheduled. Issues such as shift work, time zone change, or suspected advanced or delayed sleep phase syndrome should be taken into consideration. The study should be conducted during the patient's usual major sleep period to avoid confounding circadian rhythm factors.

When the PSG is scheduled, the patient is sent a questionnaire about his or her sleep-wake history and a sleep diary that solicits information about major sleep periods and naps for 2 weeks before the study (Appendix 9-1). Information is provided for the patient about the purpose and procedures of the sleep study. The goal—to make the patient's stay at the sleep laboratory as uncomplicated and comfortable as possible—might be facilitated if the patient brings along a favorite pillow, pajamas, or book.

The technologist should ensure that patients arriving at the laboratory are familiar with the surroundings and receive explicit information about the process. Patients should be shown through the laboratory and to a bedroom. They are informed that someone will be monitoring their sleep throughout the entire study and told how to contact the technologist if necessary.

Before the study is undertaken, a full medical and psychiatric history should be completed and made available to the technologist performing the study. Without this information, the technologist is at a loss to understand how aspects of the medical or psychiatric history may affect the study or to anticipate difficulties. Technologists must also understand what questions the study seeks to answer. This enhances their ability to make protocol adjustments when necessary, and ensures that the most pertinent information is recorded.

### Pre-Study Questionnaire

It is not uncommon for patients, particularly those with excessive sleepiness, to have a diminished capacity to evaluate their level of alertness.[18,26] In addition, many patients with difficulty initiating and maintaining sleep often report a subjective evaluation of their total sleep time and quality that is at odds with the objective data collected in the laboratory. For these reasons it is recommended that subjective data be collected systematically as part of the sleep laboratory evaluation.

The Stanford Sleepiness Scale (SSS)[28,29] (Appendix 9-2) is an instrument used to assess a patient's subjective evaluation of sleepiness before the PSG. The SSS is presented to the patient immediately before the beginning of the study. It offers a series of phrases describing various states of arousal and sleepiness. Patients respond by selecting the set of adjectives that most closely corresponds to their current state of sleepiness or alertness. The scale is used extensively in both clinical and research environments; however, it has two noteworthy limitations: It is not suitable for children who have a limited vocabulary or for adults whose primary language is not English. In these situations, a linear analog scale is recommended (Appendix 9-2). One end of the scale represents extreme sleepiness and the other end alertness. Patients mark the scale to describe their state just before testing.

Another instrument, the Epworth Sleepiness Scale,[30] measures chronic sleepiness. Patients are asked to report the likelihood of dozing in situations such as riding as a passenger in a car, watching TV, and so on.

Patients are also asked about their medication history, smoking history, any unusual events during the course of the day, their last meal before study, alcohol intake, and a sleep history for the last 24 hours, including naps. This information is critical for the study. A technologist's complete awareness of patient idiosyncrasies, in the context of the questions to be addressed by the study, ensures a good foundation for the collection of high-quality data.

### Nap Studies

A proposed alternative to nocturnal PSG has been the nap study (distinguished from the Multiple Sleep Latency Test [MSLT]). The rationale for this study is that if a patient has a sleep disorder it will be expressed during an afternoon nap as well as during a more extensive PSG. The nap study has been used most frequently for the diagnosis of sleep-related breathing disorders and was proposed in an effort to reduce the cost of a sleep laboratory evaluation. The short study in the afternoon avoids the necessity of having a technologist present for an overnight study. There are serious limitations to the use of nap studies, however, including the possibility of false-negative results or the misinterpretation of the severity of sleep-related breathing disorders if the patient is sedated or sleep deprived before the study. When a nap study is performed, it should follow the guidelines as published by the American Thoracic Society.[31,32]

Although minimal systematic data exist on the value of nap recordings, nap studies of 2–4 hours' duration may be used to confirm the diagnosis of sleep apnea, provided that all routine polysomnographic variables are recorded, that both rapid eye movement (REM) and non-REM sleep are sampled, and that the patient spends at least part of the time in the supine posture. Sleep deprivation or the use of drugs to induce a nap are contraindicated. Nap studies are inadequate to definitively exclude a diagnosis of sleep apnea.

## PREPARATION OF THE EQUIPMENT

For the purpose of this chapter we refer to the *polygraph*, an instrument in which the main component is a series of amplifiers (see also Chapter 10). Usually there is a combination of AC and DC channels. Typically, at least 12–16 channels are available for recording. The data from the amplifiers are written to a moving chart or to a computer that converts the analog signal to a digital signal. The digital data are then stored by the computer for subsequent manipulation or analysis. A complete discussion of digital systems appears in Chapter 15.

**Table 9-1.** Recommendations for Filter Settings and Sensitivity for Various Physiologic Parameters

| Channel[a] | Low-Frequency Filter (Hz) | Time Constant(s) | High-Frequency Filter (Hz) | Sensitivity (µV/cm) |
|---|---|---|---|---|
| EEG | 0.3 | 0.4 | 35 | 50 |
| EOG | 0.3 | 0.4 | 35 | 50 |
| EMG | 5[b] | 0.03 | 90–120 | 50 |
| ECG | 1.0 | 0.12 | 15 | 1 MV/cm to start; adjust as necessary |
| Airflow (AC-amp) | 0.15 | 1–2 | 15 | 50 to start; adjust as necessary |
| Effort (AC-amp) | 0.15 | 1–2 | 15 | 50 to start; adjust as necessary |

EOG = electro-oculography; EMG = electromyography; ECG = electrocardiography.
[a]EEG includes C3/A2, C4/A1, O1/A2, and O2/A1. EOG includes right outer canthus and left outer canthus referred to opposite reference.
[b]If shorter time constant or higher low-frequency filter is available, it should be used. This includes settings for all EMG channels including mentalis, submentalis, masseter, anterior tibialis, intercostal, extensor digitorum.
Source: Modified from SA Keenan. Polysomnography: technical aspects in adolescents and adults. J Clin Neurophysiol 1992;9:21.

Equipment for recording polysomnograms is produced by a number of manufacturers. Each may have a distinctive appearance and some idiosyncratic features, but there is remarkable similarity when the basic functioning of the instruments is examined.

Equipment preparation includes an understanding of how the filters and sensitivity of the amplifiers affect the data collected. The major difference between traditional clinical polysomnography and computer-based systems lies in data storage and display. It is important that all technologists, regardless of the system used, have adequate knowledge of the impact of the use of filters on the data collected during PSE.

The amplifiers used to record physiologic data are very sensitive. By using a combination of high- and low-frequency filters and appropriate sensitivity settings, we maximize the likelihood of recording and displaying the signals of interest and decrease the possibility of recording extraneous signals. Care must be taken when using the high- and low-frequency filters, however, to ensure that an appropriate window for recording specific frequencies is established and that the filters do not eliminate important data.

### Alternating Current Amplifiers

Differential AC amplifiers are used to record physiologic parameters of high frequency, such as the electroencephalogram (EEG), the electro-oculogram (EOG), the electromyogram (EMG), and the electrocardiogram (ECG). The AC amplifier has both high- and low-frequency filters. The presence of the low-frequency filter makes it possible to attenuate slow potentials not associated with the physiology of interest; these include galvanic skin response, DC electrode imbalance, and breathing reflected in an EMG, EEG, or EOG channel. Combinations of specific settings of the high- and low-frequency filters make it possible to focus on specific band widths associated with the signal of interest. For example, respiration is a very slow signal (approximately 12–18 breaths per minute) in comparison with the EMG signal, which has a much higher frequency (approximately 20–200 Hz). The choice of high- and low-frequency filter settings is driven by the frequency of the data to be displayed on the channel.

### Direct Current Amplifiers

In contrast to the AC amplifier, the DC amplifier does not have a low-frequency filter. DC amplifiers are typically used to record slower-moving potentials, such as output from the oximeter or pH meter, changes in pressure in positive airway pressure treatment, or output from transducers that record endoesophageal pressure changes or body temperature. Airflow and effort of breathing can be successfully recorded with either AC or DC amplifiers.

An understanding of the appropriate use of filters in clinical PSG is essential to proper recording tech-

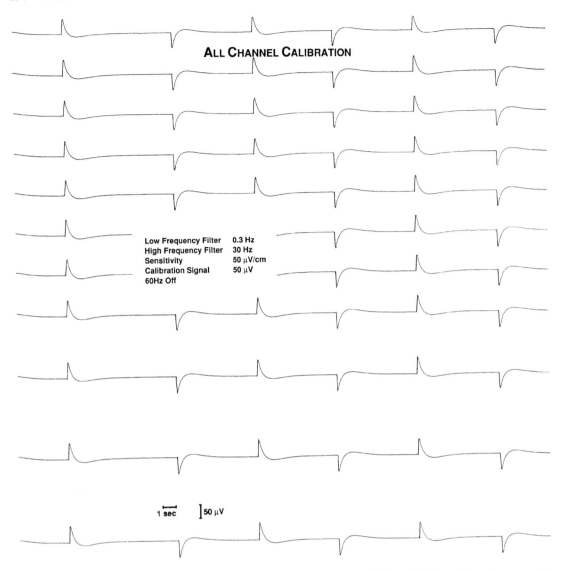

**Figure 9-1.** All channel calibration is shown. All amplifiers have the same sensitivity and high- and low-frequency filter settings.

nique.[32,33] Table 9-1 provides recommendations for filter settings for various physiologic parameters.

### *Calibration of the Equipment*

The PSG recording instrument must be calibrated to ensure adequate functioning of amplifiers and appropriate settings for the specific protocol. The first calibration is an all-channel calibration (Figure 9-1). During this calibration, all amplifiers are set to the same sensitivity, the same high- and low-frequency filter settings, and a known signal is sent through all amplifiers simultaneously. The proper functioning of all amplifiers is thus demonstrated, ensuring that all are functioning in an identical fashion.

A second calibration is performed for the specific study protocol. During this calibration, amplifiers are set with the high- and low-frequency filter, and sensitivity settings appropriate for each channel; the settings are dictated by the requirements of the specific physiologic parameter recorded on each chan-

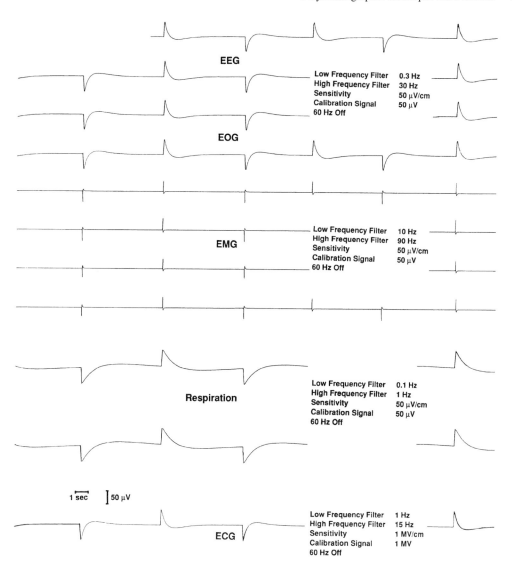

**Figure 9-2.** The montage calibration shows changes in high- and low-frequency filter settings from the all-channel calibration to accommodate the display of a variety of physiologic signals for the polysomnograph. (EOG = electro-oculogram; EMG = electromyogram; ECG = electrocardiogram.)

nel (Figure 9-2, see also Table 9-1). The protocol calibration ensures that all amplifiers are set to ideal conditions for recording the parameter of interest. Filter and sensitivity settings should be clearly documented for each channel. Paper speed and time should also be recorded for analog systems.

### Paper Speed

For analog systems, the paper speed of the instrument establishes the epoch length or the amount of

time that appears on each page of the recording. The process of sleep-stage scoring and analysis of abnormalities is accomplished by an epoch-by-epoch review of the data.

A common paper speed for traditional PSG is 10 mm per second, providing a 30-second epoch. Another widely accepted paper speed is 15 mm per second, which results in a 20-second epoch length. Significant portions of tracings at a paper speed of 30 mm per second should be used when recording patients with suspected sleep-related seizure activ-

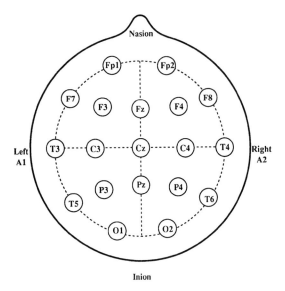

**Figure 9-3.** The complete 10-20 System of electrode placement.

ity. The increased paper speed enhances the ability to visualize EEG data, specifically the spike activity associated with epileptic discharges. In general, paper speeds slower than 10 mm per second should be avoided because they compromise an adequate display of EEG data. Data such as oxygen saturation, respiratory signals, or changes in penile circumference, however, can be more easily visualized with slower paper speeds. If a compressed time scale is required, it is possible to output the signal from the polysomnograph to a slower chart recorder. Simultaneous display of the signal on both the polysomnogram and the slower time scale chart is advantageous. The issue of selecting the appropriate paper speed becomes moot when using digital systems because of the ability to manipulate the display after data collection. This is a significant advantage of the digital systems.

## THE STUDY

### Electrode and Monitor Application Process

The quality of the tracing generated in the sleep laboratory depends on the quality of the electrode application. Before any electrode or monitor is applied, the patient should be instructed about the procedure

and given an opportunity to ask questions. The first step in the application of electrodes involves measurement of the patient's head. The 10-20 System[34] of electrode placement is used to localize specific electrode sites (Figure 9-3). The following sections address the application process for EEG, EOG, EMG, and ECG electrodes.

### Electroencephalography

Standard electrode derivations for monitoring EEG activity during sleep are C3/A2 or C4/A1, and O1/A2 or O2/A1 (see Appendix 9-4), but in many situations there may be a need for additional electrodes. For example, to rule out the possibility of epileptic seizures during sleep, or the presence of any other sleep-related EEG abnormality, it may be necessary to apply the full complement of EEG electrodes according to the 10-20 System (see Appendix 9-3).

For recording EEG, a gold cup electrode with a hole in the center is commonly used. Silver–silver chloride electrodes are also useful to record EEG, though they may have limitations such as increased maintenance (evidenced by the need for repeated chloriding) and an inability to attach these electrodes to the scalp.

The placement of C3, C4, O1, and O2 are determined by the International 10-20 System of Electrode Placement. Reference electrodes are placed on the bony surface of the mastoid process. A description of the measurement procedure appears in Appendix 9-4.

The collodion technique[35,36] has long been an accepted and preferred method of application for EEG scalp and reference electrodes. This technique ensures a long-term placement and allows for correction of high impedances (>5,000 ohms), after application. Other methods using electrode paste and conductive medium are acceptable and sometimes necessary in certain conditions.

### Electro-Oculography

The EOG is a recording of the movement of the corneoretinal potential difference that exists in the eye (see also Chapter 10). It is important to recognize that it is the movement of this dipole, not muscle activity of the eyes, that is recorded. Gold cup electrodes or silver–silver chloride electrodes can be used to monitor the EOG.

An electrode is typically applied at the outer canthus of the right eye (ROC) and is offset 1 cm above the horizontal. Another electrode is applied to the outer canthus of the left eye (LOC) and is offset by 1 cm below the horizontal. The previously mentioned A1 and A2 reference electrodes are used as follows: ROC is referred to A1 and LOC is referred to A2. Additional electrodes can be applied infraorbitally and supraorbitally for either the right or left eye. The infraorbital and supraorbital electrodes enhance the ability to detect eye movements that occur in the vertical plane and can be particularly useful in the MSLT[37] (Figure 9-4).

EOG electrodes are typically applied to the surface of the skin with an adhesive collar; this method avoids the risk of getting collodion in the patient's eyes.

*Electromyography*

A gold cup or a silver–silver chloride electrode attached with an adhesive collar is used to record EMG activity from the mentalis and submentalis muscles. At least three EMG electrodes are applied to allow for an alternative electrode, in the event that a problem develops in one. The additional electrode can be placed over the masseter muscle to allow for detection of bursts of EMG activity associated with bruxism (Figure 9-5).

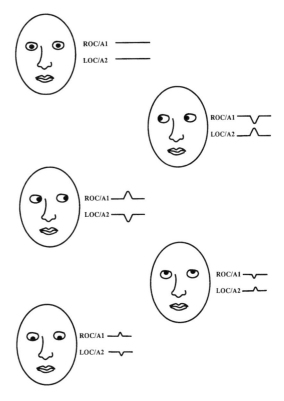

**Figure 9-4.** The recording montage for a two-channel electrooculography demonstrates out-of-phase pen deflection in association with conjugate eye movements.

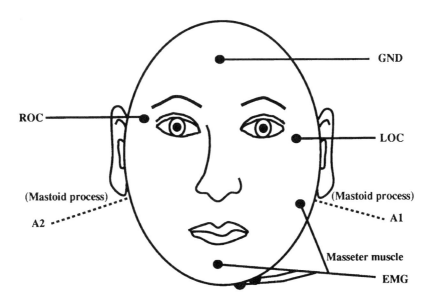

**Figure 9-5.** Schematic diagram shows placement of the electromyography (EMG) electrodes to record activity from the mental, submental, and masseter muscles. (ROC, LOC = outer canthus of the right and left eye, respectively; GND = ground [earth].)

*Electrocardiography*

A variety of approaches exist for recording the ECG during PSG. The simplest approach involves use of standard gold cup electrodes. Disposable electrodes are also available for this purpose.

ECG electrodes are applied with an adhesive collar to the surface of the skin just below the right clavicle and on the left side at the level of the seventh rib. A stress loop is incorporated into the lead wire to ensure long-term placement.

*Impedances*

Before recording, electrodes should be visually inspected to check the security of their placement and an impedance check should be obtained and documented. This requires the use of an impedance meter, which may be included within the recording system. Adjustment should be made to any EEG, EOG, ECG, or chin EMG electrode with an impedance greater than 5,000 ohms.

**Physiologic Calibrations**

Physiologic calibrations are performed after the electrode and monitor application is complete. This calibration allows for documentation of proper functioning of the electrodes and other monitoring devices, and provides baseline data for review and comparison when scoring the PSG. The following specific instructions are given to the patient for this calibration:

1. With your eyes open, look straight ahead for 30 seconds.
2. With your eyes closed, look straight ahead for 30 seconds.
3. Holding your head still, look to the left and right; now look up and down. Repeat.
4. Holding your head still, slowly blink your eyes five times.
5. Grit your teeth. Now clench your jaw or smile.
6. Inhale and exhale.
7. Hold your breath for 10 seconds.
8. Flex your right foot; now flex your left foot.
9. Flex your right hand; now flex your left hand.

As these instructions are given to the patient, the technologist examines the tracing and documents the patient's responses. When the patient stares straight ahead for 30 seconds with eyes open, the background EEG activity is examined. As the patient looks right and left, the tracing is examined for out-of-phase deflections of the signals associated with recording the EOG. Out-of-phase deflection occurs if the input to consecutive channels of the polygraph are ROC/A1 for the first EOG channel and LOC/A2 for the second. It is also important to observe the reactivity of the alpha rhythm seen most prominently in the occipital EEG (O1/A2 or O2/A1). Alpha is best visualized when the patient's eyes are closed. The patient is also asked to blink 5 times, while the technologist observes the eye movement and possible reflection of this movement in the EEG channel.

The mentalis-submentalis EMG signal is checked by asking patients to grit their teeth, clench their jaws, or yawn. The technologist documents proper functioning of the electrodes and amplifiers used to monitor anterior tibialis EMG activity by asking the patient to dorsiflex the right foot and the left foot in turn. If REM sleep behavior disorder is suspected, additional surface electrodes should be applied to record from the extensor digitorum muscle of each arm. Patients are asked to extend their wrists while the technologist examines the recording for the corresponding increase in amplitude of the extensor digitorum EMG channels.

Inhalation and exhalation allow for examination of channels monitoring airflow and breathing.[38,39] Inhalation causes a deflection of the signal and exhalation the opposite deflection. It is important that the signals on all the channels monitoring breathing are in phase with each other to avoid confusion with paradoxical breathing. The technologist should observe a flattening of the trace for the duration of a voluntary apnea.

If the 60- or 50-Hz notch filter is in use, a brief examination (2–4 seconds) of portions of the tracing with the filter in the "out" position is essential. This allows for identification of any 60- or 50-Hz interference that may be masked by the filter. Care should be taken to eliminate any source of interference and to ensure that the 60- or 50-Hz notch filter is used only as a last resort. This is most important when recording patients suspected of having seizure activity, because the notch filter attenuates the amplitude of the spike activity seen in association with epileptogenic activity. If other monitors are used, the technologist should incorporate the necessary calibrations to allow for adequate interpretation of the signs.

The physiologic calibrations enable the technologist to determine the quality of data before the PSG begins. If artifact is noted during the physiologic calibrations, it is imperative that every effort be made to correct the problem; the condition is likely to get worse through the remaining portions of the recording. The functioning of alternative (spare) electrodes should also be examined during this calibration.

When a satisfactory calibration procedure is completed and all other aspects of patient and equipment preparation are completed, lights are turned out in the patient's room and the patient is told to assume a comfortable sleeping position and attempt to fall asleep. The lights-out time should be clearly noted on the tracing.

## MONITORING AND RECORDING

Complete documentation for the PSG is essential. This includes patient identification (patient's full name and medical record number), date of recording, and a full description of the study. The name of the technologist performing the recording should be noted and any technologists involved in preparation of patient and equipment. In laboratories that use multiple pieces of equipment, the specific instrument used to generate the recording should be identified. This is particularly useful in the event that artifact is noted during the analysis portion (scoring) of the sleep study.

Specific parameters recorded on each channel should be clearly noted, as should a full description of sensitivity, filter, and calibration settings for each channel. Paper speed must also be documented to provide information or epoch length. The time of the beginning and end of the recording must be noted, as well as specific events that occur during the night. For instruments that lack automatic notation of clock time, it is important that the technologist make manual time notes at hourly intervals. Any changes made to filter and sensitivity settings or paper speed should be clearly noted on the tracing.

The technologist is also responsible for providing a clinical description of unusual events. For example, if a patient experiences an epileptic seizure during the study, the clinical manifestations of the seizure must be detailed: deviation of eyes or head to one side or the other, movement of extremities, presence of vomiting or incontinence, duration of the seizure, and postictal status. Similar information should be reported on any clinical event observed in the laboratory, such as somnambulism or clinical features of REM sleep behavior disorder. Physical complaints reported by the patient are also noted.

## TROUBLESHOOTING AND ARTIFACT RECOGNITION

In general, when difficulties arise during recording, the troubleshooting inquiry begins with the patient and follows the path of the signal to the recording device. More often than not, the problem can be identified as a difficulty with an electrode or other monitoring device. It is less likely that artifact is the result of a problem with an amplifier. If the artifact is generalized (i.e., on most channels), the integrity of the ground electrode and the instrument cable should be checked. If the artifact is localized (i.e., on a limited number of channels), the question should be which channels have this artifact in common and what is common to the channels involved. The artifact is probably the result of a problem located in an electrode or monitoring device that is common to both channels. If the artifact is isolated to a single channel, the source of artifact is limited to the input to the specific amplifier, the amplifier itself, or to the ink-writing system for the channel. Figures 9-6 through 9-14 depict some frequently encountered artifacts seen during PSG.

## ENDING THE STUDY

Clinical circumstances and laboratory protocol dictate whether the patient is awakened at a specific time or allowed to awaken spontaneously. After awakening, the patient should be asked to perform the physiologic calibrations to ensure and document that the electrodes and other monitoring devices are still functioning properly. The equipment should be calibrated at the settings used for the study, the amplifiers should be set to identical settings for high- and low-frequency filters and sensitivity, and an all-channel calibration should be performed. This is essentially the reverse of the calibration procedures mentioned for the beginning of the study.

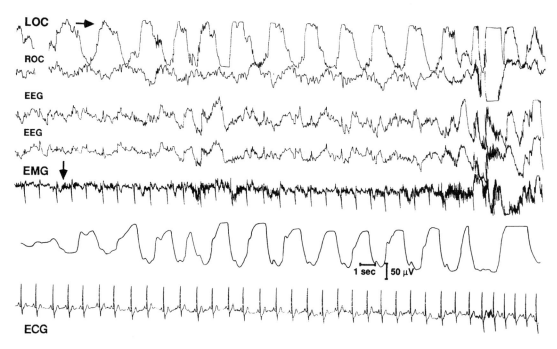

**Figure 9-6.** Artifact in the outer canthus of the left eye channel (LOC/A1) can be localized to the left outer canthus (LOC) electrode. The EEG channels in the trace are C3/A2 and O2/A1. Because the artifact does not appear in the O2/A1 channel, the artifact is localized to the LOC electrode. The electrode placement may be insecure or the patient may be lying on the electrode and producing movement of the LOC electrode in association with breathing. Additional artifact is noted in the electromyography (EMG) channel. This signal is contaminated with electrocardiography (ECG) artifact, and the intermittent slower activity as well as the wandering baseline are most likely due to a loose lead. The ECG channel also shows a pattern consistent with a loose electrode wire. (ROC = right outer canthus.)

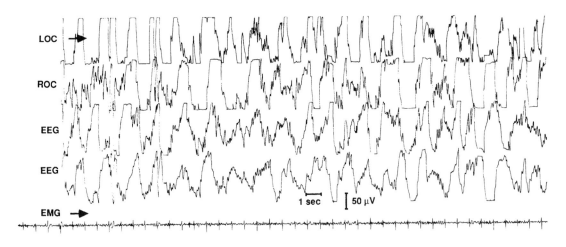

**Figure 9-7.** The blocking artifact often seen in analog tracings with inappropriate sensitivity settings is illustrated. This can be alleviated by decreasing sensitivity. If adjustments to sensitivity are made, they should be clearly noted and should be made on all channels displaying EEG data. It is common procedure to calibrate the equipment with decreased sensitivities (i.e., 100 μV/cm) for children's studies or increasing sensitivity (i.e., 30 μV/cm) for older patients. Typically, sensitivity settings are not changed frequently during the recording (as they may be in routine EEG). As a result, it is not uncommon to see this artifact when the patient enters slow-wave sleep. This is not a common problem with digital systems because of the user's ability to manipulate sensitivity after collection. (ROC, LOC = outer canthus of the right and left eye, respectively; EMG = electromyography.)

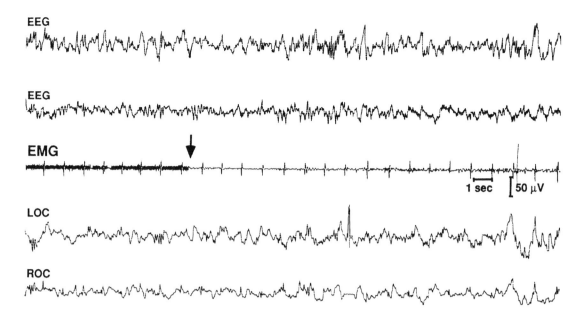

**Figure 9-8.** A 60-Hz artifact exists in the electromyography (EMG) channel in this tracing. At the arrow, the 60-Hz filter is turned on. There is continued evidence of difficulty with electrodes on this channel, however, as evidenced by the electrocardiography artifact and occasional spikelike activity. Turning on the 60-Hz filter (*arrow*) is not the correct response to eliminate the artifact. If possible, the technologist should switch to an alternative electrode or fix the one involved. (ROC, LOC = outer canthus of the right and left eye, respectively.)

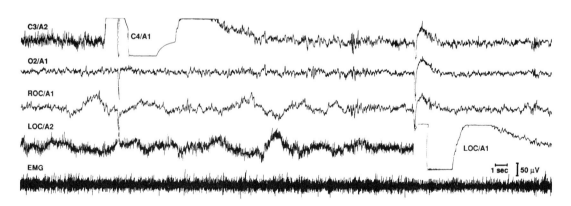

**Figure 9-9.** The high-frequency (probably electromyography [EMG]) artifact noted in the C3/A2 and the LOC/A2 channels can be localized to the A2 electrode. This problem can be solved by switching to the alternative reference (A1) electrode. A high-amplitude discharge is noted during the switch from C3/A2 to C4/A1 and LOC/A2 to LOC/A1. This can be avoided by placing the amplifier in standby mode while making the change. (ROC, LOC = outer canthus of the right and left eye, respectively.)

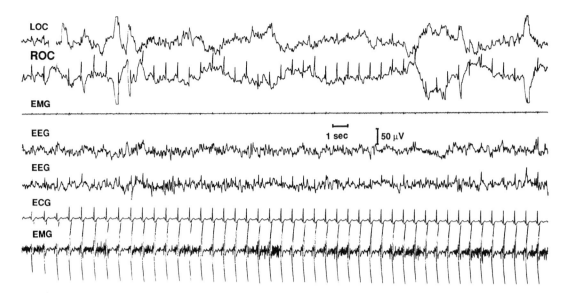

**Figure 9-10.** The outer canthus of the right eye (ROC) channel (ROC/A1) and the second EEG (O2/A1) channels are contaminated with electrocardiography (ECG) artifact. The artifact can be identified by aligning the spikelike activity noted in channels with the R wave on the ECG channel. It is localized to the A1 electrode because it is seen in both ROC/A1 and O2/A1 channels and A1 is common to both channels. It should be noted that the high-amplitude ECG artifact, seen in the electromyography (EMG) channel below the ECG channel, is unavoidable. This artifact is due to the proximity of EMG electrodes to the heart, which creates a robust signal superimposed on the intercostal EMG signal. (ROC, LOC = outer canthus of the right and left eye, respectively.)

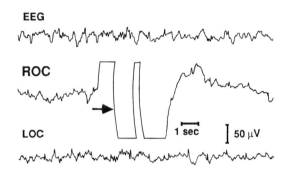

**Figure 9-11.** The high-amplitude deflection in the outer canthus of the right eye (ROC) channel (ROC/A1) is associated with an electrode artifact commonly referred to as an *electrode pop*. This can be the result of a compromised electrode placement or insufficient electroconductive gel under the electrode. When this artifact is observed, the electrode involved should not be trusted to give reliable data. (LOC = outer canthus of the left eye.)

A subjective evaluation is made by the patient. The patient is asked to estimate how long it took to fall asleep, the amount of time spent asleep, and if there were any disruptions during the sleep period.

Patients should report on quality of sleep and the level of alertness on arousal.

It is also important for the sleep laboratory staff to know how patients intend to leave the laboratory. A patient who has a severe sleep disorder should avoid driving. An arranged ride or public transportation should be used, particularly if the patient has withdrawn from stimulant medications for the purpose of the study.

## DIGITAL SYSTEMS

Within the past decade, digital systems have made it possible to manipulate data after recording and to permit extraction of otherwise inaccessible information. Digital systems have afforded greater flexibility in the manipulation of filter settings, sensitivities, and change in the display of montages after collection. The first digital EEG systems became available in the late 1980s and caused a revolution in EEG[40] and PSG. This revolution has been primarily in making the static format of analog system data more flexible.

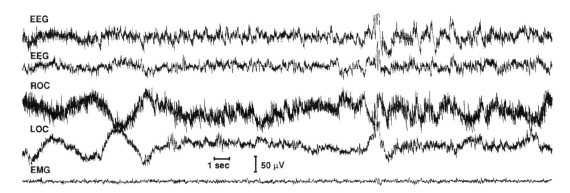

**Figure 9-12.** There is a generalized, high-frequency activity superimposed on the EEG and electro-oculography channels. This is most likely secondary to muscle activity. The electromyography (EMG) channel shows only artifact. In addition, it appears as if there is a slant to the left, particularly in channels one through four, which is probably secondary to difficulty with mechanical baseline of the pens. (ROC, LOC = outer canthus of the right and left eye, respectively.)

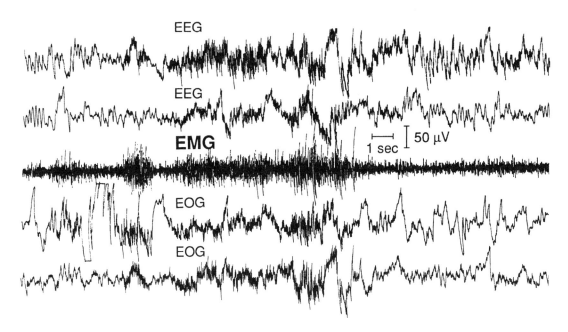

**Figure 9-13.** This burst of high-frequency artifact, superimposed on the EEG and electro-oculography (EOG) channels, is due to a brief movement on the part of the subject. As in Figure 9-14, this is a superimposition of electromyography (EMG) activity on the EEG and EOG channels. It should also be noted that in the first EOG channel there is an electrode pop. The EMG channel in this tracing is of good quality and should be compared to Figure 9-14.

Significant advantages of digital systems include auto-correction of amplifier gains, self-diagnostic tests of amplifier functions, and the software-controlled in-line impedance testing. The use of the computer has facilitated storage of data, manipulation of data after collection, and the presentation of different views of the data. Rigorous standards ensuring high-quality electrode and other sensor-application data for analog recordings are still demanded with the use of the digital system. Both analog and digital systems require that electrodes and other sensors be applied with the greatest of care. Ideally, calibration procedures should be performed to document and ensure the collection of

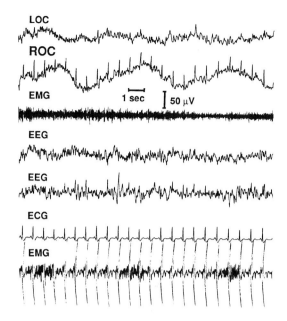

**Figure 9-14.** A high-amplitude, slow artifact is noted in the outer canthus of the right eye (ROC) channel (ROC/A1). This is most likely associated with the patient's breathing and is secondary to a loose electrode or the patient is lying on the right side and disturbing the electrode in synchrony with breathing. A relatively high-amplitude electrocardiography (ECG) artifact is also seen. The artifact can be localized to the ROC electrode. The electromyography (EMG) tracing noted at the bottom of this example is an intercostal EMG. The high-amplitude electrocardiography (ECG) spike in this channel is impossible to eliminate; however, the brief bursts of EMG activity can be noted in association with the artifact seen in the ROC/A1 channel. This lends further evidence that the artifact noted in the ROC electrode is probably associated with breathing, inasmuch as the bursts of intercostal EMG activity are seen in association with the effort of breathing. (LOC = outer canthus of the left eye.)

high-quality data at the beginning and end of the recording. Knowledge of the specifics of the equipment and of the physiology of interest are important to ensure accurate signal processing. Some of the main differences appreciated with digital systems are as follows:

- Monitor sizes vary, which affects the size of the display of the data.
- The ability to view data in retrospect during collection may not be available.
- Annotation of the recording requires the use of the mouse or a keyboard, which can be more difficult than using a pen.

- Pen noise is absent, which prevents auditory perception of movement, entry into REM sleep, or other events.

In digital systems it is rare to encounter breakdown of any mechanical component. The most frequently encountered problems are with the drives or cables. The most important things to avoid for trouble-free operation are mechanical shock, dust, or static electricity.

An important factor for understanding digital systems is the concept of *sampling rate*. Sampling rate can be understood as the frequency with which the signal is reviewed for conversion to the digital signal. EEG data are typically sampled at 200 Hz, but lower and higher sampling rates have been used. Lower sampling rates can result in a lack of fidelity to the original signal of interest. Higher sampling rates use more computer memory. The challenge is to use the sampling rate that maintains fidelity to the EEG signal but does not use excessive memory, and that avoids the confound of aliasing.

Another issue unique to digital systems is the accuracy or precision of recordings. The resolution of the signal is a function of the number of binary bits used to represent the digital values. Readers will recall that a bit is a value of 1 or 0, or "on" or "off." Eight bits is $2^8$ or 256. If an EEG voltage swing is more than 256 μV, from −128 μV to +128 μV, this would result in a resolution using an 8-bit system of 1-mV difference being represented in 1 bit of change. The 8-bit system represents the least amount of precision. A 10- or 12-bit system is usually preferred to give increased resolution. For example, at 12 bits, successive digital values represent a 0.0625-μV change. The 12-bit representation is far more precise and reflects a smaller change in the signal. The 12-bit representation is likely to appear smoother and less jagged than the 8-bit signal, and offers a signal of greater fidelity to the original wave form. Also to be considered is the display resolution, which is determined by the resolution of the monitor. Figures 9-15 through 9-18 are examples of digital data. It is interesting to note that the equivalent precision of paper tracings is approximately 6 bits. The decreased precision for analog systems is a function of the limitation in the amount of paper available for one channel and pen thickness.

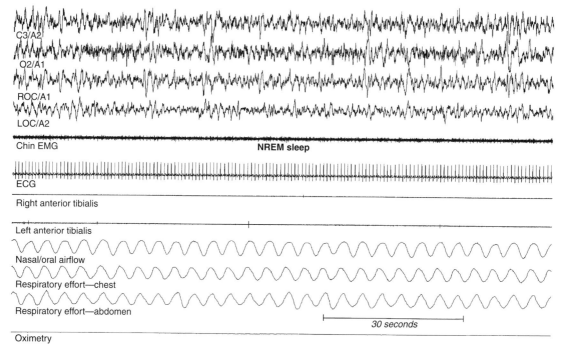

C3/A2

O2/A1

ROC/A1

LOC/A2

Chin EMG                                    **NREM sleep**

ECG

Right anterior tibialis

Left anterior tibialis

Nasal/oral airflow

Respiratory effort—chest

Respiratory effort—abdomen

|————————— *30 seconds* —————————|

Oximetry

**Figure 9-15.** Digital record sample of NREM sleep using time-scale compression. Digital data can be further compressed to display several epochs on a screen simultaneously. The sample above, and the recordings shown in Figures 9-16, 9-17, and 9-18, have been compressed to accommodate four epochs of data (2 minutes) to a page. This type of display offers the scorer or interpreter a general overview of the sleep recording, as well as a practical method of counting any prominent sleep-related events such as obstructive apneas, hypopneas, or body movements. The resolution of the data is inadequate, however, for precise EEG evaluation or sleep-stage scoring. This sample shows a normal respiratory pattern during NREM sleep, without any apparent evidence of arousal, movement, or other form of sleep disturbance. (ROC, LOC = outer canthus of the right and left eye, respectively; EMG = electromyography; ECG = electrocardiography.) (Reprinted with permission from N Butkov. Atlas of Clinical Polysomnography [Vol. I, II]. Ashland, OR: Synapse Media, 1996.)

## SUMMARY

Throughout its evolution, PSG has proved a robust tool for enhancing the understanding of sleep and its disorders. It is an essential diagnostic procedure.

PSG is complex and labor intensive. It requires specialized technical skills and knowledge of normal sleep and sleep disorders. Technologists need to be experts with sleep laboratory equipment, competent in dealing with ill patients, and capable of dealing with emergencies that may be encountered in the sleep laboratory. A registry examination is available for technologists to demonstrated competency in these skills.

Sleep specialists face many challenges. Pressure is being exerted to make PSG readily available to millions of sleep disorders patients lacking diagnosis and treatment. Cost-effectiveness in sleep health care and maintenance of the high-quality data and detailed analysis that is necessary for the formulation of accurate diagnoses remain important challenges. Digital systems can facilitate data storage, manipulation, and analysis, provided the user is knowledgeable of both instrumentation and the physiology of interest.

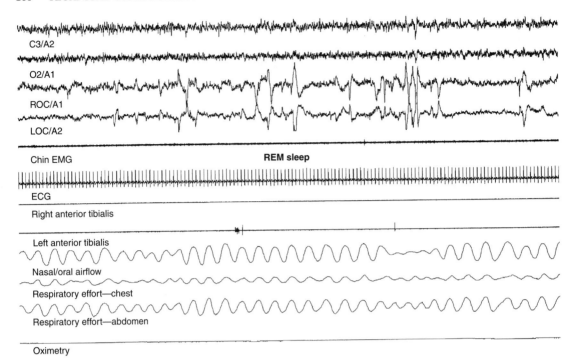

C3/A2

O2/A1

ROC/A1

LOC/A2

Chin EMG            **REM sleep**

ECG

Right anterior tibialis

Left anterior tibialis

Nasal/oral airflow

Respiratory effort—chest

Respiratory effort—abdomen

Oximetry

**Figure 9-16.** Digital record sample of REM sleep. Although altered by time-scale compression, the sleep-stage pattern seen in the above sample can readily be identified as REM. Note the mild respiratory irregularity, which is a normal variant of REM sleep physiology. (ROC, LOC = outer canthus of the right and left eye, respectively; EMG = electromyography.) (Reprinted with permission from N Butkov. Atlas of Clinical Polysomnography [Vol. I, II]. Ashland, OR: Synapse Media, 1996.)

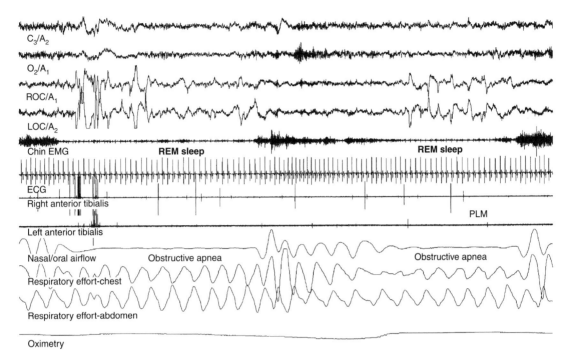

**Figure 9-17.** Digital record sample of obstructive apneas. This sample shows a compressed display of repetitive obstructive apneas, occurring during REM sleep. As noted before, these represent the extreme end of the sleep-disordered breathing continuum. In the example above, all the features of classic obstructive sleep apnea are present, including distinct paradoxic (out-of-phase) respiratory effort, instances of complete cessation of airflow, subsequent EEG arousals and cyclic $O_2$ desaturations. (ROC, LOC = outer canthus of the right and left eye, respectively; EMG = electromyography; ECG = electrocardiography.) (Reprinted with permission from N Butkov. Atlas of Clinical Polysomnography [Vol. I, II]. Ashland, OR: Synapse Media, 1996.)

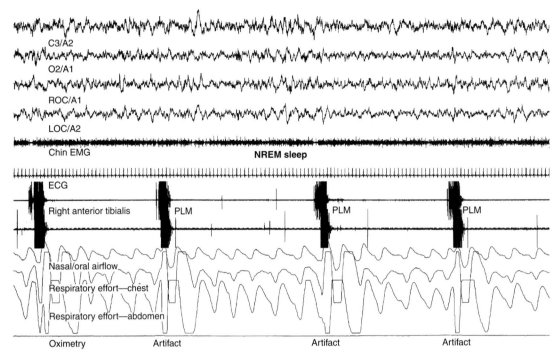

C3/A2

O2/A1

ROC/A1

LOC/A2

Chin EMG       **NREM sleep**

ECG

Right anterior tibialis      PLM      PLM      PLM

Nasal/oral airflow

Respiratory effort—chest

Respiratory effort—abdomen

Oximetry      Artifact      Artifact      Artifact

**Figure 9-18.** Digital record sample of periodic limb movements. As described previously, periodic limb movements often generate artifacts in the respiratory channels that appear similar to cyclic hypopneas. This sample shows a compressed version of the characteristic pattern of periodic limb movement (PLM), recorded by the right and left anterior tibialis electromyography (EMG). Note that the respiratory channel artifact appears almost identical to the cyclic hypopneas seen in the preceding sample. (ROC, LOC = outer canthus of the right and left eye, respectively; ECG = electrocardiography.) (Reprinted with permission from N Butkov. Atlas of Clinical Polysomnography [Vol. I, II]. Ashland, OR: Synapse Media, 1996.)

## REFERENCES

1. Holland JV, Dement WC, Raynal DM. Polysomnography: A Response to a Need for Improved Communication. Presented at the 14th Annual Meeting of the Association for the Psychophysiological Study of Sleep. Jackson Hole, WY: Association for the Psychophysiological Study of Sleep, 1974;121.

2. Broughton RJ. Polysomnography: Principles and Applications in Sleep and Arousal Disorders. In E Niedermeyer, F Lopes da Silva (eds), Electroencephalography: Basic Principles, Clinical Applications, and Related Fields (2nd ed). Baltimore: Urban & Schwarzenberg, 1987;687.

3. Coleman RM, Pollack C, Weitzman ED. Periodic movements in sleep (nocturnal myoclonus): relation to sleep-wake disorders. Ann Neurol 1980;8:416.

4. Dement WC, Kleitman N. Cyclic variations of EEG during sleep and their relation to eye movements, body motility and dreaming. Electroencephalogr Clin Neurophysiol 1957;9:673.

5. Dement WC, Rechtschaffen A. Narcolepsy: Polygraphic Aspects, Experimental and Theoretical Considerations. In H Gastaut, E Lugaresi, G Berti Ceroni (eds), The Abnormalities of Sleep in Man. Bologna: Aulo Gaggi Editore, 1968;147.

6. Dement WC, Zarcone V, Guilleminault C, et al. Diagnostic sleep recording in narcoleptics and hypersomniacs. Electroencephalogr Clin Neurophysiol 1973;35:220.

7. Dement WC. Sleep Apnea Syndromes. New York: Alan Liss, 1978;357.

8. Karacan I. Evaluation of Nocturnal Penile Tumescence and Impotence. In C Guilleminault (ed), Sleeping and Waking Disorders: Indications and Techniques. Menlo Park, CA: Addison-Wesley, 1982;343.

9. Keenan SA. Polysomnography: technical aspects in adolescents and adults. J Clin Neurophysiol 1992;9:21.

10. McGregor P, Weitzman ED, Pollack CP. Polysomnographic recording techniques used for diagnosis of sleep disorders in a sleep disorders center. Am J EEG Technol 1978;18:107.

11. Orr WC, Bollinger C, Stahl M. Measurement of Gastroesophageal Reflux During Sleep by Esophageal pH Monitoring. In C Guilleminault (ed), Sleeping and Waking Disorders: Indications and Techniques. Menlo Park, CA: Addison-Wesley, 1982;331.

12. Raynal DM. Polygraphic Aspects of Narcolepsy. In C Guilleminault (ed), Narcolepsy. New York: Spectrum, 1976;669.

13. Schenk CH, Bundlie SR, Ettinger MG, Mahowald MW. Chronic behavioral disorders of human REM sleep: a new category of parasomnia. Sleep 1986;9:293.

14. Weitzman ED, Pollack CP, McGregor P. The Polysomnographic Evaluation of Sleep Disorders in Man. In MJ Aminoff (ed), Electrodiagnosis in Clinical Neurology. New York: Churchill Livingstone, 1980; 496.

15. Martin RJ, Block AJ, Cohn MA, et al. Indications and standards for cardiopulmonary sleep studies. Sleep 1985;8:371.

16. Indications and Standards for Cardiopulmonary Sleep Studies. Am Rev Respir Dis 1989;139:559.

17. Guidelines-American Electroencephalographic Society. Polygraphic Assessment of Sleep-Related Disorders (Polysomnography), J Clin Neurophysiol 1994;14:116.

18. Thorpy MJ. The clinical use of the multiple sleep test. Sleep 1992;15:268.

19. Practice parameters for the use of portable recording in the assessment of obstructive sleep apnea. ASDA standards of practice. Sleep 1994;17:372.

20. Ferber R, Millman R, Coppola M, et al. Portable recording in the assessment of obstructive sleep apnea. ASDA standards of practice. Sleep 1994;17:378.

21. American Sleep Disorders Association, Standards Practice Committee. Practice parameters for the use of polysomnography in the evaluation of insomnia. Sleep 1995;18:55.

22. Reite M, Buysse D, Reynolds C, Mendelson W. The use of polysomnography in the evaluation of insomnia. An American Sleep Disorders Association review. Sleep 1995;18:58.

23. American Sleep Disorder Association. Practice parameters for the use of actigraphy in the clinical assessment of sleep disorders. Sleep 1995;18:285.

24. Sadeh A, Hauri PJ, Kripke DF, Lavie P. The role of actigraphy in the evaluation of the sleep disorders. An American Sleep Disorders Association review. Sleep 1995;18:288.

25. American Sleep Disorders Association. Practice parameters for the indications for polysomnography and related procedures. Sleep 1997;20:406.

26. Thorpy MJ. The clinical use of the Multiple Sleep Latency Test: the Standards of Practice Committee of the American Sleep Disorders Association. Sleep 1992:15;268. [Erratum Sleep 1992;15:381.]

27. American Sleep Disorders Association. The indications for polysomnography and related procedures. Sleep 1997;20:423.

28. Hoddes E, Dement WC, Zarcone V. The development and use of the Stanford Sleepiness Scale (SSS). Psychophysiology 1972;9:150.

29. Hoddes E, Zarcone V, Smythe H, et al. Quantification of sleepiness: a new approach. Psychophysiology 1973; 10:431.

30. Johns MW. A new method for measuring daytime sleepiness: the Epworth Sleepiness Scale. Sleep 1991;14:540.

31. American Thoracic Society. Indications and standards for cardiopulmonary sleep studies. Am Rev Respir Dis 1989;139:562.

32. Cooper R, Osselton JW, Shaw JC. EEG Technology (2nd ed). London: Butterworths, 1974.

33. Carskadon MA. Basics for Polygraphic Monitoring of Sleep. In C Guilleminault (ed), Sleeping and Waking Disorders: Indications and Techniques. Menlo Park, CA: Addison-Wesley, 1982;1.

34. Jasper HH. The ten twenty electrode system of the International Federation. Electroencephalogr Clin Neurophysiol 1958;10:371.

35. Cross C. Technical tips: patient specific electrode application techniques. Am J EEG Technol 1992;32:86.

36. Tyner FS, Knott JR, Mayer WB Jr. Fundamentals of EEG Technology. New York: Raven, 1983.

37. Carskadon MA. Measuring Daytime Sleepiness. In MH Kryger, T Roth, WC Dement (eds), Principles and Practice of Sleep Medicine (2nd ed). Philadelphia: Saunders, 1994;961.

38. Keenan Bornstein S. Respiratory Monitoring During Sleep: Polysomnography. In C Guilleminault (ed), Sleeping and Waking Disorders: Indications and Techniques. Menlo Park, CA: Addison-Wesley, 1982;183.

39. Kryger MH. Monitoring Respiratory and Cardiac Function. In MH Kryger, T Roth, WC Dement (eds), Principles and Practice of Sleep Medicine (2nd ed). Philadelphia: Saunders, 1994;984.

40. Wong PKH. Digital EEG in Clinical Practice. Philadelphia: Lippincott–Raven, 1996.

41. Butkon N. Atlas of Clinical Somnography [Vol I, II]. Ashland OR: Synapse Media, 1996.

# Chapter 9 Appendixes

## APPENDIX 9-1

For each hour of the day:

- Indicate sleep or wake time with an *X* in the appropriate box(es)
- Indicate naps with an *N* in the appropriate box(es)
- Indicate periods of extreme sleepiness with an *S* in the appropriate box(es)

**Table A9-1.** Template for 24-Hour Sleep-Wake Log.
This log should be completed by the patient for a period of 2 weeks before the study.

| Date | | | Date | | | Date | | |
|---|---|---|---|---|---|---|---|---|
| Time | Awake | Asleep | Time | Awake | Asleep | Time | Awake | Asleep |
| 12:00 | | | 12:00 | | | 12:00 | | |
| 13:00 | | | 13:00 | | | 13:00 | | |
| 14:00 | | | 14:00 | | | 14:00 | | |
| 15:00 | | | 15:00 | | | 15:00 | | |
| 16:00 | | | 16:00 | | | 16:00 | | |
| 17:00 | | | 17:00 | | | 17:00 | | |
| 18:00 | | | 18:00 | | | 18:00 | | |
| 19:00 | | | 19:00 | | | 19:00 | | |
| 20:00 | | | 20:00 | | | 20:00 | | |
| 21:00 | | | 21:00 | | | 21:00 | | |
| 22:00 | | | 22:00 | | | 22:00 | | |
| 23:00 | | | 23:00 | | | 23:00 | | |
| 24:00 | | | 24:00 | | | 24:00 | | |
| 01:00 | | | 01:00 | | | 01:00 | | |
| 02:00 | | | 02:00 | | | 02:00 | | |
| 03:00 | | | 03:00 | | | 03:00 | | |
| 04:00 | | | 04:00 | | | 04:00 | | |
| 05:00 | | | 05:00 | | | 05:00 | | |
| 06:00 | | | 06:00 | | | 06:00 | | |
| 07:00 | | | 07:00 | | | 07:00 | | |
| 08:00 | | | 08:00 | | | 08:00 | | |
| 09:00 | | | 09:00 | | | 09:00 | | |
| 10:00 | | | 10:00 | | | 10:00 | | |
| 11:00 | | | 11:00 | | | 11:00 | | |
| Exercise | | | Exercise | | | Exercise | | |
| Treatment | | | Treatment | | | Treatment | | |
| Sleep quality | | | Sleep quality | | | Sleep quality | | |
| Medications | | | Medications | | | Medications | | |
| Comments | | | Comments | | | Comments | | |

# APPENDIX 9-2. SUBJECTIVE EVALUATION OF SLEEPINESS

## *Stanford Sleepiness Scale\**

The patient is asked to make a mark on the scale that corresponds to his or her state before testing.

1. Feeling active and vital; alert; wide awake
2. Functioning at a high level, but not at peak; able to concentrate
3. Relaxed; awake; not at full alertness; responsive
4. A little foggy; not at peak; let down
5. Fogginess; beginning to lose interest in remaining awake; slowed down
6. Sleepiness; prefer to be lying down; fighting sleep; woozy
7. Almost in reverie; sleep onset soon; lost struggle to remain awake

## *Linear Analog Scale*

The patient is asked to make a mark on the scale that corresponds to his or her state before testing.

Alert                                                    Sleepy

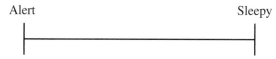

# APPENDIX 9-3. SUGGESTED EEG MONTAGES FOR RECORDING SLEEP-RELATED SEIZURE ACTIVITY

## *For a 12-Channel Study*

1. Fp1 = C3
2. C3 = O1
3. Fp2 = C4
4. C4 = O2
5. Fp1 = T3
6. T3 = O1
7. Fp2 = T4
8. T4 = O2
9. EMG—submentalis-mentalis
10. Right outer canthus—left outer canthus
11. Nasal-oral airflow
12. ECG

---

*From E Hoddes, V Zarcone, H Smythe, et al. Quantification of sleepiness: a new approach. Psychophysiology 1973;10:431.

## *For a 21-Channel Study*

1. Fp1 = F3
2. F3 = C3
3. C3 = P3
4. P3 = O1
5. Fp2 = F4
6. F4 = C4
7. C4 = P4
8. P4 = O2
9. Fp1 = F7
10. F7 = T3
11. T3 = T5
12. T5 = O1
13. Fp2 = F8
14. F8 = T4
15. T4 = T6
16. T6 = O2
17. EMG mentalis—submentalis
18. Right outer canthus/A1
19. Left outer canthus/A2
20. Nasal-oral airflow
21. ECG

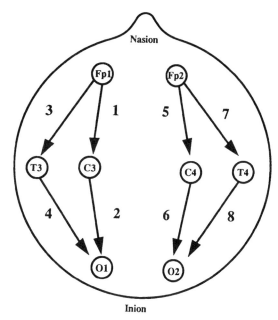

**Figure A9-1.** Suggested montage to be used to screen for possible seizure activity during sleep. Use of wide interelectrode distance affords a global view of EEG activity and conserves channels. To more adequately localize epileptogenic activity, a full complement of electrodes should be used. For a more comprehensive review of montages the reader is referred to Standard EEG Montages as proposed by American EEG Society Guidelines 1980 No. 7, Grass Instruments.

## APPENDIX 9-4. MEASURING THE HEAD FOR C3, C4, O1, AND O2

Before measuring the head, it is helpful to make an initial mark at the inion, the nasion, and the two preauricular points.

1. Measure the distance from the nasion to inion along the midline through the vertex. Make a preliminary mark at the midpoint (Cz). An electrode will not be placed on this spot, but it will be used as a landmark.
2. Center this point in the transverse plane by marking the halfway point between the left and right preauricular points. The intersection of marks from steps 1 and 2 gives the precise location of Cz.
3. Reposition the measuring tape at the midline through Cz and mark the points 10% up from the inion (Oz) and nasion (Fpz).
4. Reposition the measuring tape in the transverse plane, through Cz, and mark 10% (T3) and 30% (C3) up from the left preauricular point and 10% (T4) and 30% (C4) up from the right preauricular point.
5. Position the tape around the head through Fpz, T3, Oz, and T4. Ten percent of this circumference distance is the distance between Fp1 and Fp2 and between O1 and O2. Mark these four locations on either side of the midline.
6. The second marks for O1 and O2 are made by continuing the horizontal mark for Oz. Do this by holding the tape at T3 and T4 through Oz, and extend the horizontal mark to intersect the previous O1 and O2 marks.
7. To establish the final mark for C3, place the tape from O1 to Fp1 and make a mark at the midpoint of this line. When extended, this mark will intersect the previous C3 mark. Repeat on the right side for C4.

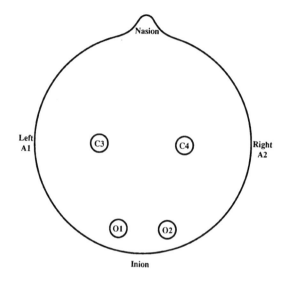

**Figure A9-2.** The International 10-20 EEG electrode placement for sleep recordings are shown.

# Chapter 10

# Electroencephalography, Electromyography, and Electro-Oculography: General Principles and Basic Technology

## Thaddeus Walczak and Sudhansu Chokroverty

The early studies of sleep typically devoted two channels to monitoring eye movement and one channel each for electromyography (EMG) and electroencephalography (EEG). This was largely due to the limited amount of channels in the machines available at that time. Although two channels probably remain sufficient for the monitoring of eye movements, multiple EEG and EMG channels should be recorded during routine night studies. Various central nervous system and metabolic disorders may result in a syndrome mimicking excessive daytime somnolence. Unusual nocturnal spells may be seizures. EEG findings during polysomnography (PSG) may be the first indication of these medical disorders. Furthermore, EEG findings associated with epilepsy may be confined solely to sleep. Thus, a fairly thorough evaluation of electrocerebral activity may be very useful during routine PSG. It follows that polysomnographers should possess a thorough knowledge of both normal and abnormal EEG patterns. Furthermore, variability in a single channel of EMG is often difficult to interpret. Multiple EMG channels help confirm that a decrease in tonic EMG is in fact physiologic.

A complete description of the technical and interpretive issues in EEG, EMG, and electro-oculography (EOG) is not possible in a single chapter. The reader is referred to several excellent monographs[1–5] for more detail. The discussion presented in this chapter starts with basic technical and safety issues. Measurement and interpretation of EOG and EMG is then briefly reviewed. The bulk

of the chapter is devoted to normal EEG findings in wakefulness and sleep as well as frequently encountered abnormalities. The discussion will be limited to findings in humans aged 2 months and older. Several useful sources are available for the reader interested in neonatal wake and sleep EEG.[1,2,4,6]

## ELEMENTARY CONCEPTS OF ELECTRICITY

It is useful to begin with a review of some elementary concepts of electricity. Electricity is largely the study of the concentration and flow of charged particles. A fundamental principle of electricity states that like charges repel and unlike charges attract. Thus, if particles of like charge are allowed to move freely, they will quickly reach a relatively uniform distribution. The flow of charged particles is called *current* (I). Various features of biological systems such as equilibrium constants of reactions or membrane permeability often result in a concentration of particles of like charge. This concentration is a store of potential energy that is released when the charged particles are allowed to move and achieve a more uniform distribution. *Voltage* (V) measures how much energy is released when a set amount of charge is allowed to move as current flow. Voltage, also known as *potential difference*, is always measured between two points. Because the concentration of charge may differ at any two points, the potential energy contained in a given concentration of charge can only be measured by relating it to the concentration of charge elsewhere. Charges experience *resistance* (R) as they move through a conducting medium. The resistance is measured in *ohms*. Current, voltage, and resistance are related by *Ohm's Law*, which states that I = V/R. The law makes intuitive sense: The higher the voltage between two points, the more flow of charge one would expect; the greater the resistance to the movement of charge, the less flow of charge one would expect.

Concentrations of charges of different polarity are often separated by a poorly conducting medium. This situation can be modeled by an electrical device known as a *capacitor*. Capacitors can be thought of as two conducting plates separated by insulation. The ability of the capacitor to store charge is measured by the capacitance, which equals the amount of charge the device can store for a given voltage. When a capacitor is connected to a source of constant voltage such as a battery, positive charges will flow from the positive pole of the battery to one plate and negative charges will flow from the negative pole of the battery to the other plate. Charges will continue flowing until the mutual repulsion of the accumulated charges on each plate equals the potential difference of the battery. At this point, current flow will cease.

The situation is different when the source of voltage varies with a predictable frequency. Voltages generated by the brain and recorded by the EEG do not stay constant but vary continuously within certain limits. In a circuit with such a voltage source and a capacitor, it can be shown that the current flow at any time equals the capacitance multiplied by the change in voltage with respect to time.* Thus, the capacitor will influence and resist the flow of current in a circuit with a varying voltage. The resistance to current flow exerted by the capacitor is measured by the *capacitative reactance* ($X_C$). It is clear that the concept of resistance must be expanded to include reactive capacitance in circuits with a voltage source that varies. *Impedance* (Z) is a measure of resistance that includes reactive capacitance and is therefore appropriate in circuits with varying voltages. In these situations, Ohm's law takes the form I = V/Z. Because cerebral voltages

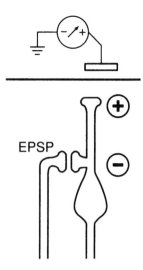

**Figure 10-1.** Scalp EEG voltage recordings resulting from an excitatory input on a deep synapse. (EPSP = excitatory postsynaptic potential.) (Modified from ER Kandel, JH Schwartz [eds]. Principles of Neural Science [2nd ed]. Amsterdam: Elsevier, 1985;642.)

vary with time, impedance is the proper measure of how well electrodes and gel transmit brain activity.

## PHYSIOLOGIC BASIS OF ELECTROENCEPHALOGRAPHY

An EEG record is essentially a measure of the changes of electrocerebral voltages over a period of time. To interpret an EEG, it is important to understand the source of the voltages recorded at the scalp and how these voltages are organized into normal cerebral rhythms.

Electrocerebral activity measured by EEG does not appear to be caused by individual or summed action potentials. Action potentials are too short (usually <1 msec) and synchronized bursts of action potentials have too limited a distribution to account for the rhythms seen in normal EEG. Excitatory and inhibitory postsynaptic potentials, on the other hand, last much longer (15–200 msec or more). These synaptic potentials induce more extensive voltage changes in extracellular space. Scalp-recorded EEG activity results from extracellular current flow induced by summated excitatory or inhibitory postsynaptic potentials.

Figure 10-1 illustrates, in a simplified fashion, how synaptic potentials induce voltage changes

---

*Capacitance* (C) is defined as the amount of charge (Q) the capacitor can store for a given voltage (V), or Q/V. Presuming that C is constant, and differentiating with respect to time (t), we find that dC/dt = 0 = –[(Q/V$^2$) (dV/dT)] + [(1/V) (dQ/dT)]. Rearranging, dQ/dt = (Q/V) (dV/dt). Current flow (I) = dQ/dt. Hence, I = C(dV/dt).

recorded at the scalp. An excitatory input on a deep dendrite causes positive ions to flow into the pyramidal neuron, resulting in a lack of positive charges, or negativity outside the neuron. Everywhere else, including the superficial dendrite, positive ions flow out of the cell into the extracellular space to complete the current loop. This results in a relative positivity in the superficial extracellular space. Because the superficial dendrite and surrounding extracellular space are closer to the scalp electrode, a positive deflection is recorded. The separation of superficial positive and deep negative charges allows one to view the pyramidal neuron as a dipole. This permits a more complete analysis of how synaptic potentials result in scalp EEG changes.[7–9]

EEG voltage recordings are rhythmic (i.e., they are regularly recurring waveforms of similar shape and duration). It is important to understand how voltage changes induced by individual neurons are organized into the widely distributed rhythms recorded with EEG. The dominant theory of EEG rhythmicity was advanced by Andersen and Andersson[10] and is based on studies of barbiturate-induced spindle activity. These investigators recorded synchronous rhythmic spindles from the cerebral cortex and thalamus. Neither removal of the cerebral cortex nor transection of the brain stem below the thalamus eliminated thalamic spindles. Ablation of the entire thalamus, however, abolished spindle activity. These findings led to the proposal that rhythmic oscillations of thalamic neurons induced synchronous synaptic excitatory or inhibitory potentials over broad areas of the cortex and thus the rhythmic voltage changes recorded with scalp EEG. Diffuse thalamocortical neuronal projections were known to exist and could mediate this thalamic influence. This model was expanded to explain most EEG rhythmic activity.

More recent work has emphasized the fact that barbiturate-induced spindles differ significantly from other cerebral rhythms.[11] The role of the thalamus in synchronizing barbiturate spindle activity over broad areas of cortex may not be relevant to other EEG rhythms. Neurons in other brain structures, including the inferior olive, hippocampus, and temporal neocortex, exhibit oscillatory behavior and may play a role in generating EEG rhythms.[12] Although widespread subcortical influences probably play an important role in organizing EEG rhythms, it is premature to conclude that all EEG rhythms are induced by oscillations of thalamic neurons.

Cerebral activity recorded at the scalp has approximately one-tenth the voltage of activity simultaneously recorded at the cortical surface. This attenuation is largely due to the cerebrospinal fluid, dura, and skull overlying the cortical surface. The area and location of the cortex generating the activity also play a role.

## COMPONENTS OF THE POLYGRAPHIC CIRCUIT

Voltages and current flows generated by the cortex, eyes, and heart during PSG studies are exceedingly small. The function of the polygraph is to transform these tiny voltages into an interpretable record. The major components necessary to accomplish this are illustrated in Figure 10-2. Each component is briefly considered in the following paragraphs.

Electrodes and conducting gel transmit biological voltages from skin or muscle to the polygraphic circuit. Various types of electrodes have been designed.[3,13] Disk electrodes are preferred for recording EEG, EOG, and ECG and may be used to record EMG as well. These are typically made of chlorided silver or noble metals such as gold or platinum.

The critical component of the conducting gel is an electrolyte, usually sodium chloride, that easily dissociates into its ionic components. The anions and cations establish a layer of positive and negative charges between the scalp and recording electrode. This charged double layer allows transmission of scalp voltage changes to the electrode and the rest of the polygraphic circuit.

The electrode-electrolyte interface is the most critical link in the polygraphic circuit. Most artifact originates here; consequently, careful technique in electrode application largely determines the quality of the recording. The impedance in any electrode pair should not exceed 10 kilo-ohms. High impedance can decrease the amount of signal the electrode presents to the amplifier. Methods to achieve low impedance are described in Chapter 9. In addition, the impedance in the two electrode inputs into the amplifier should not differ by more than 10 kilo-ohms. Higher values will degrade the ability of a differential amplifier to eliminate environmental noise and will increase artifact (see Artifacts). Impedance varies with composition and surface area of the electrode as well as with the surface area of the conducting jelly beneath the

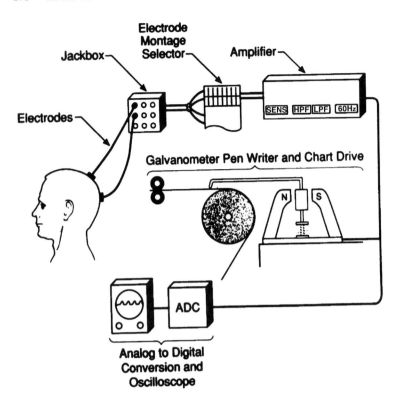

**Figure 10-2.** Components of the polygraphic circuit. (SENS = sensitivity; HPF = high-pass filter; LPF = low-pass filter; ADC = analog-to-digital converter.)

electrode. Thus, these factors should be held constant in an electrode pair attached to the same amplifier. For example, a disk electrode and needle electrode have different surface areas and conducting gel is not used with needle electrodes. Therefore impedances of the two electrodes will be significantly different. If the two electrodes are attached to the same amplifier, environmental artifact is likely to contaminate the recording.

Electrodes are attached to electrode wires, which conduct the EEG signal to the electrode box or jackbox. The electrode wires terminate in a pin which is then plugged into a receptacle in the electrode box known as a *jack*. The jacks are usually numbered or identified according to the 10-20 System. Wires from each of the jacks run together in a shielded conductor cable to the polygraph. Here, wires from each of the jacks are connected to a specific point on a multiple contact switch known as the electrode selector. The selector contains rows of switches, arranged in pairs corresponding to the two inputs of an amplifier. Depressing or otherwise activating the switches allows the technician to select which two electrodes will contribute signal to each amplifier.

The amplifiers used in polygraphic recording have several important features. *Differential* amplifiers are usually used. These amplify the *difference* in voltage between the two amplifier inputs. Figure 10-3 provides an illustration. Let us assume that T3 is connected to input 1 of an amplifier and C3 is connected to input 2 of the same amplifier. The amplifier would determine the difference between the two inputs (5 μV) and the galvanometer pen would register a deflection of 5 units. The actual amount of the deflection in millimeters would depend on the sensitivity used (see next paragraph). The fact that the differential amplifier amplifies the difference between electrode inputs rather than the absolute voltage at any electrode is a useful feature, because environmental noise, which is likely to be the same at the two electrodes, is "subtracted out" and therefore does not contaminate the recording. The *common mode rejection ratio* measures the ability of the amplifier to suppress a signal, such as noise, that is present simultaneously at both electrodes. This ratio should exceed 1,000 to 1; most contemporary polygraphic amplifiers have values that exceed 10,000 to 1.

A differential amplifier multiplies the small difference in cerebral voltages by a constant, referred to as *gain*. This multiplication is necessary because the recording galvanometer pen requires voltages much higher than those generated by the brain to generate

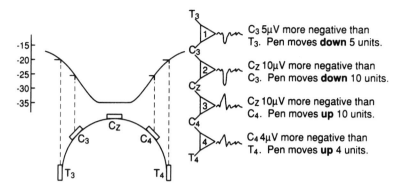

**Figure 10-3.** Scalp voltage distribution of a vertex wave. A plot of hypothetical absolute voltages at various electrode positions is shown on the left, and resulting EEG tracing with explanation is shown on the right. A transverse bipolar chain is used with amplifiers connected from left to right. The same electrode is connected to input 2 of an amplifier and input 1 of the next amplifier in the chain.

an EEG record. Analog-to-digital converters also require higher voltages to perform digitization. Amplifiers can faithfully amplify input voltages only within a certain range known as the *dynamic range*. Input voltages below the lower limit of the dynamic range are lost in noise; voltages above the upper limit result in a distorted EEG output. Flexible control of amplification within the dynamic range is achieved by manipulating the sensitivity switch. The sensitivity switch is connected to a series of voltage dividers that attenuate the amplified cerebral voltages sufficiently for the EEG record to be interpretable. *Sensitivity* is defined as the amount of voltage necessary to produce a set deflection of the pen. The usual units are microvolts per millimeter or millivolts per centimeter. One of the technologist's most important tasks is to maintain sensitivity settings low enough for the input voltage to result in a pen deflection of sufficient amplitude to be detectable. However, the sensitivity cannot be so low that the amplitude of pen deflection interferes with or "blocks" pen movements in adjacent channels. Because the voltage of electrocerebral activity varies during the study, sensitivity settings may need to be adjusted to maintain an appropriate amplitude of recorded EEG activity. Because amplitude of various waveforms is an important consideration in scoring sleep stages, these adjustments must be carefully documented. Initial recommended sensitivity settings for the biological signals routinely encountered in PSG are summarized in Chapter 9.

Whereas the sensitivity settings determine the *amplitude* of pen deflection, the polarity of the cerebral activity determines the *direction* of the pen deflection. The differential amplifier compares polarity at the two electrodes. The resulting pen deflection is determined according to the *polarity convention*. The pen moves up if input 1 is negative relative to

input 2, or if input 2 is positive relative to input 1. The pen moves down if input 1 is positive relative to input 2, or if input 2 is negative relative to input 1. It follows that *phase reversals* of EEG waveforms can be used to roughly localize the scalp distribution of those waveforms. The scalp voltage distribution of a typical vertex wave is illustrated in Figure 10-3, where hypothetical absolute voltages at several electrode positions are shown. The electrodes are linked in serial pairs from left to right. When C3 is connected to input 1 and Cz is connected to input 2 in amplifier 2, the amplifier determines that the difference between the two electrodes is 10 μV. Input 2 is more negative than input 1. Thus, the galvanometer pen recording from this amplifier registers a downward deflection of 10 units. In amplifier 3, Cz is connected to input 1 and C4 to input 2. The amplifier determines that the difference in voltages is also 10 μV. However, input 1 is now more negative than input 2. Consequently, the galvanometer pen recording from this amplifier registers an upward deflection of 10 units. The phase reversal in the adjacent channels marks the electrode where the vertex wave is most negative. This is the electrode shared by both amplifiers, Cz. Because most cerebral activity is negative at the scalp, phase reversals with the pen deflections pointing toward each other (see Figure 10-3) are encountered most commonly. Positive cerebral activity would result in a phase reversal with the pen deflections pointing away from each other at the electrode that was most positive. Note that localization by phase reversal is accurate only when electrodes spaced at relatively short distances are serially linked in adjacent amplifiers. This is known as a *bipolar montage*.

After voltages at the two inputs are subtracted and amplified, the result is passed through a series of filters. The goal of filtering is to attenuate volt-

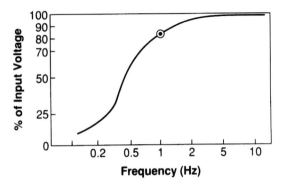

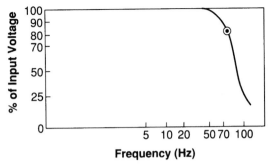

**Figure 10-4.** Frequency-response curve of a hypothetical high-pass filter with a cutoff frequency of 1 Hz and a roll-off of –6 dB per octave. (Modified with permission from F Tyner, J Kott, W Mayer Jr. Fundamentals of EEG Technology [Vol 1]. New York: Raven, 1983.)

**Figure 10-5.** Frequency-response curve of a hypothetical low-pass filter with a cutoff frequency of 70 Hz and a roll-off of –6 dB per octave. (Modified with permission from F Tyner, J Kott, W Mayer Jr. Fundamentals of EEG Technology [Vol 1]. New York: Raven, 1983.)

ages occurring at undesirable frequencies (e.g., environmental noise) without disturbing frequencies found in the biological signal of interest. A frequency response curve measures the ability of a filter to attenuate various frequencies. Frequency response curves for two types of analog filter included in many polygraphs are presented in Figures 10-4 and 10-5. A *high-pass filter*, (also known as a *low-frequency filter*), allows higher frequency activity to pass unchanged while progressively attenuating lower frequencies (see Figure 10-4). A *low-pass filter* (also known as a *high-frequency filter*), allows lower frequencies to pass unchanged while progressively attenuating higher frequencies (see Figure 10-5). Analog filters are defined by *cutoff frequency* and *roll-off*. The filter with a given cutoff frequency will attenuate voltage of that frequency by 20%* (e.g., the high-pass filter in Figure 10-4 has a cutoff frequency of 1 Hz, so a 100-µV, 1-Hz wave passed through this filter will have an amplitude of 80 µV). Attenuation of frequencies above the cutoff frequency is more or less linear for the high-pass filter. Attenuation of frequencies below the cutoff frequency is progressively more severe as lower frequencies are encountered. This progressively more severe attenuation is defined by the filter's roll-off. Roll-off for most EEG filters is

–6 dB per octave. For the high-pass filter, this means that the voltage of activity is decreased by half for every halving of the frequency.

The *60-Hz* or *notch* filter is also present in most polygraphic amplifiers.[†] This filter is designed to attenuate mains frequency very harshly while attenuating activity of surrounding frequencies less extensively.[3] Because electrical mains are ubiquitous, 60-Hz artifact may easily contaminate an EEG recording. The notch filter should be used sparingly for at least two reasons. First, some biological signals of interest to the polysomnographer have waveforms with important components in the range of 40–80 Hz. Examples include myogenic activity and epileptiform spikes, both of which may be significantly attenuated by the notch filter. For example, use of the notch filter in the chin EMG channel may result in a false impression that tonic EMG has significantly decreased. In addition, the capability of the differential amplifier to reject common signals (see Components of the Polygraphic Circuit) should be sufficient to suppress 60-Hz artifact in most cases. Thus, the appearance of 60 Hz usually signals a problem somewhere in the polygraphic circuit that needs to be resolved. Most often the culprit is high impedance at the electrode-scalp interface. Less frequently, defects in the amplifier or grounding of the polygraph are responsible. In these cases, addressing the cause of the 60 Hz rather than using the notch filter is the appropriate course. There

---

*In electrophysiology, a widely used convention dictates that voltage at the cutoff frequency is attenuated by 20%. In electrical engineering, voltage at the cutoff frequency is attenuated by approximately 30%.

---

[†]Because mains frequency is 50 Hz, a 50-Hz notch filter is widely available.

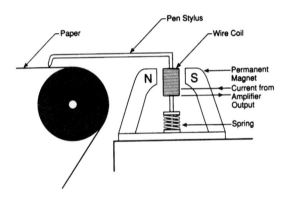

**Figure 10-6.** Hypothetical galvanometer pen writer unit (not to scale). (Modified with permission from F Tyner, J Kott, W Mayer Jr. Fundamentals of EEG Technology [Vol 1]. New York: Raven, 1983.)

are circumstances in which a nearby source of 60 Hz (e.g., a critical piece of medical equipment that cannot be disconnected) renders the EEG uninterpretable. Use of the 60-Hz filter may be justified in these circumstances but must be clearly documented.

The preceding paragraphs discuss analog filters, which consist of various arrays of resistors and capacitors. Computerization has allowed routine on-line digitization of the amplified EEG waveform, which can then be subjected to digital filtering. Digital filters are computer algorithms that transform digitized EEG by filtering out designated frequencies. Digital filtering can be performed in the frequency domain by computing the Fourier transform of a segment of EEG, replacing coefficients at the frequency one wishes to eliminate by zero, and then reconstituting the EEG by computing the inverse Fourier transform.[14] Digital filtering can also be performed in the time domain by using a moving average method.[14] Such finite impulse response[11] filters are increasingly used in digital EEG machines and allow filtering without phase distortion, an advantage over traditional analog filters. See Spectral Analysis, later in this chapter, for an introductory discussion of digitization and Fourier analysis.

A writer unit transforms the amplified and filtered signal into a written record. The writer unit consists of an oscillograph and chart drive. A *galvanometer pen unit* is a widely used oscillograph (Figure 10-6). A specially designed coil of wire and a pen stylus are mounted on a rod. The coil of wire is placed between the two poles of a permanent

magnet. Current flow from the amplifier enters the coil and induces a magnetic field. The induced magnetic field interacts with the field of the permanent magnet resulting in a deflection of the pen stylus on the paper. The amount of deflection is proportional to the magnetic field, which is proportional to the current from the amplifier, which in turn is proportional to the biological signal. A spring attached to the rod returns the pen stylus back to baseline after the current responsible for the deflection has ceased. This spring, together with the friction of the pen stylus against the paper and the inertia of the galvanometer, are collectively known as *damping* and resist the pen movement. Very rapid signal changes (high-frequency signal) require very rapid galvanometer movement increasing disproportionately the amount of energy necessary to overcome damping. Because more energy is required to write out high-frequency signals, the galvanometer pen unit, in effect, acts as a high-frequency filter. Galvanometer pen writer units usually do not faithfully reproduce signals with frequencies higher than 80–90 Hz.

The *chart drive* pulls the paper below the pens at a constant speed to provide a continuous record of pen deflections (voltage changes) over time. Paper speeds slower than 10 mm per second save paper but cannot be recommended because resolution of faster waveforms necessary for scoring sleep stages is impossible. When suspicious waveforms such as epileptiform spikes are noted, increasing paper speed to 30 mm per second can aid interpretation.

Many currently available polygraphic systems avoid the need for paper writeout by digitizing amplifier output and storing it on various nonpaper media. These signals can be processed and subsequently displayed on a video monitor. Digitization and magnetic or optical storage have several advantages. Interpreters are not limited to the settings chosen by the technologist and can review stored EEG segments with whatever filter, sensitivity, or montage deemed appropriate. Selected portions can be printed out but the entire record can be stored on optical or magnetic disk. Storage of records requires less space and ultimately costs less. Digitization is performed by analog-to-digital conversion. Analog-to-digital conversion consists of assigning a numerical value, which corresponds to the amplitude of the continuous analog waveform, at identical brief intervals (intersample interval). Number of intervals in a period of time is called the *sampling rate*; for example, a sampling rate of 256 per second means that the voltage of the waveform is sampled (assigned a numerical value) at each serial interval of 1 per 256 seconds. This inter-sample interval indicates the horizontal (time) resolution. If the digitized signal is to reflect the analog signal faithfully, the sampling rate must be at least two times the highest frequency in the analog signal. Frequencies in the analog signal exceeding half the sampling rate will appear in the digitized signal at frequencies below the sampling rate. This is known as *aliasing* because the faster frequencies in the analog signal appear under the "alias" of a lower frequency in the digitized signal. The number of discrete numerical levels that the voltage of the analog signal can potentially be assigned indicates the vertical resolution. Vertical resolution of the analog-to-digital converter is measured in "bits" or powers of 2. For example, a 10-bit converter can assign $2^{10}$, or 1,024, levels to the voltage of a signal at any point in time. Vertical resolution of the converter should be higher than the noise level of the amplifier so that all signals exceeding noise level can be represented. Because noise level of contemporary amplifiers is approximately 1 μV, a 10-bit converter is usually adequate for EEG signals. A 10-bit converter would allow amplitude at any point in an analog signal to be assigned a value in 1-μV steps from –511 to +512 μV. This range encompasses the vast majority of EEG voltages recorded from the scalp. Twelve-bit converters are used in many contemporary digital polygraphic systems.

## SPECTRAL ANALYSIS

Spectral analysis is probably the most widely used computerized analysis of digitized EEG.[14–16] Spectral analysis is based on the Fourier theorem, which states that any waveform can be decomposed into a sum of sine waves at different frequencies with different amplitudes and different phase relationships. When summed, these waves reconstitute the original waveform. The Fourier transformation is a mathematical operation that provides the frequency, amplitude, and phase parameters of each of these component sine waves. Fourier coefficients represent the amplitude and phase relationship at each of the component sine-wave frequencies. Squaring and summing the Fourier coefficients at each frequency provides the power at that frequency. A plot of power

at each of the component frequencies is called the *power spectrum*. The power spectrum allows determination of relative amounts of given frequencies in the waveform over the time segment analyzed.

The fast Fourier transform algorithm[17] allows real-time spectral analysis with contemporary personal computers. Commercially available software packages offer straightforward presentation of the power contained in the traditional frequency bands during a set period of EEG. This allows detection and quantification of frequencies not detected with visual inspection. However, there are many potential pitfalls.[15,16] Theoretically, the power spectrum is a faithful representation of the original signal only if the original signal is stationary (has stable statistical properties). The EEG signal is clearly not stationary over long periods, although it appears reasonably stationary over brief epochs.[18] In practice this means that the EEG segment selected for analysis should not include obvious changes such as those due to alerting or drowsiness. In addition, the Fourier theorem assumes that an infinitely long sample is available for analysis. Because even long samples are clinically impractical, tapering or "windowing" of the end points of the sample is necessary to attenuate the spurious frequencies (leakage) arising from the segmentation of the signal. Windowing is never completely successful—some leakage is unavoidable. This may affect clinical interpretation when power is displayed in the traditional frequency bands; for example, a reasonable amount of alpha power may leak to the theta band or beta bands. Nonsinusoidal rhythms, such as "spiky alpha" are common in routine EEG. Fourier analysis of a nonsinusoidal rhythm of a set frequency often show a large peak at that frequency with smaller peaks at harmonics of the frequency. These smaller, higher-frequency peaks may lead the interpreter to conclude that cerebral activity at the higher frequency is actually present. The most common pitfall in interpreting power spectra is artifact. Artifact is ubiquitous, often subtle, and can take an almost infinite variety of forms. The computer cannot separate artifact from EEG and includes artifact in the computation of the power spectrum. This can lead to significant misinterpretation. Artifact is much more difficult to recognize in the power spectrum than in the unprocessed EEG. It is therefore very important to review EEG before spectral analysis or interpretation of the power spectrum to prevent analysis of segments contaminated by artifact.

Despite these limitations, spectral analysis can play a useful role in the operating room and in routine scoring of sleep studies (see Chapter 15). A basic understanding of the principles of signal processing and thorough experience in the appearance of various cerebral activities after spectral analysis is necessary. The unprocessed EEG must always be reviewed. Spectral analysis has not demonstrated any consistent clinical utility in routine EEG despite almost two decades of active research. Because the potential for misinterpretation and abuse is high, the major neurologic and neurophysiologic professional organizations have taken strong positions against the use of spectral analysis during routine EEG.[19,20]

## ELECTRICAL SAFETY

Contemporary polygraphic and EEG studies are very safe procedures. Nevertheless, the possibility of electrical injury exists whenever a patient is connected to an electrical apparatus. Thus, technicians performing studies and physicians supervising sleep laboratories must understand the basic principles of electrical safety.

Electrical injury is caused by excessive current flow through biological tissue. Such electrical injury includes burns, seizures, and irreversible damage to nervous tissue. When excessive current flows through the heart, ventricular arrhythmias, including ventricular fibrillation, may occur. The amount of current necessary to induce ventricular fibrillation is dependent on skin impedance, the mass of tissue the current must traverse before reaching the heart, the health of the heart, and the general health of the patient, among other factors. In a healthy adult with dry intact skin, 100–300 mA delivered at 60 Hz will induce fibrillation (macroshock).[3] Smaller amounts of current (microshock) will induce fibrillation in electrically susceptible patients. These include patients with wet skin or wounds, as well as patients with pacemaker electrodes inserted in the ventricular myocardium. Dry intact skin offers high impedance to current flow, as technicians well appreciate. Moisture on the skin or extensive interruption of the skin significantly reduces this impedance, allowing current to flow toward the heart more readily. Pacemaker wires allow the current to flow directly into the vulnerable myocardium rather than through the high imped-

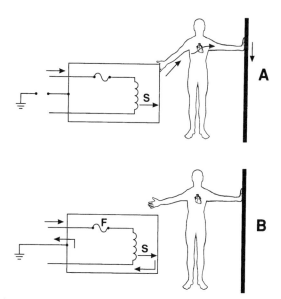

**Figure 10-7. (A)** Technician touches polygraph chassis and water pipe. Polygraph chassis is ungrounded because of interruption in ground wire. A short circuit (S) in the power supply unit allows current to flow to the chassis, through the technician's heart, and to the water pipe. Arrows trace path of current flow. **(B)** A short circuit in the polygraph with an intact chassis ground. A short circuit (S) in the power supply allows current to flow to the chassis. The low-resistance chassis ground allows unimpeded flow of current to building ground. The current surge blows a fuse (F), quickly stopping further current flow. Bystanders are safe unless they touch the chassis at the moment of the short circuit.

ance offered by the chest wall and pleural cavities. When a 60-Hz current is applied directly to the heart, intensities as low as 100 µA will result in fibrillation although higher values are necessary in most cases.[21–23]

Current flow requires a source of current and the formation of a complete circuit. Thus, electrical safety has two goals: (1) The polygraph must not become a source of excessive current, and (2) the polygraph and patient (or technician) must not form a complete circuit through which excessive current may flow and cause electrical injury. Proper maintenance, proper grounding, and use of isolation devices accomplish these goals.

The power unit of the polygraph is a potential source of excessive current. A fault in the power unit may result in a short circuit that would allow a *fault current* to flow to the polygraph chassis (Figure 10-7A). If the machine ground was disabled and the patient was touching a pipe or some other conducting substance, current would flow through the electrodes and the patient to the pipe possibly causing electrical injury. Current would also flow through a technician touching the polygraph and a conducting substance. To guard against this possibility, the chassis of the polygraph is connected to the building ground through a three-pronged outlet (Figure 10-7B). Should a current-bearing element contact the chassis, the current would be shunted through machine ground to the building ground because this path has the least resistance. The sudden high-current flow would blow a fuse in the power unit or open a circuit breaker stopping further current flow. A brief period is necessary for the excessive current to blow the fuse and if the patient is touching a conducting substance during this period, current will still flow through the patient. The duration of the current flow would be briefer, however, and the danger to the patient decreased.

It follows that the connection between the polygraph and building ground must not be compromised. Electrical outlets powering appliances connected to patients must have documented secure connection to building ground. Technicians should ensure good contact between the ground pin of the power cord and the outlet. Three- and two-pronged adapters do not provide secure contact with building ground and must not be used. Resistance of the ground circuit in the polygraph should be checked periodically to detect interruptions. Fuses should never be defeated (i.e., short-circuited). Repeatedly blown fuses may indicate fault currents and potential danger to the technician and patient. Finally, regular maintenance may prevent potentially dangerous fault currents.

Even in the absence of a fault, the complicated circuitry of the polygraph generates lower-intensity currents known as *leakage currents*. *Stray capacitance* is a major source of leakage current. Any circuit with current flow that is insulated from other conducting substances can be viewed as a capacitor. The current-carrying circuit can be considered one plate of a capacitor, the insulation and surrounding space can be considered the dielectric, and the other conducting substances can be considered the other plate of the capacitor. Alternating current flowing through any insulated circuit will therefore generate currents in other conducting substances in the area. One pertinent example is the power cord of the polygraph. AC current flow in the insulated

"hot" wire of the power cord will induce a lower amount of current flow in the neutral and ground wires. Although leakage currents are much smaller than fault currents, they can cause injury in electrically susceptible patients. Acceptable limits for leakage currents have been defined.[3,24] Adequate grounding protects both patient and technician in this circumstance. The leakage current is shunted to the low-resistance machine ground and then to building ground. Extension cords increase stray capacitance and thus leakage currents and should never be used during PSG. Isolation jackboxes that limit the amount of possible current flow through electrodes are available. These offer additional protection in electrically susceptible patients.

Current flow can also occur when machinery attached to the patient draws power from different outlets or when multiple grounds are attached to the patient. The voltage of the ground contact at different outlets may be quite different, resulting in current flow. Multiple grounds can result in a *ground loop*, which can act as a secondary coil of a transformer and generate current flow. A ground loop also acts as an antenna that will pick up ubiquitous environmental electromagnetic radiation and will increase artifact. These potentially dangerous situations can be avoided by plugging in all machinery attached to the patient to the same outlet cluster and using only one patient ground.

## ELECTRO-OCULOGRAPHY

The electrical field generated by the eye approximates a simple dipole (Figure 10-8A) with a posterior negativity centered at the retina and a relative positivity probably centered at the cornea. Eye movements change the orientation of this dipole. Polygraphic recording from strategically placed electrodes can detect these changes and can therefore be used to monitor eye movements. The standard sleep scoring manual[25] recommends that an EOG use at least two channels (Figure 10-8B). One electrode is placed 1 cm superior and lateral to the outer canthus of one eye. This electrode is input 1 to an amplifier; input 2 to this amplifier is an electrode attached to one ear or mastoid. Another electrode is placed 1 cm inferior and lateral to the outer canthus of the other eye. This electrode forms input 1 to a second amplifier; input 2 to this amplifier is

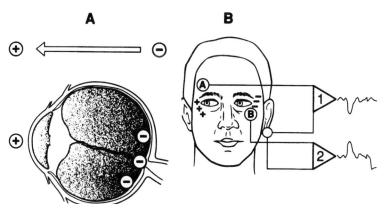

**Figure 10-8. (A)** The voltage field generated by the eye can be represented by a simple dipole, the cornea being positive and the retina negative. **(B)** Use of two polygraphic channels to detect conjugate eye movements according to the scheme suggested in the sleep scoring manual.[18] Eye movements result in out-of-phase potentials in the two channels.

attached to the same ear as input 2 of the first amplifier. This placement scheme will detect conjugate horizontal and vertical eye movements. For example, when the eyes look to the right (see Figure 10-8B), the cornea of the right eye approaches electrode A and electrode A becomes positive relative to the inactive ear. According to the polarity convention, amplifier 1 will register a downward deflection. Simultaneously, the retina of the left eye approaches electrode B. Consequently, electrode B becomes negative relative to the inactive ear and amplifier 2 registers an upward deflection. The out-of-phase deflections in the two adjacent channels indicate that a conjugate eye movement has occurred. Similarly, an upward eye movement results in an downward deflection in amplifier 1 and a upward deflection in amplifier 2. Eye blinks will produce an identical pattern because eye closure results in an upward rotation of the eyeball (Bell's phenomenon). (See also Chapter 9.)

Some laboratories attach electrodes to both ears and refer the periocular electrodes to the contralateral ear (e.g., right upper canthus to left ear and left lower canthus to right ear). This minor change has several advantages. The longer interelectrode distances increase the amplitude of the deflections. The amplitude of the deflections generated by the movement of each eye is more likely to be equal because the interelectrode distances are equal. Finally, if one of the ear electrodes comes off during the study, the technician can refer both periocular electrodes to the remaining ear electrode and avoid waking the patient. Whereas these montages detect both horizontal and vertical eye movements, they cannot distinguish between them. This can be easily accomplished by

recording inputs from supraorbital and infraorbital electrodes with a third amplifier.[3,13]

Several varieties of eye movements are recorded during routine PSG. Although the patient is awake, saccadic eye movements as well as eye blinks are noted. Saccadic eye movements are rapid and can point in any direction. Eye blinks produce the same EOG pattern as vertical eye movement. One of the first signs of drowsiness is the cessation of any eye movements. Somewhat later in drowsiness slow eye movements are seen. These usually have a frequency of less than 0.5 Hz,[26] are most consistently recorded in the horizontal axis, gradually increase in amplitude as background alpha activity drops out, and usually disappear in stage II sleep. Rapid eye movements (REM) occur during REM sleep. Movements along the horizontal axis are the most common, although oblique and vertical movements occur as well. REM typically occur in bursts and may be preceded by characteristic sawtooth waves on the EEG. There is no widely accepted definition of REM that would serve to distinguish these from slow eye movements. Parameters useful for computerized quantification of REM have been reported,[27] but these are not directly applicable to visual scoring. Radtke[28] has suggested a reasonable, clinically applicable definition for REM, namely that the duration of the initial pen deflection is less than 200 msec and that the duration of the entire waveform is less than 1 second.

In a study of drowsiness in normal subjects, Santamaria and Chiappa[26] recorded eye movements with a sensitive motion transducer attached over the globe as well as with the traditional EOG. They found two types of eye movements not previously reported. What were named *small fast irregular eye movements* were found in 60% of normal subjects in early drowsiness, before the occurrence of slow eye movements. They did not appear in the routine EOG channels. What were called *small fast rhythmic eye movements* were found in 30% of normal subjects, usually associated with the traditional slow eye movements. These occasionally appeared in the routine EOG channels, although usually with a very low amplitude. If confirmed, these findings could be useful for determination of early stages of drowsiness.

## ELECTROMYOGRAPHIC RECORDINGS IN SLEEP DISORDERS

EMG activities are important physiologic characteristics that need to be recorded for diagnosis and classification of a variety of sleep disorders. EMG represents electrical activities of muscle fibers resulting from depolarization of the muscles after transmission of nerve impulses along the nerves and neuromuscular junctions.[5] EMG could represent tonic, phasic, and rhythmic activity. Physiologically, there is a fundamental tone in the muscles, at least throughout the period of wakefulness and non-REM (NREM) sleep, but it is markedly diminished or absent in major muscle groups during REM sleep. Maintenance of muscle tone is a complex physiologic phenomenon that depends on suprasegmental, segmental, and peripheral afferent mechanisms.[29] Tone, therefore, may be influenced by a variety of extrinsic and intrinsic stimuli. After a nerve impulse, the resting muscle membrane potential is altered, and when it reaches a threshold level, depolarization of the muscle results from a change in the external and internal ionic balance and muscle calcium channel alterations.[5] The threshold depolarization causes an action potential to develop in the muscle. A compound muscle action potential represents summation of the action currents in many muscle fibers. Surface EMG recordings are of many muscle fibers, bundles, and groups; needle EMGs record approximately 15–20 muscle fibers near the needle tip.[5] Phasic EMG represents activities related to some physiologic alterations, either spontaneous or induced. Examples of phasic EMGs are EMG activities phasically related to inspiratory bursts and myoclonic muscle bursts that occur spontaneously or in response to some stimuli. If there are rhythmic activities, for example tremor, EMG bursts have a rhythm. In sleep disorders medicine, the tonic and phasic EMG bursts are usually the most important ones. As sometimes happens, however, rhythmic EMG bursts are noted in certain sleep disorders, such as patients with restless legs syndrome (see Chapter 26).

### Method of Recording

EMG recordings from submental muscles using surface electrodes are routinely performed in PSG and multiple sleep latency tests. Electrodes placed in this area record mostly the activities of the mylohyoid and the anterior belly of the digastric muscles. The electrodes also record some activities from the genioglossus and hyoglossus muscles by volume conduction. This recording is important for identifying the presence or absence of muscle tone for sleep stage scoring.

In a patient suspected of restless legs syndrome, tibialis anterior muscles must be recorded, preferably bilaterally, because sometimes the periodic movements of legs alternate between the two legs. Ideally, the recording should also include one or two EMG channels from the upper limb muscles, as occasionally movements are noted in the upper limbs.

To understand the pathophysiology of sleep apnea, it is important to record the respiratory muscle activities (see also Chapter 12). These should include not only the intercostal muscles but also the diaphragmatic muscle, a variety of upper airway muscles, and the facial muscles. The true diaphragmatic activities are typically recorded by intraesophageal bipolar electrodes, which can also quantitate the diaphragmatic EMG activity.[30–32] This technique as well as esophageal pressure recording by inserting an esophageal balloon transnasally (which provides respiratory muscle mechanical activity) are invasive and uncomfortable. The noninvasive technique of placing surface electrodes to the right or left of the umbilicus or over the anterior costal margin may also pick up diaphragmatic activity, but the admixture of intercostal muscle activity makes this noninvasive technique unreliable for quantitative assessment of diaphragmatic EMG.[33] The intercostal EMG recorded from the seventh to the ninth intercostal space[34] with active electrodes on the anterior axillary line and the reference electrodes on the midaxillary line may record some diaphragmatic muscle activity in addition to the intercostal activity. Sharp et al.[35] compared data from chest wall surface electrodes (surface electrodes over the sixth and seventh intercostal space just above the right costal margin) with simultaneous data obtained from a swallowed bipolar electrode double-balloon catheter similar to that described by Onal and coworkers.[36] After performing power spectral analysis of diaphragmatic EMGs from surface electrodes and esophageal electrodes, Sharp et al.[35] concluded that thoracic surface recordings of the diaphragmatic EMG do not accurately reflect frequency information. Esophageal balloon manometry is important for a definite diagnosis of upper airway resistance syndrome.[37] In this condition, a narrowed upper airway results in increased work necessary to move air through a constricted airway but does not cause apneas or hypopneas.[37,38] Esophageal balloon manometry in this condition documents abnormally increased negative intrathoracic pressure during inspiration associated with repeated arousals and fragmentation of sleep that are responsible for daytime hypersomnolence. Esophageal balloon manometry has been superseded by the use of a thinner and better-tolerated water-filled catheter connected to a transducer.[38,39]

An important muscle for recording respiratory activity is the alae nasi muscle.[34] This muscle picks up not only inspiratory activity but also some expiratory activity. Many upper airway muscles are accessory muscles of respiration. All the facial muscles, including the masseter muscles, show inspiratory bursts during the recordings.[34] To show the decrease of tone in the genioglossus and other oropharyngeal and laryngeal muscles, it is important to record EMGs from them. Intramuscular electrodes in humans are typically used to record inspiratory-related genioglossal muscle activity.[40–42] For many of these upper airway muscles, however, recordings can be made in a noninvasive manner by means of intraoral surface electrodes.[34,43] For some laryngeal muscles, an invasive technique using fine-wire electrodes is required.[40] To record the muscle activity from an individual muscle only, wire electrodes must be inserted into that particular muscle only.

For patients with suspected REM behavior disorder, multiple muscle EMGs from all four limbs are essential—there is often dissociation in the activities between upper and lower limb muscles with these patients. Hence, if upper limb EMGs are not included in the recording, REM sleep without atonia may be missed in some cases.[44]

In patients with nocturnal paroxysmal dystonia, which is thought to be a form of frontal lobe seizure disorder, multiple muscle EMGs including all four limbs are required. In this condition, the patient displays dystonic-choreoathetoid movements; surface EMGs in addition to the video recordings are necessary to record these activities.

### *Clinical Significance of EMG Recording*

EMG shows decreasing tone from wakefulness through stages I–IV of NREM sleep. In REM sleep, the EMG tone is markedly diminished or absent. It is important to use the appropriate filters and very high gain at the beginning of the recording to appreciate the decreasing muscle tone during REM sleep. In certain pathologic conditions (e.g., REM behavior disorder), the EMG tone may persist or phasic muscle bursts may be seen repeatedly during REM sleep. This may also happen in patients being treated for narcolepsy, and may represent a medication side effect.

EMG recordings of the tibialis anterior muscles are essential for the diagnosis of periodic limb movements of sleep, which are seen in most of the cases of restless legs syndrome; a variety of other sleep disorders; and normal individuals, particularly older ones. Characteristics of the EMG bursts in periodic limb movements of sleep are described in Chapter 26. In upper airway obstructive apnea, the EMG of the upper airway muscles shows marked decrease of tone during the apneic episodes, whereas the diaphragmatic and intercostal muscle activity persists.[34] During REM sleep, however, intercostal and even diaphragmatic EMGs show marked diminution of the tonic activity.[45]

In certain neurodegenerative diseases such as the Shy-Drager syndrome, laryngeal EMG recording may be important to detect vocal cord paralysis causing upper airway obstructive apnea.[46]

Multiple muscle EMG recordings are also important in patients with restless legs syndrome because of the presence of a variety of EMG activity in these patients, including periodic limb movements of sleep, myoclonic bursts both during wakefulness and sleep, and a mixture of myoclonic and dystonic EMG bursts during wakefulness and occasionally during sleep (see Chapter 26).

## ELECTROENCEPHALOGRAPHY

EEG is recorded in sleep studies mostly to assist scoring of sleep stages. Obviously, EEG can provide other useful information as well. Routine diagnostic EEGs usually sample at most 1 hour of electrocerebral activity. The PSG records EEG activity for much longer periods, increasing the likelihood that abnormalities will be recorded. Consequently, the polysomnographer must be familiar with the broad range of normal EEG findings and the abnormalities encountered in the various age groups. The following is at best an incomplete review of some of the major patterns encountered in routine EEG.

### Normal Waking Rhythms

Individual waves recorded on the EEG can be characterized by their frequency (i.e., how many of that wave would be required to occupy a given period of time, typically 1 second). Frequency of EEG activity has been divided into four bands, assigned the Greek letters beta, alpha, theta, and delta. Scoring of sleep is largely based on the amplitude and frequency of EEG waves. Human electrocerebral activity is better characterized, however, by the broader concept of EEG *rhythms*. EEG rhythms can be defined as sustained periods of electrocerebral activity of similar frequency with a stereotyped distribution, reactivity, symmetry, and synchrony, and are associated with specific physiologic states. These rhythms have also been assigned Greek letters that correspond, in part, to the letters assigned to frequency.

Several rhythms characterize the awake adult EEG. The most obvious is the *alpha* rhythm. Alpha rhythm frequency varies between 8 and 13 Hz. This rhythm is distributed over the parieto-occipital regions bilaterally. A normal alpha rhythm is synchronous and symmetric over the two hemispheres. Frequency of the rhythm should not vary by more than 1 Hz, and amplitude should not vary by more than 50%. The alpha rhythm is best seen during quiet alertness with eyes closed. Various maneuvers cause alpha rhythm to react or decrease in amplitude. The most effective is opening the eye, but any

sort of intense stimulation produces some degree of amplitude attenuation. Up to 10% of normal adults will show no alpha rhythm during quiet wakefulness. The low-voltage EEG in these subjects is characterized by poorly sustained beta and theta frequencies with amplitudes between 10 and 20 μV. Occasionally, hyperventilation elicits a typical alpha rhythm in such patients. Low-voltage EEGs have not been recorded in normal subjects less than 10 years old.

*Beta rhythms* are present in virtually all adults, although they are usually less striking than alpha rhythms. Frequency of the beta rhythm is by definition above 13 Hz but typically ranges between 18 and 25 Hz. There are probably at least two beta rhythms, one distributed over the frontal and central regions and the other with a more diffuse distribution. Beta rhythms are present during wakefulness and drowsiness. They may appear more persistent during drowsiness, drop out during deeper sleep, and reappear during REM sleep. Amplitude over the two hemispheres should not vary by more than 50%. Amplitude of beta activity is less than 20 μV in 98% of normal drug-free subjects. A persistent beta rhythm with higher amplitude suggests use of sedative-hypnotic medications because most such medications increase amplitude of beta activity.

*Mu rhythms* are recorded in approximately 20% of routine daytime EEGs and are most common in young adults. This rhythm consists of brief trains of 7–11 Hz waves over the central regions, often with phase reversals over C3 or C4. The waves have a wicket or arciform shape (Figure 10-9). Mu may occur synchronously or independently over the two hemispheres. This rhythm shows a characteristic reactivity. Active or passive movement of the limbs or even an intention to move a limb attenuates mu activity. Mu is seen during wakefulness and may become more prominent during stages I and II of NREM sleep. It typically disappears in slow-wave sleep and may reappear during REM sleep.[47] Direct EEG recordings from human motor cortex have demonstrated superharmonics of mu activity that react to limb movement.[48] This has led to the conclusion that mu is an "ubiquitous rhythm of the sensorimotor cortex at rest."[49]

*Lambda rhythm* is present in approximately 75% of young adults and becomes somewhat less common as individuals age. Lambda consists of a diphasic or triphasic waveform with the most prominent phase being a positivity at O1 or O2. The

**Figure 10-9.** Mu rhythm in the left parietal region (P3). Note phase reversal of the 7- to 8-Hz comblike rhythm at P3 with spread of activity to C3.

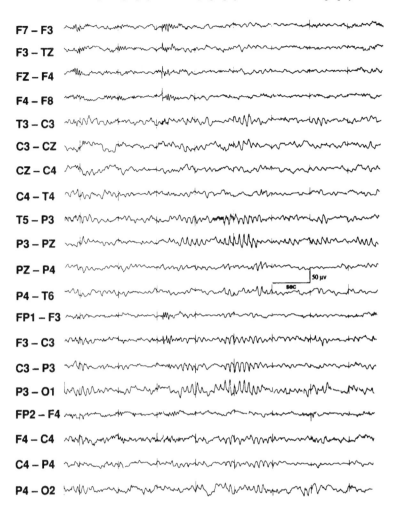

lambda rhythm is elicited by saccadic eye movements and appears to be an evoked response. It is present only during wakefulness with eyes open.

EEG in infants and children undergoes significant evolution with increasing age. This paragraph emphasizes a few major points; the reader is referred to other sources for details.[50–52] A sustained parieto-occipital, alpha-type rhythm is not seen until approximately 3 months of age. At that time, reactive 3-Hz waves are recorded during wakefulness. Frequency of the parieto-occipital rhythm increases rapidly over the next several years, reaching adult values in most children by 3 years of age. *Polyphasic slow waves* (slow waves of youth) are found in the occipital regions bilaterally after 2 years in as many as 10% of normal subjects. Prevalence is highest at approximately age 10 and gradually decreases afterwards. These waveforms rarely occupy more than 25% of the record, and they do not significantly exceed amplitude of other background rhythms. Polyphasic slow waves react to eye opening in the same manner as does alpha rhythm; these waves are in fact considered a variant of the alpha rhythm. Greater amounts of random frontocentral theta are seen in children than in adults, but this decreases as the child ages. Brief runs of more sustained low-amplitude (<15 μV) frontal 6- to 7-Hz waves are seen in as many as 35% of adolescents. This rhythm is present during quiet wakefulness with eyes open and may be related to affective arousal.

In the elderly, frequency of the alpha rhythm slows somewhat from a population mean of approximately 10.5 Hz to approximately 9 Hz. However, an alpha rhythm with a dominant frequency of less than 8 Hz is abnormal in adults. Focal temporal theta is seen in as many as 35% of asymptomatic individuals older than 50 years. Such activity is more commonly noted over the left temporal regions and should probably occupy no more than 5% of the tracing. Lower frequency or more prevalent temporal slowing is considered abnormal by the authors. The exact point at which temporal slowing in the elderly can be considered unequivocally abnormal, however, remains controversial.[53–55]

### Sleep Electroencephalography in Adults

The Standard Scoring Manual[25] divides sleep into four stages. EEG findings in each of these stages are discussed in this section.

Drowsiness or stage I sleep is used to designate the transition between wakefulness and stage II sleep and beyond. Stage I sleep is also briefly seen after arousals from other sleep stages and often transiently precedes and follows periods of REM sleep. Because this is a transitional sleep stage, it occupies a relatively small percentage of a normal night's sleep, generally less than 5%.[56]

A number of studies have emphasized the fact that EEG activity recorded during the transition between wakefulness and stage II sleep is variable and complex. EEG and physiologic changes that are inconsistent with wakefulness clearly occur before stage I as defined in the sleep scoring manual. Santamaria and Chiappa[26] identified several phases of drowsiness and more than 20 distinct EEG patterns in a careful study of 55 normal adults. The patterns of drowsiness varied in different subjects and varied in the same subject at different times. An early phase was characterized by changes in the alpha rhythm that persisted throughout this phase. Alpha may shift from its characteristic parieto-occipital distribution to the frontocentral or temporal regions. Amplitude of alpha activity may either increase or decrease and frequency of the alpha rhythm may slow. Slower theta and delta frequencies may be superimposed in the central or temporal regions. These may have a paroxysmal or sharpish character and be confused with epileptiform potentials. Paroxysmal theta bursts may predominate in one temporal region and be misinterpreted as the temporal sharp waves often associated with complex partial seizures. Criteria for distinguishing these benign potentials from genuine focal epileptiform discharges have been outlined.[57]

As the alpha rhythm disappears, bursts of frontocentral beta and generalized delta slowing may appear. Frankly paroxysmal but nonetheless benign patterns are occasionally seen in normal adults at this time as well. *Benign epileptiform transients of sleep* (BETS) are seen in 5–24% of normal subjects.[26,58] These are spiky, often diphasic transients with a broad field of distribution, usually involving both hemispheres. They typically shift from side to side and become less frequent during deeper sleep stages. Although BETS may superficially resemble epileptiform spikes, they are not associated with seizure disorders. White and coworkers[58] have outlined useful criteria distinguishing BETS from genuine epileptiform discharges. Less frequently, paroxysms of 6-Hz spike and wave (Figure 10-10) may be noted in either the frontal or temporal regions. The spike component usually has a relatively low amplitude, whereas the following slow wave is more prominent. Paroxysms of such activity rarely last longer than 3 seconds,[59] have an evanescent quality, and are less common during deeper sleep. Despite their paroxysmal quality, they are not associated with seizures either.[59]

Eventually, the alpha rhythm disappears altogether. *Vertex waves* are now frequently present. These are high-voltage sharp transients, surface negative, followed by a lower-voltage, surface-positive component. They have maximal voltage at the Cz electrode. Mild asymmetry between the two hemispheres and extension of the field to Fz, or less frequently Pz, is not uncommon. Vertex waves occur spontaneously or in response to stimuli that are insufficient to fully arouse the subject. *Positive occipital sharp waves of sleep* (POSTS) appear in post-transitional stage I, although these potentials are more common in deeper sleep stages (Figure 10-11). These are diphasic or triphasic sharp waves with a predominant positive phase at the occipital electrodes. They have a triangular appearance similar to lambda waves. POSTS are noted synchronously over the two hemispheres and may occur singly or in runs. Occasional shifting amplitude asymmetry is noted in normal controls; however, persistent significant asymmetry should raise suspicion of a posterior lesion. Because these potentials have a paroxysmal sharpish appearance, they may be confused with epileptiform discharges.

To summarize, drowsiness, or stage I, is a transitional state with many shifting and variable EEG

**Figure 10-10.** Spike and wave of 6 Hz (phantom spike and wave) seen in the last four channels.

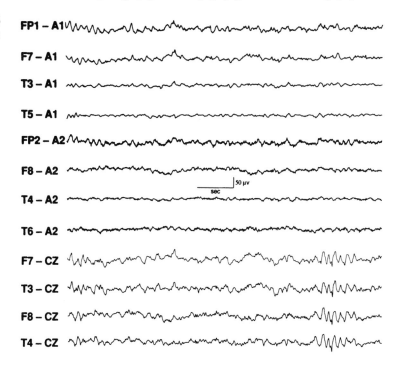

**Figure 10-11.** Positive occipital sharp transients (T5-O1, T6-O2, P3-O1, P4-O2 channels) during stage I NREM sleep.

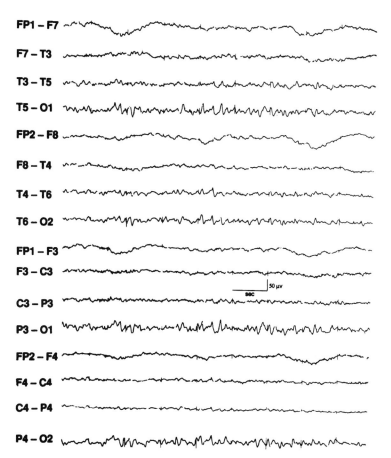

patterns. Some of these resemble abnormal patterns and determining whether an individual potential is normal may be difficult with the limited EEG montages typically used in PSG. It is important not to overinterpret. If there is uncertainty, routine EEG with a full complement of electrodes and multiple montages often clarifies the issue.

The standard sleep scoring manual defines stage II sleep by the presence of sleep spindles of at least 0.5 second's duration or K complexes, as well as the absence of the features of stage III or IV sleep. Stage II sleep (see Figure 2-3) comprises the bulk of a normal night's sleep (approximately 50% in normal adults).[56] Sleep spindles consist of a sequence of 12- to 14-Hz sinusoidal waves typically lasting a second or more. Voltage is usually maximal over the central regions. There is a high degree of symmetry and synchrony between the two hemispheres in normal subjects older than 1 year. Some investigators have proposed a classification of spindles based on topography and frequency[49,60,61] but it is not clear that this has clinical utility at this time.

K complexes have been defined differently by sleep disorder specialists and electroencephalographers, which may confuse those trained in both disciplines. The sleep scoring manual[25] defines the K complex as a well-delineated negative sharp wave followed by a positive component. The K complex must exceed 0.5 seconds in duration and may or may not be accompanied by sleep spindles. Vertex waves are not specifically defined in the manual or the sleep disorders glossary of terms.[62] Most polysomnographers accept that vertex waves have a duration of less than 0.5 seconds and distinguish vertex waves from K complexes on the basis of duration, although this may be difficult at the slow paper speeds often used. This distinction is important when scoring sleep because K complexes, even without spindles, are sufficient for scoring stage II sleep, whereas vertex waves alone do not allow the scoring of stage II sleep. Glossaries of EEG terminology,[63] on the other hand, insist that K complexes always have associated sleep spindles and do not specify a duration.

EEG in NREM sleep stages III and IV (see Figures 2-4 and 2-5) is marked by the high-amplitude slow waves. The sleep scoring manual[25] requires that more than 20% of any epoch be occupied by slow waves slower than 2 Hz and greater than 75 μV for stage III and that more than 50% of any epoch

be occupied by slow waves with these characteristics for stage IV. Computerized analyses indicate that sleep spindles, vertex waves, and POSTS[64,65] are abundant in stages III and IV, although they may be less discernible to the interpreter's eye because of the abundant slow activity.

During REM sleep (see Figure 2-6), the background EEG is characterized by low-voltage, mixed-frequency activity similar to early stage I. Alpha frequencies are often present and may be more persistent than in stage I. The alpha frequencies are usually 1–2 Hz less than the subject's waking rhythm.[66] Vertex waves, sleep spindles, and K complexes are absent. Characteristic *sawtooth waves* are frequently recorded. These are 2- to 3-Hz sharply contoured triangular waves, usually occurring serially for a duration of several seconds with highest amplitude over the Cz and Fz electrodes. A series of sawtooth waves typically precedes a burst of REM.[67,68] REM sleep occupies 20–25% of a night's sleep in a normal subject.[56] Brief periods of stage I sleep typically precede and follow a period of REM sleep. Detailed rules for demarcating onset and termination of REM in these and other circumstances have been outlined in the sleep scoring manual.[25]

Various atypical PSG patterns have been described. These usually occur in various sleep pathologies or when sleep has been significantly disrupted in normal individuals. *Alpha-delta sleep* (see Figures 16-5 and 29-1) is characterized by persistence of alpha activity during stages III and IV. Excessive alpha intrusion may be seen in stage II as well, and the abundance of spindles appears to be decreased. This pattern appears to be associated with nonrestorative sleep and is seen in a variety of conditions.[69,70] It may signal the fibromyalgia syndrome. Moldovsky and Scarisbrick[71] have elicited this EEG pattern in normal subjects by selectively depriving them of stage IV sleep. Deprivation of stage IV sleep also elicited complaints of diffuse arthralgias, myalgias, and fatigability, similar to the complaints of the fibromyalgia syndrome. *REM-spindle sleep* (Figure 10-12) is characterized by the intrusion of sleep spindles into portions of the PSG that otherwise meet all criteria for REM sleep. This pattern may be seen in 1–7% of normal subjects[72] but is more common when sleep is disrupted and after the first night of continuous positive airway pressure treatment. Broughton[73] reviewed other

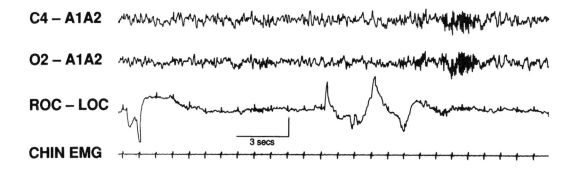

C4 – A1A2

O2 – A1A2

ROC – LOC

CHIN EMG

3 secs

**Figure 10-12.** REM-spindle sleep. Note intrusion of sleep spindles in the EEG channels of a portion of a polysomnography that meet all criteria for REM sleep. REM is present in the eye channel—outer canthus of the right and left eye (ROC – LOC)—and atonia in the chin electromyography (EMG). Calibration (*vertical bar*) is 50 μV for the top three channels and 20 μV for the bottom channel.

atypical patterns that occasionally occur during REM sleep.

### *Normal Sleep Electroencephalography in Pediatrics*

The transition from neonatal to infantile EEG sleep patterns occurs between 1 and 3 months. Even after this period, there is a great deal of change in the electroencephalographic patterns until the adult patterns are reached. The major points are emphasized in the following paragraphs; the reader is referred elsewhere for more detailed discussion (see also Chapter 2).[50–52,74]

Drowsiness in the pediatric age group differs from the adult patterns in several ways. Before 8 months of age, drowsiness is marked by a progressive slowing of EEG frequencies until delta waves predominate. After 8 months, the onset of drowsiness is marked by long runs of continuous, generalized, high-voltage, rhythmic theta or delta, which have been called *hypnagogic hypersynchrony*. Three types have been described in normal subjects.[51,52,74] In the most common type, the rhythmic slow waves have highest amplitude in the frontal and central regions. The continuous rhythmic slowing may persist for several minutes. Less commonly, amplitude is highest in the parieto-occipital regions. Finally, a paroxysmal type occurs in approximately 10% of normal children. With this pattern, the alpha rhythm is gradually replaced by mixed frequencies. Diffuse

bursts of 2- to 5-Hz slow waves, a few seconds in duration, then appear intermittently. Occasionally, random, poorly developed, sharpish waveforms are noted amidst the slow waves. These may be random, superimposed alpha transients and should not be confused with epileptiform spike and wave. The first two types of hypnagogic hypersynchrony are rarely recorded after age 10. The paroxysmal type persists into the midteens or, rarely, into adulthood.[51,52] In infancy and early childhood, 20- to 25-Hz beta is also a prominent feature of drowsiness. The beta may have maximum voltage anteriorly or posteriorly or have a diffuse distribution. The amplitude may reach 60 μV. This pattern appears at 6 months and is seen most frequently from 12 to 18 months. Prevalence decreases subsequently, and prominent beta during drowsiness is rarely seen after 7 years.[74]

Vertex waves and K complexes appear at age 6 months. These potentials are rather blunt and may reach amplitudes exceeding 200 μV in infancy and early childhood. By age 5, both vertex waves and K complexes have an increasingly spiky configuration. Mild asymmetry is quite common. They may occur repetitively in brief bursts.

Sleep spindles appear at approximately 3 months of age. Between 3 and 9 months of age, spindles occur in wicketlike trains often exceeding several seconds. These potentials are common at this age, occupying 14% of stage II sleep. Asynchrony between the hemispheres is the rule, with only half of the trains demonstrating interhemispheric synchrony at 6 months.[75,76] Interhemispheric syn-

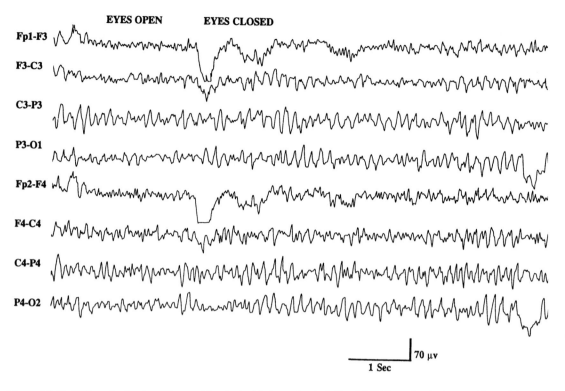

**Figure 10-13.** Diffuse slowing in a 67-year-old patient with dementia. Activity of 6–7 Hz predominates over the parieto-occipital regions. Although it is reactive to eye closure, the frequency of this rhythm is abnormally slow. Calibration: vertical bar = 70 μv, horizontal bar = 1 sec. (Reproduced with permission from RE Emerson, TS Walczak, CA Turner. EEG and Evoked Potentials. In LP Rowland [ed], Merritt's Textbook of Neurology [Update 9]. Philadelphia: Lea & Febiger, 1992;3.)

chrony increases to 70% by 12 months and the duration and frequency of the spindle bursts gradually decrease. By 2 years of age, virtually all spindle trains are synchronous; however, spindles are much less frequent, occupying only 0.5% of stage II sleep.[75,76] Spindles remain infrequent until approximately 5 years of age.[76]

Stages III and IV sleep are marked by high-amplitude, slow activity, as in adults. However, amplitude of the slow activity is usually higher. An occipitofrontal gradient is often present with the very high–amplitude, slower frequencies predominating posteriorly and lower-amplitude, faster frequencies predominating anteriorly.[77] This gradient becomes less striking with age, so that by 5 years, the slow waves are distributed more diffusely.

EEG during REM sleep in infants and children is characterized by a greater amount of slow activity than is seen in adults. The mature desynchronized EEG with scattered alpha emerges during the mid-

teens.[78] The percentage of a normal night's sleep occupied by REM gradually decreases from 40% at age 3–5 months to 30% at age 12–24 months and then gradually assumes adult values after puberty.[79] REM onset latency gradually lengthens over the first year of life as well.

### Abnormal Electroencephalograph

Many abnormal EEG patterns have been described. Only frequently encountered abnormalities are discussed in this section. *Diffuse slowing of background activity* (Figure 10-13) is probably the most commonly recorded EEG abnormality. It can take several forms. One may see slowing of the parieto-occipital, alpha-type rhythm to a frequency below that allowable for the patient's age. Alternatively, frequency of the alpha-type rhythm may be normal but excessive, diffuse theta and delta activity may be recorded. Finally, one

**Figure 10-14.** Focal left hemispheric slowing in a 67-year-old (y/o) patient with a large left hemispheric infarction. Left hemispheric alpha rhythm is also attenuated. (Courtesy of Dr. Timothy Pedley.)

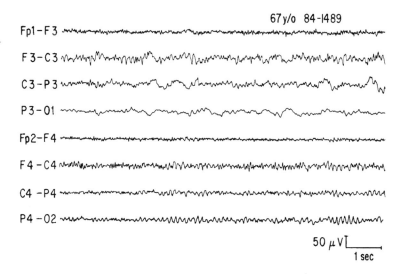

may see both a slowing of the alpha-type rhythm and excessive, diffuse slower frequencies. Before concluding that an EEG has excessive slowing of background frequencies, the polysomnographer must consider the patient's age and state of alertness. More diffuse theta is seen in normal children than is acceptable for adults. Frequency of background rhythms must be assessed while the patient is clearly awake. As noted earlier, both slowing of alpha-type rhythms and diffuse slower frequencies are commonly found in drowsiness in normal subjects. Consequently, the polysomnographer must be certain that the background frequencies are slow during wakefulness. Unfortunately, diffuse slowing of background frequencies is a very nonspecific pattern. It is commonly interpreted as being consistent with a variety of diffuse encephalopathies, including toxic, metabolic, and degenerative encephalopathies, among others.

*Focal slowing* (Figure 10-14) means that slow frequencies predominate over one region of the brain. Electrocerebral activity elsewhere is normal or the slowing is relatively mild. In experimental models, focal slowing is produced by focal white matter lesions, even when the cerebral cortex remains intact.[80] Focal cerebral lesions often involve both white matter and cortex, however, so the usefulness of this distinction is blurred in practice. A structural lesion must always be suspected when persistent focal slowing is recorded. Not all patients with focal slowing, however, will have neuroradiologically demonstrable lesions.[81] Patients with transient ischemic attacks or focal epilepsy

often have focal EEG slowing even with normal neuroradiologic investigations. In epilepsy patients, this slowing may be due to ongoing local inhibitory phenomena or may be a transient postictal finding.

*Focal attenuation of background rhythms* means that frequencies in one region of the brain have significantly lower amplitude than elsewhere. In experimental models, focal attenuation of background is produced when the gray matter is lesioned and the underlying white matter remains intact.[80] Consequently, focal attenuation is often interpreted as indicating focal cortical dysfunction. In practice, attenuation of background frequencies is usually seen in combination with focal slowing (see Figure 10-14). Neuroradiologic investigations usually reveal large lesions involving both cortex and white matter.[82,83] Any fluid collection between the cortex and the recording electrode attenuates the recorded EEG activity. Thus, subdural fluid collections and subgaleal hematomas may result in a focal attenuation of background, although the cortex may not be damaged.

The detection of *epileptiform discharges* is important because these potentials have close association with epilepsy. Pedley[84] suggested that an epileptiform discharge should meet several criteria: (1) It must be paroxysmal, which means that it must clearly stand out from the background. (2) An epileptiform discharge must be spiky, which means that the transition from ascending to descending phase is abrupt and the duration of the discharge is short (by convention, <200 msec). (3) It must have a clear field—that is, it should not be confined to one electrode. (4) It should

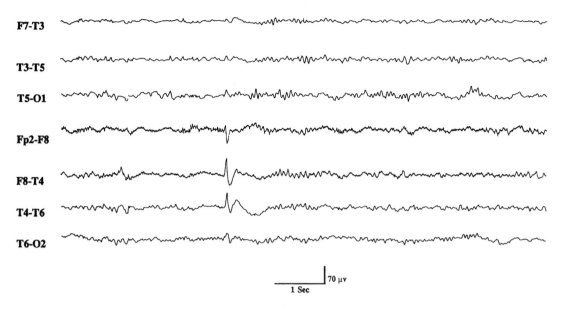

**Figure 10-15.** Right temporal interictal epileptiform discharge in a 32-year-old patient with complex partial seizures. Calibration: vertical bar = 70 μv, horizontal bar = 1 sec. (Reproduced with permission from RE Emerson, TS Walczak, CA Turner. EEG and Evoked Potentials. In LP Rowland [ed], Merritt's Textbook of Neurology [Update 9]. Philadelphia: Lea & Febiger, 1992;3.)

have negative polarity because epileptiform discharges with positive polarity are uncommon.* (5) Finally, a slow wave often follows an epileptiform discharge. Several varieties of epileptiform discharges have been described and associated with epilepsy syndromes.[84,85] A basic distinction is made between generalized and focal epileptiform discharges. Generalized epileptiform discharges indicate that the patient's seizure is likely to start simultaneously throughout the brain. An example is the generalized 3-Hz spike and wave (see Figure 34-2) that is characteristic of petit mal absence seizures. Focal epileptiform discharges indicate that the patient's seizure is likely to start in a restricted area of the brain, although it may subsequently spread. An example is the anterior temporal sharp wave that is characteristic of complex partial seizures of temporal lobe origin (Figure 10-15). This is an important distinction because the treatment and prognosis in these two epilepsy syndromes are very different.[85] Approximately 90% of adults with epileptiform discharges will have a his-

tory of seizures[86,87] and incidental epileptiform discharges are very uncommon in normal adults.[88] The association of epileptiform discharges with seizures in the pediatric age group is not as strong and varies with patient age and type of epileptiform discharge.[89]

The polysomnographer must be able to recognize *electrographic seizures* (see Figure 34-10). These may occur in patients with epilepsy or in patients with sleep apnea during severe hypoxia. The EEG patterns associated with seizures are extremely variable. In general, an electrographic seizure has abrupt onset, sustained and rhythmic evolution of frequencies, spreads to contiguous areas of the brain, and terminates abruptly, often followed by irregular postictal slowing. Typically, faster frequencies are seen at seizure onset and these gradually decrease in frequency as the seizure continues. Seizures associated with hypoxia usually have a generalized onset. A good deal of experience is necessary to recognize the various EEG patterns that can occur during a seizure. In practice, any sustained and evolving rhythm with an abrupt onset raises concern about electrographic seizures. However, the polysomnographer must recall that drowsiness and arousal responses may begin abruptly and have rhythmic, sustained characteristics as well, especially in children.

---

*Positive rolandic sharp waves are occasionally recorded in premature infants with intraventricular hemorrhage or periventricular leukomalacia. Otherwise, positive sharp waves are very uncommon in older patients.

**Figure 10-16.** Periodic lateralized epileptiform discharges at a rate of 0.8 per second arising from the left parietal and posterior temporal regions (P3, T5) in a 72-year-old woman with a history of confusion and falling episodes.

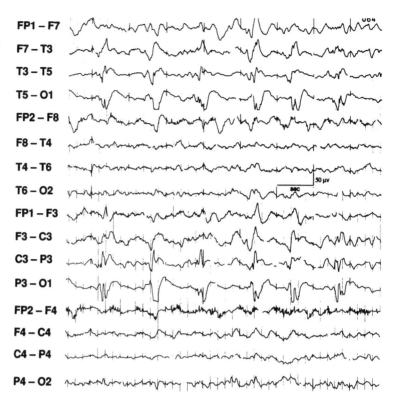

*Periodic lateralizing epileptiform discharge* (PLED) is another important pattern to recognize. In this pattern, epileptiform discharges are recorded continuously over a given region (Figure 10-16). The epileptiform discharges occur at regular intervals, usually every 1–2 seconds, and are thus labelled periodic.[90,91] Background activity is usually significantly attenuated on the side with the discharges, and excessive slow frequencies are often seen bilaterally.[90,91] This pattern is usually associated with an acute focal cerebral insult. In a review of 586 cases reported in the literature,[92] 35% were related to an acute cerebral infarction, 26% to other sorts of mass lesions, and the remainder to infection, anoxia, or other causes. Clinically, PLED is associated with obtundation, seizures, and focal neurologic deficits. Seventy to 90% of patients with PLED have seizures during the acute stage of their illness.[90–92] Twenty-five to 40% of patients with this pattern die in the hospital or shortly after discharge. Mortality may be especially high in patients with acute stroke and PLED.[90,91,93] PLED is almost always a transient phenomenon. The discharges become less frequent and lower in amplitude over

the 2 weeks after the acute insult and are gradually replaced by focal delta slowing.[94]

### Artifacts

The polygraph is designed to record the relatively small voltages generated by the human brain, muscle, eye, and heart. Unfortunately, the remainder of the human body and the surrounding environment are not electrically silent. These generate abundant electrical activity that may obscure the biological signals of interest. This extraneous electrical activity is called *artifact* (see also Chapter 9).[1–4] Making the distinction between the signal of interest and artifact is a central task for the polysomnographer and the task is most difficult when interpreting EEG. Because high sensitivities are required to record the relatively low voltages generated by the brain, extraneous voltage sources are especially likely to contaminate the EEG recording.

Four sources of artifact exist: (1) irrelevant physiologic signals, (2) environmental signals, (3) aberrant signals due to faulty or improperly applied electrodes, and (4) aberrant signals produced by the polygraph. More than one of these sources can contribute to a particular artifact. The following discussion summarizes frequently encountered artifacts and is by no means exhaustive.

### Irrelevant Physiologic Signals

Irrelevant signals may contaminate recording of biological signals of interest, especially EEG. *Myogenic potentials* originating from scalp muscles may obscure EEG recording (see Figures 9-9 and 9-12). Myogenic activity may be difficult to distinguish from electrocerebral activity in the beta-frequency range, especially at slow paper speeds. It may obscure lower-amplitude electrocerebral activity.

*Head movement* also causes artifacts, frequencies of which are usually in the delta range (see Figure 9-13). These artifacts are due to changes in electrode impedance, together with spurious static and capacitative potentials. Head movement artifacts are induced by slight movement of the electrodes on the scalp and the swaying of wires. The head movements associated with respiration often elicit movement artifact on the EEG, especially when the patient is lying on the recording electrodes. Correlating the spurious delta waves on the EEG with a respiratory monitor establishes their artifactual source. This may be important because these spurious potentials should not be used to score slow-wave sleep.

*Sweating* may result in very slow frequencies and changes in baseline, especially when direct current amplifiers are used in the polygraph. The salt content of sweat changes the ionic composition of the conducting gel, resulting in this particular artifact. Potentials that arise from the sweat glands also play a role. Sweating may be asymmetric, and the resulting EEG asymmetry may mislead the interpreter.

*Pulse artifact* occurs when an electrode is placed on one of the scalp arteries. The electrode movement caused by the pulsations produces a delta wave. The regular relationship of the delta wave to ECG indicates the extracerebral origin of this activity.

The electrical fields generated by *ECG* and eye movements are commonly recorded from scalp electrodes (see Figure 9-10) and may be confused with electrocerebral activity. Again, referring to the channels that are recording ECG and eye movements demonstrates whether suspicious activity recorded at the scalp is caused by these extracerebral sources.

### Environmental Signals

The hospital environment contains many sources of electrical signals that may mimic electrocerebral or other physiologic activity. The *circulation of moistened air* through a respirator tube may induce bursts of alpha or theta frequencies at scalp electrodes. The electrostatic charges on drops entering an intravenous cannula—*intravenous drop artifacts*—may cause periodic spikelike artifacts. *Intravenous infusion pumps* can cause bursts of spiky transients followed by slower components. These artifacts are thought to be due to electromagnetic (rather than electrostatic) sources. *Telephones and pager systems* are among the other potential sources of environmental artifacts. The interpreter relies on the technician to correlate unusual recorded potentials with specific events in the environment, thereby establishing the artifactual nature of the potentials.

*Sixty-hertz* electromagnetic radiation due to alternating current in power lines is ubiquitous in the hospital environment and may contaminate the recording (in Europe, mains frequency is 50 Hz). The resulting 60-Hz artifact may be impossible to distinguish from myogenic activity at the slow paper speeds commonly used for PSG. The presence of this artifact in EMG leads may persuade the interpreter that tonic EMG activity is at a high level when it is actually low. The 60-Hz artifact is verified when 60 cycles are counted in 1 second of recording. Usually, paper speed must be increased to at least 60 mm per second to distinguish adjacent potentials of this frequency and count them accurately. After the presence of 60 Hz is verified, the technician should proceed systematically to determine the source of the artifact. First, the technician must ensure that both of the involved electrodes are in fact attached to the patient, plugged into the jackbox, and connected to the relevant amplifier. The integrity of the patient ground must be similarly ensured. Next, the technician should check the impedances of the involved electrodes and the patient ground. Impedances in any electrode pair should not exceed 10 kilo-ohms and the impedances of the two electrodes should be roughly equal. Only

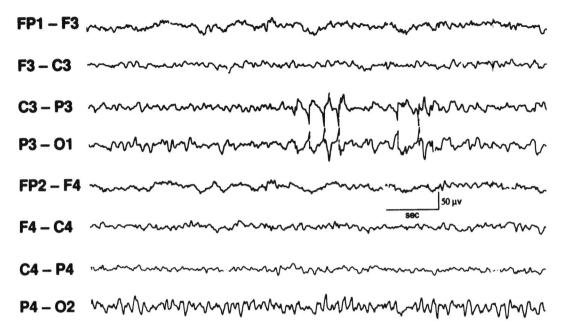

**Figure 10-17.** Electrode pops at P3 electrode.

then can the technician conclude that the electrode-scalp interface is probably not the source of the artifact. At this point, the technician should search for 60-Hz sources in the environment. A "dummy patient," consisting of two leads shorted with a 10 kilo-ohm resister, may be carried around the room until the 60-Hz artifact reaches maximal amplitude and the source is identified. Finally, the technician should remember that faults with instrument ground may result in 60-Hz activity as well.

*Aberrant Signals from Faulty Electrodes*

Improperly applied electrodes or electrode faults may result in other sorts of artifact.

*Electrode "pops"* are the most common electrode artifact. These are abrupt vertical transients (Figure 10-17), usually of positive polarity, that are confined to one electrode. They are superimposed on but do not modify ongoing recording. Pops are due to abrupt changes in impedance and usually indicate either that the electrode is not securely attached or that electrolyte gel is insufficient. When confronted with a popping electrode, the technician should reset the electrode and apply more gel. If popping persists, the electrode needs to be changed.

Occasionally the electrode impedances change more gradually, mimicking slow activity. Again, the observation that the slow activity is confined to one electrode indicates that the electrode, rather than the body, is the source of the potential.

*Other electrode faults* may result in artifact even if the electrode-scalp interface is intact. An interruption in the plating of the electrode may result in battery potentials, which can appear as bizarre, high-amplitude discharges confined to the faulty electrode. A similar artifact may occur when electrode gel connects the disk electrode and the wire lead, which are usually made of different metals.

*Aberrant Signals from the Polygraph*

Finally, the polygraph can be a source of artifact. Random fluctuation of charges in any complicated recording instrument results in some spurious output. In a well-built polygraphy, this *instrument noise* is infrequent and has low amplitude. It should not contaminate recording at standard sensitivities but may occasionally appear when sensitivities greater than 2 μV/mm are required.

*Corrosion or loosening of contacts* in switches or wires may cause abrupt changes in voltage or sudden loss of signal. The nonphysiologic nature of such potentials is usually readily apparent, but finding the source in the instrument may be difficult, especially if the artifact is intermittent.

A meticulous, alert, and experienced technician is the first and best defense against artifact. The critical importance of properly applied and gelled electrodes cannot be overemphasized for PSG, because adjusting or changing electrodes usually means waking the patient. The technician should be on the lookout for bizarre potentials and seek to determine whether these are physiologic or artifactual. Observation of the patient and environment, correlations with the recorded activity, and careful documentation are critical. The technician must then decide whether the artifact significantly interferes with recording of the signal of interest. Deciding whether to change an electrode and possibly wake the patient, or allow a partially interpretable recording to continue requires seasoned judgment. Technicians should be aware of the major issues involved in interpreting a PSG so they can make these on-the-spot decisions wisely.

## CONCLUSION

The interpretation of a PSG can be considered a pattern-recognition task. The EEG is the most complicated and variable recording the polysomnographer interprets. Several issues continuously preoccupy the polysomnographer when interpreting the EEG. One question is whether the recorded signal is a true cerebral potential or whether it represents artifact. Another is whether the signal is present throughout the scalp or whether it is confined to a single region of the scalp. The use of multiple channels for EEG recording allows the polysomnographer to answer these questions with greater certainty. Unfortunately, EEG recorded during routine PSG is often limited to a single channel. Limited montages and slow paper speeds often do not allow confident interpretation of unusual activity. This is especially unfortunate because EEG abnormalities important to the patient's care are more likely to occur during the longer PSG recordings than during routine EEG. The cost of a few additional EEG channels is more than repaid by the greater certainty in interpretation and the greater likelihood that important abnormalities will be found. Sometimes a confident decision regarding the nature of suspicious potentials cannot be made, even when several EEG channels are available. It is important not to overinterpret suspicious events. The polysomnographer should not be afraid to admit uncertainty in a situation in which data are insufficient. Referral for routine sleep EEG is usually appropriate in these circumstances. The full complement of scalp EEG channels often provides the necessary information. Similarly, information from additional EMG and EOG channels often clarify ambiguities. Equivocal changes are often interpreted more confidently when more data are available.

## REFERENCES

1. Daly DD, Pedley TA (eds). Current Practice of Clinical EEG (2nd ed). New York: Raven, 1990.
2. Neidermeyer E, Lopes da Silva F (eds). Electroencephalography. Basic Principles, Clinical Applications and Related Fields (2nd ed). Baltimore: Urban & Schwarzenberg, 1987;687.
3. Tyner F, Knott J, Mayer W Jr. Fundamentals of EEG Technology (Vol 1). New York: Raven, 1983.
4. Fisch BJ. Spehlman's EEG Primer (2nd ed). Amsterdam: Elsevier, 1991.
5. Kimura J. Electrodiagnosis in Diseases of Nerve and Muscle: Principles and Practice. Philadelphia: FA Davis, 1983.
6. Werner SS, Stockard JE, Bickford RG. Atlas of Neonatal Electroencephalography. New York: Raven, 1977.
7. Kandel ER, Schwartz JH (eds). Principles of Neural Science (2nd ed). Amsterdam: Elsevier, 1985;642.
8. Creutzfeldt O, Houchin J. Neuronal Basis of EEG Waves. In O Creutzfeldt (ed), Handbook of Electroencephalography and Clinical Neurophysiology (Vol 2C). Amsterdam: Elsevier, 1974;5.
9. Li CL, Cullen C, Jasper HH. Laminar microelectrode studies of specific somato-sensory cortical potentials. J Neurophysiol 1956;19:111.
10. Andersen P, Andersson SA. Physiological Basis of the Alpha Rhythm. New York: Appleton-Century-Crofts, 1968.
11. Steraide M, Gloor P, Llinas RR, et al. Basic mechanisms of cerebral rhythmic activities—report of IFCN committee on basic mechanisms. Electroencephalogr Clin Neurophysiol 1990;76:481.
12. Pedley TA, Traub RD. Physiological Basis of the EEG. In DD Daly, TA Pedley (eds), Current Practice of Clinical EEG (2nd ed). New York: Raven, 1990;107.
13. Geddes LA, Baker LE. Principles of Applied Biomedical Instrumentation. New York: Wiley, 1968.
14. Oppenheim AV, Schaefer R. Digital Signal Processing. Englewood Cliffs, NJ: Prentice-Hall, 1975.
15. Gotman J. The Use of Computers in Analysis and Display of EEG and Evoked Potentials. In DD Daly, TA

Pedley (eds), Current Practice of Clinical EEG (2nd ed). New York: Raven, 1990.

16. Gevins A, Remond A (eds). Handbook of Electroencephalography and Clinical Neurophysiology (Vol I): Methods of Analysis of Brain Electrical and Magnetic Signals. Amsterdam: Elsevier, 1986.

17. Cooley WJ, Tukey JW. An algorithm for the machine calculation of complex Fourier series. Math Comput 1965;19:297.

18. Oken BS, Chiappa KH. Short-term variability in EEG frequency analysis. Electroencephalogr Clin Neurophysiol 1988;69:191.

19. American Electroencephalographic Society. American Electroencephalographic Society statement on the clinical use of quantitative EEG. J Clin Neurophysiol 1987;4:75.

20. American Academy of Neurology Therapeutic and Technology Subcommittee. Assessment: EEG brain mapping. Neurology 1989;39:1100.

21. Whalen RE, Starmer CF, McIntosh HD. Electrical hazards associated with cardiac pacemaking. Ann N Y Acad Sci 1964;3:922.

22. Starmer CF, McIntosh HD, Whalen RE. Electrical hazards and cardiovascular function. N Engl J Med 1971;284:181.

23. Geddes LA, Baker LE. Electrical safety in hospitals. J AAMI 1971;6:27.

24. Cooper R, Osselton JW, Shaw JC. EEG Technology. London: Butterworths, 1980.

25. Rechstaffen A, Kales A. A Manual of Standardized Terminology, Techniques and Scoring System for Sleep Stages of Human Subjects. Washington, DC: U.S. Government Printing Office, 1968.

26. Santamaria J, Chiappa KH. The EEG of Drowsiness. New York: Demos, 1987.

27. McPartland RJ, Kupfer DJ. Computerized measures of EOG activity during sleep. Int J Biomed Comput 1978;9:409.

28. Radtke RA. Sleep Disorders. In DD Daly, TA Pedley (eds), Current Practice of Clinical EEG (2nd ed). New York: Raven, 1990;561.

29. Lance JW. The control of the muscle tone, reflexes and movement. The Robert Wartenberg lecture. Neurology 1980;30:1303.

30. Lourenco RV, Mueller EP. Quantification of electrical activity in the human diaphragm. J Appl Physiol 1967;22:598.

31. Lopata M, Evanich MJ, Lourenco RV. Quantification of diaphragmatic EM response to $CO_2$ rebreathing in humans. J Appl Physiol 1977;43:262.

32. Lopata M, Zubillaga G, Evanich MJ, et al. Diaphragmatic EMG response to isocapnic hypoxia and hyperoxic hypercapnia in humans. J Lab Clin Med 1978;91:698.

33. Lopata M, Lourenco RV. Evaluation of respiratory control. Clin Chest Med 1980;1:33.

34. Chokroverty S, Sharp JT. Primary sleep apnoea syndrome. J Neurol Neurosurg Psychiatry 1981;44:970.

35. Sharp JT, Hammond MD, Aranda AU, Rocha RD. Comparison of diaphragm EMG centroid frequencies: esophageal versus chest surface electrodes. Am Rev Respir Dis 1993;147:764.

36. Onal E, Lopata M, Gimsburg A, O'Connor T. Diaphragmatic EMG and transdiaphragmatic pressure measurements with a single catheter. Am Rev Respir Dis 1981;124:563.

37. Guilleminault C, Stoohs R, Clerk A, et al. A cause of excessive daytime sleepiness: the upper airway resistance syndrome. Chest 1993;104:781.

38. Chervin RD, Guilleminault C. Obstructive sleep apnea and related disorders. Neurol Clin 1996;14:583.

39. Baydur A, Behraks PK, Zin WA, et al. A simple method for assessing the validity of the esophageal balloon technique. Am Rev Respir Dis 1982;129:788.

40. Horner RL. Motor control of the pharyngeal musculature and implications for the pathogenesis of obstructive sleep apnea. Sleep 1996;19:1827.

41. Sauerland EK, Mitchell SP. Electromyographic activity of the human genioglossus muscle in response to respiration and to positional changes of the head. Bull LA Neurol Soc 1970;35:69.

42. Sauerland EK, Mitchell SP. Electromyographic activity of intrinsic and extrinsic muscles of the human tongue. Techs Rep Biol Med 1975;33:445.

43. Leiter JC, Daubenspeck JA. Selective reflex activation of the genioglossus in humans. J Appl Physiol 1990;68:2581.

44. Mahowald M, Schenck CH. REM Sleep Behavior Disorder. In MH Kryger, T Roth, WC Dement (eds), Principles and Practice of Sleep Medicine. Philadelphia: Saunders 1994;574.

45. Phillipson EA, Bowes G. Control of Breathing During Sleep. In AF Fishman, AS Cherniack, JG Widdicombe (eds), Handbook of Physiology (Sect 3), The Respiratory System (Vol II, Part 2). Bethesda, MD: American Physiological Society, 1986;649.

46. Guindi GM, Bannister R, Gibson W, et al. Laryngeal electromyography in multiple system atrophy with autonomic failure. J Neurol Neurosurg Psychiatry 1981;44:49.

47. Yamada T, Kooi KA. Level of consciousness and the mu rhythm. Clin Electroencephalogr 1975;6:80.

48. Jasper HH, Penfield W. Electrocorticograms in man: effect of voluntary movement upon electrical activity of precentral gyrus. Arch Psychiatry 1949;183:163.

49. Kellaway P. An Orderly Approach to Visual Analysis: Characteristics of the Normal EEG of Adults and Children. In DD Daly, TA Pedley (eds), Current Practice of Clinical EEG (2nd ed). New York: Raven, 1990;139.

50. Blume WT. Atlas of Pediatric Electroencephalography. New York: Raven, 1982.

51. Eeg-Olofsson O, Petersen I, Sellden U. The development of the EEG in normal children from the age of 1 to 15 years: paroxysmal activity. Neuropadiatrie 1971;4:375.

52. Eeg-Olofsson O. The development of the electroencephalogram in normal adolescents from the age of 16 through 21 years. Neuropadiatrie 1971;3:11.

53. Obrist WD. The electroencephalogram of normal aged adults. Electroencephalogr Clin Neurophysiol 1954;6:235.

54. Katz RI, Horowitz GR. Electroencephalogram in the septuagenerian: studies in a normal geriatric population. J Am Geriatr Soc 1982;30:273.

55. Torres F, Faoro A, Loewenson R, Johnson E. The electroencephalogram of elderly subjects revisited. Electroencephalogr Clin Neurophysiol 1983;56:391.

56. Williams RL, Karacan I, Hursch CJ. Electro-Encephalography of Human Sleep: Clinical Applications. New York: Wiley, 1974.

57. Reiher J, Lebel M. Wicket spikes: clinical correlates of a previously undescribed EEG pattern. Can J Neurol Sci 1977;4:39.

58. White JC, Langston JW, Pedley TA. Benign epileptiform transients of sleep; clarification of the small sharp spike controversy. Neurology 1977;27:1061.

59. Thomas JE, Klass DW. Six per second spike and wave pattern in the electroencephalogram. A reappraisal of its clinical significance. Neurology 1968;18:587.

60. Gibbs F, Gibbs E. Atlas of Electroencephalography (Vol 1). Cambridge, MA: Addison-Wesley, 1951.

61. Deebenham P. Sleep spindle symposium—introduction. Sleep 1981;4:384.

62. Association of sleep disorders centers and association for the psychophysiological study of sleep. Glossary of terms used in the sleep disorders classification. Sleep 1979;2:123.

63. Dutertre F. Catalogue of the Main EEG Patterns. In A Remond (ed), Handbook of Electroencephalography and Clinical Neurophysiology (Vol 11A). Amsterdam: Elsevier, 1977;40.

64. Vignaendra V, Matthews RL, Chatrian GE. Positive occipital sharp transients of sleep: relationships to nocturnal sleep cycle in man. Electroencephalogr Clin Neurophysiol 1974;37:239.

65. Gaillard J, Blois R. Spindle density in sleep of normal subjects. Sleep 1981;4:385.

66. Johnson LC, Nute C, Austin MT, Lubin A. Spectral analysis of the EEG during waking and sleeping. Electroencephalogr Clin Neurophysiol 1967;23:80.

67. Schwartz RA. EEG et mouvements oculaires dans le sommeil de nuit. Electroencephalogr Clin Neurophysiol 1962;14:126.

68. Berger RJ, Olley P, Oswald I. The EEG, eye movements and dreams of the blind. Q J Exp Psychol 1962;14:183.

69. Hauri P, Hawkins DR. Alph-delta sleep. Electroencephalogr Clin Neurophysiol 1973;34:233.

70. Moldofsky H, Lue FA. The relationship of alpha and delta EEG frequencies to pain and mood in fibrositis patients treated with chlorpromazine and L-tryptophane. Electroencephalogr Clin Neurophysiol 1980;50:71.

71. Moldofsky H, Scarisbrick P. Induction of neurasthenic muskuloskeletal pain syndrome by selective sleep stage deprivation. Psychosom Med 1976;38:35.

72. Snyder F. Toward an evolutionary theory of dreaming. Am J Psychiatry 1966;123:121.

73. Broughton RJ. Polysomnography: Principles and Applications in Sleep and Arousal Disorders. In E Neidermeyer, F Lopes da Silva (eds), Electroencephalography. Basic Principles, Clinical Applications and Related Fields (2nd ed). Baltimore: Urban & Schwarzenberg, 1987;687.

74. Kellaway P, Fox BJ. Electroencephalographic diagnosis of cerebral pathology in infants during sleep. Its rationale, technique and the characteristics of normal sleep in infants. J Pediatr 1952;41:262.

75. Lenard HG. The development of sleep spindles during the first two years of life. Neuropaediatrie 1970;1:264.

76. Tanguay PE, Ornitz EM, Kaplan A, Bozzo ES. Evolution of sleep spindles in childhood. Electroencephalogr Clin Neurophysiol 1975;38:175.

77. Slater GE, Torres F. Frequency-amplitude gradient. A new parameter for interpreting pediatric sleep EEGs. Arch Neurol 1979;36:465.

78. Niedermeyer E. Maturation of the EEG: Development of Waking and Sleep Patterns. In E Neidermeyer, F Lopes da Silva (eds), Electroencephalography. Basic Principles, Clinical Applications and Related Fields (2nd ed). Baltimore: Urban & Schwarzenberg, 1987;687.

79. Roffwarg H, Muzio J, Dement W. Ontogenic development of the human sleep-dream cycle. Science 1966;152:604.

80. Gloor P, Ball G, Schaual N. Brain lesions that produce delta waves in the EEG. Neurology 1977;27:326.

81. Marshall DW, Brey RL, Morse MW. Focal and/or lateralized plymorphic delta activity. Association with either 'normal' or 'nonfocal' computed tomographic scans. Arch Neurol 1988;45:33.

82. Schaul N, Green L, Peyster R, Gotman J. Structural determinants of electroencephalographic findings in acute hemispheric lesions. Ann Neurol 1986;20:703.

83. Ottonello GA, Regesta G, Tanganelli P. Correlation Between Computerized Tomography and EEG Findings in Acute Cerebrovascular Disorders. In H Lechner, A Aranibar (eds), EEG and Clinical Neurophysiology. Amsterdam: Excerpta Medica, 1980;148.

84. Pedley TA. Interictal epileptiform discharges: discriminating characteristics and clinical correlations. Am J Electroencephalogr Technol 1980;20:101.

85. Roger J, Dravet C, Bureau M, et al. Epileptic Syndromes in Infancy, Childhood, and Adolescence. Amsterdam: John Libbey Eurotext, 1985.

86. Ajmone-Marsan C, Zivin LS. Factors related to the occurrence of typical paroxysmal abnormalities in the EEG records of epileptic patients. Epilepsia 1970;11:361.

87. Salinsky M, Kanter R, Dasheiff RM. Effectiveness of multiple EEGs in supporting the diagnosis of epilepsy: an operational curve. Epilepsia 1987;28:331.

88. Zivin L, Ajmone Marsan C. Incidence and prognostic significance of 'epileptiform activity' in the EEG of non-epileptic subjects. Brain 1968;91:751.

89. Kellaway P. The Incidence, Significance and Natural History of Spike Foci in Children. In CE Henry (ed),

Current Clinical Neurophysiology. Update on EEG and Evoked Potentials. North-Holland: Elsevier, 1980;150.

90. Chatrian GE, Shaw C, Leffman H. The significance of periodic lateralized epileptiform discharges in EEG: an electrographic, clinical and pathological study. Electroencephalogr Clin Neurophysiol 1964; 17:177.

91. Markand ON, Daly DD. Pseudoperiodic lateralized paroxysmal discharges in electroencephalogram. Neurology 1971;21:975.

92. Snodgrass SM, Tsuburaya K, Ajmone-Marsan C. Clinical significance of periodic lateralized epileptiform discharges, relationship to status epilepticus. J Clin Neurophysiol 1989;6:159.

93. Walsh JM, Brenner RP. Periodic lateralized epileptiform discharges—long term outcome in adults. Epilepsia 1987;28:533.

94. Schwartz MS, Prior PF, Scott DF. The occurrence and evolution in the EEG of a lateralized periodic phenomenon. Brain 1973;96:613.

# Chapter 11

# Electrocardiographic Recognition of Cardiac Arrhythmias

## Daniel M. Shindler and John B. Kostis

A wealth of information is available about cardiac rate and rhythm disturbances during sleep. Twenty-four-hour ambulatory electrocardiography (ECG) has made it possible to study cardiac rhythm in both awake and sleeping subjects. For most practical purposes, it is possible to think about cardiac rhythm during sleep in the same way as during wakefulness, although the average heart rate is slower during sleep. As a result, escape-type arrhythmias may appear or become more frequent. One should first be familiar with the normal behavior of the heart and subsequently become familiar with a simple classification of cardiac arrhythmias.

## NORMAL CARDIAC RHYTHM

The normal cardiac rhythm is defined as a normal sinus rhythm—that is, the cardiac rate is between 60 and 100 bpm and the cardiac impulse originates in the sinus node. This is best confirmed by identifying a normal-looking P wave that is followed by a normal and constant PR interval and is always succeeded by a single QRS complex. It is quite normal for cardiac cycle length (RR interval) in a given patient to be somewhat variable. This is referred to as *sinus arrhythmia* (Figure 11-1).[1–3] The heart rate of children and infants is faster than the heart rate of adults. The rate of the sinus node is influenced by the autonomic nervous system.

## CARDIAC ARRHYTHMIAS

Arrhythmias are due to disturbances of impulse formation, impulse conduction, or a combination of the two. Arrhythmias can be separated into two large groups. Those that originate in the sinus node, atria, or atrioventricular (AV) node are referred to as *supraventricular arrhythmias*; those that originate in the ventricles are classified as *ventricular arrhythmias*. Figures 11-2 to 11-18 illustrate a variety of cardiac arrhythmias.

### Supraventricular Arrhythmias

When the QRS complex is narrow, the arrhythmia is, with few exceptions, supraventricular. Unfortunately, when the QRS complex is wide, it is often impossible to determine conclusively whether an arrhythmia is supraventricular or ventricular. Inspection of the ECG is the first step in evaluating an arrhythmia. If the arrhythmia is considered potentially life threatening, a specialized electrophysiologic study may be required to further assess its significance.

### Sinus Tachycardia

The most common rhythm disturbance (which may not be abnormal), sinus tachycardia, is an acceleration of the sinus heart rate above 100 bpm.[4] In most

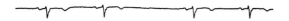

**Figure 11-1.** Normal sinus rhythm with sinus arrhythmia.

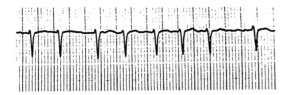

**Figure 11-2.** Atrial fibrillation.

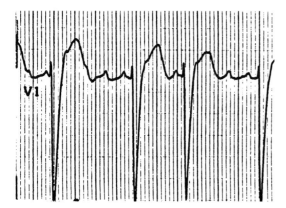

**Figure 11-3.** Atrial flutter with variable ventricular response.

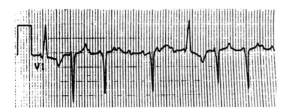

**Figure 11-4.** Atrial flutter. The first and fifth QRS complexes are aberrantly conducted.

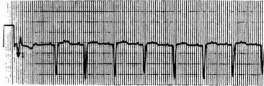

**Figure 11-5.** Atrial tachycardia with 2-to-1 block.

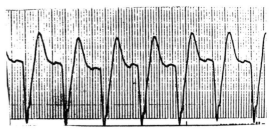

**Figure 11-6.** Undetermined wide complex rhythm, rate 100 bpm.

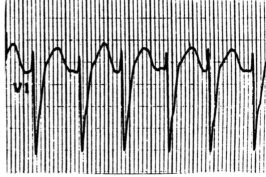

**Figure 11-7.** Undetermined wide complex tachycardia, rate 145 bpm.

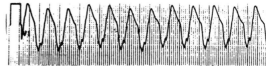

**Figure 11-8.** Ventricular tachycardia.

cases sinus tachycardia does not exceed 180 bpm. Sinus tachycardia is best diagnosed by identifying P waves, determining that they are of normal morphology, subsequently establishing that the PR interval is normal and constant, and determining that each QRS complex is preceded by the P wave and each P wave is followed by a normal QRS. In the course of normal daily activity, the heart rate rises in a gradual fashion and subsides in a gradual fashion.[5] Sinus tachycardia can occur during REM sleep. Yet, patients

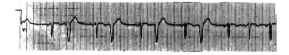

**Figure 11-9.** Normal sinus rhythm. Premature ventricular contractions in bigeminy.

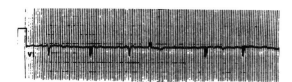

**Figure 11-10.** Atrial fibrillation. Premature ventricular contraction.

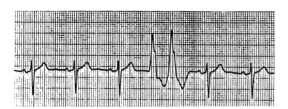

**Figure 11-11.** Normal sinus rhythm. Premature ventricular couplet.

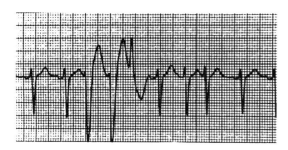

**Figure 11-12.** Normal sinus rhythm. Three-beat multifocal ventricular tachycardia salvo. The eighth QRS complex is a premature atrial contraction.

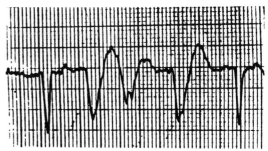

**Figure 11-13.** Three-beat ventricular salvo resembling baseline artifact. Artifacts do not have T waves.

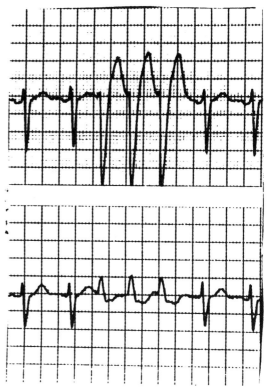

**Figure 11-14.** Three-beat ventricular salvo demonstrated in two simultaneous leads.

suffering from REM sleep behavior disorder can have violent body movements without an increase in the heart rate due to the absence of autonomic arousal.

### Sinus Bradycardia

The opposite boundary of normal heart rate is sinus bradycardia. Sinus bradycardia is defined as a rate

slower than 60 bpm.[6] Again, it is manifested by a normal P wave appearance; a normal and constant PR interval; and a normal relationship of the P wave to the QRS complex, with a one-to-one sequence similar to that of sinus tachycardia. One observational pitfall in the patient with sinus bradycardia is the fact that, at times, U waves become very prominent and can easily be confused with P waves. As a

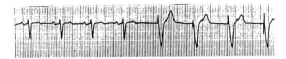

**Figure 11-15.** Sinus rhythm with a demand pacemaker taking over in the last four beats. Note the disappearance of P waves.

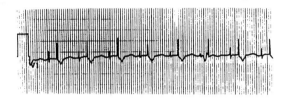

**Figure 11-16.** AV sequence pacemaker. The sixth QRS complex is a native nonpaced premature beat. The pacemaker is programmed to deliver a ventricular pacing spike anyway.

result, blocked premature atrial contractions can be misdiagnosed. Beta blockers can slow the heart rate as well as cause nightmares and sleep disruption.

### Sinus Arrhythmia

Sinus arrhythmia is especially easy to notice with slowing of the heart rate during sleep. The P wave morphology usually does not change. If it does change, the changes are phasic and the P waves do not appear retrograde. There should be a 10% difference between the maximum and minimum cardiac cycle length. Atrioventricular conduction is normal. This is manifested as a PR interval greater than 120 msec. A shorter PR interval with an abnormal P wave would indicate that the beats are not of sinus origin. The variations in sinus cycle length may be phasic

**Figure 11-17.** Aberrant conduction.

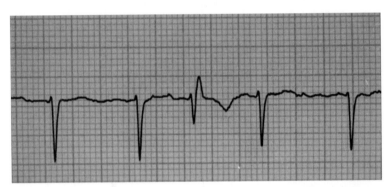

**Figure 11-18.** Torsades de pointes.

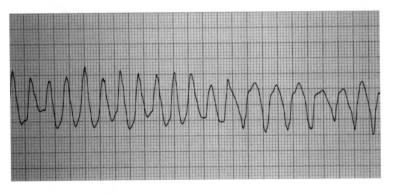

with respiration becoming shorter with inspiration due to reflex inhibition of vagal tone. This form of sinus arrhythmia disappears with apnea.

### Premature Atrial Contractions

Premature atrial contractions are observed frequently in normal subjects and patients with a variety of diseases. They are manifested as an interruption in the heart rhythm with a premature beat having a narrow QRS complex. Because the origin of the atrial impulse is ectopic, the appearance of the P wave is abnormal, denoting its abnormal early origin. There is quite a wide spectrum in the incidence and frequency of premature atrial contractions. Their nature is classified as follows: If the premature atrial contractions occur singly, they are classified according to their incidence per period of time. Therefore, an ambulatory ECG report commonly describes how many premature atrial contractions were observed in a given time, such as an hour, a minute, or 24 hours, according to how common they are. When premature atrial contractions are frequent, it is customary to further describe their nature (cyclic or noncyclic) and rate. For example, when premature atrial contractions occur cyclically, they may show a bigeminal pattern.

### Multifocal Atrial Tachycardia

A variant of frequent premature atrial contractions is tachycardia, which is called *multiform atrial tachycardia* or *chaotic atrial tachycardia*.[7] This is a rhythm disturbance with definite clinical significance. It is identified by an irregular heart rhythm with narrow QRS complexes and rates in excess of 100 bpm. As the name implies, it is multifocal: The atrial beats originate in multiple sites in the atria. Consequently, the appearance of the P waves varies with the point of origin. There is variability in both the P wave morphology and the PR interval. Multifocal atrial tachycardia is an arrhythmia that may have significant consequences. It is particularly common in patients with significant lung disease. These same patients often suffer sleep disorders. When analyzing ECG recordings, multifocal atrial tachycardia should not be confused with atrial fibrillation.

### Atrial Fibrillation

Atrial fibrillation is a very common rhythmic disturbance that is important to diagnose, as the initial heart rate can be quite fast and drug therapy (usually digitalis) may be required to slow it down. Patients with chronic atrial fibrillation are at increased risk for thromboembolic phenomena and are therefore often admitted to the hospital for further management when this rhythm is diagnosed.[8] The ECG hallmark of atrial fibrillation is a completely random and irregular heart rhythm with no reproducible RR interval. Because the atria are fibrillating at a rate of 500 bpm, there are no P waves. The ECG baseline may appear irregular and erratic. This should not be confused with the variable P waves of chaotic atrial tachycardia or with U waves, as mentioned earlier. The ventricular rate in patients with atrial fibrillation tends to be fast when it first occurs. The rate may range around 150 bpm. A clue to underlying conduction system disease is a slow ventricular rate. In this case, caution needs to be exercised with therapeutic modalities, because therapy with an agent such as digitalis may produce undesirable AV conduction problems.[9,10]

### Atrial Flutter

A variant of atrial fibrillation is a rhythm disturbance known as *atrial flutter*.[11] Atrial flutter differs in that atrial activity can be diagnosed as occurring 300 times per minute. At this rate, the ECG hallmark is a characteristic sawtooth pattern at a rate of 300 bpm. The usual presentation of atrial flutter is an atrial rate of 300 bpm with some degree of block between the atria and ventricles (the usual block is 2 to 1). Therefore, it is quite typical to recognize atrial flutter by the presence of sawtooth baseline with a ventricular response of 150 bpm. The therapeutic goal in atrial flutter (similar to atrial fibrillation) is to slow down the ventricular response when it is fast. Again, caution is exercised when the initial ventricular response (with no medication) is an unduly slow rate with a conduction block of 4 to 1 or greater.

### Automatic Versus Re-Entrant Tachycardia

The rhythm disturbances referred to earlier are classified as automatic rhythm disturbances. If properly diagnosed, they can be classified as disorders of cardiac automaticity. The warmup phenomenon (gradual, nonabrupt increase in heart rate) is a hallmark of automatic tachycardia. Usually, an automatic tachycardia requires a search for its cause, which is then treated. For example, multifocal atrial tachycardia is typically seen in patients with lung disease, and improvement of hypoxemia often results from the return of the cardiac rhythm to normal. Sinus tachycardia frequently indicates a metabolic disturbance such as fever, thyrotoxicosis, or hypovolemia. Again, therapy of the cause is the proper approach rather than addressing the mechanism of the rhythm disturbance itself.[12,13] Conversely, a group of tachycardias referred to as *re-entrant* are treated by addressing the mechanism of re-entry. When this is corrected, the rhythm is restored to normal.

### Paroxysmal Atrial Tachycardia

Paroxysmal atrial tachycardia is the classical re-entrant tachycardia treated with medications that interrupt the mechanism of re-entry.[14] As the name implies, a paroxysmal atrial tachycardia begins abruptly. There is no warmup phenomenon, and the heart rate instantly increases to between 140 and 180 bpm. It may cease spontaneously and, just as abruptly, return to sinus rhythm. It is quite common to observe these salvos of atrial tachycardia in patients, whether they are awake or asleep. When paroxysmal atrial tachycardia is persistent, it warrants treatment because of the unduly fast heart rate. Several maneuvers that increase vagal tone, such as Valsalva's maneuver or carotid sinus massage, can break the arrhythmia.[15] When these are ineffective, it becomes necessary to use medication. The calcium channel blocker verapamil is quite useful for this purpose. More recently, an agent that causes complete but very transient AV block, called *adenosine*, has emerged as the modality of choice.[16]

### Sick Sinus Syndrome

Various combinations of tachycardia with bradycardia may suggest the diagnosis of sick sinus syndrome. Ambulatory ECG monitoring may be required to demonstrate the presence of sinus node dysfunction.[17–20]

### Aberrant Supraventricular Conduction

A transient delay in intraventricular (IV) conduction can be seen in patients with supraventricular tachycardias. If the P waves are not clearly identifiable, the rhythm may be misdiagnosed as ventricular tachycardia (see Ventricular Tachycardia, later). QRS complex morphology may be useful in making the correct diagnosis. The initial aberrant conduction occurs in the QRS, which terminates a short cardiac cycle immediately preceded by a long cardiac cycle.[21,22]

## VENTRICULAR ARRHYTHMIAS

The next group of rhythm disturbances, the ventricular arrhythmias, may be more hemodynamically significant and can be associated with clinically important heart disease. They can also be seen in normal patients.

### Premature Ventricular Contractions

A very common rhythm disturbance often felt by patients is the premature ventricular contraction. It is most commonly an early beat that is easily recognized on the ECG as a wide QRS complex with abnormal repolarization.[23] The incidence on 24-hour ECG monitoring can be reported according to how often this finding is present; therefore, premature ventricular contractions are reported as occurring a certain number of times per hour. If rare, they are classified by how many times they occur in 24 hours; if very common, they may be classified in terms of occurrence per minute.[24]

### Ventricular Bigeminy

A very common rhythm disturbance is a sustained rhythm, especially at night, consisting of an alternating normally conducted QRS complex with a premature ventricular contraction followed by a pause and a resumption of the sequence. This is referred to as *ventricular bigeminy*. It is benign for most practical purposes, but it has some clinical implications. For example, a patient taking a pulse may notice only the normally conducted beats. The pulse deficit might then result in a mistaken diagnosis of bradycardia.

### Ventricular Tachycardia

The finding of three or more premature ventricular contractions in a row (at a heart rate faster than 100 bpm) is referred to as *ventricular tachycardia*,[25] and it may be brief or sustained.[26] The most important distinction that needs to be made when ventricular tachycardia is suspected is the alternate diagnosis of supraventricular tachycardia with aberrant ventricular conduction. The diagnostic approach to this critical differential diagnosis is multifaceted. The diagnosis begins at the bedside. If the patient is hemodynamically decompensated, it is necessary to act rapidly.[27,28] Multiple ECG leads should be used to identify P waves that mark atrial activity. Atrial P waves that are unrelated to ventricular QRS complexes make ventricular tachycardia more likely than aberrant conduction. The appearance of the QRS complex has been useful in the recognition of a ventricular origin for tachycardia. Sustained ventricular tachycardia often degenerates into ventricular fibrillation, resulting in death.[29]

### Ventricular Fibrillation

Ventricular fibrillation is a lethal terminal dysrhythmia that requires immediate electrical defibrillation.[11] There are no identifiable QRS complexes. It may begin on a T wave (this is referred to as *R on T*). It may also be seen in association with a unique ventricular tachyarrhythmia called *torsades de pointes*.

### Torsades de Pointes

The morphology of torsades de pointes is unique. The points of the ventricular complexes vary in their height, appearing to turn around a central axis, the baseline of the ECG tracing. It is important to measure the QT interval. QT prolongation can be caused by electrolyte disturbances, antiarrhythmic drugs, or central nervous system or congenital disease.[30–34]

### Accelerated Idioventricular Rhythm

The law of the heart states that the fastest pacemaker is the one that governs the heart. Accelerated idioventricular rhythm (AIVR) is a slow ventricular rhythm that captures the heart because the sinus rate is even slower. The rate of AIVR is less than 100 bpm. It is usually faster than the typical 40-bpm ventricular escape rate (thus the term *accelerated* ). This is typically an escape rhythm that should not be suppressed with antiarrhythmic agents such as lidocaine. AIVR is often short-lived and has no hemodynamic consequences. In this setting, it does not require treatment. When AIVR is sustained and hypotension is observed, an agent such as atropine may be useful in overdriving the AIVR by accelerating the sinus node. The ECG diagnosis of AIVR consists of establishing the ventricular origin of the rhythm.

## PACEMAKER RHYTHM

Pacemaker rhythms are identified by the pacemaker spike preceding the wide QRS complex. It is necessary to determine proper capture as well as proper sensing. Dual-chamber pacemakers are designed to restore the normal sequence of AV contraction. They are also associated with pacemaker-induced arrhythmias.[35] Some patients may have a pacemaker or defibrillator implanted to treat life threatening ventricular arrhythmias.[36,37]

## INTRACARDIAC RECORDINGS

Certain patients may be referred for electrophysiologic study to further evaluate their arrhythmia. The tracings obtained during those studies may demonstrate ECG information about the heart that is unobtainable from surface ECG studies. It is possible to record the electrical activity of the bundle of His. This may help decide which patients require a permanent pacemaker. The sinus node recovery time can be measured in patients with sick sinus syndrome. Ventricular arrhythmias can be induced to assess efficacy of antiarrhythmic therapy.[38]

## SIGNAL-AVERAGED ELECTROCARDIOGRAM

It is possible to amplify the electrocardiographic complex by as much as 1,000 times with the use of signal averaging. The signal-averaged ECG can demonstrate the presence of late potentials (high-frequency, low-amplitude signals). Their absence is associated with a more favorable prognosis after myocardial infarction.

## MANAGEMENT OF ARRHYTHMIAS DETECTED DURING SLEEP

The sophisticated monitoring equipment available today permits detection of cardiac arrhythmias and conduction disturbances as they occur during sleep. Sustained ventricular arrhythmias require immediate attention. The patient needs to be awakened, and blood pressure and mental status must be determined. If the ventricular arrhythmia causes hypotension or the patient is unarousable, emergency measures may be required, but this is extremely rare. Nonsustained ventricular arrhythmias are a more common finding. Typically, by the time the patient is aroused, blood pressure is normal. The patient needs to be monitored, however, for recurrence of the arrhythmia. Conduction disturbances can also be detected. Sinus arrest is manifested by the disappearance of P waves and an area other than the sinus node taking over the cardiac rhythm. This can be a junctional, ectopic atrial, or ventricular rhythm. It is important to ascertain by ECG whether arrhythmias are, as mentioned, sustained or nonsustained. It is also worthwhile to determine whether a newly detected rhythm disturbance is a consequence of a conduction abnormality followed by an escape mechanism, rather than a premature mechanism for arrhythmia initiation such as a premature ventricular contraction. The hemodynamics, as measured by blood pressure, are the most important indicators of the significance of an arrhythmia as it is occurring. It is also important to take into account the underlying cardiac status of the particular patient in whom the arrhythmia is observed.

## REFERENCES

1. Rawles JM, Pai GR, Reid SR. A method of quantifying sinus arrhythmia: parallel effect of respiration on PP and PR intervals. Clin Sci 1989;12:954.
2. de Marneffe M, Jacobs P, Haardt R, et al. Variations of normal sinus node function in relation to age: role of autonomic influence. Eur Heart J 1986;7:662.
3. Gomes JA, Winters SL. The origins of the sinus node pacemaker complex in man: demonstration of dominant and subsidiary foci. J Am Coll Cardiol 1987;9:45.
4. Coelho A, Palileo E, Ashley W, et al. Tachyarrhythmias in youth athletes. J Am Coll Cardiol 1986;7:237.
5. Yeh SJ, Lin FC, Wu DL. The mechanisms of exercise provocation of supraventricular tachycardia. Am Heart J 1989;117:1041.
6. Northcote RJ, Canning GP, Ballantyne D. Electrocardiographic findings in male veteran endurance athletes. Br Heart J 1989;61:155.
7. Scher DL, Arsura EL. Multifocal atrial tachycardia: mechanisms, clinical correlates and treatment. Am Heart J 1989;118:574.
8. Wolf PA, Abbott RD, Kannel WB. Atrial fibrillation: a major contributor to stroke in the elderly. The Framingham Study. Arch Intern Med 1987;147:1561.
9. Fananapazir L, German LD, Gallagher JJ, et al. Importance of pre-existed QRS morphology during induced atrial fibrillation to the diagnosis and location of multiple accessory pathways. Circulation 1990;81:578.
10. Kopecky SL, Gersh BJ, McGoon MD, et al. The natural history of lone atrial fibrillation. A population-based study over 3 decades. N Engl J Med 1987;317:669.
11. Waldo AL, Carlson MD, Henthorn RW. Atrial Flutter: Transient Entrainment and Related Phenomena. In DP Zipes, J Jalife (eds), Cardiac Electrophysiology: from Cell to Bedside. Philadelphia: Saunders, 1990;530.
12. Simpson RJ Jr, Amara I, Foster JR, et al. Thresholds, refractory periods, and conduction times of the normal and diseased human atrium. Am Heart J 1988; 116:1080.
13. Villain E, Vetter VL, Garcia JM, et al. Evolving concepts in the management of congenital junction ectopic tachycardia. Circulation 1990;81:1544.
14. Pritchett EL, McCarthy EA, Lee KL. Clinical behavior of paroxysmal atrial tachycardia. Am J Cardiol 1988;62:30.
15. Morady F, Krol RB, Nostrant TT, et al. Supraventricular tachycardia induced by swallowing: a case report and review of the literature. Pacing Clin Electrophysiol 1987;10:133.
16. Rankin AC, Oldroyd KG, Chong E, et al. Value and limitations of adenosine in the diagnosis and treatment of narrow and broad complex tachycardias. Br Heart J 1989;62:195.
17. Bharati S, Lev M. Cardiac Conduction System in Unexplained Sudden Death. Mt. Kisco, NY: Futura, 1990.
18. Choi YS, Kim JJ, Oh BH, et al. Cough syncope caused by sinus arrest in a patient with sick sinus syndrome. Pacing Clin Electrophysiol 1989;12:883.
19. Sasaki Y, Shimotori M, Akahane K, et al. Long-term follow-up of patients with sick sinus syndrome: a comparison of clinical aspects among unpaced, ventricular inhibited paced, and physiologically paced groups. Pacing Clin Electrophysiol 1988;11:1575.
20. Schuger CD, Tzivoni D, Gottlieb S, et al. Sinus node and atrioventricular nodal function in 220 patients recovering from acute myocardial infarction. Cardiology 1988;75:274.

21. Akhtar M, Shenasa M, Jazayeri M, et al. Wide QRS complex tachycardia. Reappraisal of common clinical problem. Ann Intern Med 1988;109:905.

22. Miles WM, Zipes DP. Electrophysiology of wide QRS tachycardia. Prog Cardiol 1988;1/2:77.

23. Moulton KP, Medcalf T, Lazzara R. Premature ventricular complex morphology. Circulation 1990;81:1245.

24. Funck-Brentano C, Coumel P, Lorente P, et al. Rate dependence of ventricular extrasystoles: computer identification and quantitative analysis. Cardiovasc Res 1988;22:101.

25. Akhtar M. Clinical spectrum of ventricular tachycardia. Circulation 1990;82:1561.

26. Wilber DJ, Olshansky B, Moran JF, et al. Electrophysiological testing and nonsustained ventricular tachycardia. Circulation 1990;82:350.

27. Lucente M, Rebuzzi AG, Lanza GA, et al. Circadian variation of ventricular tachycardia in acute myocardial infarction. Am J Cardiol 1988;62:670.

28. Steinman RT, Herrera C, Schuger CD. Wide QRS tachycardia in the conscious adult. Ventricular tachycardia is the most frequent cause. JAMA 1989;261:1013.

29. Trappe HJ, Brugada P, Talajic M, et al. Prognosis of patients with ventricular tachycardia and ventricular fibrillation: role of the underlying etiology. J Am Coll Cardiol 1988;12:166.

30. Jackman WM, Friday KJ, Clark M, et al. The long QT syndromes: a critical review, new clinical observations and unifying hypothesis. Prog Cardiovasc Dis 1988;31:115.

31. Laks MM. Long QT interval syndrome. A new look at an old electrophysiologic measurement-power of the computer. Circulation 1990;82:1539.

32. Nguyen PT, Scheinman MM, Seger J. Polymorphous ventricular tachycardia: clinical characterization, therapy, and the QT interval. Circulation 1986;74:340.

33. Opie LH. Forum on torsades de pointes: introduction. Cardiovasc Drugs Ther 1990;4:1167.

34. Rosen MR, Danilo P Jr, Robinson RB, et al. Sympathetic neural and alpha-adrenergic modulation of arrhythmias. Ann N Y Acad Sci 1988;533:200.

35. Levander-Lindgren M, Lantz B. Bradyarrhythmia profile and associated diseases in 1,265 patients with cardiac pacing. Pacing Clin Electrophysiol 1988;11:2207.

36. Rosenthal ME, Josephson ME. Current status of antitachycardia devices. Circulation 1990;82:1889.

37. Winkle RA, Mead RH, Ruder MA, et al. Long-term outcome with the automatic implantable cardioverter-defibrillator. J Am Coll Cardiol 1989;13:1353.

38. Zipes DP, Akhtar M, Denes P, et al. ACC/AHA guidelines for clinical intracardiac electrophysiologic studies. J Am Coll Cardiol 1989;14:1827 and Circulation 1989;80:1925.

# Chapter 12

# Respiration and Respiratory Function: Technique of Recording and Evaluation

Richard A. Parisi

## EVALUATION OF RESPIRATORY FUNCTION IN PATIENTS WITH SLEEP DISORDERS

A critical part of the initial medical evaluation of all patients with sleep disorders is the assessment of respiratory function. The reason for the importance of this assessment is straightforward: Many of the most common and potentially serious sleep disorders (e.g., sleep apnea syndromes, nocturnal asthma, and sleep-related hypoventilation) are respiratory in nature and may be associated with respiratory abnormalities also evident in the awake state. Although a detailed discussion of the diagnostic evaluation of respiratory disease is beyond the scope of this volume, a general approach is presented here, emphasizing systematic assessment of the key components of the respiratory system.

### Lung Diseases Associated with Sleep Disorders

Individuals with previously diagnosed lung diseases are often referred for evaluation of sleep complaints. Patients with chronic obstructive pulmonary disease (COPD) present with symptoms of insomnia related to frequent awakenings.[1] Hypersomnia may also occur, particularly in patients who exhibit sleep-related hypoventilation. Many patients with asthma experience exacerbations of this disorder during sleep. Like patients with COPD, asthmatics

often describe episodic arousals associated with dyspnea, cough, or wheezing.[2] Lung diseases that produce a restrictive (rather than obstructive) pattern of pulmonary dysfunction, such as pulmonary fibrosis, may also be associated with poor, fragmented sleep.[3] Another important group of patients are those with chronic respiratory neuromuscular diseases. Symptoms of nocturnal respiratory insufficiency, including frequent arousals often associated with dyspnea, cough, choking, or morning headache, are frequently among the earliest signs of impending respiratory failure.[4] A related but distinct group of patients in whom sleep-disordered breathing is common are those with altered central neural respiratory drive. Such individuals may exhibit hypoventilation syndromes while awake that are exacerbated by sleep.

### Physiologic Testing

Formal testing of pulmonary mechanics, respiratory muscle strength, gas exchange, and central respiratory drive may be indicated for selected patients with clinical sleep disorders, although none of these tests should be a routine part of a sleep evaluation.

Spirometry is the most commonly performed clinical test of pulmonary function and is readily available at most centers and in many physicians' offices. It is relatively inexpensive and simple to perform, and it provides a quantitative assessment of intrathoracic airway obstructive disease. Spirometry is also a moderately sensitive screening test for restrictive mechanical processes such as interstitial lung disease and respiratory muscle weakness. Although weakness of the diaphragm and other respiratory muscles usually causes reduction of the forced vital capacity as measured by spirometry, the most sensitive clinical test for muscle strength is measurement of maximal inspiratory and expiratory pressures generated at the mouth against an occluded airway. When restriction of vital capacity is evident on spirometry, more complete measurement of lung volumes in the pulmonary function laboratory is indicated to evaluate the pattern of restriction. For example, interstitial lung diseases generally decrease all lung volumes symmetrically, whereas extrapulmonary processes such as respiratory muscle weakness primarily reduce vital capacity without affecting functional residual capacity.

Arterial blood gases of most patients referred to a sleep disorders center need not be measured, although this test provides valuable information in some patients with sleep-disordered breathing. This is particularly true for those individuals found by pulse oximetry, performed during an office consultation or at the time of polysomnography, to be hypoxemic while awake. Most patients with the obstructive sleep apnea syndrome have normal blood gases while awake. In contrast, patients with the obesity-hypoventilation syndrome are characteristically hypercapnic during wakefulness as well as sleep, as are patients with advanced COPD or chronic neuromuscular diseases.

The obstructive sleep apnea syndrome typically is not associated with overt abnormalities of respiratory drive.[5] When chronic waking hypercapnia is present in a patient with sleep-disordered breathing, a primary impairment of respiratory drive should be considered. In the absence of chronic lung disease or neuromuscular weakness, chronic hypercapnia may be attributed to reduced respiratory $CO_2$ sensitivity, as in the central alveolar hypoventilation syndrome. Patients with moderate ventilatory impairment, whose respiratory $CO_2$ drive is suspected to be abnormal, present a diagnostic challenge. In such cases, the change in $Paco_2$ during a brief period (2 minutes) of maximal voluntary hyperventilation may be measured.[6] Hypercapnia due primarily to mechanical factors is usually not correctable through volition, whereas central hypoventilation can be overcome during a brief period of conscious effort. A blunted ventilatory response to hypercapnia and hypoxia, measured by standard techniques,[7,8] can confirm this clinical impression. The value of these tests in an individual patient is limited by the considerable variability of normal responses and by the confounding effect of mechanical ventilatory impairment, however, which may also decrease the measured responses.

## RESPIRATORY MONITORING DURING SLEEP

### General Principles

It should be evident from the following discussion that a wide array of methods is available to monitor respiratory output during sleep in the clinical setting. Clearly, the number and type of monitoring devices used are dependent on the purpose of the study to be performed. For some purposes, a single measure that assesses adequacy of gas exchange, such as pulse oximetry, is sufficient. Detection of subtle changes in airflow due to increased upper airway resistance requires more sensitive techniques. In discussing various modalities, an effort has been made to convey which are generally considered part of "standard" polysomnography.

### Monitoring Respiratory Mechanical Output Airflow and Snoring

Clinically applicable sensors can be classified as direct or indirect and as quantitative or semiquantitative (Table 12-1). For most clinical purposes, semiquantitative indirect methods, such as an oronasal thermistor, are sufficient to identify disordered breathing events.

Quantitative measurement of airflow or tidal volume usually requires a sealed mask placed over the nose or the nose and mouth, connected to a calibrated pneumotachograph. Although this technique provides the accuracy necessary for some research applications, the method can be cumbersome and intrusive, thus limiting its value for clinical monitoring. One setting in which direct quantitative airflow monitoring is not only possible but preferable is during application of nasal continuous positive airway pressure (CPAP). Several commercially

**Table 12-1.** Methods for Monitoring Airflow During Sleep

| Method | Principle | Signal Characteristics | Comments |
|---|---|---|---|
| Pneumotachygraph | Direct | Excellent; quantitative and easily integrated to yield tidal volume | Requires sealed face mask<br>Can be incorporated into nasal CPAP systems |
| Thermistor/thermo-couple | Indirect; detects increased temperature of expired air | Semiquantitative; only directional changes are reliable | Inexpensive, easy to use<br>Signal quality reduced during nasal CPAP treatment |
| Capnograph | Indirect; detects increased $CO_2$ in expired air | Semiquantitative for airflow; significant time delay because air is sampled continuously for remote analysis | Easy to use<br>Signal quality reduced during nasal CPAP treatment |
| Respiratory inductance plethysmograph | Indirect; senses change in thoracic and abdominal cross-sectional areas; sum of these compartments is proportional to airflow | Good when properly calibrated | Least intrusive (no sensor near face)<br>Calibration errors due to slippage or position changes a common problem |
| Tracheal sound | Indirect; airflow through trachea produces sound audible via microphone | Good; sound amplitude increases during snoring or partial upper airway obstruction | Inexpensive<br>Can be used to quantitate snoring |
| Intranasal pressure | Indirect; pressure changes reflect airflow | Excellent dynamic response to airflow profile | Capable of detecting inspiratory flow limitation |

CPAP = continuous positive airway pressure.

available laboratory models of nasal CPAP systems provide flow and volume outputs directly from the remote CPAP control. By examining the dynamic profile of the inspiratory airflow signal, the presence of inspiratory flow limitation can be easily detected (Figure 12-1), indicating the need for an increase in the therapeutic CPAP level.[9] These signals are also useful because the more commonly used semiquantitative sensors, such as thermistors or $CO_2$ meters, require placement under the nasal mask seal, potentially causing discomfort or pressure leakage. Moreover, respiratory-related temperature and $P_{CO_2}$ changes at the nose may be damped considerably by the bias flow of room air required to maintain positive pressure in the nasal airway. Monitoring of the inspiratory upper airway pressure profile has been shown to be a practical and valuable method for detecting airflow limitation using nonoccluding nasal cannulae placed inside the nares and connected to a pressure transducer.[10]

Snoring is an airflow-related phenomenon, although most measures of flow are not very sensitive to it. Many sleep laboratories document snoring through notes detailing the observation of a polysomnographic technician. Quantitative assessment of snoring can be obtained with relative ease by placing a microphone near the patient and using a sound-level meter. Several studies have documented that sound detected by a microphone or piezoelectric transducer placed over or near the cervical trachea can be used as a semiquantitative indicator of airflow as well as snoring.[11,12]

### Respiratory Muscle Activity

The principal purpose of monitoring respiratory muscle activity, commonly described as "respiratory effort," is to detect disparities between these measures and airflow. The most commonly used methods are indirect, semiquantitative, or nonquantitative techniques that detect changes in circumference of the thorax and abdomen, including inductive plethysmography, magnetometers, and strain gauges (Table 12-2). Figure 12-2 illustrates the manner in which these devices, used in tandem, respond to normal tidal breathing and respiratory muscle contractions against an obstructed upper airway. Although paradoxical expansion of the thorax and abdomen may occur under other circumstances,

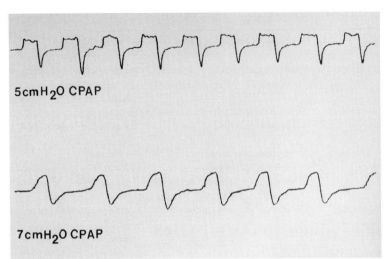

**Figure 12-1.** Recordings of airflow taken from polysomnography performed for the purpose of nasal continuous positive airway pressure (CPAP) titration are shown. The upper tracing shows airflow limitation at 5 cm $H_2O$ CPAP as indicated by the truncated inspiratory airflow profile. The tracing below shows a normal, nonlimited airflow profile at 7 cm $H_2O$ CPAP.

**Table 12-2.** Methods for Monitoring Respiratory Muscle Activity During Sleep

| Method | Principle | Signal Characteristics | Comments |
|---|---|---|---|
| Esophageal pressure | Direct; esophageal pressure equivalent to intrathoracic pressure generated by respiratory muscles | Excellent; reliable; quantitative | Invasive<br>Requires transnasal insertion<br>Uncomfortable for patient or subject |
| Diaphragmatic; electromyogram | Direct; measures neural activation rather than mechanical output | Quantitative; poor signal-to-noise ratio with surface electrodes | Electrocardiography artifact<br>Nonrespiratory muscle electromyography difficult to eliminate |
| Inductance plethysmography/strain gauge/magnetometer | Indirect; senses changes in thoracic and abdominal cross-sectional areas due to respiratory muscle contraction | Semiquantitative | Easy to use<br>Amplitude decreases during obstructive apnea/hypopnea (despite increased effort)<br>Paradoxical motion of thorax and abdomen during obstructive apnea/hypopnea |

such as with fatigue or paralysis of the diaphragm, periodic reversal of this pattern is quite useful in detecting intermittent upper airway obstruction during sleep. In addition, calibration of the relative thoracic and abdominal compartmental volume changes allows summation of the two impedance signals to obtain an indirect and potentially quantitative measure of lung volume changes and airflow.[13] These indirect techniques are noninvasive and simple to use. One disadvantage, however, is that volume changes do not reflect muscle activity when upper airway impedance changes. For exam-

ple, respiratory motion of the chest wall invariably decreases during obstructive apnea or hypopnea despite increasing muscle activity.

Direct monitoring of respiratory muscle activity, either electrical or mechanical, has some advantages over the more commonly used indirect methods, in that such methods continue to accurately reflect activity in the presence of partial or complete upper airway obstruction. Diaphragm or parasternal electromyography is limited, in that reliable recordings are often difficult to obtain from the diaphragm using surface electrodes, and inter-

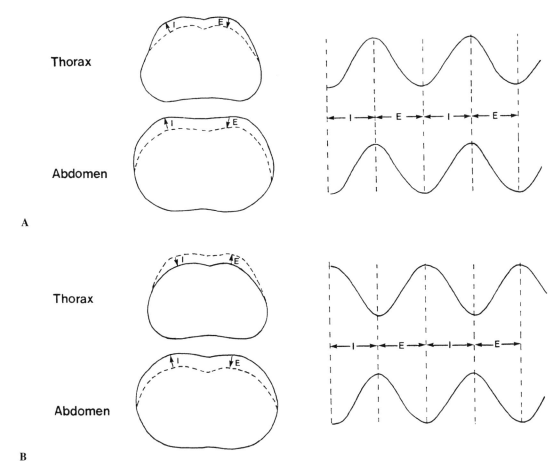

**Figure 12-2.** The diagrams illustrate changes in a cross-sectional area of the thoracic and abdominal compartments during inspiration (I) and expiration (E), and the resultant appearance of polygraph recordings from a respiratory inductive plethysmograph placed around each compartment. **(A)** Normal synchronous inflation. **(B)** Paradoxical respiratory motion in the presence of upper airway obstruction.

costal electromyography typically is inhibited during rapid eye movement sleep. Esophageal pressure provides a reliable, quantitative, and sensitive measure of respiratory muscle mechanical activity, and this method has been favored by some clinical laboratories because of the sensitivity of the finding of increased negative inspiratory pressures with subtle increases in upper airway resistance. The requirement for transnasal insertion of a pressure catheter is sufficiently uncomfortable and invasive for most laboratories performing polysomnography to use the indirect methods described above. Water-filled catheters connected to pressure transducers, however, which are relatively small and flexible, have made this technique less difficult than it was

in the past, and do not significantly disturb sleep architecture.[14,15]

### Monitoring Gas Exchange Pulse Oximetry

It is well-known that oxyhemoglobin and deoxyhemoglobin differ in their absorption spectra for visible light. This principle underlies the technique of oximetry, which can be used to measure the degree of hemoglobin saturation by oxygen through transillumination of an accessible structure such as the earlobe or fingertip. Pulse oximetry is the simplest and most reliable noninvasive method for assessing adequacy of pulmonary gas exchange and has

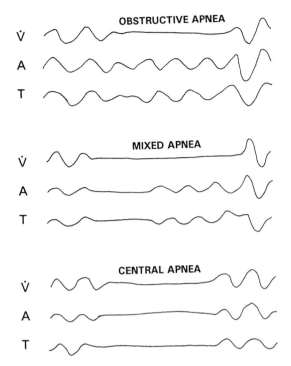

**Figure 12-3.** Simultaneous recordings of airflow ($\dot{V}$) monitored with a thermistor, and motion of the abdomen (A) and thorax (T) recorded with a pair of circumferential inductive plethysmographic sensors during an obstructive apnea, a mixed apnea, and a central apnea. Note the paradoxical abdominal and thoracic motion during the obstructive apnea and obstructive portion of the mixed apnea.

become an essential part of polysomnographic assessment of respiratory disorders of sleep.

### Carbon Dioxide Monitoring

By sampling expired air at the nose, $CO_2$ concentration can be monitored. Under optimal circumstances, end-tidal $P_{CO_2}$ reflects alveolar $P_{CO_2}$ and, thus, arterial $P_{CO_2}$. End-tidal $P_{CO_2}$ measurements should be interpreted with caution, however, because dilution of the sampled expired gas with room air (gas is typically sampled at flow rates of 50–150 ml per minute) systematically reduces the measured $P_{CO_2}$. Transcutaneous monitoring of $P_{CO_2}$ has been used in some studies of adults with sleep-disordered breathing, but its use is more established in neonatal monitoring.[16] Because transcutaneous $P_{CO_2}$ may vary unpredictably from $Pa_{CO_2}$, and because of the long response times

of the measurements, it is primarily useful as a semi-quantitative index of trends in alveolar ventilation.

### Classification of Disordered Breathing Events During Sleep

Although respiratory events are identified and classified in various ways by different sleep disorders centers, the most common method requires concurrent measurement of respiratory airflow, respiratory muscle activity, and, in some cases, arterial oxygen saturation. More limited monitoring may be performed in some instances, such as during unattended home monitoring, but the identification of subtypes of respiratory dysrhythmia with these methods may be less reliable and are not yet considered standard.

### Apneas

In adults, apnea is defined as the absence of airflow for 10 seconds or more.[17–19] Apneas are classified as central, obstructive, or mixed by the concurrent pattern of respiratory muscle activity, as shown in Figure 12-3. Central apneas are due to absence of respiratory effort, and thus any measure of respiratory muscle activity will be absent. During obstructive apneas, respiratory efforts continue (and increase) while airflow is prevented by upper airway obstruction. Mixed apneas are a variant of obstructive apneas during which respiratory effort is absent for several seconds after the onset of upper airway occlusion. By far, obstructive apneas are the most commonly seen type in patients with a clinically significant sleep apnea syndrome. Arterial oxygen saturation characteristically declines during apneas, although the degree of desaturation varies considerably among patients.

### Hypopneas

A hypopnea may be defined as a transient decrease in respiratory airflow of sufficient magnitude to cause significant hypoxemia or an arousal from sleep. Precise criteria defining such events have been a matter of disagreement, and several different methods have been in common use.[20] One method requires a reduction in airflow of one-half or two-thirds, although such precision is difficult to apply if a semiquantitative, nonlinear method is used to monitor flow. Other methods use decreased respiratory excursions,[21] a decrease in arterial oxygen saturation of 4%,[22] or some combination of these criteria. In the absence of a clear and measurable decline in airflow or significant arterial oxygen desaturation, hypopnea may be identified by changes in the inspiratory flow profile consistent with flow limitation followed closely by an electroencephalographic arousal.

More uncertainty surrounds the question of how to differentiate hypopneas, which are predominantly central or obstructive. The most reliable way to achieve this is with a direct measurement of respiratory muscle activity, such as esophageal pressure, which decreases during central hypopnea and increases during an obstructive event. Paradoxical motion of the thorax and abdomen is also more common during obstructive than central hypopneas.

## REFERENCES

1. Fleetham J, West P, Mezon B, et al. Sleep, arousals, and oxygen desaturation in chronic obstructive pulmonary disease. Am Rev Respir Dis 1982;126:429.
2. Cattarall JR, Douglas NJ, Calverley PM, et al. Irregular breathing and hypoxaemia during sleep in chronic stable asthma. Lancet 1982;1:301.
3. Perez-Padilla R, West P, Lertzman M, Kryger MH. Breathing during sleep in interstitial lung disease. Am Rev Respir Dis 1985;132:224.
4. Smith PEM, Calverley PMA, Edwards RHT, et al. Practical problems in the respiratory care of patients with muscular dystrophy. N Engl J Med 1987;316:1197.
5. Garay SM, Rapoport D, Sorkin B, et al. Regulation of ventilation in the obstructive sleep apnea syndrome. Am Rev Respir Dis 1981;124:451.
6. Skatrud JB, Dempsey JA, Bhansali P, Irvin C. Determinants of carbon dioxide retention and its correction in humans. J Clin Invest 1980;65:813.
7. Hirshman CA, McCullough RE, Weil JV. Normal values for hypoxic and hypercapnic ventilatory drives in man. J Appl Physiol 1975;38:1095.
8. Rajagopal KR, Abbrecht PH, Tellis CJ. Control of breathing in obstructive sleep apnea. Chest 1984;85:174.
9. Condos R, Norman RG, Krishnasamy I, et al. Flow limitation as a noninvasive assessment of residual upper airway resistance during continuous positive airway pressure therapy of obstructive sleep apnea. Am J Respir Crit Care Med 1994;150:475.
10. Hosselet JJ, Norman RG, Rapoport DM. Detection of flow limitation with a nasal cannula/pressure transducer system. Am J Respir Crit Care Med 1997;155:A129.
11. Cummiskey JM, Williams TC, Krumpe PE, Guilleminault C. The detection and quantification of sleep apnea by tracheal sound recordings. Am Rev Respir Dis 1982;126:221.
12. Peirick J, Shepard JW Jr. Automated apnea detection by computer: analysis of tracheal breath sounds. Med Biol Eng Comput 1983;21:632.
13. Sackner MA. Monitoring of Ventilation Without a Physical Connection to the Airway. In MA Sackner (ed), Diagnostic Techniques in Pulmonary Disease. New York: Marcel Dekker, 1980;503.
14. Asher MI, Coates AL, Collinge JM, Milic-Emili J. Measurement of pleural pressure in neonates. J Appl Physiol 1982;52:491.
15. Chervin RD, Aldrich MS. Effects of esophageal pressure monitoring on sleep architecture. Am J Respir Dis 1997;156:881.
16. McLellan PA, Goldstein RS, Ramcharan V, Rebuck AS. Transcutaneous carbon dioxide monitoring. Am Rev Respir Dis 1981;124:199.
17. Martin RJ, Block AJ, Cohn MA, et al. Indications and standards for cardiopulmonary sleep studies. Sleep 1985;8:371.
18. Kurtz D, Krieger J. Analysis of Apnea in Sleep Apnea. In C Guilleminault, WC Dement (eds), Sleep Apnea Syndromes. New York: Liss, 1978;145.
19. American Thoracic Society Consensus Conference. Indications and standards for cardiopulmonary sleep studies. Am Rev Respir Dis 1989;139:559.
20. Moser NJ, Phillips BA, Berry DT, Harbison L. What is hypopnea, anyway? Chest 1994;105:426.
21. Whyte KF, Allen MB, Fitzpatrick MF, Douglas NJ. Accuracy and significance of scoring hypopneas. Sleep 1992;15:257.
22. Block AJ, Boysen PG, Wynne JW, Hunt LA. Sleep apnea, hypopnea, and oxygen desaturation in normal subjects: a strong male predominance. N Engl J Med 1979;300:513.

# Chapter 13

# Measurement of Sleepiness and Alertness: Multiple Sleep Latency Test

## Thomas Roth, Timothy A. Roehrs, and Leon Rosenthal

Daytime sleepiness as a consequence of inadequate sleep the previous night is a common experience for most adults. Because of the universality of the acute experience of daytime sleepiness, it is typically minimized as a health problem within the general population; in a 1997 Gallup Poll of Americans, only 6% of those reporting impairing sleepiness considered it medically serious.[1] Although minimized by lay people, increasingly chronic excessive daytime sleepiness is recognized as an important and significant symptom in medicine. Furthermore, excessive daytime sleepiness can and should be distinguished from fatigue, tiredness, and lassitude, although many patients may not make such distinctions themselves unless they are carefully queried.

Representative surveys of the populations of industrialized countries have found that between 11% and 32% of respondents report that sleepiness interferes with activities almost daily.[1–5] Sleepiness is associated with a number of medical, behavioral, and pharmacologic causes, and, regardless of its cause, has serious social and medical consequences. Nearly half of the patients with excessive sleepiness seen at sleep disorders centers report automobile accidents; more than half report occupational accidents, some life threatening; many have lost jobs because of their sleepiness; and the impact of sleepiness on family life is disruptive.[6] Information on traffic and industrial accidents in the general population suggests a link between sleepiness and life-threatening events. For example, the highest rate of automobile accidents occurs in the early morning

hours, which is remarkable because fewer automobiles are on the road during these hours.[7] Shift workers, a particularly sleepy subpopulation, have the poorest job performance and the highest rate of industrial accidents among all workers.[8]

Problems in assessing sleepiness became evident during early research on the daytime consequences of sleep loss before the clinical significance of sleepiness was recognized. Sleep loss compromises daytime functions. Virtually all individuals experience dysphoria and reduced performance when they do not sleep adequately. The majority of performance tasks are insensitive to the effects of sleep loss,[9] but long and monotonous tasks are reliably sensitive to changes in the quantity and quality of nocturnal sleep. Using various measures of mood, including factor analytic scales, the most consistent and systematic response to sleep loss is increased sleepiness. Among the various subjective measures of sleepiness, the Stanford Sleepiness Scale (SSS) is the best validated.[10] Yet clinicians have found that patients may rate themselves alert on the SSS even as they are falling asleep.[11]

Normal and pathologic variations in daytime sleepiness and alertness can now be directly assessed and quantified by the Multiple Sleep Latency Test (MSLT), a test of the rapidity with which a subject falls asleep in a standardized, sleep-conducive setting, repeated at 2-hour intervals throughout the day. The MSLT uses standard sleep recording methods to document both the rate of sleep onset and the appearance of rapid eye movement (REM) episodes at sleep onset. Other procedures that have been used to quantify sleepiness and alertness (but because of a variety of shortcomings are not widely used), including pupillometery, subjective rating scales, and tests of vigilance or reaction time, are all correlated to some extent with the MSLT. The MSLT has become the standard method in clinical sleep disorders medicine for documenting complaints of excessive daytime sleepiness and to document treatment success. It is also used to document sleep-onset REM periods, a diagnostic sign of narcolepsy. Since the development of the MSLT by Carskadon and Dement[12] in the late 1970s, enormous progress has been made in the scientific investigation and understanding of both normal and pathologic variations in sleepiness and alertness.

## MULTIPLE SLEEP LATENCY TEST METHODS

### Recording Montage

General and specific technical guidelines for the administration of the MSLT have been published.[13] Briefly, the guidelines require that the standard Rechtschaffen and Kales recording montage be used in performing the MSLT.[14] The montage includes the referential electroencephalogram (EEG) from a central (C3 or C4) placement, two horizontal referential electro-oculograms (EOGs) from right and left outer canthi, and a mental or submental electromyogram. Also helpful in the determination of sleep onset is a referential occipital EEG lead, which shows alpha activity in relaxed wakefulness with eyes closed and is followed by a characteristic change to mixed-frequency EEG activity at the onset of sleep. An EOG recording with filters set to allow visualization of slow rolling eye movements (e.g., 250 msec) is another sign of sleep onset.

### General Procedures

As indicated in the guidelines, to ensure a reliable and valid MSLT, a number of general procedures are necessary.[13] A 1- or 2-week sleep diary recorded before the test that includes information on usual bedtime, time of arising, napping, and drug use (i.e., caffeine, alcohol, illicit and licit drugs) is very helpful. Deviations from the subject's habitual sleep behavior should be noted, because sleep time accumulated or lost over the week before an MSLT can significantly affect the result. Central nervous system (CNS)-active drugs, as well as their discontinuation, can alter sleep and REM latencies and therefore should be discontinued sufficiently well in advance of the test. The sleep of the night preceding an MSLT should be documented with a standard nocturnal sleep recording. This nocturnal sleep recording should be scheduled to coincide with the timing and amount of the subject's usual sleep, as revealed in the diary.

The reliability of the MSLT is based on multiple determinations of sleep latency, as the studies discussed in the following sections have shown. Consequently, as indicated in the guidelines, four or five tests of sleep latency at 2-hour intervals throughout the day should be conducted.[13] Testing should be initiated from 1.5 to 3 hours after the nocturnal sleep period has been terminated, typically at 9:30 or 10:00 AM. The MSLT should be conducted in a sleep-conducive environment that is quiet, dark, and controlled at a comfortable temperature. Any potentially arousing stimuli should be removed from the test area.

### Specific Procedures

The following procedures are specified by the guidelines for conducting the MSLT[13]: After arising from nocturnal sleep, the subject should toilet, dress in street clothes, and eat the usual breakfast (avoiding caffeinated beverages). Between the latency tests the subject should be kept out of the bed and monitored by technical staff to assure that no napping occurs. Preparations before each latency test include smoking cessation 30 minutes before lights out, bedtime preparation (removing shoes and restrictive clothes such as belts or neckties) at 10 minutes before lights out, all electrode connections and calibrations completed at 5 minutes before lights out, and the instructions to relax and fall asleep given 5 seconds before lights out.

### Ending a Test

According to the guidelines, if sleep does not occur, each test is concluded 20 minutes after lights out.[13]

For the clinical version of the MSLT, in which the occurrence of REM sleep is at question, the test is concluded 15 minutes after the first 30-second epoch of sleep. In a research version of the MSLT, the test is concluded after three consecutive 30-second epochs of stage I sleep or one 30-second epoch of another sleep stage. When the recording is equivocal, it is safer to allow clearer signs of sleep (i.e., spindles and K complexes) to emerge rather than to terminate the test prematurely.

### Scoring and Interpretation

Criteria for scoring sleep onset differ from criteria for test termination.[13] There has been some confusion in the MSLT literature in this regard. Furthermore, it should be noted that the MSLT sleep latency criteria differ from the typical definition of nocturnal sleep onset (stage II sleep or 10 continuous minutes of sleep) in much of the all-night sleep literature. MSLT sleep latency is the elapsed time in minutes from lights out to the first 30-second epoch scored as sleep. According to the scoring criteria of Rechtschaffen and Kales,[14] this implies that 16 seconds of sleep (i.e., >50% on a given epoch of the recording) is sufficient to score a sleep onset. REM sleep latency in a clinical test is scored as minutes from sleep onset (as defined earlier) to the first epoch of REM sleep.

Average sleep latency (in minutes) for the four or five latency tests is the parameter typically used to express the level of sleepiness. In some of the clinical literature, the MSLT result is expressed as a median sleep latency or a sleepiness index, which is merely the average latency subtracted from 100 and multiplied by 100% (and corrected if fewer than five tests are conducted). The occurrence of REM sleep within 10–15 minutes of sleep onset is generally defined as a sleep-onset REM period (SOREMP), and the frequency of such SOREMPs is also tabulated.

### Sources of Error

The level of sleepiness (defined as the average sleep latency) observed on the MSLT is affected by the sleep of the previous night and weeks. Any deviation from the subject's habitual sleep schedule (as revealed in the sleep diary) and sleep quality (as seen in the nocturnal sleep recording and the individual's estimate of its consistency with usual sleep) is likely to overestimate or underestimate the usual level of daytime sleepiness. Similarly, the timing of the nocturnal sleep and daytime MSLT assessment relative to the subject's circadian phase is a potential source of error that is an issue in studying shift and night workers. Out-of-phase sleep is likely to be disturbed and associated with shorter MSLT latencies. Moreover, sleep latency itself varies as a function of circadian phase.

Sedating or alerting effects of drugs or discontinuation of long-term drugs use can also be a source of error in documenting sleepiness. For some patients, a urine drug screen may be necessary to confirm the absence of drugs. A noisy or stimulating test environment invalidates an MSLT result. Instructions given to the subject at the initiation of the test are also important. Subjects should be aware that they are to close their eyes, lie still, and allow sleep to occur. Excessive tossing and turning are to be avoided. It should be recognized that the instruction "relax and fall asleep" may be emotionally loaded for patients with insomnia. This issue is discussed under Validity.

Finally, a "last test" effect might be observed (this has not yet been systematically studied). In anticipation of going home for the day, subjects remain awake for the 20 minutes of the last latency test. This last test effect could elevate the average sleep latency for the day. It can be avoided by scheduling other nonarousing activities after the last latency test. Scheduling a patient-feedback session with the clinician, either before or after the last test, can be disruptive to that test and should be avoided.

REM sleep can occur during the MSLT. Many drugs suppress REM sleep, and discontinuing them increases the likelihood of SOREMPs on an MSLT. The circadian-phase timing of the MSLT is also important with respect to the occurrence of REM sleep. REM sleep can occur on early morning latency tests in a person who is a late-morning sleeper. Excessive disturbance of the sleep of the previous night also has the potential to result in REM sleep on early morning latency tests. For example, it has been suggested that apnea patients with highly fragmented sleep may have more SOREMPs than the general population. Thus, SOREMPs should be re-evaluated in patients suspected of narcolepsy, but who show apneas in the nocturnal sleep recording. It is rare for sleep restriction the week previous to an MSLT to alter REM occurrence on the MSLT.

## RELIABILITY AND VALIDITY

### Reliability

Several studies of the reliability of the MSLT have been conducted. In healthy normals who maintained consistent sleep-wake schedules, the test-retest reliability of a four-test MSLT was 0.97 over a 4- to 14-month test-retest interval.[15] The test-retest interval (≤6 months vs. >6 months) and the level of sleepiness (average latency of ≤5 minutes vs. ≥15 minutes) did not affect this MSLT reliability. The *number* of latency tests did alter MSLT reliability: The coefficient dropped to 0.85 for three tests and 0.65 for two tests. Another study of patients with insomnia over an interval of 3–90 weeks found a test-retest correlation of 0.65 on a five-test MSLT.[16]

There has also been interest in the test-retest reliability of SOREMPs in patients with narcolepsy. The current criteria require two or more SOREMPs out of five possible sleep onsets. In the only study done to date, 28 of 30 patients had two or more SOREMPs when retested ($\kappa = 0.93$, $P < .05$). Of particular interest is the finding that the REM latency on SOREMPs during the initial evaluation was also correlated to that during retesting ($r = 0.64$, $P < .02$).[17]

### Validity

#### Determinants of Daytime Sleepiness

A number of different causes of pathologic sleepiness have been identified. The degree of daytime sleepiness is directly related to the amount of nocturnal sleep. Partial or total sleep deprivation in normal subjects is followed by increased sleepiness the following day, which can reach pathologic levels.[18] Furthermore, modest sleep deprivation (as little as 1 hour per night) accumulates over time to progressively increase daytime sleepiness, again to pathologic levels.[19]

In normal young adults, however, increased sleep time—extending time in bed beyond the usual 7 or 8 hours per night—produces increased alertness (i.e., reduction in sleepiness).[20]

Daytime sleepiness also relates to the quality and continuity of a previous night's sleep. Sleep in patients with a number of sleep disorders is punctuated by frequent, brief arousals of 3–15 seconds' duration. The arousals typically do not result in awakening, as judged by either Rechtschaffen and Kales sleep staging criteria or behavioral indicators, and the arousals recur in some conditions as often as one to four times per minute.[14] The arousing stimulus differs in the various disorders and can be identified in some cases (e.g., apneas, leg movements, pain). The critical point is that the arousals generally do not result in shorter sleep, but rather in fragmented or discontinuous sleep, and this fragmentation produces daytime sleepiness.

Correlational evidence suggests a relationship between sleep fragmentation and daytime sleepiness.[21] Fragmentation, as indexed by the number of brief EEG arousals, number of shifts from other sleep stages to stage I sleep or wake, and the percentage of stage I sleep, correlates with excessive sleepiness in various patient groups.[22] Experimental fragmentation of the sleep of healthy normals has been produced by inducing arousal with an auditory stimulus. Studies have shown that subjects aroused at various intervals during the night demonstrate performance decrements and increased sleepiness on the following day.[23–26]

CNS-depressant drugs, as might be expected, increase sleepiness. The benzodiazepine hypnotics hasten sleep onset at bedtime and shorten the latency to return to sleep after an awakening during the night, as demonstrated in a number of objective studies.[27,28] If taken at bedtime, long-acting benzodiazepines continue to shorten sleep latency on the MSLT the next day.[29] Ethanol administered at bedtime and during the day reduces sleep latency as measured by the MSLT.[30,31] One of the most commonly reported side effects associated with the use of $H_1$ antihistamines is daytime sleepiness, and studies with objective measurement of sleepiness have confirmed the effect.[32,33]

Disorders of the CNS are assumed to be another determinant of daytime sleepiness. An unidentified CNS disturbance is thought to cause excessive sleepiness in patients with narcolepsy.[34]

Another sleep disorder associated with excessive sleepiness and thought to be due to an unknown disorder of the CNS is idiopathic CNS hypersomnolence.[35] In both conditions, although the pathophysiology has not been definitively established, excessive sleepiness has been well-documented.[36,37]

A number of case series have presented MSLT results in patients with complaints of excessive daytime sleepiness.[38] These series have clearly shown that patients experiencing difficulties with excessive sleepiness can be differentiated from healthy normals based on the MSLT results. These patients typically have average sleep latencies of 8 minutes or less, whereas normals usually have average latencies of 10 minutes or more. (Deviations from the norm in healthy adults are discussed later.) In addition, SOREMPs are rarely seen in normal individuals, whereas the occurrence of two or more is considered specific to narcolepsy. Furthermore, the data have shown that differences in the severity of some sleep disorders are reflected in different levels of sleepiness on the MSLT. For example, patients with obstructive sleep apnea syndrome who have 40 or more apneas per hour of nocturnal sleep usually have average sleep latencies of 5 minutes or less, whereas those with fewer apneas per hour (20–40) have average latencies of 5–8 minutes and sometimes more. Finally, among sleep disorders associated with excessive daytime sleepiness, a differentiation in levels of sleepiness and frequency of SOREMPs can be seen. Patients with chronic insufficient sleep usually have a more moderate level of sleepiness (5–8 minutes) than do patients with narcolepsy or severe obstructive sleep apnea syndrome (no more than 5 minutes). Among sleep disorders patients, only those with narcolepsy show two or more SOREMPs.

The relationship between nocturnal sleep and daytime sleepiness (i.e., MSLT scores) in insomnia patients is not as clearly established. Insomnia patients do not necessarily complain of daytime sleepiness as the consequence of their perceived inadequate nocturnal sleep. Often the complaint is fatigue, tiredness, and dysphoria. In fact, some data suggest that insomnia patients may be hyperalert.[39] Although showing shortened nocturnal sleep compared to age-matched, healthy controls, this group of insomnia patients has unusually high average sleep latencies (i.e., >15 minutes).

*Evaluation of Therapeutic Interventions*

A number of studies have shown that MSLT levels in various sleep disorders are improved after appropriate therapeutic intervention. Two current treatments of obstructive sleep apnea syndrome are continuous positive airway pressure (CPAP) and uvulopalatopharyngoplasty (UPPP). CPAP provides a pneumatic splint of the airway, eliminating the upper airway obstructions and thus the brief arousals that fragment sleep. This improved sleep is associated with normalization of the MSLT.[40] UPPP, a surgical treatment aimed at removing excess upper airway tissue and thus establishing a patent airway, is less consistently successful. In those patients who benefit from the surgery, apneas are reduced, sleep is improved, and the MSLT level of sleepiness is normalized[41]; but in patients whose apnea does not improve, the MSLT result remains at presurgery levels, even though patients perceive a subjective improvement in alertness. This once again indicates the inaccuracy of subjective assessments of sleepiness and alertness.

## MODIFICATIONS OF THE MULTIPLE SLEEP LATENCY TEST

The basic MSLT procedure has been modified in various ways, with no clear improvement. The first such modification was a change in the instructions to "try and stay awake" while lying in bed in a quiet, dark room.[42] The instruction does produce longer sleep latencies, but the change did not increase sensitivity of the MSLT.[43] A subsequent variation, the Maintenance of Wakefulness Test (MWT), instructs the subject to stay awake while seated in a chair.[44] Again, longer sleep latencies result from the change, but improvement in sensitivity over the MSLT has not been documented. Finally, the Modified Assessment of Sleepiness Test (MAST) has been offered as an alternative to the MSLT.[45] It consists of three standard sleep latency tests (with a "try to sleep" instruction) alternating with two tests of the subject's ability to remain awake while seated in a chair reading a book. As indicated above, MSLT reliability begins to decline as the number of tests is reduced; this is also found with the MAST. Improved sensitivity has not been established for the MAST.

The intent of the MSLT modifications is to measure a subject's ability to remain awake. It is argued that, clinically, the patient's problem is remaining awake (which adds a certain face validity to the instruction to remain awake). The ability to stay awake is a function of many factors that can momentarily override the underlying physiologic state, including the motivation to remain awake, presence of competing motives, the environment, and time of day. Consequently, the ability to maintain wakefulness varies significantly between individuals and hour to hour within an individual. No single laboratory test is generalizable to the variety of circumstances under which wakefulness is to be maintained. The MSLT attempts to remove the confounding factors and measure the underlying physiologic state, thus defining the patient's maximal risk.

Correlations among the standard MSLT and these modified versions of the MSLT and also with two widely used subjective measures of sleepiness, the Epworth Sleepiness Scale and the Sleep-Wake Activity Inventory, are relatively weak.[46,47] This has led some to argue that there are different types of or dimensions to sleepiness. A more parsimonious and valid explanation, however, is that the methodologies differ in sensitivity. Another more plausible explanation is that rather than different kinds of sleepiness, there are different levels of ability to detect sleepiness, different environmental demands for alertness, and different abilities to counteract sleepiness. Additional constructs have utility and become meaningful when the same variable affects the constructs in different ways. This has not been demonstrated for the various versions of the MSLT.

## MULTIPLE SLEEP LATENCY TEST NORMS

Enough data on the MSLT have now been collected in normal and patient populations to describe the range of normal and abnormal values. In several reports of healthy, noncomplaining adults using a four-test MSLT, younger subjects aged 21–35 years had an average daily sleep latency of 10 minutes, adults aged 30–49 years had an average latency of 11–12 minutes, and subjects 50–59 years old averaged a latency of 9 minutes.[48,49] For the older subjects, nocturnal sleep efficiency was lower than that of the other age groups, and periodic leg movements during sleep were observed in 50% of the sample. In samples of healthy, normal individuals, some have latencies in the pathologic range (no more than 5 minutes), but they differ from sleep disorders patients in that the sleepiness is not persistent. With adequate sleep over a number of nights, the average daily sleep latency increases, reaching the population norm.[50]

Evidence for pathologic sleepiness is considered to be an average daily sleep latency of no more than 5 minutes. An average latency of 5–8 minutes is considered borderline pathologic. Latencies of 9 minutes and greater are considered normal.

## REFERENCES

1. National Sleep Foundation. Sleepiness in America. Princeton, NJ: Gallup Organization, 1997.
2. Hublin C, Kaprio J, Partinen M, et al. Daytime sleepiness in the Finnish population. J Intern Med 1996;239:417.
3. Lavie P. Sleep habits and sleep disturbances in industrial workers in Israel: main findings and some characteristics of workers complaining of excessive daytime sleepiness. Sleep 1981;4:147.
4. Bixler ED, Kales A, Soldatos CR, et al. Prevalence of sleep disorders in the Los Angeles metropolitan area. Am J Psychol 1979;136:1257.
5. Lugaresi E, Cirignotta F, Zucconi M, et al. Good and Poor Sleepers: An Epidemiological Survey of the San Marino Population. In C Guilleminault, E Lugaresi (eds), Sleep/Wake Disorders: Natural History, Epidemiology, and Long-Term Evolution. New York: Raven, 1983;2.
6. Navelet Y, Anders T, Guilleminault C. Narcolepsy in Children. In C Guilleminault, WC Dement, P Passouant (eds), Narcolepsy. New York: Spectrum, 1976;171.
7. Pack AL, Pack AM, Radgman E, et al. Characteristics of crashes attributed to the driver having fallen asleep. Accid Anal Prev 1995;27:769.
8. Folkard S. Shiftwork and Performance. In LC Johnson, DI Tepas, WJ Colquhoun, MJ Colligan (eds), The Twenty-Four Hour Workday: Proceedings of a Symposium on Variations in Work-Sleep Schedules. DHHS Publication No. 81-127. Washington, DC: US Government Printing Office, 1981;347.
9. Webb WB. Sleep Deprivation: Total, Partial and Selective. In MH Chase (ed), The Sleeping Brain. Los Angeles: UCLA Brain Information Service/Brain Research Institute, 1972;323.
10. Hoddes E, Zarcone VP, Smythe H, et al. Quantification of sleepiness: a new approach. Psychophysiology 1973;10:431.
11. Dement WC, Carskadon MA, Richardson GS. Excessive Daytime Sleepiness in the Sleep Apnea Syndrome. In C Guilleminault, WC Dement (eds), Sleep Apnea Syndromes. New York: Liss, 1978;23.

12. Carskadon MA, Dement W. The multiple sleep latency test: what does it measure? Sleep 1982;5:S67.

13. Carskadon MA, Dement WC, Mitler M, et al. Guidelines for the Multiple Sleep Latency Test (MSLT): a standard measure of sleepiness. Sleep 1986;9:519.

14. Rechtschaffen A, Kales A. A Manual of Standardized Techniques and Scoring System for Sleep Stages of Human Sleep. Los Angeles: UCLA Brain Information Service/Brain Research Institute, 1968.

15. Zwyghuizen-Doorenbos A, Roehrs T, Schaefer M, et al. Test-retest reliability of the MSLT. Sleep 1988;11:562.

16. Seidel WF, Dement WC. The Multiple Sleep Latency Test: test-retest reliability. Sleep Res 1981;10:105.

17. Folkerts M, Rosenthal L, Roehrs T, et al. The reliability of the diagnostic features in patients with narcolepsy. Biol Psychiatry 1996;40:208.

18. Carskadon MA, Dement WC. Nocturnal determinants of daytime sleepiness. Sleep 1982;5:S73.

19. Carskadon MA, Dement WC. Cumulative effects of sleep restriction on daytime sleepiness. Psychophysiology 1981;18:107.

20. Roehrs T, Shore E, Papineau K, et al. A two-week sleep extension in sleepy normals. Sleep 1996;19:576.

21. Carskadon MA, Brown E, Dement WC. Sleep fragmentation in the elderly: relationship to daytime sleep tendency. Neurobiol Aging 1982;3:321.

22. Stepanski E, Lamphere J, Badia P, et al. Sleep fragmentation and daytime sleepiness. Sleep 1984;7:18.

23. Bonnet MH. The effect of sleep disruption on performance, sleep, and mood. Sleep 1985;8:11.

24. Bonnet MH. Performance and sleepiness as a function of the frequency and placement of sleep disruption. Psychophysiology 1986;23:263.

25. Roehrs T, Merlotti L, Petrucelli N, et al. Experimental sleep fragmentation. Sleep 1994;17:438.

26. Levine B, Roehrs T, Stepanski E, et al. Fragmenting sleep diminishes its recuperative value. Sleep 1987;10:590.

27. Roth T, Zorick F, Wittig R, Roehrs T. Pharmacological and medical considerations in hypnotic use. Sleep 1982;5:S46.

28. Nicholson AN. The use of short- and long-acting hypnotics in clinical medicine. Br J Clin Pharmacol 1981;11:615.

29. Roth T, Roehrs T. Determinants of residual effects of hypnotics. Accid Anal Prev 1985;17:291.

30. MacLean A, Cairns J. Dose-response effects of ethanol on the sleep of young men. J Stud Alcohol 1982;43:433.

31. Zwyghuizen-Doorenbos A, Roehrs T, Lamphere J, et al. Increased daytime sleepiness enhances ethanol's sedative effects. Neuropsychopharmacology 1988;1:279.

32. Roehrs T, Tietz E, Zorick F, Roth T. Daytime sleepiness and antihistamines. Sleep 1984;7:137.

33. Nicholson AN, Stone BM. Antihistamines: impaired performance and the tendency to sleep. Eur J Clin Pharmacol 1986;30:27.

34. Kilduff TS, Bowersox SS, Kaitin KI, et al. Muscarinic cholinergic receptors and the canine model of narcolepsy. Sleep 1986;9:102.

35. American Sleep Disorders Association. The International Classification of Sleep Disorders: Diagnostic and Coding Manual (rev ed). Rochester, MN: American Sleep Disorders Association, 1997;46.

36. Zorick F, Roehrs T, Koshorek G, et al. Patterns of sleepiness in various disorders of excessive daytime somnolence. Sleep 1982;5:S165.

37. Coleman R, Roffwarg H, Kennedy S, Guilleminault C. Sleep-wake disorders based upon a polysomnographic diagnosis—a national cooperative study. JAMA 1981;247:997.

38. Roth T, Roehrs T, Carskadon M, Dement W. Daytime Sleepiness and Alertness. In M Kryger, T Roth, WC Dement (eds), Principles and Practice of Sleep Medicine. Philadelphia: Saunders, 1989;14.

39. Stepanski E, Zorick F, Roehrs T, et al. Daytime alertness in patients with chronic insomnia compared with asymptomatic control subjects. Sleep 1986;11:54.

40. Lamphere J, Roehrs T, Wittig R, et al. Recovery of alertness after CPAP in apnea. Chest 1989;96:1364.

41. Zorick F, Roehrs T, Conway W, et al. Effects of uvulopalatopharyngoplasty on the daytime sleepiness associated with sleep apnea syndrome. Bull Eur Pathophysiol Res 1983;19:600.

42. Hartse KM, Roth T, Zorick FJ. Daytime sleepiness and daytime wakefulness: the effect of instruction. Sleep 1982;5:S107.

43. Hilloker NAJ, Muehlbach MJ, Schweitzer PK, et al. Sleepiness/alertness on a simulated night shift schedule and morningness-eveningness tendency. Sleep 1992;15:430.

44. Mitler MM, Gujavarty KS, Browman CP. Maintenance of wakefulness test: a polysomnographic technique for evaluating treatment efficacy in patients with excessive somnolence. Electroencephalogr Clin Neurophysiol 1982;53:658.

45. Erman MK, Beckham B, Gardner DA, Roffwarg HP. The modified assessment of sleepiness test (MAST). Sleep Res 1987;16:550.

46. Johns MW. A new method for measuring daytime sleepiness: the Epworth Sleepiness Scale. Sleep 1991;14:540.

47. Rosenthal L, Roehrs TA, Roth T. The Sleep Wake Activity Inventory: a self-report measure of daytime sleepiness. Biol Psychiatry 1993;34:810.

48. Levine B, Roehrs T, Zorick F, Roth T. Daytime sleepiness in young adults. Sleep 1988;11:39.

49. Roehrs T, Zorick F, McLeaghan A, et al. Sleep and MSLT norms for middle adults. Sleep Res 1984;13:87.

50. Roehrs T, Timms V, Zwyghuizen-Dorrenbos A, et al. Sleep extension in sleepy and alert normals. Sleep 1989;12:449.

# Chapter 14

# Maintenance of Wakefulness Test

Karl Doghramji

The maintenance of wakefulness test (MWT) is a polysomnographic procedure used to evaluate the extent of daytime somnolence. It assesses an individual's ability to successfully resist the urge to fall asleep (i.e., the ability to remain awake) during soporific circumstances and provides, therefore, an objective measure of *wake tendency*. The instructions to the patient comprise a key difference between this procedure and the multiple sleep latency test (MSLT) (see Chapter 13), which is also used for the evaluation of daytime somnolence. Whereas during the MWT patients are instructed to resist the urge to fall asleep, during the MSLT they are instructed to yield to this urge. It follows that the MSLT measures an individual's ability to fall asleep, or *sleep tendency*. Therefore, the MWT and the MSLT differ substantially in the functions that they assess.

## HISTORICAL OVERVIEW

Daytime nap studies have been used extensively as a way of assessing the extent of daytime somnolence.[1–5] The first procedure to be used extensively for clinical purposes was the MSLT introduced by Richardson and his colleagues in 1978.[6] Initially, its primary application had been the confirmation of the diagnosis of narcolepsy by the demonstration of pathologic levels of physiologic daytime sleepiness. It was soon applied to other disorders of excessive somnolence as well, most notably obstructive sleep apnea syndrome,[7] both at baseline and after treat-

ment. Concerns were expressed, however, that the MSLT did not accurately measure the clinical function of greatest interest in sleepy patients. Whereas the MSLT assesses how easily patients succumb to sleep, the function of greater relevance is how successful they are in resisting this urge, given that the latter more closely reflects the challenge patients face in the soporific situations of everyday life such as driving and reading. Hartse and colleagues[8] noted that sleep latency on a multiple nap study did increase by changing instructions from "try to sleep" to "try to stay awake" in normal subjects. Accordingly, Mitler and colleagues[9,10] developed the MWT and reported both the methodology and results in ten narcoleptics and eight controls. Mean sleep latency differed significantly between narcoleptics and controls (9.9 vs. 17.9 minutes, respectively). Narcoleptics exhibited an average of 3.2 sleep-onset REM episodes over the five sessions versus none for the controls. Sleep latency increased by 300% when instructions were changed from "try to sleep" to "try to remain awake." Nevertheless, eight narcoleptics who were retested after treatment did not exhibit a significant increase in MWT sleep latency. In the intervening years, the MWT has been used clinically to quantify the extent of daytime somnolence, to assess the effects of treatment in sleepy patients, and to determine patients' suitability for performing tasks at home and in the workplace.

Despite diversity in methodology over the years, the core aspects of the test have remained constant.

After a night of polysomnography, and while being monitored polysomnographically, patients are given four to five opportunities, at 2-hour intervals, to remain awake while comfortably reclining in a bed or armchair. The first trial begins at 10:00 AM. Patients are instructed to remain awake as long as possible. Depending on the application, trials are terminated either at sleep onset or after a constant period of sleep. The sleep latency is calculated for each wakefulness opportunity and an average sleep latency score is reported. The sleep latency score is regarded as being inversely proportional to the extent of daytime somnolence.

Methodologic diversity has existed in various areas. These include polysomnographic montage, illuminance level, seating position, room temperature, meal timing, and patient instructions. Methodologic uniformity is clearly important, so that results of various trials can be compared and so that individual patient results can be assessed in the context of normative data. The two methodologic areas of greatest concern are the definition of sleep onset and duration of each wakefulness opportunity. The initial studies of Mitler and colleagues[9,10] used a stringent definition of sleep onset (three 30-second epochs of stage I or one epoch of any other sleep stage). Later studies with obstructive sleep apnea patients by Sangal and colleagues[11,12] used a more lenient definition of sleep onset (one 30-second epoch of any sleep stage). The former, stricter definition of sleep onset would be expected to yield longer sleep latency scores than the latter. Similarly, wakefulness opportunity durations have varied between 20 and 40 minutes. Scores for the 40-minute trial would be expected to be longer.

## NORMATIVE DATA

Doghramji and colleagues[13] obtained normative data for the MWT using various criteria for trial duration and definition of sleep onset. They adhered to uniform MWT procedural conditions, however, including polysomnographic montage, illuminance level, seating position, room temperature, meal timing, and subject instructions. The study was conducted across six centers and included 64 healthy subjects (27 men and 37 women) with ages ranging between 30 and 70 years. On the day after nocturnal polysomnography, subjects were given four 40-minute MWT trials at 2-hour intervals, with the first trial beginning at 10:00 AM. Bedrooms were dimly lit and illuminance was measured at 0.10–0.13 lux at the corneal level. Subjects sat up in bed with their backs and heads supported by a cushion. Ambient temperature was kept at 72°F. Meals were given 1 hour before the first MWT trial and immediately after the termination of the noon trial. Subjects were given the following instructions: "Please sit still and remain awake for as long as possible. Look ahead of you, and do not look directly at the light." Subjects were not allowed to maintain wakefulness by using extraordinary measures such as slapping the face or singing.

In the study by Doghramji and colleagues,[13] each wakefulness trial was terminated either at the first onset of sleep or, if sleep onset was not achieved, after a maximum in-bed duration of 40 minutes. Sleep onset was defined as the first occurrence of sustained sleep (three consecutive 30-second epochs of stage I or any single 30-second epoch of another sleep stage—II, III, IV, or REM). An effort was made to compare results of this normative trial with those of earlier trials that had used different methods. Therefore, sleep latency scores were calculated on the basis of a sleep onset defined as the first epoch of any sleep stage. Similarly, although the study was conducted with a maximum wakefulness trial duration of 40 minutes, sleep latency scores were also calculated on the basis of 20-minute trial durations. Therefore, the trial not only yielded normative data, but also allowed for comparison of these data to those of previous trials using various methods. The results were obtained using the following four protocols:

1. SUSMWT40: 40-minute MWT trials with sleep onset defined as three continuous epochs of stage I sleep or any single epoch of another sleep stage
2. MWT40: 40-minute MWT trials with sleep onset defined as the first epoch of any sleep stage
3. SUSMWT20: 20-minute MWT trials with sleep onset defined as three continuous epochs of stage I sleep or any single epoch of another sleep stage
4. MWT20: 20-minute MWT trials with sleep onset defined as the first appearance of any sleep stage

Normative data obtained from the trial are summarized in Tables 14-1 and 14-2. As anticipated, longer maximum trial durations yielded longer sleep latency scores. It is also of interest that for the 20-

**Table 14-1.** Individual and Average Maintenance of Wakefulness Test Sleep Latency Scores[a] for the SUSMWT40[b] Protocol

|                 | Trial 1 | Trial 2 | Trial 3 | Trial 4 | Mean |
|-----------------|---------|---------|---------|---------|------|
| Mean            | 36.3    | 34.0    | 34.2    | 36.5    | 35.2 |
| Standard deviation | 9.2  | 12.0    | 11.5    | 8.8     | 7.9  |
| Minimum         | 3.0     | 4.5     | 3.5     | 1.2     | 7.1  |
| Maximum         | 40.0    | 40.0    | 40.0    | 40.0    | 40.0 |
| 10th percentile | 18.2    | 9.6     | 11.5    | 25.4    | 21.7 |
| 25th percentile | 40.0    | 40.0    | 40.0    | 40.0    | 32.8 |
| 50th percentile | 40.0    | 40.0    | 40.0    | 40.0    | 40.0 |
| 75th percentile | 40.0    | 40.0    | 40.0    | 40.0    | 40.0 |
| 90th percentile | 40.0    | 40.0    | 40.0    | 40.0    | 40.0 |

[a]Sleep latency scores are in minutes.
[b]40-minute maintenance of wakefulness test trials with sleep onset defined as three continuous epochs of stage I sleep or any single epoch of another sleep stage.
Source: Reprinted with permission from K Doghramji, M Mitler, RB Sangal, et al. A normative study of the maintenance of wakefulness test (MWT). Electroencephalogr Clin Neurophysiol 1997;103:554.

minute protocols, normal cutoff scores were close to the corresponding score of 10 minutes for the MSLT,[14] which also uses a 20-minute maximum trial duration. Although the normal MWT scores are based on empirical data and a statistical definition of normality, however, the normal MSLT cutoff of 10 minutes is consensus based.

## CLINICAL APPLICATIONS

Normative data allow clinicians to determine whether a given individual is "normal" in terms of wake tendency during soporific daytime tasks. Cutoff points for normality are often considered to be two standard deviations from the mean.[15] Applying this definition to the normative data of Doghramji and colleagues[13] yields low limits for normality (Table 14-3). Depending on the protocol used, therefore, individuals scoring below these cutoff points would be considered "too sleepy."

An example of the application of these threshold values is their comparison to the MWT results of 258 patients with complaints of sleepiness reported by Sangal and colleagues.[11] Nineteen percent had mean sleep latency scores of less than 10.9 minutes on the MWT20, and the same number had scores of less than 12.9 minutes on the MWT40. Thus, 19% of these patients can be considered to be "too sleepy" by these criteria.

The MWT has also been used clinically in various disorders associated with excessive daytime somnolence such as narcolepsy and sleep apnea syndrome, as summarized in Table 14-2.[11,12,16–18] Its main application in these studies has been the evaluation of the extent of impairment in daytime wakefulness through comparison with healthy controls. As is evident in Table 14-2, regardless of the protocol used, normative data exhibit scores that are significantly higher than those of patients with disorders of excessive somnolence. These results strongly support the MWT's usefulness in differentiating groups with normal daytime alertness from those with impaired ability. The MWT has also proven to be sensitive in assessing treatment efficacy of continuous positive airway pressure in obstructive sleep apnea syndrome[12] and various pharmacologic agents in narcolepsy.[19-21] It has proven less useful than the MSLT as a diagnostic test for narcolepsy,[16] however, because it is less likely to capture REM sleep episodes.

The MWT has been effectively used in the following applications:

1. Assessing whether a given individual is "normal" in terms of wake tendency during soporific daytime tasks
2. Differentiating groups with normal daytime alertness from those who are impaired
3. Determining the efficacy of treatment in disorders of excessive somnolence

**Table 14-2.** Comparison of Maintenance of Wakefulness Test (MWT) Normative with Clinical Data

| Study | Sample | N | Sleep Onset Criteria | Trial Duration[a] | Protocol | Mean Sleep Latency | P[b] |
|---|---|---|---|---|---|---|---|
| Doghramji et al., 1997[13] | Normals | 64 | A | 40 | SUSMWT40 | 35.2 ± 7.9 | |
| | | | A | 20 | SUSMWT20 | 18.7 ± 2.6 | |
| | | | B[c] | 40 | MWT40 | 32.6 ± 9.9 | |
| | | | B[c] | 20 | MWT20 | 18.1 ± 3.6 | |
| Poceta et al., 1992[18] | OSA | 322 | A | 40 | SUSMWT40 | 25.9 ± 11.8 | <.0001 |
| Sangal et al., 1992[11] | Excessive daytime sleepiness | 258 | B | 20[d] | MWT20[d] | 15.9 ± 5.0 | <.001 |
| | Excessive daytime sleepiness | 258 | B | 40 | MWT40 | 26.5 ± 12.4 | <.001 |
| Browman et al., 1986[17] | Narcolepsy | 11 | A | 20 | SUSMWT20 | 10.7 ± 5.3 | <.001 |
| | Normals | 11 | A | 20 | SUSMWT20 | 19.0 ± 1.5 | >.05 |
| Browman et al., 1983[16] | Narcolepsy | 12 | A | 20 | SUSMWT20 | 11.0 ± 5.6 | <.001 |
| | OSA | 12 | A | 20 | SUSMWT20 | 11.0 ± 4.8 | <.001 |
| | Normals | 10 | A | 20 | SUSMWT20 | 18.3 ± 4.0 | >.05 |
| Mitler et al., 1982[9] | Narcolepsy | 10 | A | 20 | SUSMWT20 | 9.9 ± 6.1 | <.001 |
| | Normals | 8 | A | 20 | SUSMWT20 | 17.9 ± 4.4 | >.05 |

A = three 30-second epochs of stage I or one epoch of any other sleep stage; B = one 30-second epoch of any sleep stage; SUSMWT40 = 40-minute MWT trials with sleep onset defined as three continuous epochs of stage I sleep or any single epoch of another sleep stage; MWT40 = 40-minute MWT trials with sleep onset defined as the first epoch of any sleep stage; SUSMWT20 = 20-minute MWT trials with sleep onset defined as three continuous epochs of stage I sleep or any single epoch of another sleep stage; MWT20 = 20-minute MWT trials with sleep onset defined as the first appearance of any sleep stage; OSA = obstructive sleep apnea.
[a]Trial durations are in minutes and mean sleep latency scores in minutes ± standard deviation.
[b]Compared with corresponding measure of sleep latency in K Doghramji, M Mitler, RB Sangal, et al. A normative study of the maintenance of wakefulness test (MWT). Electroencephalogr Clin Neurophysiol 1997;103:554.
[c]Or 10 seconds of microsleep.
[d]Data based on a 40-minute protocol were recalculated for the 20-minute protocol.
Source: K Doghramji, M Mitler, RB Sangal, et al. A normative study of the maintenance of wakefulness test (MWT). Electroencephalogr Clin Neurophysiol 1997;103:554.

## RELATIONSHIP WITH THE MULTIPLE SLEEP LATENCY TEST

That the MSLT and the MWT assess separate functions is supported by the lack of a consistent relationship between the two when applied to the same patient groups.[11,17] Therefore, each may have a unique set of clinical applications. Various studies have indicated that, whereas the MSLT is not particularly sensitive in detecting treatment effects in patient groups, the MWT is.[12,22] The MWT is also sensitive in detecting the effects of the manipulation of the previous night's sleep quality and quantity on daytime alertness.[23] It stands to reason that the MWT may be more accurate in assessing the risk of falling asleep unintentionally during soporific activities when individuals are attempting to stay awake, such as driving, reading, and other activities of daily life. However, no such comparisons between the two tests have been yet performed. Clearly, more study is needed to explore the reasons for the discordance between the two tests and the relative usefulness of each.

## CONCLUSIONS AND RECOMMENDATIONS

As noted above, various definitions of sleep onset and trial duration have been used for the MWT

**Table 14-3.** Lower Limits for Normality as Assessed by Two Standard Deviations Lower than the Mean for Various Maintenance of Wakefulness Test Protocols

| Protocol | Lower Limit* | % Subjects Scoring Less than Lower Limit |
|----------|--------------|------------------------------------------|
| SUSMWT40 | 19.4 | 8 |
| MWT40 | 12.9 | 9 |
| SUSMWT20 | 13.5 | 6 |
| MWT20 | 10.9 | 8 |

*Mean minus two standard deviations in minutes.
Source: K Doghramji, M Mitler, RB Sangal, et al. A normative study of the maintenance of wakefulness test (MWT). Electroencephalogr Clin Neurophysiol 1997;103:554.

since its introduction. Regardless of definition, however, the MWT appears to be capable of separating sleepy from nonsleepy individuals. Therefore, the determination of which of these protocols should be used in each case can be based on the specific clinical need and the nature of practical constraints. For example, if the sample being tested is likely to have subjects with a low level of sleepiness, it may be desirable to maximize the test's sensitivity by using the 40-minute trial duration and the first appearance of any epoch of sleep. The same protocol may be best suited for assessing treatment response. If diagnostic accuracy is critical, however, as in medico-legal settings, or if test results are to be used to establish the presence or absence of an illness, the more stringent definition of sleep onset (three epochs of stage I or one epoch of any other sleep stage) may be preferred. Practical, economic limitations may favor the use of the 20-minute duration.

For routine clinical applications, Doghramji and colleagues[13] recommend use of the 20-minute protocol with sleep latency measured to the onset of any sleep stage. They note that the 20-minute protocols are more cost-effective and, unlike the 40-minute protocol, are not affected by age. Following are their recommendations:

1. The room should be maximally insulated from external light. The light source should be positioned slightly behind the subject's head, so that it is just out of his or her field of vision, and should produce an illuminance of 0.10–0.13 lux at the corneal level. (In Doghramji and colleagues,[13] a 7.5-W night light was used, positioned 1 foot from the floor and 3 feet laterally removed from the subject's head.)

2. The subject should sit in bed, with his or her back and head supported by a cushion or pillow that prevents the neck from being uncomfortably flexed or extended during sleep.

3. Room temperature should be as close to 22°C (72°F) as possible. Temperature should be recorded at the beginning of each trial.

4. The subject should eat a light breakfast at least 1 hour before the first nap and a light lunch immediately after the termination of the noon nap.

5. Subjects should be given the following instructions: "Please sit still and remain awake for as long as possible. Look directly ahead of you, and do not look directly at the light." Subjects should not be allowed to use extraordinary measures to stay awake, such as slapping the face or singing.

6. The following monitoring montage should be used: C3/A2, O1/A2, electromyography, electrooculography.

7. Sleep onset should be defined as the first occurrence of one epoch of any stage of sleep.

8. Trials should be performed at 2-hour intervals, the first beginning at 10:00 AM.

9. A trial should be terminated at sleep onset or after 20 minutes in bed if sleep onset is not achieved.

10. Sleep latency should be defined as the time from trial onset to the first epoch of any sleep stage.

11. Sleep latency, total sleep time, total wake time, and stages of sleep achieved should be recorded for each trial.

12. Impairment in wake tendency exists if the mean sleep latency is less than 11 minutes.

## REFERENCES

1. Tepas D. Evolved brain response as a measure of human sleep and wakefulness. Aerospace Med 1967;38:148.
2. Weitzman E, Nogeire C, Perlow M, et al. Effects of a prolonged three-hour sleep-wake cycle on sleep stages, plasma cortisol, growth hormone and body temperature in man. J Clin Endocrinol Metab 1974;38:1018.
3. Carskadon M, Dement W. Effects of total sleep loss on sleep tendency. Percept Mot Skills 1979;48:495.

4. Moses J, Hord D, Lubin A, et al. Dynamics of nap sleep during a 40-hour period. Electroencephalogr Clin Neurophysiol 1975;39:627.

5. Webb W, Agnew H. Sleep efficiency for sleep-wake cycles of varied length. Psychophysiology 1975;12:637.

6. Richardson G, Carskadon M, Flagg W, et al. Excessive daytime sleepiness in man: multiple sleep latency test measurements in narcoleptic vs. control subjects. Electroencephalogr Clin Neurophysiol 1978;45:621.

7. Roth T, Hartse KM, Zorick F, Conway W. Multiple naps in the evaluation of daytime sleepiness in patients with upper airway sleep apnea. Sleep 1980;3:425.

8. Hartse K, Roth T, Zorick F, Zammit G. The effect of instruction upon sleep latency during multiple daytime naps of normal subjects. Sleep Res 1980;9:123.

9. Mitler MM, Gujavarty KS, Browman CP. Maintenance of wakefulness test: a polysomnographic technique for evaluating treatment efficacy in patients with excessive somnolence. Electroencephalogr Clin Neurophysiol 1982;53:658.

10. Mitler MM, Gujavarty KS, Sampson MG, Browman CP. Multiple daytime nap approaches to evaluating the sleepy patient. Sleep 1982;5:S119.

11. Sangal RB, Thomas L, Mitler MM. Maintenance of Wakefulness Test and Multiple Sleep Latency Test. Measurement of different abilities in patients with sleep disorders. Chest 1992;101:898.

12. Sangal RB, Thomas L, Mitler MM. Disorders of excessive sleepiness: treatment improves ability to stay awake but does not reduce sleepiness. Chest 1992;102:699.

13. Doghramji K, Mitler M, Sangal RB, et al. A normative study of the maintenance of wakefulness test (MWT). Electroencephalogr Clin Neurophysiol 1997;103:554.

14. Carskadon MA. Guidelines for the multiple sleep latency test (MSLT): a standard measure of sleepiness. Sleep 1986;9:519.

15. American Electroencephalographic Society guidelines in electroencephalography evoked potentials, and polysomnography. J Clin Neurophysiol 1994;11:1.

16. Browman CP, Gujavarty KG, Sampson MG, Mitler MM. REM sleep episodes during the maintenance of wakefulness test in patients with sleep apnea and narcolepsy. Sleep 1983;6:23.

17. Browman CP, Gujavarty KS, Yolles S, Mitler MM. Forty-eight hour polysomnographic evaluation of narcolepsy. Sleep 1986;9:183.

18. Poceta JS, Timms RM, Jeong D, et al. Maintenance of wakefulness test in obstructive sleep apnea syndrome. Chest 1992;101:893.

19. Fry JM, Pressman MR, DiPhillipo MA, Frost-Paulus M. Treatment of narcolepsy with codeine. Sleep 1986;9:269.

20. Mitler MM, Hajdukovic RM, Erman M, Koziol JA. Narcolepsy. J Clin Neurophysiol 1990;7:93.

21. Mitler MM, Shafor R, Hajdukovich R, et al. Treatment of narcolepsy: objective studies on methylphenidate, pemoline, and protriptyline. Sleep 1986;9:260.

22. Gaddy JR, Doghramji K. Daytime sleepiness after nCPAP treatment. Sleep Res 1991;20:245.

23. Sugarman JL, Walsh JK. Physiological sleep tendency and ability to maintain alertness at night. Sleep 1989;12:106.

# Chapter 15
# Computerized and Portable Sleep Recording

## Max Hirshkowitz and Constance A. Moore

Computerized systems have revolutionized the way many of us perform our work in the field of sleep disorders research. This is most apparent in office applications; however, embedded microprocessors probably have even more influence. Equipment design incorporates digital technology, making machines "smarter" and easier to operate. Often, the cost is less flexibility. For tasks that are performed hundreds or thousands of times in precisely the same manner, computerization is a natural extension of applied technology. The more standardized the task, the more amenable it is to automation. This applies to procedures in which all judgment points can be identified and criteria can be operationalized. Difficulties arise when controversy surrounds judgment criteria at a decision point. Unfortunately, sometimes technologies are accepted in the interest of expediency rather than on the basis of sound reasoning.

In the 1970s, the small computer was the single most flexible piece of laboratory equipment available. The laboratory computer served as a programmable analytic and data collection tool. It is ironic, therefore, that computers now seem so inflexible. This is the result of the decline in locally available programming resources. *End users*, rather than programmers, now serve as the principal operators of computerized systems and their knowledge is usually limited to parameters of particular commercially available programs.

Complex programs (now called *systems*) characteristically require pseudoprogramming for opera-tion. Specific instruction sets exist for these systems. Computerized polysomnographic systems have elaborate instruction sets often presented to the end user as menu selections. In some ways, operating instruction sets are taking the place of programming languages. Systems may support macro instructions, batch-processing routines, profile settings, and option sets in addition to menu-driven selection. Modern complex systems can incorporate a dazzling array of options. Learning to use a program often amounts to learning what options are available and how to apply them. It is common for an end user to understand and use only a small percentage of the available options. In computer jargon, an adept end user who achieves a fairly complete command of available options is called a *power user*. This individual typically serves as the work environment's computer guru.

The essential difference between end users and programmers affects a laboratory's technical environment. An end user tells the programming what to do, whereas a programmer tells the computer what to do. The programming directs computer operations. If programming does not contain the desired procedure in its instruction repertoire, however, it may select a procedure that is similar but incorrect. Alternatively, the programming may fail to perform the requested procedure, display an error message, or both.

Some difficulty arises from ambiguity in natural language. The vast majority of words have more than one meaning. The meaning can be either systematically related or unrelated. This underlies part of the reason that communication problems occur so frequently. Consider the term *arousal*. Until recently, there existed no standardized guideline for recording or scoring brief arousals from sleep. When an end user requests arousal scoring, the computerized system may provide tabulation of arousals scored according to increased electromyography (EMG) activity rather than American Sleep Disorders Association (ASDA) criteria. It could be argued that having some index of arousal is better than none. Because it is easier to enter a few keystrokes than to manually review a polysomnogram and identify each electroencephalography (EEG) arousal, expediency becomes a major factor. Herein lies one danger associated with computerized polysomnography: *the sloth factor.*

Computers seduce us into taking an easy avenue. The impressive graphics and reams of printout can enamor one to the point of becoming amnestic about the original misgivings concerning the computational procedure. When this happens, the end user has succumbed to form over content. Seeming efficiency should never be confused with cost-effectiveness, especially because cost-effectiveness is the first in the triad of good reasons for using a computerized system.

## REASONS TO USE A COMPUTER

Basically, there are three good reasons to use a computer: (1) cost-effectiveness, (2) standardization and accuracy, and (3) opening new horizons. The commercial success of automation largely derives from its cost-effectiveness. Word processors are much more efficient than typewriters for creating and revising manuscripts. Computerized telephone switching has replaced legions of switchboard operators. Standardization is a natural byproduct of automation. Form entry systems require a rigorously systematic approach for appropriate operation. For numerical data, computerized system accuracy is unparalleled (assuming correct programming). Accuracy is so well-recognized that we have come to consider computers infallible with respect to arithmetic operations.

The most exciting computer applications are those that allow us to expand our horizons. In sleep disorders research, waveform analysis provides the opportunity to explore sleep in a manner not feasible with manual scoring. Two analytic approaches commonly used for sleep research include power spectral analysis (PSA) and period amplitude analysis. PSA most commonly relies on fast Fourier transform (FFT) for waveform decomposition. FFT uses phase and amplitude information to calculate power (voltage × time) at each frequency. Power can be grouped according to frequency ranges occurring during the course of an epoch. We refer to this as a *frequency domain analysis*. By contrast, a *time domain analysis* calculates the amount of time spent in each frequency range. It accomplishes this by calculating frequency from time intervals between successive voltage zero crossings. High-amplitude waves commonly contain higher-frequency waveforms riding on them. For example, consider the case of sleep spindles intermixed with delta waves. The individual spindle waveforms do not necessarily cross the zero voltage point and therefore might go undetected. If zero crossing of the first derivative is determined, however, one detects changes in direction (positive to negative and vice versa). The intervals between polarity changes can be used to capture frequency of waves failing to cross the actual or averaged zero point. Amplitude can be determined by tabulating voltages at zero crossings.

When using computerized waveform analysis, adherence to certain technical standards is critical.[1] According to published guidelines, calibration is mandatory at the beginning of the recording and highly recommended at the end. The Nyquist theorem stipulates a sampling rate at minimally twice the highest frequency in the signal. If higher frequencies are not filtered out, artifactual low-frequency components (aliasing) will likely occur. An alternative is to sample four to five times faster than the high-frequency filtering rate.[2]

Some direct memory–access analogs to digital convertors can introduce nonsimultaneous sampling. For sleep studies, this is seldom a problem, unless the examiner decides to re-reference electrodes after a series of monopolar recordings are made. By contrast, artifact rejection is critical. Virtually all recordings will contain some artifact. Artifacts can completely undermine the validity of signal analysis.

In the authors' sleep research center, we have used computerized polysomnography to study sleep microarchitecture.[3,4] If performed manually, counting sleep spindles and measuring each waveform's amplitude and duration amounts to a Herculean task. Using computerized waveform analysis, we were able to compare sleep spindle activity in a standardized, objective manner for a wide variety of medications at different doses. Another fruitful application of computerized polysomnography addresses differences in sleep EEG associated with major depressive disorder. Decreased delta activity and alterations in the beta EEG are findings of particular interest.[5–7]

## STANDARD AND PARTIAL POLYSOMNOGRAPHY

Computerized polysomnography systems come in two basic varieties. The systems are designed to perform standard comprehensive polysomnography or partial polysomnography. Computer-controlled devices (e.g., actigraphs and ambulatory temperature recorders) can also record other types of activity during sleep; however, such devices fall outside the scope of this chapter.

Comprehensive polysomnography includes continuous recording of the following activity channels: EEG (one or more channels), electro-oculography (EOG) (preferably two channels), submentalis EMG, heart rhythm, airflow, respiratory effort (with rib cage and abdominal movements, intercostal EMG, or both), oxygen saturation, anterior tibialis EMG (from both legs, either on separate channels or linked), snoring sounds (optional), and some notation of body position. Most systems designed to emulate comprehensive polysomnography can be used either in the laboratory or the home. The location of use is a separate issue. Some systems provide the flexibility needed to use existing polygraph amplifiers and a wide assortment of recording equipment (e.g., pulse oximeters, nasal-oral airflow sensors, position sensors). Other automated systems require the use of specific dedicated amplifiers and ancillary recording devices.

Many ambulatory systems perform partial polysomnography, often called *screening*. The term *screening* is somewhat inappropriate in this context. Screening tests are typically inexpensive tests administered to large groups of asymptomatic individuals. Moreover, screening tests are notoriously nonreimbursable. Labeling partial polysomnography as a screening test is therefore discouraged.

**Table 15-1.** Computerized Polysomnography Usage Modes

| Usage Mode | Options |
|---|---|
| Recording | With or without paper tracings |
| Monitoring | Attended or unattended |
| Scoring | Human, computer-assisted, or automatic |

## MODES OF OPERATION

Computerized polysomnography can be classified along several dimensions. Each dimension refers to a specific mode of operation. In general, the user can choose among various options within each mode. Mathematically, there are a dozen combinations; however, few are used in actual practice. The usage modes and their options are shown in Table 15-1.

### *Recording Mode*

*Recording mode* specifies whether data are acquired and displayed on paper or on a video screen. Issues associated with choice of recording mode have been discussed in a review by Hirshkowitz and Moore.[8] A revisit of these issues with reference to currently available technology finds the situation much improved. Most systems now have adequate recording and display resolution and some provide for on-line record review.

The vastly increased microprocessor speed and the implementation of graphic accelerator cards allow for record manipulation speeds that rival paper. It still takes this author (MH) 20–30 minutes longer per record to perform a final review on the computerized system compared to paper. Nonetheless, the ability to compress the time scale to produce a graphic display similar to a slow-chart is particularly useful for record review. Viewing 5–10 minutes of respiration on one screen can give the clinician an overall sense of a patient's sleep-related breathing pattern. It also makes it easy to recognize the overall trend in response to continuous positive airway pressure. In our experience, however, we find it essential to validate sleep staging and arousal scoring before inspecting trends.

Recording mode has direct bearing on storage. The traditional problem associated with paper record storage—lack of space—has been replaced by a new and more insidious difficulty—media obsolescence. Paper tracings can be stored in their original form or can be microfilmed. By contrast, a wide assortment of computer media and media formats are available for storing digital recordings. Data stored on removable disks, magnetic tape, optical disks, and compact disks, may be unreadable by the system you are using a decade from now. Part of the reason for this is that mass storage technology is advancing so rapidly. Unless archival data are updated and preserved, one may find himself or herself with a library of records and no technique for access. The alternative is to maintain the older reading devices (like repairing your stereo's turntable because you still have 33 rpm LPs). Magnetic and some optical media decay more rapidly than most people realize. If one wants to keep computerized polysomnograms for an extended time, the specific media life should be investigated. Microfilm may be the only truly archival storage media. The 35-mm format predates Loomis and colleagues'[9] recording of the first all-night human sleep study. If Aserinsky and Kleitman[10] had microfilmed the rapid eye movement (REM) sleep discovery studies, they could be viewed today on the microfilm reader in any laboratory.

### Monitoring Mode

*Monitoring mode* signifies the procedural aspects of recording, not the act of recording. Monitoring mode refers to whether a technologist was present when data were recorded. There are theoretic advantages and disadvantages for performing unattended polysomnography, especially in the patient's home. Collecting data in a naturalistic setting, minimizing adaptation effects, and lowering costs are all attractive features. Low cost could also allow documenting of physiologic activity associated with rare events or intermittent conditions (e.g., nightmares, bruxism). The downsides are loss of control over the sleep environment, the patient engaging in maladaptive sleep habits, and interaction between the patient and his or her bed partner.

### Scoring Mode

*Scoring mode* concerns how the final information used to make clinical or scientific judgments is extracted from the polysomnogram. Traditional

**Table 15-2.** American Sleep Disorders Association Classification of Portable Recordings for Assessing Sleep-Disordered Breathing

| Level | Designation |
|-------|-------------|
| 1 | Standard polysomnography |
| 2 | Comprehensive portable polysomnography |
| 3 | Modified portable polysomnography |
| 4 | Continuous (single or dual) bioparameter recording |

paper tracings require human (manual) scoring. However, the digital recording can be analyzed with an assortment of signal processing algorithms. The mathematical product of these analytic techniques can be used directly. Alternatively, automatic detections can annotate the computer's graphic display and provide options to accept, reject, or change the scoring. In this fashion, scoring is computer assisted but the ultimate judgment remains in human hands.

### Polysomnography Classification and Guidelines

Not all sleep studies are equal. As part of the *Standard of Practice* guidelines for using portable recording to assess sleep-disordered breathing, the ASDA defines four different levels of polysomnography. Two criteria are used to categorize sleep studies. The first is based on the number of channels and derivation of signals recorded. The second is based on whether a technologist is present during data acquisition. The classification for studies is shown in Table 15-2.

The guideline stipulates three circumstances in which unattended portable recordings are acceptable: (1) in cases in which patients have severe symptoms and standard polysomnography is not readily available, (2) in patients who cannot be studied in the sleep laboratory, and (3) in follow-up studies after diagnosis was made with standard polysomnography and therapy was initiated. The ASDA also specifies data channels required for each level of polysomnography. Table 15-3 indicates recommended recording montages.

ASDA guidelines, however, do not include criteria for how the information is tabulated and analyzed. Nonetheless, for sleep center accreditation purposes, the ASDA requires that a sleep specialist review polysomnograms.

**Table 15-3.** Recommended Recording Montages for Different Levels of Portable Polysomnography

| Parameter | Level 1 | Level 2 | Level 3[a] | Level 4[a] |
|---|---|---|---|---|
| Electroencephalography | + | + | | |
| Electro-oculography | + | + | | |
| Electromyography (EMG) submentalis | + | + | | |
| Electrocardiography | + | + | + | |
| Airflow | + | + | + | |
| Respiratory effort | + | + | + | |
| Sao$_2$ | + | + | + | + |
| Body position | + | + | | |
| EMG anterior tibialis[b] | + | + | | |
| Attended | + | | | |

[a]Typical montage, but others exist.
[b]Recommended but optional for apnea studies.

## COMPUTERIZED SCORING

There are many computerized techniques used to score polysomnographic activity but there are basically two approaches used to validate results. The first is to compare computer scoring to human scoring. The other is to evaluate whether diagnostic outcome agrees between an automated system and clinical judgment based on standard polysomnography.

One difficulty peculiar to the computerized scoring literature is that information about a specific system's accuracy may be out of date by the time it is published. New system versions, updates, modifications, and software porting to more powerful computer platforms all accelerate information obsolescence. However, anyone using computer-assisted scoring soon becomes familiar with the strengths and limitations of their particular system. A user may find that many recordings are accurately computer scored but a single, easily recognized artifact can completely undermine the process. It is prudent to use a system for 6–12 months and formally index its accuracy before considering fully automated scoring. Furthermore, well thought-out and systematically applied quality control measures are critical for ongoing operation.

Published studies of computerized polysomnographic scoring accuracy can be subdivided according to several criteria, including the activity being scored, the population tested, whether the system is commercially available, whether actual patient data are presented, and the statistical approach used. Several perspectives can be taken with respect to statistical approach and they reflect fundamentally different conceptual orientations. In general, computerized polysomnography assessments either focus on diagnostic outcome or performance standard testing.

## DIAGNOSTIC OUTCOME TESTING

Outcome studies have become enormously popular in recent years. The overzealous contention that "outcome is everything" shows signs of erosion. Sophisticated readers understand that results from outcome-based treatment studies largely depend on the measures selected and the populations used. The same applies to diagnostic outcome studies. The procedure for testing new diagnostic techniques is well-established in medicine. A new test is compared with an existing standard in terms of *sensitivity* and *specificity*. The standard test is presumed to accurately make the diagnosis. A new test's sensitivity is the percentage of the time that the new test detects the pathology when it is in fact present according to the standard test. In other words, the number of true-positive (TP) tests is divided by the sum of TPs and false-negatives (FNs). The specificity of a test is the percentage of time that the test is negative, given that the disease is absent. That is, the number of true-negatives (TN) is divided by the sum of TNs and false-positives (FPs). Table 15-4 shows the computational procedures for these metrics.

It is critical to note that there has been misuse of this terminology in the sleep literature. Although it is unclear why, the 1994 ASDA review paper[11] presents tables with sensitivity and specificity defined as TN/(TP + FN) and TP/(TN + FP), respectively. However, it also appears that the labeling of sensitivity and specificity columns may

**Table 15-4.** Testing New Diagnostics

|  |  | Disease Status | |
|---|---|---|---|
|  |  | **Present** | **Absent** |
| **Test result** | **Positive** | True-positive (TP) | False-positive (FP) |
|  | **Negative** | False-negative (FN) | True-negative (TN) |

Sensitivity = TP/(TP + FN).
Specificity = TN / (TN + FP).

be reversed on some of the tables. Therefore, the normal relationships between more stringent diagnostic criteria and changes in sensitivity and specificity do not hold true in that data review.

In general, as the diagnostic criteria are made more stringent, sensitivity will decline; however, the specificity will increase. This was clearly demonstrated in the paper published by Douglas and colleagues.[12] In their study, 200 patients were tested with polysomnography and oximetry. To determine the accuracy of oximetry alone for diagnosing sleep apnea, the number of 4% desaturations per hour in bed was calculated. Several desaturation index criteria were presented. Table 15-5 shows the sensitivity and specificity calculated from their data.

Sensitivity and specificity statistics are particularly popular for evaluating partial polysomnographic systems. More often than not, these systems focus on sleep-related breathing. Although such systems may not assess sleep stages, leg movements, or arousals, they are touted to accurately detect, classify, and quantify respiratory events.

There are several issues to address concerning this statistical approach. First, should one completely rely on the new test for diagnosing sleep-disordered breathing? Second, should treatment be

initiated without directly confirming the pathophysiology? If the answers to these questions are yes, then what criteria are set? If the answers are no, then how will patients be studied further?

One school of thought asserts that the value of partial testing relates directly to the TP rate because negative tests waste resources, time, and money. Thus, individuals with positive tests should then be studied in the laboratory and treated. However, a compelling case can be made that individuals with negative tests are the ones in greater need of standard laboratory polysomnography because their symptoms are unexplained. This raises the main question: *If* one thinks a laboratory study is needed when a partial test is positive and that a laboratory study is also needed when a partial test is negative, *then* what function does the test serve? In many cases, the usefulness of the test lies in selecting different assessment protocols based on test findings. At our center, a partial test indicating moderate to severe obstructive sleep apnea will result in ordering a split-night protocol instead of a full-night baseline study.

## PERFORMANCE STANDARD TESTING

The traditional engineering approach to testing new equipment is assessing reliability and validity against an existing standard. Variability represents an obstacle that must be considered when evaluating data for performance standard testing. Variability can exist in the standard itself, in the application of that standard, in the samples used for testing, in the experimental rigor (e.g., scorer blinding), and the statistical technique.[8] Finally, performance standard testing may focus on specific event detection, specific classification accuracy, or global conglomerate indices of performance.

To do performance standard testing, one must have standards. The *Manual of Standardized Termi-*

**Table 15-5.** Sensitivity and Specificity of Overnight Oximetry for Diagnosing Sleep-Disordered Breathing

| Diagnostic Criteria* | True-Positive | False-Negative | True-Negative | False-Positive | Sensitivity | Specificity |
|---|---|---|---|---|---|---|
| >5 | 61 | 30 | 100 | 9 | 67 | 92 |
| >10 | 48 | 43 | 106 | 3 | 53 | 97 |
| >15 | 37 | 54 | 106 | 3 | 41 | 97 |
| >20 | 33 | 58 | 108 | 1 | 36 | 99 |

*4% desaturations per hour. Source: Data from NJ Douglas, S Thomas, MA Jan. Clinical value of polysomnography. Lancet 1992;339:347.

*nology, Techniques and Scoring System for Sleep Stages of Human Subjects* [13] specifies standards for recording and scoring sleep stages. Common departures from this standard include classifying sleep stages using other than central EEG, referencing EOG to frontal pole, and relying on a single-channel EOG tracing. Standardized ASDA guidelines also exist for recording and scoring periodic leg movements[14] and EEG arousals.[15] Methods for collecting and detecting other polysomnographic data are less consistent. Although no official standards exist for scoring sleep-related breathing or penile erections, procedures are detailed in *Sleeping and Waking Disorders: Indications and Techniques*[16] and in the methodology section of *Principles and Practice of Sleep Medicine.*[17] These guidelines serve as de facto standards in clinical polysomnography.

Applying the standard or de facto standard may vary between individuals. Variability between human scorers is well-documented.[18–20] This variability must be considered when interpreting human versus computer scoring discrepancies.

Polysomnographic data from sleep studies are scored in three basic ways. Some scoring entails classifying time-based intervals (epochs) such as sleep stages. Another type involves detecting events (e.g., obstructive apnea episodes). Finally, some scoring is merely tabulation of activity level (e.g., oxygen saturation). For epoch-classified and event-detected data, measures can derive from a single data point (e.g., REM sleep latency) or be calculated from many epochs or events (e.g., sleep efficiency and apnea index).

Paired comparisons on the mean or median and correlations are the most often used statistics for comparing human and computer-scored data. These statistics are quite appropriate for contrasting single-point data; however, difficulties arise when they are used to compare conglomerate indices. The finding of no differences between mean values for night summary parameters (e.g., REM sleep percentage) can occur because of large variance or overall regression to the mean effects. In fact, two polysomnograms in which there was never agreement between the human and computer on any individual epoch of REM sleep could have identical means. Thus, the lack of significant differences does not necessarily indicate that the computerized analysis is accurate. For different reasons, correlation coefficients do not provide information concerning absolute level of

agreement. This statistic quantifies the relative association between pairs of variables. Consistent, additive, systematically inflated (or deflated) computer scores will not alter the coefficient; however, a nonzero Y-axis intercept indicates a problem. Thus, very good correlations can be found between human and computer scoring when the computer consistently overscores or underscores a parameter.

The only foolproof way to test computerized polysomnographic system performance is to examine elemental data. The agreement rate for individual epoch classifications or individual event detections provides the most useful information. For inferential testing, kappa coefficients are appropriate. Correlations and paired comparisons are helpful on single-point data; however, Y-axis intercept, scaling, and variance must be cautiously inspected.

If the purpose of polysomnography is to document and quantify pathophysiology, then accurate scoring is required. If it is unacceptable for a person to "make up" the numbers then it is equally unacceptable to have a computer do this. Every instrument has intrinsic variability, and an intelligent user will develop a sense of a tool's limitation. Consider the following example: Computerized polysomnographic system X is known to have a 5–10% disagreement rate (*margin of error*) with human scorers under a wide variety of conditions. In a patient with severe sleep-disordered breathing (e.g., apnea index >60), the margin of error may be small relative to the level of pathology. In such a case, the data may be acceptable. By contrast, when a patient's computer-scored apnea plus hypopnea index is close to treatment threshold (e.g., apnea + hypopnea index = 20), the margin of error figures prominently into the course of action. A prudent clinician would hand-score such a polysomnogram.

## CURRENT STATE OF KNOWLEDGE AND CONCLUSIONS

It is difficult to compare specific systems, because available information is inadequate. At present, such comparison would amount to little more than opinion. Hardware and software are in constant flux. Since 1995, we have seen major changes: the emergence of Windows '95, multiple software revisions, faster computer platforms, and incorporation of network concepts into computerized polysomno-

**Table 15-6.** Mean Number of Citations per Year in Different MEDLINE Databases Using a Variety of Search Terms

| Database Used | Sleep Computer Scoring | Sleep Computer Apnea | Sleep Computer Scoring Human | Sleep Computer Apnea Human |
|---|---|---|---|---|
| 1966–1975 | 0.10 | 0.00 | 0.10 | 0.00 |
| 1976–1980 | 0.80 | 0.40 | 0.60 | 0.40 |
| 1981–1986 | 1.33 | 1.00 | 1.33 | 1.00 |
| 1987–1992 | 3.33 | 3.50 | 3.00 | 3.50 |
| 1993 to present | 5.08 | 6.61 | 4.16 | 6.31 |

graphic systems. These advances greatly change the market landscape.

Published information concerning computerized polysomnography steadily increases. MEDLINE searches using text words *computer* and *sleep* produced only 29 citations in the 1966–1975 database. The number of citations for other databases were as follows: 48 in 1976–1980, 68 in 1981–1986, 146 in 1987–1992, and 118 in 1993 to present. Table 15-6 shows the mean number of citations per year in different MEDLINE databases using a variety of search strategies. The trends indicate not only an increase in the number of papers but also in the proportion focused on computerized scoring and sleep apnea. In fact, the number focused on sleep-disordered breathing has recently surpassed those indexed on computer scoring. There seems little doubt that computerized polysomnography is the wave of the future. The important questions that remain are how accurate are the particular systems and how will they be used and by whom.

# REFERENCES

1. Pivik RT, Broughton RJ, Coppola R, et al. Committee report: guidelines for the recording and quantitative analysis of electroencephalographic activity in research contexts. Psychophysiology 1993;30:547.
2. Oken BS, Chiappa KH. Statistical issues concerning computerized analysis of brain wave topography. Ann Neurol 1986;19:493.
3. Hirshkowitz M, Thornby JI, Karacan I. Sleep pharmacology and automated EEG analysis. Psychiatry Ann 1979;9:510.
4. Hirshkowitz M, Thornby JI, Karacan I. Sleep spindles: pharmacological effects in humans. Sleep 1982;5:85.
5. Borbely AA, Tobler I, Loepfe M, et al. All-night spectral analysis of the sleep EEG in untreated depression and normal controls. Psychiatr Res 1984;12:27.
6. Kupfer DJ, Ulrich F, Coble PA, et al. Application of automated REM and slow wave sleep analysis: 1. normal and depressed subjects. Psychiatry Res 1984;13:325.
7. Armitage R. Microarchitectural findings in sleep EEG in depression: diagnostic implications. Biol Psychiatry 1995;37:72.
8. Hirshkowitz M, Moore CA. Issues in computerized polysomnography. Sleep 1994;17:105.
9. Loomis AL, Harvey EN, Hobart GA III. Cerebral states during sleep, as studied by human brain potentials. J Exp Psychol 1937;21:127.
10. Aserinsky E, Kleitman N. Regular occurring periods of eye motility, and concomitant phenomena, during sleep. Science 1953;188:273.
11. Ferber R, Millman R, Coppola M, et al. ASDA Standards of Practice. Portable recording in the assessment of obstructive sleep apnea. Sleep 1994;17:378.
12. Douglas NJ, Thomas S, Jan MA. Clinical value of polysomnography. Lancet 1992;339:347.
13. Rechtschaffen A, Kales A (eds). A Manual of Standardized Terminology, Techniques and Scoring System for Sleep Stages of Human Subjects. NIH Publication No. 204. Washington, DC: U.S. Government Printing Office, 1968.
14. Bonnet M, Carley D, Guilleminault C, et al. ASDA report. Recording and scoring leg movements. Sleep 1993;16:748.
15. Bonnet M, Carley D, Carskadon M, et al. ASDA report. EEG arousals: scoring rules and examples. Sleep 1992;15:173.
16. Guilleminault C (ed). Sleeping and Waking Disorders: Indications and Techniques. Menlo Park, CA: Addison-Wesley, 1982.
17. Kryger MH, Roth T, Dement WC (eds). Principles and Practice of Sleep Medicine (2nd ed). Philadelphia: Saunders, 1994.
18. Bliwise D, Bliwise NG, Kraemer HC, Dement WC. Measurement error in visually scored electrophysiological data: respiration during sleep. J Neurosci Methods 1984;12:49-56.
19. Bliwise DL, Keenan S, Burnburg D, et al. Inter-rater reliability for scoring periodic leg movements in sleep. Sleep 1991;14:249.
20. Karacan I, Orr WC, Roth T, et al. Establishment and implementation of standardized sleep laboratory data collection and scoring procedures. Psychophysiology 1978;15:173.

# Chapter 16
# Sleep Scoring Technique

Merrill M. Mitler, J. Steven Poceta, and Barbara G. Bigby

Continuous recordings of electroencephalographic (EEG), electro-oculographic (EOG), and electromyographic (EMG) activity are required for the modern classification of wakefulness, rapid eye movement (REM) sleep, and non-REM (NREM) sleep.

Since the first days of EEG recordings, EEG potentials were thought to depend somehow on electrical activity generated by brain cells. Exactly what brain cell activity and the mechanisms by which electrical signals are picked up at the site of an electrode, however, are not yet completely understood. It is now certain that the relatively brief action potentials generated when a neuron fires are not significantly involved. Rather, EEG waves are thought to represent volume-conducted summations of the excitatory and inhibitory post-synaptic potentials (EPSPs and IPSPs) that constantly occur on cells of the cerebral cortex closest to the recording electrode. The most common neurons involved are thought to be the pyramidal cells found in layers III and V of the cerebral cortex. Pyramidal neurons have long apical dendritic structures projecting from above the cell body as well as axons projecting below the cell body. Desynchronized or activated EEG patterns, then, are produced when the numbers of simultaneous EPSPs and IPSPs are relatively equal, yielding small and rapid changes in the voltages as recorded from the scalp. Synchronized or deactivated EEG patterns, by contrast, arise when the numbers of simultaneous EPSPs and IPSPs yield large, slow changes in the voltages as recorded from the scalp. In contrast to standard EEG procedures, polysomnographic (PSG) scoring into wakefulness, NREM sleep stages I–IV, and REM sleep usually requires only the C3/A2 or C4/A1 and O1/A2 or O2/A1 derivations of the many derivations defined by the 10-20 System.

The EOG recording depends on the retinocorneal potential. That is, the back of the eye (retina) is electronegative relative to the front of the eye (cornea). When the eyeball moves, it is as if a battery (dipole) is moving in space. If the cornea is moving toward an electrode, it will register a positive potential and vice versa. Typical EOG electrode placement for the active electrode in PSG is at the outer canthi and, perhaps, above and below each orbit. The usual reference electrode is the opposite ear lobe or mastoid (A1 or A2).

The EMG recording depends on the summation of electrical potentials generated when individual muscle fibers contract. For sleep staging in PSG, selection of the muscle group to record is based on the presence of appropriate levels of muscle tone during NREM sleep, against which loss of tone can be documented during REM sleep. Other factors important in selection include ease of access and comfort for the patient. The best choice is the group of muscles just below the chin—that is, the digastric and submental muscles. Because of unreliable tonus during NREM sleep, the group of muscles in the back of the neck is a poor second choice for humans. The EMG recordings in PSG are usually bipolar with both electrodes positioned 2–4 cm apart over the muscle group to be recorded.

## EARLY APPROACHES TO ELECTROENCEPHALOGRAPHY STAGING

Soon after bioelectric potentials were recorded from the human scalp, attention was directed at how the patterns of EEG potentials correlate with behavior. Early investigators focused on EEG changes as humans went from wakefulness to sleep, and were unaware of the existence of REM sleep. Loomis' group at Harvard University and Blake's group at the University of Chicago each devised a system to categorize EEG patterns by using the frequency and amplitude of brain activity.[1,2] Gibbs and Gibbs also categorized the EEG along the dimension of depth.[3]

The discovery of REM sleep, previously referred to as *paradoxical sleep*, led to the routine recording of eye movements and muscle tension when monitoring sleep, and required a restructuring and reconceptualization of the sleep staging. For example, the notion of sleep depth could no longer be linked to EEG amplitude and frequency. Rather, depth of sleep had to be operationally defined along some dimension of the intensity of the arousing stimulus, and measures had to be taken in both NREM and REM sleep.

## SCORING SYSTEMS

In 1968, Rechtschaffen and Kales published guidelines for the standardization of terminology and sleep staging methods in humans.[4] This technique has since served as the standard by which sleep is analyzed. The Rechtschaffen and Kales scoring system uses the international EEG 10-20 System of electrode placement.[5,6] Based on EEG, chin muscle EMG, and EOG, the following stages can be recognized, as well as their prominent features:

- Stage wakefulness: EEG with alpha activity (8–13 Hz) or low-voltage, mixed-frequency activity
- Stage I: a relatively low-voltage, mixed-frequency EEG without REM
- Stage II: relatively low-voltage, mixed-frequency EEG background with 12- to 14-Hz sleep spindles and K complexes (see later, under Clinical Methodology and Sleep Staging)

- Stage III: moderate amounts of high-amplitude, slow-wave activity (see later)
- Stage IV: large amounts of high-amplitude, slow-wave activity (see later)
- Stage REM: a relatively low-voltage, mixed-frequency EEG in conjunction with episodic REM and low-amplitude EMG

*NREM sleep* refers to stages I–IV. Some laboratories use the term *movement time* to refer to portions of the record where movement (muscle) artifact obscures the underlying brain potentials. Many laboratories that deal only with adult subjects consider such periods as wakefulness.

For the details of the technical aspects, the reader is referred to the Rechtschaffen and Kales manual.[4] The EEG recording should use a paper speed of at least 10 mm per second; most laboratories use this speed, although 15 mm per second and 30 mm per second allow for greater analysis of rapid EEG waveforms, especially epileptiform activity. Filter settings must allow an adequate pen response, and sensitivities should allow for a pen deflection of 7.5–10.0 mm for a 50-μV signal. The manual bases the sleep stages in part on EEG waveform amplitudes, and thus a standard electrode array must be used, such as a central electrode (C3 or C4) referenced to the opposite ear lobe (mastoid, A2 or A1). An occipital lead is useful for optimal recognition of the alpha rhythm. Bipolar montages and recording from other areas of the brain have specific applications, but are not needed in the routine scoring of sleep stages. Chapters 9 and 10 discuss in detail the technical aspects of recording.

The Rechtschaffen and Kales system is an epoch-by-epoch approach to the scoring of human sleep. An epoch is a given amount of time chosen to be both convenient and realistic. Usually, an epoch is one page, and this one page may represent 20 or 30 seconds, depending on the paper speed (15 or 10 mm per seconds, respectively). In general, epochs are scored as one stage depending on the majority of the epoch. Thus, short-lived stage changes may not enter into the analysis at all. For example, a person who is having repetitive arousals lasting for 5 seconds and occurring every 25 seconds would be scored as having continuous sleep, thus underestimating the total amount of time spent in wakefulness. Alternatively, a patient could show sleep records for 12 seconds and then arouse or move for 18 seconds, and all epochs would show wake, thus underestimating the total time spent asleep. These are more than just technical points, because these short-lived stage changes clearly have meaning for the restorative aspects of sleep. The Rechtschaffen and Kales method cannot adequately analyze them, however, as this method was developed using normal sleep as the model. When pathologic processes are present, certain modifications are necessary. Simply staging sleep does not give all the necessary information. The concept of *transitional sleep* has been proposed in an effort to quantify periods of sleep with very frequent sleep stage transitions.[7] This method is not in common use, but has the advantage of avoiding the rigidness of a fixed epoch scored as only one stage. Our laboratory also gives attention to short-lived sleep stage changes, primarily by counting the number and type of arousals and noting their relation to various other aspects of the PSG, such as stage preference and body position.

## COMPUTERIZED METHODS OF ELECTROENCEPHALOGRAPHY ANALYSIS AND SLEEP STAGE SCORING

Computerized methods have attempted to manage the large amount of analog data an overnight sleep study generates, as well as to minimize the amount of time required to accurately score and analyze a PSG (see also Chapter 15). Several commercially available systems appear adequate for the routine sleep staging of relatively normal sleepers but manual sleep scoring is preferred. When sleep EEG is disrupted by pathology, however, such as sleep apnea or drug-related spindling and fast activity, hand scoring is the only reliable method for sleep staging.

One important development is the broadening availability of quantified EEG technology.[8] Using analog-to-digital conversion followed by Fourier transformation, the power of the EEG signal is mapped into various frequency bands. Quantified EEG permits the detailed analysis of the EEG power attributable to, for example, alpha activity or delta activity. Several groups are exploring the usefulness of quantified EEG to compare sleep data from night to night, from treatment condition to treatment condition, from patient to patient, and even from electrode to electrode.

## PORTABLE MONITORING TECHNIQUES

Efforts to reduce health care costs and to use newly available microcomputer technology have produced an increased interest in portable recording devices. Such devices are available for performing, in the patient's home or at any other location, essentially complete clinical PSG or selected components of PSG such as continuous measurement of respiratory parameters. This topic has been reviewed recently by Broughton et al.[9] and is the subject of Chapter 15 in this volume.

Our laboratory has had firsthand experience with several portable recording devices and found them to be reliable for PSG data acquisition and recording. We have also examined the automatic sleep-scoring capabilities of the SensorMedics Somnostar system[10] (Sensor Medics, Yorba Linda, CA) and the Medilog 9200 system (Oxford Medical Instruments, Largo, FL).[11] Our conclusions are that for undisturbed sleep, automated sleep scoring methods can produce results that are comparable to those of a trained technician. For disturbed sleep such as that associated with sleep apnea or periodic leg movements, however, the automated scoring routines produce results that are not comparable to those of a trained technician. Under circumstances of disturbed sleep, the scoring parameters related to resumption of sleep after an awakening and the duration of various sleep stages are discrepant from those produced by a trained technician. On the positive side, for the quantification of selected events such as apneas or leg movements, automated scoring routines can reduce the tedium of the scoring technician's job with minimal loss of accuracy.

## CLINICAL METHODOLOGY AND SLEEP STAGING

At our center, most PSGs are hand scored for both sleep stages and for pathologic events such as apneas, periodic leg movements, abnormal REM structure, or unusual arousals.

We follow the Rechtschaffen and Kales guidelines exactly, and have summarized them in the following paragraphs. We hand score the records in 30-second epochs. The scorer uses a worksheet preprinted with the epoch numbers, with two spaces next to the epoch number for recording both the sleep stage and any pathologic event. The scorer records the sleep stage each time there is a change and any event, such as an arousing apnea. Occasionally, when the record shows a pattern of repetitive apneas, we simply score a representative portion of the record for events only and do not perform formal staging. The portions of the record scored, perhaps 60–120 minutes, should contain all sleep stages seen in the patient and, when possible, all sleeping positions.

As is generally accepted, sleep is "staged" into 20- or 30-second epochs, and these epochs are considered both independently and in the context of preceding and succeeding epochs. Sleep is a continuous and dynamic process, with very few patterns that change suddenly. Thus, our delineation of sleep into 30-second epochs is somewhat artificial from the outset, but a practical and reasonably realistic means of describing the physiologic process.

Stage W, or wakefulness, is scored when the EEG shows either an alpha rhythm or a lower-voltage, mixed-frequency EEG, perhaps with beta potentials (>13-Hz activity). The stage can also usually be recognized because of the high chin-EMG tone, frequent rapid eye movements and blinks, and sometimes frequent body movements. Sometimes the alpha rhythm is prominent and of high voltage; at other times it can barely be discerned. The major problem in those subjects without a well-defined alpha rhythm is deciding when to score stage I. Usually, some slowing of the EEG can be seen in combination with rolling eye movements and lessening of the chin EMG.

Stage I sleep is scored when, by definition, there is a relatively low-voltage, mixed-frequency EEG with a prominence of activity in the range of 2–7 Hz. This stage occurs most often in the transition from wakefulness to other sleep stages, or after body movements or arousals. Usually, this stage is short-lived (1–10 minutes). Vertex sharp waves and higher-voltage theta activity can be recognized, usually near the end of this stage, but scoring of stage I requires an absence of K complexes and sleep spindles. Slow (rolling) eye movements are often recognized, both during drowsiness or wakefulness when an alpha rhythm is present, and during early stage I. Sometimes these movement are "fast," but they should never be truly saccadic, as in REM sleep or wakefulness. Usually, stage I is a transition stage from wakefulness to stage II or REM sleep, and is scored when more than 50% of the epoch is characterized by the stage I criteria. Typically, one observes rolling eye

movements and mild decreases in EMG muscle tone as the alpha rhythm breaks up and yields to the slower, lower-voltage theta patterns of stage I sleep.

Stage II sleep is defined by the presence of sleep spindles or K complexes and the absence of high-amplitude slow waves sufficient to define stages III and IV. By definition, a sleep spindle requires 12- to 14-Hz activity occurring for at least 0.5 second. K complexes are triphasic potentials defined as well-delineated, negative sharp waves followed by a positive component and lasting more than 0.5 second. Some definitions of the K complex require it to be immediately followed by spindle frequencies, but this is not part of the Rechtschaffen and Kales criteria. The K complex is maximal in the vertex region and is often associated with a potentially arousing stimulus such as a noise. Other EEG patterns that may be identified during this stage include lambdoid waves, more commonly known as *positive occipital sharp transients of sleep* (POSTS), which may also be seen during other NREM stages. The occurrence of K complexes is not specific to stage II and may be seen during NREM stages III and IV.

Because of the transient nature of the sleep spindle and K complex, long periods may occur between these events, and the definition of stage II sleep allows for up to 3 minutes of stage I epochs between spindles or K complexes. If more than 3 minutes of EEG patterns consistent with stage I sleep occur, the interval should be scored as stage I. If an arousal occurs during the 3 minutes between spindles or K complexes, the epochs up to the arousal are scored as stage II, and the epochs after the arousal are scored independently (usually as wake or stage I). This rule and similar guidelines for scoring REM sleep in long periods between eye movements typify the fact that not all epochs can be scored independently, but often depend on their context.

Stage III and stage IV sleep, also known as *slow-wave sleep* or *delta sleep*, take their definition from delta waves. These are EEG waveforms that usually begin later in stage II and are 2 Hz or slower with a minimum amplitude of 75 µV (peak-to-peak). They must be distinguished from K complexes. Stage II contains less than 20% delta activity. Stage III is scored when an epoch contains from 20% to 50% delta waves, and stage IV is scored when the epoch has greater than 50% delta waves. In borderline epochs, it is often necessary to actually measure (perhaps by underlining) the slow waves present in the epoch. The definition refers to actual time during the slow waves, not lower-amplitude portions between slow waves. Sleep spindles and K complexes may or may not be present in these stages.

When carefully performed, there is a fairly high interscorer reliability reported for scoring slow-wave sleep, but in actual practice, we find that the reliable scoring of stage III often depends on the experience of the scorer. It is not always practical to measure all borderline epochs, and thus within each laboratory, a standardized norm develops, which is hopefully close to the published Rechtschaffen and Kales guidelines. Another area that causes confusion is the amplitude criteria. It is well-known that a variety of conditions will affect the measured amplitude of EEG signals. Some of these conditions include the local biophysical properties of the skull. In addition, in aging, there is a tendency for a decrement in amplitude of the slow waves seen in sleep, due at times to both pathologic and nonpathologic processes. If the minimum amplitude criterion is not applied, significantly more slow-wave sleep might be scored, as in the case of elderly persons with some cerebral atrophy. The Rechtschaffen and Kales committee decided for a variety of reasons to retain the minimum amplitude criterion, in part to remain consistent with previous research, and in part to force a more explicit and exact definition of these sleep stages. This does not disallow others from analyzing studies with other criteria, but such differences must be specifically noted.

Stage REM is scored by the appearance of a relatively low-voltage, mixed-frequency EEG, low chin EMG, and rapid (saccadic) eye movements. The EEG pattern resembles that of stage I, although there should not be as many vertex sharp waves or other high-voltage waveforms. Notched theta waves, appearing in bursts (called *sawtooth waves*) are characteristic. Alpha activity may occur, and may be more prominent than in stage I.

The chin-EMG level often causes problems in scoring REM. Obviously, this measurement is not quantitative. Thus, relative levels are assessed. Ideally, chin tone is highest in waking, lower in stage I, even lower in stages II–IV, and very low in stage REM. Sometimes this is not true, and chin tone can increase in sleep (e.g., as a result of bruxism and tension headaches), but to score REM sleep, the *chin EMG cannot be relatively elevated*. That is, it must be as low or lower than the EMG seen elsewhere in the record. Technically, a problem often develops if the gain setting is such that the chin EMG appears too low during wakefulness or NREM. In that case, one may not be able to see the drop in tone that should occur during REM. Thus, it is important to keep the gain on the chin-EMG amplifier as high as practically possible during any NREM stage. This often necessitates changing gain just after the patient falls asleep to minimize pen damage and ink splattering. With increasing use of digital (paperless) EEG and sleep equipment, questions of pen damage and ink spattering are increasingly irrelevant.

Problems may occur while scoring the beginning and ending of REM periods, sleep spindles, long periods without eye movements, and arousals within a REM period. With regard to sleep spindles, the Rechtschaffen and Kales manual states that any section of record contiguous with stage REM in which the EEG shows relatively low-voltage mixed frequency is scored REM, regardless of whether the characteristic eye movements are present, provided the EMG remains at the REM level and there are no intervening arousals. If two spindles occur with no intervening eye movements, however, and if the amount of time between spindles is sufficient to influence a full epoch or epochs, then that portion of the record between the spindles can be considered stage II and is scored as such. The problem with the beginning and end of REM periods is that the three determinants of the stage—EEG, EOG, and EMG—do not change simultaneously. Several possibilities exist, therefore, and are illustrated in detail in the manual.

## SLEEP EEG SCORING IN RELATION TO PATHOLOGIC EVENTS

The basic rules of Rechtschaffen and Kales pertain to the scoring of sleep stages even if pathologic events such as apneas occur. Epochs are still scored according to the majority of the epoch. In general, we only score pathologic events during sleep, although clearly some events, particularly periodic leg movements, may occur during wakefulness. These events must be noted by the technician and taken into account when formulating a final diagnosis and treatment plan, but they are not counted by the technician or used in calculating indices (e.g., respiratory disturbance index).

### Respiratory Events

When respiratory events such as apneas and hypopneas occur, the patient is usually sleeping, although we have clearly seen snoring and events while the EEG continues to show alpha activity, albeit with rolling eye movements. Occasionally, the apneas are brief enough that an entire epoch cannot be scored as sleep, despite repetitive apnea. This is a special situation about which one cannot make rules, and that requires the judgment of a polysomnographer.

A respiratory event is scored when there is a decrease or cessation of airflow for 10 seconds or longer. In our laboratory, we consider the total loss of airflow to be apnea, and a decrease of any other amount (subtotal) to be hypopnea. Most definitions require a decrease of at least 50% of resting, prehypopnea airflow, but we find this too strict for two reasons. First, neither a thermistor nor end-tidal $CO_2$ is a calibrated or quantitative measure of airflow. Second, even minimal decreases in airflow, especially if associated with a decline in oxyhemoglobin saturation or arousal, may be clinically significant. Both hypopneas and apneas are considered respiratory events, and are used to calculate a respiratory disturbance index (apnea-hypopnea index). We do not usually consider the significance of apneas to be different from that of hypopneas in terms of effect on sleep disruption or desaturation, for example. There might be significant physiologic differences between them in certain patients, however—for example, a patient with cardiomyopathy in whom a greater negative intrapleural pressure swing from an apnea would increase left ventricular transmural pressure (and work). Also, experience with nasal bilevel positive airway pressure has illustrated the importance of distinguishing between apneas and hypopneas for purposes of adjusting applied pressures while the patient sleeps. Again, any airflow, such as that which would produce a snoring noise, prohibits the use of the term *apnea*, and is therefore considered hypopnea.

Events are considered obstructive when respiratory effort continues during the decrement in airflow. Depending on the means by which one is measuring respiratory effort, and whether the event is apnea or hypopnea, the effort may be increased or decreased. (Bands around the chest measure chest wall excursion, not effort. In an apnea, for example, strong diaphragmatic contraction might be occurring, but if no air can come into the chest, there will be little thoracic expansion.) Usually, obstructive events have associated snoring and a "breakthrough" breath, which is the larger-amplitude hyperpnea at the start of the postapneic breathing. Paradoxic effort is a good indicator of intensified respiratory effort and upper airway resistance (occlusion), but paradoxing may often be observed in normals during REM sleep. When normal, the paradoxing should not be associated with discrete respiratory events, arousals, or desaturation. The use of intrapleural (endoesophageal) pressure monitoring with a catheter or balloon allows for investigation of the negative pressure generated within the thorax, and is the most sensitive measure of "respiratory effort." When combined with a measure of flow, total upper airway resistance can be calculated.[12] The upper airway resistance syndrome[13] is marked by increased upper airway resistance but without frank obstructive hypopneas or apneas, desaturation, and perhaps even without snoring in some patients. The resistance is observed to increase over a short period (20–60 seconds) leading to arousal. Depending on technique, the investigator usually can monitor only the intrapleural pressure breath by breath, and sees an increase in negative pressure with succeeding breaths leading to the arousal. Arousals preceded by such pressure changes can be scored as respiratory arousals.

Obstructive apneas, by definition, have respiratory effort throughout the entire period of decreased airflow. Mixed apneas have a central component at the beginning of the event, followed by obstructive elements. In our experience, however, most *obstructive* apneas (defined clinically and pathophysiologically) begin with a brief period of cessation in respiratory effort. This may be due to hypocapnia, which occurs at the end of the resuscitative breathing, or may in part be a pharyngeal reflex. Therefore, we do not bother to score as mixed those apneas that have a brief central component followed by typical obstructive features. That is, we score apneas in which the central component at the beginning of the apnea is less than 25% the time of the total apnea as obstructive. We score an apnea as mixed when the central component is predominant, but several breaths of obviously obstructive effort then occur before the arousal. Thus, mixed apneas are those with a central component ranging from approximately 25% to 90% of the apnea, followed by clear signs of obstruction before

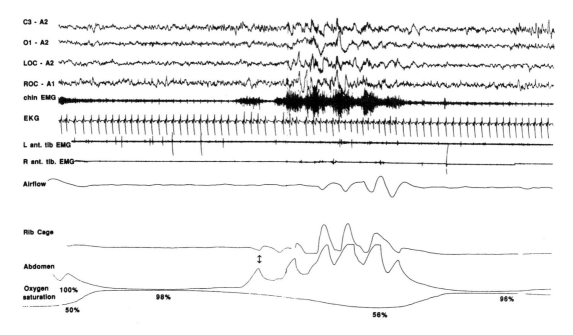

**Figure 16-1.** A 60-second excerpt from a nocturnal polysomnogram showing mixed apnea. Note significant central component (absence of respiratory effort) at onset of apnea and paradoxing of rib cage and abdomen near end of apnea (*arrows*). Paper speed = 10 mm per second; EEG and electro-oculography calibration = 75 μV/cm (*vertical extent of double arrow*). Other gain settings are not standardized in our laboratory because they are adjusted for clarity throughout the night. (LOC, ROC = left and right outer canthus of the eye; EMG = electromyography; EKG = electrocardiography.)

the apnea ends (Figure 16-1). This is somewhat arbitrary, but our clinical experience overwhelmingly supports the idea that there is a gradual transition in grading apneas from obstructive to mixed to central.

A central (sometimes called *diaphragmatic*) apnea is one in which neither respiratory effort nor airflow occurs. Central apneas can often be recognized as one of two types. One has waxing and waning effort, commonly called *Cheyne-Stokes respiration* (CSR), with no evidence at all of an obstructive component. CSR, with gradual onset and offset of respiratory effort, is easily recognized, and usually associated with cardiac or central nervous system disease. The other type of central apnea appears more like a mixed apnea, but with minimal or no terminal obstructive phase. We score this type of apnea as central when most of the apnea contains no respiratory effort at all, the terminal phase with effort is nonexistent or very short (one or two breaths at the most), and paradoxing is not evident. The offset and onset of breathing may be abrupt, and the breathing phase (as opposed to the apnea phase) is usually shorter than in CSR.

There is sometimes uncertainty in the scoring of central apneas, and hard and fast rules about central versus obstructive events should not be made. It is different to define these events pathophysiologically versus descriptively (for purposes of scoring). The pathophysiology and the scoring should coincide, but this is not always possible. We have seen patients who have central apneas only when supine, and others who have predominantly central apnea yet respond well to nasal CPAP, as if upper airway obstruction could trigger a central apnea.[14] We allow for some component of measured obstruction when scoring central apneas because even in a person in whom the upper airway structure and function do not produce frank apneas, a long central apnea might produce some minor upper airway floppiness and occlusion. Thus, when the central drive returns, some evidence of the upper airway resistance may be seen (perhaps some snoring). We encountered another example when a 35-year-old man with a history of loud snoring but no apnea developed a severe viral cardiomyopathy with congestive heart failure and CSR. His predisposition to snoring made many

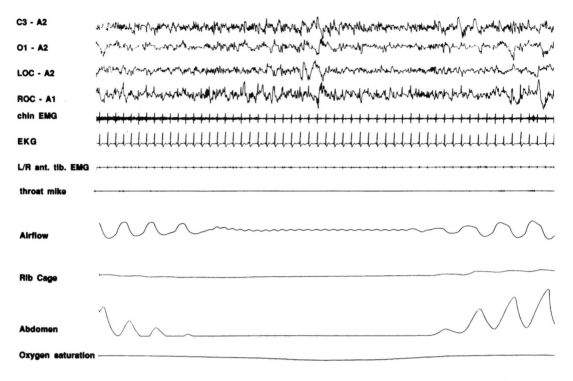

**Figure 16-2.** A 60-second excerpt from a nocturnal polysomnogram showing central apnea. Note the absence of respiratory effort. The sinusoidal variation in the airflow channel during the apnea is cardiac artifact. Each heartbeat displaces a small amount of air which is detected by the nasal thermistor. The fact that cardiogenic air movement is present in the upper airway further substantiates the assumption that the upper airway is patent, supporting the characterization of this event as a central apnea. Calibration as in Figure 16-1. (LOC, ROC = left and right outer canthus of the eye; EMG = electromyography; EKG = electrocardiography.)

of the respiratory events appear as mixed or obstructive, but with the application of nasal CPAP the "pure" central apneas (Figure 16-2) were evident. The measurement of intrapleural pressure with an endoesophageal catheter and intercostal EMG can be helpful in determining the degree to which a respiratory disturbance is caused by decreased effort or increased upper airway resistance. Until a clear understanding of the pathophysiology of respiration and sleep emerges and can account for the wide variety of clinical phenomena observed, much of our scoring and labeling are somewhat contrived.

Respiratory events can cause arousals. The arousals may be of different types, as discussed under Arousals, later in this chapter. We divide all respiratory events into one of three categories based on the type and duration of the arousal: (1) no EEG change, (2) EEG changes without awakening, and (3) EEG changes with awakening. The first category is obvious and is characterized by events that

do not appear to affect the EEG or produce other signs of arousal (such as significant chin muscle tension). The second category refers to those arousals characterized as a change in stage of sleep (such as from stage III to stage I) or those with a change to alpha rhythm that lasts less than 15 seconds. The last category refers to a waking EEG pattern that lasts longer than 15 seconds.

In summary, all respiratory events are recorded both by type (obstructive, mixed, or central), and by arousal (none, <15 seconds, or waking).

### Leg Movements

One can measure the electrical activity of many muscles, but in routine sleep recordings, both anterior tibialis muscles are typically monitored. One can see potentials occur from these muscles in many different circumstances. For example, with

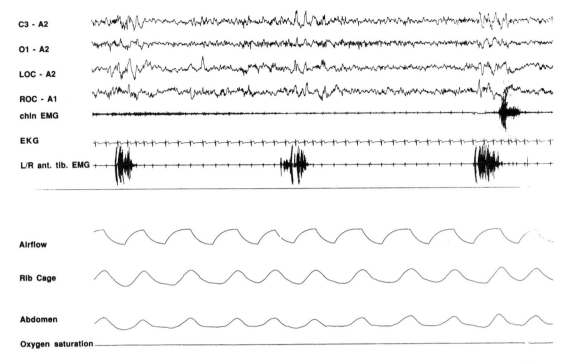

**Figure 16-3.** A 60-second excerpt from a nocturnal polysomnogram showing typical nocturnal myoclonus. We would score the final leg jerk as arousing because of the evident change in the EEG. Calibration as in Figure 16-1 except that signals from the right and left legs are combined. (LOC, ROC = left and right outer canthus of the eye; EMG = electromyography; EKG = electrocardiography.)

almost any bodily movement of the patient during wake or sleep, a potential is seen. Our laboratory follows the criteria originally outlined by Coleman to score periodic leg movements (nocturnal myoclonus).[15] Figure 16-3 illustrates periodic leg movements in sleep.

Leg jerks are scored when a potential occurs in one or both anterior tibialis channels and cannot be attributed to an arousal from some other cause. To be scored as a leg jerk, a potential must have a duration of at least 0.5 second. We do not score potentials that occur during wakefulness.

Leg movements may occur randomly or in episodes with a periodicity. For the purposes of calculating movement indices, we consider only those potentials that occur in episodes. We divide all leg potentials into one of three categories, as we do for respiratory events: (1) no EEG changes, (2) EEG changes without awakening, and (3) EEG changes with awakening.

When leg movements occur in an episode, the arousal may precede, occur simultaneously, or fol-

low the beginning of the leg potential.[16] During an obvious episode, therefore, we do not try to make a fine distinction between which comes first, the arousal or the leg movement. For arousals not in episodes, however, we do try to differentiate between a spontaneous arousal and one that is caused by a leg jerk. When scoring random arousals, if the leg potential occurs before the initial signs of arousal, we score this as an arousing leg jerk. If the K complex or other sign of arousal occurs before the leg potential, it is scored as a spontaneous arousal.

### Arousals

There are many types of arousals. Usually, one defines arousals based on the EEG. Thus, although an increase in heart rate or respiratory rate may constitute a physiologic arousal in response to some event, these are not usually scored. One tries to describe both the nature and the cause of the arousal. We discussed some of the causes of arousal earlier, including respiratory events and leg movements. Often, however, arousals appear to be spontaneous with no discernible cause. Not all arousals are pathologic. For the purposes of sleep stage scoring and analysis, however, an attempt should be made to identify the cause of as many arousals as possible. In some cases of apparently spontaneous arousals, one can presume that the cause is an event in a system not being monitored, such as occult gastroesophageal reflux. Many spontaneous arousals are caused by intrinsic brain activity alone and are not triggered by any particular peripheral factor.

Careful analysis of each arousal is necessary before concluding that the arousal is spontaneous (produced entirely by the central nervous system). For example, snoring can cause repetitive arousals in the absence of frank apneas, and even in the absence of hypopneas. For this reason, we routinely record from a snoring microphone taped onto the neck. Increased upper airway resistance even in the absence of snoring can cause arousals. Similarly, very slight fluctuations in oxygen saturation can provoke arousal. In other instances, review of the videotape may reveal noise coming from adjoining rooms.

In general, we do not score as an arousal a simple sleep stage shift, such as a shift from stage III to stage II, unless there is some accompanying behavioral or neurophysiologic change. For example, an abrupt change from stage IV to stage I with an increase in muscle tone and a light cry from the patient is probably significant and should be scored. In addition, when a patient is just entering sleep and is drowsing from wakefulness toward stage I, we usually do not score arousals. Only if a very long period of shifts from stage I to wakefulness occurs do we describe these arousals as pathologic.

A commonly encountered arousal may take the form of a sudden return to a waking record such as the alpha rhythm. There may be an increase in chin muscle tone, and evidence of movement. The arousal may be short-lived or produce wakefulness. The arousals may be predominant during a certain stage of sleep and may be absent during another. They may be periodic or random. Such factors and patterns of arousals are necessary to note, in addition to simply scoring the number of arousals.

As mentioned earlier, a certain number of arousals from various causes are normal in sleep and are always encountered when scoring a record. The scorer must have an appropriate threshold for scoring arousals, which must be determined by the laboratory staff. For example, the K complex is often considered to be a brain response to some internal arousing stimulus, but obviously one cannot score all K complexes as arousals. At the other extreme, a scorer must not overlook brief arousals that might not be sufficient to cause stage changes, but are sufficient to affect sleep in other ways.

A report from a task force of the American Sleep Disorders Association has provided some rules for the scoring of EEG arousals.[17] In the system, an EEG arousal is defined as an abrupt shift in EEG frequency, which may include theta, alpha, or frequencies greater than 16 Hz but not spindles, subject to various conditions, some of which will be mentioned later. Subjects must be asleep, a state defined as 10 or more continuous seconds of an indication of any stage of sleep before an EEG arousal can be scored. Thus, arousal scoring is independent of the Rechtschaffen and Kales procedure for epoch scoring. At least 10 continuous seconds of intervening sleep is necessary to score a second arousal. The EEG frequency shift must last 3 seconds or more to be scored as an arousal. Arousals in NREM sleep can occur without any increase in chin muscle tone, whereas arousals in REM sleep can be scored only if accompanied by an increase in submental EMG amplitudes. Arousals are not scored on the basis of chin muscle tone or on changes in respiration or heart rate alone. In addition, K complexes or delta waves are not considered arousals unless there is also the abrupt shift to higher frequencies, seen in at least one derivation.

Our laboratory uses these criteria, described in greater detail in the report,[17] with the addition of a few modifying rules to assist the technicians. First, the word *abrupt* is very important, because fast frequencies are often seen in various stages of sleep that should not be counted as arousals. Thus, we have had to emphasize that arousals need to be distinguishable from the background rhythm of the concurrent stage. Second, we prefer to score some arousals that are mostly in the form of K complexes. A series of high-voltage waves, probably representing K complexes, is a common response to any arousing stimulus. Such complexes are increasingly recognized as clinically significant entities, especially when they occur in a periodic fashion or are associated with nonrestorative sleep.[18] A possibly related phenomenon is the epileptic K complex, in which sharp waves are intermingled with a series of K complexes.[19]

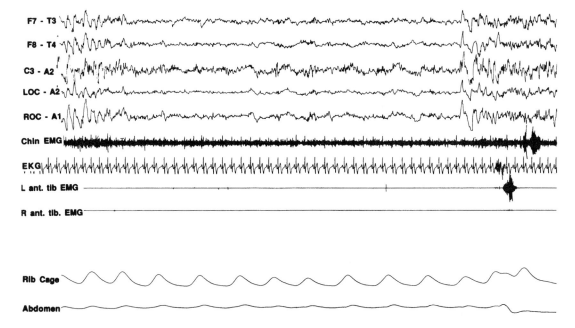

**Figure 16-4.** A 60-second excerpt from a nocturnal polysomnogram showing periodic K-alpha arousals in a 45-year-old man who had frequent nocturnal awakenings and complained of daytime sleepiness. He was successfully treated with carbamazepine (Tegretol). Calibration as in Figure 16-1. (LOC, ROC = left and right outer canthus of the eye; EMG = electromyography; EKG = electrocardiography.)

The task force recommendations require fast activity as a prerequisite to scoring an arousal. We consider as an arousal a series of at least three or four K-like complexes, especially if they occur in association with some identifiable event such as a contraction of the anterior tibialis muscle, an increase in chin EMG, or intrusion of alpha activity (Figure 16-4). Even if no events are associated with these complexes, however, such as EMG changes, we are more likely to score them and to consider them clinically significant if the complexes are periodic.

### Alpha-Delta Sleep

Another common pattern of sleep EEG is delta sleep with alpha frequencies superimposed on or interspersed with the slower delta waves.[20] This pattern is often seen in patients with chronic musculoskeletal pain and other patients with the complaint of nonrestorative sleep. An epoch of alpha-delta sleep consists of 5–20% of delta activity interspersed with prominent alpha activity. Neither the frequency nor the cortical distribution of alpha activity during sleep is identical to the alpha activity

seen during relaxed wakefulness.[21] In our hands, this alpha activity is usually approximately 1 Hz slower than the alpha rhythm typical of quiet waking. We score the record as stage III or IV, but make note of the overriding alpha activity (Figure 16-5).

### Sleep Stage Scoring in Patients with a Disease of the Central Nervous System

Often, one must score the record of a patient with a brain disease that is likely to disrupt the normal patterns of activity described earlier. This is particularly true in patients with head injuries, degenerative neurologic diseases, previous brain surgery, or metabolic encephalopathy. One could also consider patients with REM behavior disorder in this category. Often, there is no identifiable alpha rhythm, because the waking state is characterized by diffuse theta and delta activity. Sleep onset and offset are thus very difficult to delineate. Such cases require a revision of the normal rules. For example, one must note rapid eye movements at the beginning of the record, coupled with frequent body movements and a high chin EMG to determine that

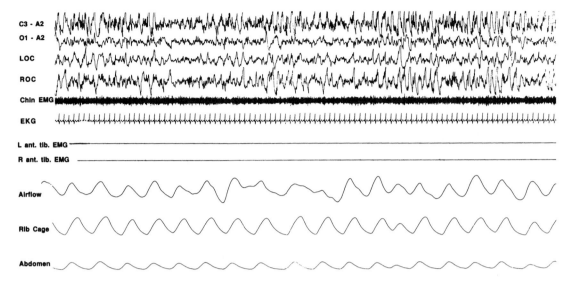

**Figure 16-5.** A 60-second excerpt from a nocturnal polysomnogram showing alpha-delta sleep. Note that both alpha and delta frequencies are evident. Calibration as in Figure 16-1. (LOC, ROC = left and right outer canthus of the eye; EMG = electromyography; EKG = electrocardiography.)

the EEG represents wakefulness. One can then determine the onset of sleep through other means, including behavioral correlates from the videotape, regularization of respiration, or the presence of rolling eye movements. At this time, the EEG will usually slow or increase in voltage, and this represents the person's initial sleep. Stage III or IV sleep can be overscored in such patients because of an underlying tendency for (pathologic) delta activity. We have seen patients with a monotonous tendency for similar EEG patterns in waking and sleeping, and often the usual landmarks of stage II sleep are completely absent. All such patients must be recorded and scored on an ad hoc basis.

REM behavior disorder should no longer cause major problems in scoring REM, but we have encountered patients with Parkinson's disease who had almost no identifiable REM. On close review of the record (already complicated by the problems discussed earlier) of these patients, we could identify probable REM of very short duration (less than one to two epochs), aborted by muscle activity and movement. The onset of REM periods in patients with REM behavior disorder can be identified, but they are frequently interrupted by muscle artifact, arousals, and waking rhythms. The scorer must make special note of these arousals, and score them within the REM period as necessary.

## SLEEP STUDIES IN NEWBORNS

The development of sleep and wakefulness begins in utero and continues throughout the perinatal period.[22] During this same period, sleep begins to differentiate into two distinct states that are consistent with REM and NREM sleep stages. Because of these developmental changes, sleep studies in newborn infants require a unique set of interpretative tools that are outlined in the infant counterpart of Rechtschaffen and Kales, by Anders and coworkers.[23] In this manual, four states of sleep and wakefulness are recognized in newborn infants: awake, active-REM sleep, quiet sleep, and indeterminate sleep. Assigning sleep states in the infant requires consideration of external factors such as light, sound, and temperature, which have profound physiologic effects in the newborn. In addition, respiratory monitoring is crucial because the pattern of breathing is the single most useful characteristic for sleep state scoring. The remainder of this section lists and describes useful categories to aid in coding observed behavior and PSG data.[23]

### *Respiration*

Breathing is called *regular* if the respiratory rate varies less than 20 cycles per minute; breathing is called *irregular* if the respiratory rate varies more than 20 cycles per minute.

### Eye Movements

Eye movements are coded positive (+) if at least one REM occurs in the epoch, and negative (−) if none occurs.

### Electromyogram

The muscles near the chin are recommended for recording EMGs. Muscle tone is called *high* if more than half the epoch shows *tonic* muscle activity; muscle tone is called *low* if more than half the epoch shows suppression.

### Patterns of Electroencephalographic Activity

The technician should look for the following patterns of EEG activity when coding data in sleep studies of newborns:

- Low-voltage, irregular (LVI): Voltage ranges from 14 to 35 μV, usually 20–30 μV. The record is dominated by theta activity (5–8 Hz), but slow waves (1–5 Hz) do occur.
- Tracé alternant (TA): Bursts of high-voltage, slow waves with occasional rapid, low-voltage waves superimposed, and sharp waves of 2–4 Hz interspersed with periods of relative quiescence between the slow waves.
- High-voltage, slow (HVS): Continuous, moderately rhythmic, moderately high-voltage waves with an amplitude of 50–150 μV and a frequency of 0.5–4.0 Hz.
- Mixed (M): Both low- and high-voltage, slow components.

### Miscellaneous

The category of miscellaneous behavior includes penile erections, sneezes, coughs, hiccups, yawns, burps, regurgitations, and flatus.

### Disruptions

External events that disturb the infant and may change the sleep recording include feedings and diaper changes.

Behavioral scales have been developed to supplement PSG findings because of the difficulty in determining sleep stage using EEG alone. One such scale, developed by Prechtl and Beintema,[24] identifies five behavioral states:

- State 1: eyes closed, regular respiration, no gross movements
- State 2: eyes closed, irregular respiration
- State 3: eyes open, no gross movement
- State 4: eyes open, gross movements
- State 5: eyes open or closed, vocal

### Criteria for Sleep State Scoring in Infants

In practice, sleep state scoring in infants involves assessment of behavioral state along with EMG, EEG, and EOG recordings.[23–25]

To score an epoch as *awake*, at least three of the following criteria must be fulfilled:

1. Sustained tonic EMG with active bursts
2. Eyes open
3. Within a given minute, breathing-rate variation is greater than 45 breaths per minute as measured by a respiratory tachometer
4. Vocalization
5. Sustained gross movement

### Active REM Sleep

Active REM sleep in infants is defined as the absence of chin EMG (EMG is coded as *low*) plus at least three of the following criteria:

1. At least one eye movement, independent of chin and gross body movement (EOG is positive)
2. Within a given minute, breathing rate variation greater than 20 breaths per minute as measured by a respiratory tachometer (respiration is *irregular*)
3. Presence of twitches and brief head movements
4. Absence of EEG spindles or TA (EEG is usually LVI or M)

Other observations that help establish the state of REM sleep include frequent facial movements, including grimaces, frowns, and bursts of sucking; limb movements and gross body movement; penile erections; and brief vocalizations such as grunts and whimpers.

### Quiet Sleep

For quiet sleep, all of the following criteria must be fulfilled:

1. Within a given minute, breathing variation is less than 20 breaths per minute (respiration is *regular*)

2. Eyes closed; no more than one isolated eye movement (EOG is negative)
3. Sustained EMG tonus (EMG is *high*) and EEG spindles, TA, or both (EEG is HVS, TA, or M)
4. No gross body movements

### Indeterminate Sleep

Indeterminate sleep is defined as epochs in which the criteria for any stage are not fulfilled, or epochs at sleep onset, sleep state change or on arousal.

### Sleep Scoring in Older Infants and Children

By approximately 3 months of age, the rudimentary forms of REM and NREM sleep stages are present, allowing the use of a modified adult scoring system.[26] In children older than 2 years, the adult equipment setup can be used with little or no modification, and the Rechtschaffen and Kales methodology can be applied.[4]

## TABULATION AND REPORT

Modern clinical practice of sleep disorders medicine is now so uniform that a standard format is the norm for sleep laboratory findings. At minimum, nocturnal sleep parameters should be tabulated to present clearly time in bed, total sleep time, and standard parameters relating to sleep structure (i.e., time spent in various stages and selected latencies). After the tabulation of sleep parameters, a narrative summary (often with tabular presentation of selected data) is prepared that incorporates relevant cardiopulmonary and movement data. Appendix 16-1 contains a sample report from our laboratory that is representative of the standards of practice observed in North America. The sleep data are dictated into our template by the clinician relying on a computer program that reduces sleep stage data previously entered in the form of page numbers and technologist-scored sleep staging. Many programs of this type are commercially available. The narrative conclusion of the report aims to relate all sleep laboratory findings to a final diagnosis.

It is important to prepare the sleep laboratory report as a document that is distinct from the sleep disorders center consultation, which sets forth the clinical history, diagnosis, and treatment recommendations or management plan. In fact, many of our sleep laboratory reports are prepared by a physician who has no clinical knowledge of the patient. It is the consultation (rather than the sleep laboratory report) that should conform to local standards of medical practice regarding treatment recommendations and applicable laws regarding reporting of disability and driving impairment.

## REFERENCES

1. Davis H, Davis P, Loomis A. Human brain potentials during the onset of sleep. J Neurophysiol 1939;1:24.
2. Blake H, Gerard R. Brain potentials and depth of sleep. Am J Physiol 1937;119:692.
3. Gibbs F, Gibbs E. Atlas of Electroencephalography. I. Methodology and Normal Controls. Cambridge, MA: Addison-Wesley, 1950.
4. Rechtshaffen A, Kales A. A Manual of Standardized Terminology, Techniques and Scoring System for Sleep Stages of Human Subjects. Los Angeles: UCLA Brain Information Service/Brain Research Institute, 1968.
5. Jasper HH. The ten twenty electrode system of the International Federation. Electroencephalogr Clin Neurophysiol 1958;10:371.
6. Brazier MAB, Cobb W, Fischgold H, et al. Preliminary proposal for an EEG terminology by the Terminology Committee of the International Federation of Electroencephalography and Clinical Neurophysiology. Electroencephalogr Clin Neurophysiol 1961;13:646.
7. McGregor P, Snyder M, Schmidt-Nowara W, Thorpy M. T-sleep: a new method for scoring breathing-disordered sleep. Sleep Res 1989;18:395.
8. American Psychiatric Association Task Force on Quantitative Electrophysiological Assessment. Quantitative electroencephalography: a report on the present state of computerized EEG techniques. Am J Psychiatry 1991;148:961.
9. Broughton R, Fleming J, Fleetham J. Home assessment of sleep disorders by portable monitoring. J Clin Neurophysiol 1996;13:272.
10. Lessnau JM, Erman M, Mitler MM. Scoring reliability among the SensorMedics somnostar system and two experienced polysomnographic technologists. Sleep Res 1991;20:430.
11. Wylie D, Miller JC, Shultz T, et al. Technical Report: Commercial Driver Fatigue, Loss of Alertness, and Countermeasures. FHWA-MC-97-001. Washington, DC: U.S. Department of Transportation, 1996.
12. Dawson A, Bigby BG, Poceta JS, Mitler MM. Effect of bedtime alcohol on inspiratory resistance and respira-

tory drive in snoring and nonsnoring men. Alcohol Clin Exp Res 1997;21:183.

13. Strollo PJ Jr, Sanders MH. Significance and treatment of nonapneic snoring. Sleep 1993;16:403.

14. Issa FG, Sullivan CE. Reversal of central sleep apnea using nasal CPAP. Chest 1986;90:165.

15. Coleman RM. Periodic Movements in Sleep (Nocturnal Myoclonus) and Restless Legs Syndrome. In C Guilleminault (ed), Sleeping and Waking Disorders. Indications and Techniques. Menlo Park, CA: Addison-Wesley, 1982;265.

16. Kotagal P, Ferber RA, Mograss M. Relationship of EEG changes to periodic leg movements. Sleep Res 1990;19:224.

17. Sleep Disorders Atlas Task Force of the American Sleep Disorders Association (preliminary report). EEG arousals: scoring rules and examples. Sleep 1992;15:174.

18. Hoelscher TJ, Ware JC, McBrayer RH. Insomnia with periodic EEG arousals in the absence of apnea and myoclonus. Sleep Res 1989;18:245.

19. Peled R, Lavie P. Paroxysmal awakenings from sleep associated with excessive daytime sleepiness: a form of nocturnal epilepsy. Neurology 1986;36:95.

20. Wittig RM, Zorick FJ, Blumer D, et al. Disturbed sleep in patients complaining of chronic pain. J Nerv Ment Dis 1982;170:429.

21. Fredrickson PA, Krueger BR. Insomnia Associated with Specific Polysomnographic Findings. In M Kryger, T Roth, WC Dement (eds), Principles and Practice of Sleep Medicine (2nd ed). Philadelphia: Saunders, 1994;523.

22. Guilleminault C (ed). Sleep and Its Disorders in Children. New York: Raven, 1987.

23. Anders T, Emde R, Parmelee A. A Manual of Standardized Terminology, Techniques and Criteria for Scoring of Stages of Sleep and Wakefulness in Newborn Infants. Los Angeles: UCLA Brain Information Service, NINDS Neurological Information Network, 1971.

24. Prechtl HFR, Beintema D. The Neurological Examination of the Full Term Newborn Infant. In Clinics in Developmental Medicine (no. 12), Spastics International Medical Publications. Philadelphia: Lippincott, 1964;74.

25. Hoppenbrouwers T. Electronic Monitoring in the Newborn and Young Infant: Theoretical Considerations. In C Guilleminault (ed), Sleeping and Waking Disorders. Indications and Techniques. Menlo Park, CA: Addison-Wesley, 1982;17.

26. Coons S. Development of Sleep and Wakefulness During the First 6 Months of Life. In C Guilleminault (ed), Sleep and Its Disorders in Children. New York: Raven, 1987;17.

# Chapter 16 Appendix
# Clinical Polysomnography Report

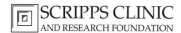 SCRIPPS CLINIC
AND RESEARCH FOUNDATION

*Division of Sleep Disorders*
*Sleep Disorders Center*

## DIAGNOSIS: SLEEP APNEA

## PROCEDURES

Polysomnography was conducted on the night of 3/24/91. Recording began at 2211 and ended at 0635 for a total recording of 504 minutes.

Medical parameters monitored throughout the night were left and right central electroencephalogram, left and right electro-oculogram, digastric muscle electromyogram (EMG), respiratory air flow from sensors placed at the nasal and buccal orifices, and respiratory effort from sensors placed around the thorax and around the abdomen. Cardiac rhythm was monitored from electrodes placed on either clavicle, producing an all-night (8–12 hours) electrocardiographic waveform similar to V2. An all-night audio and visual record of events was kept by means of continuous monitoring with an infrared video camera, a low-level microphone, and a videocassette recorder. A microphone was fixed on the neck to record respiratory sounds.

Additional parameters for the specific diagnostic purposes of this recording included EMG from both anterior tibialis muscles and oxygen saturation by all-night, quantified pulse oximetry.

## PARAMETRIC ANALYSIS

See Table 16A-1.

## QUALITATIVE DESCRIPTION

The patient reported that the quality and quantity of sleep was much better than usual. He did not awaken with his hangover-headachy feeling. He did not awaken with nasal congestion. Respiratory sounds were heard as occasional snores. Respiratory air flow and effort measures disclosed 39 obstructive hypopneas, all of which caused arousal. Interestingly, the patient had significant desaturations in REM sleep, which were not associated with discrete apneas or hypopneas, although there may have been a slight decrease in tidal volume over long periods during his REM periods leading to desaturation. The study was not typical for obstructive sleep apnea syndrome, although occasional hypopneas were seen. Baseline oxygen saturation was 95%. The mean overnight was 92%, and the lowest value was 76%. The computer counted 44 desaturation events. The pattern of oximetry shows long desaturations to about 80% during each REM period, some of which are repetitive but many are simply stable desaturations. This pattern suggests that the patient is on the steep part of the oxyhemoglobin dissociation curve and has limited pulmonary reserve, and that changes in tidal volume, although difficult to measure, were occurring during REM sleep. The steady-state heart rate was approximately 70 without significant change. The blood pressure was 170/70

**Table 16A-1.** Parametric Analysis

| Sleep Parameter | Observed Value | Laboratory Norms |
|---|---|---|
| Sleep latency (3 epochs stage I sleep) | 1 min | 0–60 mins |
| Patient's estimate of sleep latency | 60 mins | 5–60 mins |
| Estimation error for sleep latency | +59 mins | −5 to +20 mins |
| Sleep duration | 332 mins | 300–420 mins |
| Patient's estimate of sleep duration | 420 mins | 300–450 mins |
| Estimation error for sleep duration | +88 mins | −60 to +30 mins |
| Sleep efficiency (% of time asleep) | 65.9% | 80–93% |
| Percentage of stage I NREM sleep | 7.7% | 7–16% |
| Percentage of stage II NREM sleep | 60.5% | 47–87% |
| Percentage of stage III NREM sleep | 11.5% | 0–5% |
| Percentage of stage IV NREM sleep | 5.4% | 0 |
| Percentage of stage REM sleep | 14.9% | 13–29% |
| Latency from first sleep to REM sleep | 75 mins | 11–210 mins |

mm Hg (hs) and 140/80 mm Hg (AM). The EMG recordings from both legs disclosed 215 contractions of the anterior tibialis muscle organized into several episodes, mostly in the middle and late portions of the night. These occurred during non-REM sleep and were absent in REM sleep. The potentials have a period of about 30 seconds. Review of the videotape reveals mild movements of the ankles and knees, the details of which are obscured by the bed covers. The leg movements significantly fragmented sleep and contributed to more than 150 arousals.

Sleep structure was abnormal for this 80-year-old man. Sleep was deep at times but frequently fragmented. He had long periods of waking time. REM sleep in particular was fragmented. For reasons that were not quite clear, there was more slow-wave activity than expected.

## CONCLUSION

The nocturnal polysomnographic data and accompanying audiovisual recording demonstrate the following:

1. Periodic limb movements of sleep (nocturnal myoclonus). This is moderately severe with a movement index of 39 and a movement arousal index of 27.
2. REM hypoxemia. This is not definitely obstructive in nature and appears to be on the basis of a central decrease in tidal volume in association with limited pulmonary reserve. The lowest saturation value obtained was 76% and the patient spent 9% of the sleeping time with a saturation of under 90%. The mean saturation overnight was 92%.
3. Occasional obstructive hypopneas. Number is borderline for the diagnosis of obstructive sleep apnea. The respiratory disturbance index is 7.
4. Subjectively, an extremely good night of sleep with the patient awakening without his usual headachy feeling and his usual sinus congestion. This could be due to the different sleeping environment.

# Chapter 17

# Techniques for the Assessment of Sleep-Related Erections

## Max Hirshkowitz and Constance A. Moore

## SLEEP-RELATED ERECTIONS: DEFINITION AND DESCRIPTION

Sleep-related erections (SREs) occur cyclically during sleep in all sexually potent men. SREs are naturally occurring, involuntary episodes of penile tumescence that are closely associated with rapid eye movement (REM) sleep. In healthy normal young adults, SREs persist during a REM sleep episode and detumescence proceeds when non-REM sleep re-emerges. SREs were originally called *nocturnal penile tumescence*, a term coined by Karacan in deference to his advisors' suggestion that "penile erections in sleep" was too explicit.[1] Polysomnographic (PSG) technique provides an opportunity to noninvasively index erectile function. Because SREs occur with great consistency and can be objectively quantified, they represent an unparalleled approach for research and clinical assessment of human erectile function.

## SLEEP-RELATED ERECTIONS, REM SLEEP, AND DREAMING

In the early 1960s, two research groups independently demonstrated the close temporal relationship between REM sleep and SREs. Long before either Karacan[1] or Fisher and associates[2] documented the relationship between REM sleep and SREs, Aserinsky[3] hypothesized that there was such a relationship. The existence of an erection cycle during sleep

had previously been described by Ohlmeyer and associates.[4]

When dreaming was found to occur mainly during REM sleep, laboratory sleep studies were conceptualized as a tool to investigate the "royal road to the unconscious mind."[5] The coupling of SREs and REM sleep revived interest in Freud's postulated underlying psychosexual nature of dreaming. A case series published by Fisher and colleagues[6] described sudden increases in SREs correlated with overtly erotic dream content. In contrast, a systematic study by Karacan[1] did not find a relationship between sexual dream content and SREs. It is worth noting that laboratory dream reports seldom contain erotic content.[7,8] In fact, McCarley and Hoffman[9] found no erotic content in 104 dreams from 14 subjects they studied.

## SLEEP-RELATED ERECTIONS AND THE DIAGNOSIS OF IMPOTENCE

Motivated by the desire to find an objective biological marker to distinguish psychogenic from organic impotence, Karacan[10] proposed using SRE testing to differentially diagnose erectile dysfunction. Concurrent development of surgical interventions for treating erectile failure increased the need for reliable diagnostic techniques.

Inability to volitionally attain a rigid erection can result from either psychogenic or organic factors. Erectile capacity is confirmed if the patient can have an erection of normal circumference increase and rigidity. Because impotence, regardless of etiology, often results in psychosocial complications, psychometric evaluation does not rule out organicity. Some practitioners have their patients view sexually explicit videotapes to assess erectile responsiveness. If fantasy or erotica fail to elicit an adequate erection, however, the cause of impotence remains obscure. Situational factors in the clinical setting can inhibit erection in some men, especially those with performance anxiety. Therefore, sleep studies provide another opportunity to examine erectile capacity. It is of interest to note that presleep sexual activity or arousal does not alter SRE patterns. In addition, sexual abstinence in healthy volunteer subjects is not associated with changes in SRE patterns.[11,12]

Under the veil of sleep, wakefulness-related sexual inhibition fades. Parasympathetic activity during REM sleep is conducive to erectile activity. Central nervous system, vascular, and endocrine mechanisms engage and SREs occur. Documenting a penile erection of normal size and rigidity accompanying REM sleep establishes erectile capability. It must be emphasized, however, that PSG studies of SREs do not obviate the need for a thorough sexual history, genital neurovascular examination, psychometrics, medical history, and physical examination. In some cases, endocrine and nerve conduction studies are also required.

---

## TRADITIONAL POLYSOMNOGRAPHIC TECHNIQUE FOR SLEEP-RELATED ERECTIONS

### Overview

The traditional approach for evaluating SREs includes standard PSG with additional channels for penile circumference increase (PCI). Measuring PCI involves placing mercury-filled strain gauges around the penis. During an erection, the strain gauge tubing elongates and narrows, thereby increasing the circuit's electrical resistance. This change in resistance is transduced to direct current voltage by a bridge amplifier. The bridge amplifier output, when connected to the polygraph pen driver input, provides a continuous tracing of circumference change. Placing gauges at both the penile base and the coronal sulcus

offers several advantages compared to a single gauge placed at midshaft. Advantages include redundancy, improved reliability, and greater sensitivity to erectile anomalies.

Research indicates that men with erectile dysfunction have a high prevalence of sleep apnea and periodic limb movement disorder.[13,14] Therefore, current sleep laboratory protocols for assessing SREs should include monitoring respiration and leg movement. These data assist the clinician interpreting SRE recordings and help avoid false-positive tests (incorrectly diagnosing organic impotence).

### Gauge Size and Calibration

Accurate SRE recording requires properly fitting gauges. A loose gauge allows circumferential expansion that is not registered by polygraphic pen deflection. The result is PCI underestimation and in extreme cases, SRE episodes may go undetected. A gauge that is too tight may produce distorted output. Transduction amplifiers have an optimal range in which the input-output response is linear. Significantly elevated baseline input from a tight gauge can drive the bridge amplifier beyond its linear range when an erection occurs. In addition, a tight gauge may break during body movement. Consequently, valid SRE testing begins with accurate penile circumference measurement and selecting a properly sized gauge. Gauges should be carefully inspected before and after placement around the penis to assure a snug but not tight fit. Furthermore, kinking or rolling the gauge must be avoided.

Because electrical characteristics differ among gauges, each gauge requires individual, nightly calibration. The ultimate purpose of calibration is to establish an invariant relationship between actual circumference increase and the amplitude of pen deflection on the polygraph. One can attain this goal using different calibration procedures; however, I will describe the one used at our sleep disorders center.

To simulate a 20-mm PCI, we use a calibration block consisting of two short cylinders differing in circumference and mounted concentrically, one atop the other. The circumference of the larger cylinder (called the *large end*) exceeds the smaller by precisely 20 mm. We maintain a selection of calibration blocks to calibrate different size gauges. Blocks are named according to the circumference of the smaller of the two cylinders (*small end*) and range from 50 to 150 mm, in increments of 5 mm.

Calibration involves four steps. First, the gauge is placed around the small end and the bridge amplifier's electrical baseline is adjusted until it aligns with the desired polygraphic baseline. Second, the gauge is carefully moved to the large end and the amplifier's gain is adjusted so that the polygraph pen deflects 15 mm above pen baseline. We use a 20 to 15 mm (actual size to pen-deflection) ratio to avoid pen blocking during robust erections (recorded from research volunteers). Many laboratories prefer the more intuitive 1 to 1 ratio, especially if they perform only clinical evaluations. Third, the gauge is moved back to the small end and the examiner checks to make sure the pen returns to baseline. If the pen fails to return to baseline, the procedure must be repeated. Finally, the large end is re-examined to ensure a 15-mm deflection. To expedite calibration, gauges should be handled carefully (to avoid damage) and properly sized calibration blocks should be used.

After the calibrated, properly fitting gauges are placed on the patient, the pen should deflect several millimeters above baseline (assuming the patient does not have an erection). If the pen is below baseline, the gauge is too loose and should be replaced. If the pen has a large deflection, the gauge is too tight and likewise should be replaced. With a properly fitting gauge, the small initial pen deflection can be adjusted to baseline mechanically or with the balance control. Gain should never be altered after calibration.

### *Measuring Rigidity*

The minimum amount of force applied to the glans capable of buckling the penile shaft indexes axial rigidity (penile buckling resistance). Circumference increase alone is not sufficient to achieve vaginal penetration. Although PCI and penile rigidity are correlated under normal circumstances, dissociation occurs in a significant number of patients with erectile failure.[15] Therefore, penile rigidity during an erection is arguably the most important parameter when assessing erectile competence.

To measure rigidity, we awaken the patient during a representative SRE and quickly apply a calibrated force to the tip of the penis. If no buckling occurs with forces of up to 1,000$g$, we terminate the

procedure and assign the value 1,000$g$. In the older literature, buckling was sometimes measured in pressure (0–300 mm Hg). Devices used are typically electronic or spring-loaded force meters.

At the time rigidity is measured, the technologist photographs the erect penis, obtains a patient estimate of the percentage of full erection, and rates the erection for percentage of fullness. The photograph helps document abnormalities in penile size and shape (e.g., the curvature associated with Peyronie's disease). For patients electing prosthetic implantation, the photograph may aid surgeons in selecting the size of the prosthesis. The photograph also helps validate rigidity measures.

## WHAT CAN BE MEASURED?

### *Scoring Sleep-Related Erections*

Each tumescence episode is scored for three phases of activity. The first phase scored is called *T-up*. During T-up, arterial inflow produces penile swelling and increased intracorporeal pressure. T-up plateaus at maximum circumference increase (MCI) in normal individuals. The second phase, during which circumference remains at the maximum plateau, is called *T-max*. The third phase is detumescence (*T-down*) and is initiated by venous outflow and decreasing penile circumference. *T-zero* marks the point at which the T-down phase ends. For detailed scoring rules, see Ware and Hirshkowitz.[16]

### *Quantity, Quality, and Architecture of Erections*

Like most physiologic phenomena, SREs can be quantified along three dimensions: frequency, magnitude, and duration. The number of SRE episodes represents frequency. Magnitude is indexed by overall nightly MCI and the mean MCI per episode. Total tumescence time is the most common measure of duration.

Penile rigidity is used to objectively quantify erectile quality. Subjective estimates of erectile quality derive from patient and technician estimates of the percentage of full erection. Exaggerated patient underestimation suggests a psychogenic component in the erectile impotence.

SRE architectural measures provide numerical information about the overall erectile pattern. These include the slopes of increasing tumescence (T-up) and the swiftness of detumescence (T-down). Duration of sustained maximal erection (T-max) is especially important because many patients specifically complain about an inability to sustain erection during intercourse. Abnormal phase durations help characterize pathophysiology. Abnormal concordance between circumferential expansion at the penile base and at the coronal sulcus suggests vascular problems.

### Coordination between Sleep and Erections

To properly appreciate a patient's SRE pattern, data concerning SRE and REM sleep coordination are essential. The frequency, periodicity, and duration of SREs largely depend on REM sleep. For between-patient and normative data comparisons, it is useful to normalize SRE measures according to the amount of sleep or REM sleep. Study validation requires sleep staging to rule out SRE decreases secondary to sleep fragmentation or insufficient REM sleep. Frequent NREM sleep erections should alert the clinician to possible neurogenic problems.

## OTHER RECORDING DEVICES AND WHAT THEY MEASURE

### Home Monitoring Devices

The need to objectify diagnostic techniques fueled enthusiasm for using SRE testing in clinical practice. The cost and intensive labor associated with laboratory sleep studies encouraged development of less expensive, nonlaboratory alternatives.[17–24] One of the earliest alternative techniques was the *stamp test*.[17] This test involved encircling the penis with postage-type stamps at bedtime and instructing the patient to note in the morning if separation had occurred at the perforations between stamps. Stamp ring breakage was attributed to SREs and an intact ring was thought to verify organic impotence. In the original study, 22 potent men broke the stamp ring on 58 of 62 nights compared to only one stamp breakage observed among 11 impotent patients tested for 30 nights. Subsequent studies by other investigators reported less consistent results.[25,26] Stamp tests and snap gauges may detect SREs; however, they provide no data about frequency, magnitude, or duration. More elaborate SRE detection devices include felt gauges and expandable tubes. Again, initial validation study successes for some of these devices were followed by mixed results.[27] Some of these devices can produce false-negative results (finding normal SREs when the patient is organically impaired) due to movement artifact.[26,28]

More sophisticated SRE recorders are also available for home use. Most of them record penile circumference change, but not brain and eye movement activity. If SREs occur, the frequency, magnitude, and duration can be inspected and often quantified. The presence of a normal SRE pattern provides potentially useful diagnostic information. By contrast, the absence of an erection cycle may indicate organic impotence, equipment failure, improper gauge placement, or disturbed sleep. Without information concerning the presence or absence of REM sleep, false-positive tests (finding reduced SREs that are not produced by organic impotence) is a critical concern, especially in candidates for surgical intervention.

### Penile Buckling Resistance versus Penile Compressibility

Some portable erection monitors purport to measure rigidity. However, they derive the value from penile compressibility rather than buckling resistance. For example, RigiScan (Dacomed, Minneapolis, MN) assesses compressibility by tightening its penile loops and measuring penile resistance to compression. Snap gauges have embedded calibrated filaments that break upon reaching certain outward pressure. Felt gauges expand when the penis exceeds specific noncompressible expansion. It should be noted that the original literature emphasizing the importance of penile rigidity refers specifically to penile buckling resistance, not compressibility.

## VALUE OF SLEEP-RELATED ERECTION TESTING

Laboratory sleep studies provide the most complete data characterizing SREs, including visual

**Table 17-1.** Sleep-Related Erection (SRE) Recording Devices and What They Measure

| | Laboratory Sleep Studies | Bedside Monitors | Stamps, Snap, and Felt Gauges |
|---|---|---|---|
| SRE presence | Yes | Yes | Yes |
| SRE frequency | Yes | Yes | No |
| SRE magnitude | Yes | Yes | Yes* |
| SRE duration | Yes | Yes | No |
| SRE architecture | Yes | Yes | No |
| SRE–REM sleep coordination | Yes | No | No |
| Penile buckling resistance | Yes | No | No |

*Stamp rings and snap gauges do not provide SRE magnitude data.

**Table 17-2.** Comparison of Nonlaboratory and Laboratory Recording Procedures for Susceptibility to Artifact and Tampering

| | Laboratory Sleep Studies | Bedside Monitors | Stamps, Snap, and Felt Gauges |
|---|---|---|---|
| Body movement artifact | OK | OK | FN |
| Reflex erection (spasm) | OK | OK | FN |
| Disrupted REM sleep | OK | FP | FP |
| Significant sleep disorder | OK | FP | FP |
| Tampering/faking good | OK | OK* | FN |
| Tampering/faking bad | OK | FP | FP |

Note: A false-positive (FP) test erroneously supports the diagnosis of organic impotence. A false-negative (FN) test erroneously supports the diagnosis of psychogenic impotence.
*Careful inspection of tracings by an experienced scorer looking for sudden baseline changes can help avoid FN conclusions. However, research has shown that the addition of simultaneous electromyographic tracings improves overall accuracy.
Source: M Hirshkowitz, CA Moore, I Karacan. NPT/Rigidometry. In RS Kirby, CC Carson, GD Webster (eds), Impotence Diagnosis and Management of Male Erectile Dysfunction. Oxford: Butterworth–Heinemann, 1991.

inspection and penile buckling resistance measures. Critical reviews of SRE testing frequently intermix laboratory PSG evaluations and nonlaboratory, nonpolygraphic procedures. This fuels the controversy concerning the reliability and validity of SRE testing for the differential diagnosis of impotence. Table 17-1 summarizes parameters obtained from different recording devices. Most portable monitors continuously monitor penile circumference change; however, they provide no information concerning sleep status. The expandable and felt gauges can detect tumescence episodes and record the nightly maximum circumference increase. Finally, the least expensive device (stamp rings) will, at best, only reveal whether an erection has occurred during the sleep period. Like stamp rings, snap gauges may detect SREs and provide a crude measure of compressibility.

As nonlaboratory techniques became readily available, the referral pattern changed. PSG SRE study referrals now frequently involve three special types of clinical cases. The first includes those difficult cases with complex, confusing histories. The second consists of legal cases in which compensation or guilt hinges on erectile status. Finally, physicians, other health care workers, foreign dignitaries, and celebrities needing erectile function assessment are routinely referred for sleep studies at our center. The selection of when and for whom laboratory SRE studies are ordered may reflect less clinical confidence in nonlaboratory techniques. Table 17-2 summarizes the susceptibility of various techniques to false-positive and false-negative interpretations.

Over the years, we have encountered a significant number of patients who attempted to manipulate test outcome. Their motivations ranged from psychopathology to intent to defraud. Men with psychiatric disorders (e.g., somatoform disorder, hypochondriasis, Munchausen's syndrome) seeking surgical procedures and psychogenically impotent men seeking a surgical *quick fix* can easily produce false-positive test results when non-PSG techniques are used. Patients intentionally not wearing snap gauges or stamp rings, incorrectly reporting results of expandable gauges, or avoiding sleep by using stimulants represent real problems to diagnosis using non-PSG evaluations. A patient accused of sexual assault may claim innocence based on erectile impotence. Others may seek compensation for job-related injury. By contrast, patients have intentionally broken gauges (*faking good*) to avoid surgery. With proper sleep laboratory evaluation, maneuvers to produce false-positive or false-negative tests do not succeed.

## INTERPRETING SLEEP-RELATED ERECTIONS

### *Age-Related Normative Data*

Studies indicate a general decline in erectile function with advancing age. It is not known if these changes are secondary to pathology, a natural consequence of aging, or both. The use of medication known to adversely affect potency becomes more common with aging. Most available information derives from self-report and clinical observations. Karacan[10] first championed the idea that SRE testing could provide an objective basis for diagnosing male impotence. He immediately recognized that to achieve this goal, normative data were required. Therefore, data were gathered in young boys, young adults, middle-aged men, and the elderly.[29,30] Several other research groups have also described the relationship between aging and SREs in sexually potent men.[31,32]

The studies conducted at our laboratories[29,30] excluded individuals with significant mental or physical disease; therefore, the oldest groups (60–69 and 70–79 years) represent a "super-normal" sample of the senior population. Our primary finding was that all sexually potent men had SREs. Modest but statistically reliable declines were found for total tumescence time, duration of REM sleep–related tumescence, and number of REM-erection episodes with aging. Schiavi and colleagues[32] found greater SRE decline in their oldest group (age 65–74 years). Their sample included men with intermittent erectile failure, however, a problem that afflicted more men in the older groups. The research team lead by Reynolds[31] found a small age-related decline in the number of episodes, the ratio of tumescence to sleep duration, and the proportion of REM sleep with tumescence. These authors indicate that age accounted for less than 15% of variance in their measures of SREs. Moreover, they found no age-related decline in penile buckling resistance. The empirical data from these investigations demonstrate the ubiquity of SREs and their persistence, notwithstanding aging, in healthy, sexually potent men.

Comparing an individual's results to normative data requires caution. Normative values derive from multinight PSGs from men selected for good health and normal sleep. Patients referred for SRE assessments often have significant sleep disturbance. The close association between REM sleep and SREs may necessitate interpolation of normative values when sleep is disturbed. Normalizing SRE measures using REM sleep time or total sleep time can help; however, severely disturbed or fragmented sleep may render a study uninterpretable. The most common REM sleep disturbance results from *first night* adaptation to the laboratory setting. Additional nights usually remedy this nuisance. For patients with sleep pathology, therapeutic intervention (e.g., sleep-restriction therapy to consolidate sleep) typically improves interpretability. Nonetheless, some studies may prove inconclusive, which, although disappointing, is certainly preferable to false-positive or false-negative test interpretations. With proper technical procedures and interpretive skill, however, the percentage of inconclusive studies is very low.

As previously mentioned, penile rigidity is the most important measure obtained during SRE testing. The rationale for its use comes from several studies. To achieve penetration, female volunteers performing vaginal insertions with various-sized, lubricated, Lucite rods needed an average minimum force of $500g$.[33] In another study, men were asked during rigidity measurement if their erection was adequate for sexual intercourse. We found that erections with buckling resistance below $500g$ were seldom rated as sufficient to achieve penetration.

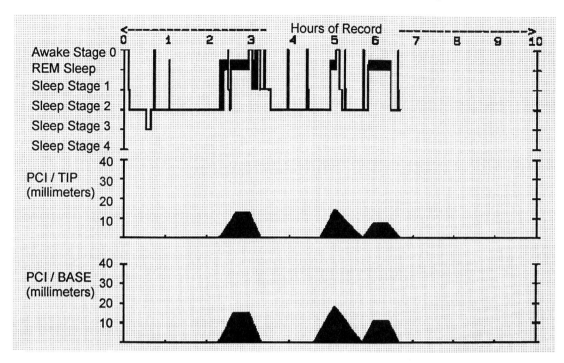

**Figure 17-1.** Sleep stages and sleep-related erections recorded from a 56-year-old man with psychogenic impotence. Sleep-related erections are well coordinated with REM sleep and normal with respect to frequency, magnitude, and duration. Rigidity measured during the first erectile episode was 880 g. The patient grossly underestimated his percentage of a full erection (30%) compared to the technician's rating (70%). There was no evidence of pelvic steal syndrome. The patient's medical history is significant for alcohol abuse, duodenal ulcers, hypertension (treated with hydrochlorothiazide), and depression (after death of first wife). Currently there are no sleep-wake complaints; however, combat-related nightmares associated with post-traumatic stress disorder were noted in the past. (PCI = penile circumference increase.)

Finally, groups of sexually potent men, regardless of age, have rigidities averaging well above 500$g$.[31] These data have led most clinicians to regard a buckling resistance of 500–600$g$ as the critical minimum *cutting score* for erectile capacity.

### Interpreting Normal Sleep-Related Erections

Normal SREs with adequate rigidity suggest functional erectile capacity. Figure 17-1 illustrates sleep stages and SREs recorded from a patient with psychogenic impotence. Before diagnosing psychogenic impotence in a man with normal SREs, the clinician should consider four conditions: (1) Peyronie's disease, (2) pelvic steal syndrome, (3) somatic nerve lesion or neuropathy, and (4) acute androgen deficiency. Although rare, these are organic conditions in which normal SRE profiles may occur. However,

misdiagnosis can be avoided by performing a neurovascular genital examination and a proper rigidity measure.

Peyronie's disease results in abnormal penile curvature that can impair penetration, notwithstanding normal circumferential expansion. Surprisingly, some men are unaware of their condition. Visual observation and photographing the erection during the rigidity measurement procedure documents penile curvature and provides the basis for proper diagnosis. *Pelvic steal syndrome* refers to the loss of an erection due to shunting of blood away from the pelvis during leg movement and thrusting. Measuring the consequence of deep knee bends on Doppler penile arterial blood pressure help detect pelvic steal syndrome. Large, rapid blood pressure drops immediately after this procedure alert the clinician to the need for further urologic assessment. Similarly, neurovascular genital examination of ascending sensory

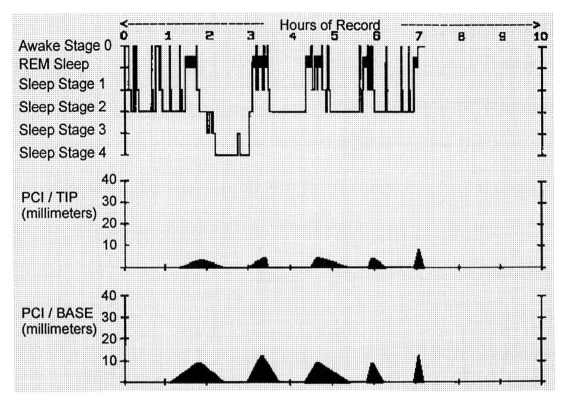

**Figure 17-2.** Sleep stages and sleep-related erections recorded from a 64-year-old man with organic impotence. Notwithstanding a normal number of tumescence episodes, well coordinated with REM sleep, circumference increase and rigidity were below normal. Maximum rigidity, measured during the patient's best erection, was 220*g*. The other recording night had a similar sleep-related erection profile. Past health was significant for insulin-dependent diabetes. We found borderline prolonged bulbocavernosus reflex latency and reduced penile arterial blood pressures on the right side. Sleep efficiency (91%) and REM percent (16%) were within normal limits. REM sleep latency was 73 minutes (43 minutes on night one) and all slow-wave sleep followed the first REM episode (also on night 1); however, we found no history or indication of depression. Significant periodic leg movements in sleep, for which the patient was subsequently treated, were revealed by polysomnography. Although the patient had a small oropharynx and low-set soft palate, sleep-related breathing was normal. (PCI = penile circumference increase.)

pathways may be needed to rule out neural lesions. Although men with long-term androgen deficiency have markedly diminished SREs,[34] men with acute deficiency (<2 months) may continue to have values in the normal range.[35] There exists a short but critical time frame during which endocrine evaluation is needed to rule out acute androgen deficiency in patients with normal SREs.

If normal SREs occur and Peyronie's disease, pelvic steal syndrome, penile-nerve problems, and acute androgen deficiency are ruled out, psychogenic erectile dysfunction is diagnosed. It is incorrect to assume, however, that psychopathology will invariably accompany psychogenic impotence; psychometric testing may be completely normal.

The erectile failure may arise from specific behavioral or relationship problems. Conversely, men with impotence of organic etiology are not immune to intrapsychic or relationship problems. We commonly find significant psychopathology in men with clearly organic impotence.

### *Interpreting Diminished Sleep-Related Erections*

PSGs with below normal SREs require special attention. The clinician must consider sleep integrity, drug effects, and comorbidity factors. Figure 17-2 illustrates sleep stages and SREs in a man with organic impotence.

Reasonably consolidated REM sleep of adequate duration is required to properly interpret diminished SREs. Sleep pathologies are common in men referred for evaluation of erectile impotence. We reviewed PSG data recorded from 768 consecutively evaluated impotent men and found that 54% had 15 or more leg movements per hour of sleep.[13] Many of these patients had disrupted sleep and repeated leg movement–related REM sleep interruptions. In some instances, therapeutic intervention reduced movement arousals sufficiently to permit SRE interpretation. In others cases, the high night-to-night variability in leg movements permitted interpretation of repeat recordings made on nights when the number of leg movements was fortuitously low.

We also investigated sleep-related breathing in 1,025 men complaining of erectile dysfunction.[14] Forty-four percent had sleep apnea (five or more episodes per hour of sleep) and 20% had moderate to severe sleep apnea (15 or more apnea episodes per hour). These two large-scale studies confirm previously reported high prevalence of leg movement and apnea disorders in men suffering from impotence.[36] Direct evidence that occult sleep disorders can impede interpretation of simple penile circumference recordings is provided by Pressmen and colleagues.[37] Thus, in patients with concurrent sleep pathology, PSG is crucial for interpretation.

Nasal continuous positive airway pressure (CPAP) therapy for management of sleep-related breathing disorders is now generally available. CPAP affords the sleep center a unique opportunity to advance diagnostic technique for impotence in men with sleep apnea. In our current impotence assessment protocol, we routinely titrate CPAP if PSG reveals significant respiratory disturbance. In patients with apnea-related reductions in REM sleep, REM-rebound sometimes unmasks normal SREs. Thus, SREs are sometimes normalized by CPAP therapy (Figure 17-3); moreover, self-reported erectile function may also improve.

Many drugs reportedly cause impotence.[38,39] The widespread use of antihypertensives makes them highly visible in the sexual dysfunction clinic. Prevalence estimates of sexual dysfunction range upward to 66% for beta blockers, 42% for α-adrenergics, and 36% for diuretics. Antidepressants, especially tricyclics with strong anticholinergic properties, produce erectile failure. Clinical reports also indicate impotence related to antipsychotic medications,

most notably haloperidol and chlorpromazine. Finally, we frequently encounter an assortment of other impotence-producing drugs, including anti-androgens, cancer chemotherapy agents, cimetidine, digoxin, disulfram, and atropine. Segraves and associates[38] provide an extensive review of the association between erectile dysfunction and pharmacologic agents.

Aside from their detrimental effects on sexual potency, some drugs adversely affect REM sleep. If a medication significantly suppresses or abolishes REM sleep, SRE testing may be inconclusive. Therefore, acquiring a thorough drug history is essential. Selective serotonin-reuptake inhibitors, tricyclic antidepressants, monoamine oxidase inhibitors, amphetamines, cocaine, barbiturates, and some benzodiazepines are particularly troublesome. When possible, we arrange for abstinence or reduction in medication, leading up to and during sleep evaluations. In some cases, data from the later portion of the night provide adequate information. For example, we occasionally see patients treated with antihypertensives who have no erections associated with their early REM sleep episodes. Toward morning, however, when drug levels declined, normal REM sleep–related tumescence occurred. Ware[40] reports a similar profile in his patients treated with cardiovascular medications.

The clinical literature associates erectile impotence with a wide variety of cardiovascular, endocrine, genitourinary, neurologic, psychiatric, and other conditions. Those most often encountered at our clinic include diabetes, hypertension, genital or pelvic trauma, hypogonadism, myocardial infarction, obstructive sleep apnea, chronic obstructive pulmonary disease, prostate conditions, chronic alcoholism, renal failure, spinal cord injury, multiple sclerosis, epilepsies, Parkinson's disease, opiate and cocaine abuse, and major depressive disorders. Evidence for whether a disease is causally related to impotence varies. Abnormal SREs have been associated with several conditions. Investigators have studied men with diabetes,[41–43] hypogonadism,[34,35] chronic obstructive pulmonary disease,[44] alcoholism,[45] spinal lesions,[46–48] end-stage renal disease,[49] hypertension,[50,51] and depression.[52]

In an early report by Karacan and colleagues,[53] data were presented indicating that sleep erections were diminished by dream anxiety. This finding is often cited as evidence for SRE responsiveness to

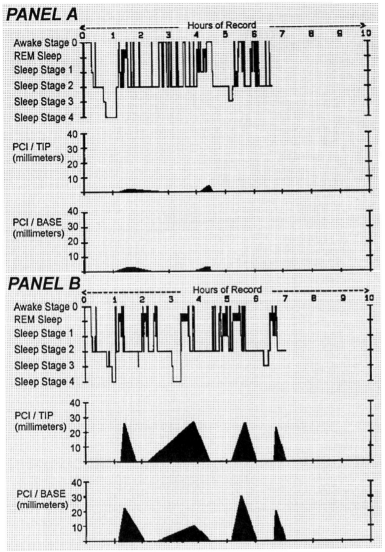

**Figure 17-3.** Sleep stages and sleep-related erections recorded from a 48-year-old man with erectile failure and obstructive sleep apnea. **(A)** The baseline night during which apnea + hypopnea (AHI) was 29 episodes per hour of sleep. **(B)** The histogram for a night recorded during continuous positive airway pressure (CPAP) treatment (7 cm $H_2O$ pressure); AHI was reduced to four episodes per hour. Sleep architecture, REM sleep, and sleep-related erections improved. The value of apnea detection and CPAP intervention as part of the diagnostic protocol are evident. (PCI = penile circumference increase.)

psychogenic phenomena. In the original study, however, dream reports were subjected to content analysis and indexed according to anxiety descriptor scores. Dreams were either associated with normal erections, irregular erections, or no erections. Anxiety index scores did not differ between dreams associated with the different types of tumescence. By contrast, content analysis scores for anxiety were statistically higher in dreams with predominantly irregular erections. Irregular erections were those in which circumference fluctuated or detumescence began before the awakening made to gather dream reports. Irregular erection, in this

study, by no means indicated that SREs were below normal limits.[54]

### Clinical Importance of Proper Diagnosis

Years ago when treatment options were limited, differential diagnosis was less crucial. With the advent of treatment options ranging from psychotherapy to surgical intervention, however, information concerning etiology became more important. The development of an implantable penile prosthesis intensified the need for more accurate diagnostic techniques.

Currently, therapeutic options for impotence include individual psychotherapy, marriage counseling, behavior therapy, psychiatric treatment of depression, revascularization surgery, penile arterial bypass, prosthetic implantation, androgen replacement therapy, external vacuum device, medication, and vasodilator injection or insertion into the urethra.

As it is one of the basic biological drives, the importance of sexuality should never be underestimated. It is well-known that patients may be noncompliant when a medication's side effects include impotence.[56,57] For some men, sexual potency fills an essential psychological need. Self-image, job performance, and interpersonal adjustment can all be adversely affected by impotence. An erroneous diagnosis of psychogenic impotence can lead to ineffective psychological treatment. The resulting increase in frustration level can make a bad situation worse. Misdiagnosis of organic impotence may lead to unnecessary surgical procedures that destroy normal penile physiology.

Erectile failure affects not only the patient but also the patient's sexual partner. Improper treatment of impaired sexual function can provoke frustration, guilt, and marital discord. In contrast, seeing the dramatic improvement in mental outlook among couples for whom accurate diagnosis led to proper treatment is tremendously gratifying.

## REFERENCES

1. Karacan I. The Effect of Exciting Presleep Events on Dream Reporting and Penile Erections During Sleep (ScD thesis). Brooklyn, NY: State University of New York, Downstate Medical Center, 1965.
2. Fisher C, Gross J, Zuch J. Cycle of penile erection synchronous with dreaming (REM) sleep. Arch Gen Psychiatry 1965;12:29.
3. Aserinsky E. Ocular Motility During Sleep and Its Application to the Study of Rest-Activity Cycles and Dreaming (doctoral dissertation). Chicago: University of Chicago, 1953.
4. Ohlmeyer P, Brilmayer H, Hullstrung H. Periodische Vorgange im Schlaf. Pflugers Arch 1944;248:559.
5. Freud S. The Interpretation of Dreams. New York: Random House, 1950.
6. Fisher C. Dreaming and Sexuality. In RM Loewenstein, LM Newman, M Schur, AJ Solnit (eds), Psychoanalysis—A General Psychology. New York: International Universities Press, 1966;537.
7. Snyder F. The Phenomenology of Dreaming. In L Madow, LH Snow (eds), The Psychodynamic Implications of the Physiological Studies on Dreams. Springfield, IL: Thomas, 1970.
8. Gaillard JM, Moneme A. Modification of dream content after preferential blockade of mesolimbic and mesocortical dopaminergic systems. J Psychiatr Res 1977;13:247.
9. McCarley RW, Hoffman E. REM sleep dreams and the activation-synthesis hypothesis. Am J Psychiatry 1981;138:904.
10. Karacan I. Clinical value of nocturnal erection in the prognosis and diagnosis of impotence. Med Aspects Hum Sex 1970;4:27.
11. Karacan I, Williams RL, Salis PJ. The effect of sexual intercourse on sleep patterns and nocturnal penile erections. Psychophysiology 1970;7:338.
12. Karacan I, Ware JC, Salis PJ, et al. Sexual arousal and activity: effect on subsequent nocturnal penile tumescence patterns. Sleep Res 1979;8:61.
13. Hirshkowitz M, Karacan I, Arcasoy MO, et al. The prevalence of periodic limb movements during sleep in men with erectile dysfunction. Biol Psychiatry 1989;26:541.
14. Hirshkowitz M, Karacan I, Arcasoy MO, et al. Prevalence of sleep apnea in men with erectile dysfunction. Urology 1990;36:232.
15. Wein AJ, Fishkin R, Carpiniello VL, Mallory TB. Expansion without significant rigidity during nocturnal penile tumescence: a potential source of misinterpretation. J Urol 1981;126:343.
16. Ware JC, Hirshkowitz M. Monitoring Penile Erections During Sleep. In MH Kryger, T Roth, WC Dement (eds), Principles and Practice of Sleep Medicine (2nd ed). Philadelphia: Saunders, 1994;967.
17. Barry JM, Blank B, Boileau M. Nocturnal penile tumescence monitoring with stamps. Urology 1980; 15:171.
18. Kenepp D, Gonick P. Home monitoring of penile tumescence for erectile dysfunction. Initial experience. Urology 1979;14:261.
19. Procci WR, Martin DJ. Preliminary observations of the utility of portable NPT. Arch Sex Behav 1984;13:569.
20. Bradley WE, Timm GW, Gallagher JM, Johnson BK. New method for continuous measurement of nocturnal penile tumescence and rigidity. Urology 1985;26:4.
21. Virag R, Virag H, Lajujie J. A new device for measuring penile rigidity. Urology 1985;25:80.
22. Bertini J, Boileau MA. Evaluation of nocturnal penile tumescence with Potentest. Urology 1986;27:492.
23. Bradley WE. New techniques in evaluation of impotence. Urology 1987;29:383.
24. Slob AK, Blom JHM, van der Werff ten Bosch JJ. Erection problems in medical practice: differential diagnosis with relatively simple method. J Urol 1990;143:46.
25. Imagawa A, Kawanishi Y. NPT monitoring with stamps: actual intracavernous pressure at separation. Impotence 1986;1:64.
26. Morales A, Condra M, Reid K. The role of penile tumescence monitoring in the diagnosis of impotence: a review. J Urol 1990;143:441.

27. Allen R, Brendler CB. Snap-gauge compared to a full nocturnal penile tumescence study for evaluation of patients with erectile impotence. J Urol 1990; 143:51.

28. Morales A, Marshall PG, Surridge DH, Fenemore J. A new device for diagnostic screening of nocturnal penile tumescence. J Urol 1983;129:288.

29. Karacan I, Williams RL, Thornby JI, Salis PJ. Sleep-related penile tumescence as a function of age. Am J Psychiatry 1975;132:932.

30. Karacan I, Salis PJ, Thornby JI, Williams RL. The ontogeny of nocturnal penile tumescence. Waking Sleeping 1976;1:27.

31. Reynolds CF, Thase ME, Jennings JR, et al. Nocturnal penile tumescence in healthy 20- to 59-year olds: a revisit. Sleep 1989;12:368.

32. Schiavi RC, Schreiner-Engel P, Mandeli J, et al. Healthy aging and male sexual function. Am J Psychiatry 1990;147:766.

33. Karacan I, Moore CA, Sahmay S. Measurement of pressure necessary for vaginal penetration. Sleep Res 1985;14:269.

34. Cunningham GR, Karacan I, Ware JC, et al. The relationships between serum testosterone and prolactin levels and nocturnal penile tumescence (NPT) in impotent men. J Androl 1982;3:241.

35. Cunningham GR, Hirshkowitz M, Korenman SG, Karacan I. Testosterone replacement therapy and sleep-related erections in hypogonadal men. J Clin Endocrinol Metab 1990;70:792.

36. Schmidt HS, Wise HA. Significance of impaired penile tumescence and associated polysomnographic abnormalities in the impotent patient. J Urol 1981;126:348.

37. Pressman MR, DiPhillipo MA, Kendrick JI, et al. Problems in the interpretation of nocturnal penile tumescence studies: disruption of sleep by occult sleep disorders. J Urol 1986;136:595.

38. Segraves RT, Madsen R, Carter CS, Davis JM. Erectile Dysfunction Associated with Pharmacological Agents. In RT Segraves, HW Schoenberg (eds), Diagnosis and Treatment of Erectile Disturbances: A Guide for Clinicians. New York: Plenum, 1985;23.

39. Murray FT, Klimberg IW, Cohen MS. Organic Impotence. In JP Kassirer (ed), Current Therapy in Internal Medicine (Vol 3). Philadelphia: Decker, 1991;1375.

40. Ware JC. Suppression of NPT during the first REM sleep period. Sleep Res 1984;13:71.

41. Karacan I, Scott FB, Salis PJ, et al. Nocturnal erections, differential diagnosis of impotence, and diabetes. Biol Psychiatry 1977;12:373.

42. Karacan I, Salis PJ, Ware JC, et al. Nocturnal penile tumescence and diagnosis in diabetic impotence. Am J Psychiatry 1978;135:191.

43. Hirshkowitz M, Karacan I, Rando KC, et al. Diabetes, erectile dysfunction, and sleep-related erections. Sleep 1990;13:53.

44. Fletcher EC, Martin RJ. Sexual dysfunction and erectile impotence in chronic obstructive pulmonary disease. Chest 1982;81:413.

45. Snyder S, Karacan I. Effects of chronic alcoholism on nocturnal penile tumescence. Psychosom Med 1981;43:423.

46. Karacan I, Dimitrijevic M, Lauber A, et al. Nocturnal penile tumescence (NPT) and sleep stages in patients with spinal cord injuries. Sleep Res 1977;6:52.

47. Karacan I, Dervent A, Salis PJ, et al. Spinal cord injuries and NPT. Sleep Res 1978;7:261.

48. Halstead LS, Dimitrijevic M, Karacan I, Aslan C. Impotence in spinal cord injury: neurophysiological assessment of diminished tumescence and its relation to supraspinal influences. Curr Concepts Rehab Med 1984;1:8.

49. Karacan I, Dervent A, Cunningham G, et al. Assessment of nocturnal penile tumescence as an objective method for evaluating sexual functioning in ESRD patients. Dialysis Transpl 1978;7:872.

50. Karacan I, Salis PJ, Hirshkowitz M, et al. Erectile dysfunction in hypertensive men: sleep-related erections, penile blood flow, and musculovascular events. J Urol 1989;142:56.

51. Hirshkowitz M, Karacan I, Gurakar A, Williams RL. Hypertension, erectile dysfunction, and occult sleep apnea. Sleep 1989;12:223.

52. Thase ME, Reynolds CF, Glanz LM, et al. Nocturnal penile tumescence in depressed men. Am J Psychiatry 1987;144:89.

53. Karacan I, Goodenough DR, Shapiro A, Starker S. Erection cycle during sleep in relation to dream anxiety. Arch Gen Psychiatry 1966;15:183.

54 Kaya N, Moore C, Karacan I. Nocturnal penile tumescence and its role in impotence. Psychiatr Ann 1979;9:426.

55. Goldstein I, Lue TF, Padma-Nathan H, et al. Oral Sildenfil in the treatment of erectile dysfuncion. N Engl J Med 1998;338:1397.

56. Gillin JC, Horowitz D, Wyatt RJ. Pharmacologic Studies of Narcolepsy Involving Serotonin, Acetylcholine, and Monoamine Oxidase. In C Guilleminault, WC Dement, P Passouant (eds), Narcolepsy. New York: Spectrum, 1976;585.

57. Hogan MJ, Wallin JD, Baer RM. Antihypertensive therapy and male sexual dysfunction. Psychosomatics 1980;21:234.

# Part III
## Clinical Aspects

# Chapter 18

# Approach to the Patient with Sleep Complaints

## Sudhansu Chokroverty

Several epidemiologic studies have clearly shown that sleep complaints are very common in the general population.[1-14] Two important multiple-center studies were conducted by Coleman and his colleagues.[8,9] The first study,[8] conducted over a 2-year period (1978–1980), included 4,698 patients, each of whom underwent a polysomnographic (PSG) study. The proportions of diagnostic categories in those with sleep complaints, after those evaluated for impotency are excluded, are 51% with hypersomnia, 31% with insomnia, 15% with parasomnia, and 3% with sleep-wake schedule disorders. A subsequent report by Coleman[9] on 3,085 patients over a 1-year period (1981–1982) showed remarkable consistency with the results of the first study. The most frequent disease categories included in these surveys were sleep apnea, narcolepsy, and insomnia related to psychiatric or psychophysiologic disorders. The 1979 Institute of Medicine[7] study concluded that about one-third of all adults in the United States experienced some sleep disturbances. A survey conducted more recently[11-14] confirmed the 1979 Institute of Medicine[7] findings. Approximately 35% of adults aged 18–79 years reported difficulty in the preceding year falling asleep, staying asleep, or both.[11] In the Gallup survey of 1991,[12] 36% of adults reported some sleep problem (9% considered the problem chronic and 27% occasional). In the survey conducted between 1981 and 1985 by the U.S. National Institute of Mental Health Epidemiologic Catchment Area Study, 10% reported difficulty sleeping for 2 weeks or longer in

the preceding 6 months, for which no medical or psychiatric cause could be found. Therefore, in all of these studies, there is a prevalence of sleep complaints in about one-third of the adult population. Some important epidemiologic factors identified in various studies include old age, female gender, poor education and socioeconomic status, recent stress, and alcohol or drug abuse.[15] It is important for physicians to be aware of this high prevalence of sleep disturbances, which cause considerable physical and psychological stress.

An approach to a sleep complaint must begin with a clear understanding of the various sleep disorders listed in the *International Classification of Sleep Disorders*[16] (see also Chapter 19). Briefly, this classification includes four categories: (1) dyssomnias, (2) parasomnias, (3) medical or psychiatric sleep disorders, and (4) proposed sleep disorders.

Dyssomnias include intrinsic, extrinsic, and circadian rhythm sleep disorders. Intrinsic disorders result from causes within the body; extrinsic disorders are secondary to external causes. Circadian rhythm disorders result from disruption of sleep-wake circadian rhythm.

The two major sleep complaints in the category of dyssomnia are insomnia and hypersomnia. Insomnia includes idiopathic and psychophysiologic insomnia, insomnia with central sleep apnea syndrome, and insomnia with restless legs syndrome–periodic limb movement in sleep disorder (RLS-PLMS).

Hypersomnia includes narcolepsy, obstructive sleep apnea syndrome (OSAS), central sleep apnea syndrome, alveolar hypoventilation syndrome, idiopathic, recurrent, and post-traumatic hypersomnia, and sometimes RLS-PLMS.

Parasomnias are disorders of arousals and sleep-wake transition disorders that are not primary sleep disorders but intrude into sleep. These consist of arousal and sleep-wake transition disorders, rapid eye movement (REM)-related parasomnias, and others.

Medical or psychiatric sleep disorders include disorders secondary to medical, psychiatric, and neurologic disorders.

Proposed sleep disorders include those about which we have inadequate information.

Physicians should also have an understanding of the severity of the two major sleep complaints. Sleepiness (hypersomnia) and sleeplessness (insomnia) can be mild, moderate, or severe.[16] Multiple Sleep Latency Tests (MSLTs) show a mean sleep onset latency of 10–15 minutes for mild hypersomnia, 5–10 minutes for moderate hypersomnia, and less than 5 minutes for severe hypersomnia. Mild insomnia causes little or no functional impairment, moderate insomnia mild to moderate impairment, and severe sleeplessness severe impairment. An understanding of the severity of hypersomnia and insomnia is important for designing of tests, therapeutic intervention, follow-up, and prognosis.

## CLINICAL CHARACTERISTICS OF THE TWO MAJOR COMPLAINTS

More detailed discussion of hypersomnia and insomnia is provided in several chapters (19, 22–30, and 32–34) of this volume. The following sections summarize these two complaints.

### Insomnia

The general complaints of insomnia may include all or some of the following[15]: difficulty falling asleep, frequent awakening, early morning awakening, insufficient or total lack of sleep, daytime fatigue, tiredness or sleepiness, lack of concentration, irritability, anxiety, and sometimes depression and forgetfulness. Some patients may be preoccupied with psychosomatic symptoms such as aches and pains.

### Hypersomnia

Hypersomnolent patients may complain of excessive daytime sleepiness (EDS), falling asleep in an inappropriate place and under inappropriate circumstances (e.g., while driving, at school, at work, at social activities), a lack of relief of symptoms after additional sleep at night, daytime fatigue, morning headache, inability to concentrate and remain alert, impairment of motor skills and cognition, and listlessness. Additional symptoms that may help make an etiologic diagnosis include snoring, cessation of breathing at night as reported by the bed partner, and waking up at night fighting for breath as noted in OSAS. Attacks of cataplexy, hypnagogic hallucinations, sleep paralysis, and automatic behavior may be observed in patients with narcolepsy.

## ETIOLOGIC DIAGNOSIS

Insomnia and hypersomnia are symptoms and do not constitute a specific diagnosis. Every attempt should be made to find a cause for these complaints. The causes are described in several chapters in this book (19, 22–30, 32–34) and are briefly enumerated here.

Insomnia may be secondary to a variety of psychiatric (e.g., depression, anxiety), psychological, medical, or neurologic disorders; pain anywhere in the body; drug or alcohol abuse; or associated with RLS-PLMS. It may be a manifestation of circadian rhythm sleep disorders (e.g., jet lag, delayed sleep phase syndrome, irregular sleep-wake schedule disorders). Shift workers may suffer sleep disturbances at night and daytime fatigue and sleepiness. For some, insomnia is a lifelong condition and no cause is found (idiopathic insomnia). Other patients have subjective complaints of sleeplessness but no objective evidence (i.e., normal PSG findings).

The etiologic differential diagnosis of hypersomnia may include the following conditions: OSAS; central sleep apnea and primary alveolar hypoventilation syndrome; narcolepsy; a variety of psychiatric, medical, and neurologic illnesses; drug or alcohol abuse; idiopathic hypersomnia; and periodic somnolence (e.g., Kleine-Levin syndrome, menstrual cycle-associated). Occasionally, patients with RLS-PLMS complain of EDS.

For patients complaining of abnormal movements and behavior during sleep, the differential diagnosis should include non-REM (NREM) para-somnias (confusional arousals, sleepwalking, and sleep terror); REM sleep parasomnias (REM sleep behavior disorder, nightmares); sleep-wake transition disorders (rhythmic movement disorder, sleep talking); diffuse parasomnias without any state preference (bruxism or tooth grinding and neonatal sleep myoclonus); nocturnal seizures including nocturnal paroxysmal dystonia, which is thought to be a type of frontal lobe seizure; and the common movement disorders seen during the daytime that may sometimes persist or emerge during sleep stage transitions.

## METHOD OF CLINICAL EVALUATION

A physician equipped with this background knowledge should attempt to make a clinical diagnosis based on the history and physical examination of a patient who complains of sleep disturbance. PSG study, MSLT, and other laboratory tests must be confirmatory and secondary to the clinical diagnosis, which depends on a multifactorial analysis of many facets of a sleep complaint.

### History

The first step in the diagnosis and assessment of a sleep-wakefulness disturbance is a careful evaluation of the sleep complaints. The history should seek information on sleep habits, drugs and alcohol consumption, psychiatric, medical, and neurologic illnesses, history of previous illness, and family history.[17–20]

### Sleep History

The sleep history[17–20] is fundamentally important and is the first step in identifying the nature of the sleep disorder. Symptoms during the entire 24 hours should be evaluated, not just those that occur at sleep onset or during sleep at night. In addition to intrinsic and extrinsic dyssomnias, 24-hour symptomatic evaluation helps diagnose and manage circadian rhythm sleep disorders. The clinician should pay attention to symptoms that occur in the early evening or at sleep onset (e.g., paresthesias and uncontrollable limb movements

of RLS), during sleep at night (e.g., repeated awakenings, snoring, and cessation of breathing in OSAS), on awakening in the morning (e.g., feeling exhausted and sleepy as in OSAS), or in late morning and afternoon (e.g., daytime fatigue and excessive somnolence as in OSAS and irresistible desire to have brief sleep as in narcolepsy). Early morning awakening may be noted in insomnia due to depression. Abnormal motor activities may be associated with REM behavior disorder and other parasomnias and found in patients with seizures.

In evaluating sleep history, Kales and coworkers[17–19] enumerated six important principles: (1) Define the specific sleep problem; (2) assess the clinical course; (3) differentiate between various sleep disorders; (4) evaluate sleep-wakefulness patterns; (5) question the bed partner; and (6) evaluate the impact of the disorder on the patient.

One should analyze the onset, frequency, duration, and severity of the sleep complaint; its progression, evolution, and fluctuation over time; and any events that could have initiated it.[21] An analysis of these factors may differentiate transient disorders from persistent ones. The physician should inquire about the patient's functional status and mood during the day, any medicines and their effects on the sleep complaint, and sleep hygiene.

Finally, psychological, social, medical, and biological factors and their interactions should be considered, to understand the patient's problem.[21] An interview with the bed partner, caregiver, and, in the case of a child, a parent, is important for diagnosis of abnormal movements (PLMS or other body movements), abnormal behavior (parasomnias, nocturnal seizures), and breathing disorders during sleep. The bed partner may also be able to answer questions about the patient's sleeping habits, history of drug use, psychosocial problems (e.g., stress at home, work or school), and changes in sleep habits.

### Sleep Questionnaire

A sleep questionnaire containing a list of pertinent questions relating to sleep complaints; sleep hygiene; sleep patterns; medical, psychiatric, and neurologic disorders; and drug or alcohol use may be filled out by the patient to save time in obtaining the history.

*Sleep Log or Sleep Diary*

A sleep log kept over a 2-week period is a valuable indicator of sleep hygiene and can also be used to monitor progression following therapeutic intervention. Such a log should include notations of bedtime, arising time, daytime naps, amount of time needed to go to sleep, number of night-time awakenings, total sleep time, and feelings on arousal (e.g., refreshed or drowsy).

*Drug and Alcohol History*

The physician should inquire about drugs that could cause insomnia (e.g., central nervous system [CNS] stimulants, bronchodilators, beta blockers, corticosteroids, sedative-hypnotics) or hypersomnolence. In addition, the physician should have information about alcohol consumption and dependence as well as about insomnia related to drug withdrawal (e.g., intermediate- or short-acting benzodiazepines, nonbenzodiazepine hypnotics).[17–19] Caffeine consumption and smoking should also be considered as contributing factors to insomnia.

*Psychiatric History*

Attention should be paid to signs of possible psychiatric or psychophysiologic disorders (e.g., depression, anxiety, psychosis, obsession, life stress, personality traits).[17–20] If sleep disorders are secondary to a psychiatric illness, treating it alleviates the sleep disturbance in most cases. If the sleep complaint persists after such treatment, an additional cause or a primary sleep disorder should be suspected.

*Medical and Neurologic History*

The physician should question the patient about any reported symptom that has been associated with a variety of medical and neurologic illnesses (see Chapters 27 and 29). These symptoms direct attention to secondary sleep disorders.

*History of Illnesses*

The patient history might contain information about past medical, psychiatric, or neurologic disorders that could be responsible for the present sleep disturbance. It is also important to learn and evaluate the premor-

bid personality of the patient. Finally, a history of a drug or alcohol habit or use of street drugs may reveal the role of these agents in the sleep complaint.

*Family History*

In certain sleep disorders, family history is very important.[17] A family history is found in about one-third of patients with narcolepsy and RLS. OSAS, with or without obesity, has also been described in other family members. There is a high prevalence of sleepwalking, sleep terrors, and primary enuresis in other family members. Many neurologic disorders, including fatal familial insomnia, have a family history. Currently, an intensive search is going on for a gene specific for narcolepsy and RLS.

**Physical Examination**

It is essential to conduct a thorough physical examination of every patient with a sleep complaint. It may uncover clues to important medical disorders, such as those involving respiratory, cardiovascular, gastrointestinal, or endocrine systems, or neurologic disease, especially one affecting the neuromuscular system, cervical spinal cord, or the brain stem region, which may cause sleep-related breathing disorders as well as insomnias. In OSAS, physical examination may uncover upper airway anatomic abnormalities, which may need surgical correction if medical and continuous positive airway pressure (CPAP) treatment fail to relieve the symptoms. Examination may reveal systemic hypertension, which is a risk factor for sleep apnea.

## CLINICAL PHENOMENOLOGY

Clinical characteristics of some common sleep disorders are briefly described in the following sections. More detailed discussion can be found in several chapters of this volume (19, 22–34).

**Obstructive Sleep Apnea Syndrome**

OSAS is much more common in men than women, and onset of symptoms generally occurs after age 40 years. The symptoms are of two kinds: (1) those that occur during sleep and (2) those that occur during the waking hours (see Chapter 22). Nocturnal sleep symptoms can include loud snoring, choking during sleep, cessation of breathing, sitting up to fight for breath, abnormal motor activities during sleep disruption, esophageal reflux, nocturia and nocturnal enuresis (noted mostly in children), and profuse sweating at night. The daytime symptoms include excessive daytime somnolence, which is characterized by sleep attacks lasting 0.5–2.0 hours and occurring mostly when the patient is sitting down (e.g., watching television). The prolonged duration and the nonrefreshing nature of the sleep attacks differentiate them from narcoleptic sleep attacks. The other diurnal events include personality changes such as impairment of memory, irritability, impairment of motor skills, morning headache, sometimes hypnagogic hallucinations, and automatic behavior with retrograde amnesia. In men, impotence is often associated with severe and long-standing cases of OSAS. Physical examination may reveal obesity in approximately 70% of cases, in addition to anatomic abnormalities in the upper airway. In severe cases, polycythemia and evidence of cardiac failure, pulmonary hypertension, and cardiac arrhythmias may be noted.

## Narcolepsy

The sleep attacks of narcolepsy generally begin in the second or third decade of life, and in approximately 30% of cases a family member has a history of similar attacks. The classic sleep attack begins with an irresistible desire to fall asleep at inappropriate times. The resulting sleep period lasts from a few minutes to as long as 20–30 minutes. These attacks are often accompanied by cataplexy, during which there is transient loss of tone in the somatic muscles, and are often triggered by an emotional outburst. The patient may momentarily fall to the ground or simply slump forward for a few seconds. Three additional manifestations (e.g., hypnagogic hallucinations, sleep paralysis, and disturbed night sleep) are part of the narcolepsy pentad. It is a lifelong condition and is generally less severe in the elderly. Patients with narcolepsy occasionally also have sleep apnea (central, obstructive, or mixed).

## Idiopathic Hypersomnia

Idiopathic hypersomnia is a condition of excessive somnolence that has no known cause, although a CNS cause has been suspected. The International Classification of Sleep Disorders defines idiopathic hypersomnia as a disorder of presumed CNS cause that is associated with a normal or prolonged major sleep episode consisting of prolonged NREM sleep episodes and excessive sleepiness.[16] The disease develops gradually and generally manifests between the ages of 15 and 30 years. Idiopathic hypersomnia closely resembles narcolepsy. Patients with idiopathic hypersomnia generally sleep for hours, but the sleep is not refreshing. The patient does not give a history of snoring. The condition is generally life long and is disabling. MSLTs show evidence of pathologic sleepiness without sleep-onset REM.

## Insomnia

Insomnia, difficulty initiating or maintaining sleep, may occur at any age. A large percentage of insomnia patients suffer from psychiatric illness, and a common cause of insomnia is depression. In this condition, early morning awakening is characteristic. Insomnia may be associated with a variety of psychiatric, medical, and neurologic illnesses or may be drug-induced. It is sometimes the case that no cause can be found.

## Restless Legs Syndrome

The fundamental problem in RLS is a complex sensorimotor disorder involving predominantly the legs. RLS is marked by intense, disagreeable, creeping sensations (paresthesias or dysesthesias), motor restlessness, presence of symptoms or worsening of symptoms at rest or repose with relief by motor activity, and worsening of the symptoms in the evening and nightfall, suggesting a possible circadian variability.[22] There are additional diagnostic criteria, including involuntary movements (myoclonic jerks or dystonic movements) during relaxed wakefulness in some patients and PLMS in greater than 80% of patients. Sleep disturbance, in particular sleep-onset insomnia, is a major problem associated with the disorder. RLS may begin at any age but often presents in childhood or adolescence. The condition continues throughout life, with periodic fluctuations. RLS sometimes becomes severe in patients older than 50 years of age. Approximately one-third of patients give a family history of a similar condition, suggesting a dominant mode of inheritance.

## Parasomnias

Parasomnias are a variety of abnormal movements and behaviors that occur during sleep.

### Sleepwalking

Somnambulism, or sleepwalking, is common in children and begins with abrupt onset of motor activity arising out of slow-wave sleep (stages III and IV of NREM sleep) during the first third of the night. The episode generally lasts less than 10 minutes. Occasionally, injuries and violent activities are reported, but usually individuals can negotiate their way around the room. Triggering factors include sleep deprivation, fatigue, concurrent illness, and sedative-hypnotics.

### Sleep Terror

Sleep terror, or pavor nocturnus, also occurs during NREM sleep stages III and IV. Sleep terror is common in childhood, and somnambulism and sleep terror may occur together. Again, patients have no or only vague recollection of the events. The attacks accompany intense autonomic and motor components. The patients are completely confused and fearful.

### Confusional Arousals

Similar to sleepwalking and sleep terror, confusional arousals are episodes, arising out of slow-wave sleep, during which the patient is disoriented and confused. Confusional arousals occur primarily before the age of 5 years, and are typically benign and require no treatment.

### Nightmares

Nightmares—intense, frightening dreams followed by awakening and vivid recall—occur during REM sleep. The most common time of occurrence, there-fore, is from the middle to the late part of the night. Nightmares are typically normal phenomena. Approximately 50% of children have nightmares beginning at 3–5 years of age. The incidence of nightmares continues to decrease as one grows older and the elderly have very few or no nightmares. Nightmares are common after sudden withdrawal of REM-suppressant drugs and can also occur as side effects of certain medications, such as antiparkinsonian drugs, anticholinergics, and beta blockers.

### Rapid Eye Movement Behavior Disorder

REM behavior disorder is common in elderly persons and occurs during REM sleep. A characteristic feature of this syndrome is the intermittent loss of REM-related muscle hypotonia and appearance of a variety of abnormal motor activities during REM sleep. The violent motor behavior during sleep may pose a risk to the bed partner. The condition may be idiopathic or may be secondary to some neurologic disorder, particularly Parkinson's disease.

### Rhythmic Movement Disorder

Rhythmic movement disorder (head banging or jactatio capitis nocturna) is characterized by rhythmic forward and backward or lateral head and body movements lasting approximately 1 hour. It is most common in infants and may occur at any stage of sleep.

## LABORATORY INVESTIGATIONS

### Polysomnography

PSG is an invaluable laboratory test for the diagnosis and treatment of sleep disorders, particularly in patients with hypersomnia. All-night PSG, rather than a single-nap daytime study, is required for accurate diagnosis of many sleep disorders. A daytime single-nap study generally misses REM sleep, and most severe cases of OSAS are noted during REM sleep. Maximum oxygen desaturation also occurs at this stage. With a daytime study, the severity of symptoms cannot be assessed. Because treatment—and particularly treatment with CPAP—might be adversely affected, an all-night sleep study is essential.

The American Sleep Disorders Association (ASDA) Standards of Practice Committee Task

Force has provided the following recommendations for the practice of sleep medicine in North America regarding the PSG and its role in the diagnosis of sleep disorders.[23] The task force recommendations for sleep-related breathing disorders may be summarized as follows:

- PSG is routinely indicated for the diagnosis of sleep-related breathing disorders. This should be an all-night, attended PSG study.
- PSG is indicated for CPAP titration in patients with sleep-related breathing disorders.
- PSG should be routinely performed to document the presence of OSAS in patients before they undergo laser-assisted uvulopalatopharyngoplasty.
- PSG is indicated to ensure therapeutic benefit (after good clinical response) after oral appliance treatment or surgery for patients with OSAS and for patients whose symptoms return after surgery.
- A follow-up PSG is indicated for assessment of treatment if the patient has lost or gained substantial weight, when the clinical response is insufficient, or when symptoms return despite a good initial response to treatment with CPAP.
- For the diagnosis of suspected narcolepsy, an overnight PSG followed by MSLT the next day is routinely indicated.

For parasomnias, the task force made the following recommendations: PSG is indicated for evaluating sleep-related behaviors that are violent or otherwise potentially injurious to the patient or others, as well as for patients who have unusual or atypical behaviors during sleep. PSG may also be indicated in situations with forensic considerations. However, PSG is not routinely indicated for typical and uncomplicated parasomnias.

PSG is not routinely indicated to diagnose or treat RLS. PSG is indicated when a diagnosis of PLMS is considered as a result of a complaint by the patient or bed partner of repetitive limb movements during sleep, frequent awakenings, difficulty maintaining sleep, or excessive daytime somnolence.

PSG is not routinely indicated for diagnosis of circadian rhythm sleep disorders or depression.

Indications for PSG in patients with insomnia are somewhat controversial. The diagnosis of insomnia is basically clinical. The ASDA Standards of Practice Committee Guidelines[24] do not list PSG for routine evaluation of transient or chronic insomnia. PSG may be useful, however, when the cause of insomnia is uncertain or when behavioral or pharmacologic treatment is unsuccessful. If a patient with insomnia is suspected of having a sleep-related breathing disorder or PLMS, PSG is indicated as outlined earlier.

### Multiple Sleep Latency Test

The MSLT is essential for documenting pathologic sleepiness and for diagnosing narcolepsy (see Chapter 13).

### Video-Polysomnographic Study

Parasomnias are generally diagnosed on the basis of clinical history, but sometimes PSG, and particularly video-PSG,[23,25] is required to document the condition. Because certain parasomnias mimic seizure disorders, PSG or video-PSG is essential when a seizure disorder is suspected.[23,25] To document nocturnal epilepsy, video-PSG using multiple-channel electroencephalography (EEG) and multiple montages is required. If sleep epilepsy is suspected, the video-PSG recording should have the capability for EEG analysis at the standard EEG speed of 30 mm per second to identify epileptiform discharges.[23,25]

### Standard Electroencephalographic Study

EEG is necessary to investigate suspected epilepsy.

### Ambulatory Electroencephalography or Polysomnography

Ambulatory EEG or PSG is sometimes useful for patients with suspected sleep epilepsy, for understanding circadian variation, and for studying circadian rhythm sleep disorders. However, technical problems associated with unattended recording are serious limitations.

### Actigraphy

Actigraphy is an activity monitor or a motion detector developed to record activities during sleep and waking.[26] Actigraphs complement the sleep diary or sleep log data. Actigraphy is very useful in the diagnosis of circadian rhythm sleep disorders, sleep state misperception, and other types of insomnia. It is not useful, however, for the assessment of breathing-related sleep disorders.

### Neuroimaging Study

Neuroimaging is essential when a neurologic illness is suspected of causing a sleep disturbance (see Chapter 27).

### Other Laboratory Tests

Blood and urinalysis, electrocardiography (ECG), Holter ECG, chest radiography, and other investigations to rule out gastrointestinal, pulmonary, cardiovascular, endocrine, and renal disorders should be conducted when diagnosing insomnia or hypersomnia, because both can result from a variety of medical disorders. For rare cases in which autonomic failure causes a sleep disturbance or sleep-related breathing disorder, autonomic function tests may be required to diagnose the primary condition. With some patients suspected of having a sleep disturbance of psychiatric or psychological cause, the Minnesota Multiphasic Personality Inventory may be required.

## SUMMARY AND CONCLUSION

This chapter outlines the approach to a patient with a sleep complaint. The approach should begin with a careful clinical analysis of the patient's symptoms, keeping in mind the *International Classification of Sleep Disorders* and its pertinent manifestations along with the underlying basic science foundations of such disorders. The detailed history should consist of sleep history (including night sleep complaints and daytime sleepiness), as well as family, psychiatric, medical (including neurologic), drug, and alcohol histories. Physical examination should include neurologic and general medical and other organ system examination. A sleep diary or log is often very useful. The patient history and physical examination should provide information about the patient's quality of life and how sleep disturbances are affecting the daily activities, including those associated with the patient's professional, family,

and social lives. An occasional sleep complaint (insomnia or sleepiness) is common, but if the symptoms are persistent or frequent and are interfering with daily life, professional advice should be sought. In most cases, diagnosis can be made on clinical grounds with minimal laboratory investigation, minimizing the patient's suffering and expenses. In this way, we honor the Hippocratic oath by comforting patients and causing no harm. Most of the time, patients with sleep complaints seek the advice of their primary care physician, who may decide, based on the patient history and physical examination, that a patient's sleep complaints are due to a medical, psychiatric, or neurologic condition. The next step would be for the primary care physician either to treat the condition causing the sleep disturbance, or to refer the patient to an appropriate specialist. For primary sleep disorders, it is advisable to refer the patient to a sleep specialist, who may then decide to conduct further laboratory tests (e.g., PSG, MSLT, actigraphy, video-PSG) and provide treatment.

## REFERENCES

1. McGhie A, Russell SM. The subjective assessment of normal sleep patterns. J Ment Sci 1962;108:642.
2. Hammond EC. Some preliminary findings on physical complaints from a prospective study of 1,064,004 men and women. Am J Public Health 1964;54:11.
3. Tune G. Sleep and wakefulness in 509 normal adults. Br J Med Psychol 1969;42:75.
4. Johns MWW, Egan P, Gay TJ, et al. Sleep habits and symptoms in male medical and surgical patients. BMJ 1970;2:509.
5. Karacan I, Thornby JI, Anch M, et al. Prevalence of sleep disturbance in a primarily urban Florida county. Soc Sci Med 1976;10:239.
6. Bixler EO, Kales A, Soldatos CR, et al. Prevalence of sleep disorders in the Los Angeles metropolitan area. Am J Psychiatry 1979;136:1257.
7. Institute of Medicine. Sleeping Pills, Insomnia and Medical Practice. Washington, DC: National Academy of Sciences, 1979.
8. Coleman RM, Roffwarg HP, Kennedy SJ, et al. Sleep-wake disorders based on a polysomnographic diagnosis. A national cooperative study. JAMA 1982;247:997.
9. Coleman RM. Diagnosis, Treatment and Follow-Up of About 8000 Sleep/Wake Disorder Patients. In C Guilleminault (ed), Sleep/Wake Disorders: Natural History, Epidemiology and Long-Term Evaluation. New York: Raven, 1983;87.

10. Gislason T, Almqvist M. Somatic diseases and sleep complaints: an epidemiological study of 3201 Swedish men. Acta Med Scand 1987;221:475.

11. Mellinger GD, Balter MB, Uhlenhuth EH. Insomnia and its treatment; prevalence and correlates. Arch Gen Psychiatry 1985;42:225.

12. National Sleep Foundation. Sleep in America: A National Survey of U.S. Adults. Princeton, NJ: Gallup Organizations, 1991.

13. Ford DE, Kamerow DB. Epidemiologic study of sleep disturbances and psychiatric disorders. JAMA 1989;262:1479.

14. Costa E, Silva JA, Chase M, et al. Special report from a symposium held by the World Health Organization and the World Federation of Sleep Research Societies: an overview of insomnias and related disorders—recognition, epidemiology, and rational management. Sleep 1996;19:412.

15. Aldrich MS. Cardinal Manifestations of Sleep Disorders. In MN Kryger, T Roth, WC Dement (eds), Principles and Practice of Sleep Medicine (2nd ed). Philadelphia: Saunders, 1994;418.

16. American Sleep Disorders Association. The International Classification of Sleep Disorders (revised). Diagnostic and Coding Manual. Rochester, MN: American Sleep Disorders Association, 1997.

17. Kales A, Soldatos CR, Kales JD. Taking a sleep history. Am Fam Physician 1980;22:101.

18. Kales A, Kales JD. Evaluation and Treatment of Insomnia. New York: Oxford University Press, 1984.

19. Kales JD, Carvell M, Kales A. Sleep and Sleep Disorders. In CK Cassel, DE Riesenberg, LB Sorensen, et al. (eds), Geriatric Medicine. New York: Springer, 1990;562.

20. Hauri PJ. Evaluating Disorders of Initiating and Maintaining Sleep (DIMS). In C Guilleminault (ed), Sleeping and Waking Disorders: Indications and Techniques. Menlo Park, CA: Addison-Wesley, 1982;225.

21. Liebmann RC, et al. The Assessment of Sleep-Wakefulness. In JH Peter, T Podszus, P Von Wichert (eds), Sleep-Related Disorders and Internal Diseases. New York: Springer, 1987;30.

22. Walters A, and The International Restless Legs Syndrome Study Group. Toward a better definition of the restless legs syndrome. Mov Disord 1995;10:634.

23. Indications for Polysomnography Task Force, American Sleep Disorders Association Standards of Practice Committee. Practice parameters for the indication for polysomnography and related procedures. Sleep 1997;20:406.

24. Standards of Practice Committee of the American Sleep Disorders Association. Practice parameters for the use of polysomnography in the evaluation of insomnia. Sleep 1995;18:55.

25. Aldrich M, Jahnke B. Diagnostic value of video-EEG polysomnography. Neurology 1991;41:1060.

26. Saadeh A, Hauri P, Kripke DF, Lavie P. The role of actigraphy in the evaluation of sleep disorders. Sleep 1995;18:288.

# Chapter 19

# Classification of Sleep Disorders

Michael J. Thorpy

The past symptom-based classifications of sleep disorders formed the basis for modern classifications. In 1990, the widely used *International Classification of Sleep Disorders* (*ICSD*) was produced after a lengthy 5-year process initiated by the American Sleep Disorders Association (Table 19-1).[1–150] The *ICSD* was developed in association with the three major international sleep societies—the European Sleep Research Society, the Japanese Society of Sleep Research, and the Latin American Sleep Society—resulting in the comprehensive text, the *ICSD Diagnostic and Coding Manual*.[151] A revised version of the *ICSD* with minor revisions to the text was produced in 1997.[152]

The *ICSD* lists 84 sleep disorders, each with descriptive details and specific diagnostic, severity, and duration criteria. In addition, there is coding information for clinical and research purposes. The *ICSD* has four major categories: (1) dyssomnias, disorders of initiating and maintaining sleep and of excessive sleepiness; (2) parasomnias, disorders that primarily do not cause a complaint of insomnia or excessive sleepiness; (3) disorders associated with medical or psychiatric disorders; and (4) *proposed* sleep disorders—that is, disorders for which insufficient information is available to confirm their acceptance as definitive sleep disorders. The proposed sleep disorders category was required because of the rapid advances in sleep medicine, which have resulted in the discovery of several new sleep disorders.

## DYSSOMNIAS

The dyssomnias, disorders that produce either insomnia or excessive sleepiness, are the sleep disorders primarily associated with either disturbed nighttime sleep or impaired wakefulness.

The dyssomnias contain a heterogeneous group of sleep disorders that have their origin in different body systems. For example, a disorder of the central nervous system (CNS) is believed to be the cause of narcolepsy,[7,8] whereas a physical obstruction in the upper airway may be the sole cause of obstructive sleep apnea syndrome (OSAS).[14,15]

The dyssomnias are divided into three major groups: the intrinsic sleep disorders, the extrinsic sleep disorders, and the circadian rhythm sleep disorders. The divisions are based, in part, on pathophysiologic mechanisms. Because the circadian rhythm sleep disorders share a common chronophysiologic basis, they are kept as a single group. Both intrinsic and extrinsic factors may be involved in some of the circadian rhythm sleep disorders, so some of them, such as delayed sleep phase syndrome, are subdivided into intrinsic and extrinsic types.

### Intrinsic Sleep Disorders

The intrinsic sleep disorders are primary sleep disorders that originate or develop in the body or arise from causes in the body. This section contains only those disorders that are included in the definition of

**Table 19-1.** The *International Classification of Sleep Disorders*

| Disorder | ICD-9-CM Number |
|---|---|
| **Dyssomnias** | |
| Intrinsic sleep disorders | |
| Psychophysiologic insomnia[1,2] | 307.42-0 |
| Sleep state misperception[3,4] | 307.49-1 |
| Idiopathic insomnia[5,6] | 780.52-7 |
| Narcolepsy[7,8] | 347 |
| Recurrent hypersomnia[9,10] | 780.54-2 |
| Idiopathic hypersomnia[11,12] | 780.54-7 |
| Post-traumatic hypersomnial[13] | 780.54-8 |
| Obstructive sleep apnea syndrome[14,15] | 780.53-0 |
| Central sleep apnea syndrome[16,17] | 780.51-0 |
| Central alveolar hypoventilation syndrome[18,19] | 780.51-1 |
| Periodic limb movement disorder[20,21] | 780.52-4 |
| Restless legs syndrome[21,22] | 780.52-5 |
| Intrinsic sleep disorder NOS | 780.52-9 |
| Extrinsic sleep disorders | |
| Inadequate sleep hygiene[23,24] | 307.41-1 |
| Environmental sleep disorder[25,26] | 780.52-6 |
| Altitude insomnia[27,28] | 993.2 |
| Adjustment sleep disorder[3,29] | 307.41-0 |
| Insufficient sleep syndrome[30,31] | 307.49-4 |
| Limit-setting sleep disorder[32] | 307.42-4 |
| Sleep-onset association disorder[33] | 307.42-5 |
| Food allergy insomnia[34,35] | 780.52-2 |
| Nocturnal eating (drinking syndrome)[36,37] | 780.52-8 |
| Hypnotic-dependent sleep disorder[38,39] | 780.52-0 |
| Stimulant-dependent sleep disorder[40,41] | 780.52-1 |
| Alcohol-dependent sleep disorder[42] | 780.52-3 |
| Toxin-induced sleep disorder[43] | 780.54-6 |
| Extrinsic sleep disorder NOS | 780.52-9 |
| Circadian rhythm sleep disorders | |
| Time zone change ( jet lag syndrome)[44,45] | 307.45-0 |
| Shift work sleep disorder[46,47] | 307.45-1 |
| Irregular sleep-wake pattern[48,49] | 307.45-3 |
| Delayed sleep phase syndrome[50,51] | 780.55-0 |
| Advanced sleep phase syndrome[52,53] | 780.55-1 |
| Non–24-hour sleep-wake disorder[54,55] | 780.55-2 |
| Circadian rhythm sleep disorder NOS | 780.55-9 |
| **Parasomnias** | |
| Arousal disorders | |
| Confusional arousals[56,57] | 307.46-2 |
| Sleepwalking[57,58] | 307.46-0 |
| Sleep terrors[57,59] | 307.46-1 |
| Sleep-wake transition disorders | |
| Rhythmic movement disorder[60,61] | 307.3 |
| Sleep starts[62,63] | 307.47-2 |
| Sleep talking[64,65] | 307.47-3 |
| Nocturnal leg cramps[66,67] | 729.82 |
| Parasomnias usually associated with REM sleep | |
| Nightmares[68,69] | 307.47-0 |
| Sleep paralysis[70,71] | 780.56-2 |
| Impaired sleep-related penile erections[72,73] | 780.56-3 |
| Sleep-related painful erections[74,75] | 780.56-4 |

| Disorder | ICD-9-CM Number |
|---|---|
| REM sleep–related sinus arrest[76] | 780.56-8 |
| REM sleep behavior disorder[77,78] | 780.59-0 |
| Other parasomnias | |
| Sleep bruxism[79,80] | 306.8 |
| Sleep enuresis[81,82] | 780.56-0 |
| Sleep-related abnormal swallowing syndrome[83] | 780.56-6 |
| Nocturnal paroxysmal dystonia[84,85] | 780.59-1 |
| Sudden unexplained nocturnal death syndrome[86,87] | 780.59-3 |
| Primary snoring[88,89] | 780.53-1 |
| Infant sleep apnea[90,91] | 770.80 |
| Congenital central hypoventilation syndrome[92,93] | 770.81 |
| Sudden infant death syndrome[94,95] | 798.0 |
| Benign neonatal sleep myoclonus[96,97] | 780.59-5 |
| Other parasomnia NOS | 780.59-9 |
| **Sleep disorders associated with medical or psychiatric disorders** | |
| Associated with mental disorders | 290-319 |
| Psychoses[98,99] | 292-299 |
| Mood disorders[100,101] | 296-301 |
| Anxiety disorders[102,103] | 300 |
| Panic disorder[104,105] | 300 |
| Alcoholism[106,107] | 303 |
| Associated with neurologic disorders | 320-389 |
| Cerebral degenerative disorders[108] | 330-337 |
| Dementia[109,110] | 331 |
| Parkinsonism[111,112] | 332-333 |
| Fatal familial insomnia[113,114] | 337.9 |
| Sleep-related epilepsy[115,116] | 345 |
| Electrical status epilepticus of sleep[117,118] | 345.8 |
| Sleep-related headaches[119,120] | 346 |
| Associated with other medical disorders | |
| Sleeping sickness[121,122] | 086 |
| Nocturnal cardiac ischemia[123,124] | 411-414 |
| Chronic obstructive pulmonary disease[125,126] | 490-494 |
| Sleep-related asthma[127,128] | 493 |
| Sleep-related gastroesophageal reflux[129,130] | 530.1 |
| Peptic ulcer disease[131,132] | 531-534 |
| Fibrositis syndrome[133,134] | 729.1 |
| **Proposed sleep disorders** | |
| Short sleeper[135,136] | 307.49-0 |
| Long sleeper[135,136] | 307.49-2 |
| Subwakefulness syndrome[137] | 307.47-1 |
| Fragmentary myoclonus[138] | 780.59-7 |
| Sleep hyperhidrosis[139,140] | 780.8 |
| Menstruation-associated sleep disorder[141,142] | 780.54-3 |
| Pregnancy-associated sleep disorder[143,144] | 780.59-6 |
| Terrifying hypnagogic hallucinations[145] | 307.47-4 |
| Sleep-related neurogenic tachypnea[146] | 780.53-2 |
| Sleep-related laryngospasm[147,148] | 780.59-4 |
| Sleep choking syndrome[149,150] | 307.42-1 |

NOS = not otherwise specified.

Source: Reproduced by permission of the American Sleep Disorders Association from Diagnostic Classification Committee. MJ Thorpy, Chairman. International Classification of Sleep Disorders: Diagnostic and Coding Manual. Rochester, MN: American Sleep Disorders Association, 1990.

dyssomnias. Some sleep disorders due to processes in the body are listed in the Parasomnias, Medical-Psychiatric, or Proposed Sleep Disorders sections.

The intrinsic sleep disorders include various types, some of which, such as psychophysiologic insomnia,[12] sleep state misperception,[32] restless legs syndrome,[21,22] and idiopathic insomnia,[5,6] are primarily disorders that produce insomnia. Psychophysiologic insomnia, a common form of insomnia, is a disorder of somatized tension and learned sleep preventing associations that result in a complaint of insomnia and associated decreased functioning during wakefulness. *Sleep state misperception* is a relatively new term for a disorder in which a complaint of insomnia or excessive sleepiness occurs in the absence of objective evidence of sleep disturbance. Restless legs syndrome is well-known, but the term *idiopathic insomnia* indicates a lifelong inability to obtain adequate sleep that presumably is due to an abnormality of the neurologic control of the sleep-wake system.

Narcolepsy,[7,8] recurrent hypersomnia,[9,10] idiopathic hypersomnia,[11,12] and post-traumatic hypersomnia[13] are principally disorders of excessive sleepiness. Narcolepsy is a disorder of unknown cause that is characterized by excessive sleepiness typically associated with cataplexy and other rapid eye movement (REM) sleep phenomena such as sleep paralysis and hypnagogic hallucinations. In recurrent hypersomnia, recurrent episodes of hypersomnia typically occur weeks or months apart. One form of this disorder is the Kleine-Levin syndrome. Idiopathic hypersomnia, which can be confused clinically with narcolepsy, is a disorder of presumed CNS cause that is associated with a normal or prolonged major sleep episode and excessive sleepiness during the day with prolonged (1- to 2-hour) sleep episodes of non-REM (NREM) sleep. Post-traumatic hypersomnia is hypersomnia that occurs as a result of a traumatic event involving the CNS.

The next four disorders, OSAS,[14,15] central sleep apnea syndrome,[16,17] central alveolar hypoventilation syndrome,[18,19] and periodic limb movement disorder,[20,21] are sleep-related breathing disorders that can produce a complaint of either insomnia or excessive sleepiness.

The term *intrinsic* implies that the primary cause of the disorder is an internal (endogenous) physiologic abnormality. It is clear, however, that for some disorders, external factors are important in either precipitating or exacerbating the disorder. The following examples are given to help explain the rationale for organizing the disorders under the group heading of *intrinsic*.

Post-traumatic hypersomnia[13] is an example of an intrinsic disorder that could not exist without an external event (in this case, one that produces a head injury). The primary cause of the hypersomnia, however, is of CNS origin, and because the disorder persists after the traumatic event has terminated, it is considered intrinsic. OSAS can be induced by an external event such as consumption of alcohol, but the syndrome would not be possible without the internal factor of upper airway obstruction and a physiologic predisposition to develop the disorder.

### Extrinsic Sleep Disorders

The extrinsic sleep disorders include those that originate or develop from causes outside the body. External (exogenous) factors are integral in producing these sleep disorders, and removal of the external factors leads to resolution of the sleep disorder. Internal factors may be important in the development or maintenance of the sleep disorder, just as external factors can be important in the development or maintenance of an intrinsic sleep disorder. The internal factors would not, by themselves, have produced the sleep disorder in the absence of an external factor.

Although there appears to be overlap between some disorders, such as alcohol-dependent sleep disorder,[42] environmental sleep disorder,[25,26] and inadequate sleep hygiene,[23,24] the *ICSD* text and diagnostic criteria highlight the differences. Some explanation may be helpful.

Inadequate sleep hygiene[23,24] is a sleep disorder due to daily habits that are inconsistent with the maintenance of good quality sleep and full daytime alertness. It is a sleep disorder that develops out of normal behavior that for another person usually would not disturb sleep. For example, an irregular bedtime or waketime that might not be associated with sleep disturbance in one person may produce a sleep disturbance in another. Although environmental factors can produce a disorder of inadequate sleep hygiene, the diagnosis of an environmental sleep disorder is made only when the environmental factors are particularly abnormal and not under the patient's control, such as excessive noise or extreme lighting effects that would produce sleep disturbance in most people. Caffeine consumed in coffee or sodas can produce a disorder of inadequate sleep hygiene if the amount consumed is within the limits of common use, whereas taking stimulants in amounts considered excessive by normal standards can lead to a diagnosis of a stimulant-dependent sleep disorder.[40,41] Similarly, sleep that is disrupted by drinking what would be considered a socially normal amount of alcohol can lead to a diagnosis of inadequate sleep hygiene, whereas sleep disrupted by drinking what most people consider an excessive amount of alcohol taken primarily to induce sleep can lead to a diagnosis of alcohol-dependent sleep disorder.[42]

Altitude insomnia,[27,28] also known as *acute mountain sickness*, is an acute insomnia usually accompanied by headache, loss of appetite, and fatigue, that follows ascent to high altitudes. Insomnia may be the sole manifestation of altitude insomnia, whereas the term *acute mountain sickness* usually applies when other physiologic disturbances predominate.

Some extrinsic sleep disorders have internal factors that are important for the expression of the sleep disturbance. When they are removed, the sleep disturbance is resolved. For example, the extrinsic disorder *adjustment sleep disorder*[3,29] represents sleep disturbance that is temporarily related to acute stress, conflict, or environmental change that causes emotionally induced arousal. Because it is due to psychologically stressful factors, it could be considered internally generated, but an external factor causes the sleep disturbance and if this factor is removed the disorder resolves. If the sleep disorder continues after removal of the external factor, an intrinsic sleep disorder may have developed, such as psychophysiologic insomnia.[1,2]

Limit-setting sleep disorder[32] is primarily a childhood disorder characterized by inadequate enforcement of bedtime by a caretaker, with resultant stalling or refusal to go to bed at an appropriate time. Another sleep disorder that primarily affects children is sleep-onset association disorder,[33] which occurs when sleep onset is impaired by the absence of a certain object or set of circumstances, such as sucking on a pacifier.

## Circadian Rhythm Sleep Disorders

The circadian rhythm sleep disorders comprise the third section of the dyssomnias and are grouped together because they share an underlying chronophysiologic basis. The major feature of these disorders is a misalignment between the timing of the patient's sleep pattern and that which is desired or regarded as the societal norm. The underlying problem in the majority of circadian rhythm sleep disorders is that the patient cannot sleep when sleep is desired, needed, or expected. The waking hours can occur at undesired times as a result of sleep episodes that occur at inappropriate times. Therefore, the patient may complain of insomnia or excessive sleepiness. For several of the circadian rhythm sleep disorders, once sleep is initiated the major sleep episode is of normal duration and has normal REM-NREM cycling. Intermittent sleep episodes can occur in some disorders, such as the irregular sleep-wake pattern.[48,49]

The first two circadian rhythm sleep disorders, time zone change syndrome (jet lag)[44,45] and shift-work sleep disorder,[46,47] are disorders in which the sleep episodes occur at a time that is not synchronized with the underlying circadian rhythms of such measures as temperature or biochemical variables. Delayed sleep phase syndrome,[50,51] advanced sleep phase syndrome,[52,53] and non–24-hour sleep-wake syndrome[54,55] are disorders in which the timing of sleep is synchronized with underlying circadian rhythms. Delayed sleep phase syndrome is a disorder in which the major sleep episode is delayed in relation to the desired clock time, a delay that results in symptoms of sleep-onset insomnia or difficulty awakening at the desired time. Advanced sleep phase syndrome is similar, but the sleep episode is advanced in relation to the desired clock time with symptoms including intense evening sleepiness, early sleep onset, and awakening earlier than desired. The non–24-hour sleep-wake syndrome is a rare disorder that consists of a chronic steady pattern of 1- to 2-hour daily delays in sleep onset and awaking times.

It should be pointed out that the appropriate timing of sleep within the 24-hour day can be disturbed in many other sleep disorders, particularly those associated with the complaint of insomnia. Patients with narcolepsy[7,8] can have a pattern of sleepiness identical to that caused by an irregular sleep-wake pattern.[48,49] Because the primary sleep diagnosis is narcolepsy, however, the patient should not receive a second diagnosis of a circadian rhythm sleep disorder unless the disorder is unrelated to the narcolepsy. For example, a diagnosis of time zone change (jet lag) syndrome could be stated along with a diagnosis of narcolepsy, if appropriate. Similarly, patients with mood disorders[100,101] or psychoses[98,99] can, at times, have a sleep pattern similar to that of delayed sleep phase syndrome.

Some disturbance of sleep timing is a common feature in patients who have a diagnosis of inadequate sleep hygiene.[23,24] Only if the timing of sleep is the predominant cause of the sleep disturbance, and is outside the societal norm, is the diagnosis circadian rhythm sleep disorder. Limit-setting sleep disorder[32] is also associated with an altered time of sleep within the 24-hour day, but the timing of sleep in this disorder is not within the patient's control, nor is it intrinsically induced. If the setting of limits is a function of the caretaker, then the sleep disorder is more appropriately diagnosed within the extrinsic subsection of the dyssomnias—that is, as a limit-setting sleep disorder.[32]

Three circadian rhythm sleep disorders have intrinsic and extrinsic subtypes: delayed sleep phase syndrome, advanced sleep phase syndrome, and non–24-hour sleep-wake syndrome. These disorders can be socially or environmentally induced or can be due to an abnormal circadian pacemaker or its entrainment mechanism.

## PARASOMNIAS

The parasomnias consist of sleep disorders that are not abnormalities of the processes responsible for sleep and wakefulness per se but are undesirable phenomena that occur predominantly during sleep. The parasomnias are disorders of arousal, partial arousal, and sleep stage transition. Many of the parasomnias are manifestations of CNS activation. Autonomic nervous system changes and skeletal muscle activity are the predominant features. The parasomnias are subdivided into the arousal disorders, the sleep-wake transition disorders, the parasomnias associated with REM sleep, and other parasomnias.

The arousal disorders consist of the classic disorders of sleepwalking[57,58] and sleep terrors[57,59] as well as a more recently described disorder, confusional arousals.[56,57]

The sleep-wake transition disorders include those that occur in the transition from wakefulness to sleep or from sleep to wakefulness, such as sleep starts[62,63] and sleep talking.[64,65] This group does not include

disorders that are clearly associated with REM sleep, such as sleep paralysis.[70,71] Although some of the sleep-wake transition disorders can occur during sleep or even in wakefulness, such as rhythmic movement disorder (jactatio capitis nocturna),[60,61] the most typical occurrence of these disorders is in the transition from wakefulness to sleep. Restless legs syndrome[21,22] could be considered a sleep-wake transition disorder, but it is not a parasomnia, as it is associated primarily with a complaint of insomnia and therefore is listed in the dyssomnias.

The parasomnias usually associated with REM sleep include six disorders that have a close association with the REM sleep stage. The fourth subsection contains parasomnias that are not classified in the previous three sections. *Other parasomnias* include disorders such as sleep bruxism[79,80] and sleep enuresis.[81,82] Infant sleep-related breathing disorders are listed here, as they do not produce complaints of insomnia or excessive sleepiness and are most typically regarded as parasomnias. Sudden infant death syndrome (SIDS) is listed in this section, as it most commonly occurs during sleep and appears likely to have a sleep-related mechanism.

### Disorders of Arousal

The disorders of arousal are disorders associated with impaired arousal from sleep. Onset in slow-wave sleep is a typical feature. Confusional arousals[56,57]—more recently described although they were alluded to in the original description of the disorders of arousal—consist of confusion during and after arousal from sleep, most typically from deep sleep in the first part of the night. These episodes are more prevalent in children who sleepwalk[57,58] or have sleep terrors[57,59] and may be partial manifestations of those disorders. Confusional arousals can occur as an isolated sleep disorder.

### Sleep-Wake Transition Disorders

Sleep-wake transition disorders occur in the transition from wakefulness to sleep, sleep to wakefulness, or, more rarely, at sleep stage transitions. All commonly occur in otherwise healthy individuals and thus are regarded as physiologic alterations rather than pathologic conditions. Each can occur with exceptionally high frequency or severity that can lead to discomfort, pain, embarrassment, anxiety, or disturbance of a bed partner's sleep.

Rhythmic movement disorder[60,61] is the preferred term for head banging or jactatio capitis nocturna, as several forms of rhythmic activity can occur without head banging as the predominant characteristic. Although this disorder occurs in sleep stages, it more commonly is associated with drowsiness during sleep onset or in the transition from wakefulness to sleep. Rhythmic movement disorder can occur during full wakefulness and alertness, particularly in persons who are mentally retarded. Sleep starts (hypnic jerks)[62,63] are included as a disorder because they can cause sleep onset insomnia. Sleep talking[64,65] does not usually have any direct consequence for the patient, though it can be embarrassing and disturb the sleep of the bed partner.

### Parasomnias Usually Associated with Rapid Eye Movement Sleep

The parasomnias associated with REM sleep are grouped together because some common pathophysiologic mechanism related to REM sleep may underlie all of them.

The term *nightmares* applies to REM sleep phenomena. Thus, there is little chance of confusing this disorder with that associated with slow-wave sleep, sleep terror.[57,59] Two recently described sleep disorders are included in this section: REM sleep–related sinus arrest[76] and REM sleep behavior disorder.[77,78] REM sleep–related sinus arrest is a rare cardiac rhythm disorder that is characterized by sinus arrest during REM sleep in otherwise healthy persons. REM sleep behavior disorder is characterized by the intermittent loss of REM sleep electromyographic atonia and by the appearance of elaborate motor activity associated with dream mentation. This disorder is being recognized more often, particularly in elderly persons and those with neurologic disorders, and sometimes in association with other sleep disorders such as narcolepsy.

### Other Parasomnias

The terms *sleep bruxism*[79,80] and *sleep enuresis*[81,82] are preferred over the terms *nocturnal bruxism* and

*nocturnal enuresis* used previously, as they denote the association with sleep rather than time of day. A new entry, primary snoring,[88,89] is included because snoring may be associated with altered cardiovascular status, and can be a forerunner to the development of the OSAS.[14,15] Primary snoring can lead to impaired health, can be a cause of social embarrassment, and can disturb the sleep of a bed partner. Snoring associated with OSAS is not diagnosed as primary snoring. The sleep-related abnormal swallowing syndrome[83] is retained in this classification, though it is noted that there have been few additional reports since it was first described. Nocturnal paroxysmal dystonia[84,85] is characterized by repeated dystonia or dyskinetic (ballistic, choreoathetoid) episodes that are stereotyped and occur during NREM sleep. A sleep-related frontal lobe epileptic focus is considered to be responsible for the disorder in some patients. Because this disorder is solely a sleep phenomenon, it is classified here rather than as a sleep disorder associated with neurologic disease.

Sudden unexplained death syndrome[86,87] is also a relatively recently described syndrome that has a specific association with sleep and therefore is classified here. Benign neonatal sleep myoclonus[96,97] is a disorder of muscle activity that occurs solely during sleep in infants.

Included in this group are SIDS[94,95] and the infant sleep-related breathing disorders infant sleep apnea[90,91] and congenital central hypoventilation syndrome.[92,93] Insomnia or excessive sleepiness is not a predominant complaint, and usually the disorders are associated with a sudden event that occurs during sleep. Thus, they are listed in the parasomnias section. The inclusion of these infant breathing disorders as sleep disorders requires further explanation. Newborns and young infants sleep a great portion of the day, and the majority of apneas and related respiratory disorders are observed during sleep. Apnea, hypoventilation, and periodic breathing are intrinsic features of infancy, reflecting immaturity of the respiratory system rather than disease. The respiratory instability during sleep may predispose some infants to SIDS.[94,95] The majority of SIDS cases happen while the infant is presumed to be asleep, but even though infant sleep apnea has been implicated as a precursor to SIDS, there is no definitive evidence of a direct link. SIDS is therefore discussed separately.

# MEDICAL OR PSYCHIATRIC
# SLEEP DISORDERS

Many medical and psychiatric disorders are associated with disturbances of sleep and wakefulness. The division into medical and psychiatric is somewhat arbitrary. This section is divided into three subsections. The first is a listing of the psychiatric disorders commonly associated with disturbed sleep or wakefulness, the second indicates the importance of neurologic disorders and their effect upon the sleep and wakefulness states, and the third is a list of disorders that fall into other medical specialty areas.

Only medical disorders commonly seen in the practice of sleep disorders medicine are listed in the medical-psychiatric section. It is recognized that a large number of medical and psychiatric disorders are associated with disturbances of sleep and wakefulness, but an exhaustive list is not provided in the classification.

## Sleep Disorders Associated
## with Mental Disorders

Although most psychiatric disorders can have an associated sleep disturbance, the psychoses,[98,99] mood disorders,[100,101] anxiety disorders,[102,103] panic disorders,[104,105] and alcoholism[106,107] are presented here because they are common in patients who present with sleep complaints and they need to be considered in the differential diagnosis. Panic disorder,[104,105] one of the anxiety disorders, can produce only a sleep complaint.

## Sleep Disorders Associated
## with Neurologic Disorders

Neurologic disorders commonly associated with sleep disturbance are cerebral degenerative disorders,[108] dementia,[109,110] and Parkinson's disease.[111,114] Fatal familial insomnia[113,114] is a rare progressive disorder that begins with difficulty initiating sleep and leads within a few months to total lack of sleep and later to spontaneous lapses from quiet wakefulness into a sleep state with enacted dreams (oneiric stupor). This disorder is associated with autonomic and thalamic degeneration and ultimately leads to death.

Epilepsy can be exacerbated by a sleep disturbance and there can be epileptic phenomena that occur predominantly during sleep, thus the term *sleep-related epilepsy*.[115,116] Because of its pure association with NREM sleep, electrical status epilepticus of sleep[117,118] is listed separately. Electrical status epilepticus of sleep is characterized by continuous and diffuse spike- and slow-wave complexes that persist throughout NREM sleep.

Some forms of headache, particularly migraine and cluster headaches, can occur predominantly in sleep and are listed under sleep-related headaches.[119,120]

## Sleep Disorders Associated
## with Other Medical Disorders

A variety of additional medical disorders have features that occur during sleep or cause sleep disturbance. Sleeping sickness[121,122] is included, as it is common in Africa. Encephalitis lethargica is not included because it rarely occurs.

Cardiac ischemia during sleep can lead to myocardial infarction or cardiac arrhythmias and may not be symptomatic. Nocturnal cardiac ischemia[123,124] is presented in the classification because of its importance to the health of the population and in the hope of stimulating further research on its causes. Myocardial infarction during sleep is not listed, as it rarely is seen in the practice of sleep medicine and rarely needs to be included in the differential diagnosis of a sleep complaint.

Chronic obstructive pulmonary disease[125,126] and sleep-related asthma[127,128] are common enough in the population to warrant inclusion. Other pulmonary disorders can have sleep-related features but rarely present because of sleep disturbances. Many respiratory disorders produce disturbed breathing during sleep that can lead to the development of the central sleep apnea syndrome.[16,17]

Two gastrointestinal disorders are included in this section: sleep-related gastroesophageal reflux[129,130] and peptic ulcer disease.[131,132] The discomfort associated with peptic ulcer disease commonly occurs during the major sleep episode. Although the incidence of peptic ulcer disease appears to be declining in the United States, in some countries, notably Japan, it is very high.

Fibrositis syndrome,[133,134] also known as *fibromyalgia syndrome*, is included because it is associated with disturbed sleep and an abnormal electroencephalographic pattern during sleep called *alpha-delta sleep*.

## PROPOSED SLEEP DISORDERS

The fourth section of the *ICSD* lists proposed sleep disorders, disorders for which insufficient information is available to substantiate unequivocally the existence of the disorder. Some of these disorders are newly described, such as sleep-related laryngospasm,[147,148] and some are the subject of controversy as to whether they are disorders in their own right or are at the extreme end of the range of normal physiology, such as short sleeper.[135,136]

Short sleepers and long sleepers[135,136] are persons whose sleep episodes are either shorter or longer than is considered normal, but whose sleep is not disturbed. They present with either an inability to sleep or excessive sleepiness, and thus are important in the differential diagnosis of these symptoms. It is necessary to describe the symptoms to provide appropriate diagnostic information for clinical purposes.

The subwakefulness syndrome,[137] also known as the *subvigilance syndrome*, has been described for many years, although it is little known. It consists of a complaint of inability to sustain alertness despite the fact that evidence of nocturnal sleep disruption or severe excessive sleepiness cannot be documented by polysomnography. It is unclear whether this is a variant of another disorder of excessive sleepiness, such as idiopathic hypersomnia,[11,12,137] or represents a manifestation of a psychological state.

Fragmentary myoclonus,[138] a disorder associated with excessive sleepiness, consists of frequent brief myoclonic jerks that occur during NREM sleep at random in many muscle groups. It may be a variant of the normal phasic muscle activity that typically is seen at sleep onset, but insufficient information is currently available to determine this.

Sleep hyperhidrosis[139,140] or night sweats can be due to a variety of underlying disorders, such as neurologic disease and the OSAS. An idiopathic form of this disorder occurs, but it has rarely been described in the literature.

Sleep disturbance characterized by either insomnia or excessive sleepiness can be associated with the menstrual cycle and menopause (menstrual-associated sleep disorder)[141,142] or pregnancy (pregnancy-associated sleep disorder).[143,144] Although well-recognized as common, reports of the sleep characteristics of these states are rare and the underlying cause of the sleep disturbances is unclear. Whether these disorders are due to a specific and primary effect on sleep mechanisms or to another disorder, such as premenstrual stress syndrome or back pain related to pregnancy, is not known.

Terrifying hypnagogic hallucinations[145] are intensely frightening hallucinatory phenomena that occur at sleep onset. Although sometimes associated with other sleep disorders such as narcolepsy,[74] they can occur in an idiopathic form. Terrifying hypnagogic hallucinations have rarely been described, and they have not been clearly differentiated from unpleasant sleep-onset dreams.

Sleep-related neurogenic tachypnea[146] is characterized by a sustained increase in respiratory rate during sleep. It occurs at sleep onset, is maintained throughout sleep, and reverses immediately on return to wakefulness. Although it is rarely described as an idiopathic form of tachypnea, it can be associated with an underlying neurologic disorder.

Sleep-related laryngospasm[147,148] and sleep choking syndrome are associated with a complaint of sleep-related breathing difficulty. Sleep-related laryngospasm is an episode of abrupt awakening from sleep with an intense sensation of inability to breathe and stridor. The sleep choking syndrome is a disorder of unknown cause characterized by frequent episodes of awakening with a choking sensation. Patients with these disorders present because of symptoms similar to those of the OSAS.[14,15]

The proposed sleep disorders are described in anticipation that additional information will be forthcoming in the medical literature to establish their nature more clearly.

## REFERENCES

1. Hauri PJ, Fischer J. Persistent psychophysiological (learned) insomnia. Sleep 1986;9:38.
2. Reynolds CF, Taska LS, Sewitch DE, et al. Persistent psychophysiologic insomnia: preliminary research diagnostic criteria and EEG sleep data. Am J Psychiatry 1984;141:804.
3. Beutler LE, Thornby JI, Karacan I. Psychological Variables in the Diagnosis of Insomnia. In RL Williams, I

Karacan (eds), Sleep Disorders: Diagnosis and Treatment. New York: Wiley, 1978;61.

4. Carskadon M, Dement W, Mitler M, et al. Self-report versus sleep laboratory findings in 122 drug free subjects with the complaint of chronic insomnia. Am J Psychiatry 1976;133:1382.

5. Hauri PJ, Olmsted E. Childhood onset insomnia. Sleep 1980;3:59.

6. Regestein QR, Reich P. Incapacitating childhood onset insomnia. Compr Psychiatry 1983;24:244.

7. Guilleminault C. Narcolepsy and Its Differential Diagnosis. In C Guilleminault (ed), Sleep and Its Disorders in Children. New York: Raven, 1987;181.

8. Mitler MM, Hajdukovic R, Erman M, et al. Narcolepsy. J Clin Neurophysiol 1990;7:93.

9. Reynolds CF, Kupfer DJ, Christianson CL. Multiple sleep latency test findings in Kleine-Levin syndrome. J Nerv Ment Dis 1984;172:41.

10. Takahashi Y. Clinical studies of periodic somnolence. Analysis of 28 personal cases. Psychiatr Neurol Jpn 1965;10:853.

11. Billiard M. Other Hypersomnias. In MJ Thorpy (ed), Handbook of Sleep Disorders. New York: Marcel Dekker, 1990;353.

12. Poirier G, Montplaisir J, Lebrun A, et al. HLA antigens in narcolepsy and idiopathic hypersomnolence. Sleep 1986;9:153.

13. Guilleminault C, Faull KM, Miles L, et al. Posttraumatic excessive daytime sleepiness: a review of 20 patients. Neurology 1980;33:1584.

14. Brouillette RT, Fernbach SK, Hunt CE. Obstructive sleep apnea in infants and children. J Pediatr 1982;100:31.

15. Guilleminault C. Clinical Features and Evaluation of Obstructive Sleep Apnea. In MH Kryger, T Roth, WC Dement (eds), Principles and Practice of Sleep Medicine. Philadelphia: Saunders, 1989;552.

16. Guilleminault C, Kowall J. Central Sleep Apnea in Adults. In MJ Thorpy (ed), Handbook of Sleep Disorders. New York: Marcel Dekker, 1990;337.

17. Guilleminault C, Quera-Salva MA, Nino-Murcia G, et al. Sleep apnea and partial obstruction of the airway. Ann Neurol 1987;21:465.

18. Plum F, Leigh RJ. Abnormalities of Central Mechanisms. In TF Hornbein (ed), Regulation of Breathing, Part II. Lung Biology in Health and Disease. New York: Marcel Dekker, 1981;17:989.

19. Sullivan CE, Issa FG, Berthon-Jones M, et al. Pathophysiology of Sleep Apnea. In NA Saunders, CE Sullivan (eds), Sleep and Breathing. Lung Biology in Health and Disease. New York: Marcel Dekker, 1984;21:299.

20. Coleman R. Periodic Movements in Sleep (Nocturnal Myoclonus) and Restless Legs Syndrome. In C Guilleminault (ed), Sleeping and Waking Disorders: Indications and Techniques. Menlo Park, CA: Addison-Wesley, 1982;265.

21. Coccagna G. Restless Legs Syndrome/Periodic Leg Movements in Sleep. In MJ Thorpy (ed), Handbook of Sleep Disorders. New York: Marcel Dekker, 1990;457.

22. Ekbom KA. Restless legs syndrome. Neurology 1960; 10:868.

23. Bootzin RR, Nicassio PM. Behavioral Treatments for Insomnia. In M Hersen, RM Eisler, PM Miller (eds), Progress in Behavior Modification. New York: Academic, 1978;6:1.

24. Spielman AJ. Assessment of insomnia. Clin Psychol Rev 1986;6:11.

25. Haskell EH, Palca JW, Walker JM, et al. The effects of high and low ambient temperatures on human sleep stages. Electroencephalogr Clin Neurophysiol 1981;51:494.

26. Thiessen GJ, Lapointe AC. Effect of continuous traffic noise on percentage of deep sleep, waking, and sleep latency. J Acoust Soc Am 1983;73:225.

27. Nicholson AN, Smith PA, Stone BM, et al. Altitude insomnia: studies during an expedition to the Himalayas. Sleep 1988;11:354.

28. Weil JV. Sleep at High Altitude. In M Kryger, T Roth, WC Dement (eds), Principles and Practice of Sleep Disorders Medicine. Philadelphia: Saunders, 1989;269.

29. Agnew H, Webb W, Williams RL. The first night effect: an EEG study of sleep. Psychophysiology 1966;7:263.

30. Carskadon M, Dement W. Effects of total sleep loss on sleep tendency. Percept Mot Skills 1979;48:495.

31. Roehrs T, Zorick F, Sickelsteel R, et al. Excessive daytime sleepiness associated with insufficient sleep. Sleep 1983;6:319.

32. Ferber R. Sleeplessness in the Child. In MH Kryger, T Roth, WC Dement (eds), Principles and Practice of Sleep Medicine. Philadelphia: Saunders, 1989;633.

33. Ferber R. Sleeplessness in Children. In R Ferber, MH Kryger (eds), Principles and Practice of Sleep Medicine in the Child. Philadelphia: Saunders, 1985;79.

34. Kahn A, Mozin MJ, Casimir G, et al. Insomnia and cow's milk allergy in infants. Pediatrics 1985;76:880.

35. Kahn A, Mozin MJ, Rebuffat E, et al. Difficulty in initiating and maintaining sleep associated with cow's milk allergy in infants. Sleep 1987;10:116.

36. Ferber R. The Sleepless Child. In C Guilleminault (ed), Sleep and Its Disorders in Children. New York: Raven, 1987;141.

37. Stunkard AJ, Grace WJ, Wolfe HG. The night eating syndrome. Am J Med 1955;7:78.

38. Gillin JC, Spinwebber CL, Johnson LC. Rebound insomnia: a critical review. J Clin Psychopharmacol 1989;9:161.

39. Kales A, Soldatos CR, Bixler EO, et al. Rebound insomnia and rebound anxiety: a review. Pharmacology 1983;26:121.

40. Oswald I. Sleep and Dependence on Amphetamines and Other Drugs. In A Kales (ed), Sleep: Physiology and Pathology. Philadelphia: Lippincott, 1969;317.

41. Watson R, Hartmann E, Shildkraut J. Amphetamine withdrawal: affective state, sleep patterns and MHPG excretion. Am J Psychiatry 1972;129:263.

42. Pokorny AD. Sleep Disturbances, Alcohol, and Alcoholism: A Review. In RL Williams, I Karacan (eds),

Sleep Disorders: Diagnosis and Treatment. New York: Wiley, 1978;233.

43. Friedman PA. Poisoning and Its Management. In E Braunwald, KJ Isselbacher, RG Peterdorf, LD Wilson, et al. (eds), Harrison's Principles of Internal Medicine (11th ed). New York: McGraw-Hill, 1987.

44. Graeber RC. Sleep and wakefulness international aircrew. Aviat Space Environ Med 1986;57:S12.

45. Winget CM, DeRoshio CW, Markley CL, et al. A review of human physiological and performance changes associated with desynchronosis of biological rhythms. Aviat Space Environ Med 1984;55:1085.

46. Torsvall L, Akerstedt T. Sleepiness on the job: continuously measured EEG changes in train drivers. Electroencephalogr Clin Neurophysiol 1987;66:502.

47. Walsh JK, Tepas DL, Moss PD. The EEG Sleep of Night and Rotating Shift Workers. In LC Johnson, DI Tepas, WP Colquhoun, et al. (eds), Biological Rhythms, Sleep and Shift Work. New York: SP Medical, 1981;347.

48. Okawa M, Takahashi K, Sasaki H. Disturbance of circadian rhythms in severely brain-damaged patients correlated with CT findings. J Neurol 1986;233:274.

49. Wagner D. Circadian Rhythm Sleep Disorders. In MJ Thorpy (ed), Handbook of Sleep Disorders. New York: Marcel Dekker, 1990;493.

50. Thorpy MJ, Korman E, Spielman AJ, et al. Delayed sleep phase syndrome in adolescents. J Adolesc Health Care 1988;9:22.

51. Weitzman ED, Czeisler CA, Coleman RM, et al. Delayed sleep phase syndrome, a chronobiological disorder with sleep-onset insomnia. Arch Gen Psychiatry 1981;38:737.

52. Kamei R, Hughes L, Miles L, et al. Advanced-sleep phase syndrome studied in a time isolation facility. Chronobiologia 1979;6:115.

53. Moldofsky H, Musisi S, Phillipson EA. Treatment of advanced sleep phase syndrome by phase advance chronotherapy. Sleep 1986;9:61.

54. Kokkoris CP, Weitzman ED, Pollak CP, et al. Long-term ambulatory monitoring in a subject with a hypernychthemeral sleep-wake cycle disturbance. Sleep 1980;2:347.

55. Weber AL, Cary MS, Conner N, et al. Human non–24-hour sleep-wake cycles in an everyday environment. Sleep 1980;2:347.

56. Ferber R. Sleep Disorders in Infants and Children. In TL Riley (ed), Clinical Aspects of Sleep and Sleep Disturbance. Boston: Butterworths, 1985;113.

57. Thorpy MJ. Disorders of Arousal. In MJ Thorpy (ed), Handbook of Sleep Disorders. New York: Marcel Dekker, 1990;531.

58. Kales A, Soldatos CR, Bixler EO, et al. Hereditary factors in sleep walking and night terrors. Br J Psychiatry 1980;137:111.

59. Fisher C, Kahn E, Edwards A, et al. A psychophysiological study of nightmares and night terrors: physiological aspects of the stage 4 night terror. J Nerv Ment Dis 1973;157:75.

60. Sallustro F, Atwell CW. Body rocking, head banging and head rolling in normal children. J Pediatr 1978;93:704.

61. Thorpy MJ. Rhythmic Movement Disorder. In MJ Thorpy (ed), Handbook of Sleep Disorders. New York: Marcel Dekker, 1990;609.

62. Broughton R. Pathological Fragmentary Myoclonus, Intensified Sleep Starts and Hypnagogic Foot Tremor: Three Unusual Sleep-Related Disorders. In WP Koella (ed), Sleep 1986. Stuttgart: Fischer, 1988;240.

63. Oswald I. Sudden bodily jerks on falling asleep. Brain 1959;82:92.

64. Aarons L. Evoked sleep talking. Percept Mot Skills 1970;31:27.

65. Arkin AM. Sleep talking: a review. J Nerv Ment Dis 1966;143:101.

66. Jacobsen JH, Rosenberg RS, Huttenlocher PR, et al. Familial nocturnal cramping. Sleep 1986;9:54.

67. Weiner IH, Weiner HL. Nocturnal leg muscle cramps. JAMA 1980;244:2332.

68. Fisher CJ, Byrne J, Edwards T, et al. A psychophysiological study of nightmares. J Am Psychoanal Assoc 1970;18:747.

69. Hartmann E. The Nightmare. New York: Basic Books, 1984.

70. Goode GB. Sleep paralysis. Arch Neurol 1962;6:228.

71. Hishikawa Y. Sleep Paralysis. In C Guilleminault, WC Dement, P Passouant (eds), Narcolepsy. New York: Spectrum, 1976;97.

72. Fisher C, Schavi RC, Edwards A, et al. Evaluation of nocturnal penile tumescence in the differential diagnosis of sexual impotence: a quantitative study. Arch Gen Psychiatry 1979;36:431.

73. Karacan I, Howell W. Impaired Sleep-Related Penile Tumescence. In MJ Thorpy (ed), Handbook of Sleep Disorders. New York: Marcel Dekker, 1990;631.

74. Karacan I. Painful nocturnal penile erections. JAMA 1971;215:1831.

75. Matthews BJ, Crutchfield MB. Painful nocturnal penile erections associated with rapid eye movement sleep. Sleep 1987;10:184.

76. Guilleminault C, Pool P, Motta J, et al. Sinus arrest during REM sleep in young adults. N Engl J Med 1984;311:1006.

77. Schenck CH, Bundlie SR, Ettinger MG, Mahowald MW. Chronic behavioral disorders of human REM sleep: a new category of parasomnia. Sleep 1986; 9:293.

78. Mahowald MW, Schenck CH. REM Sleep Behavior Disorder. In MJ Thorpy (ed), Handbook of Sleep Disorders. New York: Marcel Dekker, 1990;567.

79. Funch DP, Gale EN. Factors associated with nocturnal bruxism and its treatment. J Behav Med 1980;3:385.

80. Ware JC, Rugh J. Destructive bruxism: sleep stage relationship. Sleep 1988;11:172.

81. Mikkelsen EJ, Rapoport JL. Enuresis: psychopathology, sleep stage, and drug response. Urol Clin North Am 1980;7:361.

82. Brown L. Nocturnal Enuresis. In MJ Thorpy (ed), Handbook of Sleep Disorders. New York: Marcel Dekker, 1990;595.

83. Guilleminault C, Eldridge FL, Phillips JR, et al. Two occult causes of insomnia and their therapeutic problems. Arch Gen Psychiatry 1976;33:1241.

84. Lugaresi E. Nocturnal Paroxysmal Dystonia. In MJ Thorpy (ed), Handbook of Sleep Disorders. New York: Marcel Dekker, 1990;551.

85. Lugaresi E, Cirignotta F, Montagna P. Nocturnal paroxysmal dystonia. J Neurol Neurosurg Psychiatry 1986;49:375.

86. Baron RC, Thacker SB, Gorelkin L, et al. Sudden death among Southeast Asian refugees. JAMA 1983;250:2947.

87. Otto CM, Tauxe RV, Cobb LA, et al. Ventricular fibrillation causes sudden death in Southeast Asian immigrants. Ann Intern Med 1984;100:45.

88. Lugaresi E, Cirignotta F, Montagna P. Snoring: Pathogenic, Clinical, and Therapeutic Aspects. In MH Kryger, T Roth, WC Dement (eds), Principles and Practice of Sleep Medicine. Philadelphia: Saunders, 1989;494.

89. Waller PC, Bhopal RS. Is snoring a cause of vascular disease? An epidemiological review. Lancet 1989;1:143.

90. Durand M, Cabal L, Gonzalez F, et al. Ventilatory control and carbon dioxide response in preterm infants with idiopathic apnea. Am J Dis Child 1985;139:717.

91. Henderson-Smart DJ. The effect of gestational age on the incidence and duration of recurrent apnea in newborn babies. Aust Paediatr J 1985;17:273.

92. Fleming PJ, Cade D, Bryan MH, et al. Congenital central hypoventilation and sleep state. Pediatrics 1980;66:425.

93. Paton JY, Swaminathan S, Sargent CW, et al. Hypoxic and hypercapnic ventilatory responses in awake children with congenital central hypoventilation syndrome. Am Rev Respir Dis 1989;140:368.

94. Hoppenbrouwers T, Hodgman JE. Sudden infant death syndrome (SIDS): an integration of ontogenetic, pathologic, physiologic and epidemiologic factors. Neuropediatrics 1982;13:36.

95. Merritt TA, Valdes Dapena M. SIDS research update. Pediatr Ann 1984;13:193.

96. Coulter DL, Allen RJ. Benign neonatal sleep myoclonus. Arch Neurol 1982;39:191.

97. Resnick TJ, Moshe SL, Perotta L, et al. Benign neonatal sleep myoclonus: relationship to sleep states. Arch Neurol 1986;43:266.

98. Ganguli R, Reynolds CF, Kupfer DJ. EEG sleep in young, never-medicated, schizophrenic patients: a comparison with delusional and nondelusional depressives and with healthy controls. Arch Gen Psychiatry 1987;44:36.

99. Zarcone VP. Sleep and Schizophrenia. In RL Williams, J Karacan, CA Moore (eds), Sleep Disorders: Diagnosis and Treatment. New York: Wiley, 1988;165.

100. Gillin JC, Duncan W, Pettigrew KD, et al. Successful separation of depressed, normal, and insomniac subjects by EEG sleep data. Arch Gen Psychiatry 1979;36:85.

101. Reynolds CF, Kupfer DJ. Sleep research in affective illness: state of the art circa 1987. Sleep 1987;10:199.

102. Reynolds CF, Shaw DM, Newton TF, et al. EEG sleep in outpatients with generalized anxiety: a preliminary comparison with depressed outpatients. Psychiatry Res 1983;8:81.

103. Rosa RR, Bonnett MM, Kramer M. The relationship of sleep and anxiety in anxious subjects. Biol Psychol 1983;16:119.

104. Hauri PJ, Friedman M, Ravaris CL. Sleep in patients with spontaneous panic attacks. Sleep 1989;12:323.

105. Mellman TA, Unde TW. Electroencephalographic sleep in panic disorder. Arch Gen Psychiatry 1989;46:178.

106. Porkny AD. Sleep Disturbances, Alcohol and Alcoholism: A Review. In RL Williams, I Karacan (eds), Sleep Disorders: Diagnosis and Treatment. New York: Wiley, 1978;389.

107. Wagman A, Allen R. Effects of Alcohol Ingestion and Abstinence on Slow Wave Sleep of Alcoholics. In MM Gross (ed), Alcohol Intoxication and Withdrawal, II. New York: Plenum, 1975;453.

108. Aldrich M. Sleep and Degenerative Neurological Disorders Involving the Motor System. In MJ Thorpy (ed), Handbook of Sleep Disorders. New York: Marcel Dekker, 1990;673.

109. Evans LK. Sundown syndrome in institutionalized elderly. J Am Geriatr Soc 1987;35:101.

110. Vitiello MV, Prinz PN. Sleep/Wake Patterns and Sleep Disorders in Alzheimer's Disease. In MJ Thorpy (ed), Handbook of Sleep Disorders. New York: Marcel Dekker, 1990;703.

111. Mouret J. Difference in sleep in patients with Parkinson's disease. Electroencephalogr Clin Neurophysiol 1975;38:563.

112. Nausieda PA. Sleep in Parkinson's Disease. In MJ Thorpy (ed), Handbook of Sleep Disorders. New York: Marcel Dekker, 1990;719.

113. Lugaresi E, Medori R, Montagna P, et al. Fatal familial insomnia and dysautonomia with selective degeneration of thalamic nuclei. N Engl J Med 1986;315:997.

114. Lugaresi E. Fatal Familial Insomnia. In MJ Thorpy (ed), Handbook of Sleep Disorders. New York: Marcel Dekker, 1990;479.

115. Degan R, Niedermeyer E (eds). Epilepsy, Sleep and Sleep Deprivation. Amsterdam: Elsevier, 1984.

116. Montplaisir J. Epilepsy and Sleep: Reciprocal Interactions and Diagnostic Procedures Involving Sleep. In MJ Thorpy (ed), Handbook of Sleep Disorders. New York: Marcel Dekker, 1990;643.

117. Patry G, Lyagoubi S, Tassinari CA. Subclinical "electrical status epilepticus" induced by sleep in children. Arch Neurol 1971;24:242.

118. Tassinari CA, Bureau M, Dravet C, et al. Epilepsy with Continuous Spikes and Waves During Sleep. In J Roger, C Dravet, M Bureau, et al. (eds), Epileptic Syndromes in Infancy, Childhood and Adolescence. London: John Libbey Eurotext, 1985;194.

119. Dexter JD. Relationship Between Sleep and Headaches. In MJ Thorpy (ed), Handbook of Sleep Disorders. New York: Marcel Dekker, 1990;663.

120. Kayed K, Godtlibsen OB, Sjaastad O. Chronic paroxysmal hemicrania IV: "REM sleep locked" nocturnal headache attacks. Sleep 1978;1:91.

121. Bert J, Collomb H, Fressy J, Gastaut H. Etude Electrographique du Sommeil Nocturne. In H Fischgold (ed), Le Sommeil de Nuit Normal et Pathologique. Paris: Masson, 1965;334.

122. Schwartz BA, Escande C. Sleeping sickness: sleep study of a case. Electroencephalogr Clin Neurophysiol 1970;3:83.

123. Muller J, Ludmer PL, Wellick SN, et al. Circadian variation in the frequency of sudden cardiac death. Circulation 1987;75:131.

124. Nowlin JB, Troyer WG Jr, Collins WS, et al. The association of nocturnal angina pectoris with dreaming. Ann Intern Med 1965;63:1040.

125. Fleetham J, West P, Mezon B, et al. Sleep, arousals and oxygen desaturation in chronic obstructive pulmonary disease. The effect of oxygen therapy. Am Rev Respir Dis 1982;126:429.

126. Flenley C. Chronic Obstructive Pulmonary Disease. In MH Kryger, T Roth, WC Dement (eds), Principles and Practice of Sleep Medicine. Philadelphia: Saunders, 1989;601.

127. Douglas NJ. Asthma. In MH Kryger, T Roth, WC Dement (eds), Principles and Practice of Sleep Medicine. Philadelphia: Saunders, 1989;591.

128. Montplaisir J, Walsh J, Malo JL. Nocturnal asthma features of attacks, sleep and breathing patterns. Am Rev Respir Dis 1982;125:18.

129. Orr WC. Gastrointestinal Disorders. In MH Kryger, T Roth, WC Dement (eds), Principles and Practice of Sleep Medicine. Philadelphia: Saunders, 1989;622.

130. Orr WC, Johnson LF, Robinson MG. The effect of sleep on swallowing, esophageal peristalsis, and acid clearance. Gastroenterology 1984;86:814.

131. Segawa K, Nakazawa S, Tsukamoto Y, et al. Peptic ulcer is prevalent among shift workers. Dig Dis Sci 1987;32:449.

132. Stacher G, Presslich B, Starker H. Gastric acid secretion and sleep stages during natural night sleep. Gastroenterology 1975;68:1455.

133. Moldofsky H, Saskin P, Lue FA. Sleep and symptoms in fibrositis syndrome after a febrile illness. J Rheumatol 1988;15:1701.

134. Saskin P, Moldofsky H, Lue FA. Sleep and posttraumatic rheumatic pain modulation disorder (fibrositis syndrome). Psychosom Med 1986;48:319.

135. Hartmann E, Baekeland F, Zwilling GR. Psychological differences between short and long sleepers. Arch Gen Psychiatry 1972;26:463.

136. Webb WB. Are short and long sleepers different? Psychol Rep 1979;44:259.

137. Roth B. Narcolepsy and Hypersomnia. Basel: Karger, 1980.

138. Broughton R, Tolentino MA, Krelina M. Excessive fragmentary myoclonus in NREM sleep: a report of 38 cases. Electroencephalogr Clin Neurophysiol 1985;61:123.

139. Geschickter EH, Andrews PA, Bullard RW. Nocturnal body temperature regulation in man: a rationale for sweating in sleep. J Appl Physiol 1966;21:623.

140. Lea MJ, Aber RC. Descriptive epidemiology of night sweats upon admission to a university hospital. South Med J 1985;78:1065.

141. Billiard M, Guilleminault C, Dement WC. A menstruation-linked periodic hypersomnia. Neurology 1975; 25:436.

142. Ho A. Sex hormones and the sleep of women. Sleep Res 1972;1:184.

143. Errante J. Sleep deprivation or postpartum blues? Top Clin Nurs 1985;6:9.

144. Karacan I, Williams RL, Hursh CJ, et al. Some implications of the sleep pattern of pregnancy for postpartum emotional disturbances. Br J Psychiatry 1969;115:929.

145. Broughton R. Neurology and dreaming. Psychiatr J Univ (Ottawa) 1982;7:101.

146. Willmer JP, Broughton RJ. Neurogenic sleep related polypnea—a new disorder? Sleep Res 1989;18:322.

147. Kryger MH, Acres JC, Brownell L. A syndrome of sleep, stridor and panic. Chest 1981;80:768.

148. Thorpy MJ, Aloe F. Sleep-related laryngospasm. Sleep Res 1989;18:313.

149. Arnold GE. Disorders of Laryngeal Function. In MM Paparella, DA Shumrick (eds), Otolaryngology. Philadelphia: Saunders, 1973;3:638.

150. Thorpy MJ, Aloe FS. Choking during sleep. Sleep Res 1989;18:314.

151. Diagnostic Classification Steering Committee. International Classification of Sleep Disorders. Diagnostic and Coding Manual. Rochester, MN: American Sleep Disorders Association, 1990.

152. American Sleep Disorders Association. International Classification of Sleep Disorders (Revised). Diagnostic and Coding Manual. Rochester, MN: American Sleep Disorders Association, 1997.

# Chapter 20

# Epidemiology of Sleep Disorders

Maurice M. Ohayon and Christian Guilleminault

The epidemiology of sleep disorders is still a fledgling discipline encompassing a broad range of phenomena, such as insomnia, hypersomnia, parasomnias, and sleep apnea. Surveys in the field remain scarce, and existing figures are difficult to compare owing primarily to the considerable shift that sleep disorder classifications have undergone over the years. This in itself may account in large part for the wide variance in prevalence rates between the earliest and the most recent studies. Methodologic differences and sample size are other factors warranting scrutiny. In addition, the interpretation of results is limited by the nearly exclusive reliance on self-reported data. Consequently, the picture of sleep disorders in the general population remains hazy. A sharper resolution is in the offing, however, as the literature steadily grows and improves.

This chapter provides a general review of the epidemiologic surveys into sleep disorders since the 1970s. The discussion is divided into four main sections covering the phenomena most commonly investigated in the general population: (1) insomnia and associated syndromes, (2) excessive sleepiness, (3) sleep-disordered breathing, and (4) parasomnias.

## INSOMNIA AND ASSOCIATED SYNDROMES

The epidemiology of insomnia has suffered from the absence of an operational definition among health care authorities and in official classifications. In 1979, the American Institute of Medicine equated *insomnia* with "unsatisfactory sleep."[1] The Association of Sleep Disorders Centers defined insomnia for the first time in 1979 as a "heterogeneous group of conditions . . . considered to be responsible for inducing disturbed sleep or diminished sleep."[2] The 1990 edition of its classification system, now called the *International Classification of Sleep Disorders,* or *ICSD-90,* delineates insomnia with greater precision by taking into account severity, frequency of symptoms, and impact on social and occupational functioning.[3] The 1992 *International Classification of Diseases,* or *ICD-10,* specifies that insomnia manifests itself through difficulty initiating sleep (DIS) or difficulty maintaining sleep (DMS)—be it in the form of disrupted sleep (DS) or early morning awakenings (EMA)— occurring at least three times a week, accompanied by worry over the lack of sleep and its consequences, and causing either distress or daytime repercussions.[4] Finally, the American Psychiatric Association included a definition of insomnia for the first time in its revised third edition of the *Diagnostic and Statistical Manual of Mental Disorders,* or *DSM-III-R.*[5] In this classification, insomnia required the presence of DIS, DMS, or nonrestorative sleep lasting at least 1 month, occurring at least three times a week, and causing either distress or daytime repercussions. In its fourth edition, the *DSM-IV,* the criteria for insomnia have been harmonized with those of the *ICSD-90*—that is, the definition includes the presence of DIS, DMS, or nonrestorative sleep lasting at least 1 month and causing either distress or daytime consequences.[3,6]

## EPIDEMIOLOGY OF INSOMNIA COMPLAINTS

### North America

One of the earliest epidemiologic surveys on insomnia complaints (Table 20-1) was carried out in 1972 in the metropolitan area of Los Angeles.[7] Of the 1,006 subjects aged 18 or older queried, 32.2% reported insomnia complaints (DIS: 14.4%; DS: 22.9%; and EMA: 13.8%), with higher rates among women, the elderly, lower income earners, and the less educated. Half of the insomniacs reported recurrent or persistent health problems or multiple health problems (17.3% of the entire sample). Insomnia complaints were also found to be related to loneliness, depression, and stress.

Karacan et al.[8] undertook the first of their two surveys in Florida with 1,645 participants 18 years or older. Defined as "trouble with sleep often or all the time," insomnia complaints were reported by 10.9% of men and 15.4% of women. The second study was conducted in Houston with 2,347 subjects aged 18 years or older.[9] In this sample, DMS occurring "often or always" was twice as common as DIS in men and slightly higher in women. DMS and EMA increased with age in both genders, whereas DIS remained relatively unchanged over time.

In the large-scale epidemiologic study carried out by Welstein et al.[10] in the San Francisco Bay area, 31% of the 6,340 subjects ranging in age from 6 to 103 years perceived themselves as insomniacs and reported DIS, DS, EMA, or any combination of these three.

The 1979 study by Mellinger et al.[11] involved 3,161 individuals 18–79 years of age. Insomnia complaints were assessed for both a 12-month period and lifetime. The 12-month prevalence for DIS or DMS was 35%; however, only 17% of respondents reported being bothered "a lot" by their sleep problem. A higher proportion of women and the elderly reported being bothered by their sleep problem. These subjects were more likely to be depressed or anxious. It was also found that insomnia complaints affected more than half of the subjects with two health problems or more.

Analyzing data on 2,187 individuals aged 18 years or older from the Tucson, Arizona, epidemiologic study of obstructive airway diseases, Klink and Quan[12] computed the prevalence of DIS or DMS to be 37.8%. The rate was found to be higher for women and increased with age. Insomnia complaints also proved to be related to obstructive airway diseases, especially concurrent asthma and chronic bronchitis.

Ford and Kamerow[13] used data collected within the framework of the National Institute of Mental Health Epidemiological Catchment Area study between 1981 and 1985, which involved 7,954 respondents 18 years of age or older. Their definition of insomnia complaints was narrower than that of other studies and, consequently, the 6-month prevalence of insomnia was comparatively lower (10.2%) in their sample. They found a high co-occurrence of insomnia complaints and mental disorders (40%). Insomnia complaints were associated with a higher risk (odds ratio, 39.8) of developing a new major depressive illness if they persisted over two interviews within a 12-month interval, but were not a significant factor if they were not present by the second interview.

In a study of 1,722 subjects 15–100 years of age from the Montréal metropolitan area,[14] the prevalence of insomnia symptoms was found to be 29%. However, only 11.2% of the sample claimed to be dissatisfied with sleep or took medication to enhance sleep. These subjects made greater use of health care services and were more likely to have a physical illness; more than half of them presented with a concomitant psychiatric disorder. Primary insomnia was found in one-fifth of complainers.

A Mexican survey of 1,000 subjects aged 18–84 years was performed in 1986–1987 in the Monterrey metropolitan area by Téllez-Lòpez et al.[15] DIS, DMS, and EMA were measured on 3-point scales for severity (none, sometimes, frequent) and duration (<1 month, >1 month but <1 year, >1 year). Occasional or frequent insomnia was observed in 36.1% of the sample. Frequent insomnia was reported by 16.4% of respondents. Insomnia complaints increased with age among women. DMS and EMA were significantly higher in women than in men.

### Western Europe

From 1976 to 1979, Lugaresi et al.[16] surveyed 5,713 individuals aged 3 years or older in the Republic of

**Table 20-1.** Prevalence of Insomnia Symptoms in the General Population of America, Western Europe, and Australia

| Authors Location | N | Age (years) | Sample | Interview | Description | Prevalence (%) (M/F) |
|---|---|---|---|---|---|---|
| Karacan et al., 1976[8] Alachua County, FL, U.S. | 1,645 | ≥18 | Random | Household | Trouble with sleep often or all the time | 10.9/15.4 |
| Bixler et al., 1979[7] Los Angeles, CA, U.S. | 1,006 | ≥18 | Random stratified | Household | DIS, DMS, or EMA | 32.2 |
| Karacan et al., 1983[9] Houston, TX, U.S. | 2,347 | ≥18 | Random | Household | DIS or DMS, often or always | DIS: 6.0/11.2 DMS: 12.9/17.4 |
| Welstein et al., 1983[10] San Francisco, CA, U.S. | 6,340 | ≥6 | Random | Telephone | Insomnia, DIS, DMS | 31.1/42.1 |
| Mellinger et al., 1985[11] U.S. | 3,161 | ≥18 | Probability | Household | Bothered frequently by DIS, DMS, or EMA | 14.0/20.0 |
| Klink and Quan, 1987[12] Tucson, AZ, U.S. | 2,187 | ≥18 | Random stratified | Self-administered questionnaire | DIS, DMS, or EMA | 31.1/42.1 |
| Ford and Kamerow, 1989[13] Baltimore, MD; Durham, NC; Los Angeles, CA, U.S. | 7,954 | ≥18 | Household probability | Household | DIS, DMS, or EMA lasting ≥2 weeks; problems with sleep interfere significantly with daily activities; professional consultation; sleep-enhancing medication | 7.9/12.1 |
| Téllez-Lòpez et al., 1995[15] Monterrey, Mexico | 1,000 | ≥18 | Not specified | Household | Bothered frequently by DIS, DMS, or EMA | 16.4 |
| Ohayon et al., 1997[14] Montreal, Canada | 1,722 | ≥15 | Two stages: random stratified and household probability | Telephone | DIS, DMS, or EMA; sleep dissatisfaction | 8.7/13.2 |
| Lugaresi et al., 1983[16] San Marino, Italy | 5,713 | ≥3 | Representative | Household | Poor sleep always or almost always | 9.9/16.8 |
| Gislason and Almqvist, 1987[18] Uppsala, Sweden | 3,201 men | 30–69 | Random | Postal questionnaire | Major complaints of DIS or DMS | DIS: 6.9 DMS: 7.5 |
| Liljenberg et al., 1988[19] Gävleborg and Kopparberg Counties, Sweden | 3,557 | 30–65 | Random | Postal questionnaire | Problems with DIS or DMS great or very great | DIS: 5.1/7.1 DMS: 7.7/8.9 |
| Janson et al., 1995[20] Reykjavik, Iceland; Uppsala and Göteborg, Sweden; Antwerp, Belgium | 2,202 | 20–45 | Two stages: random from general population and random from stage one population | Stage one: postal questionnaire; stage two: structured interview and self-administered questionnaire | DIS or EMA at least three times/week | DIS: 6–9 EMA: 5–6 |

**Table 20-1.** *continued*

| Authors Location | N | Age (years) | Sample | Interview | Description | Prevalence (%) (M/F) |
|---|---|---|---|---|---|---|
| Husby and Lingjaerde, 1992[17] Tromsø, Norway | 14,667 | 20–54 | Entire population of 20–54 years | Self-administered questionnaire | Sleeplessness | 29.9/41.7 |
| Quera-Salva et al., 1990[21] France | 1,003 | ≥16 | Representative stratified | Household | DIS, DMS, or EMA | 48 |
| Ohayon, 1996[22] France | 5,622 | ≥15 | Two stages: random stratified and household probability | Telephone | DIS, DMS, or EMA; sleep dissatisfaction | 15.6/24.4 |
| Ohayon et al., 1995[24] U.K. | 4,972 | ≥15 | Two stages: random stratified and household probability | Telephone | DIS, DMS, or EMA; sleep dissatisfaction | 6.8/10.6 |
| Brabbins et al., 1993[25] Liverpool, U.K. | 1,070 | ≥65 | Random | Household | DIS, DMS, or EMA, lasting 1 month | 35 |
| Henderson et al., 1995[26] Canberra and Queanbeyan, Australia | 874 | ≥70 | Stratified | Household | DIS or EMA nearly every night in the past 2 weeks | 12.6/18.0 |
| Foley et al., 1995[27] East Boston (MA), New Haven (CT), Iowa and Washington Counties (FL), U.S. | 9,282 | ≥65 | Random | Household | DIS, DMS, or EMA, most of the time; insomnia (DIS or EMA most of the time) | DIS, DMS, or EMA: 29.1–43.4/38.3–47.4 Insomnia: 19.5–29.4/ 25.4–36.4 |
| Blazer et al., 1995[28] NC, U.S. | 3,976 | ≥65 | Random | Household | DIS, DMS, or EMA most of the time | DIS: 14.8 DMS: 26.6 EMA: 14.3 |

DIS = difficulty initiating sleep; DMS = difficulty maintaining sleep; EMA = early morning awakening.

San Marino. A total of 13.4% reported poor sleep "always" or "almost always." The prevalence of poor sleep was higher in women and increased with age. In a Norwegian study performed in the Tromsø municipality in 1979–1980[17] involving 14,667 participants aged 20–54 years, 41% of women and 29.9% of men reported being bothered by sleeplessness. Prevalence of complaints of sleepiness increased with age. Although insomnia was more frequent during the winter months, it was not associated with a specific time of the year for approximately 16% of the sample.

In 1984–1985, Gislason and Almqvist[18] studied sleep complaints in a sample of 3,201 Swedish men aged 30–69 years. Symptom severity was assessed on a 5-point scale ranging from absence of symptoms to severe symptoms. They found a prevalence of 6.9% for severe DIS and 14.3% for moderate DIS. Severe DMS was observed in 7.5% of the sample and moderate DMS in 14.9%. Obstructive pulmonary disease was associated with DMS, and rheumatic disease and untreated hypertension with DIS and DMS.

Another Swedish study[19] surveyed 3,557 individuals aged 30–65 years. Frequency of insomnia symptoms was assessed on a 5-point scale ranging from "no problems" to "very often." DIS was first considered present if the subject reported a sleep latency greater than 30 minutes, and DMS was considered present if the time awake during the night exceeded 30 minutes. Three additional criteria were included to confirm the presence of DIS or DMS: too little sleep, daytime sleepiness, and a perceived sleep deficit exceeding 1 hour. The prevalence of DIS dropped from 7.1% to 1.1% in women and from 5.1% to 0.5% in men after the addition of confirming criteria. Likewise, DMS diminished from 8.9% to 1.1% in women and from 7.7% to 1.1% in men.

Another study performed by Janson et al.[20] investigated four municipalities in three European countries (Iceland, Sweden, Belgium). A total of 2,202 subjects 20–45 years of age completed sleep questionnaires between 1990 and 1993. Insomnia symptoms were assessed on a 5-point frequency scale ranging from "never" to "almost every night." DIS occurring at least three times per week was reported by 6–9% of the sample; EMA occurring at least three times per week was reported by 5–6%. Nocturnal awakenings and EMA increased with age.

Quera-Salva et al.[21] interviewed a representative sample of the French population comprising 1,003 individuals aged 16–91 years about insomnia complaints and hypnotic drug use. They found the overall prevalence of sleep problems to be 48%. DIS was found in 17.1% of subjects, DS in 11.7%, and EMA in only 3.8%. Rates were higher among women and increased with age. Sleep complaints were associated with a higher score on a depression-anxiety scale.

Another nationwide French survey performed in 1993 on a sample of 5,622 subjects[22] showed that insomnia complaints accompanied by sleep dissatisfaction or sleep-enhancing drug use were common (20.1%) in the population and more prevalent among women and the elderly. However, only 5.6% of the sample had insomnia according to the *DSM-IV* diagnosis of insomnia disorder.[23] Approximately half of the insomnia subjects were found to have a concomitant mental disorder.

In a nationwide general population study performed in the United Kingdom,[24] 36.2% of the 4,972 subjects surveyed reported at least one insomnia symptom. These subjects were then divided into those satisfied and dissatisfied with sleep. The presence of an insomnia symptom accompanied by sleep dissatisfaction occurred in 8.7% of the sample. These subjects had a longer duration of insomnia complaints and almost unanimously reported daytime consequences of insomnia; 35.5% suffered from a *DSM-IV* psychiatric disorder. *DSM-IV* primary insomnia was found in 4.2% of the sample. Based on the *ICSD-90*, psychophysiologic insomnia was identified in 2.2% of the sample and idiopathic insomnia in 0.4%.

### Insomnia in the Elderly

Most epidemiologic surveys have included elderly subjects in their samples. The majority of these studies have shown that insomnia complaints are more prevalent in persons aged 65 years or older, when compared with surveys of younger individuals. Several epidemiologic inquiries, however, have focused specifically on insomnia complaints in the elderly. For example, Brabbins et al.[25] interviewed 1,070 noninstitutionalized elderly individuals (≥65 years) living in Liverpool (U.K.). They found a prevalence of 35% for insomnia complaints, with the rate twice as high for women as for men. In Canberra and Queanbeyan (Australia), Henderson et al.[26] interviewed 874 noninstitutionalized individuals 70 years of age or older and 59 institutionalized elderly individuals. Using "nearly every night over the last 2 weeks" as the basis for the presence of insomnia complaints, they found a prevalence of 16.2% in the community and 12.2% in the institutionalized population. Insomnia complaints were associated with depression, pain, and poor health.

In an epidemiologic survey begun in 1982 and involving 9,282 elderly individuals (65 years or older) from four U.S. communities, Foley et al.[27] found the prevalence of DIS or DMS to be 42.7% and the prevalence of insomnia (DMS or EMA most of the time) to be 28.7%. Insomnia complaints were associated with respiratory symptoms, physical disabilities, over-the-counter medication use, depressive symptoms, and the perception of poor health. The same research team also studied a sample of 3,976 elderly individuals from a community in North Carolina.[28] On the basis of "most of the time," DIS was reported by 14.8% of subjects, DMS by 26.6%, and EMA by 14.3%. Again, the rate was higher among women and increased with age. Insomnia complaints were also associated with white race, high depression score, cognitive impairment, chronic health conditions, and perception of poor health.

In summary, the definition of insomnia symptoms varies considerably across studies, as do the time frame considered and the wording of questions. Most investigations assessed DMS, DIS, and EMA, but defined these terms differently. Few specifically addressed the daytime consequences or distress accompanying insomnia symptomatology.[13,14,19,23,24] The mental health status of insomnia complainers was rarely explored[11,13,14,23,24] despite the fact that it is the most frequently associated factor observed in sleep clinics.[29–31]

## EXCESSIVE SLEEPINESS

Excessive sleepiness unfortunately receives less attention than insomnia, although its consequences can be severe. For instance, sleepiness is involved in approximately 16% of motor vehicle accidents in England.[32] Moreover, it has been suggested that half of work-related accidents and one-fourth of household accidents are caused by sleepiness.[33]

Existing studies (Table 20-2) can be divided into two main categories: those measuring hyper-

somnia symptoms and those assessing excessive daytime sleepiness (EDS). In the former, participants are generally queried regarding perceived sleep excess or daytime naps. In the latter, daytime sleepiness refers to sleep propensity in situations of diminished attention. The terms *hypersomnia* and *excessive daytime sleepiness* are often used interchangeably, however, and EDS is defined differently across surveys.

## EPIDEMIOLOGY OF EXCESSIVE SLEEPINESS

### *North America*

Hypersomnia rates have been reported in four U.S. studies. Karacan et al.[8] found a rate of 0.3%, Bixler et al.[7] 4.2%, and Ford and Kamerow[13] reported a 6-month prevalence of 3.2%. In this last study, subjects were asked whether they had gone a period of 2 weeks or more in which they slept too much (hypersomnia). No gender difference was observed and the rate was highest in the youngest age group (18- to 24-year-olds). Using the same criteria as Ford and Kamerow, Breslau et al.[34] found a lifetime prevalence of hypersomnia of 16.3% in their young adult sample (21–30 years of age). Klink and Quan[11] measured EDS by asking participants whether they fell asleep during the day. They found an overall prevalence of 12%. The rate increased with age but was not gender related. In their study, Téllez-Lòpez et al.[15] found a rate of hypersomnia (defined as "getting too much sleep") of 9.5% and a rate of EDS (defined as "a strong need to sleep in the day") of 21.5%. In both cases, rates decreased with age for women.

Hays et al.[35] assessed the mortality risk associated with EDS in an elderly sample of 3,962 subjects living in the community. Measuring EDS on the basis of self-reported napping, they reported a rate of 25.2%. They found that elderly persons who napped most of the time and made two or more errors on a cognitive status test had a higher mortality rate by a factor of 1.73. Frequent daytime nappers were more likely to be men, to be overweight, and to report insomnia complaints and depressive symptoms. They were also more limited in their physical activity and had more functional impairment. The study by Kripke et al.[36] revealed that long

**Table 20-2.** Prevalence of Excessive Sleepiness in the General Population of America and Western Europe

| Authors Location | N | Age (years) | Sample | Interview | Description | Prevalence (%) (M/F) |
|---|---|---|---|---|---|---|
| Karacan et al., 1976[8] Alachua County, FL, U.S. | 1,645 | ≥18 | Random | Household | Hypersomnia | 0.3 |
| Bixler et al., 1979[7] Los Angeles, CA, U.S. | 1,006 | ≥18 | Random stratified | Household | Sleeping too much | 4.2 |
| Klink and Quan, 1987[12] Tucson, AZ, U.S. | 2,187 | ≥18 | Random stratified | Self-administered questionnaire | Falling asleep during the day | 12.3/11.7 |
| Ford and Kamerow, 1989[13] Baltimore, MD; Durham, NC; Los Angeles, CA, U.S. | 7,954 | ≥18 | Household probability | Household | Sleeping too much for ≥2 weeks, professional consultation, sleep-enhancing medication, problems with sleep interfere significantly with daily activities | 2.8/3.5 |
| Téllez-López et al., 1995[15] Monterrey, Mexico | 1,000 | ≥18 | Not specified | Household | Getting too much sleep or strong need to sleep during the day | Too much sleep: 9.5 Daytime need to sleep: 21.5 |
| Hays et al., 1996[35] NC, U.S. | 3,962 | ≥65 | Random | Household | Frequent feeling of sleepiness and need to take a nap during the day or evening | 25.2 |
| Lugaresi et al., 1983[16] San Marino, Italy | 5,713 | ≥3 | Representative | Household | Sleepiness independent of meal times | 8.7 |
| Gislason and Almqvist, 1987[18] Uppsala, Sweden | 3,201 men | 30–69 | Random | Postal questionnaire | Moderate or severe daytime sleepiness | Moderate: 16.7 Severe: 5.7 |
| Liljenberg et al., 1988[19] Gävleborg and Kopparberg Counties, Sweden | 3,557 | 30–65 | Random | Postal questionnaire | Daytime sleepiness often or very often | 5.2/5.5 |
| Martikainen et al., 1992[39] Tampere, Finland | 1,190 | 36–50 | Random stratified | Postal questionnaire | Self-described as more clearly tired than others, daily desire to sleep during normal activities, or tired every day | 9.8 |
| Hublin et al., 1996[40] Finland | 11,354 | 33–60 | Twin cohort | Postal questionnaire | Daily or almost daily daytime sleepiness | 6.7/11.0 |
| Janson et al., 1995[38] Reykjavik, Iceland; Uppsala and Göteborg, Sweden; Antwerp, Belgium | 2,202 | 20–45 | Two stages: random from general population and random from stage 1 population | Stage 1: postal questionnaire; stage 2: structured interview and self-administered questionnaire | Daytime sleepiness experienced ≥3 days/week | 11–21 |
| Enright et al., 1996* Forsyth (NC), Sacramento (CA), Washington (MD), Pittsburgh (PA) Counties, U.S. | 5,201 | ≥65 | Random from the Health Care Finance Administration Medicare eligibility lists | Self-administered questionnaire and clinical examination | Usually sleepy during day | 17.0/15.0 |

**Table 20-2.** *Continued*

| Authors Location | N | Age (years) | Sample | Interview | Description | Prevalence (%) (M/F) |
|---|---|---|---|---|---|---|
| Asplund, 1996[41] Västerbotten and Norrbotten, Sweden | 6,143 | ≥65 | None | Postal questionnaire | Often sleepy or naps during the day | Sleepy: 32.0/23.2 Naps: 29.4/14.4 |
| Ohayon et al., 1997[42] U.K. | 4,972 | ≥15 | Two stages: random stratified and house-hold probability | Telephone | Feeling greatly or moderately sleepy during the day for ≥1 month | Greatly: 4.4/6.6 Moderately: 21.5/17.9 |

*PL Enright, AB Newman, PW Wahl, et al. Prevalence and correlates of snoring and observed apneas in 5,201 older adults. Sleep 1996;19:531.

sleep (>9 hours per night) and short sleep (<4 hours per night) were associated with a mortality risk 1.8 times higher at a 6-year follow-up compared with the rest of the population. A similar study performed in California by Wingard et al.[37] found that among people who slept either more than 9 hours or less than 6 hours per night, the mortality risk for men and women, respectively, was 1.7 and 1.6 times as high as for the general population.

### Western Europe

Most of the epidemiologic surveys focusing on the phenomenon of excessive sleepiness in the general population have been conducted in the Nordic countries (Iceland, Finland, Sweden). Gislason and Almqvist[18] reported a moderate EDS prevalence of 16.7% in their sample of men and a major EDS prevalence of 5.7%. Both significantly decreased with age. Another study was performed by Janson et al.[38] on a young adult population from three countries (20–44 years of age). They found a prevalence of daytime sleepiness, occurring at least 1 day per week, of approximately 40%; daily sleepiness occurring in the daytime was observed in approximately 5% of the sample.

Martikainen et al.[39] assessed 1,190 Finnish subjects aged 36–50 years. They found that 9.8% of the sample considered themselves "clearly more tired than others," experienced a "daily desire to sleep in the course of normal activities," or felt "very tired daily." Hublin et al.[40] found a prevalence of daytime sleepiness occurring daily or almost daily in 9% of their Finnish twin cohort. Indicators of moderate or severe depression were observed in one-fourth of those complaining of sleepiness, and narcolepsy in 0.3%. Subjects with daytime sleepiness were more likely to report snoring, most notably among men. Approximately one-tenth of the subjects with daytime sleepiness complained of insufficient sleep.

A Swedish study investigated daytime sleepiness in 6,143 elderly people living in the community.[41] The mean age of participants was 73 years. It was found that 32.0% of men and 23.2% of women reported being "often sleepy during the day." Napping was reported by 24.4% of men and 14.9% of women. Both these sleepiness measures increased in frequency with age and were associated with poor health status, somatic disease, and poor sleep.

In their U.K. study, Ohayon et al.[42] assessed daytime sleepiness on a severity scale. Severe daytime sleepiness was observed in 5.5% of their sample, and moderate daytime sleepiness in 15.2%. Severe daytime sleepiness was more frequent in women and in middle-aged subjects, whereas moderate daytime sleepiness was higher among the elderly. Both severe and moderate daytime sleepiness were associated with a variety of *ICSD-90* diagnoses, the most common being, in decreasing order, mood disorder associated with sleep disturbance, psychophysiologic insomnia, obstructive sleep apnea syndrome, restless legs syndrome, and insufficient sleep syndrome. Narcolepsy was identified in 0.04% and idiopathic hypersomnia in 0.20%.

A number of conclusions can be drawn from these general population surveys. Unlike insomnia symptoms, excessive sleepiness is generally not gender related. Absence of consistent definitions of EDS brings an unacceptable variability for proper prevalence related to age.[12,18] These epidemiologic surveys have also confirmed that EDS can be the primary symptom of idiopathic hypersomnia or narcolepsy. These two disorders registered prevalence rates of only 0.026–0.040% in the samples studied.[43–45]

In addition, EDS has been shown to be induced by several lifestyle factors: work conditions,[42] poor sleep hygiene,[40,42] and psychotropic drug consumption.[40,42] EDS is also associated with sleep-disordered breathing,[38,40,42] various psychiatric disorders, depression (in particular),[13,34,35,40,42] and physical illnesses.[18,38,42] In other words, excessive sleepiness is often caused by specific factors that can be easily identified by physicians.

## SLEEP-DISORDERED BREATHING

### Snoring

Snoring is a symptom indicating that at least a partial airway occlusion occurs during sleep. Epidemiologic surveys assessing this phenomenon (Table 20-3) unanimously report that the prevalence is higher among men and increases with age. In their San Marino survey, Lugaresi et al.[46] found that 19% of their overall sample were habitual snorers; 24.1% of these were men and 13.8% women. The rate was 60% in subjects aged 60 years or older. A Danish survey involving 1,504 subjects aged 30–60 years[47]

**Table 20-3.** Prevalence of Snoring in the General Population of America, Western Europe, and Australia

| Authors Location | N | Age (years) | Sample | Interview | Description | Prevalence (%) (M/F) |
|---|---|---|---|---|---|---|
| Lugaresi et al., 1981[46] San Marino, Italy | 5,713 | ≥3 | Representative | Household | Habitual snoring | 24.1/13.8 |
| Fitzpatrick et al., 1993[48] Lerwick, Thurso, Aberdeen, Ayr, Leeds, Coventry, Southampton, and St. Helier, U.K. | 1,478 | ≥18 | Two stages: random and youngest adult (≥18)[a] | Postal questionnaire | Snoring ≥4 nights/week | 23.0/9.0 |
| Gislason et al., 1993[49] Reykjavik, Iceland | 1,505 women | 40–59 | Random | Postal questionnaire | Intermittent (1–5 nights/week) or habitual (6–7 nights/week) snoring | Intermittent: 21.7 Habitual: 11.2 |
| Jennum and Sjol, 1994[47] Copenhagen, Denmark | 1,504 | 30–60 | Random | Clinical interviews | Nightly snoring | 19.1/7.9 |
| Martikainen et al., 1994[53] Tampere, Finland | 1,190 | 36–50 | Random stratified | Postal questionnaire | Habitual snorers (nightly or almost nightly) | 18.9–38.9/6.8–13.3 |
| Koskenvuo et al., 1994[50] Finland | 3,750 men | 40–59 | Twin cohort | Postal questionnaire | Habitual (almost always) Frequent snorers (often) Occasional snorers (sometimes) | Habitual: 8.8 Frequent: 20.4 Occasional: 60.4 |
| Bearpark et al., 1995[51] Busselton, Australia | 294 men | 40–65 | All male[b] | Clinical and portable device recording | Snoring >10% of the night Snoring >50% of the night | >10%: 81 >50%: 22 |
| Janson et al., 1995[38] Reykjavik, Iceland; Uppsala and Göteborg, Sweden; Antwerp, Belgium | 2,202 | 20–45 | Two stages: random from general population and random from stage 1 population | Stage 1: postal questionnaire; stage 2: structured interview and self-administered questionnaire | Snoring every night | 5/2–3 |
| Jennum et al., 1995[52] Copenhagen, Denmark | 2,937 men | 54–74 | None | Self-administered questionnaire, clinical interviews | Snoring always or often | 49.9 |
| Enright et al., 1996[c] Forsyth (NC), Sacramento (CA), Washington (MD), Pittsburgh (PA), Counties, U.S. | 5,201 | ≥65 | Random from the Health Care Finance Administration Medicare eligibility list | Self-administered questionnaire and clinical examination | Loud snoring | 33.0/19.0 |
| Ohayon et al., 1997[d] U.K. | 4,972 | ≥15 | Two stages: random stratified and household probability | Telephone | Regular snoring | 47.7/33.6 |

[a] In the household, the youngest adult aged 18 years or over completed the questionnaire.
[b] Busselton residents aged 40–65 years on the volunteer register.
[c] PL Enright, AB Newman, PW Wahl, et al. Prevalence and correlates of snoring and observed apneas in 5,201 older adults. Sleep 1996;19:531.
[d] MM Ohayon, C Guilleminault, RG Priest, M Caulet. Snoring and breathing pauses during sleep: telephone interview survey of a United Kingdom population sample. BMJ 1997;314:860.

found that the prevalence of habitual male and female snorers was, respectively, 19.1% and 7.9%, and that the rate increased with age for both genders. Fitzpatrick et al.[48] assessed the prevalence of snoring in a random sample of 1,478 British subjects aged 18 years or older. They obtained an overall rate of 37% in their sample; the rate for frequent snorers alone was 11%. Again, frequent snoring was more prevalent in men (16% compared with 7% for women) and increased with age.

In a study undertaken in Iceland in 1988[49] with 1,505 women aged 40–59 years, intermittent snoring was reported by 21.7% of the participants and habitual snoring by 11.2%. The prevalence of snoring increased with age and weight. In Finland, Koskenvuo et al.[50] studied 3,750 men aged 40–59 years from a Finnish twin cohort. They found that 8.8% were habitual snorers and 20.4% were frequent snorers. Only 10% reported never snoring. Habitual or frequent snoring was associated with a body mass index (BMI) greater than 27 kg/m$^2$ (i.e., overweight or obese), smoking, physical inactivity, hostility, and morning tiredness.

In Australia, 294 men aged 40–65 years were recruited for home monitoring (MESAM IV) in the Busselton health survey.[51] The sample represented 18% of the total male population in this age group in this town. They found that 81% snored more than 10% of the night, and 22% more than half the night. The best predictors of snoring at least half the night were a BMI greater than 30 kg/m$^2$, sleeping supine 50% or more of the time, and smoking.

Follow-up surveys are essential to identify the potential long-term consequences of diseases and symptoms. Two studies have explored the course of snoring and the mortality risks for snorers. A prospective Danish survey spanning a 6-year period was conducted by Jennum et al.[52] with 2,937 men aged 54–74 years. Of these, 49.9% reported snoring "always" or "often." The authors did not find a higher mortality in snorers than in nonsnorers, and both groups had the same risk of suffering from ischemic heart disease. A Finnish 5-year follow-up study was performed with 1,190 participants at year 1 and 626 at year 5.[53] Subjects were aged 36–50 years at the start. At both assessments, the prevalence of habitual snoring increased with age and was higher in men. At follow-up, the highest increase in snoring (up by 10%) was reported by the younger age group (36 years) of men. At year 1,

they found a higher incidence of "doze-offs" at the wheel among habitual snorers (22%) compared with nonsnorers (14.8%). In 1990, they found a slightly higher rate of snorers involved in traffic accidents due to sleepiness.

### Sleep Apnea

Sleep apnea is characterized by repeated breathing cessation during sleep lasting at least 10 seconds. The number of apnea and hypopnea events (respiratory disturbances) per hour, called the *respiratory disturbance index* (RDI) or *apnea/hypopnea index* (AHI), is used to determine whether breathing patterns are abnormal. Usually, an AHI of 5 or more is considered an abnormal number of sleep respiratory disturbances. When a sleep apnea syndrome is suspected, polysomnographic recordings are necessary to confirm the diagnosis. Obstructive sleep apnea syndrome is associated with a high number of obstructive and mixed events. This criterion can be misleading in the general population, however, as the severity of this sort of sleep-disordered breathing tends to be unimodally distributed.[54] It is not surprising, then, that few surveys have attempted to estimate the prevalence of sleep apnea syndrome or obstructive sleep apnea syndrome in community-based samples (Table 20-4).

One of the oldest studies of obstructive sleep apnea was performed in Israel by Lavie[55] with 300 working men, of which 78 were examined polysomnographically. He found that 2.7% of the sample had an AHI greater than or equal to 10 and that 0.7% had an AHI greater than or equal to 20. In the Finnish twin cohort study, Telakivi et al.[56] did polysomnographic recordings on 25 snorers and 27 nonsnorers selected from among 278 men aged 41–50 years. They estimated that 0.4% of this population had an AHI greater than or equal to 20 and that 1.4% had an AHI greater than or equal to 10, with an oxygenation desaturation index (ODI) of at least 4%.

Gislason et al.[57] assessed 3,201 Swedish men aged 30–60 years and carried out polysomnographic recordings on 61 of these men who complained of sleepiness and who snored. Based on their polysomnographic findings, the researchers estimated that 0.9% of this population had an AHI greater than or equal to 10 and that 1.4% had an AHI greater than or equal to 5. Gislason et al.[49]

**Table 20-4.** Prevalence of Sleep Apnea Syndrome in Selected Samples

| Authors Location | N | Age (years) | Sample | Interview | Description | Prevalence (%) (M/F) |
|---|---|---|---|---|---|---|
| Lavie, 1983[55] Israel | 1,502 (78) | 32–67 | Male workers | Questionnaire and PSG | AI ≥10 | 0.89 |
| Gislason et al., 1988[57] Uppsala, Sweden | 3,201 (61) | 30–69 | Men, general population | Postal questionnaire; PSG for snorers complaining of sleepiness | AHI ≥30 and daytime sleepiness | 1.3 |
| Cirignotta et al., 1989[58] Bologna, Italy | 1,170 (40) | 30–69 | Men, general population | Postal questionnaire; PSG for nightly snorers | AHI ≥10 | 2.7 |
| Martikainen et al., 1994[53] Tempere, Finland | 1985: 1,190 1990: 626 (22) | 36–50 | General population | (1) Postal questionnaire (2) PSG for male habitual snorers | (1) ODI ≥4% >5/hr (2) ODI ≥4% >10/hr | (1) 1.8 (2) 1.1 |
| Ancoli-Israel et al., 1991[a] San Diego, CA, U.S. | 615 (427) | 65–95 | General population | Home PSG | AI ≥5; RDI ≥10 | AI: 24.0; RDI: 62.0 |
| Stradling and Cosby, 1991[b] Oxford, U.K. | 1,001 (893) | 35–65 | Men, age-sex register of a group general practice | Oximetry | (1) ODI ≥4% >5/hr (2) ODI ≥4% >10/hr (3) ODI ≥3% >10/hr and symptoms | (1) 5.0 (2) 1.0 (3) 0.8 |
| Gislason et al., 1993[49] Reykjavik, Iceland | 1,505 (35) | 40–59 | Women, general population | Postal questionnaire and PSG for snorers complaining of sleepiness | AHI ≥30 and daytime sleepiness | 2.5 |
| Young et al., 1993[59] U.S. | 3,513 (625) | 30–60 | State employees | Questionnaire and PSG for snorers | AHI ≥5 | 4.0 (men) 2.0 (women) |
| Olson et al., 1995[60] Australia | 2,202 (441) | 35–69 | General population | Questionnaire and respiratory measurement, overrepresentation of snorers and sleep complainers | AHI ≥10 | 5.7 (men) 1.2 (women) |
| Bearpark et al., 1995[51] Busselton, Australia | 486 (294) | 40–65 | Men, general population | (1) Questionnaire (2) PSG | (1) RDI ≥5 and at least occasional daytime sleepiness (2) RDI ≥5 and at least often daytime sleepiness | (1) 12.2 (2) 3.1 |

AI = apnea index; AHI = apnea/hypopnea index; ODI = oxygen desaturation index; RDI = respiratory disturbance index; PSG = polysomnography.
[a] S Ancoli-Israel, DF Kripke, MR Klauber, et al. Sleep-disordered breathing in community-dwelling elderly. Sleep 1991;14:486.
[b] JR Stradling, JH Crosby. Predictors and prevalence of obstructive sleep apnoea and snoring in 1001 middle aged men. Thorax 1991;46:85.

conducted a similar survey with 1,505 Icelandic women 40–59 years of age, performing polysomnographic recordings on 35 snorers with EDS. It was estimated that approximately 2.5% of this population was affected with a sleep apnea syndrome (daytime sleepiness accompanied by an AHI ≥5).

Cirignotta et al.[58] recorded 156 men recruited from a sample of 1,510 Italian men aged 30–69 years. They estimated that 4.8% of this population had an AHI greater than 5 and 3.2% an AHI greater than 10. The 5-year follow-up survey by Martikainen et al.[53] found that the prevalence of symptoms (the combination of snoring and breathing pauses during sleep) indicating possible sleep apnea rose 2.3% over the study period, from 4.7% in 1985 to 7% in 1990. They also found that being overweight and gaining weight were the best predictors of an AHI greater than 5 and an ODI equal to or greater than 4%. Self-reported snoring and breathing pauses were found to be the best predictors of an AHI greater than 10 and an ODI equal to or greater than 4%.

The Wisconsin sleep cohort study[59] surveyed 3,513 workers aged 30–60 years. They invited all habitual snorers and 25% of the nonhabitual snorers to a one-night polysomnographic recording. In all, 625 subjects accepted. For women, 18.9% of the habitual snorers and 5% of the nonhabitual snorers had an AHI of 5 or greater. For men, the corresponding figures were 34% and 16.1%, respectively. Based on these findings, the prevalence of sleep apnea syndrome (daytime sleepiness or nonrestorative sleep and an AHI ≥5) was estimated at 4% among men and 2% among women.

The Busselton health survey[51] found that 12.2% of men aged 40–65 years had at least five respiratory disturbances per hour of sleep (RDI ≥5) along with "at least occasional" daytime sleepiness, and that 3.1% had an RDI greater than or equal to 5 along with "at least often" daytime sleepiness. Another Australian survey[60,61] involved 2,202 subjects aged 35–69 years, of which 441 subjects who complained about their sleep or snored were monitored polysomnographically. It was estimated that the rate of obstructive sleep apnea syndrome (based on an AHI ≥15) was 3.6% in the sample population (5.7% among men vs. 1.2% among women).

Unlike snoring and other sleep disorder symptoms, obstructive sleep apnea syndrome has not been the subject of any sound epidemiologic survey in the general population. None of the studies to date used a true random sample of subjects to be monitored polysomnographically. Most were cohort studies. This is a major flaw in this field of research, despite many claims to the contrary.

## PARASOMNIAS

Parasomnias include a group of sleep disorders characterized by abnormal behavioral or physiologic events occurring at different sleep stages or during sleep-wake transitions. The *ICSD*[3] divides parasomnias into four subgroups: (1) arousal (confusional arousals, sleepwalking, and sleep terrors), (2) sleep-wake transition (rhythmic movement disorder, sleep starts, sleep talking, and nocturnal leg cramps), (3) REM sleep disorders (nightmares, sleep paralysis, REM sleep behavior disorder), and (4) a residual group.

Parasomnias have seldom been investigated in the adult general population. Arousal parasomnias occur primarily in childhood and normally cease by adolescence. In the adult general population, a study by Bixler et al.[7] set the prevalence of sleepwalking at 3%. Téllez-Lòpez et al.[15] reported a prevalence of 1.9% in their Mexican survey. In the Finnish twin cohort study, Hublin et al.[62] obtained a prevalence of 0.7% among adult men and of 0.5% among adult women (with at least one episode per month). Infrequent episodes (less than monthly) were reported by 3.2% of men and 2.6% of women.

These studies showed that sleepwalking is not gender related but is more common among younger subjects (<25 years) and almost never reported by elderly persons. The most dramatic consequence of this parasomnia is the harm that sleepwalkers can inflict on themselves or others. Cases of murder during sleepwalking episodes have been documented.[63] The prevalence of sleep terrors and confusional arousals in adulthood is not known. In children, the prevalence of sleep terrors ranges from 1.0% to 6.5%.[64–66]

Epidemiologic data on the sleep-wake transition parasomnias are scarce. Téllez-Lòpez et al.[15] reported a prevalence rate of 21.3% for sleep talking and 3% for frequent sleep talking. Again, this phenomenon is more frequent in the younger age group (≤30 years). The prevalence of nocturnal leg cramps is not well-documented, but certain studies have suggested that they are quite frequent among the elderly.[67] In their U.K. study, Ohayon et al.[42] reported that nocturnal leg cramps are more frequently observed in subjects with severe daytime sleepiness (4.7%) compared with nonsleepy subjects (0.5%). Regarding the group of REM sleep disorder parasomnias, nightmares have been reported to occur at least once a week in 5% of the adult population.[68]

Sleep paralysis is one of the symptoms mainly associated with narcolepsy. Téllez-Lòpez et al.[15] found a sleep paralysis prevalence (occurring at least sometimes) of 11.3%. REM sleep behavior disorders were first described in the late 1970s by Japanese researchers[69] and labeled by Schenck et al.[70] These disorders are characterized by "injuries or disruptive behaviors emerging during REM sleep, which ordinarily exhibits a generalized skeletal muscle atonia."[70] However, in REM sleep behavior disorder a characteristic finding is REM sleep without muscle atonia. The prevalence of these disorders in the general population is not well-documented.

## CHALLENGES FOR THE EPIDEMIOLOGY OF SLEEP DISORDERS

### Insomnia and Associated Syndromes

Since the 1980s, research into insomnia symptomatology has established that sleep complaints are common in the general population and affect primarily women and the elderly. Epidemiologists must now distinguish between the various subtypes of insomnia. Few surveys present insomnia complaints as a whole when assessing their causes and consequences.[14,24] Moreover, epidemiologic data on transient and seasonal patterns of insomnia are nonexistent. Longitudinal epidemiologic data on the evolution and consequences of insomnia complaints are still lacking. To date, only two surveys have addressed this specific subject in the general population.[13,34]

### Excessive Sleepiness

A uniform operational definition of excessive sleepiness is still missing. Although many surveys have been undertaken on the topic, differences in definition and the variance in results do not make it possible to reach any definite conclusions. As is the case for insomnia complaints, the causes and consequences of excessive sleepiness are rarely presented as a whole. The prevalence of transient or seasonal patterns of symptoms is not known, nor is its longitudinal evolution in the general population.

### Sleep-Disordered Breathing

The study of obstructive sleep apnea syndrome in the general population suffers primarily from a subsample selection bias. Few studies have drawn subjects for polysomnographic recordings in true random fashion. Most surveys used a sleep questionnaire to screen potential subjects with obstructive sleep apnea. Consequently, certain categories are likely to be underrepresented, such as individuals unaware of their symptoms. In addition, many of these studies did not record enough cases to reach a 95% level of precision, thus undermining the validity of results. Prevalence, therefore, has likely been underestimated.

## REFERENCES

1. Institute of Medicine. Sleeping Pills, Insomnia, and Medical Practice. Washington, DC: National Academy of Sciences, 1979.
2. Association of Sleep Disorders Centers. Diagnostic classification of sleep and arousal disorders. Sleep 1979;2:5.
3. Diagnostic Classification Steering Committee, Thorpy MJ, Chairman. International Classification of Sleep Disorders: Diagnostic and Coding Manual (ICSD). Rochester, MN: American Sleep Disorders Association, 1990.
4. World Health Organization. The ICD-10 Classification of Mental and Behavioural Disorders: Clinical Descriptions and Diagnostic Guidelines. Geneva: World Health Organization, 1992.
5. American Psychiatric Association. Diagnostic and Statistical Manual of Mental Disorders (3rd ed) (rev ed). Washington, DC: American Psychiatric Association, 1987.
6. American Psychiatric Association. Diagnostic and Statistical Manual of Mental Disorders (4th ed). Washington, DC: American Psychiatric Association, 1994.
7 Bixler EO, Kales A, Soldatos CR, et al. Prevalence of sleep disorders in the Los Angeles metropolitan area. Am J Psychiatry 1979;136:1257.
8. Karacan I, Thornby JI, Anch M, et al. Prevalence of sleep disturbance in a primarily urban Florida county. Soc Sci Med 1976;10:239.

9   Karacan I, Thornby JI, William R. Sleep Disturbance: A Community Survey. In C Guilleminault, E Lugaresi (eds), Sleep/Wake Disorders: Natural History, Epidemiology, and Long-Term Evolution. New York: Raven, 1983;37.

10. Welstein L, Dement WC, Redington D, Guilleminault C. Insomnia in the San Francisco Bay Area: A Telephone Survey. In C Guilleminault, E Lugaresi (eds), Sleep/Wake Disorders: Natural History, Epidemiology, and Long-Term Evolution. New York: Raven, 1983;29.

11. Mellinger GD, Balter MB, Uhlenhuth EH. Insomnia and its treatment: prevalence and correlates. Arch Gen Psychiatry 1985;42:225.

12. Klink M, Quan SF. Prevalence of reported sleep disturbances in a general adult population and their relationship to obstructive airways diseases. Chest 1987;91:540.

13. Ford DE, Kamerow DB. Epidemiologic study of sleep disturbances and psychiatric disorders. An opportunity for prevention? JAMA 1989;262:1479.

14. Ohayon MM, Caulet M, Guilleminault C. Complaints about nocturnal sleep: how a general population perceives its sleep, and how this relates to the complaint of insomnia. Sleep 1997;20:715.

15. Téllez-Lòpez A, Sánchez EG, Torres FG, et al. Hábitos y trastornos del dormir en residentes del área metropolitana de Monterrey. Salud Mental 1995;18:14.

16. Lugaresi E, Cirignotta F, Zucconi M, et al. Good and Poor Sleepers: An Epidemiological Survey of the San Marino Population. In C Guilleminault, E Lugaresi (eds), Sleep/Wake Disorders: Natural History, Epidemiology, and Long-Term Evolution. New York: Raven, 1983;1.

17. Husby R, Lingjaerde O. Prevalence of reported sleeplessness in northern Norway in relation to sex, age and season. Acta Psychiatr Scand 1990;542.

18. Gislason T, Almqvist M. Somatic diseases and sleep complaints: an epidemiological study of 3201 Swedish men. Acta Med Scand 1987;221:475.

19. Liljenberg B, Almqvist M, Hetta J, et al. The prevalence of insomnia: the importance of operationally defined criteria. Ann Clin Res 1988;20:393.

20. Janson C, Gislason T, De Backer W, et al. Prevalence of sleep disturbances among young adults in three European countries. Sleep 1995;18:589.

21. Quera-Salva MA, Orluc A, Goldenberg F, Guilleminault C. Insomnia and use of hypnotics: study of a French population. Sleep 1991;14:386.

22. Ohayon M. Epidemiological study on insomnia in the general population. Sleep 1996;19(3):S7.

23. Ohayon MM. Prevalence of DSM-IV diagnostic criteria of insomnia: distinguishing between insomnia related to mental disorders from sleep disorders. J Psychiatr Res 1997;31:333.

24. Ohayon MM, Caulet M, Priest RG, Guilleminault C. DSM-IV and ICSD-90 insomnia symptoms and sleep dissatisfaction. Br J Psychiatry 1997;20:1082.

25. Brabbins CJ, Dewey ME, Copeland JRM, et al. Insomnia in the elderly: prevalence, gender differences and relationships with morbidity and mortality. Int J Geriatr Psychiatry 1993;8:473.

26. Henderson S, Jorm AF, Scott LR, et al. Insomnia in the elderly: its prevalence and correlates in the general population. Med J Aust 1995;162:22.

27. Foley DJ, Monjan AA, Brown SL, et al. Sleep complaints among elderly persons: an epidemiologic study of three communities. Sleep 1995;18:425.

28. Blazer DG, Hays JC, Foley DJ. Sleep complaints in older adults: a racial comparison. J Gerontol A Biol Sci Med Sci 1995;50:M280.

29. Buysse DJ, Reynold CF, Kupfer DJ, et al. Clinical diagnoses in 216 insomnia patients using the international classification of sleep disorders (ICSD), DSM-IV and ICD-10 categories: a report from the APA/NIMH DSM-IV field trial. Sleep 1994;17:630.

30. Coleman RM, Roffwarg HP, Kennedy SJ, et al. Sleep-wake disorders based on a polysomnographic diagnosis: a national cooperative study. JAMA 1982;247:997.

31. Tan TL, Kales JD, Kales A, et al. Biopsychobehavioral correlates of insomnia, IV: diagnosis based on DSM-III. Am J Psychiatry 1984;141:357.

32. Horne JA, Reyner LA. Sleep-related vehicle accidents. BMJ 1995;310:565.

33. Leger D. The cost of sleep-related accidents: a report for the national commission on sleep disorders research. Sleep 1994;17:84.

34. Breslau N, Roth T, Rosenthal L, Andreski P. Sleep disturbance and psychiatric disorders: a longitudinal epidemiological study of young adults. Biol Psychiatry 1996;39:411.

35. Hays JC, Blazer DG, Foley DJ. Risk of napping: excessive daytime sleepiness and mortality in an older community population. J Am Geriatr Soc 1996;44:693.

36. Kripke DF, Simons RN, Garfinkel L, Hammond EC. Short and long sleep and sleeping pills. Is increased mortality associated? Arch Gen Psychiatry 1979;36:103.

37. Wingard DL, Berkman LF. Mortality risk associated with sleeping patterns among adults. Sleep 1983;6:102.

38. Janson C, Gislason T, De Backer W, et al. Daytime sleepiness, snoring and gastro-oesophageal reflux amongst young adults in three European countries. J Intern Med 1995;237:277.

39. Martikainen K, Hasan J, Urponen H, et al. Daytime sleepiness: a risk factor in community life. Acta Neurol Scand 1992;86:337.

40. Hublin C, Kaprio J, Partinen M, et al. Daytime sleepiness in an adult, Finnish population. J Intern Med 1996;239:417.

41. Asplund R. Daytime sleepiness and napping amongst the elderly in relation to somatic health and medical treatment. J Intern Med 1996;239:261.

42. Ohayon MM, Caulet M, Philip P, et al. How sleep and mental disorders are related to complaints of daytime sleepiness. Arch Intern Med 1997;157:2645.

43. Dement W, Carskadon M, Ley R. The prevalence of narcolepsy II. Sleep Res 1973;2:147.

44. Dement W, Zarcone V, Varner V, et al. The prevalence of narcolepsy. Sleep Res 1972;1:148.

45. Hublin C, Kaprio J, Partinen M, et al. The prevalence of narcolepsy: an epidemiological study of the Finnish twin cohort. Ann Neurol 1994;35:709.

46. Lugaresi E, Coccagna G, Cirignotta F, Piana C. Snoring: Some Epidemiological Data. In I Karacan (ed), Psychophysiological Aspects of Sleep. Park Ridge, NJ: Noyes Medical, 1981;106.

47. Jennum P, Sjol A. Snoring, sleep apnoea and cardiovascular risk factors—the MONICA-II study. Int J Epidemiol 1993;22:439.

48. Fitzpatrick MF, Martin K, Fossey E, et al. Snoring, asthma and sleep disturbance in Britain—a community-based survey. Eur Respir J 1993;6:531.

49. Gislason T, Benediktsdottir B, Bjornsson JK, et al. Snoring, hypertension, and the sleep apnea syndrome—an epidemiologic survey of middle-aged women. Chest 1993;103:1147.

50. Koskenvuo M, Partinen M, Kaprio J, et al. Snoring and cardiovascular risk factors. Ann Med 1994;26:371.

51. Bearpark H, Elliott L, Grunstein R, et al. Snoring and sleep apnea—a population study in Australian men. Am J Respir Crit Care Med 1995;151:1459.

52. Jennum P, Hein HO, Suadicani P, Gyntelberg F. Risk of ischemic heart disease in self-reported snorers—a prospective study of 2,937 men aged 54 to 74 years—the Copenhagen male study. Chest 1995;108:138.

53. Martikainen K, Partinen M, Urponen H, et al. Natural evolution of snoring—a 5-year follow-up study. Acta Neurol Scand 1994;90:437.

54. Davies RJO, Stradling JR. The epidemiology of sleep apnoea. Thorax 1996;51(Suppl 2):65.

55. Lavie P. Incidence of sleep apnea in a presumably healthy working population: a significant relationship with excessive daytime sleepiness. Sleep 1983;6:212.

56. Telakivi T, Partinen M, Koskenvuo M, et al. Periodic breathing and hypoxia in snorers and controls: validation of snoring history and association with blood pressure and obesity. Acta Neurol Scand 1987;76:69.

57. Gislason T, Almqvist M, Erikson G, et al. Prevalence of sleep apnea syndrome among Swedish men—an epidemiological study. J Clin Epidemiol 1988;41:571.

58. Cirignotta F, D'Alessandro R, Partinen M, et al. Prevalence of every night snoring and obstructive sleep apneas among 30–69 year old men in Bologna, Italy. Acta Neurol Scand 1989;79:366.

59. Young T, Palta M, Dempsey J, et al. The occurrence of sleep-disordered breathing among middle-aged adults. N Engl J Med 1993;328:1230.

60. Olson LG, King MT, Hensley MJ, Saunders NA. A community study of snoring and sleep-disordered breathing—prevalence. Am J Respir Crit Care Med 1995;152:711.

61. Olson LG, King MT, Hensley MJ, Saunders NA. A community study of snoring and sleep-disordered breathing—health outcomes. Am J Respir Crit Care Med 1995;152:717.

62. Hublin C, Kaprio J, Partinen M, et al. Prevalence and genetics of sleepwalking: a population-based twin study. Neurology 1997;48:177.

63. Broughton R, Billings R, Cartwright R, et al. Homicidal somnambulism: a case report. Sleep 1994;17:253.

64. Klackenberg G. Sleep behaviour studied longitudinally. Data from 4–16 years on duration, night-awakening and bed-sharing. Acta Paediatr Scand 1982; 71:501.

65. Salzavulo P, Chevalier A. Sleep problems in children and their relationship with early disturbances of the waking-sleeping rhythms. Sleep 1983;6:47.

66. Simonds JF, Parraga H. Prevalence of sleep disorders and sleep behaviors in children and adolescents. J Am Acad Child Psychiatry 1982;21:383.

67. Jacobsen JH, Rosenberg RS, Huttenlocher PR, et al. Familial nocturnal cramping. Sleep 1986;9:54.

68. Hartmann E. The Nightmare. New York: Basic Books, 1984.

69. Hishikawa Y, Sugita Y, Teshima Y, et al. Sleep Disorders in Alcoholic Patients with Delirium Tremens and Transient Withdrawal Hallucinations—Reevaluation of the REM Rebound and Intrusion Theory. In I Karacan (ed), Psychophysiological Aspects of Sleep. Park Ridge, NJ: Noyes Medical 1981;109.

70. Schenck CH, Bundlie SR, Ettinger MG, Mahowald MW. Chronic behavioral disorders of human REM sleep: a new category of parasomnia. Sleep 1986;9:293.

# Chapter 21

# Human and Animal Genetics of Sleep and Sleep Disorders

## Emmanuel Mignot

Sleep is a vital function of uncertain phylogeny.[1,2] Animals die if totally deprived of sleep.[3,4] Both the universal and irrevocable nature of sleep and the preservation of slow-wave sleep (SWS) and rapid eye movement (REM) in mammals and birds imply that phylogenetically old constitutional factors are involved in generating sleep. Major phenotypic differences in sleep organization between species, strains, and individuals suggest the existence of polymorphic genetic factors. These facts, together with the rapid advance of reverse and forward genetic techniques, offer a unique path to uncover new information on the physiology of sleep and its associated pathologies. In this chapter, the involvement of genetic factors in the regulation of normal and abnormal sleep and the potential of the emerging field of animal and human genetics in sleep are discussed.

## GENETIC FACTORS AND NORMAL HUMAN SLEEP: TWIN STUDIES

Research in the area of animal and human genetics in sleep consists mostly of questionnaire studies comparing sleep habits (duration of sleep, patterns and quality of sleep, frequency of napping) in monozygotic and dizygotic twins.[5–8] For most of the variables analyzed, correlations are higher for monozygotic versus dizygotic twins. This finding remains significant even when twins do not live in the same environment,[6] and it is not explained by correlations in depressive or anxious symptoms.[9] However, environmental factors do contribute significantly to the variance.[6,7] Measures of the residual variance between monozygotic twins $(1-r_{mz})$ quantify the influence of environmental factors specific to each twin pair.[10] In all studies, correlations barely reach 0.60, thus suggesting that half of the variance is associated with environmental factors. Because twins typically live in similar environments, this difference probably corresponds to short-term environmental variance.

Very few authors have studied sleep in monozygotic and dizygotic twins using polygraphic techniques.[11–14] These studies generally confirm the results obtained with questionnaires, but sample sizes are always small. Linkowski et al.,[13,14] studying 26 twin pairs during three consecutive nights, demonstrated significant differences between monozygotic and dizygotic twin–pair correlations for all stages of sleep but REM sleep. Vogel's[15] work with resting wake EEG suggests dominant alpha-occipital rhythms, in turn suggesting that EEG genetic variations are not only quantitative but also qualitative[15]; a linkage marker for low-voltage alpha EEG has now been identified on human chromosome 20q.[16,17]

Most of these early studies did not take into account the fact that sleep is independently regulated by circadian and homeostatic factors. Linkowski et al.[18,19] tried to address this issue by measuring cortisol and prolactin hormonal levels in twins. Results suggest that genetic factors play a major role in the regulation of cortisol secretion but not of prolactin. Drennan et al.[8] used the Horne-

Ostberg questionnaire to examine diurnal preference in 238 twin pairs and found higher correlations in monozygotic pairs, thus suggesting the existence of human circadian genetic factors. Such studies could certainly be extended. There has been no twin study measuring SWS or REM sleep homeostasis nor circadian rhythm properties under optimal experimental conditions.

## GENETIC INFLUENCES AND NORMAL ANIMAL SLEEP

Animal sleep studies support the theory that there are genetic influences on sleep. Major differences in the amount and proportion of SWS versus REM sleep can be observed within the same species; these differences are resistant to prolonged manipulations such as forced immobilization or sleep deprivation.[20–23] Significant variations in sleep-wake architecture and EEG profiles are also observed between rodent inbred strains.[21–27] C57BL or C57BR strains are characterized by long REM sleep episodes, short SWS episodes, and significant circadian variation under light/dark conditions.[22,26] At the opposite end of the spectrum, BALB/c is characterized by a very short duration of REM sleep episodes and poor diurnal rhythm, whereas DBA is intermediary for these characteristics.[22,26] The free-running period is also 50 minutes longer in C57BL/6J than in BALB/cByJ.[28] Qualitative differences in EEG signals are also observed. CBA and BALB/c (but not C57BR) display high-amplitude spindles, whereas REM sleep–associated theta frequency varies significantly between strains.[22,26]

The phenotypic differences discussed earlier are genetically transmitted. Diallelic methods,[24] simple segregation analysis in a backcross setting,[26] and recombinant inbred strain studies[28,29] suggest that many genes are involved in the expression of each trait.[23–25,28,29] The interactions observed are complex and not strictly additive; the hybrids of inbred strains occasionally present important deviations when compared to the average of parental strains.[24]

## PHARMACOGENETIC APPROACHES IN RODENTS

The basis of the pharmacogenetic approach in rodents is the selection of animal strains relatively sensitive or resistant to pharmacologic agents (e.g.,

ethanol,[30–32] benzodiazepines,[33] barbiturates,[34] or cholinergic compounds[35,36]). These models can then be studied pharmacologically, physiologically, and genetically. For example, mice that have been selected for their hypersensitivity to cholinergic compounds display an increase in paradoxical sleep,[36] which confirms the role of acetylcholine in REM sleep regulation.

The long-sleep (LS) and short-sleep (SS) mouse strains have been the most extensively studied.[32,37] These mouse strains were created in the 1970s by selecting mice more or less sensitive to ethanol's sedative effects, measured as the duration of loss of the righting reflex (*sleep time*) after ethanol.[30] After 18 generations of selection, the resulting strains now present an average sleep time of 10 minutes (SS) or 2 hours (LS) after ingestion of a similar dose of ethanol. These animals are useful for two reasons. First, it is well-established that there is pharmacologic overlap between anesthetics—that is, ethanol and most benzodiazepine and barbituric hypnotics. Partial or total cross-tolerance is observed for numerous pharmacologic properties,[38,39] thus suggesting that all these compounds act directly or indirectly through the γ-aminobutyric acid (GABA)-ergic system. Studying the differential sensitivity of the LS and SS strains to various hypnotics or anesthetic agents thus allows exploration of the question of whether genetic control of these compounds overlaps with that of ethanol.[40–46] Studies in this area have concluded that there is some overlap for the hypnotic effect of the less liposoluble anesthetic compounds (e.g., urethane and trifluoroethanol) with ethanol. In contrast, liposoluble anesthetics such as barbiturates seem to produce similar effects in SS and LS strains,[44] thus suggesting independent genetic control.[34] A preferred interaction between the effects of ethanol and cholinergic[35,43,47] and dopaminergic[32] transmission has also been suggested.

The second reason the SS and LS mouse strains are of interest is for purely genetic studies. A detailed phenotypic comparison of the SS and LS strains, as well as other strains hypersensitive to ethanol, suggests that the various pharmacologic effects of ethanol (e.g., sedation, hypothermy, toxicity) are controlled by different genes.[32,41,42] Traditional segregation studies and phenotypic analysis of SS × LS hybrids suggest that at least seven or eight genes are involved in the hypnotic effects of ethanol.[48,49] Analysis of quantitative trait loci

(QTL) has been performed in recombinant inbred strains and multiple QTL have been identified.[38,51]

The relations between these pharmacogenetic models and the genetic control of sleep remain uncertain. Indeed, as of this writing, LS and SS animals have not been studied for sleep and circadian rhythms using either polygraphic recordings or wheel running. Moreover, the effects of benzodiazepines and alcohol on sleep seem to be indirect and dependent on previously accumulated sleep debt.[51–54] A better analysis of the physiology of these models, specifically addressing circadian rhythms and sleep during baseline conditions and after sleep deprivation, are needed.

## CIRCADIAN CONTROL IN *DROSOPHILA*, *NEUROSPORA*, AND OTHER ORGANISMS: IS GENE REGULATION GENERATING THE CLOCK?

Circadian rhythmicity is an almost universal property that can be observed in most organisms, some of them unicellular.[56] Multiple independent genetic mutations have been reported to alter circadian rhythmicity in *Drosophila*, *Neurospora*, and *Arabidopsis*.[56,57] Thanks to the relative genetic simplicity of these organisms, research in this field has led to the isolation of two genes in *Drosophila* (loci *period* [*per*] and *timeless* [*tim*]) and one gene in *Neurospora* (*frequency* [*frq*]), whose mutations can suppress, decrease, or increase circadian free-running period.[55,58–60] The exact mechanism of action of these genes is debated,[61] but likely involves transcription-translation autoregulatory feedback loops.[55] In *Drosophila*, per protein and *per* mRNA fluctuates with a 3- to 4-hour difference in phase, and tim is necessary for these fluctuations to occur. It is hypothesized that tim interacts with per to enter into the nuclei, where tim directly or indirectly regulates the transcription of the *per* locus, thus creating 24 hours of rhythmicity.[59–61]

## CIRCADIAN RHYTHMICITY IN MAMMALS AND THE SUPRACHIASMATIC NUCLEI

Genetic research in mammals is facilitated by the fact that most circadian rhythms are generated in a discrete region of the hypothalamus, the suprachiasmatic nuclei (SCN); for review, see Klein et al.[62] A lesion of these nuclei suppresses all rhythmic behavior in absence of time cues. Transplanting fetal hypothalamic tissue in lesioned animals restores circadian fluctuations. Mouse strains and mutant hamsters with abnormal free-running periods (too long or too short) have been isolated.[62] Transplanting mutant SCN tissue in the third ventricle of a normal animal whose SCN have been lesioned induces an abnormal rhythmicity in the transplanted animal.[62] Neuronal, metabolic, and neurochemical activity of these nuclei's tissue also varies with a circadian periodicity in vitro.[62] The mechanism by which the SCN generate rhythmicity is still debated. The transplanted SCN probably generate rhythmicity independently of any synaptic connection with the host tissue. Rhythmicity within the nuclei also seems independent of the existence of synaptic connections as individual neurons and glial cells can generate circadian fluctuations independently. These results parallel knowledge accumulated from the study of avian pineal glands and retinae and in the marin mollusc *Bulla*.[55] Based on what is known about lower organisms, it is likely that transcription-translation mechanisms within individual cells make up a core phenomenon initiating overall behavioral circadian rhythmicity across the animal kingdom. Synaptic organization in the SCN may thus coordinate and relay, rather than generate, rhythmicity.

## CLONING MUTATIONS AFFECTING CIRCADIAN RHYTHMICITY IN MAMMALS

It is generally assumed that the genetic control of circadian rhythmicity is polygenic in mammals, as it is in lower organisms; several mutations with a strong effect on free-running period have been reported.[55,63–65] One of these phenotypes is a spontaneous semidominant mutation in the golden hamster, *Tau*,[63] which induces a shorter free-running period and no other apparent abnormalities. Two other phenotypes, *Clock* and *Wheel*, are dominant mutations in mice that were produced with germline mutagens using *N*-ethyl-*N*-nitrosourea. *Wheel* is a complex neurologic mutation that associates a complex array of abnormal behaviors such as circling, hyperactivity, and abnormal circadian rhythmicity and was mapped to mouse chromosome 4.[65] *Clock* is a pure circadian mutation associated with a long free-running period that was mapped to the midportion of mouse chromosome 5 in a region syntenic to human chromosome 4. The mutation has been localized within a 150-kb bacterial artificial chromosome genomic segment that has been shown to rescue the mutation using transgenic technology.[66] It was cloned and shown to share some homology with the *Drosophila* PER gene. [67]

## PERSPECTIVES ON CLONING SLEEP AND CIRCADIAN GENES IN MAMMALS USING RODENT MODELS

Even for a relatively simple, anatomically localized function such as the regulation of circadian rhythmicity in mammals, multiple genes are involved. The situation is thus likely to be even more complex for normal and abnormal sleep regulation. A number of genes may cause pathologic phenotypes in animals and humans, whereas others may be more involved in explaining interindividual or interspecies variations.

Mouse models are likely to be one of the best paths to discovering sleep-related genes.[68] High-density marker maps, such as the Whitehead Institute/MIT map, are now available for the mouse, and the rodent model is easy to breed and study. One possible approach, used in the study of circadian rhythmicity, is to use mutagenesis to produce mutants with sleep or circadian abnormalities and to positionally clone and isolate these mutations. The feasibility of this approach is limited by the relatively large number of animals (200–1,000) that need to be screened to find a mutation of interest,[55] but this is clearly one of the most promising avenues for future study. Another approach is to use QTL analysis and inbred mouse strains. This would involve first studying recombinant inbred strains to identify possible genetic effects and phenotypes of interest and then verifying the QTL through breeding experiments, genetic typing, and building congenic lines. This approach has been used successfully for numerous other multifactorial traits from autoimmune diabetes in nonobese (nod) mice[69] to drug response for addiction research.[50,70] Candidate QTL for circadian rhythmicity in mice have been reported using available recombinant inbred strains.[29,71] One important limitation of the QTL approach is that genetic effects may be weak or very dependent on their genetic background. This makes the next step, gene isolation, extremely difficult—if not impossible in many cases. An advantage of the QTL technique is that it may lead to the isolation of naturally polymorphic factors that are involved in phenotypic variations; it is thus a complementary technique to mutagenesis.

Another approach consists of studying directly "candidate" genes in animal strains phenotypically distinct. Korpi et al.,[33] for example, demonstrated that a strain of rats particularly more resistant to benzodiazepines and alcohol presented a specific mutation of the subunit $\alpha_6$ of the $GABA_A$ receptor. This result supports the idea that sensitivity to alcohol and to benzodiazepines proceeds from a common GABAergic mechanism. Other genes and factors also seem to be involved, however, because this mutation is not found in other models of rodents sensitive to sedatives or to alcohol.[33] This approach will become more feasible as more genes are isolated and sequenced. It is likely to be most powerful for humans, as gene isolation and sequencing is moving forward at a faster pace than in mice and human disorders offer a more extensive field of investigation.

Another research path that looks promising uses animal strains (transgenic or *knockout*) that have been genetically manipulated.[72,73] This approach uses mouse strains whose genetic inheritance has been modified either by adding extra copies of a given gene (transgenic), or by "knocking out" a specific gene. If the animal is viable, the analysis of the obtained phenotype provides information on the normal function of the modified gene. An example of this research path was provided by the study of the prion knockout mouse.[74] Mice with a null mutation in the prion protein gene, a gene associated with fatal familial insomnia and Creutzfeldt-Jakob disease, displayed alterations in both circadian activity and sleep patterns,[74] thus suggesting a role for the prion protein in sleep regulation. This technique should be used widely in the future, because new mouse strains manipulated for one or several candidates genes (e.g., neuroreceptors and enzymes, human candidate disease genes) are being developed in various laboratories. Ultimately, sleep and circadian rhythms will also be studied in these mutants, and conclusions will be drawn regarding the involvement of a given system in the control of sleep.

Genetic research will soon lead to the identification of numerous genetic factors involved in the physiologic control of sleep in rodents. The clinical implications are difficult to predict. Only a fraction of the genes isolated in rodents will play a role in human disease, and, as mentioned earlier, gene isolation is likely to proceed more rapidly in humans. However, the rodent model will be an attractive model for the design of better-controlled behavior and genetic studies.

## GENETIC ASPECTS OF PATHOLOGIC HUMAN SLEEP

Numerous sleep pathologies including narcolepsy, fatal familial insomnia, sleep paralysis, hypnagogic hallucinations, sleep apnea, and restless legs syndrome (RLS) are well-known to recur in certain families with a high frequency.[7,75–81] This fact supports the suggestion that there is a group of genes whose function is specifically related to sleep. The identification of pathologic factors by genome screening in sleep disorders is therefore another possible research path.

### Molecular Genetics and Narcolepsy with Cataplexy

Narcolepsy with cataplexy is characterized by excessive daytime sleepiness and abnormal symptoms of dissociated REM sleep (cataplexy, sleep paralysis, and hypnagogic hallucinations). Narcolepsy with cataplexy affects 0.02–0.18% of the general population, across all ethnic groups.[82–86] Since its description in 1880 by Gélineau, familial cases have been reported by numerous authors,[80,87–91] thus suggesting a genetic basis to narcolepsy. This pathology thus offers a unique opportunity to discover genes involved in the control of sleep.

More recent studies, however, suggest that narcolepsy with cataplexy is not simply a genetic disorder (see Mignot et al.[86] for a review). The development of human narcolepsy involves environmental factors on a specific genetic background, and only 25–31% of monozygotic twins reported in the literature are concordant for narcolepsy.[86] One of the predisposing genetic factors for narcolepsy is located in the major histocompatibility complex (MHC) DQ

region. Approximately 90–100% of all narcoleptic patients with cataplexy share a specific HLA allele, HLA-DQB1*0602 (most often in combination with HLA-DR2) versus 12–38% of the general population across ethnic groups.[92–96] The finding of an HLA association in narcolepsy, together with the fact that HLA-DQB1*0602 is likely to be the actual HLA narcolepsy susceptibility gene,[97] suggests that narcolepsy might be an autoimmune disorder. All attempts to demonstrate an immunopathology in narcolepsy have failed, however, and the mode of action of HLA-DQB1*0602 is still uncertain.[98–103]

Approximately 12–38% of the general population carries HLA-DQB1*0602, but only a small fraction of the general population has narcolepsy; DQB1*0602 is thus a weakly penetrant genetic factor ($\mu_{HLA} = 2$), despite its high association with the disorder. Other genetic factors, possibly more penetrant than HLA, are likely to be involved. Approximately 1–2% of the first-degree relatives of a patient with narcolepsy with cataplexy are affected by the disorder, versus 0.02–0.18% in the general population across ethnic groups, a $\lambda_{siblings}$ of 20- to 40-fold increase.[80,86,91] Familial aggregation cannot be explained by the sharing of HLA haplotypes alone[86] and some families are non–HLA-DQB1*0602 positive,[80] thus suggesting the importance of non-HLA susceptibility genes that could be positionally cloned using genome screening approaches in human multiplex families or isolated populations.

Studies using a canine model of narcolepsy also illustrate the importance of non-MHC genes. In this model, narcolepsy with cataplexy is transmitted as a single autosomal recessive trait with full penetrance, *canarc-1*.[104–106] This high-penetrance narcolepsy gene is not linked to MHC class II but cosegregates with a DNA segment with high homology to the human immunoglobulin μ-switch sequence.[107] This linkage marker is located very close to the actual narcolepsy gene (the current logarithm of odds score is 15.3 at 0% recombination) and gene isolation is ongoing in both canines and in the corresponding human syntenic region.

### Genetics and Dissociated REM Sleep Events

Sleep paralysis and hypnagogic hallucinations, two symptoms of dissociated REM sleep, occur commonly in the general population independently of narcolepsy.[108,109] Sleep paralysis presents a high familial incidence and an autosomal dominant transmission, in some cases.[76,88,110,111] Twin studies suggest a much higher concordance in monozygotic versus dizygotic twins for sleep paralysis,[112] which may be more common in the black population.[111] There is no association with HLA-DQB1*0602.[108]

In REM-sleep behavior disorder (RBD), automatic behavior arises during REM sleep and disturbs sleep continuity.[113] RBD is commonly associated with other pathologies, such as narcolepsy, but also occurs in isolation.[113] Whether isolated RBD is familial has not been established but the disorder may be weakly associated with HLA-DQ1.[114]

Cataplexy without sleepiness is exceptional[85] but some rare familial cases have been described with or without associated sleep paralysis.[115–117] In the clearly isolated cases of cataplexy, for which there is no other symptom from the tetrad (i.e., sleepiness, sleep paralysis, and hypnagogic hallucinations), clinical presentation seems to differ quite significantly from narcolepsy with cataplexy and cataplexy occurring in the first months of life.[116,117] HLA typing was not done for these families.

### Molecular Genetics and Fatal Familial Insomnia

Fatal familial insomnia is a rare neurologic condition characterized by severe insomnia, neurovegetative symptoms, and intellectual deterioration.[79,118–120] Insomnia is an early sign of the disorder and sleep disruption is associated with a disappearance of stage II sleep and SWS, although brief episodes of REM sleep are usually maintained. Neuropathologic lesions are mostly limited to degeneration of the anterior, ventral, and mediodorsal thalamic nuclei and of the inferior olive.[120] This pathology is typically associated with a mutation of the codon 178 in the prion protein gene but a codon 200 mutation has been detected.[121] These same mutations are also found in some forms of dementia, including Creutzfeldt-Jakob disease, but a polymorphism on codon 129 seems to determine the phenotypic expression into fatal familial insomnia.[119,121]

The prion protein is encoded by a gene located on human chromosome 20. The normal function of the protein is unknown but the gene is expressed in neurons. Mice homozygous for mutations disrupting the prion protein gene are behaviorally normal but may display sleep abnormalities.[74] Prions are involved in a group of human and animal disorders (spongiform encephalopathies) with more or less anatomically confined spongiose degeneration and neuronal atrophy. A proteinase-resistant form of the prion protein is probably involved in the pathology.[122] These diseases can appear either in a familial or infectious context, with the prion protein (or an agent that cannot be distinguished from the proteic element) acting as the transmitting agent. The mechanism by which certain isoforms of the protein are infectious is debated.[123,124]

How a simple additional polymorphism on codon 129 can alter the symptomatology from Creutzfeldt-Jakob disease to fatal familial insomnia is not understood, but molecular studies are under way to evaluate the effect of these mutations on the metabolism of the protein.[125] The differences in symptomatology are probably due to a different anatomic localization of the lesions. In fatal familial insomnia, degeneration is mostly localized in the anterior, ventral, and mediodorsal thalamic nuclei, whereas lesions are much more diffuse in Creutzfeldt-Jakob disease.[123,126] The well-established role of the thalamus (mostly the intralaminar thalamus) and its cortical projections in the generation of the cortical synchronization of SWS and sleep spindles[127] suggests that thalamic lesions may cause the insomnia in fatal familial insomnia.[126] However, no study has convincingly demonstrated that the destruction of these nuclei can produce a fatal insomnia in animal models. Bilateral lesions of these nuclei produce a persistent insomnia that is not fatal.[128] Other, more discrete anatomic lesions or a distinct pathophysiologic mechanism could thus also play a role. Mice carrying transgenes with the human prion allele specific for fatal familial insomnia have now been generated and are being studied.

The implication of the thalamus in the physiopathology of fatal familial insomnia suggests that this brain structure may be involved in the genesis of other, more common insomnias. Insomnia is a common complaint that affects at least 10% of the general population.[129,130] Many insomnias appear to be constitutional[131] and genetic factors involving the thalamus and homeostatic abnormalities in the regulation of sleep could be involved in some cases. Additional genetic factors, such as those regulating circadian rhythmicity at the level of the SCN, could be involved in some cases.

## Genetic Aspects of Restless Legs Syndrome and Periodic Limb Movements

RLS affects 2–5% of the general population.[132–135] The syndrome worsens with age and affects both sexes. RLS is almost always associated with periodic leg movements (PLMs) during sleep. RLS is best defined as uncomfortable or painful sensations in the legs that force a patient to get up several times during a night.[135,136] PLMs are brief, repetitive muscular jerks of the legs, occurring mostly during stage II sleep.[135] When these movements increase in strength and frequency, sleep is affected. RLS is highly familial; up to one-third of the reported cases may transmit the condition as an autosomal dominant trait[75,137–142] with possible genetic anticipation.[142] There has been no twin study of the disorder and both the prevalence and the proportion of familial cases seem to vary widely according to the geographic origin of the population studied. These differences may reflect founder effects (e.g., in Quebec, one finds a high proportion of familial cases[135] and a higher prevalence[143]) or the influence of local environmental factors.

Population-based risk estimations for first- and second-degree relatives are not available for RLS. In one study (published only as an abstract), risk to first- and second-degree relatives was 19.9% and 4.1%, respectively.[144] This compared to 3.5% and 0.5% for first- and second-degree relatives of control subjects and suggested a $\lambda_{siblings}$ of approximately 5.[144] Linkage studies using microsatellite markers or candidate genes in multiplex families are being undertaken with the goal of identifying the gene(s) involved in RLS[145] (Montplaisir, personal communication, 1997). Possible candidate genes are enzymes and receptors of the dopaminergic and enkephalinergic metabolisms, two neurotransmitters involved in the pharmacologic treatment of the syndrome.

## Genetic Aspects of Parasomnias

Sleepwalking, sleep talking, and night terrors generally occur during SWS (sleep stages III and IV).[146] They are usually grouped together and considered to share a common or related physiopathologic mechanism,[147] although this is not universally accepted.[146] The prevalence of these symptoms is approximately 3% in children and only rarely requires a medical consultation. Symptoms generally disappear in the adult phase.[146,148]

The familial nature of these symptoms has been recognized by most authors[76,149–151] but the exact mode of transmission is uncertain. Twin studies have shown a high degree of concordance for sleepwalking and sleep terrors (50% for monozygotes, 10–15% for dizygotes).[112,152,153] The genetic predisposition of sleepwalking, sleep talking, and, to a lesser degree, night terrors, may overlap. Some studies have suggested that the frequency of sleep terrors, for example, might be more common in families with somnambulism.[76,149,151] This suggests a related physiopathologic mechanism and a similar genetic control. No molecular study of these pathologies has been initiated.

## Obstructive Sleep Apnea Syndrome and Related Breathing Abnormalities During Sleep

Obstructive sleep apnea syndrome (OSAS) is a complex syndrome in which the upper airway collapses repetitively during sleep, thus blocking breathing.[154] Snoring is one of the cardinal symptoms of this syndrome. Repeated apneas prevent the patient from sleeping soundly, and the patient is frequently excessively sleepy the next day. Ultimately, OSAS leads to high blood pressure and increased risk for cardiovascular problems.[155–157] Approximately 4–5% of the general population has OSAS[158,159] and there may be increased vulnerability in blacks.[160]

Twin studies of OSAS are lacking but two studies have shown higher concordance in monozygotic versus dizygotic twins for habitual snoring.[112,161] Multiplex families of patients suffering from OSAS have been reported in the literature[81,162–169] and one study found a substantial increase of HLA-A2 and HLA-B39 in Japanese patients with OSAS.[170] Familial aggregation is generally explained by the fact that most risk factors involved in the physiopathology of sleep apnea, including obesity, alcoholism, soft facial tissue, and particular bone anatomy, are genetically determined.[81,167,169,171,172] In some cases, the genetic factor primarily involves abnormal ventilatory control by the central nervous system.[81,163] A possible genetic overlap between OSAS and sudden infant death syndrome,[163,164,173] and the high degree of concordance in chemoreceptor responses observed in monozygotic twins,[174,175] suggest the importance of genetic factors regulating the central control of ventilation in OSAS.

A number of genetic factors is likely to correspond to the multifactorial aspect of OSAS. A genetic linkage approach in OSAS would thus be facilitated by a careful phenotypic analysis (e.g., studying sleepy vs. nonsleepy subjects, obese vs. nonobese OSAS patients,[171] or subjects with selected morphologic features).[176]

### *Chromosomal and Genetic Abnormalities and Sleep Disturbances*

The coincidental association of specific chromosomal breakpoints with specific pathologies can be very helpful to localize susceptibility gene(s). In practice, however, karyotypes are rarely requested when a sleep disorder is the primary abnormality and very few sleep studies have been performed in patients with chromosomal or genetic abnormalities. Such abnormalities frequently produce behavioral and medical problems that have secondary effects on sleep, in general disturbed nocturnal sleep, so it may be difficult to identify a disease-specific sleep phenotype.[177] Despite these limitations, fragile X subjects have been reported to experience sleep disturbances and low melatonin levels,[178,179] whereas subjects with Norrie disease (genetic alterations in a region encompassing the monoamine oxidase genes at Xp11.3) or Neiman-Pick disease type C (18q11–q12) may experience cataplexy and sleep disturbances.[180,181] A family with autosomal-dominant cerebellar ataxia, deafness, normal karyotype, and clinically defined narcolepsy with cataplexy has been described and shown to be non–HLA-DR2 associated.[182] OSAS is also commonly observed as a result of anatomic malformations, adenotonsillar enlargement, or morbid obesity.[177,183,184] In a few instances, however, polygraphic studies suggest that central factors are involved in addition to or independently of abnormal breathing during sleep. This may be the case for the Prader-Willi and Angelman syndromes (del[15q])[184–186] or the Smith Magenis syndrome (del[17][p11.2]).[187,188]

Despite their relatively high-population frequency, sex chromosomal aneuploidies have been only marginally studied. XXY subjects, however, may display increased 24-hour sleep time.[189] These issues should be investigated more thoroughly because narcolepsy often starts with adolescence and puberty is associated with established changes in sleep needs.[190] In two cases, narcolepsy started at the age of 6—one of these cases concerned a patient with Turner syndrome (XO)[191] and in the other the onset of narcolepsy coincided with precocious puberty.[192]

### *Other Sleep Pathologies*

Insomnia, OSAS, narcolepsy, PLM, RLS, the parasomnias discussed in this chapter, and circadian disorders are the most common sleep pathologies. There are few or no studies on other forms of hypersomnias or parasomnias. One twin study suggests increased frequency of bruxism in monozygotic versus dizygotic twins[112] and bruxism has been reported in a multiplex context.[193] Familial forms of essential hypersomnia,[88] hypersomnias associated with dystrophia myotonica[194] or sleep-responsive extrapyramidal dystonias,[195,196] and jactatio capitis nocturna[197] have also been reported. A possible association between idiopathic hypersomnias and HLA-Cw2 and between hypersomnia in dystrophia myotonica with DR6 have also been found,[194,198] but need independent confirmation.

## PERSPECTIVES IN HUMAN GENETIC RESEARCH IN SLEEP DISORDERS

The complexity of sleep as a physiologic phenomenon is exemplified by a vast number of pathologies. Most of these pathologies are multifactorial and, to a large extent, genetically determined. Molecular genetics enables researchers to undertake a purely genetic approach to understanding the pathophysiology of these disorders. This approach will lead to the identification of genes involved in etiologically homogeneous sleep disorders such as narcolepsy. Genome screening studies in more common and complex sleep disorders such as OSAS and RLS are feasible but require the inclusion of a large number of multiplex families. Examination of these disorders may also benefit from studies of isolated populations or association studies using very large numbers of single-case families, a study design that could be used for secondary candidate gene studies. These studies are likely to become more viable research options as more and more genes are cloned and positioned on the human map and possible candidate genes are isolated in mouse models.

# REFERENCES

1. Zepelin H. Mammalian Sleep. In MH Kryger, T Roth, WC Dement (eds), Principles and Practice of Sleep Medicine (2nd ed). Philadelphia: Saunders, 1994;69.
2. Siegel JM. Phylogeny and the function of REM sleep. Behav Brain Res 1995;69:29.
3. Rechtschaffen A, Gilliland MA, Bergmann BM, et al. Physiological correlates of prolonged sleep deprivation in rats. Science 1983;221:182.
4. Kushida CA, Bergman BM, Rechtschaffen A. Sleep deprivation in the rat. IV. Paradoxical sleep deprivation. Sleep 1989;12:22.
5. Gedda L, Brenci G. Twins living apart test: progress report. Acta Genet Med Gemellol (Roma) 1983;32:17.
6. Partinen M, Kaprio J, Koskenvuo M, et al. Genetic and environmental determination of human sleep. Sleep 1983;6:179.
7. Heath A, Kendler KS, Eaves LJ, et al. Evidence for genetic influences on sleep disturbance and sleep patterns in twins. Sleep 1990;13:318.
8. Drennan MD, Shelby J, Kripke DF, et al. Morningness/eveningness is heritable [abstract]. Soc Neurosci 1992;8:196.
9. Kendler KS, Heath AC, Martin NG, et al. Symptoms of anxiety and symptoms of depression: same genes, different environments? Arch Gen Psychiatry 1987;122:451.
10. Hrubec Z, Robinette CD. The study of human twins in medical research. N Engl J Med 1984;310:435.
11. Webb WB, Campbel SS. Relationship in sleep characteristics of identical and fraternal twins. Arch Gen Psychiatry 1983;40:1093.
12. Hori A. Sleep characteristics in twins. Jpn J Psychiatr Neurol 1986;40:35.
13. Linkowski P, Kerhofs M, Hauspie R, et al. EEG sleep patterns in man: a twin study. Electroencephalogr Clin Neurophysiol 1989;73:279.
14. Linkowski P, Kerkhofs M, Hauspie R, et al. Genetic determinants of EEG sleep: a study in twins living apart. Electroencephalogr Clin Neurophysiol 1991;79:114.
15. Vogel F. Brain Physiology: Genetics of the EEG. In F Vogel, AG Motulsky (eds), Human Genetics. New York: Springer, 1986;590.
16. Anokhin A, Steinlein O, Fischer, et al. A genetic study of the human low-voltage electroencephalogram. Hum Genet 1992;90:99.
17. Steinlein O, Anokhin A, Yping M, et al. Localization of a gene for low-voltage EEG on 20q and genetic heterogeneity. Genomics 1992;12:69.
18. Linkowski P, Kerhofs M, Van Cauter E. Sleep and biological rhythms in man: a twin study. Clin Neuropharmacol 1992;15(Suppl 1):A42.
19. Linkowski P, Van Onderbergen A, Kerkhofs M, et al. Twin study of the 24-h cortisol profile: evidence for genetic control of the human circadian clock. Am J Physiol 1993;264:E173.
20. Webb WB, Friedmann JK. Attempts to modify the sleep patterns of rats. Physiol Behav 1971;6:459.
21. Kitahama K, Valatx JL. Instrumental and pharmacological paradoxical sleep deprivation in mice: strain differences. Neuropharmacology 1980;19:529.
22. Valatx JL. Genetics as a model for studying the sleep-waking cycle. Exp Brain Res 1984;(Suppl 8):135.
23. Rosenberg RS, Bergmann BM, Son HJ, et al. Strain differences in the sleep of rats. Sleep 1987;10:537.
24. Friedmann JK. A diallel analysis of the genetic underpinnings of mouse sleep. Physiol Behav 1974;12:169.
25. Valatx JL, Buget R, Jouvet M. Genetic studies of sleep in mice. Nature 1972;238:226.
26. Valatx JL, Buget R. Facteurs génétiques dans le déterminisme du cycle veille-sommeil chez la souris. Brain Res 1974;69:315.
27. Van Twyver H, Webb WB, Dube M, et al. Effects of environment and strain differences on EEG and behavioral measurement of sleep. Behav Biol 1973;9:105.
28. Schwartz WJ, Zimmerman P. Circadian time keeping in BALB/c and C57BL/6 inbred mouse strains. J Neurosci 1990;10:3685.
29. Hofstetter JR, Mayeda AR, Possidented B, et al. Quantitative trait loci for circadian rhythms of locomotor activity in mice. Behav Genet 1995;25:545.
30. McClearn GE, Kakihana R. Selective breeding for ethanol sensitivity in mice. Behav Genet 1973;3:409.
31. Morzorati S, Lamishaw B, Lumeng L, et al. Effects of low dose ethanol on the EEG of alcohol-preferring and nonpreferring rats. Brain Res Bull 1988;21:101.
32. Phillips TJ, Feller DJ, Crabbe JC. Selected mouse lines, alcohol and behavior. Experientia 1989;45:805.
33. Korpi ER, Kleingoor C, Kettenmann H, et al. Benzodiazepine-induced motor impairment linked to point mutation in cerebellar GABA-A receptor. Nature 1993;361:356.
34. Stino FKR. Divergent selection for pentobarbital-induced sleeping times in mice. Pharmacology 1992;44:257.
35. Overstreet DH, Rezvani AH, Janowsky DS. Increased hypothermic responses to ethanol in rats selectively bred for cholinergic supersensitivity. Alcohol Alcohol 1990;25:59.
36. Shiromani PJ, Velazquez-Moctezuma J, Overstreet D, et al. Effects of sleep deprivation on sleepiness and increased REM sleep in rats selectively bred for cholinergic hyperactivity. Sleep 1991;14:116.
37. Markel PD, Fulker DW, Bennet B, et al. Quantitative trait loci for ethanol sensitivity in the LS×SS recombinant inbred strains: interval mapping. Behav Genet 1996;26:447.

38. Khanna JM, Kalant H, Shah G, et al. Tolerance to ethanol and cross-tolerance to pentobarbital and barbital in four rat strains. Pharmacol Biochem Behav 1991;39:705.

39. Khanna JM, Kalant H. Effects of chronic treatment with ethanol on the development of cross-tolerance to other alcohols and pentobarbital. J Pharmacol Exp Ther 1992;263:480.

40. Marley RJ, Freund RK, Whener JM. Differential response to flurazepam in long-sleep and short-sleep mice. Pharmacol Biochem Behav 1988;31:453.

41. Erwin VG, Jones BC, Radcliffe R. Further characterization of LS×SS recombinant inbred strains of mice: activating and hypothermic effects of ethanol. Alcohol Clin Exp Res 1990;14:200.

42. Phillips TJ, Dudek BC. Locomotor activity responses to ethanol in selectively bred long- and short-sleep mice, two inbred mouse strains, and their F1 hybrids. Alcohol Clin Exp Res 1991;15:255.

43. De Fiebre CM, Collins A. Classical genetic analyses of responses to nicotine and ethanol in crosses derived from long- and short-sleep mice. J Pharmacol Exp Ther 1992;261:173.

44. De Fiebre CM, Marley RJ, Miner LL, et al. Classical genetic analyses of responses to sedative-hypnotique drugs in crosses derived from long-sleep and short-sleep mice. Alcohol Clin Exp Res 1992;16:511.

45. Wehner JM, Pounders JI, Bowers BJ. The Use of Recombinant Inbred Strains to Study Mechanisms of Drug Action. In Behavioral and Biochemical Issues in Substance Abuse. London: Haworth, 1991.

46. Wehner JM, Pounders JI, Parham C, et al. A recombinant inbred strain analysis of sleep-time responses to several sedative-hypnotics. Alcohol Clin Exp Res 1992;16:522.

47. Erwin VG, Korte A, Jones BC. Central muscarinic cholinergic influences on ethanol sensitivity in long-sleep and short-sleep mice. J Pharmacol Exp Ther 1988;247:857.

48. Dudek BC, Abbott ME. A biometrical genetic analysis of ethanol response in selectively bred long-sleep and short-sleep mice. Behav Genet 1984;14:1.

49. DeFries JC, Wilson JR, Erwin VG, et al. LS × SS recombinant inbred strains of mice: initial characterization. Alcohol Clin Exp Res 1989;13:196.

50. Crabbe JC, Belknap J, Buck KJ. Genetic animal models of alcohol and drug abuse. Science 1994;264:1715.

51. Roehrs T, Zwyghuizen-Doorenbos A, Timms V, et al. Sleep extension, enhanced alertness and the sedating effects of ethanol. Pharmacol Biochem Behav 1989;34:321.

52. Zwyghuizen-Doorenbos A, Rohers T, Timms V, et al. Individual differences in the sedating effects of ethanol. Alcohol Clin Exp Res 1990;14:400.

53. Edgar DM, Seidel WF, Martin CE, et al. Triazolam fails to induce sleep in suprachiasmatic nucleus-lesioned rats. Neurosci Lett 1991;125:125.

54. Mignot E, Edgar DM, Miller JD, et al. Strategies for the Development of New Treatments in Sleep Disorders Medicine. In J Mendelwicz, G Racagni (eds), Target Receptors for Anxiolytics and Hypnotics: From Molecular Pharmacology to Therapeutics. New York: Karger, 1992;129.

55. Takahashi JS. Molecular neurobiology and genetics of circadian rhythms in mammals. Annu Rev Neurosci 1995;18:531.

56. Dunlap JC. Genetic analysis of circadian clocks. Annu Rev Physiol 1993;55:683.

57. Millar AJ, Carré IA, Strayer CA, et al. Circadian clock mutants in arabidopsis identified by luciferase imaging. Science 1995;267:1161.

58. Hall JC. Tripping along the trail to the molecular mechanism of biological clocks. Trends Neurosci 1995;18:230.

59. Dunlap JC. The genetic and molecular dissection of a prototypic circadian system. Annu Rev Genet 1996;30:579.

60. Sehgal A, Ousley A, Hunter-Ensor M. Control of circadian rhythms by a two component clock. Mol Cell Neurosci 1996;7:165.

61. Hall JC. Are cycling gene products as internal zeitgebers no longer the *Zeitgeist* of chronobiology? Neuron 1996;17:799.

62. Klein D, Moore RY, Reppert SM. Suprachiasmatic Nucleus (The Mind's Clock). New York: Oxford University Press, 1991;467.

63. Ralph MR, Menaker M. A mutation of the circadian system in golden hamsters. Science 1988;241:1225.

64. Vitaterna MH, King DP, Chang AM, et al. Mutagenesis and mapping of a mouse gene clock, essential for circadian behavior. Science 1994;264:719.

65. Nolan P, Sollars PJ, Bohne BA, et al. Heterozygosity mapping of partially congenic lines; mapping of a semidominant neurological mutation, wheels, on mouse chromosome 4. Genetics 1995;140:L245.

66. Antoch MP, Song E-J, Chang A-M, et al. Functional identification of the mouse circadian *Clock* gene by transgenic *BAC* rescue. Cell 1997;89:655.

67. King DD, Zhao Y, Sangoram AM, et al. Positional cloning of the mouse circadian *Clock* gene. Cell 1997;89:641.

68. Takahashi JS, Pinto LH, Vitaterna MH. Forward and reverse genetic approaches to behavior in the mouse. Science 1994;264:1724.

69. Todd JA, Aitman TJ, Cornall RJ, et al. Genetic analysis of autoimmune type 1 diabetes mellitus in mice. Nature 1991;351:542.

70. Dudek BC, Tritto T. Classical and nonclassical approaches to the genetic analysis of alcohol-related phenotypes. Alcohol Clin Exp Res 1995;19:802.

71. Maeda AR, Hofstetter JR, Belknap JR, Nurnberger JI Jr. Hypothetical quantitative trait loci (QTL) for circadian period of locomotor activity in C×B recombinant inbred strains of mice. Behav Genet 1996;26:505.

72. Roemer K, Johnson PA, Friedmann T. Knock-in and knock-out. Transgenes, development and disease. N Biol 1991;3:331.

73. Travis J. Scoring a technical knockout in mice. Science 1992;256:1392.

74. Tobler I, Gauss SE, Deboer T, et al. Altered circadian activity rhythms and sleep in mice devoid of prion protein. Nature 1996;380:639.

75. Bornstein B. Restless leg syndrome. Psychiatr Neurol 1961;141:165.

76. Roth B, Bruhova S, Berkova L. Familial sleep paralysis. Arch Suisse Neurol Neurochir Psychiatr 1968;102:321.

77. Kales A, Soldatos CR, Bixler EO, et al. Hereditary factors in sleepwalking and night terrors. Br J Psychiatry 1980;137:111.

78. Montplaisir J, Godbout R, Boghden D, et al. Familial restless legs with periodic movements in sleep. Electrophysiological, biochemical, and pharmacological study. Neurology 1985;35:130.

79. Lugaresi E, Medori R, Montagna P, et al. Fatal familial insomnia and dysautonomia with selective degeneration of thalamic nuclei. N Engl J Med 1986;315:997.

80. Guilleminault C, Mignot E, Grumet FC. Familial patterns of narcolepsy. Lancet 1989;335:1376.

81. El Bayadi S, Millman RP, Tishler PV, et al. A family study of sleep apnea. Anatomic and physiologic interactions. Chest 1990;98:554.

82. Dement WC, Carskadon M, Ley R. The prevalence of narcolepsy II. Sleep Res 1973;2:147.

83. Honda Y. Consensus of narcolepsy, cataplexy and sleep life among teenagers in Fujisawa city. Sleep Res 1979;8:191.

84. Solomon P. Narcolepsy in Negroes. Dis Nerv Syst 1945;6:179.

85. Aldrich M. Narcolepsy. Neurology 1992;42(Suppl 6):34.

86. Mignot E. Genetic and familial aspects of narcolepsy. Neurology 1997;50(Suppl 1):516.

87. Daly D, Yoss R. A family with narcolepsy. Proc Staff Meet Mayo Clin 1959;34:313.

88. Nevsimalova-Bruhova S. On the problem of heredity in hypersomnia, narcolepsy and related disturbance. Acta Univ Carol [Med] (Praha) 1973;18:109.

89. Kessler S, Guilleminault C, Dement WC. A family study of 50 REM narcoleptics. Acta Neurol Scand 1979;50:503.

90. Singh S, George CFP, Kryger MH, et al. Genetic heterogeneity in narcolepsy. Lancet 1990;335:726.

91. Billiard M, Pasquie-Magnetto V, Heckman M, et al. Family studies in narcolepsy. Sleep 1994;17:S54.

92. Honda Y, Asaka A, Tanaka Y, et al. Discrimination of narcolepsy by using genetic markers and HLA. Sleep Res 1983;12:254.

93. Honda Y, Matsuki K. Genetic Aspects of Narcolepsy. In MJ Thorpy (ed), Handbook of Sleep Disorders. New York: Marcel Dekker, 1990;217.

94. Matsuki K, Grumet FC, Lin X, et al. DQ (rather than DR) gene marks susceptibility to narcolepsy. Lancet 1992;339:1052.

95. Rogers AE, Meehan J, Guilleminault C, et al. HLA DR15(DR2) and DQB1*0602 typing studies in 188 narcoleptic patients with cataplexy. Neurology 1997; 48:1550.

96. Mignot E, Hayduk R, Black J, et al. HLA DQBI*0602 is associated with cataplexy in 509 narcoleptic patients. Sleep 1997;20:1012.

97. Mignot E, Kimura A, Lattermann A, et al. Extensive HLA class II studies in 58 non DRB1*15 (DR2) narcoleptic patients with cataplexy maps susceptibility to the coding region of DQA1*0102 and DQB1*0602. Tissue Antigens 1997;49:329.

98. Matsuki K, Juji T, Honda Y. Immunological Features in Japan. In Y Honda, T Juji (eds), HLA and Narcolepsy. New York: Springer, 1988;58.

99. Rubin RL, Hajdukovic RM, Mitler MM. HLA DR2 association with excessive somnolence in narcolepsy does not generalize to sleep apnea and is not accompanied by systemic autoimmune abnormalities. Clin Immunol Immunopathol 1988;49:149.

100. Fredrikson S, Carlander B, Billiard M, et al. CSF immune variable in patients with narcolepsy. Acta Neurol Scand 1990;81:253.

101. Carlander B, Eliaou JF, Billiard M. Autoimmune hypothesis in narcolepsy. Neurophysiol Clin 1993; 23:15.

102. Mignot E, Tafti M, Dement WC, Grumet FC. Narcolepsy and immunity. Adv Neuroimmunol 1995;5:23.

103. Tafti M, Nishino S, Aldrich MS, et al. Narcolepsy is associated with increased microglia expression of MHC class II molecules. J Neurosci 1996;16:4588.

104. Baker TL, Dement WC. Canine Narcolepsy-Cataplexy Syndrome: Evidence for an Inherited Monoaminergic-Cholinergic Imbalance. In DJ McGinty, R Drucker-Colin, A Morrisson (eds), Brain Mechanisms of Sleep. New York: Raven, 1985;199.

105. Mignot E, Guilleminault C, Dement WC, et al. Genetically Determined Animal Models of Narcolepsy, A Disorder of REM Sleep. In P Driscoll (ed), Genetically Defined Animal Models of Neurobehavioral Dysfunction. Cambridge, MA: Birkhaüser Boston, 1992;90.

106. Mignot E, Nishino S, Hunt-Sharp L, et al. Heterozygosity at the canarc-1 locus can confer susceptibility for narcolepsy: induction of cataplexy in heterozygous asymptomatic dogs after administration of a combination of drugs acting on monoaminergic and cholinergic systems. J Neurosci 1993;13:1145.

107. Mignot E, Wang C, Rattazzi C, et al. Genetic linkage of autosomal recessive canine narcolepsy with an immunoglobulin μ chain switch-like segment. Proc Natl Acad Sci U S A 1991;88:3475.

108. Dalhitz M, Parles JD, Vaughan R, et al. The sleep paralysis-excessive daytime sleepiness syndrome. J Sleep Res 1992;1(Suppl 1):52.

109. Oyahon MM, Priest R, Caulet M, et al. Hypnagogic and hypnopompic hallucinations: pathological phenomena? Br J Psychiatry 1996;169:459.

110. Goode GB. Sleep paralysis. Arch Neurol 1962;6:228.

111. Bell GC, Dixie-Bell DD, Thompson B. Further studies on the prevalence of isolated sleep paralysis in black subjects. J Natl Med Assoc 1986;78:649.

112. Hori A, Hirose G. Twin studies on parasomnias. Sleep Res 1995;24A:324.

113. Mahowald MW, Schenk CH. REM Sleep Behavior Disorder. In MH Kryger, T Roth, WC Dement (eds), Principles and Practice of Sleep Medicine (2nd ed). Philadelphia: Saunders, 1994;574.

114. Schenck CH, Garcia-Rill E, Segall M, et al. HLA class II genes associated with REM sleep behavior disorder. Ann Neurol 1996;39:261.

115. Gelardi JAM, Brown JW. Hereditary cataplexy. J Neurol Neurosurg Psychiatry 1967;30:455.

116. Vela Bueno A, Campos Castello JC, et al. Hereditary cataplexy: is it primary cataplexy? Waking Sleeping 1978;2:125.

117. Hartse KM, Zorick FJ, Sicklesteel JM, et al. Isolated cataplexy: a family study. Henry Ford Hosp Med J 1988;36:24.

118. Julien J, Vital C, Deleplanque B, et al. Athrophie thalamique subaigue familiale. Troubles amnésiques et insomnie totale. Rev Neurol (Paris) 1990;146:173.

119. Goldfarb LG, Petersen RB, Tabaton M. Fatal familial insomnia and familial Creutzfeldt-Jakob disease: a disease phenotype determined by a DNA polymorphism. Science 1992;258:806.

120. Manetto V, Medori R, Cortelli P, et al. Familial fatal insomnia: clinical and pathological study of five new cases. Neurology 1992;42:312.

121. Chapman J, Arlazoroff A, Goldfarb LG, et al. Fatal insomnia in a case of familial Creutzfeldt-Jakob disease with codon 200(lys) mutation. Neurology 1996;46:758.

122. Prusiner SB. Molecular biology of prion diseases. Science 1991;252:1515.

123. Weissman C. A "unified theory" of prion propagation. Nature 1991;352:679.

124. Mestel R. Putting prions to the test. Science 1996;273:184.

125. Petersen RB, Parchi P, Richardson SL, et al. Effect of the D178N mutation and the codon 129 polymorphism on the prion protein. J Biol Chem 1996;271:12661.

126. Lugaresi E. The thalamus and insomnia. Neurology 1992;42(Suppl 6):28.

127. Stériade M. Basic mechanisms of sleep generation. Neurology 1992;42(Suppl 6):9.

128. Marini G, Imeri L, Mancia M. Changes in sleep waking cycle induced by lesions of medialis dorsalis thalamic nuclei in the cat. Neurosci Lett 1988;85:223.

129. National Institute of Mental Health. Consensus development conference: drugs and insomnia: the use of medications to promote sleep. JAMA 1984;251:2410.

130. Angst J, Vollrath M, Koch R, et al. The Zurich study. VII. Insomnia: symptoms, classification and prevalence. Eur Arch Psychiatry Neurol Sci 1989;238:285.

131. Hauri P. Primary Insomnia. In MH Kryger, T Roth, WC Dement (eds), Principles and Practice of Sleep Medicine (2nd ed). Philadelphia: Saunders, 1994;494.

132. Ekbom K. Restless legs syndrome. Neurology 1960;10:868.

133. Strang PG. The symptom of restless legs. Med J Aust 1967;1:1211.

134. Cirignotta F, Zucconi M, Mondini D, et al. Epidemiological data on sleep disorder. Sleep Res 1982;11:211.

135. Montplaisir J, Godbout R, Pellettier G, et al. Restless Legs Syndrome and Periodic Movements During Sleep. In M Kryger, T Roth, WC Dement (eds), Principles and Practice of Sleep Medicine. Philadelphia: Saunders, 1994;589.

136. Walters AS and the International RLS Study Group. Toward a better definition of the restless legs syndrome. Mov Disord 1995;10:634.

137. Ambrosetto C, Lugaresi E, Coccagna G, et al. Clinical and polygraphic remarks on the restless leg syndrome. Rev Pathol Nerv Ment 1965;86:244.

138. Montagna P, Coccagna G, Cirignotta F, et al. Familial Restless Leg Syndrome. In C Guilleminault, E Lugaresi (eds), Sleep/Wake Disorders: Natural History, Epidemiology and Long Term Evolution. New York: Raven, 1983;231.

139. Jacobsen JH, Rosenberg RS, Huttenlocher PR, et al. Familial nocturnal cramping. Sleep 1986;9:54.

140. Walters A, Picchieti D, Hening W, et al. Variable expressivity in familial restless legs syndrome. Arch Neurol 1990;47:1219.

141. Walters AS, Picchietti D, Ehrenberg BL, et al. Restless legs syndrome in childhood and adolescence. Pediatr Neurol 1994;1193:241.

142. Trenkwalder C, Colladoso-Seidel V, Gasser T, Oertel WH. Clinical symptoms and possible anticipation in a large kindred of familial restless legs syndrome. Mov Disord 1996;11:389.

143. Lavigne G, Montplaisir J. Restless legs syndrome and sleep bruxism: prevalence and association among Canadians. Sleep 1994;17:739.

144. Labuda MC. Epidemiology, Family Patterns, and Genetics of Restless Legs Syndrome. In RLS Foundation Conference Abstract Book. Washington, DC, 1997;7.

145. Johnson W, Walter A, Lehner T, et al. Affected only linkage analysis of autosomal dominant restless legs syndrome. Sleep Res 1992;21:214.

146. Keefauver SP, Guilleminault C. Sleep Terrors and Sleep Walking. In M Kryeger, T Roth, WC Dement (eds), Principles and Practice of Sleep Medicine (2nd ed). Philadelphia: Saunders, 1994;567.

147. Broughton RJ. Sleep disorders: disorders of arousal? Science 1968;159:1070.

148. Abe K, Shimakawa M. Genetic and developmental aspects of sleeptalking and teeth-grinding. Acta Paedopsychiatr 1966;33:339.

149. Debray P, Huon H. A propos de trois cas de somnambulisme familial. Ann Méd Interne (Paris) 1973;124:27.

150. Hälstrom T. Night terror in adults through three generations. Acta Psychiatr Scand 1972;48:350.

151. Abe K, Amatomi M, Oda N. Sleepwalking and recurrent sleeptalking in children of childhood sleepwalkers. Am J Psychiatry 1984;141:800.

152. Bakwin H. Sleepwalking in twins. Lancet 1970;2:466.

153. Hublin C, Kaprio J, Partinen M, et al. Prevalence and genetics of sleepwalking: a population based twin study. Neurology 1997;48:177.

154. Gastaut H, Tassinari C, Duron B. Etude polygraphique des manifestations épisodiques (hypniques et respiratoires) diurnes et nocturnes du syndrome de Pickwick. Rev Neurol (Paris) 1965;112:573.

155. Guilleminault C, Eldridge FL, Simmons FB. Sleep apnea syndrome: can it induce hemodynamic changes? West J Med 1975;123:7.

156. Koskenvuo M, Kaprio J, et al. Snoring as a risk for hypertension and angina pectoris. Lancet 1985;1:893.

157. Hall MJ, Bradley TD. Cardiovascular disease and sleep apnea. Curr Opin Pulm Med 1995;1:512.

158. Partinen M, Telakivi T. Epidemiology of obstructive sleep apnea syndrome. Sleep 1992;15:51.

159. Young T, Palta M, Dempsey J, et al. The occurrence of sleep-disordered breathing among middle-aged adults. N Engl J Med 1993;328:1230.

160. Redline S, Tishler PV, Hans MG, et al. Racial differences in sleep-disordered breathing in African-Americans and Caucasians. Am J Respir Crit Care Med 1997; 155:186.

161. Ferini-Strambi L, Calori G, Oldani A, et al. Snoring in twins. Respir Med 1995;89:337.

162. Strohl KP, Saunders NA, Feldman NT, et al. Obstructive sleep apnea in family members. N Engl J Med 1978;229:969.

163. Adickes ED, Buehler BA, Sanger WG. Familial sleep apnea. Hum Genet 1986;73:39.

164. Oren J, Kelly DH, Shannon DC. Familial occurrence of sudden infant death syndrome and apnea of infancy. Pediatrics 1987;80:355.

165. Manon-Espaillat R, Gothe B, Adams N, et al. Familial "sleep apnea plus" syndrome: report of a family. Neurology 1988;38:190.

166. Wittig RM, Zorick FJ, Roehrs TA, et al. Familial childhood sleep apnea. Henry Ford Hosp Med J 1988;36:13.

167. Mathur R, Douglas NJ. Family study in patients with the sleep apnea-hypopnea syndrome. Ann Intern Med 1995;122:174.

168. Pillar G, Lavie P. Assessment of the role of inheritance in sleep apnea syndrome. Am J Respir Crit Care Med 1995;151:688.

169. Redline S, Tishler PV, Tosteson TD, et al. The familial aggregation of obstructive sleep apnea. Am J Respir Crit Care Med 1995;151:682.

170. Yoshizawa T, Akashiba T, Kurashina K. Genetics and obstructive sleep apnea syndrome. Intern Med 1993; 32:94.

171. Guilleminault C, Partinen M, Hollman K, et al. Familial aggregates in obstructive sleep apnea syndrome. Chest 1995;107:1545.

172. Kronholm E, Aunola S, Hyyppa MT, et al. Sleep in monozygotic twin pairs discordant for obesity. J Appl Physiol 1996;80:14.

173. Tishler PV, Redline S, Ferrette V, et al. The association of sudden unexpected infant death with obstructive sleep apnea. Am J Respir Crit Care Med 1996; 153:1857.

174. Kawakami Y, Yamamoto H, Yoshikawa T, Shida A. Chemical and behavioral control of breathing in twins. Am Rev Respir Dis 1982;129:703.

175. Thomas DA, Swaminathan S, Beardsmore CS, et al. Comparison of peripheral chemoreceptor responses: monozygotic and dizygotic twin infants. Am Rev Respir Dis 1993;148:1605.

176. Kushida CA, Guilleminault C, Mignot E, et al. Genetics and craniofacial dysmorphism in family studies of obstructive sleep apnea. Sleep Res 1996;25:275.

177. Carskadon MA, Pueschel SM, Millman RP. Sleep-disordered breathing and behavior in three risk groups: preliminary findings from parental reports. Childs Nerv Syst 1993;9:452.

178. O'Hare JP, O'Brien IA, Arendt J, et al. Does melatonin deficiency cause the enlarged genitalia of the fragile-X syndrome? Clin Endocrinol 1986;24:327.

179. Staley-Gane MS, Hollway RJ, Hagerman MD. Temporal sleep characteristics of young fragile X boys. Am J Hum Genet 1996;59:A105.

180. Challamel MJ, Mazzola ME, Nevsimalova S, et al. Narcolepsy in children. Sleep 1994;17:S17.

181. Vossler DG, Wyler AR, Wilkus RJ, et al. Cataplexy and monoamine oxidase deficiency in Norrie disease. Neurology 1996;46:1258.

182. Melberg A, Hetta J, Dahl N, et al. Autosomal dominant cerebellar ataxia, deafness and narcolepsy. J Neurol Sci 1995;124:119.

183. Goldberg R, Fish B, Ship A, et al. Deletion of a portion of the long arm of chromosome 6. Am J Med Genet 1980;5:73.

184. Kaplan J, Frederickson PA, Richardson JW. Sleep and breathing in patients with the Prader-Willi syndrome. Mayo Clin Proc 1991;66:1124.

185. Summers JA, Lynch PS, Harris JC, et al. A combined behavioral/pharmacological treatment in sleep-wake schedule disorder in Angelman syndrome. Dev Behav Pediatrics 1992;13:284.

186. Vgontzas An, Kales A, Seip J, et al. Relationship of sleep abnormalities in Prader-Willi syndrome. Am J Hum Genet 1996;67:478.

187. Greenberg F, Guzzetta V, Montes de Oca-Luna R, et al. Molecular analysis of the Smith-Magenis syndrome: a possible contiguous syndrome associated with del(17)(p11.2). Am J Hum Genet 1991;49:1207.

188. Fischer H, Oswald HP, Duba HC, et al. Constitutional interstitial deletion of 17 (p11.2) (Smith Magenis syndrome): a clinically recognizable microdeletion syndrome. Report of two cases and review of the literature. Klin Padiatr 1993;205:162.

189. Higurashi M, Kawai H, Segawa M, et al. Growth, psychologic characteristics, and sleep-wakefulness cycle of children with sex chromosomal abnormalities. Birth Defects 1986;22:251.

190. Carskadon MA. Patterns of sleep and sleepiness in adolescents. Pediatrician 1990;17:1.

191. George CF, Singh SM. Juvenile onset narcolepsy in an individual with Turner syndrome. A case report. Sleep 1991;14:267.

192. Chilshlom RC, Brooks CJ, Harrison GF, et al. Prepubescent narcolepsy in a six year old girl. Sleep Res 1985;15:113.

193. Hartman E. Bruxism. In M Kryger, T Roth, WC Dement (eds), Principles and Practice of Sleep Medicine. Philadelphia: Saunders, 1989;385.

194. Manni R, Zucca C, Martinetti M, et al. Hypersomnia in dystrophia myotonica: a neurophysiological and immunogenetic study. Acta Neurol Scand 1991;84:498.

195. Byrne E, White O, Cook M. Familial dystonic choreoathetosis with myokymia: a sleep responsive disorder. J Neurol Neurosurg Psychiatry 1991;54:1090.

196. Ishikawa A, Miyatake T. A family with hereditary juvenile dystonia-parkinsonism. Mov Disord 1995;10:482.

197. Thorpy MJ, Glovinsky PB. Headbanging (Jactatio Capitis Nocturna). In M Kryger, T Roth, WC Dement (eds), Principles and Practice of Sleep Medicine. Philadelphia: Saunders, 1989;648.

198. Poirier G, Montplaisir J, Decary F, et al. HLA antigens in narcolepsy and idiopathic central nervous system hypersomnolence. Sleep 1986;9:153.

# Chapter 22
# Obstructive Sleep Apnea Syndrome

## Anstella Robinson and Christian Guilleminault

Obstructive sleep apnea syndrome (OSAS) is a condition characterized by repeated episodes of upper airway closure during sleep. It is associated with a constellation of symptoms and objective findings.[1] The most common presenting complaints are loud, disruptive, interrupted snoring, associated with unrefreshing sleep and excessive daytime sleepiness (EDS) or fatigue. OSAS may long remain undetected because the breathing disturbances occur at night, but the consequences are reflected in impairment of daytime function. Amazingly, many patients with even severe sleep apnea of many decades' duration remain unaware of the cause of their difficulties. Bed partners are invaluable informants, describing frightening cessations of breathing, choking sounds, and stridorous gasps when breathing resumes. The course is a slowly progressive one. Thus, the patient's daytime performance becomes insidiously more impaired, until the patient eventually decompensates and presents to the health care system, either volitionally or as a result of one of the complications of sleep apnea. Sleepiness is typically misperceived as a natural consequence of aging. There is a disparity between the prevalence of OSAS in the community and recognition among medical professionals of the frequency and impact of OSAS; this disparity is particularly sizable among primary care providers and health system managers.[2]

Complete obstruction of the upper airway is termed *obstructive apnea* and partial closure is referred to as *hypopnea*. When measured by polysomnographic (PSG) recording, obstructive apneas are defined as total cessation of airflow at the nose and mouth, lasting at least 10 seconds, associated with ongoing thoracic and abdominal efforts to inspire. Hypopneas are seen as greater than 50% decreases in airflow, lasting at least 10 seconds, associated with continued respiratory efforts. Hypopneas are usually associated with a drop in blood oxygen saturation.[1] Gould and coworkers[3] have suggested defining hypopnea differently by focusing more on thoracoabdominal effort. If inductive plethysmography is used, hypopnea is defined as a decrease in thoracoabdominal effort of at least 50%.[3] More advanced technology has shown that a small decrease in tidal volume ($V_T$) may involve only one breath (or respiratory cycle) and lead to a transient, electroencephalography (EEG)-defined arousal, when associated with increased respiratory efforts while asleep. The current, noninvasive means of measuring oxygen saturation in arterial blood ($Sao_2$) do not indicate a recognizable drop in $Sao_2$ in association with this $V_T$ decrease. If repeated, however, the short arousal will have an impact on sleep continuity—that is, lead to sleep fragmentation. In the strictest sense of the term, a short arousal is a hypopnea and some sleep specialists do not limit the term *hypopnea* to the definitions outlined earlier. This may be appropriate, given that very short events can have pathophysiologic consequences and impair well-being, as with the upper airway resistance syndrome.[4,5] Both apneas and hypopneas are terminated with a large inspiratory breath. Central apneas are seen on PSG as episodes of cessation of thoracic and abdominal respiratory efforts as well as nasal-oral airflow, lasting at least 10 seconds. Long-standing obstructive apnea may result in disturbances of central and peripheral respiratory reflexes, in turn causing central apneas. Moreover, the effort associated with obstructive events may be detectable only with esophageal manometry. Because this diagnostic tool is not in common use in sleep laboratories, these events are often interpreted as central apneas. Mixed apneas are comprised of central and obstructive components.

The number of apneas and hypopneas are separately totaled, then divided by the hours of total sleep time to yield an apnea index (AI) and hypopnea index (HI). The AI and HI are summed to determine the respiratory disturbance index (RDI), which is the average number of respiratory disturbances per hour of sleep.[6]

The minimum RDI and AI required to constitute a mild disorder is debated.[7] The symptomatology that is produced by a given objective amount of respiratory disturbance varies from individual to individual. As the AI or RDI increases, however, so does the severity of symptoms. The correlation between RDI severity and long-term morbidity is not precisely delineated. This complex relationship is confounded by nightly fluctuations in the RDI, the amount of oxygen desaturation, and the percentage of time spent with reduced oxygen saturation. For clinical purposes, an RDI higher than 5 is most commonly considered to be in the pathologic range.[8,9]

OSAS lies along a continuum of sleep disordered breathing. This continuum ranges (in order of increasing severity) from pure snoring without daytime sleepiness, to upper airway resistance syndrome, through progressive degrees of obstructive apnea based on RDI and oxyhemoglobin desaturations. The upper airway resistance syndrome may be present without associated snoring and is associated with daytime sleepiness or fatigue.[4,5]

The specific pathophysiology of these syndromes is discussed later in this chapter. As the incidence and prevalence of upper airway resistance syndrome have not been characterized, most of the presentation focuses on the well-known OSAS.

## EPIDEMIOLOGY

The risk of developing OSAS increases with age and is strongly correlated with obesity and the male gender.[10–13] Menopausal women develop OSAS at a similar rate to that of men. Prevalence reaches a maximum between the fifth and seventh decades.[14] Some minority populations appear to have a higher prevalence of sleep disordered breathing, indicating that race may be a risk factor. Two such populations are Pacific Islanders[15] and Mexican-Americans,[16] although there have been no studies that control for comorbid conditions found more frequently in these populations than in whites. As data from the Cleveland Family Study indicate, blacks may be at increased risk for sleep apnea.[17] In this study, the increased prevalence was not accounted for by differences in exposure to alcohol or tobacco or differences in body mass index (BMI). Moreover, this effect was most apparent in individuals younger than 25 years of age. Variable age of puberty, speed of development of secondary sexual characteristics, and mucosal enlargement associated with hormonal surge may have biased these findings. Familial aggregates of OSAS clearly indicate that risk factors for the development of this condition may exist very early in life.[18–20]

Initial studies that attempted to define rates of OSAS were limited by biases that tended to underestimate actual prevalence. Early studies by Lavie[21] in Israel and Gislason[22] in Sweden assessed the prevalence of OSAS in the adult male population to be 7% and 1.3%, respectively. More recent studies of large, comprehensive population samples suggest a prevalence rate of OSAS at least two times higher than those early estimates.[23,24] In 1993, Young and colleagues published a large community-based study of adults 30–60 years of age that found, if OSAS was defined as having an AHI greater than 5, a prevalence of 9% in women and 24% in men.[9] If the AHI of greater than 5 was associated with symptoms of excessive sleepiness, however, the prevalence was 2% and 4% in women and men, respectively.[9]

OSAS has been associated with mortality both from vascular complications and from highway and industrial accidents. A retrospective study by He and colleagues[25] found an increased mortality rate for patients with OSAS, particularly in those younger than 50 years of age. As previously stated, OSAS is underdiagnosed. Untreated OSAS is a cause of death and serious injury on the road and in the workplace.[26–29] Work by Findley[29] suggests that the accident rate for OSAS patient is seven times that of the general population.

## MORBIDITY: CARDIOVASCULAR SYSTEM

Systemic and pulmonary hemodynamics undergo acute and chronic changes as a consequence of obstructive apnea, most of which reverse on successful treatment of the upper airway obstruction. Significant increases in systemic arterial pressure occur cyclically with episodes of apnea, with maximal elevations occurring after the resumption of ventilation. In a study of 10 moderate to severe apneics, systolic and diastolic pressures rose approximately 25% from their baseline values during apneas (i.e., from 126 to 159 mm Hg systolic and from 65 to 83 mm Hg diastolic).[30] When apneas occur continually throughout the night, often in association with very severe oxygen desaturations, elevations may be extreme, exceeding 200 mm Hg systolic and 120 mm Hg diastolic.[31]

Evidence implicates several mechanisms that contribute to cyclic increases in blood pressure. A fall in $Pao_2$ and an increase in acidosis signal the carotid chemoreceptors to trigger vasomotor center–mediated arteriolar constriction, which leads to increased systemic vascular resistance. Increased ventilatory effort against a closed upper airway in the face of air trapping leads to significant right-to-left bowing of the interventricular septum and decreased cardiac output.[32] Left ventricular collapse can occur with very negative inspiratory pressures.[33] With resumption of ventilation, and the abrupt shift from sleep to wake, there is a release of vagal predominance and heightened sympathetic tone. Pulmonary stretch reflexes induce tachycardia, which increases cardiac output. Changes in preload and afterload due to the repetitive Müller's and, at times, Valsalva's maneuvers are also factors in the cardiac output changes. Elevated sympathetic nervous system activity is evidenced by increased urinary catecholamine levels, which return to normal after treatment of apnea.[34]

Untreated OSAS is associated with a prevalence of chronic hypertension in excess of 40%,[8] whereas approximately 30% of all idiopathic hypertensives have OSA.[35–38] Although a direct causal role for OSA in the development of chronic hypertension has not been proved, hypertension improves after treatment of apnea.[34,39] The ameliorative effect of treatment has been found after upper airway surgery[40] and nasal continuous positive airway pressure (CPAP).[41] The relationship between the apnea-hypopnea index and blood pressure remained significant even after the effects of obesity were evaluated and controlled in a number of studies.[42–44] Chemoreflex and baroreflex activation mediate hypoxia-induced increases in sympathetic tone in OSAS. This contributes to increases in blood pressure along with arousals associated with apneic events and increased intrathoracic pressure differentials.[45,46]

Increased release of atrial natriuretic peptide (ANP) during sleep has been found in sleep apnea, with concomitant increases in urine and sodium output.[47] ANP suppresses the renin-angiotensin-aldosterone system, and plasma renin activity curves have been found to be abnormally flattened in apneics during sleep.[48] These changes lower blood volume and blood pressure and may play a protective or compensatory role against blood pressure increases in OSAS. Treatment of apnea normalizes ANP, thereby diminishing diuresis and natriuresis, and increases renin and aldosterone release.

Moderate to severe increases in pulmonary arterial pressure occur with each apneic episode. Maximal pulmonary pressures are generated during rapid eye movement (REM) sleep. They coincide with maximal hypoxemic and hypercapnic values[39] and probably reflect hypoxic pulmonary vasoconstriction. When pressure gradients between the pulmonary artery lumen and thoracic cavity are evaluated, transpulmonary arterial pressure decreases during the first 25 seconds of apnea, then increases until breathing returns and transiently rises more rapidly.[49] Another hemodynamic change consists of reductions in cardiac output of up to one-third of baseline values in apneas longer than 35 seconds.[50]

The development of persistent pulmonary hypertension and cor pulmonale may be caused by severe hypoxemia during sleep[51,52] but is more likely in daytime hypoxemia.[53] Treatment of apnea improves pulmonary artery hypertension and right heart failure.[54,55]

Cardiac arrhythmias that occur exclusively during sleep are common in apneics. Sinus arrhythmia accompanies each obstructive respiratory cycle, in which rate diminishes with the cessation of airflow and accelerates when breathing resumes. These changes can be mild or severe, resulting in repetitive cycles of bradycardia and tachycardia fluctuating from fewer than 30 to more than 120 bpm.[56] Severe sinus bradycardia (fewer than 30 beats per second) affects approximately 10% of sleep apneics and is usually seen with severe hypoxemia.[57–59]

These aberrations of rate combined with hypoxemia predispose to conduction defects, malignant arrhythmias, and perhaps sudden death. Asystoles of up to 13 seconds, second-degree atrioventricular (AV) block, premature ventricular contractions, and runs of ventricular tachycardia are among documented apnea-related abnormalities.

Proposed mechanisms for bradycardia, Mobitz I AV block, and asystole involve vagal nerve activation due to both Müller's maneuver and hypoxemic carotid body stimulation. EEG arousal with airway reopening and lung expansion triggers cardiac acceleration. Increased sympathetic tone due to hypoxemia and acidosis may be expressed after vagal influence is withdrawn, leading to premature ventricular contractions (PVCs), sinus tachycardia, and ventricular tachycardia. PVC frequency and other ventricular arrhythmias have been shown to correlate with severity of oxygen desaturation, increasing threefold with desaturations lower than 60% (as compared to 90%).[60]

From a global perspective, many of these physiologic changes to asphyxia may be viewed as an attempt to preserve perfusion to the critical cerebral and coronary systems. Increased systemic pressure selectively perfuses these critical central vessels, whereas bradycardia decreases myocardial oxygen consumption. As bradycardia becomes more profound, however, myocardial perfusion may become more impaired, because the perfusion gradient drops as diastole is prolonged. Coronary ischemia may result in ventricular arrhythmia. On return of ventilation, cardiac rate and output arise in the setting of sympathetic dominance and decreased systemic resistance. The demand for myocardial oxygen to accomplish this work outweighs the supply of reperfused blood, rendering the myocardium vulnerable to malignant arrhythmias.[61]

Surprisingly, in spite of the strong cerebral vasodilating effects of hypercapnia and the "protective" mechanisms discussed earlier, cerebral blood flow during sleep is more decreased in apneics than in normals.[62,63] Especially interesting is the finding that global and regional cerebral perfusion is decreased in apneics during wakefulness.[63,64] This suggests altered cerebral autoregulatory mechanisms.

Sleep apnea and even snoring have been epidemiologically linked to increased incidences of myocardial infarction and stroke.[65,66] Spriggs and coworkers[67] looked at risk factors for stroke in approximately 400 individuals with OSAS who had been matched with controls for sex and age and found an odds ratio of 3.2 for symptoms of snoring. Another study found an increased odds ratio even after adjustment for ethanol use, hypertension, and heart disease. The ratio increased approximately fourfold if obesity, observed apneas, and a subjective sense of EDS were present.[68] In a study comparing cumulative survival after 5 years of untreated versus treated patients with an AI greater than 20, cumulative survival was approximately 75% in the untreated group as compared to almost 100% for the treated group.[69] Cardiovascular death was also significantly increased compared to the general U.S. population data in another study. Peak age of death in sleep apneics was between 55 and 64 years compared to a peak mortality rate in a general male U.S. population at 72 years of age.[70]

Other systemic abnormalities that cause morbidity in association with OSAS include early renal dysfunction characterized by an increased incidence of proteinuria.[71] Proteinuria was found in 26% of 50 patients with an RDI higher than 5 compared with zero in an equal number of patients with other types of sleep disorders.[72]

## PATHOPHYSIOLOGY

It is in the regions made up of soft tissues of the upper airway that most airway obstructions occur during sleep. In the early 1970s, there was disagreement as to whether decreased patency of the upper airway during sleep was related to an active contraction at the velopharyngeal sphincter[73] or to inability of the upper airway muscles to oppose a sucking maneuver during inspiration.[74] Weitzman et al.[73] presented videotapes indicating that occlusion occurred mainly at the velopharyngeal "sphincter," a finding recently re-emphasized by Remmers et al.[75] with fiberoptic endoscopy. The Stanford team (Hill et al.[74] and Guilleminault et al.[76]) performed similar fiberoptic evaluations, however, continuously filming and simultaneously recording the electromyographic (EMG) activities of many different upper airway muscles. These authors concluded that there was no active contraction. At sleep onset, they found a decrease in EMG activity in the upper airway muscles, not only at the level of the velopharyngeal sphincter but also in many dilator muscles.

The first breaths after sleep onset or a return to sleep after arousal were associated with a closure of the upper airway, as indicated by endoscopy.

Since this early work, the pathophysiology of upper airway occlusion during sleep has been elucidated. The size of the pharyngeal upper airway is dependent on a balance of forces between the upper airway dilators, which maintain upper airway patency, and the negative pharyngeal intraluminal pressure created during thoracic expansion as a result of inspiration. Skeletal factors also play a role. Thus upper airway patency requires the coordination of upper airway dilators and inspiratory muscles. Bernoulli's principle dictates that narrowing of any segment while airflow is maintained causes an increased velocity of airflow in that segment. In sleep, the stage (REM vs. non-REM [NREM]) also influences upper airway patency. This decreases intraluminal pressure and further narrows the segment favoring upper airway collapse. Lack of coordination between inspiratory muscles and upper airway dilators leads to upper airway occlusion during sleep. This was reported as early as 1978 by Guilleminault and Motta[77] in an investigation of patients with postpoliomyelitis syndrome who had been treated with a cuirass ventilator. These patients developed a negative intrathoracic pressure that could not be counteracted by the upper airway dilators and that led to the development of OSAS. These findings were later confirmed by Hyland et al.[78] and by Simmonds and Branthwaite.[79] A lack of coordination in reflexes, however, does not seem to be the first step in most cases of OSAS.

It has been demonstrated that with sleep onset in adult men there is an increase in resistance due to a decrease in upper airway muscle tone.[80] This increase in upper airway resistance has no known consequences. In snorers, however, there is a further increase with each snore. In response to this increased resistance, many subjects are able to increase their inspiratory effort and maintain normal $V_T$. Increased effort is demonstrated by esophageal pressure (Pes) monitoring,[81] which may reach peak inspiratory nadirs of −12 to −15 cm $H_2O$. The effort is constant over time, without any impact on sleep EEG or oxygen saturation. In other cases,[81] however, the upper airway dilators are unable to oppose the negative pharyngeal intraluminal pressure sufficiently to maintain minute ventilation and normal gas exchange. In these cases, inspiratory effort is increased. This increase is reflected by an increase in Pes nadir. With increasing inspiratory efforts, there is a decrease in the width of the upper airway, as upper airway dilators are unable to exactly match the inspiratory negative pressure.

Several mechanisms can be used by the subject to maintain normal minute ventilation. One well-demonstrated method consists of a prolongation of inspiratory time associated with a decrease in expiratory time. (The total respiratory cycle is unchanged.[81]) At some point, however, an abnormally negative Pes pressure is reached, $V_T$ is reduced for one to three breaths due to the further narrowing of the upper airway passage, and an arousal response is triggered. This response is transient and short-lived (as short as 2 seconds with visual EEG scoring).

The transient EEG arousal response leads to a reopening of the upper airway. It also fragments sleep.[81] Initially, these intermittent changes are not recognized as OSAS, due to monitoring techniques. However, sleep deprivation has been shown to slowly blunt the responses of many reflexes. In addition, this initial, intermittent sleep fragmentation probably plays a role in the progressive development of full-blown OSAS.

It is interesting to note that a large percentage of OSAS patients present subtle craniofacial abnormalities, such as a highly arched hard palate; a long soft palate with low placement and redundant tissues; and a moderately retroplaced mandible.[82] It has been suggested that these abnormalities are responsible for obstructive apnea during the first weeks of life in certain subjects.[83] These abnormalities are related to genetic factors, and we have investigated several families in which a small upper airway has been passed down for generations.[84]

As stated previously, the upper airway begins at the nares and includes the nasal vestibule, nasopharynx, oropharynx, and hypopharynx. The pharynx is an especially vulnerable portion of the upper airway because it serves both digestive and respiratory functions. It must be sufficiently floppy to contract and guide food into the esophagus, while alternately maintaining sufficient muscle dilation to keep from being sucked closed.

Nasal obstruction from any cause, including allergic congestion, inflamed lymphoid tissue, or septal deviation, can initiate obstructive nocturnal respiratory pathology by converting breathing from the nasal to the oral route. Oral breathing predisposes to abnormal airway dynamics favoring pharyngeal collapse and backward displacement of the base of the tongue. The dilating genioglossus and geniohyoid muscles become mechanically disadvantaged and airway resistance is increased.

The next potential level of obstruction arises at the nasal and oropharynx due to enlarged adenoidal, tonsillar, and soft palate tissues. Enlargement of these tissues is secondary to hereditary and acquired factors. Allergies and recurrent upper respiratory infections can cause hyperplasia and scarring of lymphoid tissue. Snoring renders the uvula more edematous due to suction and trauma, which further compromises the small oropharyngeal space. Macroglossia may be due in part to obesity and is implicated in OSAS.[85]

As mentioned earlier, a constellation of jaw malformations are associated with OSAS, including a highly arched hard palate and class II dental occlusion (overjet). The position of the mandible relative to the maxilla determines the posterior extension of the tongue. Because the genioglossus muscle inserts on the mandible, with retrognathia or micrognathia the genioglossus originates on a backwardly displaced mandible and thus extends further posteriorly, predisposing to hypopharyngeal obstruction. During sleep in the supine position, gravity pulls the tongue further into the pharyngeal lumen, and varying degrees of decreased muscle tone additionally relax the tongue dorsally.

Chronic nasal obstruction during childhood that results in oral breathing may induce craniofacial changes predisposing to sleep apnea later in life. This has been shown in rhesus monkeys with experimentally partially occluded nostrils who developed mandibular deficiency relative to paired controls. Oral breathing changed EMG activity in facial muscle groups, leading to altered forces on the developing facial skeleton.[86–88] Partial improvement in these changes occurred if the obstruction was relieved early enough. Upper airway obstruction from enlarged adenoids in children has been shown to lead to decreased mandibular size and retrognathia, among other craniofacial changes.[89–93]

Adiposity compromises the upper airway not only because the "double chin" externally compresses the pharynx in the supine position, but also through internal infiltration of parapharyngeal structures (i.e., the adipose tissue alters and reduces airspace). Pharyngeal dilator muscle mechanics may be compromised by this loading.[94]

Testosterone may contribute to obstruction by inducing more parapharyngeal muscle bulk and more centripetal fat distribution. This might explain the fact that snoring often begins at puberty or during the immediate postpubertal period. It should be emphasized that morbid obesity is not a requirement for the development of OSAS. Even a few kilograms of excessive weight can tip the balance toward upper airway obstruction in anatomically vulnerable patients.

Morbid obesity degrades waking and sleeping ventilation in addition to its impact on upper airway dynamics. Adipose deposition around the abdomen, diaphragm, and ribs reduces thoracic cage compliance, requiring increased work to breathe.[95] Functional residual capacity is decreased and atelectasis of dependent airways may create ventilation and perfusion mismatch with hypoxemia.[96] In the supine position, the abdominal weight creates additional load, which increases hypoxemia.[97] During REM sleep, muscle atonia renders accessory respiratory muscles such as the intercostals and upper airway dilators functionally paralyzed. Thus, the diaphragm contributes mostly to inspiration against the load created by the heavy chest mass, leading to the profound oxygen desaturations seen during REM sleep in some obese patients.

## Summary

Partial or complete upper airway occlusion is related to the development of greater subatmospheric intrathoracic pressure during inspiration. This subatmospheric pressure is transmitted to the pharyngeal region, creating a "suction" on the soft tissues, which are the major constituents of the pharyngeal airway. To prevent closure, reflexes are normally activated at least 500 msec before the beginning of inspiration to activate the contraction of upper airway dilator muscles in opposition to this subatmospheric intrathoracic pressure.

During sleep, many of the upper airway dilator muscles have much less contractile power than the diaphragm. The genioglossus and geniohyoid muscles are particularly affected. This physiologic change allows the development of abnormal inspiratory upper airway resistance, which may result in partial or complete occlusion. If abnormalities of the upper airway, either anatomic or physiologic, reduce size to a level lower than critical or limit the capabilities of upper airway dilator muscles, a more or less pronounced collapse will occur during sleep in this very flexible region.

The obesity hypoventilation syndrome with increased $Paco_2$ has been described during the awake state. It is felt to result from reduced hypoxic and hypercapnic ventilatory drives and is not attributed to weight-related mechanical factors.[98]

Neural factors that relate to state changes from wakefulness to sleep, as well as changes across sleep stages, play an adjunctive role in the anatomic considerations of the genesis of OSAS. During sleep, the wake-related contribution to ventilatory drive is lost. This *wakefulness stimulus*[99] consists of factors that are independent of metabolic and voluntary components. With sleep onset, autonomic integration of acid-base and oxygen homeostasis is believed to occur in the medulla. Inputs to this regulator include peripheral chemoreceptors for $Pco_2$ and $Po_2$; central chemoreceptors for pH and $Pco_2$; and stretch receptors in the lung, thoracic wall, and upper airway. Ventilatory responses to both hypercapnia and hypoxia are decreased in all stages of sleep,[100,101] with more profound decrements usually occurring during phasic REM than in NREM sleep states. A REM sleep–related obesity hypoventilation syndrome may be seen, however, indicating that state-related changes produce further blunting of hypoxic and hypercapnic drives. REM sleep–related decrements in muscle tone leading to changes in thoracoabdominal mechanics with distortion of the thoracoabdominal wall will be further increased in obesity. During sleep, $Po_2$, $V_T$, and minute ventilation are decreased, whereas $Pco_2$ increases by 2–6 mm Hg. These changes are attributed to a resetting of the carbon dioxide ($CO_2$) set point and a depressed ventilatory drive per given level of $Pco_2$ compared to wakefulness. For unknown reasons, males have a reduced ventilatory response to $CO_2$ compared to females.[102]

The upper airway dilator muscles are accessory respiratory muscles, which are partially controlled by chemoreceptors for arterial blood gases. They also receive input from thoracic, mouth, and jaw proprioceptors. Upper airway obstruction possibly occurs when there is a mismatch in timing between neural signals triggering the inspiratory pump muscles (of which the diaphragm predominates), and those activating the upper airway dilator muscles.[103]

Diaphragmatic inspiratory effort before activation of the dilator muscles would tend to "suck" the upper airway closed. Such a phenomenon is seen experimentally when normal sleeping humans are passively hyperventilated and then allowed to resume spontaneous breathing. Hypocapnia causes a transient central apnea that may be terminated with an obstructive apnea.[104]

With sleep onset, sensitivity of the central $CO_2$ set point to the peripheral chemoreceptors is reduced. This results in a central apnea or a reduction in diaphragmatic effort and a decrease in $V_T$ (central hypopnea), which allows $Pco_2$ to rise. If resumption of breathing induces obstruction by the mismatched timing mechanism discussed earlier, then a brief arousal may be triggered. Arousal resets the $Pco_2$ to the awake set point and increases ventilation. With the resumption of sleep, a cycling of central apnea, obstructive apnea, and arousal will occur.[105] This is commonly observed in the mixed apneas typically seen in obstructive sleep apneics. Any cause of sleep fragmentation, such as periodic limb movements, may bring about the unstable respiratory state in predisposed individuals that produces this common type of sleep-onset apneas.

In addition to the chemoreceptor influences described earlier, pressure-sensitive reflexes exert a more rapid influence on upper airway patency. Located throughout the upper airway,[106] pressure-sensitive reflexes coordinate the interplay of forces between inspiratory pump muscles and dilator muscles in a breath-to-breath fashion. When suction pressure produced by the diaphragm is registered, these reflexes increase genioglossus muscle activity, moving the tongue anteriorly and prolonging the duration of inspiration. Longer inspiratory times reduce the peak suction pressure, facilitating patency of the airway.

These reflexes are normally reduced during sleep but may be defective or ineffectual in patients with sleep apnea. Sullivan and coworkers[107] found upper airway closure to occur at abnormally low inspiratory pressures in patients with sleep apnea during a study where the nasal airway was occluded. Even when peripheral chemoreceptor drive was added, which should facilitate patency, there was no augmentation in activation of the dilator muscles, as measured by closing pressure.

The degree of hypercapnia in sleep apnea is influenced by input from the peripheral chemoreceptors on upper airway dilators and the inspiratory pump as well as the ability of these reflexes to trigger arousal with resumption of ventilation. Most OSAS patients are normocapnic while awake. A limited population of severe sleep apneics display hypercapnia while awake, however, which is not attributable to pulmonary disease or obesity. The hypercapnia in these patients indicates hypoventilation due to downward resetting of chemoreceptor reflex sensitivity. Sullivan's group[107] showed that these patients had decreased carotid body responses to hypoxemia and failed to develop normal augmentation of response to superimposed arterial hypercarbia. Elevated levels of $CO_2$ were required to produce a ventilatory response. These patients demonstrated long periods of obstructive apnea or hypopnea, concomitant with sustained arterial oxygen desaturations and arterial $CO_2$ elevations.

Resetting of chemoreceptors may allow the endurance of longer apneic events while asleep without producing arousals. Because the chemoreceptor responses are depressed, they do not lead to increased inspiratory efforts—as would normally occur with sensitive reflexes—thereby preventing the partially occluded upper airway from being sucked entirely closed. Diminished inspiratory efforts through a narrow upper airway cause reduced total ventilation, with oxyhemoglobin desaturation and $CO_2$ elevation. Tracheostomy or nightly treatment with nasal CPAP normalizes awake hypercapnia, suggesting that sleep apnea is a major factor in its development.

### Snoring

Snoring is a noise produced when vibration occurs at several levels of the upper airway. It may be associated with various degrees of upper airway resistance. It may be heard after a complete airway obstruction; with a significant hypopnea; or with hypoventilation, leading to a cohort of symptoms. It may be associated with a limited and intermittent drop in $V_T$ and be associated with isolated sleepiness. It may be present with no other clinical symptoms. The notion that snoring itself may engender cardiovascular risk is in question. Studies that suggested this probably failed to separate out subpopulations with upper airway resistance syndrome (discussed later), or situational apneics based on

such behavior elicitors as alcohol or sedative use. Although more research is required, it is likely that chronic heavy snorers eventually become patients with clinically significant syndromes of obstruction.[76] As already mentioned, however, snoring is not a prerequisite for partial upper airway occlusion leading to clinical symptoms.

### Upper Airway Resistance Syndrome

Upper airway resistance syndrome[4,5] (Figure 22-1) causes a chronic complaint of EDS that is objectively confirmed by abnormal scores on the Multiple Sleep Latency Test (MSLT). A retrospective study selected 54 patients previously diagnosed at Stanford University with idiopathic hypersomnolence based on pathologic MSLT scores, who were also snorers. The mean group MSLT score was 6.1 minutes, with abnormal scores defined as less than 8 minutes. These patients did not fit standard criteria for OSAS in terms of RDI, significant oxygen desaturations, or both.

In 14 patients (nine women, five men), nocturnal sleep showed fragmentation with repetitive 3- to 14-second alpha EEG arousals, with a mean of $49 \pm 11$ arousals per hour of sleep. When studied by esophageal balloon manometry (a technique reflecting intrathoracic inspiratory efforts as negative "suction" pressure) and a pneumotachometer with face mask to quantify airflow, a pattern emerged. Increasing inspiratory efforts were demonstrated by excessively negative Pes nadirs between –13 and –51 cm $H_2O$ (normal is >–8), accompanied by decreasing peak flows and $V_T$s one to three breaths before the arousals. These sequences were punctuated by repetitive arousals. Because the arousals and snoring would have been the only abnormalities identifiable by standard PSG recordings, these patients would not have met standard criteria for OSAS based on oxygen desaturation or apneas and hypopneas.

These 14 patients underwent CPAP titration to eliminate the snoring and alpha arousals. At a 3-week follow-up, subjective complaints of EDS were eliminated in all 14 patients, MSLT scores normalized to a group mean of $13 \pm 3$ minutes, and arousals were reduced to eight per hour of sleep.

In a prospective study of patients presenting with EDS, 48 patients fulfilling PSG and MSLT criteria

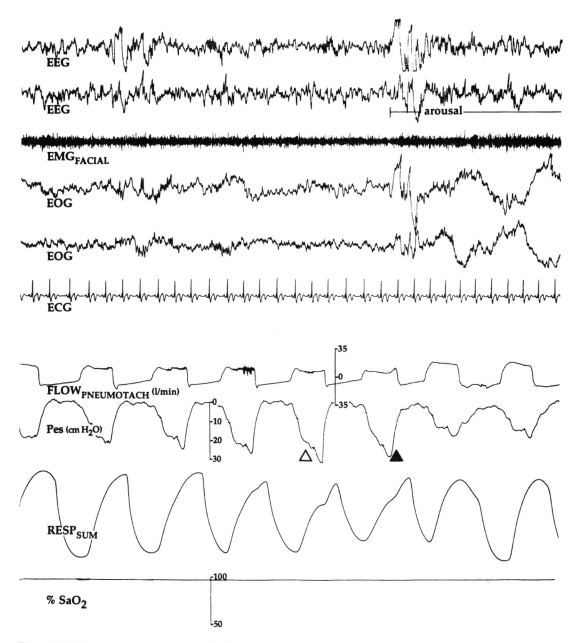

**Figure 22-1.** Polysomnographic recording showing an example of upper airway resistance syndrome. Note peak increase in effort (indicated by the solid arrowhead) is associated with a small drop in peak flow and tidal volume triggering a transient electroencephalographic arousal. ($EMG_{FACIAL}$ = facial muscle electromyogram; EOG = electro-oculogram (right and left); ECG = electrocardiogram; $FLOW_{PNEUMOTACH}$ = pneumotachometer to quantify airflow; Pes = esophageal manometry to record esophageal pressure; $RESP_{SUM}$ = respiratory effort; $SaO_2$ = saturation with oxygen.)

for idiopathic hypersomnia (RDI <5 and MSLT ≤8) were studied with home ambulatory monitoring including evaluation of snoring, several nocturnal PSG recordings, and subsequent nocturnal Pes polygraphic monitoring. Fifteen subjects (eight women, seven men) with sleep fragmentation and peak Pes nadirs lower than –12 cm $H_2O$ were restudied with Pes in conjunction with quantitative airflow measurement via pneumotachometer and face mask. Mean BMI was $22.7 \pm 2.1$ kg/m$^2$ for the women and $24.3 \pm 4.0$ kg/m$^2$ for the men. Snoring was continuous in 10 subjects, intermittent in three, and absent in two. Mean RDI was $2.1 \pm 1.7$. Mean Sao$_2$ nadir was $91.4 \pm 2.1\%$. These patients showed abnormal breathing periods during which progressive increases of Pes nadir, associated with decreases in peak flow and V$_T$, were interrupted by alpha EEG arousal.

These subjects were adapted to nasal CPAP for two nights. On the second night, optimum CPAP pressure eliminated the abnormal Pes nadirs, snoring, and sleep fragmentation. Follow-up MSLT results showed an improved mean of $13.5 \pm 2.1$ with subjective disappearance of EDS. Thus, approximately one-third of patients diagnosed in a standard manner at a major sleep disorders center as having idiopathic hypersomnia had a treatable form of upper airway obstruction.

### Secondary Apnea

A variety of medical conditions and craniofacial malformations are commonly associated with OSAS. Patients with congenital syndromes of micrognathia such as the Pierre Robin, Crouzon, Hunter's, and Treacher Collins syndromes, present in childhood; children with cleft palates repaired by a pharyngeal flap have developed iatrogenic obstruction. Cranial base abnormalities associated with OSAS include achondroplasia, Arnold Chiari, and Klippel-Feil malformations. Down syndrome patients have large tongues and retrognathia predisposing to upper airway obstruction. Children with Prader-Willi syndrome may suffer OSAS due to morbid obesity.

Endocrine abnormalities causing OSAS include hypothyroidism with myxedema, which causes macroglossia and parapharyngeal tissue infiltration. Acromegaly is a known cause of macroglossia.

Neurologic disorders associated with OSAS include the Shy-Drager syndrome of multisystem degeneration (central and obstructive apnea) and neuromuscular diseases involving facial and thoracoabdominal musculature such as polio and myotonic and muscular dystrophies. Secondary kyphoscoliosis will worsen nocturnal respiratory function.

Lesions of the temporomandibular condyle leading to retrognathia may be developmental or acquired due to rheumatoid arthritis, osteomyelitis, or trauma.

## EVALUATION

### History

Pertinent symptoms of OSAS fall into daytime and nocturnal categories. Loud guttural snoring, at its worst in the supine position, punctuated by choking sounds and followed by cessation of breathing, is virtually pathognomonic. Although snoring commonly starts around the time of puberty, presentation to a physician is typically prompted by a recent increase in snoring intensity associated with weight gain. The sleep of the bed partner is compromised by the patient's high-amplitude snoring and restless sleep. The volume may be so loud as to exceed standards set by the Occupational Safety and Health Administration for workplace safety.[108] The apneic phase can last from seconds to more than a minute. These respiratory cessations may be frightening to bed partners who often remain vigilant to wake the patient to resume breathing. Commonly, partners begin sleeping in separate rooms, which may create stress in the relationship.

Restless sleep in large part stems from sleep fragmentation caused by airway obstruction. Repetitive EEG arousals lasting seconds may terminate apneic episodes, thereby causing a regain of "wakeful" muscle tone observed on the chin EMG. This facilitates a restorative breath, allowing the cycle to repeat. Behavioral arousals accompany some of these EEG arousals, resulting in position changes, abrupt raising of the upper torso from the bed, and large flailing limb movements. Some of these movements appear to be agitated, with concomitant groaning or crying out of short dysphoric phrases. The vast majority of brief arousals are not consciously recalled on awakening, although the patient may appreciate that the quality of sleep has been poor. Clues to restless sleep are obtained by asking the patient how disturbed bedcovers are by morning, and how many times he or she awoke during the night.

It is surprisingly infrequent for the patient to awaken with actual awareness of an asphyxial sensation such as choking or gasping. When this does occur, it may be accompanied by a "feeling of dying," and the patient may run to the window or sit up at the edge of the bed. Rarely, patients are still unable to draw an inspiratory breath upon awakening, but usually can do so after coughing. It is believed that this may be due to adhesion of the uvula to the posterior pharynx.

There appears to be a subpopulation of sleep apneics in whom the presenting complaint is sleep maintenance insomnia. Some of their arousals trigger full awakenings that last at least several minutes. Because they remain unaware of the respiratory antecedents of these awakenings, OSAS should be considered among the differential diagnoses in evaluating patients with chronic difficulties maintaining sleep.

The clinician should ask about symptoms related to snoring, such as the presence of a dry mouth or sore throat on awakening. Morning headaches that resolve within an hour of awakening should also be asked about, as they may be clues to nocturnal hypercarbia and increased intracranial pressure. These headaches are typically generalized or bifrontal in nature. The occurrence of nocturnal confusional spells, such as going to the refrigerator and watering the plants with milk, may be due to either hypoxemia or slow-wave sleep (SWS) parasomnia triggered by respiratory-induced arousal.

Multiple episodes of nocturia have been related to elevated plasma levels of ANP and catecholamines.[109,110] After the first night of treatment with nasal CPAP, a return to normal levels with concomitant decrease in urinary volume to approximately 50% of pretreatment amounts has been reported. This helps explain why enuresis is more common in children with OSAS and was reported in 7% of 120 apneic adults seen successively at Stanford in 1992. Confusion and increased intra-abdominal pressure from inspiratory attempts against a closed upper airway may also contribute to enuresis.

Symptoms of nocturnal esophageal acid reflux and heartburn are facilitated when excessively negative intrathoracic pressure exerts upward suction on abdominal contents, and increased abdominal pressure expels the contents. The patient may also complain of nocturnal aspiration.

Bruxism may be noted and may be a clue to dental malocclusion resulting from the common jaw misalignment etiologically related to OSA. A history of orthodontia to correct an overjet is common. The patient may have a history of wisdom tooth extraction secondary to impaction. These individuals may also manifest morning headaches or dysfunction of the temporomandibular joint.

History of seasonal or environmental allergies should be sought, as these are common causes of nasal obstruction in adults and adenotonsillar enlargement in children. Studies of rhesus monkeys with chronic and temporary nasal obstruction suggest that nasal obstruction with mouth breathing during childhood is etiologically related to subsequent mandibular growth insufficiency.[87,88] We have documented craniofacial abnormalities with cephalometric radiography that were not appreciated on clinical examination.[89]

Nocturnal diaphoresis may be seen in association with the increased effort required to inspire against resistance during the night. Increased caloric expenditures to breathe may also account for a subpopulation of sleep apneics who have difficulty gaining weight.

Ethanol or other sedatives used before bedtime worsen OSAS by at least two mechanisms. They greatly diminish the contraction of the upper airway dilators, as well as interfering with the organization of reflexes coordinating upper airway dilators with the contraction of inspiratory muscles.[111] A history of increased snoring or development of any of the symptoms discussed earlier in association with sedating substances should raise the index of suspicion for OSAS. In elderly patients with AI greater than 5, sedative use or sleep deprivation may escalate the AI into the pathologic range.[112]

The cardinal daytime symptom of OSAS is EDS, which manifests as a tendency to inadvertently fall asleep during quiet or passive activities, to take intentional naps, or to experience short but repetitive attention lapses while doing monotonous tasks. Such sleepiness is the consequence of sleep fragmentation. Patients usually misperceive the act of dozing off as being caused by the characteristics of the situation (i.e., boredom), rather than by their abnormal intrinsic degree of somnolence. It helps to inform patients that quiet settings do not produce sleepiness, but merely unmask it. Patients often forget or deny episodes of daytime sleepiness, which may better be elicited from household members who frequently observe the patient dozing while watching television or reading. Momentary lapses into sleep while driving are a potentially lethal consequence of somnolence and history of this should always be sought by inquiring about motor vehicle accidents due to sleepiness or inadvertently dozing at the wheel or swerving into another lane. Such incidents are particularly likely on long or monotonous trips. Affirmative answers require rapid treatment interventions.

Cognitive complaints resulting from EDS are common, and may be the only clue to EDS in those who misperceive their sleepiness. Symptoms include poor memory and difficulties concentrating or making decisions. Automatic behavior, when an action is performed without subsequent recall, is an extreme manifestation of such cognitive impairment. Increased errors and poor judgment may place patients at risk of losing their jobs.[8] Severe morning confusion and disorientation, termed *sleep drunkenness*, may be a sequela of preceding hypoxemia.

Sleep fragmentation may produce personality changes that are often first noted by family members. These include irritability, anxiety, aggression, and depression. More marked personality changes involving irrational behavior, jealousy, and paranoia have been reported.[8] Sleepy patients report less enjoyment from previously engaging activities. They are typically misperceived as unmotivated or lazy, descriptors they come to believe if the underlying etiology remains undiscovered. Diminished libido or impotence is not uncommon, even in nonelderly patients.

In taking the medical history, inquiries regarding systemic sequelae must be sought. These include the existence and duration of borderline or elevated blood pressure; angina; symptoms of right heart failure, including peripheral edema; and transient cerebrovascular ischemic symptoms.

### Examination

Patient evaluation begins with observing the patient in the waiting room for sleeping or snoring. The height and weight provide a BMI (expressed in $kg/m^2$) from which to assess the degree of obesity, with the upper limit of normalcy being 25 $kg/m^2$ for American males. The distribution of weight should be noted, as more midline depositions favor nocturnal respiratory pathology. In particular, adiposity or muscularity of the neck predisposes to upper airway

obstruction, and severe abdominal obesity may also predispose to alveolar hypoventilation. A nasal voice is a clue to nasal obstruction, and mild hoarseness is often noted in heavy snorers. The lateral facial profile should be inspected for retrognathia or micrognathia, keeping in mind that the relevant site is the indentation below the lip that identifies the genial tubercle, where the tongue takes insertion on the mandible. The patient should bite down to demonstrate dental occlusion. Overjet is recorded in millimeters, and underbite should be noted as well. Palpate the temperomandibular joint with wide jaw opening for subluxation or a click for further evidence of jaw misalignment. The oral cavity is inspected for dental prostheses, size of tongue, and soft palate tissue size and appearance. Soft palate edema and erythema may be due to snoring. A soft palate inferiorly positioned behind the tongue may be due to chronic excessive suction from snoring. Tonsillar hypertrophy is noted. The hard palate is checked for a high arch, which has been found to correlate with OSAS.

Evidence of upper airway obstruction is obtained by evaluating breathing in the supine position with the jaw slackened slightly open and nares occluded, to simulate oral breathing during sleep. If snoring or labored breathing results, this is good evidence that even greater difficulties will occur during sleep.

The nose should be assessed for septal deviation, polyps, flaring of the nostrils, and patency of either vestibule with the opposite naris occluded. The thyroid should be examined for evidence of enlargement.

Blood pressure and pulse are measured and a general physical examination is performed, bearing in mind signs of dysrhythmia or heart failure. Lung auscultation provides clues of pulmonary pathology that would exacerbate oxygen desaturation caused by upper airway obstruction. A complete neurologic evaluation may uncover neuromuscular disorders impacting on upper airway patency and respiratory muscle function. A complete physical examination can eliminate the presence of generalized diseases, particularly those inducing lymph node enlargement or mucosal infiltration, that may reduce the upper airway lumen.

History and evaluation should reveal possible secondary causes of OSAS. This includes a search for a local tumor in the upper airway. Suspicion is raised in the presence of rapid emergence of obstructive symptoms not associated with weight gain, throat pain, constant hoarseness or other vocal cord dysfunction, prominent difficulty swallowing, or nasal regurgitation. Such symptoms should prompt otolaryngologic evaluation.

### Laboratory Evaluation

*Polysomnography*

A full-night PSG study in the sleep laboratory is the main method of evaluation. The study devotes various channels to the EEG (i.e., C4-A1, C3-A2, O1-O2), electro-oculogram, chin and limb (usually anterior tibialis) noninvasive EMG, qualitative measurements of oronasal airflow, thoracic and abdominal respiratory efforts, electrocardiogram, and pulse oximetry. An entire night of study is recommended, as opposed to a partial night, because substantial changes in respiratory disturbance typically occur from one sleep cycle to another across the night. Because REM sleep predominates toward the end of the night, REM sleep–related respiratory disturbances might easily be missed without a full night of study.

PSG allows quantification of various factors disturbed in sleep apneics, including the RDI, oxygen desaturation, sleep-stage percentages, and sleep efficiency. Sleep fragmentation can be assessed as variable length awakenings or EEG arousals lasting only several seconds. PSG helps determine the causes of arousals as due to apnea or unsuspected factors such as periodic limb movements or primary insomnia.

Associations between sleep stage and positional influences on respiratory disturbance can be made. Cardiac dysrhythmias and their relationship to oxygen desaturation and sleep stage can be identified.

Relatively invasive techniques to measure upper airway pressure may have circumscribed clinical usefulness. The upper airway resistance syndrome (discussed earlier) may only be suspected based on transient alpha EEG arousals on the standard PSG, warranting additional investigation using esophageal manometry. Catheter systems allowing measurement of differential pressures at different levels of the upper airway may also help in determining the level of collapse to which surgical intervention should be addressed.[113–115]

Technologies that allow in-home sleep monitoring are rapidly emerging. Portable units range from comprehensive portable PSG (level II) to continuous single or dual bioparameter recording (level IV).[116] The American Sleep Disorders Association (ASDA) standards of practice committee recommends that portable studies be reserved for patients with severe clinical symptoms when standard PSG (level I) is not readily available and patients who are unable to be studied in the laboratory. These studies are also acceptable for follow-up evaluation of response to therapy, after the initiation of treatment, when the diagnosis has been established by standard PSG.[117] The ASDA also recommends that only level II or III equipment be used, that body position be documented during the study so that severity of disease is more accurately assessed, and that the equipment be capable of recording and storing raw data that must be reproducible.[117] Although portable studies are a convenient, cost-effective, and accessible alternative to standard PSG, there are limitations. The absence of trained personnel to intervene in the event of technical difficulty or medical emergency is one of the primary shortcomings. Concern has also been raised about the precision and accuracy of some portable units for the evaluation of more subtle cases of sleep disordered breathing, such as those with a predominance of hypopneas or upper airway resistance syndrome.[118] It is likely that these drawbacks will be circumvented in the near future.

*Multiple Sleep Latency Test*

The MSLT[119] is considered to be an objective measure of EDS. A series of daytime naps (usually five) of 20 minutes' duration at 2-hour intervals is performed to determine time to sleep onset. These sleep latencies are averaged. Scores under 8 minutes in the absence of confounding factors (e.g., insufficient preceding nocturnal total sleep time, or use of hypnotic medication) are generally regarded as abnormal. REM occurrences during naps are also noted.

Because the demonstration of EDS is not required for the diagnosis of OSAS, MSLTs are not mandatory in the evaluation of OSAS. If a PSG for suspected OSAS is negative, however, MSLT performed the subsequent day may help diagnose a different sleep disorder of excessive somnolence.

When complaints of sleepiness persist after adequate treatment is instituted, an MSLT may reveal an unsuspected second sleep disorder requiring a separate treatment approach.

*Imaging Studies*

As an adjunct to clinical evaluation, particularly when surgical treatment is contemplated, various imaging procedures can help identify the site(s) of upper airway obstruction. For a comprehensive review, the interested reader is referred to Shepard et al.[120] Imaging is also imperative when the history raises suspicion of a mass lesion as the cause of upper airway obstruction. It should be kept in mind that procedures performed on an awake patient do not reveal the actual anatomy during sleep when postural and state-related changes in muscle tone alter the awake relationships.

Cephalometric radiographs provide a midline view of relevant cranial base and facial bones with their soft tissue appendages. Maxillary or mandibular deficiency can be calculated, and awake posterior airway space measured as the distance between the base of the tongue and posterior pharyngeal wall. Soft palate and lymphoid tissue extent is identified.

Fiberoptic endoscopy of the upper airway down to the vocal cords performed in the seated and supine positions provides further assessment of the possible sites of collapse. The patient can perform Valsalva's and Müller's maneuvers to elicit collapse, although the predictive value for identifying candidates for surgical success after uvulopalatopharyngoplasty (UPPP) is limited.[121–123] Fiberoptic endoscopy should be systematically performed to eliminate secondary causes of upper airway obstruction if signs and symptoms are consistent with them.

Computed tomography (CT) scanning provides detailed surveys of cross-sectional levels of the upper airway and magnetic resonance imaging (MRI) can be used to image multiple planes. CT and MRI have mainly been used as research tools due to their expense. Newer techniques such as fast-CT scanning may prove to have prognostic clinical usefulness in selecting candidates for successful surgical outcomes. The 50-msec scan time, as compared to 2–5 seconds for conventional CT, is sufficiently rapid to show dynamic dimensional changes across various levels of the upper airway during the respiratory cycle. It can potentially be used in a sleeping patient.

Video fluoroscopy of the pharynx in anteroposterior and lateral directions offers another means for observing dynamic anatomic changes in the upper airway during ventilation. It is of limited clinical usefulness in view of its significant radiation exposure.

*Other Studies*

Pulmonary function tests including spirometry and arterial blood gases are a useful adjunct in investigation. Diminished vital capacity (VC) has been identified as a risk factor for sleep disordered breathing both in the Cleveland Family Study and in the elderly.[17,124] Although associated with excess cardiovascular morbidity, a lowered VC may be a marker for central obesity or an indicator of the presence of OSAS.[125,126] Patients with daytime hypoxemia or $CO_2$ retention due to intrinsic lung disease might be expected to show severe oxygen desaturations with the addition of obstructive sleep pathology and may require cautious addition of low-flow oxygen to nasal CPAP. Those with restrictive pulmonary dynamics based on morbid obesity might require special treatment with bilevel positive airway pressure (BIPAP) or intermittent positive pressure ventilation delivered by nasal mask. Arterial blood gases provide the most relevant information for a sleep evaluation if obtained after the patient remains supine for 20 minutes. This aids in detection of insufficient ventilation associated with the supine position.

Thyroid function screening will exclude hypothyroidism as a cause of apnea and daytime somnolence. Polycythemia without known lung disease should lead to a consideration of sleep apnea.

## TREATMENT

### Behavioral Recommendations

Once OSAS is diagnosed, treatments can be suggested based on evaluation of contributing factors and disease severity. It has long been known that weight loss in obese patients is effective in the reduction of the number of apneas, sleep fragmentation, and the extent and number of desaturations. In overweight patients without obvious fixed anatomic considerations such as retrognathia, weight loss may result in eventual cure. For most patients, nasal CPAP should be instituted along with weight loss measures. These measures include weight reduction surgery, diet with or without pharmacologic intervention, and exercise. When applicable, a program of exercise may be facilitated after daytime somnolence is ameliorated by CPAP. For those who are not completely cured by weight loss, the significant reduction in weight often allows a lower CPAP pressure requirement or increases the likelihood of a surgical cure. Patients with large losses should be retitrated to the lowest effective pressure.

Elimination of central nervous system depressants such as ethanol or sedatives from the bloodstream at bedtime decreases the severity of OSAS. If a strong positional relationship is discovered, with obstruction limited to the supine position, recommendation to remain in lateral or prone positions can be made. A sock filled with a golf or tennis ball and sewn onto the back of the pajamas or T-shirt may help patients learn to avoid the supine position. A full-length wedge pillow may also be helpful in this respect. A buzzer-type training device that sounds when the patient lies supine for a brief time has also been developed. In mild cases, attention to position may suffice.

### Pharmacologic

Tricyclic antidepressants such as protriptyline have been used to increase muscle tonus and diminish REM sleep time in cases of mild or REM sleep–related OSAS. Progesterone acts as a respiratory stimulant in obese patients but has no impact on an obstructed airway. Unfortunately, pharmacologic approaches have been largely unsuccessful.

### Continuous and Bilevel Positive Airway Pressure

An enormous advance in the treatment of OSAS began in the early 1980s with the first commercially available continuous positive pressure generators. These bedside machines compress room air and channel it through a soft vinyl or silicon nasal mask, a full-face (naso-oral) mask or endonasal cushions at a given pressure. CPAP serves as a pneumatic splint to keep the upper airway patent. Pressure requirements must be established during sleep for each patient. Optimum pressure is the lowest one that completely eliminates obstructive apneas, hypopneas, and snoring. Patients who routinely consume ethanol in the evening are most accurately titrated to CPAP after consuming their usual intake, which raises the pressure requirement.

BIPAP differs from CPAP by using separate inspiratory and expiratory pressures. The BIPAP machine (BiPAP, Respironics, Inc., Murrysville, PA) times itself to patient-initiated breathing. By reducing the pressure on expiration, it lowers the resistance against which the patient must exhale. This is advantageous for patients with severely restrictive pulmonary dynamics, such as emphysemics, the morbidly obese, and those with neuromuscular weakness. Patients with normal lungs who could not tolerate CPAP might feel more comfortable on BIPAP, especially those requiring higher CPAP pressures (approximately 13 cm $H_2O$). Those with severe discomfort due to drying of the mucosae could benefit from BIPAP because of the overall decrease in airflow relative to CPAP. BIPAP also offers a higher range of inspiratory pressures than CPAP, with maximum pressures of 40 cm $H_2O$. The newer devices with extended pressure range also have the ability to control inspiratory time (flow) and are thereby more appropriate for persons with isolated neuromuscular disease. Intermittent positive pressure ventilation may be more useful in some patients with sleep-related hypoventilation who cannot be maintained on bilevel units.

Ideally, PSG study to titrate CPAP or BIPAP pressure should be performed for one to two nights to allow adequate assessment. By the end of the first night, the optimum pressure is approximated; on the second night, this pressure can be checked for adequacy throughout all stages and positions. It is especially critical to evaluate the patient in the supine position, when the maximum pressure requirement occurs. Unfortunately, financial constraints increasingly dictate that split-night studies be performed. This method of diagnosis and treatment tends to underestimate the severity of disease because treatment takes place in the latter half of the night when apnea is usually at its worst. In severe apneics, a rebound of unusually long REM sleep and SWS that may be out of phase occurs once adequate airway patency is attained. REM sleep rebound shows unusually prominent phasic activity, whereas the SWS episodes may show exceptionally high voltages. A rare but dangerous sequela of REM rebound has been seen in severe apneics with $CO_2$ retention under slightly suboptimum pressure. Arousal is suppressed during a long rebound, and if partial upper airway closure persists, dangerous hypoxemia may result.[127]

Treatment with nasal CPAP or BIPAP offers advantages of safety and assured efficacy over surgical approaches. They offer immediate and complete treatment for OSAS and are less costly than extensive surgical approaches. They can be used temporarily while weight loss is pursued or surgery is contemplated. Positive pressure eliminates risk factors for associated morbidity along with daytime somnolence. Modern CPAP units are small, portable, and quiet. Some gradually adjust the pressure upward to the preset pressure, allowing sleep onset to occur at more comfortable lower pressures.

Disadvantages of CPAP lie in psychological resistance to ongoing nightly reliance on a machine. Poor compliance is the bane of this treatment modality. Patients may feel claustrophobic and intolerant of the restriction of their movement and may perceive the treatment as an obstacle to intimacy with their bed partner and as a reminder of their mortality. The devices are annoying to some patients, although they are continually improved. Those traveling frequently may find it inconvenient. Generally, young adults and patients who are dating find this treatment to have an unacceptable social impact.

Common physical difficulties encountered include reactive nasal congestion or rhinitis, sinusitis and epistaxis or drying of the nasal-oral mucosa, discomfort or skin trauma from a poorly fitting mask, and allergic reaction to (or contact dermatitis with) the mask. Nasal symptoms usually subside after the first few months and can be ameliorated with heated humidification and a nasal steroid inhaler. Comfort issues and dermatitis should be closely supervised and addressed with trials of various mask adaptors and styles or by altering the mode of delivery via nasal pillows or the new Monarch mask (Respironics, Inc.). Psychological distress is minimized by support from the entire sleep laboratory team, with reassurance and understanding at the time of initiation and close followup. Sleep apnea support groups exist in many areas to help with coping and compliance. Occasionally, a brief course of bedtime anxiolytics is required, with the patient's full understanding that the severity of apnea will worsen if the medication is used without their CPAP. Flow leaks through an open mouth can be minimized by use of a chin strap.

Long-term compliance has been only fair, with an estimate of 60–85% of patients using their machines regularly after 1 year.[128,129] Compliance has been associated with the severity of daytime hypersomnolence before CPAP, but not with pretreatment disease severity as indicated by the respiratory disturbance index or oxygen saturation nadir. Intellectual understanding of the benefits of nightly use (i.e., to decrease cardiovascular risk factors) appears insufficient to motivate long-term compliance.

In patients who do not wish to undergo the extensive surgeries that might be required to produce a complete cure, selective surgery to relieve nasal obstruction can reduce pressure requirements and improve CPAP tolerance.

In patients with more than mild oxygen desaturation on diagnostic testing (i.e., <85%) who choose surgical treatment, CPAP initiation may be contemplated preoperatively to decrease the postoperative risk of further desaturation due to edema. Preoperative CPAP also reduces soft palate edema due to snoring and improves overall health status. Weight loss before surgery while using CPAP increases the chance of successful cure by creating more airway space through parapharyngeal tissue reduction.

### Surgical Approaches

The first surgical treatment for OSAS was tracheostomy. This intervention is rarely needed now, because of the pervasive use of positive pressure therapy. Although used infrequently, tracheostomy provides immediate profound improvement for some individuals with severe OSAS. Maintenance of a tracheostomy is associated with excess morbidity and psychosocial implications.

Surgery is individually tailored to overcome upper airway obstruction after a thorough analysis of the three main levels of potential obstruction: the nose, soft palate, and base of the tongue. Often, more than one level must be treated, either sequentially or simultaneously. Patients must understand that surgical treatment is an extensive and more costly process with greater risks than medical treatment. In addition, surgery carries no guarantee of cure in an individual patient, with only statistical cure rates available.

Nasal obstruction can be corrected with septoplasty, polypectomy, or turbinate reduction.

Soft palate resection via UPPP or uvuloflap surgery[130] carries approximately a 50% response rate.[131] The most common postoperative adverse sequelae include severe pain for approximately 2 weeks, transient nasal reflux and nasal speech due to palatal incompetence, minor loss of taste, and tongue numbness. Major complications involve permanent nasal reflux or nasal speech due to permanent velopharyngeal incompetence and scarring with retraction leading to palatal stenosis.

Because this procedure ameliorates snoring due to vibration of the uvula without addressing potential obstruction behind the base of the tongue, a major sign of ongoing residual obstruction may be masked. It is therefore imperative to follow up all surgeries with a postoperative sleep study. Ideally, this study should be delayed at least 4 months after surgery to allow thorough resolution of edema and readjustment of respiratory reflexes. Those with moderate to severe apnea can be maintained on CPAP in the interim and withdrawn 2 weeks before study to allow expression of airway changes from potential residual obstruction.

Geniotubercle advancement via inferior sagittal osteotomy is a technique pioneered at Stanford University[132] that addresses the retroposition of the tongue by advancing the insertion point of the genioglossus. The surgeon makes a small mandibular incision at the geniotubercle, pulls the bone segment through the jaw, and allows the fracture to heal. This is usually performed in conjunction with UPPP. Common complications are minor and consist of transient dental nerve anesthesia. Mandibular fracture may occur if the incision extends into the alveolus. Hyoidotomy with subhyoid myotomy and anterior superior repositioning with a fascia graft is now commonly performed in association with geniotubercle advancement. Based on 55 patients followed up postoperatively, the combined success rate of geniotubercle advancement and inferior sagittal osteotomy with hyoid myotomy and resuspension with UPPP is approximately 70%.[133] Midface advancement involving a Le Fort I mandibular osteotomy and a maxillary osteotomy is reserved for patients for whom other treatments have failed and who do not want to be treated with nasal CPAP. Patients undergoing midface advancement have previously had the other surgeries discussed earlier and have not shown an adequate improvement at the 4- to 6-month follow-up, which includes clinical evaluation and polygraphic monitoring. A study of 30 patients undergoing such surgery revealed no significant differences in efficacy as compared to curative treatment with nasal CPAP on indices of oxygen saturation nadir, RDI, and normalization of sleep architecture.[131]

## Dental Appliances

Various types of dental devices have been used to treat OSA. These devices have the same goal as inferior sagittal osteotomy with geniotubercle advancement. However, the space gain is much more limited than that obtained by surgical procedures. The advantage over surgery is that there is no permanent change of anatomy and no surgical risk involved. The devices are worn only during sleep. The most commonly used devices are the Esmarch appliance, the bionator, and the Tongue Retaining Device (TRD Professional Positioners, Inc, Racine, WI). Objective studies reporting results at 1-year follow-up are few. In mild cases, these devices may be helpful.

## OBSTRUCTIVE SLEEP APNEA IN CHILDREN

OSA occurs in premature and full-term infants as well as in children. In very young patients, the apnea usually becomes apparent as a result of color change and bradycardia; in children, a constellation of clinical symptoms signals the condition. At different ages, different symptoms are emphasized. Postpubertal teenagers do not differ from young adults, but younger children often present a different clinical picture.

### Clinical Features

OSAS can be associated with a series of daytime and nighttime signs and symptoms that may not be obvious at an initial evaluation.[134,135] The daytime symptoms include EDS so severe that school authorities suggest medical consultation and abnormal daytime behavior ranging from aggressiveness and hyperactivity to pathologic shyness and social withdrawal. Children may exhibit learning problems, morning headaches, frequent upper airway infections, failure to thrive, or obesity. Nocturnal symptoms include difficulty breathing while asleep, heavy snoring, apneic episodes, restless sleep, heavy sweating, nightmares, night terrors, and enuresis.

Reasons for seeking consultation vary with age. In children younger than 5 years, difficulty breathing while asleep, heavy snoring, sleep apneic episodes observed by parents, restless sleep, nightmares, and night terrors are the most frequent reasons for consultation. This may be because parents check young children's sleep often and young children fall asleep early, allowing parents to note abnormal sleep behavior. In children older than 5 years, EDS (associated with complaints of tiredness and daytime fatigue), abnormal daytime behavior, learning disabilities, frequent morning headaches, nocturnal enuresis, and major discipline problems are common reasons for consultation. A few children are referred at a late stage of the syndrome. These children not only present significant failure to thrive but also may have been hospitalized for unexplained acute cardiac failure or unexplained development of systemic hypertension. The cardiac failure often will have occurred after the child had contracted a cold or bronchopneumopathy, which may not have been severe, but, in combination with the chronic nocturnal problem, nevertheless led to the acute failure.

The clinical evaluation of children should be as thorough as for adults, and suspicion of OSAS should lead to polygraphic monitoring during sleep.

### Polygraphic Testing

Although repetitive apneas may be seen in children with equal frequency as in adults, most commonly the polygraphic test indicates only intermittent apneas. Sometimes no apneas are monitored, even when a florid symptomatology exists.[136]

Prepubescent children have a greater tendency to present complete apneas during REM sleep. During NREM sleep, prepubescent children with OSAS present as loud snorers. Documented by a sonogram, snoring is commonly associated with an increase in respiratory rate. The degree of tachypnea is variable within a given age group and sometimes within a given subject during the night. The increase in breathing frequency compensates for the decrease in $V_T$ and allows maintenance of a normal minute ventilation with an appropriate level of oxygen saturation. However, partial upper airway obstruction leads to great enhancement of respiratory efforts, which is obvious when one observes

the laborious, noisy mouth breathing during sleep. Pes measures demonstrate the increase in respiratory efforts. Pes nadir may reach –35 to –40 cm $H_2O$ without induction of a complete collapse of the upper airway in children 5–6 years old. Increased efforts may also be demonstrated by monitoring of intercostal-diaphragmatic EMG. Surface electrodes placed 10 mm apart near the eighth right intercostal space, between the axillary and mamillary lines, permit collection of the EMG activity of the inspiratory muscles. The signal can be integrated, and, depending on the calibration procedures used, semiquantitative or quantitative measurements may be obtained. Measurement with surface electrodes and integration of abdominal muscle activity during expiration may demonstrate the degree of active expiratory efforts that some of these children have to perform. Despite the increase in respiratory efforts associated with snoring and increased upper airway resistance, children may not present very fragmented sleep. The short alpha EEG arousals seen with increased upper airway resistance in adults may be much more uncommon here. Breathing may appear laborious, however, and increased efforts are often demonstrated by perspiration (at the head and neck or generalized). This suggests that the daytime sleepiness observed in these children despite near normal sleep structure and absence of microarousals cannot be explained by sleep fragmentation alone.

It may be hypothesized that some changes occurring in the child's metabolism may also be involved in daytime fatigue and sleepiness. These children sometimes exhibit failure to thrive, and usually they are slim and have difficulty increasing their weight, despite a normal appetite. They also may be shorter than expected. Nocturnal secretion of growth hormone in children with repetitive apneas has been shown to be abnormally low. We have noted a similar decrease with heavy snoring. Polygraphic monitoring must thus focus not only on the presence or absence of apnea (with the knowledge that absence of apnea may be very misleading) but also on increase in respiratory effort and breathing frequency, as well as the importance of thoracoabdominal mechanical changes.

The repetitive inspiratory efforts expended during complete or, more often, partial upper airway obstruction lead to abnormal septal motion with leftward shift of the interventricular septum and the development of pulsus paradoxus.[137] Cardiac arrhythmias, particularly asystole and secondary AV block, may be seen, and intermittent increase in systolic blood pressure may be noted. Finally, systemic hypertension has been observed in association with OSAS. Systemic hypertension in prepubertal children completely disappears with tracheostomy. The only cases of systemic hypertension found to be clearly idiopathic and for which treatment of OSAS led to complete and long-term normalization of blood pressure were in prepubertal or pubertal children.

### Asthma and Upper Airway Obstruction during Sleep

In children, a relationship exists between asthma and upper airway obstruction. Allergic reactions very early in life lead to mucosal swelling and enlargement of the pharyngeal region. There is a well-known interaction between the size of the upper airway and craniofacial development, particularly development of the mandible, during early childhood. Presence of upper airway allergies will thus limit maxillomandibular growth and cause a decrease in the size of the upper airway. Small upper airways are often associated with increased upper airway resistance during sleep, leading to increased respiratory efforts and the development of snoring during sleep. Increased upper airway resistance and nocturnal snoring worsen asthma, causing increased risk of a nocturnal asthma attack.

### Orthodontic Complications and Upper Airway Obstruction during Sleep

Children with partial or complete upper airway obstruction during sleep frequently have maxillomandibular growth retardation. Abnormal orthodontic features are common. Class II malocclusion is frequently seen but is not the only orthodontic problem. As 60% of facial development is complete by 4 years of age and 90% by 11 years of age, it is important to recognize orthodontic involvement. It is also important to understand that inappropriate orthodontic treatment that further impairs maxillomandibular growth may catalyze the appearance of snoring and significantly increase upper airway resistance during sleep. Abnormal maxillomandibu-

lar development may be responsible for the nocturnal occurrence of snoring and bruxism.

### Treatment

Age has an impact on therapeutic approaches.

*Tonsillectomy and Adenoidectomy*

Nasal obstruction is rarely the only factor in the development of apnea, but it can be a contributing factor. In such cases, correcting the obstruction can alleviate, if not cure, the OSAS. If there are markedly enlarged tonsils or adenoids with no other abnormal factors, the child should undergo tonsillectomy alone or tonsillectomy and adenoidectomy. Too often, however, not enough attention is paid to problems that may be associated with enlarged tonsils and adenoids (i.e., abnormally long soft palate, retroposition of the mandible, or soft tissue infiltration behind the base of the tongue), which may explain residual apnea after tonsillectomy. Furthermore, if tonsillectomy and adenoidectomy are performed during the prepubertal years in boys, there is a chance that the extensive soft tissue growth that occurs during puberty may cause a reappearance of OSAS in those whose airway space is already compromised by a malocclusion (a mild to moderate retroposition of the lower mandible). Fiberoptic endoscopy must be performed systematically in association with one imaging test to determine the extent of soft tissue surgery needed, but the classic UPPP is not recommended in children.

*Tracheostomy*

In the past, tracheostomy was a frequent treatment when tonsillectomy and adenoidectomy were insufficient. Tracheostomy resolves the OSAS, but it may cause secondary problems such as depression in children after surgery, and families commonly have difficulty accepting the surgery and caring for the stoma. Nevertheless, tracheostomy is clearly beneficial in many cases. The need for tracheostomy can be alleviated by the use of nasal CPAP.

*Nasal Continuous Positive Airway Pressure*

Prepubertal children as young as 6 months old have been treated with nasal CPAP at Stanford since

1984,[138] and long-term treatment has been successful. Several U.S. and foreign manufacturers (Respironics, Inc.; Healthdyne, Marietta, GA; SEFAM, Vandoeuvre les Nancy, France) currently supply nasal CPAP for young children, and Respironics provides masks for infants and very young children.

The complications and problems associated with this treatment have been related to (1) the fact that the children (many of whom were mentally retarded) had difficulty understanding how the mask and CPAP equipment functioned; (2) problems with the parents' collaboration with the medical team to train the child to keep the nasal mask on his or her face; (3) air leaks at the edge of the mask causing reappearance of apnea and eye irritation; and (4) skin allergy to the masks in small children. The first two problems resulted in some children abandoning nasal CPAP treatment; the other problems, although occasionally bothersome, never led to interruption of therapy. The theoretic risk of stomach dilation due to incorrect administration or other problems has never been reported. One issue to consider is that no system has an alarm to indicate complete displacement of the mask. In very young children, hand restraint during sleep may be necessary to adapt the child to the apparatus.

*Orthodontia and Maxillomandibular Surgery*

As previously indicated, children with OSAS often have a retroposition of the mandible, a steep mandibular plane, or an abnormally arched palate. These abnormalities are not always obvious. No one can overlook a Pierre Robin syndrome, but specialists do not always appreciate a mandibular problem, and orthodontists may not be aware of the impact on the upper airway of a moderately abnormal mandible. Orthodontic approaches may help redistribute growth and, in certain children, prevent the reappearance of snoring and sleep apnea, particularly in postpubertal boys.

When maxillofacial abnormalities are clearly related to the presence of OSAS in children, maxillofacial surgery may be considered. Piecuch[139] reported a child treated with maxillofacial surgery for OSAS. Kuo et al.[140] have reported two cases and Bear and Priest[141] three cases of OSAS that were resolved by maxillofacial surgery. The most extensive series of patients (teenagers and adults) treated with maxillofacial surgery was reported by Riley et al.[132,133] Although positive results have been reported

with surgery in pubertal children, we recommend investigating orthodontic approaches before considering it as a treatment for prepubertal children.

## SUMMARY

In summary, OSAS is common and must be considered a disease with diverse, adverse systemic consequences, including cardiovascular risk. As such, inquiries into the existence of snoring and EDS should be part of a physician's general examination. Because daytime somnolence appears in many guises, such as fatigue and cognitive difficulties, a high index of suspicion for this condition must be maintained. Sleep apnea diminishes the restorative capacity of sleep, thereby degrading quality of life. Evaluation and treatment are now readily available at sleep disorders centers. Treatment recommendations can be tailored to the patient's problems, taking into consideration individual preference, age, personality, lifestyle, and objective findings with PSG.

## REFERENCES

1. American Sleep Disorders Association. Obstructive Sleep Apnea Syndrome. In The International Classification of Sleep Disorders. Diagnostic and Coding Manual. Rochester, MN: American Sleep Disorders Association. 1990;52:342.
2. Strohl KP, Redline S. Recognition of obstructive sleep apnea. Am J Respir Crit Care Med 1996;154:279.
3. Gould GA, Whyte KF, Rhind GB, et al. The sleep hypopnea syndrome. Am Rev Respir Dis 1990; 142: 295.
4. Guilleminault C, Stoohs R, Clerk A, et al. A new cause of excessive daytime sleepiness: the upper airway resistance syndrome. Chest 1993;104:781.
5. Guilleminault C, Kim YD, Stoohs R. Upper airway resistance syndrome. Oral Maxillofacial Clin North Am 1995;7:243.
6. American Sleep Disorders Association. The International Classification of Sleep Disorders. Diagnostic and Coding Manual. Rochester, MN: American Sleep Disorders Association. 1990;346.
7. Berry DTR, Webb WB, Block AJ. Sleep apnea syndrome: a critical review of the apnea index as a diagnostic criterion. Chest 1984;86:529.
8. Guilleminault C, van den Hoed J, Mitler MM. Clinical Overview of the Sleep Apnea Syndromes. In C Guilleminault, W Dement (eds), Sleep Apnea Syndromes. New York: Liss, 1978;1.

9. Young T, Palta M, Dempsey J, et al. The occurrence of sleep disordered breathing among middle aged adults. N Engl J Med 1993;328:1230.

10. Bixler E, Kales A, Soldatos C, et al. Sleep apneic activity in a normal population. Res Commun Chem Pathol Pharmacol 1982;36:141.

11. Block AJ, Boysen PG, Wynne JW, Hunt LA. Sleep apnea, hypopnea, and oxygen desaturation in normal subjects: a strong male predominance. N Engl J Med 1979;300:513.

12. Guilleminault C, Quera-Salva MA, Partinen M, Jamieson A. Women and the obstructive sleep apnea. Chest 1988; 93:104.

13. Fletcher EC, DeBehnke RD, Lovoi MS, Gorin AB. Undiagnosed sleep apnea in patients with essential hypertension. Ann Intern Med 1985;103:190.

14. Coleman RM, Roffwarg HP, Kennedy SJ, et al. Sleep wake disorders based on a polysomnographic diagnosis. A national cooperative study. JAMA 1982;247:997.

15. Grunstein RR, Lawrence S, Spies JM, et al. Snoring in paradise—the Western Samoa Sleep Survey. Eur Respir J 1989;2(Suppl 5):4015.

16. Schmid-Nowara WW, Coultas D, Wiggins C, et al. Snoring in Hispanic-American population: risk factors and association with hypertension and other morbidity. Arch Intern Med 1990;150:597.

17. Redline S, Hans M, Pracharktam N, et al. Differences in the age distribution and risk factors for sleep-disordered breathing in blacks and whites. Am J Respir Crit Care Med 1994;149:577.

18. Strohl K, Saunders NA, Feldman NT, Hallet M. Obstructive sleep apnea. N Engl J Med 1978;299:969.

19. Redline S, Tishler PV, Tosteson TD, et al. Familial aggregation of obstructive sleep apnea. Am J Respir Crit Care Med 1995;151:682.

20. Guilleminault C, Partinen M, Hollman N, et al. Familial aggregates in obstructive sleep apnea syndrome. Chest 1995;107:1545.

21. Lavie P. Incidence of sleep apnea in a presumably healthy working population: a significant relationship with excessive daytime sleepiness. Sleep 1983;6:312.

22. Gislason T, Almqvist M, Eriksson G, et al. Prevalence of sleep apnea syndrome in Swedish men—an epidemiological study. J Clin Epidemiol 1988;41:571.

23. Bresnitz EA, Goldberg R, Kosinski RM. Epidemiology of obstructive sleep apnea. Epidemiol Rev 1994;16:210.

24. Redline S, Young T. Epidemiology and natural history of obstructive sleep apnea. Ear Nose Throat J 1993; 72:20.

25. He J, Kryger M, Zorick F. Mortality and apnea index in obstructive sleep apnea. Chest 1988;89:331.

26. National Commission on Sleep Disorders Research. Wake Up America: A National Sleep Alert (Vol 1). Submitted to the U.S. Congress, 1993.

27. Findley LJ, Weiss W, Jabour ER. Drivers with untreated sleep apnea: a cause of death and serious injury. Arch Intern Med 1991;151:1451.

28. Stoohs RA, Guilleminault C, Itoi A, Dement WC. Traffic accidents in commercial long-haul truck drivers: the influence of sleep-disordered breathing and obesity. Sleep 1994;17:619.

29. Findley LJ, Unverzagt ME, Suratt PM. Automobile accidents involving patients with obstructive sleep apnea. Am Rev Respir Dis 1988;138:337.

30. Shepard JW Jr, Garrison M, Grither D, Dolan GF. Hemodynamic responses to $O_2$ desaturation in obstructive sleep apnea [abstract]. Am Rev Respir Dis 1985;131:A106.

31. Schroeder JS, Motta J, Guilleminault C. Hemodynamic Studies in Sleep Apnea. In C Guilleminault, W Dement (eds), Sleep Apnea Syndromes. New York: Liss, 1978;177.

32. Guilleminault C, Motta J, Mihm F, Melvin K. Obstructive sleep apnea and cardiac index. Chest 1988;80:331.

33. Shiomi T, Guilleminault C, Stoohs R, Schnittger I. Leftward shift of the interventricular septum and pulsus paradoxus in obstructive sleep apnea syndrome. Chest 1991;100:894.

34. Fletcher E, Miller J, Schaaf J, Fletcher J. Urinary catecholamines before and after tracheostomy in obstructive sleep apnea. Sleep Res 1985;14:154.

35. Hoffstein V. Blood pressure, snoring, obesity, and nocturnal hypoxemia. Lancet 1994;344:643.

36. Working Group on OSA and Hypertension. Obstructive sleep apnea and blood pressure—what is the relationship? Blood Press 1993;2:166.

37. Lavie P, Ben-Yosef R, Rubin AE. Prevalence of sleep apnea among patients with essential hypertension. Am Heart J 1984;107:543.

38. Williams AJ, Houston D, Finberg S, et al. Sleep apnea syndrome and essential hypertension. Am J Cardiol 1985;55:1019.

39. Coccagna G, Mantovani M, Brignani F, et al. Continuous recording of the pulmonary and systemic arterial pressure during sleep in syndromes of hypersomnia with periodic breathing. Bull Physiol Pathol Respir 1972;8:1159.

40. Lund-Johansen P, White W. Central hemodynamics and 24 hour blood pressure in obstructive sleep apnea syndrome: effects of corrective surgery. Am J Med 1990;88:678.

41. Mayer J, Becker H, Brandenberg U, et al. Blood pressure and sleep apnea: results of long term nasal continuous positive airway pressure therapy. Cardiology 1991;79:84.

42. Hla KM, Young TB, Bidwell T, et al. Sleep apnea and hypertension: a population-based study. Ann Intern Med 1994;120:382.

43. Carlson JT, Hedner JA, Ejnell H, Peterson LE. High prevalence of hypertension in sleep apnea patients independent of obesity. Am J Respir Crit Care Med 1994;150:72.

44. Kiselak J, Clark M, Pera V, et al. The association between hypertension and sleep apnea in obese patients. Chest 1993;104:775.

45. Shepard JW. Gas exchange and hemodynamics during sleep. Med Clin North Am 1985;69:1243.

46. Hedner J, Wilcox I, Laks L, et al. A specific and potent pressor effect of hypoxia in patients with sleep apnea. Am Rev Respir Dis 1992;146:1240.

47. Krieger J, Laks L, Wilcox I, et al. Atrial natriuretic peptide release during sleep in patients with obstructive sleep apnea before and during treatment with nasal continuous positive airway pressure. Clin Sci 1989;77:407.

48. Follenius M, Krieger J, Krauth MO, et al. Obstructive sleep apnea treatment: peripheral and central effects on plasma renin activity and aldosterone. Sleep 1991; 14:211.

49. Krieger J, Reitzer B, Weitzenblum E, et al. Transmural pulmonary arterial pressure during obstructive sleep apneas. Sleep Res 1987;16:375.

50. Guilleminault C, Motta J, Mihm F, Melvin K. Obstructive sleep apnea and cardiac index. Chest 1986;89:331.

51. Krieger J, Weitzenblum E. Determinants of respiratory insufficiency in obstructive sleep apnea patients. Eur Respir J 1988;1:S96.

52. Leech JA, Onal E, Givan V, et al. Right ventricular dysfunction relates to nocturnal hypoxemia in patients with sleep apnea syndrome [abstract]. Am Rev Respir Dis 1985;131:A104.

53. Bradley TD, Rutherford R, Grossman RF, et al. Role of daytime hypoxemia in the pathogenesis of right heart failure in the obstructive sleep apnea syndrome. Am Rev Respir Dis 1985;131:835.

54. Bland JW Jr, Edwards KF, Brinsfield D. Pulmonary hypertension and congestive heart failure in children with chronic upper airway obstruction. Am J Cardiol 1969;22:830.

55. Tilkian RG, Guilleminault C, Schroeder JS, et al. Hemodynamics in sleep-induced apnea. Ann Intern Med 1976;85:714.

56. Tilkian AG, Motta J, Guilleminault C. Cardiac Arrhythmias in Sleep Apnea. In C Guilleminault, W Dement (eds), Sleep Apnea Syndromes. New York: Liss, 1978;197.

57. Miller WP. Cardiac arrhythmias and conduction disturbances in the sleep apnea syndrome. Am J Med 1982; 73:317.

58. Guilleminault C, Connolly SJ, Winkle RA. Cardiac arrhythmia and conduction disturbances during sleep in 400 patients with sleep apnea syndrome. Am J Cardiol 1983;52:490.

59. Shepard JW Jr, Garrison MW, Grither DA, Dolan GF. Relationship of ventricular ectopy to nocturnal $O_2$ desaturation in patients with obstructive sleep apnea. Chest 1985;88:335.

60. Shepard JW Jr. Cardiorespiratory Changes in Obstructive Sleep Apnea. In MH Kryger, T Roth, WC Dement (eds), Principles and Practice of Sleep Medicine. Philadelphia: Saunders, 1994;657.

61. Derman S, Karacan I, Hartse KM, et al. Changes in local cerebral blood flow measured by CT scan during wakefulness and sleep in patients with sleep apnea syndrome and narcolepsy [abstract]. Sleep Res 1981;10:190.

62. Meyer JS, Sakai F, Karacan I, et al. Sleep apnea, narcolepsy and dreaming: regional cerebral hemodynamics. Ann Neurol 1980;7:479.

63. Giombetti RJ, Kneisley LW, Miller BL, et al. Waking cerebral blood flow abnormality in sleep apnea syndrome. Sleep Res 1990;19:229.

64. Kneisley LW, Daly J, Giombetti RJ, et al. Partial reversal of abnormal waking cerebral blood flow in patients with sleep apnea. Sleep Res 1990;19:243.

65. Palomaki H, Partinen M, Juvela S, Kaste M. Snoring as a risk factor for sleep related brain infarction. Stroke 1989;20:1311.

66. Lugaresi E, Cirignotta F, Coccagna G, Piana C. Some epidemiological data on snoring and cardiocirculatory disturbances. Sleep 1980;3:221.

67. Spriggs D, French JM, Murdy JM. Historical risk factors for stroke: a case control study. Age Ageing 1990; 19:280.

68. Palomaki H. Snoring and the risk of brain infarction. Stroke 1991;22:1021.

69. He J, Kryger MH, Zorck FJ, et al. Mortality and apnea index in obstructive sleep apnea. Experience in 385 male patients. Chest 1988;94:9.

70. Partinen M, Jamieson A, Guilleminault C. Long-term outcome for obstructive sleep apnea: mortality. Chest 1988;94:1200.

71. Chaudhary BA, Sklar AH, Chaudhary TK, et al. Sleep apnea, proteinuria, and nephrotic syndrome. Sleep 1988;1:69.

72. Seliger M, Mendelson WB. Renal function in obstructive sleep apnea [abstract]. APSS Annu Meet (Toronto) 1991;138.

73. Weitzman ED, Pollack CP, Borowiecki B, et al. The Hypersomnia Sleep Apnea Syndrome: Site and Mechanism of Upper Airway Obstruction. In C Guilleminault, WC Dement (eds), Sleep Apnea Syndromes. New York: Liss, 1978;235.

74. Hill MW, Guilleminault C, Simmons FB. Fiberoptic and EMG Studies in Hypersomnia Sleep Apnea Syndrome. In C Guilleminault, W Dement (eds), Sleep Apnea Syndromes. New York: Liss, 1978;249.

75. Remmers JE, Launois S, Feroah T, Whitelaw WA. Mechanics of the Pharynx in Patients with Obstructive Sleep Apnea. In FG Issa, PM Suratt, JE Remmers (eds), Sleep and Respiration. New York: Wiley, 1991;261.

76. Guilleminault C, Hill MW, Simmons FB, Dement WC. Obstructive sleep apnea: electromyographic and fiberoptic studies. Exp Neurol 1978;62:48.

77. Guilleminault C, Motta J. Sleep Apnea Syndrome as a Long-Term Sequela of Poliomyelitis. In C Guilleminault, W Dement (eds), Sleep Apnea Syndromes. New York: Liss, 1978;309.

78. Hyland RH, Hutcheon MA, Perl A, et al. Upper airway occlusion induced by diaphragmatic pacing for primary alveolar hypoventilation: implications for the pathogenesis of obstructive sleep apnea. Am Rev Respir Dis 1981;124:180.

79. Simmonds AK, Branthwaite MA. Efficiency of negative ventilatory equipment. Thorax 1985;40:213.

80. Skatrud JB, Dempsey JA. Airway resistance and respiratory muscle function in snorers during NREM sleep. J Appl Physiol 1985;59:328.

81. Stoohs R, Guilleminault C. Snoring during NREM sleep: respiratory timing, esophageal pressure behavior and EEG arousal. Respir Physiol 1991;85:151.

82. Jamieson A, Guilleminault C, Partinen M, Quera-Salva MA. Obstructive sleep apneic patients have craniomandibular abnormalities. Sleep 1986;9:469.

83. Guilleminault C, Stoohs R. From "apnea of infancy" to obstructive sleep apnea syndrome in the young child. Chest 1992;102:1065.

84. Guilleminault C, Heldt G, Powell N, Riley R. Small upper airway: a familial risk for apnea in near-miss SIDS and their parents. Lancet 1986;1:402.

85. Larsson S-G, Gislason T, Lindholm C-E. Computed tomography of the oropharynx in obstructive sleep apnea. Acta Radiol 1988;29:401.

86. Vargervik K, Miller AJ, Chierici G, et al. Morphologic response to changes in neuromuscular patterns induced by altered modes of respiration. Am J Orthod 1984; 85:115.

87. Miller AJ, Vargervik K, Chierici G, Harvold E. Experimentally induced neuromuscular changes during and after nasal airway obstruction. Am J Orthod 1984; 85:385.

88. Vargervik K, Harvold E. Experiments on the interaction between orofacial function and morphology. Ear Nose Throat J 1987;66:201.

89. Partinen M, Guilleminault C, Quera-Salva MA, Jamieson A. Obstructive sleep apnea and cephalometric roentgenograms: the role of anatomic upper airway abnormalities in the definition of abnormal breathing during sleep. Chest 1988;93:1199.

90. Linder-Aronson S. Adenoids. Their effect on mode of breathing and nasal airflow and their relationship to characteristics of the facial skeleton and the dentition. Acta Otolaryngol Suppl 1970;265:1.

91. Solow B, Siersbaek-Nielsoen S, Greve E. Airway adequacy, head posture, and craniofacial morphology. Am J Orthod 1984;86:214.

92. Harvold EP. Neuromuscular and Morphological Adaptation in Experimentally Induced Oral Respiration. In RA McNamara (ed), Naso-Respiratory Function and Craniofacial (Monozygotic) [Cranio-Facial Growth Series]. Ann Arbor, MI: University of Michigan Center for Human Growth and Development, 1979;149.

93. Cooper BC. Naso-respiratory function and oro-facial development. Otolaryngol Clin North Am 1989;22:413.

94. Harmon E, Wynne JW, Block AJ. Sleep disordered breathing and oxygen desaturation in obese patients. Chest 1981;79:256.

95. Naimark A, Cherniack RM. Compliance of the respiratory system and its components in health and obesity. J Appl Physiol 1960;15:377.

96. Holley HS, Milic-Emili J, Becklake MR, Bates DV. Regional distribution of pulmonary ventilation and perfusion in obesity. J Clin Invest 1967;46:475.

97. Tucker DH, Sieker HO. The effects of change in body position on lung volumes and intrapulmonary gas mixing in patients with obesity, heart failure and emphysema. J Clin Invest 1960;39:787.

98. Zwillich CW, Sutton FO, Pierson DJ, et al. Decreased hypoxic ventilatory drive in the obesity-hypoventilation syndrome. Am J Med 1975;59:343.

99. Fink BR. Influence of cerebral activity in wakefulness on regulation of breathing. J Appl Physiol 1961;16:15.

100. Berthon-Jones M, Sullivan CE. Ventilatory and arousal responses to hypoxia in sleeping humans. Am Rev Respir Dis 1982;125:632.

101. Douglas NJ. Control of ventilation during sleep. Chest Clin N Am 1985;6:563.

102. Weill J, White DP, Douglas NJ, Zwillich CW. Ventilatory Control During Sleep in Normal Humans. In JB West, S Lahini (eds), High Altitude and Man. Bethesda, MD: American Physiological Society, 1984;91.

103. Hwang JC, St John WM, Bartlett D Jr. Afferent pathways for hypoglossal and phrenic responses to changes in upper airway pressure. Respir Physiol 1984;55:341.

104. Skatrud JB, Dempsey JA. Interaction of sleep state and chemical stimuli in sustaining rhythmic ventilation. J Appl Physiol 1983;55:813.

105. Dempsey JA, Skatrud JB. A sleep-induced apneic threshold and its consequences. Am Rev Respir Dis 1986;133:1163.

106. Widdicombe J, Sant'Ambrogio G, Mathew OP. Nerve Receptors of the Upper Airway. In OP Mathew, G Sant'-Ambrogio (eds), Respiratory Function of the Upper Airway. New York: Marcel Dekker, 1988;193.

107. Sullivan CE, Grunstein RR, Marrone O, Berthon-Jones M. Sleep Apnea—Pathophysiology: Upper Airway and Control of Breathing. In C Guilleminault, M Partinen (eds), Obstructive Sleep Apnea Syndrome. Clinical Research and Treatment. New York: Raven, 1990;49.

108. Lugaresi E, Cirignotta F, Coccagna G, Montagna P. Clinical Significance of Snoring. In NA Saunders, CE Sullivan (eds), Sleep and Breathing. New York: Marcel Dekker, 1984;283.

109. Guilleminault C. Obstructive sleep apnea syndrome: a review. Psychiatr Clin North Am 1987;4:607.

110. Baruzzi A, Riva R, Cirignotta F, et al. Atrial natriuretic peptide and catecholamines in obstructive sleep apnea syndrome. Sleep 1991;1:83.

111. Issa FG, Sullivan CE. Alcohol, snoring and sleep apnea. J Neurol Neurosurg Psychiatry 1982;45:353.

112. Guilleminault C, Silvestri R, Mondini S, Coburn S. Aging and sleep apnea: action of benzodiazepine acetazolamide, alcohol and sleep deprivation in a healthy elderly group. J Gerontol 1984;39:655.

113. Hudgel DW. Variable site of airway narrowing among obstructive sleep apnea patients. J Appl Physiol 1986;61:1403.

114. Chaban R, Cole P, Hoffstein V. Site of upper airway obstruction in patients with idiopathic obstructive sleep apnea. Laryngoscope 1988;98:641.

115. Shepard JW Jr, Thawley SE. Localization of upper airway collapse during sleep in patients with obstructive sleep apnea. Am Rev Respir Dis 1990;141:1350.

116. Ferber R, Millman R, Coppola M, et al. Portable recording in the assessment of sleep apnea: ASDA standards and practice. Sleep 1994;17:378.

117. Standards of Practice Committee of the American Sleep Disorders Association. Practice parameters for the use of portable recording in the assessment of obstructive sleep apnea. Sleep 1994;17:372.

118. Stiller RA, Strollo PJ, Sanders MH. Unattended recording in the diagnosis and treatment of sleep-disorder breathing: unproven accuracy, untested assumptions, and unready for routine use. Chest 1994;105:1306.

119. Carskadon MA, Dement WE, Mitler MM, et al. Guidelines for the Multiple Sleep Latency Test (MSLT): a standard measure of sleepiness. Sleep 1986;9:519.

120. Shepard JW, Gefter WB, Guilleminault C, et al. Evaluation of the upper airway in patients with obstructive sleep apnea. Sleep 1991;4:361.

121. Sher AE, Thorpy MJ, Shprintzen RJ, et al. Predictive value of Mueller maneuver in selection of patients for uvulopalatopharyngoplasty. Laryngoscope 1985; 95:1483.

122. Wittig R, Fujita S, Fortier J, et al. Results of uvulopalatopharyngoplasty in patients with both oropharyngeal and hypopharyngeal collapse on Muller maneuver. Sleep Res 1988;17:269.

123. Katsantonis GP, Maas CS, Walsh JK. The predictive efficacy of the Muller maneuver in uvulopalatopharyngoplasty. Laryngoscope 1989;99:677.

124. Bliwise DL, Bliwsie NG, Partinen M, et al. Sleep apnea and mortality in an aged cohort. Am J Public Health 1988;78:544.

125. Marcus EB, Curb JD, MacClean CJ, et al. Pulmonary function as a predictor of coronary heart disease. Am J Epidemiol 1989;129:97.

126. Enzi G, Vianello A, Baggio MB. Respiratory Disturbances in Visceral Obesity. In Y Oomura, S Tarui, S Inoue, T Shimazu (eds), Progress in Obesity Research. London: Libbey 1991;335.

127. Krieger J, Weitzenblum E, Manassier JP. Dangerous hypoxemia during continuous positive airway pressure treatment of obstructive apnea. Lancet 1983; 2:1429.

128. Waldhorn RE, Herrick TW, Nguyen MC, et al. Long-term compliance with nasal continuous positive airway pressure therapy of obstructive sleep apnea. Chest 1990;97:33.

129. Nino-Murcia G, McCann CC, Bliwise DL, et al. Compliance and side effects in sleep apnea patients treated with nasal continuous positive airway pressure. West J Med 1989;150:165.

130. Powell N, Riley R, Guilleminault C, Troell R. A reversible uvulopalatal flap for snoring and sleep apnea syndrome—short report: surgical technique. Sleep 1996;19:593.

131. Riley RW, Powell NB, Guilleminault C. Maxillofacial surgery and nasal CPAP. A comparison of treatment for obstructive sleep apnea syndrome. Chest 1990;98:1421.

132. Riley R, Powell NB, Guilleminault C, Nino-Murcia G. Maxillary, mandibular, and hyoid advancement: an alternative to tracheostomy in obstructive sleep apnea syndrome. Otolaryngol Head Neck Surg 1986;94:584.

133. Riley RW, Powell NB, Guilleminault C. Maxillofacial surgery and obstructive sleep apnea: review of 80 patients. Otolaryngol Head Neck Surg 1989;101:353.

134. Guilleminault C, Eldridge FL, Simmons FB, et al. Sleep apnea in eight children. Pediatrics 1976;58:28.

135. Guilleminault C, Korobkin K, Winkle R. A review of 50 children with obstructive sleep apnea syndrome. Lung 1981;159:275.

136. Guilleminault C, Winkle R, Korobkin R, et al. Children and nocturnal snoring: evaluation of the effects of sleep-related respiratory resistive load and daytime functioning. Eur J Pediatr 1982;139:165.

137. Guilleminault C, Shiomi T, Stoohs R, Schnittger I. Echocardiographic Studies in Adults and Children Presenting with Obstructive Sleep Apnea or Heavy Snoring. In C Gaultier, P Escourrou, L Curzi-Dascalova (eds), Sleep and Cardio-Respiratory Control (Vol 217). Paris: Collogue INSERM/Libbey, 1991;95.

138. Guilleminault C, Nino-Murcia G, Heldt G, et al. Alternative treatment to tracheostomy in obstructive sleep apnea: nasal CPAP in children. Pediatrics 1986; 78:797.

139. Piecuch JF. Costo-Chondral Drafts to Temporo-Mandibular Joints. In Abstracts and Proceedings of the Annual Meeting of the American Association of Oral and Maxillofacial Surgeons (Abstract 38). Chicago, 1978.

140. Kuo PC, West RR, Bloomquist DS, et al. The effect of mandibular osteotomy in 3 patients with hypersomnia sleep apnea. Oral Surg 1979;48:385.

141. Bear SE, Priest JH. Sleep apnea syndrome: correction with surgical advancement of the mandible. J Oral Surg 1980;35:543.

# Chapter 23

# Positive Airway Pressure in the Treatment of Sleep-Related Breathing Disorders

Mark H. Sanders, Patrick J. Strollo, Jr., and Ronald A. Stiller

## NASAL POSITIVE AIRWAY PRESSURE FOR OBSTRUCTIVE SLEEP APNEA AND HYPOPNEA

The application of nasal continuous positive airway pressure (CPAP) for the treatment of obstructive sleep apnea (OSA) in adults was first described in 1981.[1] Since that time, it has become the medical therapy of choice for obstructive sleep apnea or hypopnea (OSA/H).

In essence, conventional CPAP systems used to treat OSA/H patients consist of a blower unit that generates airflow and directs it downstream to the patient. Positive pressure is generated by variations in delivered airflow and resistance within the system. This pressure, delivered to the patient through one of several types of interfaces (discussed later), pressurizes and pneumatically splints the upper airway so that it remains patent. The splinting effect constitutes the primary mechanism of therapeutic action.[2] Some authors have speculated that nasal CPAP maintains upper airway patency during sleep by virtue of reflex augmentation of dilator muscle tone. This reflex was postulated to be mediated through increased end-expiratory lung volume accompanying CPAP administration.[3–5] Alternatively, it has been postulated that the direct relationship between lung volume and upper airway patency could be due to traction on mediastinal and upper

airway structures created during lung inflation.[6,7] Although upper airway resistance does vary directly with lung volume, this effect is relatively small.[8] Furthermore, Sériès and coworkers[2] have demonstrated that there is no significant alteration in the impact of CPAP on upper airway resistance when the increase in lung volume is prevented by the concomitant application of positive extrathoracic pressure. Controversy regarding the degree to which lung inflation contributes to the therapeutic effect of CPAP still exists, however. Sériès et al.[5] reported a patient in whom obstructive apnea was virtually eliminated during sleep in a poncho-type negative pressure ventilatory device that increased functional residual capacity by 0.5 liters during wakefulness. Although apneas were eliminated, the apnea-hypopnea index (AHI) remained substantially elevated, consistent with persistent hypopneas. Abbey et al.[9] observed that CPAP substantially reduced the respiratory event index in four patients, whereas application of continuous negative extrathoracic pressure did not, despite comparably increased lung volume. Finally, several investigators have demonstrated that the administration of nasal CPAP depresses electromyographic activity of the upper airway dilator muscles, which is evidence against a reflex-mediated reduction in upper airway resistance.[10–12] Regardless of the mechanism, nasal CPAP has documented effectiveness in eliminating obstructive and mixed apneas.[13] Some "central" apneas, particularly those observed in patients with predominantly obstructive events, are also elimi-

Supported in part by Department of Veterans Affairs Medical Center and NHLBI Training Grant NHLBI2T32HL0756311A2.

nated by nasal CPAP.[13,14] This finding strongly supports the contention of Sanders and coworkers[15,16] that the central portion of mixed apneas and many central apneas may actually represent delayed inspiratory effort due to prolongation of the preceding expiration. These investigators hypothesized that this increase in expiratory time is related to expiratory upper airway instability with augmented upper airway resistance and slowing of expiratory airflow.

Within a short time after the initiation of nasal CPAP therapy during sleep, most OSA/H patients report increased daytime alertness, relief of morning headaches, decreased nocturnal awakenings, improved temperament, increased ability to focus their attention, and a sense of well-being.[17-19] There is also improvement in objective measures of daytime sleepiness (assessed by the Multiple Sleep Latency Test [MSLT]), the ability to enforce wakefulness, and perceived sleepiness or alertness after introduction of CPAP therapy.[18-24] Reduced subjective daytime sleepiness has been reported after just one night of nasal CPAP therapy.[25] However, Lamphere and coworkers[26] reported that progressive increases in daytime alertness, objectively assessed by MSLT, may occur over several weeks after initiation of therapy. It is possible, however, that suboptimal nightly compliance contributed to the gradual nature of improvement, given that objective measures of patient use of CPAP were not used. Nonetheless, the progressive nature of the improvement in symptoms highlights the importance of recognizing that patients may not be sufficiently alert to fully resume daily activities (especially those who must operate vehicles or perform potentially dangerous tasks) within the first several days of treatment. To better assess the improvement in symptoms of daytime sleepiness, the health care provider should have follow-up contact with the patient soon after the initiation of therapy. Close follow-up will facilitate evaluation of the patient's ability to perform activities that require alertness as well as to assess therapeutic compliance (see later discussion).

Clinical experience indicates that nasal CPAP maintains upper airway patency and acceptable oxygenation during sleep in the overwhelming majority of patients with OSA. Some individuals continue to have alveolar hypoventilation and oxyhemoglobin desaturation on the basis of persistent partial upper airway obstruction, despite maximal achievable or tolerable levels of CPAP. Under these circumstances, supplemental oxygen can be added to the CPAP system, either directly into the mask or into the tubing that leads to the mask.[27-30] Other patients continue to have episodic reductions in oxyhemoglobin saturation or reset their baseline saturation to unacceptably low levels on nasal CPAP, despite elimination of discrete apneas and hypopneas.[31] These individuals often have underlying lung or chest wall abnormalities that impair gas exchange during wakefulness. Such abnormalities take on greater physiologic significance during sleep, when there is a reduction in ventilatory chemosensitivity, alteration of ventilatory muscle function, and "load" compensation.[32-37] In these patients, initiation of noninvasive positive-pressure ventilation, rather than CPAP, may be useful for augmenting ventilation to prevent hypercapnia and desaturation during sleep, as well as to promote normalization of awake $Paco_2$ (see later discussion). After the awake $Paco_2$ approaches a normal value, CPAP may provide sufficient nocturnal therapy.[31]

The literature suggests that OSA/H contributes, at least modestly, to diurnal systemic arterial hypertension.[38] It is conceptually appealing to speculate that CPAP application would have a beneficial impact on hypertension, given that this modality of positive-pressure therapy has reduced sympathetic activation[39-41] and atrial natriuretic peptide secretion in OSA/H patients during sleep. Unfortunately, there are only limited published data addressing the impact of CPAP on hypertension in OSA/H patients. Suzuki et al.[42] observed a decrease in daytime systolic pressure from 152.3 to 141.2 mm Hg ($P = .08$) and a decrease in diastolic pressure from 91.8 to 85.1 mm Hg ($P = .14$) in hypertensive patients after initiation of CPAP therapy during sleep. Specifically during sleep, systolic pressure decreased from 133.9 to 125.9 ($P = .04$) and diastolic pressure decreased from 76.8 to 73.7 mm Hg ($P = .08$) for patients on CPAP therapy. The relatively slight reduction in blood pressure may be attributable to the mild degree of baseline hypertension in the study population. In 14 patients who were compliant with CPAP therapy, Wilcox and coworkers[43] observed a statistically significant reduction in mean systolic and diastolic pressures over a 24-hour period (systolic pressure = 141 ± 18

**Table 23-1.** Side Effects of Nasal Continuous Positive Airway Pressure (CPAP)

| Side Effect | Management Measures[a] |
|---|---|
| Mask-related | |
| Skin abrasion or rash | Optimize mask fit from wide selection of commercially available types of masks (select nonallergenic material)[46]; protective skin covering; customized mask; reinforce hygienic care of device |
| Conjunctivitis from air leak | Eye patch |
| Pressure or airflow-related | |
| Chest discomfort | Pressure ramp; reduce pressure with bilevel positive airway pressure[29]; try to reduce requisite pressure using oral appliance and CPAP |
| Aerophagia | |
| Sinus discomfort | |
| Smothering sensation | |
| Difficulty exhaling | |
| Difficulty initiating or maintaining sleep | |
| Pneumothorax or pneumo-mediastinum | |
| Pneumoencephalus | |
| Problems related to the nasal route | |
| Rhinorrhea | Heated humidification[57,58]; saline nasal spray; topical nasal steroid preparation; consider trial of nasal aerosol of ipratropium bromide solution; chin-strap for oral dryness; oronasal mask interface[52,53]; desensitization over time[51]; oronasal mask interface[52,53] |
| Nasal congestion, nasal or oral dryness | |
| Epistaxis (may be massive, especially in anticoagulated patients) | |
| Other | |
| Noise | Longer tubing to move device further from bedside |
| Cumbersomeness or inconvenience | Intensify education of patient and spouse |
| Spousal intolerance | Recommend attending a patient support group[b] |

[a]Reference provided when available.
[b]Contact A.W.A.K.E. Network of the American Sleep Apnea Association.

$\rightarrow 134 \pm 19$ mm Hg, $P <.02$; diastolic pressure = $89 \pm 11 \rightarrow 85 \pm 13$ mm Hg, $P <.05$, mean $\pm$ SD). It should be noted that these investigators excluded morbidly obese patients (>150% ideal body weight) from the study. When considering the modest nature of the changes in blood pressure after initiation of therapy, it is important to recognize that hypertension in most OSA/H patients is probably multifactorial with a substantial contribution from obesity and genetic influences. In addition, it is likely that hypertension in these individuals is a chronic problem, and the degree to which it is reversible through nonpharmacologic intervention is uncertain. Similarly, it is not known if a favorable impact of CPAP on blood pressure requires a minimum duration of therapy to become evident. In this context, it has been hypothesized that vascular remodeling, with uncertain reversibility, may occur over time in hypertensive patients.[44] Further studies are needed

to establish our expectations of CPAP treatment in terms of simplifying antihypertensive therapy in OSA/H patients.

### Side Effects of Continuous Partial Airway Pressure Therapy

Like most treatment interventions, nasal CPAP is associated with a variety of generally minor but troublesome side effects (Table 23-1).[18,21,24,45–50] These are most often attributable to either the patient-device interface or the sensation of high airflow or pressure. Rather than complaining of side effects, some patients simply find that nasal CPAP is too cumbersome and interferes with their lifestyle to an unacceptable degree.[3,46,48] Such individuals are often, but not invariably, younger patients who are unable to envision indefinite nasal CPAP therapy. On the other hand, most clinicians have patients who consider nasal CPAP an inconvenience worth enduring.

Occasionally, patients complain of claustrophobia in conjunction with enforced breathing through a nasal mask or nasal prongs.[47,48,51] One alternative is to use an oronasal mask, which permits breathing through either the oral or nasal route (see later).[52–54] Another approach to the claustrophobic patient is a desensitization program used to acclimatize the patient to nasal CPAP.[51] Although further study will be required to determine effectiveness and the optimal method, it is possible that desensitization will be helpful in selected patients.

Problems with skin abrasion or leakage of air directed into the eyes, with or without consequent conjunctivitis,[55] may result from a poor mask fit. Mask leaks have been reported to increase in prevalence once CPAP exceeds 12 cm $H_2O$.[45,46,56] These difficulties can generally be overcome by trying different sizes of commercially available masks, with use of a protective skin barrier, or by fabrication of a customized mask.[46] Other complaints related to the nasal route of breathing include nasal dryness, congestion, and rhinorrhea. The reported prevalence of such effects varies from 25% to 65%.[45,46,56] Nasal dryness and congestion can occasionally be treated simply with either administration of saline nasal spray at bedtime or with a room humidifier. More commonly, but not invariably, a topical nasal steroid is effective. Addition of a low-resistance humidifier to the CPAP system may also be extremely helpful for certain patients. Richards et al.[57] documented increased nasal airway resistance in the presence of high nasal flow, such as occurs when there is a mouth leak during nasal CPAP application. Incorporation of a heated, but not an unheated, humidifier into the CPAP system minimized the increase in nasal resistance, presumably by increasing the relative humidity of the inspired gas and reducing release of inflammatory mediators. The superiority of heated humidifiers to cold, passover humidifiers in restoring relative humidity to inhaled air was confirmed in a study by Fleury et al.[58] Although routine use should be discouraged, occasional administration of a vasoconstrictive nasal spray may be helpful when nasal congestion is related to a self-limited condition such as an upper respiratory tract infection.

Although nasal dryness is rarely a serious problem, a case of massive epistaxis was reported in a patient with sleep apnea, right ventricular dysfunction, and a coagulopathy.[56] The authors believed that mucosal dryness contributed to the epistaxis, which did not recur after placement of a humidifier in the CPAP system. In light of this report, it seems prudent to treat patients with bleeding tendencies who are on nasal CPAP with particular care and to consider humidifying the delivered air from the outset of therapy.

We have found rhinorrhea to be a more difficult problem to solve. Although this is a significant complaint in only approximately 5% of our patients, it was present in approximately 10–35% of cases reported in the literature.[3,24,46] The cause of the rhinorrhea is uncertain. Although it may be related to drying of the airways, we have not found cold-water humidification to be of noteworthy benefit. Similarly, Pépin et al.[46] did not observe a beneficial effect from humidification, but it is uncertain if a heated humidifier was used. Therefore, it may be worth trying a heated water-bath humidifier, as described earlier, for the treatment of rhinorrhea. It is also possible that this problem is related to stimulation of pressure-sensitive nasal mucosal receptors.[59] We have found the administration of cromoglycate or anticholinergic nasal sprays such as ipratropium bromide to be variably effective among patients with rhinorrhea. As noted previously, nasal steroids have been observed to provide more consistent benefit.

When providing positive-pressure therapy, the clinician must always consider the potential for barotrauma. Surprisingly, pneumomediastinum and pneumothorax are not prevalent in OSA/H patients receiving CPAP, at least as assessed by review of the literature. Pneumocephalus has been reported in one OSA patient with a cerebrospinal fluid leak who was placed on nasal CPAP.[60] Pneumocephalus has been described as a complication of CPAP application with a full-face mask in patients with head trauma and should be considered when any patient using CPAP therapy develops a nasal discharge or neurologic signs and symptoms, including headache, seizures, dizziness, or cranial nerve palsy.

A small number of patients complain of chest discomfort on nasal CPAP therapy.[13,50,59] This is probably related to increased end-expiratory pressure and the consequent elevation of resting lung volume,[10] which stretches the chest wall muscles and cartilaginous structures, creating a sensation of chest wall pressure that persists through the hours of wakefulness. Although the complaint of chest discomfort should be completely evaluated in any patient, if a cardiopulmonary workup in the OSA/H patient on CPAP is nondiagnostic, efforts should be made to reduce the expiratory pressure, if necessary by using bilevel positive airway pressure (BIPAP) (discussed later). Similarly, a certain proportion of patients feel discomfort when exhaling against positive expiratory pressure.[18] If the level of CPAP cannot be satisfactorily reduced, a trial of BIPAP should be considered (see later).

Although it is usually beneficial to patients with OSA/H, administration of nasal CPAP may be associated with negative effects on arterial blood gases and oxyhemoglobin saturation. Krieger and colleagues[61] reported severe oxyhemoglobin desaturation during nasal CPAP therapy in a hypercapnic sleep apnea patient with cor pulmonale. Similarly, Piper and Sullivan[31] reported persistent desaturation despite CPAP administration with supplemental oxygen to hypercapnic OSA/H patients. Although the cause of this desaturation is not certain, it may be due to one or more of the following factors: (1) worsening hypoventilation related to the added mechanical impedance to ventilation associated with exhalation against increased pressure, (2) increased dead-space ventilation,[62] and (3) a decrease in venous return and cardiac output due to increased intrathoracic pressure during CPAP administration in patients with impaired right or left ventricular function and inadequate filling pressure. With regard to the potential contribution of alveolar hypoventilation to nocturnal oxyhemoglobin desaturation during CPAP therapy, Fukui et al.[63] noted that nasal CPAP failed to reduce sleep-related hypercapnia during non–rapid eye movement sleep in OSA/H patients. Although clinical situations such as this are not common, it highlights the prudence of conducting CPAP trials under monitored conditions in patients at high risk for nocturnal hypoventilation, including individuals with chronic ventilatory failure (awake hypercapnia), and morbidly obese individuals.

Despite the above caveats and troublesome experiences, nasal CPAP administration has also been reported to improve awake arterial blood gases in sleep apnea patients with hypercapnia and cor pulmonale.[64–66] The mechanism responsible for augmented alveolar ventilation during wakefulness in these persons has not been clearly defined. Berthon-Jones and Sullivan[67] reported a leftward shift in the ventilatory response to carbon dioxide ($CO_2$) without a change in the slope of the line describing the relationship between $CO_2$ tension and ventilation. This reinforced the results of an earlier study by Guilleminault and Cummiskey,[68] demonstrating augmented ventilatory responsiveness to $CO_2$ after tracheostomy. These data are consistent with a reduction in the chemoreceptor set-point to $Paco_2$ after initiation of therapy. Although the question was not specifically addressed by these investigators, this alteration of the ventilatory response to $CO_2$ might be related to reduced serum buffering capacity as a result of relief from apnea and decreased $CO_2$ retention during sleep while on CPAP. The data of Fukui et al.[63] and others, however, suggest that CPAP does not reduce $Paco_2$ during sleep.[62] Alternatively, enhanced chemosensitivity to $CO_2$ during wakefulness may be due to relief of hypoxic depression of central nervous system respiratory centers or sleep deprivation.[69] Improved ventilation during wakefulness could also be due to improved ventilatory muscle function. Further studies are needed before conclusions can be made with confidence.

### Acceptance and Compliance with Continuous Partial Airway Pressure Therapy

The most significant disadvantage to nasal CPAP therapy is its volitional nature. Patients must actively participate in their own treatment or CPAP will not provide effective therapy.

The acceptance rate of nasal CPAP varies across a number of studies. Nineteen of the 115 patients (17%) reported by Waldhorn et al.[50] were either unable to sleep with CPAP, unable to complete a nocturnal trial in the laboratory, or refused to use CPAP at home. In a study by Rauscher and coworkers,[70] 72% of 65 patients accepted home CPAP therapy after a full-night titration. Krieger et al.[19] reported that 153 (21%) of 728 OSA/H patients (AHI >15) who underwent a full-night CPAP titration refused home therapy. The reasons for nonacceptance include difficulties falling asleep, frequent nocturnal awakenings, and mask discomfort. Acceptors of CPAP therapy were more likely to complain of greater tiredness as well as episodes of falling asleep at undesirable times.[70] These investigators noted that the patients who refused CPAP therapy had less severe OSA/H, were less obese, and had less objectively measured sleepiness as assessed by the MSLT than those who accepted therapy.

In recent years, there has been increasing application of "split-night" polysomnography (PSG), in which the initial portion of the night is used in performing a diagnostic evaluation for OSA/H.[71–76] If the diagnosis of OSA/H is established during the initial portion of the night, a therapeutic titration of CPAP is undertaken. The impact of this paradigm has begun to be explored. In a study by Fleury et al.,[74] 75% of patients who underwent a split-night diagnostic evaluation and CPAP titration accepted therapy. In contrast, the data reported by Strollo et al.[76] from our laboratory reflected acceptance by only 62–67% of patients (depending on whether patients who were lost to follow-up were considered nonacceptors). Although the different results may be related to the fact that the patients in the latter study had a lower AHI ($27.1 \pm 40.6$) than those evaluated by Fleury et al. (AHI, $63.6 \pm 20.5$), the data provide some level of concern that abbreviated titration regimen may impact on patient willingness to accept CPAP treatment. This issue requires further study.

Once a patient has "accepted" CPAP therapy, he or she must be compliant with it. Until relatively recently, patient compliance with chronic CPAP therapy was assessed using subjective reporting of patient use.[27,28,50,77–79] Studies indicated that compliance varies from approximately 65% to 85%. Investigators and clinicians currently objectively monitor patient compliance with meters (incorporated into the CPAP devices) that record the duration of time that the device has been running. This enables calculation of the average daily hours of CPAP use over a given time interval. It is now known that subjective patient reports overestimate time of use.[24,46,48,80] It might be preferable to know not only the number of hours that the machine is turned on, but the number of hours that the CPAP device is actually delivering the prescribed pressure. This would not only provide information related to patient compliance, but would also add insight into how well the machine is functioning. It is of some comfort, however, to know that absolute machine run-time is highly correlated with time-at-pressure[21,48,80]; in this respect, a simple hour-meter is probably adequate, although perhaps not optimal.

**Table 23-2.** Compliance with Nasal Continuous Positive Air Pressure Therapy

| Study | Hours of Use |
|---|---|
| Fletcher and Luckett[49] | $6.1 \pm 2.2$ (SD) |
| Krieger[87] | $5.6 \pm 0.1$ (SE) |
| Kribbs et al.[48] | $4.88 \pm 2.0$ (SD) |
| Engleman et al.[21] | $4.7 \pm 0.4$ (SE) |
| Engleman et al.[22] | $3.7 \pm 0.4$ (SE) |
| Meurice et al.[24] | $6.02 \pm 2.5$ (SD) |
| Reeves-Hoché et al.[80] | 4.7 |
| Pépin et al.[46] | $6.5 \pm 3.0$ (SD) |
| Strollo et al.[76] | $5.2 \pm 2.2$ (SD) (full-night titration) |
| | $3.8 \pm 2.9$ (SD) (split-night titration) |

SD = standard deviation; SE = standard error of mean.

Information regarding the degree to which a patient is compliant with CPAP is essential for assessment of therapeutic impact. If a patient's symptoms are inadequately resolved after the initiation of CPAP treatment, it may be due to delivery of insufficient pressure to maintain upper airway patency during sleep, misdiagnosis of the etiology of the individual's symptoms, the contribution of comorbid elements to the patient's symptoms, or failure to use the device for a sufficient duration on a regular basis. Objective compliance readings can provide insight into the latter possibility. Over the last several years, a number of studies have examined patient compliance with nasal CPAP (Table 23-2). These investigations indicate that, in general, use of nasal CPAP ranges from 4 to 6 hours per day, with considerable interindividual variability. Despite the use of hour-meters, however, there are considerable gaps in our knowledge of patient compliance with this therapy. For example, although the clinician may know the average duration of daily CPAP, the *total sleep time* is not known. This information is highly desirable for optimal interpretation of the machine-use data. Four hours of CPAP use may reflect acceptable compliance if the patient is asleep for only 4.5 hours. On the other hand, 4 hours of CPAP use may represent inadequate compliance if the patient is asleep for 8 hours. It is evident that obtaining information about a patient's usual bed and sleep time is an important element of the follow-up evaluation subsequent to initiation of CPAP therapy and is essential for proper interpretation of data recorded on the CPAP device's hour-meter.[81]

Another limitation of a simple hour-meter that provides information about average daily CPAP use is that it affords no insight regarding the pattern of use. Thus, an average 5 hours of daily CPAP use inferred from the hour-meter may reflect 5 hours of use each day of the week, 8 hours on each of 4 days and 1 hour on the remaining 3 days of the week, or any other combination. New generations of CPAP devices will have software that allows the clinician to obtain a graphic illustration of the daily pattern of use, including the number of days of use per week, and the time of day that the device is used on any given day.

How much CPAP use is required to completely reverse the symptoms as well as the physiologic impact of OSA/H and prevent them from recurring? Existing data suggest that optimal relief of daytime sleepiness requires nightly use of CPAP. Both Kribbs et al.[82] and Sforza and Lugaresi[83] reported that sleeping for as little as one night without CPAP results in increased sleepiness. Is it necessary to use CPAP for the entire night, however? Hers et al.[84] observed that when CPAP was discontinued after 4 hours, there was a persistent beneficial effect on oxyhemoglobin saturation and sleep continuity for the remainder of the night. The investigators postulated that the persistent improvement results from the impact of improved sleep continuity (achieved during the initial portion of the night while on CPAP) on upper airway stability during the latter portion of the night (after CPAP was removed). This hypothesis is based on earlier data demonstrating increased upper airway collapsibility after a period of sleep fragmentation.[85] Hers and coworkers[84] as well as McNicholas[86] speculated that at least some OSA/H patients use CPAP for only part of the night because they derive a satisfactory degree of symptomatic benefit from this limited application. This speculation heightens awareness of the deficiencies in current understanding of the determinants of compliance with CPAP therapy. Greater insight into this issue would facilitate treatment modifications that would promote universal acceptance and compliance by patients.

### Determinants of Compliance and Strategies to Optimize Acceptance and Compliance

Increasing evidence suggests that the pattern of CPAP use (or nonuse) by an individual is determined within a short period after initiating home therapy, perhaps within a matter of weeks.[47,48,81,87] Despite considerable efforts by a number of investigators, however, the determinants of patient compliance remain unclear. Some reports suggest that compliance improves with increased severity of daytime sleepiness.[50,88] It should be noted that the patient's perception of daytime sleepiness (assessed using a specific questionnaire,[48] a "hypersomnia score,"[24] or the Epworth Sleepiness Scale[89]) predicts compliance with CPAP more reliably than the MSLT, which is an objective measure of sleepiness.[18,21,48] Several investigators have observed that compliant patients cannot consistently be differentiated from noncompliant patients by the frequency or variety of side effects to CPAP therapy, initial AHI, gender, weight, or the prescribed level of CPAP.[18,21,48–50,80,90] In a larger patient population reported by Krieger et al.,[87] and with the patients studied by Meurice et al.,[24] however, CPAP use was correlated with AHI and the degree of improvement during the initial titration of CPAP.

As discussed earlier, patients commonly experience side effects in conjunction with nasal CPAP therapy (see Table 23-1). Although several studies have reported that the prevalence of side effects is comparable in compliant and noncompliant patients,[48,50,88] it would be inappropriate to conclude that side effects have no impact on acceptance and compliance with therapy. It is likely that the perception of a given side effect varies across individuals, and therefore may have a different degree of impact. Thus, a simple comparison of prevalence in compliant and noncompliant patients may be misleading and could obscure the impact of a particular side effect on the compliance of individual patients. Most investigators report cessation of therapy by individual patients due to one or more of the side effects presented in Table 23-1.[18,21,24,46–48] Furthermore, it is not surprising that Engleman et al.[21] noted that patients who complained of side effects used CPAP to a lesser degree than those without complaints.

Every precaution should be taken by the clinician to minimize the side effects of positive-pressure therapy in an effort to maximize therapeutic compliance and the patient's quality of life (see Table 23-1). Several practices that may enhance patient acceptance and compliance with CPAP therapy are described in Table 23-1 as well as later in this chapter.

Appropriate patient selection for chronic CPAP therapy is an important factor. It is intuitively obvious that any patient who has been coerced into taking a nasal CPAP unit home, even after efforts have been made to explain the need for the device and the manner in which it operates, is unlikely to use it conscientiously on a long-term basis. Therefore, nasal CPAP should be provided only to patients who are receptive to using it or who are sufficiently open-minded to give it a reasonable home trial. It is also likely that the patient's initial exposure to CPAP therapy and the manner in which the level of therapeutic pressure is established play significant roles in his or her willingness to accept this treatment.

### Traditional and Evolving Methods of Initiating Continuous Partial Airway Pressure Therapy

Traditionally, patients have undergone an attended, PSG-monitored trial of nasal CPAP to establish therapeutic levels of pressure before being sent home for long-term therapy. Because the requisite level of CPAP may vary according to body position during sleep, clinicians should be certain that the delivered pressure is effective in maintaining adequate upper airway patency and oxygenation during sleep in all positions. It also provides an opportunity for the patient to examine the CPAP unit and various interfaces before retiring to sleep on positive pressure. The most comfortable and leak-free interface with the device (i.e., nasal mask, prongs, or oronasal mask) can be selected. After this selection, while the patient is still awake, positive pressure may be administered across a wide range of pressures, to permit familiarization with associated sensations. Another advantage of attended evaluation of the patient on CPAP is the immediate availability of knowledgeable and caring health care professionals who can respond to questions and allay concerns. When wearing nasal CPAP for the first time, patients have been anecdotally reported to awaken in the middle of the night disoriented and frightened by the apparatus. Under these circumstances, reassurance is readily supplied by the laboratory personnel conducting the trial.

Several other benefits have also been attributed to PSG-monitored trials of CPAP therapy. Fry and coworkers[91] observed an increased frequency of periodic leg movements (PLMs) during sleep, with and without accompanying arousals during nasal CPAP therapy. These investigators hypothesized that the improved sleep quality and architecture associated with relief of OSA/H by nasal CPAP "unmasks" PLMs. If this is the case, a patient may experience physiologic relief of OSA/H with maintenance of acceptable oxygenation on nasal CPAP but not obtain symptomatic abatement of daytime sleepiness or fatigue because of persistent sleep fragmentation attributable to the PLMs. More recent data have strongly suggested that PLMs occurring in conjunction with untreated or inadequately treated OSA/H may reflect limb movements secondary to arousals terminating unrelieved apneas, hypopneas, or episodes of increased upper airway resistance (upper airway resistance syndrome) because the arousals and the PLMs may diminish with CPAP therapy.[92,93] Thus, a monitored initial trial of CPAP addresses many issues and concerns that, if not considered, may lead to dismissal of this form of therapy as a viable therapeutic option. Attention to these factors at the outset of therapy will maximize the opportunity for a successful outcome.

### Split-Night Diagnostic and Continuous Partial Airway Pressure Titrations

The foregoing considerations notwithstanding, the current health care environment has fostered exploration of alternative means of establishing CPAP therapy for OSA/H. As noted earlier in this chapter, some clinicians are requesting that diagnostic and CPAP titrations be conducted in single, split-night studies. Although this may lead to a satisfactory CPAP prescription for many patients (a CPAP prescription consists of the pressure that maintains satisfactory upper airway patency and oxyhemoglobin saturation during sleep, while providing satisfactory sleep continuity using an interface that is well-tolerated by the patient),[71,73,74] there are many patients for whom the duration of time available for CPAP titration is too limited in the context of a split-night study to determine a satisfactory prescription.[75] In particular, patients with milder degrees of OSA/H, in whom the titration is initiated later in the night (because more prolonged monitoring was needed to establish the diagnosis of OSA/H) are more likely to have unsuccessful split-night titrations. The potential impact of such abbreviated titrations on acceptance and compliance always requires consideration. Data from an uncontrolled study by Fleury et al.[74] suggest that compliance may not be altered by a split-night methodology. As noted earlier, however, one case-controlled study suggested that acceptance is reduced after a split-night and found a trend for lower therapeutic compliance in patients who had undergone a split-night titration compared with those who had undergone a full-night titration (see Table 23-2).[76] These data do not constitute evidence for a negative impact of split-night studies but indicate the need for further study of this issue.

## Home Continuous Positive Airway Pressure Titration

Some investigators have advocated in-home initiation of CPAP therapy using both attended monitoring[94] and unattended, unmonitored titrations.[95] Waldhorn and Wood[94] described titration of CPAP by a technologist in the patient's home using a portable four-channel monitor recording heart rate, chest wall movement, CPAP pressure in the mask, and oxyhemoglobin saturation to guide CPAP adjustment. Compliance with CPAP therapy in this group of 17 patients averaged 7.23 ± 1 hour (mean ± SD) per night, which is comparable to values obtained by conventional in-laboratory titration. Whether attended in-home titration provides a cost-effective and efficient alternative to in-laboratory methodology remains to be determined.

Coppola and Lawee[95] reported experience with unattended home CPAP titration. Eleven patients experienced increases in CPAP level in response to telephone interviews between the clinician, patient, and bed partner, which revealed persistent snoring, apnea observed by the bed partner, or symptoms consistent with OSA/H. The authors reported positive subjective outcome and compliance with this technique. The applicability of this paradigm across all home environments and social conditions, as well as for patients without bed partners, remains to be determined. Similarly, larger studies addressing the impact of unattended CPAP titration

on objectively measured acceptance and compliance are needed.

## Use of Predictive Formulas to Estimate or Establish the Continuous Positive Airway Pressure Prescription

Several investigators have suggested that the requisite level of CPAP can be estimated with sufficient clinical accuracy to obviate the need for monitored titration, thus providing a starting point at which titration may begin either in the monitored environment to maximize the time available to fine-tune the final pressure prescription, or in the home setting with further adjustments made on the basis of clinical guidelines or the results of home diagnostic evaluation.[96,97] Miljeteig and Hoffstein[96] reported that the three variables that best predicted the minimal therapeutic CPAP level (defined as the level that reduced the AHI to <10) were BMI, AHI, and neck circumference. This combination accounted for approximately 67% of the variability in minimal CPAP level in a group of 38 patients ($CPAP_{min} = -5.12 + 0.13 \times BMI$ [kg/m$^2$] + 0.16 × neck circumference [cm] + 0.04 × AHI). In a subsequent data set from 129 patients, reported in the same paper, the minimal CPAP predicted from this equation was 8 ± 2.1 cm $H_2O$, and the value obtained during laboratory titration was 8.1 ± 3 cm $H_2O$ (mean ± SD). Seventy-one percent of patients had predicted values within 2.5 cm $H_2O$ of the measured values, and 95% had predicted CPAP levels within 5 cm $H_2O$ of the measured values (Figure 23-1A). The investigators pointed out that the predictive equation may not be applicable to all patients due to variability in individual responses to a given level of CPAP. In addition, it may also be important that elimination of respiratory-related arousals, as may be seen in the upper airway resistance syndrome,[98] was not included in the criteria for defining effective CPAP level. In a subsequent study of 29 patients, Hoffstein and Mateika[97] prospectively tested the predictive value of the equation. For the group as a whole, there was no significant difference between the predicted and the PSG-titrated CPAP levels. In 38% of patients, $CPAP_{predicted} = CPAP_{titrated}$; in 38% of patients, $CPAP_{predicted}$ was within 1 cm $H_2O$ of $CPAP_{titrated}$; in 15% of patients, $CPAP_{predicted}$ was within 2 cm $H_2O$ of $CPAP_{titrated}$; in 8% of patients, $CPAP_{predicted}$ was >2 cm $H_2O$ of $CPAP_{titrated}$ (Figure 23-1B). In general, $CPAP_{predicted}$ underesti-

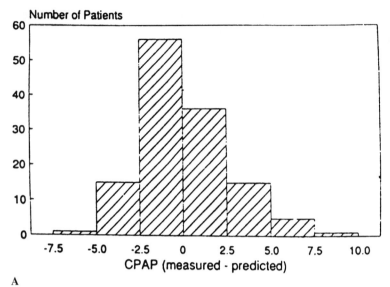

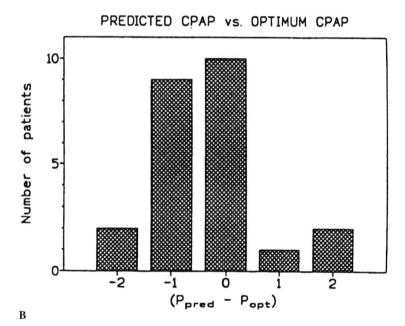

**Figure 23-1.** (**A**) Distribution of differences between predicted and actual continuous positive airway pressure (CPAP) levels. (Reprinted with permission from H Miljeteig, V Hoffstein. Determinants of continuous positive airway pressure level for treatment of obstructive sleep apnea. Am Rev Respir Dis 1993;143:1529.) (**B**) Results of prospective validation of predictive formula to predict CPAP level. Distribution of differences between predicted and actual CPAP levels. (Reprinted with permission from V Hoffstein, S Mateika. Predicting nasal continuous positive airway pressure. Am J Respir Crit Care Med 1994;150:487.)

mated $CPAP_{titrated}$. $CPAP_{predicted}$ was grossly inaccurate in 8% of the patients, being too high in one case and too low in the other. Once again, the definition of acceptable treatment did not include elimination of breathing-related arousals or snoring.

*Auto-titrating Continuous Positive Airway Pressure Devices*

Modern, fixed-level CPAP machines deliver a constant pressure to the patient throughout the applica-

**Figure 23-2.** (A) Typical inspiratory wave patterns used in one algorithm to detect upper airway dysfunction. (Reprinted with permission from M Berthon-Jones. Feasibility of a self-setting CPAP machine. Sleep 1993;16:S121.) (B) Signal used in one algorithm to detect upper airway dysfunction. (Reprinted with permission from K Behbehani, F-C Yen, JR Burk, et al. Automatic control of airway pressure for treatment of obstructive sleep apnea. IEEE Trans Biomed Eng 1995;42:1009.)

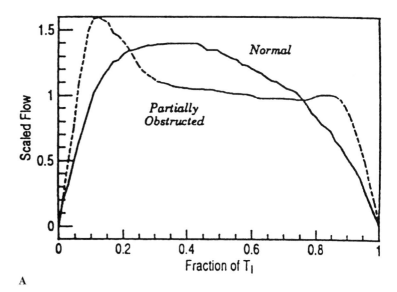

A

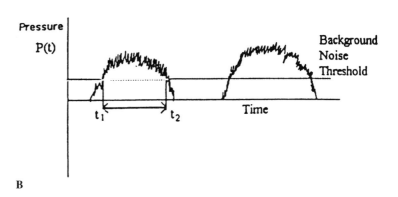

B

tion period (e.g., all night). It is well-recognized, however, that upper airway collapsibility or the pressure required to stabilize the upper airway during sleep varies with several factors, including body position.[28,99–102] Although alcohol consumption reduces upper airway stability during sleep,[103–109] there are conflicting data regarding whether there is an increase in the requisite level of CPAP after alcohol ingestion.[110,111] Evidence suggests that benzodiazepine ingestion also increases upper airway instability during sleep[105,112] and CPAP requirements may increase after administration of these agents. Upper airway collapsibility may change with sleep stage, and the level of CPAP needed to maintain upper airway patency may decrease over the months after initiation and nightly use of this ther-

apy.[113] In recognition of these issues, auto-titrating CPAP has been developed. The goal of this technology is to provide a floating level of pressure, the magnitude of which varies dynamically in response to the physiologic status of the upper airway. These devices use various algorithms to recognize if the upper airway is occluded (apnea), partially obstructed (hypopnea or snoring), or normally patent[114–117] (Figure 23-2). Having identified abnormal upper airway function, the devices respond by appropriately adjusting the pressure upward. Conversely, in the absence of algorithm-based identifiers of upper airway dysfunction for a specified time interval, the pressure is adjusted downward (Figure 23-3). Thus, unlike fixed CPAP machines that are titrated to a level that maintains upper air-

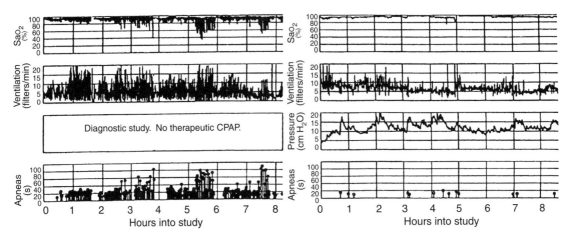

**Figure 23-3.** Patient breathing without (*left panel*) and with (*right panel*) auto-titrating continuous positive airway pressure. (Reprinted with permission from O Pollo, M Berthon-Jones, NJ Douglas, CE Sullivan. Management of obstructive sleep apnoea/hypopnoea syndrome. Lancet 1994;344:657.)

way patency under conditions of greatest collapsibility, regardless of whether these conditions exist at any given time, the auto-titrating devices are at least theoretically capable of responding to changing physiologic conditions and providing the lowest required pressure. This has potential implications for both initiation of CPAP therapy and perhaps long-term therapeutic compliance.

Several studies indicate that a variety of auto-titrating CPAP devices compare favorably with fixed CPAP devices with respect to reducing the mean AHI and arousal frequency and improving oxygenation.[114,115,117–120] Several investigators have reported that the comparable beneficial effects were obtained with lower mean overnight levels of CPAP during auto-titrating CPAP than fixed CPAP therapy.[117,120]

Before the clinician adopts a prescription of chronic auto-titrating CPAP therapy without or after an in-laboratory trial, however, several important features of the published studies should be carefully considered. Virtually all of the investigations assessing the effectiveness of auto-titrating CPAP that have been published to date in peer-reviewed journals have examined this device in an attended, monitored environment. Most of these investigations report that the technologist was permitted to intervene and adjust the mask position if significant leaks were detected, manually readjust the device in the presence of inadequate sensing or patient intolerance of pressure, or provide other assistance

to the patient.[117–121] In addition, in some instances, data collected during periods of mouth or mask leaks (this included all data obtained from one patient) were excluded from analyses, thereby potentially biasing the results.[118,119] The published literature also suggests that mouth breathing or leaks may prove particularly troublesome for auto-titrating devices.[114,115] In virtually all published studies, there have been some patients who were unable to tolerate the rapid changes in pressure[118,121] or in whom the device performed in a less than optimal manner.[115,119,120] To our knowledge, no published studies have compared the acceptance rate of auto-titrating versus fixed CPAP. One study, however, suggested that long-term compliance with auto-titrating CPAP was significantly better than with fixed CPAP (6.5 ± 1 vs. 5.1 ± 1.1 hours per night, respectively; $P = .02$).[122]

It has been suggested that one venue for auto-titrating CPAP is application in the sleep laboratory with subsequent examination of the data to determine the optimum level of CPAP to prescribe for chronic therapy with a fixed CPAP device. This would enable titration in an attended environment but without obligating the technologist to manually adjust the level of CPAP. This would reduce the technologist's responsibilities and perhaps bring down the ratio of technologists to patients (with resultant reduction in cost). In support of this proposed practice, several investigators have reported that selection of a single best therapeutic pressure by visually examining the range of CPAP delivered by an auto-titrating device across a night resulted in a pressure that was comparable to, or slightly greater than, that obtained by manual titration of fixed CPAP during PSG.[118,119]

In summary, auto-titrating CPAP is a promising technology, but its role is yet to be clearly defined. If auto-titrating CPAP is presently used, it may be most prudent to use it in a laboratory environment to establish the single best level to use as a basis for a fixed CPAP prescription. In addition, there are other components to the CPAP prescription, such as the interface, about which decisions must also be made.

### Follow-Up of Continuous Positive Airway Pressure Patients

As noted previously, it appears that an individual's pattern of CPAP use (or nonuse) is established very shortly after initiating home therapy.[47,48,81,87] It is therefore reasonable to hypothesize that early and consistent contact between the patient and the caregiver in an effort to identify and resolve problems with therapy and provide encouragement and support would facilitate compliance. In fact, the literature provides conflicting information on this subject. Two studies have suggested that positive reinforcement through periodic telephone contact with a nurse, both without or in conjunction with a program of visits by a nurse, do not favorably influence therapeutic compliance.[49,123] In contrast, considerably larger investigations have demonstrated improved compliance in conjunction with intensive education and support measures after initiation of home treatment.[19,87,124–126] A study by Chervin and coworkers[127] revealed that patients who had received educational literature regarding sleep-disordered breathing and CPAP or BIPAP use and patients who received follow-up telephone calls from health care personnel were more compliant than patients who had received neither intervention. It is also essential that a physician and staff experienced in the care of OSA/H patients act as a continuing resource for answers to questions and reassurance when uncertainties arise. At our center and others, patient support groups serve a very important function in fostering a climate of openness and sharing of information, as well as providing a forum for discussion of issues relevant to all types of sleep-disordered breathing (e.g., OSA/H, nocturnal ventilatory failure associated with neuromuscular and chest wall disorders) and overall health. Group meetings provide patients with the realization that they are not and should not be isolated by their disorder. This is crucial, because many OSA/H patients have been labeled by society as obese, lazy, or malingerers, resulting in social ostracism and low self-esteem. Many of these consequences of OSA/H are reversible by nasal CPAP therapy, with remarkable and gratifying results for all concerned. In our experience, there is no doubt that important benefits are obtained from support groups, judging from the high rate of attendance and favorable patient comments.

In summary, compliance with nasal CPAP, a treatment that entails a relatively cumbersome box at or near the bedside and an equally cumbersome (if not unappealing) interface over the nose, is surprisingly good. Compliance with CPAP compares favorably to therapies that most would consider substantially less inconvenient, such as meter-dose inhalers for asthma.[128] Undoubtedly, this relatively high rate of compliance relates to the remarkable symptomatic improvement experienced by the majority of users.

## Patient–Positive-Pressure Device Interface Options

### Nasal Prong Systems

In their initial report, Sullivan and coworkers[1] applied CPAP via nasal prongs sealed in the nares using medical-grade silicon rubber. Subsequently, self-sealing nasal masks and nasal prongs have been used as interfaces between the patient and the positive-pressure device.[64,129–131] One study (published in abstract form) suggested that there is roughly equal initial acceptance of the two interfaces.[132] It is worth noting that a relatively large number of patients in that study changed their preference after using one particular interface for a period of time. Thus, because the requisite pressures do not seem to vary,[130,132] patients should be made aware that this choice remains open to them at all times during their treatment. There have been no published studies of the impact of nasal prongs on compliance with therapy. It is likely, however, that this option favorably influences acceptance by patients who are unable or unwilling to use a mask interface.

Presently, clinicians and patients have the option of using either custom-made or commercially available nasal masks and prongs.[46,133] The nasal masks have the advantage of providing individualized and optimal fit, whereas the prongs offer the convenience of an off-the-shelf product. Clinicians also have the option to use an oronasal mask for patients who are unwilling or unable to use an exclusively nasal interface.

### Positive Airway Pressure Delivered by Oronasal Mask

Practitioners occasionally encounter patients who are either intolerant of nasal masks or prongs or unable to keep their mouth sufficiently closed during sleep to permit maintenance of adequate positive intrapharyngeal pressure. In our experience, a chin-strap is only variably helpful, and when necessary, the delivery of positive pressure via an oronasal mask should be considered. This interface has been successful for a substantial majority of the patients in whom it has been applied.[52,53] Although use in OSA/H has not been reported, Criner and coworkers[54] successfully administered positive-pressure ventilatory assistance to patients in chronic respiratory failure via a total face mask. If proven effective in OSA/H patients, without problematic increases in dead space, the oronasal mask may be a useful addition to interface options. Some patients who have proved to be intolerant of nasal masks or prongs are equally intolerant of the oronasal mask and nasal interfaces. In addition, on rare occasion, application of positive pressure via the oronasal mask fails to alleviate upper airway obstruction.

Particular care must be taken when using an oronasal mask, owing to the potential risk of aspiration of gastric contents if the patient vomits. Although this complication has not been encountered in our patients with OSA/H or neuromuscular disease who have received nocturnal positive-pressure ventilatory support via oronasal mask, it remains a concern. It is reassuring, however, that the use of prophylactic nasogastric tubes has not been recommended by other investigators as a routine precaution for critically ill patients who are receiving CPAP via oronasal mask and who did not have risk factors for

vomiting.[134,135] Patients using an oronasal mask for chronic nocturnal positive-pressure therapy should be instructed not to take anything by mouth for at least 3 hours before applying the positive pressure. Furthermore, before initiating positive-pressure therapy via an oronasal mask, patients should be instructed to notify their physician if they are experiencing nausea or vomiting from any cause.

Coverage of both the nose and mouth by an oronasal mask also raises theoretic concerns regarding the potential consequences of machine failure when airflow that can be entrained by the patient through a nonfunctional or dysfunctional device is limited or nonexistent. Safety valves should be incorporated in the circuit close to the patient to facilitate inhalation of fresh air or minimize dead space in the event of machine malfunction. Ideally, an alarm should also be present to signal power failure.

### Variations of Positive Airway Pressure Therapy for Sleep-Disordered Breathing

Some patients find the administration of positive pressure sufficiently bothersome to result in complete intolerance of therapy or unsatisfactory compliance. To minimize adverse consequences associated with the delivery of positive pressure, several therapeutic alternatives are available.

### Pressure Ramping

For some patients, the sensation of positive pressure is unpleasant enough to cause difficulty in initiating sleep. Pressure ramping of CPAP allows adjustment of the rate of rise in delivered pressure over time, from a negligible level to the target pressure required to maintain upper airway patency during sleep. This modification provides a time window during which the delivered pressure is lower than the target pressure, thereby making it easier for the patient to fall asleep (Figure 23-4). Because the level of positive pressure may be transiently below that required to maintain upper airway patency during sleep, pressure ramping may allow apnea, hypopnea, and oxyhemoglobin desaturation to occur for a variable period, until the pressure reaches the prescribed, optimal value. At the present, no published studies address the level of risk that the delay in optimal pressure delivery may pre-

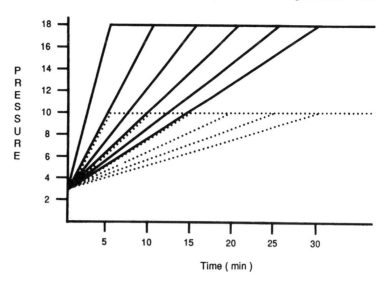

**Figure 23-4.** Pressure ramping. Pressure can be gradually increased over prescribed periods to reach target pressure (here illustrated as 10 cm $H_2O$ and 18 cm $H_2O$). (Reprinted with permission from Healthdyne Technologies Corp.)

sent to patients, nor are data available regarding the effectiveness of pressure ramping on patient compliance with CPAP therapy. Pressman and coworkers[136] described a case of "ramp abuse" in which a patient repeatedly awoke to reactivate the ramp whenever the target pressure approached. This resulted in repetitive episodes of oxyhemoglobin desaturation (because the pressure was subtherapeutic during the time that the patient was asleep) and arousals (probably due to a combination of persistent OSA/H and awakening to activate the ramp). As Pressman et al. pointed out, such abuse will not be detected if only the run time of the CPAP machine is monitored as a reflection of compliance. Monitoring run time at the prescribed pressure, however, would give the clinician insight into this activity. Thus, although pressure ramping is a conceptually attractive feature, its degree of effectiveness and safety remains to be documented, and the specific patient populations for which it might provide maximal benefit have yet to be identified.

*Bilevel Positive Airway Pressure Therapy*

As noted previously, a number of troublesome side effects associated with positive pressure can preclude adequate therapeutic tolerance or safety of CPAP administration. Some side effects, including a smothering sensation, chest wall discomfort, and bothersome nasal or sinus pressure, are related to the sensation associated with breathing against a positive pressure. In addition, some patients may be at increased risk for barotrauma because of emphysema or bullous lung disease (although a review of the literature suggests that this is not a prevalent complication of CPAP therapy for OSA/H), whereas in others, elevated expiratory pressure may be associated with a tendency toward alveolar hypoventilation.[31] One potential way to mitigate these side effects is to reduce the delivered pressure to the minimum level that maintains acceptable upper airway patency, sleep continuity, and oxyhemoglobin saturation.

Studies of the pathogenesis of OSA/H have indicated that upper airway resistance increases during expiration, despite the absence of negative intrapharyngeal pressure.[16,137,138] Sanders and coworkers[15] speculated that instability of the upper airway during expiration is the initial event in the sequence leading to obstructive apnea. Sanders and Kern[29] hypothesized that the splinting action of positive pressure in the upper airway during both inspiration and expiration was necessary to eliminate obstructive events, and that less pressure is required to maintain adequate upper airway patency during expiration than during inspiration. This was based on the hypothesis that during expiration, inherent upper airway instability represents the primary factor that favors airway closure, whereas during inspiration inadequate upper airway patency is related to two factors: the collapsing influence of negative intraluminal pressure and the inherent instability of the airway. The importance of expiratory events was subsequently demonstrated by Schwab et al.[139–141] using computed tomographic and magnetic resonance imaging to observe expiratory narrowing of the upper airway. Application of expiratory positive airway pressure by Mahadevia and colleagues[142] was associated with a reduction in apnea frequency, although these investigators postulated that the improved upper airway function was related to increased oxyhemoglobin saturation secondary to increased functional residual capacity.

Using BIPAP, which provides independently adjustable inspiratory positive airway pressure (IPAP) and expiratory positive airway pressure (EPAP), Sanders and Kern[29] observed that OSA/H patients could be treated with lower expiratory pressure than inspiratory pressure. BIPAP delivers EPAP at a level that is sufficient to prevent the upper airway from being occluded during or at end-expiration. Then, at the initiation of inspiratory effort, minimal inspiratory airflow triggers delivery of a predetermined level of IPAP before the airway can be collapsed by the developing negative intrapharyngeal pressure. The IPAP prevents generation of negative intraluminal pressure and maintains upper airway patency throughout inspiration. Over and above simply preventing complete upper airway occlusion, delivery of a sufficient level of IPAP augments upper airway patency, thus eliminating partial obstructions (hypopneas) as well as desaturations and arousals from sleep. If the airway were to become occluded during expiration, IPAP would not be triggered and the apnea would become apparent.

In a preliminary investigation of 13 patients with OSA/H in which optimal settings of nasal CPAP and BIPAP were compared, Sanders and Kern[29] noted that in each patient the EPAP delivered during BIPAP was significantly lower than the level of CPAP, and the mean value of EPAP for the group was 37% lower than the required level of CPAP ($P$ <.001). On the other hand, there was no difference between the level of IPAP during BIPAP administration and the level of CPAP. Thus, comparable relief of OSA/H was achieved using both modalities, despite the lower mean pressure during the BIPAP trial. In all patients, apnea was not relieved until a critical level of EPAP was reached, reinforcing the importance of positive-pressure delivery in maintenance of upper airway patency. However,

EPAP did not need to be as high as IPAP because persistent obstructive hypopneas were eliminated by increasing the IPAP alone. All patients considered BIPAP more comfortable than conventional CPAP, a finding attributed to greater comfort associated with exhaling against lower pressure. A number of subsequent studies have confirmed the effectiveness of BIPAP in the treatment of OSA/H in adults and children.[143–146]

It is reasonable to suspect that compliance with therapy would improve by lowering the pressure against which patients have to exhale. Indeed, patients who are intolerant of CPAP can often be successfully switched to a bilevel device.[73,147] In a prospective, randomized study, Reeves-Hoché et al.[148] compared therapeutic compliance of one group of OSA/H patients who received BIPAP treatment with another group treated with CPAP. Over a 12-month period, there was no difference in the average number of hours per day that the devices were used (5 ± 1.9 hours vs. 4.9 ± 0.23 hours, CPAP and bilevel device, respectively; mean ± SE). There was a significantly greater number of dropouts in the CPAP compared with the bilevel group, however, and the investigators speculated that this might be related to greater comfort of the latter modality. This is consistent with improved acceptance of bilevel pressure, although the study also suggests that in those patients who continue to use positive-pressure therapy in the home environment, there appears to be no difference between bilevel devices and CPAP with regard to the average number of hours used per day. The investigators further suggested that an additional study be conducted to determine the usefulness of bilevel devices as salvage therapy for CPAP failure.

Ferguson and Gilmartin[149] raised concerns about $CO_2$ rebreathing on BIPAP, particularly at EPAP levels lower than 8 cm $H_2O$. This rebreathing was related to incomplete washout of exhaled gas from the tubing that therefore acted as a reservoir. The problem was corrected with the use of specific exhalation (non-rebreathing or plateau) valves. Hill and colleagues[150] called the clinical significance of rebreathing into question when they reported no change in daytime and nocturnal $Pa_{CO_2}$ when bilevel pressure was used with any of a variety of exhalation valves. In addition, there was no effect of the type of valve on overnight heart rate, respiratory rate, or the patient's daytime symptoms.

Thus, the clinician should be aware of the possibility of $CO_2$ rebreathing and consider using a valve designed to minimize this, particularly if a suboptimal therapeutic outcome is evident.

Most BIPAP devices can be used in three modes. In one mode, IPAP can be delivered in response to a patient trigger. In another mode, the patient can trigger the delivery of IPAP and the physician can set the device so that IPAP is delivered at prescribed intervals if a spontaneously triggered delivery does not occur within that interval. This backup feature is rarely needed in the treatment of patients with OSA/H. It has been helpful in providing nocturnal ventilatory assistance to other patient groups, such as those with ventilatory muscle dysfunction owing to neuromuscular disease and nocturnal hypoventilation attributable to chest wall deformities (e.g., kyphoscoliosis) (see later). The backup feature can also be useful for patients with central sleep apnea. In these patients, spontaneous triggering facilitates tolerance of the device by the awake patient, whereas during sleep the timed BIPAP "breaths" delivered at prescribed intervals prevent the long breathing pauses between lung inflations that are characteristic of central sleep apnea.[151] It is now recognized that at least in some patients, central sleep apnea events may be associated with a closed upper airway.[152–154] Thus, it may be necessary to provide a critical level of EPAP to facilitate delivery of IPAP to the patient. Otherwise, higher levels of IPAP may be required to open the closed airway, which may disrupt sleep. Finally, in the *timed* mode, the patient cannot spontaneously trigger the delivery of IPAP, as it is administered only at the intervals prescribed by the health care professional. In our experience, use of this mode has little clinical usefulness in the treatment of OSA/H patients.

Thus, BIPAP may be a therapeutic alternative for patients who find nasal CPAP uncomfortable or for those in whom the delivery of positive airway pressure represents an unacceptable degree of risk (i.e., patients with bullous lung disease). The lower expiratory pressure also tends to minimize chest discomfort, as end-expiratory lung volume is not increased as much when the expiratory pressure is lower. This may be beneficial in certain patients. In addition, the risk of hypoventilation due to augmented mechanical impedance, which was described earlier, is probably also reduced with the lower expiratory pressures. This may be of particular advantage to patients with ventilatory muscle weakness or chest wall abnormalities and in some patients with OSA/H (discussed later). Although it is clear that a measurable number of patients prefer BIPAP to CPAP, the majority are comfortable using CPAP. Determining whether the theoretic advantages of BIPAP translate into uniformly better patient acceptance and the degree to which bilevel devices provide salvage therapy for patients who are noncompliant with CPAP awaits completion of controlled, prospective studies.

*Auto-Titrating Continuous Positive Airway Pressure*

Auto-titrating CPAP devices have been previously discussed in detail. It is anticipated that the primary application of this modality will be in the laboratory, because there are limited published studies of their effectiveness during chronic home therapy or their impact on patient acceptance and compliance.[155]

### Alcohol and Continuous Positive Airway Pressure Therapy

Specific clinical circumstances may require particular consideration and decision making with regard to therapeutic trials of positive airway pressure therapy for OSA/H. For example, it is well-established that alcohol augments upper airway instability and suppresses the arousal response, thus enhancing the frequency and duration of apneas and hypopneas.[106,109,156] On this basis, it is generally accepted that OSA/H patients should abstain from alcohol. Clinical experience indicates that this advice is often incompletely heeded by some patients. Given the adverse but transient impact of alcohol on upper airway stability, it is possible that the pressures required to maintain airway patency during sleep vary with the patient's alcohol consumption immediately before the application of the positive-pressure trial. Some reassurance to the contrary may be obtained from a report indicating that moderate alcohol consumption (1.5–2.0 ml/kg) does not significantly alter the level of positive pressure required to maintain upper airway patency during sleep in OSA patients.[111] Similarly, using an auto-titrating CPAP device, Teschler et al.[157] observed no change in median pressure or the recommended therapeutic pressure after consuming 1.5 ml/kg of vodka (40% alcohol). This does not obviate the need to advocate abstinence. Nonetheless, it is important to establish an honest relationship with patients, and if it is clear that an individual is not going to alter his or her alcohol-consumption habits, it is reasonable to conduct the evaluation of positive-pressure therapy under the prevailing, rather than artificially enforced and temporary, life circumstances. Similarly, patients who must regularly use medication that may increase the likelihood of upper airway obstruction during sleep should be allowed to maintain their usual regimen at the time of PSG evaluation.

### Altitude and Continuous Positive Airway Pressure Therapy

Most modern CPAP devices automatically compensate for changes in altitude, which are associated with changes in ambient barometric pressure. Some older machines, however, do not provide such compensation, and with increasing altitude, deliver progressively lower than prescribed pressure.[158] The clinician should consider this factor in evaluating a patient with recurrent symptoms of OSA/H who has relocated to a higher altitude from that at which the level of prescribed CPAP was determined. Conversely, this factor should be considered in assessing the patient who now complains of discomfort from the sensation of pressure after having moved to a lower altitude from that at which CPAP was prescribed.

### Other Uses for Positive Airway Pressure in Treating Sleep-Disordered Breathing

Positive airway pressure may be useful for diagnostic as well as therapeutic purposes in patients with clinical signs and symptoms consistent with OSA/H. Occasionally, patients have multiple sleep disorders, such as PLMs as well as OSA/H, both of which may contribute to sleep fragmentation and excessive daytime sleepiness. As discussed earlier, it has been demonstrated that PLMs may reflect a primary movement disorder that persists or even becomes more evident during CPAP administration[91] in some patients. In others, however, PLMs may represent a phenomenon that is secondary to breathing-related

arousals.[92,93] In individual patients, it is preferable to identify the primary pathophysiology of the PLMs to direct the initial therapeutic effort. Positive airway pressure therapy provides a noninvasive means of eliminating the OSA/H component of the patient's disorder complex and permits assessment of any residual or unmasked clinical and physiologic abnormalities. Similarly, some patients suffer from intercurrent narcolepsy and OSA/H, either of which may contribute to excessive daytime sleepiness. In patients for whom relief of excessive daytime sleepiness, rather than nocturnal oxyhemoglobin desaturation, is the primary therapeutic objective, distinguishing which (if any) is the principal causative disorder directs and simplifies treatment. For example, if elimination of OSA/H adequately relieves excessive daytime sleepiness despite coexisting narcolepsy, the latter disorder may not warrant specific pharmacologic intervention. Oral appliance therapy may offer the same noninvasive advantages. CPAP is more readily applied, however, and the effects generally can be more rapidly assessed.

As public awareness of sleep-disordered breathing increases, more patients are brought to medical attention because of concern about snoring (or socially disruptive snoring) or observed apnea during sleep. Many of these patients do not report symptoms classically associated with OSA/H. Indeed, many such persons have "low-level" abnormalities of sleep-related breathing and oxygenation that are of uncertain clinical significance. Because there are no accepted guidelines establishing the minimal level of OSA/H that is associated with adverse clinical or physiologic outcomes, it is important to document that patients with minimal OSA/H but no evident physiologic sequelae are truly asymptomatic before dismissing the need for active therapeutic intervention. Not infrequently, patients do not realize their level of impairment and believe themselves to be asymptomatic until OSA/H is relieved. Thus, a trial of nocturnal positive-pressure therapy, perhaps in conjunction with multiple sleep latency or wakefulness testing, may help determine the impact of OSA/H. Failure of positive-pressure therapy to favorably influence the patient's clinical condition or improve daytime alertness after upper airway stabilization during sleep suggests that, in fact, the nocturnal disordered breathing had no subjective impact. Unfortunately, the usefulness of positive airway pressure therapy in this context may be limited by the inability of some asymptomatic individuals with minimal OSA/H to tolerate any of the available therapeutic devices. Care must also be taken to ensure that the positive-pressure therapy does not itself induce sleep fragmentation and increase daytime sleepiness.

A trial of positive airway pressure therapy may also be informative in patients on the other end of the clinical spectrum from the patient with putative OSA/H or nonapneic snoring. These patients have symptoms disproportionately severe relative to objectively documented OSA/H (i.e., they are very symptomatic, despite relatively mild OSA/H). It is conceivable that the degree of sleep fragmentation associated with subtle degrees of upper airway dysfunction is underestimated by standard recording techniques in these individuals.[17,159,160] Such a trial may support or mitigate against a cause-and-effect relationship between OSA/H and the patient's complaints. Persistence of symptoms despite relief of OSA/H suggests the need to consider the presence of a nonpulmonary sleep-wake disorder.

## POSITIVE AIRWAY PRESSURE THERAPY OF NONAPNEIC SLEEP-DISORDERED BREATHING

### Congestive Heart Failure and Periodic Breathing (Cheyne-Stokes Respiration)

Sleep-disordered breathing is common in patients with stable congestive heart failure (CHF).[161–163] Javaheri et al.[163] observed that 45% of patients with a left ventricular ejection fraction (LVEF) had an AHI that was greater than 26 events per hour of sleep. The abnormal breathing events were predominantly central in nature (possibly reflecting Cheyne-Stokes respiration [CSR]) and the frequency of events was negatively correlated with LVEF. The presence of sleep-disordered breathing was associated with sleep fragmentation and increased nocturnal hypoxemia. This observation has several important implications: (1) There is a high prevalence of daytime sleepiness in patients with CSR in conjunction with CHF.[164] (2) Patients with CHF who also have CSR have a higher mortality than patients who have CHF without CSR. (3) CSR, AHI, and the frequency of arousals were correlated with

mortality.[165,166] It is therefore noteworthy that CPAP has been reported to have a favorable impact on sleep and breathing in patients with CHF and CSR. After 10 days to 14 weeks of nasal CPAP therapy, Takasaki and coworkers[167] observed a decrease in AHI (primarily central events) from 69.9 ± 9 to 15 ± 7 (mean ± SE, $P < .005$), an improvement in the nadir of overnight oxyhemoglobin saturation from 84 ± 3% to 91 ± 5% ($P < .025$), and less frequent arousals. Although this favorable outcome was not shared by Buckle et al.,[168] it is possible that positive-pressure therapy was not applied for an adequate time to achieve beneficial results.

Several studies have demonstrated an increase in cardiac output and stroke volume and a reduction in left ventricular wall tension during application of nasal CPAP.[169,170] In a prospective but small controlled trial, Naughton and coworkers[171] observed that patients with CHF and CSR who received 3 months of CPAP therapy had a significantly greater reduction in the number of apneas and hypopneas as well as greater improvement in fatigue than the control group. In addition, patients receiving CPAP had a significant improvement in LVEF, whereas the control group had essentially no change in this parameter of cardiac function.

It is likely that the improvement in CSR in patients with CHF is at least partly due to improved left ventricular function and cardiac output. It is also possible that CPAP-related elevation of $Paco_2$ during sleep plays a role in stabilizing the breathing pattern of these patients.[172–174]

It appears that the benefit conferred by CPAP on cardiac function during sleep in patients with CHF persists during wakefulness.[171] Although the mechanism is not well defined at this time, it may be multifactorial and related to a lasting impact of sleep-related reduction of left ventricular transmural pressure, improved oxygenation during sleep, and reduced sympathetic nervous system activation during sleep.[39,175] Elimination of OSA/H in patients with sleep-related upper airway dysfunction and CHF will also have a beneficial impact on dilated congestive cardiomyopathy.[176] These considerations notwithstanding, CPAP may be a universally appropriate addition to the therapeutic armamentarium in the care of patients with CHF. When applied to certain patients, especially those without an elevated left ventricular filling pressure and those who experience an increase in systemic vascular resistance,

CPAP can precipitate a reduction in cardiac output.[169,177,178] In addition, like OSA/H patients, not all patients with CHF tolerate nasal CPAP.[168] Centers that have reported successful outcomes have hospitalized patients for several days to facilitate acclimatization to CPAP, which was initially applied during wakefulness and then overnight, at low pressure (5 cm $H_2O$) without upward titration.[175] Over the next several days, CPAP was gradually increased by 1.0–2.5 cm $H_2O$ per day until a pressure of 10.0–12.5 cm $H_2O$ was achieved. The patient was then discharged with instructions to use CPAP for at least 6 hours per night. It is clear that this regimen requires a considerable commitment of time and resources. If long-term improvement in cardiac function, quality of life, longevity, and reduced cost of care results, however, this commitment to address a very prevalent disease that exacts a great toll in human and economic terms will be worthwhile.

There are sufficient data to be encouraged that at least in those patients who are compliant with treatment, CPAP will confer noteworthy advantages. Before CPAP can be casually administered as a standard of care for CHF patients with CSR, however, further large-scale studies are required.

### Neuromuscular and Chest Wall Disorders

A detailed discussion of noninvasive positive-pressure therapy for respiratory insufficiency that is the result of a wide variety of disorders is beyond the scope of this chapter. It is important, however, for the clinician to be aware of the increasingly recognized susceptibility of patients with compromised lung or chest wall function to significant sleep-disordered breathing, which results in substantial nocturnal hypoxemia, hypercapnia, possible worsening of pulmonary hypertension, and poor sleep quality.[179-185] Although sleep-disordered breathing in this patient population is often nonapneic in nature, health care professionals have become increasingly cognizant of the benefits of providing nocturnal ventilatory support for such patients, including improved daytime alertness, improved arterial blood gases, and perhaps reduced need for hospitalization and increased longevity.[186,187] Clinicians have the option of choosing negative pressure ventilation, using a tank-type ventilator, cuirass, or poncho, or supporting ventilation during sleep with a positive-pressure device.

**Table 23-3.** Impact of Noninvasive Positive-Pressure Therapy on $Paco_2$

| Study | Prenocturnal Ventilation $Paco_2$ (mm Hg)* | Postnocturnal Ventilation $Paco_2$ (mm Hg)* |
|---|---|---|
| Leger et al.[217] | 51 | 40 |
| Ellis et al.[207] | 61 | 46 |
| Ellis et al.[208] | 62 | 49 |
| Kerby et al.[216] | 59 | 44 |
| Carroll and Branthwaite[205] | 62 | 45 |
| Heckmatt et al.[211] | 62 | 50 |
| Gay et al.[209] | 64 | 51 |
| Goldstein et al.[210] | 62 | 62 |
| Sanders and Kern[220] | 63 | 50 |
| Waldhorn[143] | 61 | 47 |
| Hill et al.[214] | 70 | 52 |
| Jimenéz et al.[215] | 59 | 45 |
| Bach et al.[202] | 53 | 40 |
| Barbé et al.[203] | 46 | 41 |
| Sanders et al. (unpublished) | 70 | 56 |

*Mean values.

Although application of negative pressure ventilatory support is successful for many patients with neuromuscular and chest wall disorders,[188-194] the data addressing the impact on sleeping patients with chronic obstructive pulmonary disease are somewhat contradictory.[195-197] To some degree, the inconsistent results are related to the inability of these patients to sleep with this modality, variability in the patient populations among the different studies, or variability in the experimental protocols for adjusting the settings of the ventilatory assistance device. Negative-pressure ventilation during sleep has also been associated with upper airway obstruction and oxyhemoglobin desaturation in at least some patients.[198-200] Until recently, however, positive-pressure ventilation could be applied only via tracheotomy,[191,201] although noninvasive delivery of ventilatory support via nasal or oronasal mask is now virtually universally available.

A growing number of reports attest to the success of noninvasive nocturnal positive-pressure ventilatory assistance in reducing the awake $Paco_2$ in hypercapnic patients with neuromuscular and chest wall disorders (Table 23-3).[143,187,190,191,202-218] Ventilatory support may be delivered using a conventional, portable, volume-cycled or pressure-cycled device in either an assisted or fully controlled mode of ventilation.[186,187,190,191,202,203,205–208,210,211,215–217] BIPAP has also been used to provide ventilatory assistance to patients with neuromuscular and chest wall disorders in adult and pediatric patients.[212,213,219–223] Nocturnal use of these devices has been shown to reduce $Pa_{CO_2}$ during wakefulness in hypercapnic patients and to relieve symptoms indicative of nocturnal hypoxemia, hypercapnia, and disturbed sleep (e.g., morning headaches, feeling foggy-headed, personality change, and hypersomnolence).

The ideal device for providing nocturnal positive-pressure ventilatory assistance in the home should be small and portable, easy to operate, unencumbered by unnecessary alarms, and affordable. In addition, the ventilatory-assistance device should be capable of delivering the airflow demanded by the patient and permit maintenance of a physiologic breathing pattern to facilitate synchronization between patient and ventilator. Finally, a backup mechanism should be available on the device to ensure a satisfactory level of ventilation in the event of central apnea. These requirements were succinctly outlined several years ago by Branthwaite.[204] Although many authors have described the need for in-hospital acclimatization to nocturnal ventilation with conventional volume- and pressure-cycled ventilators,[205,209,216,224] we have not found this to be necessary.

Although it is evident that noninvasive nocturnal positive-pressure ventilatory assistance tends to normalize the $Pa_{CO_2}$ in hypercapnic patients with neuromuscular and chest wall disorders (see Table 23-3), the responsible mechanism is unclear. One possibility is that there is a reduction in $Pa_{CO_2}$ while the patient sleeps with positive-pressure therapy and this results in reduced blood-buffering capacity (i.e., lower serum bicarbonate), so that ventilatory chemoresponsiveness to $CO_2$ is augmented. Arguing against this, however, is our observation, as well as that of others, that awake $Pa_{CO_2}$ often falls even in persons for whom positive pressure does not reduce the $Pa_{CO_2}$ during sleep.[209,220,224] Alternatively, it is possible that nocturnal ventilatory assistance "rests" fatigued ventilatory muscles, which consequently grow stronger. Several studies have suggested that positive-pressure ventilatory assistance reduces the work performed by inspiratory muscles in patients with neuromuscular or chest wall disorders and chronic obstructive airway diseases, and that positive-pressure devices may be

more effective in doing so than negative-pressure ventilation.[225–227] Our own data indicate that the application of positive-pressure ventilatory support during sleep in some of these patients results in a variable degree of central apnea, even in the absence of respiratory alkalosis, which can be relieved by the timed delivery of positive inspiratory pressure support.[220] This observation supports the concept proposed by Rochester and colleagues[228] that the application of external ventilatory assistance to patients with increased work of breathing (or increased workload relative to the maximum capacity of the inspiratory muscles) is in some way perceived by the patient as a signal to reduce or cease the activity of the inspiratory muscles, thus permitting rest. Conversely, there is only equivocal evidence to suggest that ventilatory muscle *strength* is increased by nocturnal ventilatory assistance. Although some investigators have observed an increase in forced vital capacity and augmented maximal inspiratory pressure[208,216] after initiation of therapy, others have reported no increase in these variables or in the maximal voluntary ventilation, despite a reduction in awake $Pa_{CO_2}$.[205,209,210,217,220] Ventilatory muscle *endurance,* however, may be a more relevant factor than strength to consider as a mechanism to explain the reduction in awake $Pa_{CO_2}$ after initiation of nocturnal positive-pressure ventilatory support. Importantly, Goldstein and coworkers[210] observed a significant increase in inspiratory muscle endurance after 3 months' nocturnal therapy, but no change in respiratory muscle strength as measured by maximal inspiratory and expiratory pressures or by maximal voluntary ventilation.

In addition to central apnea, some patients with neuromuscular or chest wall disorders develop OSA/H during sleep on positive-pressure ventilation.[207,219,220,229] Unlike negative-pressure ventilation, positive-pressure ventilatory assistance is not associated with the generation of negative intrapharyngeal pressure, which could contribute to the development of upper airway obstruction, unless the patient's inspiratory flow demands are not met. The pathogenesis of upper airway collapse during positive-pressure therapy is uncertain, but it is intriguing to speculate that the upper airway dilator muscles behave in a fashion similar to the chest wall inspiratory muscles during positive-pressure ventilatory support, so that there is a loss of inspiratory activity or tone (i.e., rest). This could make the upper airway susceptible to closure even in the absence of negative intrapharyngeal pressure, if the compliance of the upper airway structures is sufficiently low.[15,16,137,138,152–154] Alternatively, Delguste and coworkers[229] suggested that hypocapnia precipitated by over-ventilation evokes glottic closure. Similar findings have been reported by Parreira et al.[230] and Jounieaux et al.[231,232] Whatever the mechanism, it is essential to maintaining upper airway patency during sleep.

### *Interfaces between Positive-Pressure Devices and Patients with Neuromuscular or Chest Wall Disorders*

Maintenance of a comfortable and leak-free interface in patients with neuromuscular or chest wall disorders who are receiving nocturnal positive-pressure ventilatory support is as important as it is in OSA/H patients receiving positive-pressure therapy. For OSA/H patients, the overriding therapeutic concern is maintenance of a patent upper airway. In non-OSA/H patients with neuromuscular or chest wall disorders who are receiving nocturnal ventilatory support, however, providing adequate minute ventilation is the critical goal (although re-establishing upper airway patency when necessary in these patients is also important). Leaks can confound the attainment of this objective and may necessitate increasing the tidal volume delivered by conventional ventilators as a compensatory maneuver. In addition, it has been shown that mask leaks may disrupt sleep quality and architecture.[233,234] It is essential to provide patients with an interface that is as leak-free and well fitted as possible. We have found that many patients obtain excellent results using commercially available nasal masks. A number of patients, particularly those with neuromuscular disorders, have a great deal of difficulty keeping their mouth sufficiently closed to avoid substantial air leakage, which can compromise therapeutic efficacy. For these patients, we have successfully delivered long-term nocturnal positive-pressure therapy via oronasal masks.[220] We have used either a large nasal mask for this purpose, or an oronasal mask. A strapless oral-nasal interface has also been suggested.[235,236] The same precautions described in the previous section on the delivery of CPAP to OSA/H patients via oronasal mask apply to the use of such an interface for any patient who requires nocturnal ventilatory support.

Another approach to the problem of providing a noninvasive interface to patients using positive-pressure devices is the use of mouthpieces. Bach and coworkers[235–238] have had substantial experience using this type of interface in postpolio and quadriplegic patients with ventilatory insufficiency. Loss of air is minimized by holding the mouthpiece in place with a commercially available lip-seal device. This technique may be ineffective, however, for those with incompetent buccopharyngeal muscles. In addition, positive-pressure ventilatory support via mouthpiece may be associated with increased risk of aspiration of gastric contents, development of bite deformities, and dry mouth.[235,237] In the presence of unacceptable nasal leakage, Bach and colleagues[237] have used nasal cotton pledgets held in place with tape. However, some patients and clinicians have expressed concern about simultaneously encumbering the oral and nasal airways.

### *Establishing Proper Ventilatory Support Settings*

Given the uncertainty about the exact mechanism(s) that reduce awake $Pa_{CO_2}$ after initiation of nocturnal ventilatory support, the diversity of approaches to determine the "correct" ventilator settings is not surprising.

Several authors have described the practice of adjusting tidal volume and inspiratory flow on conventional portable ventilators according to patient comfort,[224] whereas others report setting parameters of ventilatory assistance by monitoring end-tidal tension or $Pa_{CO_2}$, with the goal of maintaining values during sleep that approximate those during wakefulness.[216] Still others have monitored transcutaneous $CO_2$ tension ($P_{tc}CO_2$) together with diaphragm and sternocleidomastoid electromyograms using surface electrodes. In the latter studies, adequate ventilatory support during sleep is defined as a reduction in electromyogram activity by 50% with an accompanying increase in oxyhemoglobin saturation and decrease in $P_{tc}CO_2$. Unfortunately, all of these methods are imperfect. Adjusting settings to the awake patient's comfort may not ensure satisfactory support during sleep. End-tidal $CO_2$ may not be a consistently accurate reflection of $Paco_2$ during sleep, as there may be changes in dead space on the basis of delivered tidal volume, changing cardiac output, or variation in the position of the capnograph catheter in the mask.[239] Technically adequate electromyograms may be difficult to obtain in certain patients, and indeed, as we and others have found, one can silence the activity of the ventilatory muscles without appreciably changing the $Paco_2$ (although, as previously noted, the necessity of reducing the $Paco_2$ during sleep has yet to be established). There is intuitive appeal to using the $Paco_2$ as a parameter by which ventilator settings may be determined during sleep. Monitoring $Paco_2$ helps the clinician avoid the development of additional respiratory acidosis over that which exists during wakefulness as well as unacceptable respiratory alkalosis during nocturnal ventilatory support as a result of over-ventilating the patient. The latter condition may alter cerebral blood flow and enhance the likelihood of developing central and obstructive apneas,[229–232] as well as cardiac dysrhythmias. Unfortunately, peripheral arterial catheterization is currently the only accurate way to evaluate $Paco_2$ during sleep with noninvasive positive-pressure ventilatory assistance, and even the information provided in this way is not continuous. An alternative that has been proposed is $P_{tc}co_2$. Although this technique provides a continuous data readout, there are conflicts in the literature regarding its accuracy in adults. Several studies have reported a good correlation between $P_{tc}co_2$ and $Paco_2$ in hemodynamically stable adults and children,[240–243] although some of the data reflect substantial scatter in the relationship between the two variables.[241] One study indicated that there may be greater overestimation of $Paco_2$ by $P_{tc}co_2$ as the former value increases.[244] Observations from our laboratory indicate a poor correlation between $P_{tc}co_2$ and $Paco_2$ in sleeping patients with neuromuscular or chest wall disorders, both with and without noninvasive ventilatory assistance with BIPAP therapy.[239]

In our laboratory, when nocturnal ventilatory support via mask is provided by a BIPAP device or a conventional portable ventilator, the initial settings are determined both by patient comfort during wakefulness and by monitoring the $Paco_2$ during sleep via an in-dwelling arterial catheter that ensures unacceptable hyperventilation has not developed. During noninvasive positive-pressure ventilatory assistance in hypercapnic patients, IPAP is increased with the goal of keeping the $Paco_2$ within a range between the awake values and 10 mm Hg below that value, provided the pH remains at or below 7.49. On those infrequent occasions when, owing to concerns about barotrauma or patient discomfort, the IPAP level is higher than desirable, a timed backup rate is raised to increase the patient's ventilation while minimizing the applied inspiratory pressure. For patients who develop central apnea in the absence of respiratory alkalosis, a timed backup rate is instituted to provide acceptable ventilatory frequency. Finally, in the event that obstructive apneas are observed, the EPAP is increased as described earlier for OSA/H patients.

## SUMMARY

Positive-pressure ventilation via mask during sleep constitutes a safe and effective treatment for OSA/H. In addition, this treatment will be adapted as technology improves to reduce the $Paco_2$ in hypercapnic patients with neuromuscular and chest wall disorders. This modality is generally accepted as the medical therapy of choice for OSA/H. Long-term patient compliance with therapy is good, though not optimal. Further studies are needed to better define those factors that determine compliance, to assess the impact of new technologies, and to evaluate the effect of modified practice patterns for initiating therapy.

Noninvasive positive-pressure ventilatory assistance is now accepted as one standard of care for selected patients with neuromuscular respiratory failure.[245] Studies also suggest that nocturnal positive-pressure ventilation is tolerated well by the majority of patients, and that it relieves symptoms and improves quality of life. Compliance with this treatment is considerably better than in OSA/H patients.[246,247] This may be related to the potential benefits that are perceived or obtained by these patients, a better understanding of the adverse health consequences of noncompliance, or enforcement of positive-pressure therapy by caregivers.

## REFERENCES

1. Sullivan CE, Issa FG, Berthon-Jones M, et al. Reversal of obstructive sleep apnoea by continuous positive airway pressure applied through the nares. Lancet 1981;1:862.
2. Sériès F, Cormier Y, Couture J, et al. Changes in upper airway resistance with lung inflation and positive airway pressure. J Appl Physiol 1990;68:1075.

3. Hoffstein V, Zamel N, Phillipson EA. Lung volume dependence of pharyngeal cross-sectional area in patients with obstructive sleep apnea. Am Rev Respir Dis 1984;130:175.

4. Brown I, Taylor R, Hoffstein V. Obstructive sleep apnea reversed by increased lung volume? Eur J Respir Dis 1986;68:375.

5. Sériès F, Cormier Y, Lampron N, et al. Increasing the functional residual capacity may reverse obstructive sleep apnea. Sleep 1988;11:349.

6. Begle RL, Sadr S, Skatrud JB, et al. Effect of lung inflation on pulmonary resistance during NREM sleep. Am Rev Respir Dis 1990;141:854.

7. van de Graaf WB. Thoracic influence on upper airway patency. J Appl Physiol 1988;65:2124.

8. Sériès F, Cormier Y, Desmuales M. Influence of passive changes of lung volume on upper airways. J Appl Physiol 1990;68:2159.

9. Abbey NC, Cooper KR, Kwentus JA. Benefit of nasal CPAP in obstructive sleep apnea is due to positive pharyngeal pressure. Sleep 1989;12:420.

10. Alex CG, Aronson RM, Onal E, et al. Effects of continuous positive airway pressure on upper airway and respiratory muscle activity. J Appl Physiol 1987;62:2026.

11. Rapoport DM, Garay SM, Goldring RM. Nasal CPAP in obstructive sleep apnea: mechanisms of action. Bull Eur Physiopathol Respir 1983;19:616.

12. Strohl KP, Redline S. Nasal CPAP therapy, upper airway activation, and obstructive sleep apnea. Am Rev Respir Dis 1986;134:555.

13. Sanders MH. Nasal CPAP effect on patterns of sleep apnea. Chest 1984;86:839.

14. Issa FG, Sullivan CE. Reversal of central sleep apnea using nasal CPAP. Chest 1986;90:165.

15. Sanders MH, Rogers RM, Pennock BE. Prolonged expiratory phase in sleep apnea: a unifying hypothesis. Am Rev Respir Dis 1985;131:401.

16. Sanders MH, Moore SE. Inspiratory and expiratory partitioning of airway resistance during sleep in patients with sleep apnea. Am Rev Respir Dis 1983;127:554.

17. Cheshire K, Engleman H, Deary I, Douglas NJ. Factors impairing daytime performance in patients with sleep apnea/hypopnea syndrome. Arch Intern Med 1992;152:538.

18. Engleman H. Self-reported use of CPAP and benefits of CPAP therapy. A patient survey. Chest 1996;109:1470.

19. Krieger J, Kurtz D, Petiau C, et al. Long-term compliance with CPAP therapy in obstructive sleep apnea patients and in snorers. Sleep 1996;19:S136.

20. Poceta JS, Timms RM, Jeong D-U, et al. Maintenance of wakefulness test in obstructive sleep apnea syndrome. Chest 1992;101:893.

21. Engleman HM, Martin SE, Douglas NJ. Compliance with CPAP therapy in patients with the sleep apnoea/hypopnea syndrome. Thorax 1994;49:263.

22. Engleman HM, Martin SE, Deary IJ, Douglas NJ. Effect of continuous positive airway pressure treatment on daytime function in sleep apnea/hypopnea syndrome. Lancet 1994;343:572.

23. Engleman HM, Cheshire KE, Deary IJ, Douglas NJ. Daytime sleepiness, cognitive performance and mood after continuous positive airway pressure for the sleep apnoea/hypopnoea syndrome. Thorax 1993;48:911.

24. Meurice J-C, Dore P, Paquereau J, et al. Predictive factors of long-term compliance with nasal continuous positive airway pressure treatment in sleep apnea syndrome. Chest 1994;105:429.

25. Rajagopal KR, Bennett LL, Dillard TA. Overnight nasal CPAP improves hypersomnolence in sleep apnea. Chest 1986;90:172.

26. Lamphere J, Roehrs T, Wittig R, et al. Recovery of alertness after CPAP in apnea. Chest 1989;96:1364.

27. Frith RW, Cant BR. Severe obstructive sleep apnoea treated with long term nasal continuous positive airway pressure. Thorax 1985;40:45.

28. McEvoy RD, Thornton AT. Treatment of obstructive sleep apnea syndrome with nasal continuous positive airway pressure. Sleep 1984;7:313.

29. Sanders MH, Kern N. Obstructive sleep apnea treated by independently adjusted inspiratory and expiratory positive airway pressures via nasal mask. Physiologic and clinical implications. Chest 1990;98:317.

30. Demirozu MC, Steinberg N, Kiel M, et al. The effect of positive end expiratory pressure and site of oxygen entrainment on inspiratory oxygen concentration when using supplemental oxygen with nasal continuous positive airway pressure. Sleep Res 1990;19:321.

31. Piper AJ, Sullivan CE. Effects of short-term NIPPV in the treatment of patients with severe obstructive sleep apnea and hypercapnia. Chest 1994;105:434.

32. Douglas NJ, White DP, Weil JV, et al. Hypercapnic ventilatory response in sleeping adults. Am Rev Respir Dis 1982;126:758.

33. Douglas NJ, White DP, Weil JV, et al. Hypoxic ventilatory response decreases during sleep in normal men. Am Rev Respir Dis 1982;125:286.

34. White DP. Occlusion pressure and ventilation during sleep in normal humans. J Appl Physiol 1986;61:1279.

35. Skatrud JB, Dempsey JA. Interaction of sleep state and chemical stimuli in sustaining rhythmic ventilation. J Appl Physiol 1983;55:813.

36. Henke KG, Dempsey JA, Kowitz JM, et al. Effects of sleep-induced increases in upper airway resistance on ventilation. J Appl Physiol 1990;69:617.

37. Tabachnik E, Muller NL, Bryan AC, et al. Changes in ventilation and chest wall mechanics during sleep in normal adolescents. J Appl Physiol 1981;51:557.

38. Young T, Finn L, Hla KM, et al. Snoring as part of a dose-response relationship between sleep-disordered breathing and blood pressure. Sleep 1996;19(Suppl 10):202.

39. Naughton MT, Benard DC, Liu PP, et al. Effects of nasal CPAP on sympathetic activity in patients with heart failure and central sleep apnea. Am J Respir Crit Care Med 1995;152:473.

40. Waravdekar NV, Sinoway LI, Zwilich CW, Leuenberger UA. Influence of treatment on muscle sympathetic nerve activity in sleep apnea syndrome. Am J Respir Crit Care Med 1996;153:1333.

41. Hedner J, Darpo B, Ejnell H, et al. Reduction in sympathetic activity after long-term CPAP treatment in sleep apnoea: cardiovascular implications. Eur Respir J 1995;8:222.

42. Suzuki M, Otsuka K, Guilleminault C. Long-term nasal continuous positive airway pressure administration can normalize hypertension in obstructive sleep apnea patients. Sleep 1993;16:545.

43. Wilcox I, Grunstein RR, Hedner JA, et al. Effect of nasal continuous positive pressure during sleep on 24-hour blood pressure in obstructive sleep apnea. Sleep 1993;16:539.

44. Fletcher EC. The relationship between systemic hypertension and obstructive sleep apnea: facts and theory. Am J Med 1995;98:118.

45. Smith PL, Hudgel DW, Olson LG, et al. Indications and standards for use of nasal continuous positive airway pressure (CPAP) in sleep apnea syndromes. Am J Respir Crit Care Med 1994;150:1738.

46. Pépin JL, Leger P, Veale D, et al. Side effects of nasal continuous positive airway pressure in sleep apnea syndrome. Study of 193 patients in two French sleep centers. Chest 1995;107:375.

47. Hoffstein V, Viner S, Mateika S, Conway J. Treatment of obstructive sleep apnea with nasal continuous positive airway pressure. Patient compliance, perception of benefits, and side effects. Am Rev Respir Dis 1992;145:841.

48. Kribbs NB, Pack AI, Kline LR, et al. Objective measurement of patterns of nasal CPAP use by patients with obstructive sleep apnea. Am Rev Respir Dis 1993;147:887.

49. Fletcher EC, Luckett RA. The effect of positive reinforcement on hourly compliance in continuous positive airway pressure users with obstructive sleep apnea. Am Rev Respir Dis 1991;143:936.

50. Waldhorn RE, Herrick TW, Nguyen MC, et al. Long-term compliance with nasal continuous positive airway pressure therapy of obstructive sleep apnea. Chest 1990;97:33.

51. Edinger JD, Radtke RA. Use of in vivo desensitization to treat a patient's claustrophobic response to nasal CPAP. Sleep 1993;16:678.

52. Prosise GL, Berry RB. Oral-nasal continuous positive airway pressure as a treatment for obstructive sleep apnea. Chest 1994;106:180.

53. Sanders MH, Kern NB, Stiller RA. Use of an oronasal interface in the positive pressure therapy of sleep apnea. Chest 1994;106:774.

54. Criner GJ, Travaline JM, Brennan KJ, Kreimer DT. Efficacy of a new full face mask for noninvasive positive pressure ventilation. Chest 1994;106:1109.

55. Stauffer JL, Fayter NA, McClure BJ. Conjunctivitis from nasal CPAP apparatus. Chest 1984;86:802.

56. Strumpf DA, Harrop P, Dobbin J, et al. Massive epistaxis from nasal CPAP therapy. Chest 1989;95:1141.

57. Richards GN, Cistulli PA, Ungar RG, et al. Mouth leak with nasal continuous positive airway pressure increases nasal airway resistance. Am J Respir Crit Care Med 1996;154:182.

58. Fleury B, Barros VS, Rakotonanahary D, et al. Comparison of cold passover versus heated humidification during nCPAP therapy. Am J Respir Crit Care Med 1997;155:A304.

59. Sullivan CE, Grunstein RR. Continuous Positive Airways Pressure in Sleep-Disordered Breathing. In MH Kryger, T Roth, WC Dement (eds), Principles and Practice of Sleep Medicine. Philadelphia: Saunders, 1989;559.

60. Jarjour NN, Wilson P. Pneumoencephalos associated with nasal continuous positive airway pressure in a patient with sleep apnea syndrome. Chest 1989;96:1425.

61. Krieger J, Weitzenblum E, Monassier J-P, et al. Dangerous hypoxaemia during continuous positive airway pressure treatment of obstructive sleep apnoea. Lancet 1983;2:1429.

62. Martin T, Sanders M, Atwood C. Correlation between changes in $PaCO_2$ and CPAP in obstructive sleep apnea (OSA) patients. Am Rev Respir Dis 1993;147:A681.

63. Fukui M, Ohi M, Chin K, Kuno K. The effects of nasal CPAP on transcutaneous $PCO_2$ during non-REM and REM sleep in patients with obstructive sleep apnea syndrome. Sleep 1993;16:S144.

64. Rapoport DM, Sorkin B, Garay SM, et al. Reversal of the "pickwickian syndrome" by long-term use of nocturnal airway pressure. N Engl J Med 1982;307:931.

65. Sullivan CE, Berthon-Jones M, Issa FG. Remission of severe obesity-hypoventilation syndrome after shortterm treatment during sleep with nasal continuous positive airway pressure. Am Rev Respir Dis 1982;128:177.

66. Shivarum U, Cash ME, Beal A. Nasal continuous positive airway pressure in decompensated hypercapnic respiratory failure as a complication of sleep apnea. Chest 1993;104:770.

67. Berthon-Jones M, Sullivan CE. Time course of change in ventilatory response to $CO_2$ with long-term CPAP therapy for obstructive sleep apnea. Am Rev Respir Dis 1987;135:144.

68. Guilleminault C, Cummiskey J. Progressive improvement of apnea index and ventilatory response to $CO_2$ after tracheostomy in obstructive sleep apnea syndrome. Am Rev Respir Dis 1982;126:14.

69. White DP, Douglas NJ, Pickett CK, et al. Sleep deprivation and the control of ventilation. Am Rev Respir Dis 1983;128:984.

70. Rauscher H, Popp W, Wanke T, Zwick H. Acceptance of CPAP therapy for sleep apnea. Chest 1991;100:1019.

71. Iber C, O'Brien C, Schluter J, et al. Single night studies in obstructive apnea. Sleep 1991;14:383.

72. Sanders MH, Black J, Costantino JP, et al. Diagnosis of sleep-disordered breathing by half-night polysomnography. Am Rev Respir Dis 1991;144:1256.

73. Sanders MH, Kern NB, Costantino J, et al. Adequacy of prescribing positive airway pressure therapy by mask for sleep apnea on the basis of a partial-night trial. Am Rev Respir Dis 1993;147:1169.

74. Fleury B, Rakotonanahary D, Tehindrazanarivelo AD, et al. Long term compliance to continuous positive airway pressure therapy (nCPAP) set up during a split-night polysomnography. Sleep 1994;17:512.

75. Yamashiro Y, Kryger MH. CPAP titration for sleep apnea using a split-night protocol. Chest 1995;107:62.

76. Strollo PJ Jr, Sanders MH, Costantino JP, et al. Split night polysomnography does not affect compliance with positive pressure via a mask in the treatment of patients with obstructive sleep apnea. Sleep 1996;19:255.

77. Sullivan CE, Issa FG, Berthon-Jones M, et al. Home treatment of obstructive sleep apnoea with continuous positive airway pressure applied through a nose mask. Bull Eur Physiopathol Respir 1984;20:49.

78. Nino-Murcia G, McCann CC, Bliwise DL, et al. Compliance and side effects in sleep apnea patients treated with continuous positive airway pressure. West J Med 1989;150:165.

79. Sanders MH, Gruendl CA, Rogers RM. Patient compliance with nasal CPAP therapy for sleep apnea. Chest 1986;90:330.

80. Reeves-Hoché MK, Meck R, Zwillich CW. Nasal CPAP: an objective evaluation of patient compliance. Am J Respir Crit Care Med 1994;149:1494.

81. Weaver TE, Chugh DK, Maislin G, et al. Comparison of CPAP nightly duration to nocturnal sleep time. Am J Respir Crit Care Med 1997;155:A304.

82. Kribbs NB, Pack AI, Kline LR, et al. Effects of one night without nasal CPAP treatment on sleep and sleepiness in patients with obstructive sleep apnea. Am Rev Respir Dis 1993;147:1162.

83. Sforza E, Lugaresi E. Daytime sleepiness and nasal continuous positive airway pressure in obstructive sleep apnea patients: effects of chronic treatment and 1 night therapy withdrawal. Sleep 1995;18:195.

84. Hers V, Liistro G, Dury M, et al. Residual effect of nCPAP applied part of the night in patients with obstructive sleep apnoea. Eur Respir J 1997;10:973.

85. Sériès F, Roy N, Marc I. Effects of sleep deprivation and sleep fragmentation on upper airway collapsibility in normal subjects. Am J Respir Crit Care Med 1994;150:481.

86. McNicholas WT. Compliance with nasal CPAP therapy for obstructive sleep apnoea: how much is enough? Eur Respir J 1997;10:969.

87. Krieger J. Long-term compliance with nasal continuous positive airway pressure (CPAP) in obstructive sleep apnea patients and nonapneic snorers. Sleep 1992;15:S42.

88. Olson LG, Rolfe E, Saunders NA. Tolerance of nasal CPAP treatment of obstructive sleep apnea, and its effect on disease severity. Am Rev Respir Dis 1990;141:A866.

89. Johns MW. A new method for measuring daytime sleepiness: the Epworth Sleepiness Scale. Sleep 1991;14:540.

90. Engleman HM, Douglas NJ. CPAP compliance. Sleep 1993;16:S114.

91. Fry JM, DiPhillipo MA, Pressman MR. Periodic leg movements in sleep following treatment of obstructive sleep apnea with nasal continuous positive airway pressure. Chest 1989;96:89.

92. Yamashiro Y, Kryger MH. Acute effect of nasal CPAP on periodic limb movements associated with breathing disorders during sleep. Sleep 1994;17:172.

93. Atwood CW, Strollo PJ, Sanders MH, et al. Arousal producing periodic leg movements in sleep-disordered breathing pre and post treatment with positive airway pressure. Sleep Res 1994;23:220.

94. Waldhorn RE, Wood K. Attended home titration of nasal continuous positive airway pressure therapy for obstructive sleep apnea. Chest 1993;104:1707.

95. Coppola MP, Lawee M. Management of obstructive sleep apnea syndrome in the home. The role of portable sleep apnea recording. Chest 1993;104:19.

96. Miljeteig H, Hoffstein V. Determinants of continuous positive airway pressure level for treatment of obstructive sleep apnea. Am Rev Respir Dis 1993;147:1526.

97. Hoffstein V, Mateika S. Predicting nasal continuous positive airway pressure. Am J Respir Crit Care Med 1994;150:486.

98. Guilleminault C, Stoohs R. Upper airway resistance syndrome. Am Rev Respir Dis 1991;143:A589.

99. McEvoy RD, Sharp DJ, Thornton AT. The effects of posture on obstructive sleep apnea. Am Rev Respir Dis 1986;133:662.

100. George CF, Millar TW, Kryger MH. Sleep apnea and body position during sleep. Sleep 1988;11:90.

101. Cartwright RD. Effect of sleep position on sleep apnea severity. Sleep 1984;7:110.

102. Phillips BA, Okeson J, Paesani D, Gilmore R. Effect of sleep position on sleep apnea and parafunctional activity. Chest 1986;90:424.

103. Bonora M, Shields GI, Knuth SL, et al. Selective depression by ethanol of upper airway respiratory motor activity in cats. Am Rev Respir Dis 1984;130:156.

104. Krol RC, Knuth SL, Bartlett D Jr. Selective reduction of genioglossal activity by alcohol in normal human subjects. Am Rev Respir Dis 1984;129:247.

105. Dolly FR, Block AJ. Effect of flurazepam on sleep-disordered breathing and nocturnal oxygen desaturation in asymptomatic subjects. Am J Med 1982;73:239.

106. Issa FG, Sullivan CE. Alcohol, snoring and sleep apnea. J Neurol Neurosurg Psychiatry 1982;5:353.

107. Taasan VC, Block AJ, Boysen PG, Wynne JW. Alcohol increases sleep apnea and oxygen desaturation in asymptomatic men. Am J Med 1981;71:240.

108. Scrima L, Broudy M, Nay KN, Cohn MA. Increased severity of obstructive sleep apnea after bedtime alco-

hol ingestion: diagnostic potential and proposed mechanism of action. Sleep 1982;5:318.

109. Issa FG, Sullivan CE. Upper airway closing pressures in snorers. J Appl Physiol 1984;57:528.

110. Mitler MM, Dawson A, Henriksen SJ, et al. Bedtime ethanol increases resistance of upper airways and produces sleep apneas in asymptomatic snorers. Alcohol Clin Exp Res 1988;12:801.

111. Berry RB, Desa MM, Light RW. Effect of ethanol on the efficacy of nasal continuous positive airway pressure as a treatment for obstructive sleep apnea. Chest 1991;99:339.

112. St. John WM, Bartlett D, Knuth KV, et al. Differential depression of hypoglossal nerve activity by alcohol. Am Rev Respir Dis 1986;133:46.

113. Sériès F, Marc I, Cormier Y, La Forge J. Required levels of nasal continuous positive airway pressure during treatment of obstructive sleep apnoea. Eur Respir J 1994;7:1776.

114. Lofaso F, Lorino AM, Duizabo D, et al. Evaluation of an auto-nCPAP device based on snoring detection. Eur Respir J 1996;9:1795.

115. Berthon-Jones M. Feasibility of a self-setting CPAP machine. Sleep 1993;16:S120.

116. Behbehani K, Yen F-C, Burk JR, et al. Automatic control of airway pressure for treatment of obstructive sleep apnea. IEEE Trans Biomed Eng 1995;42:1007.

117. Scharf MB, Brannen DE, McDannold MD, Berkovitz DV. Computerized adjustable versus fixed nCPAP treatment of obstructive sleep apnea. Sleep 1996;19:491.

118. Lloberes P, Ballester E, Montserrat JM, et al. Comparison of manual and automatic CPAP titration in patients with sleep apnea/hypopnea syndrome. Am J Respir Crit Care Med 1996;154:1755.

119. Teschler H, Berthon-Jones M, Thompson AB, et al. Automated continuous positive airway pressure titration for obstructive sleep apnea syndrome. Am J Respir Crit Care Med 1996;154:734.

120. Sharma S, Wali S, Pouliot Z, et al. Treatment of obstructive sleep apnea with a self-titrating continuous positive airway pressure (CPAP) system. Sleep 1996;19:497.

121. Juhasz J, Schillen J, Urbigkeit A, et al. Unattended continuous positive pressure titration. Clinical relevance and cardiorespiratory hazards of the method. Am J Respir Crit Care Med 1996;154:359.

122. Meurice J-C, Marc I, Sériès F. Efficacy of auto-CPAP in the treatment of obstructive sleep apnea/hypopnea syndrome. Am J Respir Crit Care Med 1996;153:794.

123. Oliver CM, Flaherty M, Levy RD, et al. Effects of nursing intervention on patient and spouse well-being and CPAP compliance in obstructive sleep apnea (OSA). Am J Respir Crit Care Med 1997;155:A305.

124. Hoy CJ, Vennelle M, Douglas NJ. Can CPAP use be improved? Am J Respir Crit Care Med 1997;155:A304.

125. Leon C, Ballester E, Lloberes P, et al. More about the acceptable CPAP compliance in patients with sleep apnea hypopnea syndrome (SAHS). Am J Respir Crit Care Med 1997;155:A305.

126. Likar LL, Panciera TM, Erickson AD, Rounds S. Group education sessions and compliance with nasal CPAP therapy. Chest 1997;111:1273.

127. Chervin RD, Theut S, Bassetti C, Aldrich MS. Compliance with nasal CPAP can be improved by simple interventions. Sleep 1997;20:284.

128. Dekker FW, Dieleman FE, Kaptein AA, Mulder JD. Compliance with pulmonary medication in general practice. Eur Respir J 1993;6:886.

129. Sanders MH, Moore SE, Evaslage J. CPAP via nasal mask: a treatment for occlusive sleep apnea. Chest 1983;83:144.

130. Mayer LS, Kerby GR, Whitman RA. Evaluation of a new nasal device for administration of continuous positive airway pressure for obstructive sleep apnea. Am Rev Respir Dis 1989;139:A114.

131. Mayer LS, Kerby GR, Whitman RA, et al. Continued evaluation of a new nasal device for administration of continuous positive airway pressure. Am Rev Respir Dis 1990;141:A684.

132. Harris C, Daniels B, Herold D, et al. Comparison of cannula and mask systems for administration of nasal continuous positive airway pressure for treatment of obstructive sleep apnea. Sleep Res 1990;19:233.

133. Cornette A, Mougel D. Ventilatory assistance via the nasal route: masks and fittings. Eur Respir Rev 1993; 3:250.

134. Covelli HD, Weled BJ, Beekman JF. Efficacy of continuous positive airway pressure administered by mask. Chest 1982;2:147.

135. Branson RD, Hurst JM, DeHaven CB. Mask CPAP: state of the art. Respir Care 1985;30:846.

136. Pressman MR, Peterson DD, Meyer TJ, et al. Ramp abuse. A novel form of patient noncompliance to administration of nasal continuous positive airway pressure treatment of obstructive sleep apnea. Am J Respir Crit Care Med 1995;151:1632.

137. Smith PL, Wise RA, Gold AR, et al. Upper airway pressure-flow relationships in obstructive sleep apnea. J Appl Physiol 1988;64:789.

138. Schwartz AR, Smith PL, Wise RA, et al. Induction of upper airway occlusion in sleeping individuals with subatmospheric nasal pressure. J Appl Physiol 1988;64:535.

139. Schwab RJ, Gefter WB, Pack AI, Hoffman EA. Dynamic imaging of the upper airway during respiration in normal subjects. J Appl Physiol 1993;74:1504.

140. Schwab RJ, Gefter WB, Hoffman EA, et al. Dynamic upper airway imaging during respiration in normal subjects and patients with sleep disordered breathing. Am Rev Respir Dis 1993;148:1385.

141. Schwab RJ, Pack AI, Gupta KB, et al. Upper airway and soft tissue structural changes induced by CPAP in normal subjects. Am J Respir Crit Care Med 1996;154:1106.

142. Mahadevia AK, Onal E, Lopata M. Effects of expiratory positive airway pressure on sleep-induced abnor-

malities in patients with hypersomnia-sleep apnea syndrome. Am Rev Respir Dis 1983;128:708.

143. Waldhorn RE. Nocturnal nasal intermittent positive pressure ventilation with bi-level positive pressure (BiPAP) in respiratory failure. Chest 1992;101:516.

144. Geller DE, Foster JT, Wilcox JC, Howenstein MS. Bilevel CPAP (BL-CPAP) can ameliorate respiratory sleep disturbance in children. Am Rev Respir Dis 1991;143:A587.

145. Teague WG, Kervin LJ, Diwadkar VV, Scott PH. Nasal bi-level positive airway pressure (BLPAP) acutely improves ventilation and oxygen saturation in children with upper airway obstruction. Am Rev Respir Dis 1991;143:A505.

146. Padman R, Hyde C, Borkoswki W, Foster P. Efficacy of BiPAP therapy in pediatric obstructive sleep apnea syndrome. Analysis of respiratory parameters. Am J Respir Crit Care Med 1997;155:A303.

147. Becker H, Schneider H, Stamnitz A, et al. When and How to Use NBiPAP in Sleep Apnea Patients [abstract]. Lyon, France: International Conference on Home Mechanical Ventilation, 1993;19.

148. Reeves-Hoché MK, Hudgel D, Meck R, Zwillich CW. Continuous versus bilevel positive airway pressure for obstructive sleep apnea. Am J Respir Crit Care Med 1995;151:443.

149. Ferguson GT, Gilmartin M. $CO_2$ rebreathing during BiPAP ventilatory assistance. Am J Respir Crit Care Med 1995;151:1126.

150. Hill NS, Carlisle CC, Kramer NR. Does the exhalation valve really matter during bilevel nasal ventilation? Am J Respir Crit Care Med 1997;155:A408.

151. Parisi RA, England SJ, Santiago TV. Treatment of central sleep apnea with respiratory-cycled variable nasal positive pressure (BiPAP). Am Rev Respir Dis 1991; 143:A586.

152. Badr MS, Toiber F, Skatrud JB, Dempsey J. Pharyngeal narrowing/occlusion during central sleep apnea. J Appl Physiol 1995;78:1806.

153. Badr MS. Effect of ventilatory drive on upper airway patency in humans during NREM sleep. Respir Physiol 1996;103:1.

154. Morrell MJ, Badr MS, Harms CA, Dempsey JA. The assessment of upper airway patency during apnea using cardiogenic oscillations in the airflow signal. Sleep 1995;18:651.

155. Sériès F. Auto CPAP in the treatment of sleep apnea hypopnea syndrome. Sleep 1996;19:S281.

156. Block AJ, Hellard DH, Slayton PC. Effect of alcohol ingestion on breathing and oxygenation during sleep. Am J Med 1986;80:595.

157. Teschler H, Berthon-Jones M, Wessendorf T, et al. Influence of moderate alcohol consumption on obstructive sleep apnoea with and without AutoSet™ nasal CPAP therapy. Eur Respir J 1996;9:2371.

158. Fromm RE, Varon J, Lechin AE, Hirshkowitz M. CPAP machine performance and altitude. Chest 1995;108:1577.

159. Carley DW, Applebaum R, Basner RC, et al. Respiratory and electrocortical responses to acoustic stimulation. Sleep 1996;19:S189.

160. Douglas NJ, Martin SE. Arousals and the sleep apnea/hypopnea syndrome. Sleep 1996;19:S196.

161. Hanly PJ, Millar TW, Steljes DG, et al. Respiration and abnormal sleep in patients with congestive heart failure. Chest 1989;96:480.

162. Andreas S, von Breska B, Kopp E, et al. Periodic respiration in patients with heart failure. Clin Invest 1993;71:281.

163. Javaheri S, Parker TJ, Wexler L, et al. Occult sleep-disordered breathing in stable congestive heart failure. Ann Intern Med 1995;122:487.

164. Hanly P, Zuberi-Khokhar N. Daytime sleepiness in patients with congestive heart failure and Cheyne-Stokes respiration. Chest 1995;107:952.

165. Ancoli-Israel S, Engler RL, Friedman PJ, et al. Comparison of patients with central sleep apnea with and without Cheyne-Stokes respiration. Chest 1994;106:780.

166. Hanly P, Zuberi-Khokhar N. Increased mortality associated with Cheyne-Stokes respiration in patients with congestive heart failure. Am J Respir Crit Care Med 1996;153:272.

167. Takasaki Y, Orr D, Popkin J, et al. Effect of nasal continuous positive airway pressure in congestive heart failure. Am Rev Respir Dis 1989;140:1578.

168. Buckle P, Millar T, Kryger M. The effect of acute nasal CPAP on Cheyne-Stokes respiration in congestive heart failure. Chest 1992;102:31.

169. Bradley TD, Holloway RM, McLaughlin PR, et al. Cardiac output response to continuous positive airway pressure in congestive heart failure. Am Rev Respir Dis 1992;145:377.

170. Naughton MT, Rahman MA, Hara K, et al. Effect of continuous positive airway pressure on intrathoracic and left ventricular transmural pressures in patients with congestive heart failure. Circulation 1995;91:1725.

171. Naughton MT, Liu PP, Benard DC, et al. Treatment of congestive heart failure and Cheyne-Stokes respiration during sleep by continuous positive airway pressure. Am J Respir Crit Care Med 1995;151:92.

172. Hanly P, Zuberi N, Gray R. Pathogenesis of Cheyne-Stokes respiration in patients with congestive heart failure. Chest 1993;104:1079.

173. Naughton M, Benard D, Tam A, et al. Role of hyperventilation in the pathogenesis of central sleep apneas in patients with congestive heart failure. Am Rev Respir Dis 1993;148:330.

174. Naughton MT, Benard DC, Rutherford R, Bradley TD. Effect of continuous positive airway pressure on central sleep apnea and nocturnal $PCO_2$ in heart failure. Am J Respir Crit Care Med 1994;150:1598.

175. Bradley TD. Hemodynamic and sympathoinhibitory effects of nasal CPAP in congestive heart failure. Sleep 1996;19:S232.

176. Malone S, Liu PP, Halloway R, et al. Obstructive sleep apnoea in patients with dilated cardiomyopathy: effects

of continuous positive airway pressure. Lancet 1991; 338:1480.

177. Liston R, Deegan PC, McCreery C, et al. Haemodynamic effects of nasal continuous positive airway pressure in severe congestive heart failure. Eur Respir J 1995;8:430.

178. Calverley PMA. Nasal CPAP in cardiac failure: case not proven. Sleep 1996;19:S236.

179. Smith PEM, Calverly PMA, Edwards RHT. Hypoxemia during sleep in Duchenne muscular dystrophy. Am Rev Respir Dis 1988;137:884.

180. Bye PTP, Issa FG, Berthon-Jones M, et al. Studies of oxygenation during sleep in patients with interstitial lung disease. Am Rev Respir Dis 1984;129:27.

181. Perez-Padilla R, West P, Lertzman M, et al. Breathing during sleep in patients with interstitial lung disease. Am Rev Respir Dis 1985;132:224.

182. Steljes DG, Kryger MH, Kirk BW, et al. Sleep in post-polio syndrome. Chest 1990;98:133.

183. Bye PTP, Ellis ER, Issa FG, et al. Respiratory failure and sleep in neuromuscular disease. Thorax 1990;45:241.

184. Gay PC, Westbrook PR, Daube JR, et al. Effects of alterations in pulmonary function and sleep variables on survival in patients with amyotrophic lateral sclerosis. Mayo Clin Proc 1991;66:686.

185. Douglas NJ. Breathing during sleep in patients with respiratory disease. Semin Respir Med 1988;9:586.

186. Vianello A, Bevilacqua M, Salvador V, et al. Long-term nasal intermittent positive pressure ventilation in advanced Duchenne's muscular dystrophy. Chest 1994;105:445.

187. Leger P, Bedicam JM, Cornette A, et al. Nasal intermittent positive pressure ventilation. Long-term follow-up in patients with chronic respiratory insufficiency. Chest 1994;105:100.

188. Wiers PWJ, Le Coultre R, Dallinga OT, et al. Cuirass respirator treatment of chronic respiratory failure in scoliotic patients. Thorax 1977;32:221.

189. Curran FJ. Night ventilation by body respirators for patients in chronic respiratory failure due to late stage Duchenne muscular dystrophy. Arch Phys Med Rehabil 1981;62:270.

190. Garay SM, Turino GM, Goldring RM. Sustained reversal of chronic hypercapnia in patients with alveolar hypoventilation syndromes: long-term maintenance with noninvasive nocturnal mechanical ventilation. Am J Med 1981;70:269.

191. Goldstein RS, Molotiun, Skrastins R, et al. Reversal of sleep-induced hypoventilation and chronic respiratory failure by nocturnal negative pressure ventilation in patients with restrictive ventilatory impairment. Am Rev Respir Dis 1987;135:1049.

192. Kinnear W, Hockley S, Harvey J, et al. The effects of one year of nocturnal cuirass ventilation in chest wall disease. Eur Respir J 1988;9:204.

193. Splaingard ML, Frates RC, Jefferson LS, et al. Home negative pressure ventilation: report of 20 years of experience in patients with neuromuscular disease. Arch Phys Med Rehabil 1985;66:239.

194. Mohr CH, Hill NS. Long-term follow-up of nocturnal ventilatory assistance in patients with respiratory failure due to Duchenne-type muscular dystrophy. Chest 1990;97:91.

195. Zibrak JD, Hill NS, Federman EC. Evaluation of intermittent long-term negative pressure ventilation in patients with severe chronic obstructive pulmonary disease. Am Rev Respir Dis 1988;138:1515.

196. Celli B, Lee H, Criner G, et al. Controlled trial of negative pressure ventilation in patients with severe chronic airflow obstruction. Am Rev Respir Dis 1989;140:1251.

197. Shapiro SH, Ernst P, Gray-Diamond K, et al. Effect of negative pressure ventilation in severe chronic obsructive pulmonary disease. Lancet 1992;340:1425.

198. Scharf SM, Feldman NT, Goldman MD, et al. Vocal cord closure: incidence of upper airway obstruction during controlled ventilation. Am Rev Respir Dis 1978;117:391.

199. Levy RD, Bradley TD, Newman S, et al. Negative pressure ventilation: effects on ventilation during sleep in normal subjects. Chest 1989;95:95.

200. Hill NS. Clinical applications of body ventilators. Chest 1986;90:897.

201. Hoeppner VH, Cockcroft DW, Dosman JA, et al. Nighttime ventilation improves respiratory failure in secondary kyphoscoliosis. Am Rev Respir Dis 1984;129:240.

202. Bach JR, Robert D, Leger P, Langevin B. Sleep fragmentation in kyphoscoliotic individuals with alveolar hypoventilation treated by NIPPV. Chest 1995;107:1552.

203. Barbé F, Quera-Salva MA, de Lattre J, et al. Long-term effects of nasal intermittent positive-pressure ventilation on pulmonary function and sleep architecture in patients with neuromuscular diseases. Chest 1996;110:1179.

204. Branthwaite MA. Home mechanical ventilation. Eur Respir J 1990;3:743.

205. Carroll N, Branthwaite MA. Control of nocturnal hypoventilation by nasal intermittent positive pressure ventilation. Thorax 1988;43:349.

206. Ellis ER, Bye PTP, Bruderer JW, et al. Treatment of respiratory failure during sleep in patients with neuromuscular disease: positive-pressure ventilation through a nose mask. Am Rev Respir Dis 1987;135:148.

207. Ellis ER, McCauley VB, Mellis C, et al. Treatment of alveolar hypoventilation in a six-year-old girl with intermittent positive pressure ventilation through a nasal mask. Am Rev Respir Dis 1987;136:188.

208. Ellis ER, Grunstein RR, Chan S, et al. Noninvasive ventilatory support during sleep improves respiratory failure in kyphoscoliosis. Chest 1988;94:811.

209. Gay PC, Patel AM, Viggiano RW, et al. Nocturnal nasal ventilation for treatment of patients with hypercapnic respiratory failure. Mayo Clin Proc 1991;66:695.

210. Goldstein RS, De Rosie IA, Avendano MA, et al. Influence of noninvasive positive pressure ventilation on inspiratory muscles. Chest 1991;99:408.

211. Heckmatt JZ, Loh L, Dubowitz V. Night-time nasal ventilation in neuromuscular disease. Lancet 1990;335:579.

212. Herold DL, Staats BA. Symptomatic nasal CPAP treatment of bilateral diaphragm paralysis. Sleep Res 1991;20:256.

213. Hill NS, Eveloff SE, Carlisle CC, et al. Efficacy of nocturnal nasal ventilation administered by the BiPAP ventilator in restrictive pulmonary diseases. Am Rev Respir Dis 1991;143:A602.

214. Hill NS, Eveloff SE, Carlisle CC, Goff SG. Efficacy of nocturnal ventilation in patients with restrictive thoracic disease. Am Rev Respir Dis 1992;145:365.

215. Jiménez JFM, de Cos Escuin JS, Vicente CD, et al. Nasal intermittent positive pressure ventilation. Analysis of its withdrawal. Chest 1995;107:382.

216. Kerby GR, Mayer LS, Pingleton SK. Nocturnal positive pressure ventilation via nasal mask. Am Rev Respir Dis 1987;136:188.

217. Leger P, Jennequin J, Gerard M, et al. Home positive pressure ventilation via nasal mask for patients with neuromuscular weakness or restrictive lung or chest-wall disease. Respir Care 1989;34:73.

218. Segall D. Noninvasive nasal mask-assisted ventilation in respiratory failure of Duchenne muscular dystrophy. Chest 1988;93:1298.

219. Sanders MH, Black J, Stiller RA, et al. Nocturnal ventilatory assistance with bi-level positive airway pressure. Otolaryngol Head Neck Surg 1991;2:56.

220. Sanders MH, Kern NB. Long-Term Experience with BiPAP in Neuromuscular Disease Patients: Clinical and Physiologic Implications. Toyko, Japan: III World Congress for Sleep Apnea and Rhonchopathy, 1991;23.

221. Diaz CE, Deoras KS, Allen JL. Chest wall motion before and during mechanical ventilation in children with neuromuscular disease. Pediatr Pulmonol 1993;16:89.

222. Padman R, Lawless S, van Nessen S. Use of BiPAP® by nasal mask in the treatment of respiratory insufficiency in pediatric patients: preliminary investigation. Pediatr Pulmonol 1994;17:119.

223. Robertson PL, Roloff DW. Chronic failure in limb-girdle muscular dystrophy: successful long-term therapy with nasal bilevel positive airway pressure. Pediatr Neurol 1994;10:328.

224. Rodenstein DO, Stanescu DC, Delguste PM, et al. Adaptation to intermittent positive pressure ventilation applied through the nose during day and night. Eur Respir J 1989;2:473.

225. Levine S, Henson D, Levy RD. Respiratory muscle rest therapy. Clin Chest Med 1988;9:297.

226. Carrey Z, Gottfried SB, Levy RD. Ventilatory muscle support in respiratory failure with nasal positive pressure ventilation. Chest 1990;97:150.

227. Belman MJ, Soo Hoo GW, Kuei IH, et al. Efficacy of positive vs negative pressure ventilation in unloading the respiratory muscles. Chest 1990;98:850.

228. Rochester DF, Braun NMT, Laine S. Diaphragmatic energy expenditure in chronic respiratory failure. Am J Med 1977;63:223.

229. Delguste P, Aubert-Tulkens G, Rodenstein DO. Upper airway obstruction during nasal intermittent positive-pressure hyperventilation during sleep. Lancet 1991;338:1295.

230. Parreira VF, Jounieaux V, Aubert G, et al. Nasal two-level positive-pressure ventilation in normal subjects. Effects of the glottis and ventilation. Am J Respir Crit Care Med 1996;153:1616.

231. Jounieaux V, Aubert G, Dury M, et al. Effects of nasal positive-pressure hyperventilation on the glottis in normal awake subjects. J Appl Physiol 1995;79:176.

232. Jounieaux V, Aubert G, Dury M, et al. Effects of nasal positive-pressure hyperventilation on the glottis in normal sleeping subjects. J Appl Physiol 1995;79:186.

233. Robert D, Langévin B, Leger P. Mouth air leaks during noninvasive nasal intermittent positive pressure ventilation. Am Rev Respir Dis 1991;143:A587.

234. Meyer TJ, Pressman MR, Benditt J, et al. Air leak through the mouth during nocturnal nasal ventilation: effect on sleep quality. Sleep 1997;20:561.

235. Bach JR, Alba AS, Shin D. Management of alternatives for post-polio respiratory insufficiency. Am J Phys Med Rehabil 1989;68:264.

236. Bach JR, Sorter SM, Saporito LR. Interfaces for noninvasive intermittent positive pressure ventilatory support in North America. Eur Respir Rev 1993;3:254.

237. Bach JR, Alba AS, Bohatiuk G, et al. Mouth intermittent positive pressure ventilation in the management of post-polio respiratory insufficiency. Chest 1987;91:859.

238. Bach JR, Alba AS. Noninvasive options for ventilatory support of the traumatic high level quadriplegic patient. Chest 1990;98:613.

239. Sanders MH, Kern NB, Costantino JP, et al. Accuracy of end-tidal and transcutaneous $P_{CO_2}$ monitoring during sleep. Chest 1994;106:472.

240. McLellan PA, Goldstein RS, Ramacharan V, et al. Transcutaneous carbon dioxide monitoring. Am Rev Respir Dis 1981;124:199.

241. Mahutte CK, Michiels TM, Hassel KT, et al. Evaluation of a single transcutaneous $P_{O_2}$-$P_{CO_2}$ sensor in adult patients. Crit Care Med 1984;12:1063.

242. Martin RJ. Transcutaneous monitoring: instrumentation and clinical implications. Respir Care 1990;35:577.

243. Shacter EN, Rafferty TD, Knight C, et al. Transcutaneous oxygen and carbon dioxide monitoring: uses in adult surgical patients in an intensive care unit. Arch Surg 1981;116:1193.

244. Martin RJ, Beoglos A, Miller MJ, et al. Increasing arterial carbon dioxide tension: influence on transcutaneous carbon dioxide tension measurements. Pediatrics 1988;81:684.

245. Hill NS. Noninvasive positive pressure ventilation in neuromuscular disease. Enough is enough! (editorial). Chest 1994;105:337.

246. Stiller RA, Sanders MH, Walsh S, Strollo P. Compliance with noninvasive positive pressure ventilation by patients with neuromuscular respiratory failure. Am J Respir Crit Care Med 1995;151:A535.

247. Fernandes K, Sanders M, Walsh S, et al. Compliance with noninvasive positive pressure ventilation (NIPPV) in neuromuscular disease (NMD) patients: comparison with moderate and severe obstructive sleep apnea (OSA). Am J Respir Crit Care Med 1997;155:A305.

# Chapter 24

# The Clinical Interview and Treatment Planning as a Guide to Understanding the Nature of Insomnia: The CCNY Insomnia Interview

Arthur J. Spielman and Michael W. Anderson

Insomnia is common in the population and frequently chronic or recurrent in the individual.[1–3] Understandably, insomniacs and their doctors are exasperated. Furthermore, only a minority of insomnia sufferers seek treatment and those who do often encounter clinicians who prematurely conclude that the insomnia is the result of psychopathology or unavoidable stress.[4,5] As a result, the patient may receive a drug that targets the psychopathology or aims at the sleep disturbance itself, rather than its cause. The resulting prescription for an antidepressant or a hypnotic, for example, may be of help, but often does not comprehensively address the problem. Such unidimensional approaches are limited and reveal that the clinician does not appreciate that chronic insomnia is the product of multiple determinants.[6–8] A thorough evaluation of insomnia should include assessment of the myriad mechanisms known to produce or sustain disturbed sleep and effective treatment should have multiple components.[9]

This chapter takes the perspective of the clinician, not the theoretician. The emphasis is on clinical observations and what clinicians think and do. Theory, although in the background, plays a prominent role in what clinical material is considered important and an understanding of how the features of insomnia fit into a clinical formulation. Throughout this chapter, we have aimed at assisting the clinician in understanding case material and enhancing the effectiveness of clinical decision making. With this purpose in mind, we have organized this chapter in the form of the clinical evaluation of adult patients with chronic insomnia. Instead of the details of the case, the reader is presented with the features of insomnia that need to be assessed and the understanding that such information yields. Furthermore, the order in which the material is presented reflects the sequence we recommend the clinician follow in the course of the evaluation of the patient. In the typical workup, diagnostic possibilities are formulated and tested throughout the evaluation. It is the framework of this ongoing problem-solving process that we have used to organize the diagnostic entities. Therefore, descriptions of the different insomnia disorders are presented in association with the material from the evaluation that will confirm or exclude that particular diagnosis. Because a plan for treatment is developed at the end of the clinical evaluation, the discussion of treatment approaches is at the end of the chapter.

The purpose of this mode of presentation is didactic. Although all clinicians are familiar with the structure of the clinical encounter, many may be less well-versed in the multiple causes of insomnia. The aim of this chapter is to improve diagnostic reasoning by forging the connection between the interview and the multifaceted nature of insomnia. To further this aim, in the chapter appendix we present a semi-structured interview that schematically summarizes our approach. Generally, the headings and subheadings in this chapter correspond to the headings and subheadings in the interview. Although this chapter is not meant to be a manual for the City College of New York (CCNY) Insomnia Interview, the organization and content of this exposition constitute a primer on the manner in which to conduct the interview. We hope that it will facilitate the understanding and treatment of patients with insomnia.

## IDENTIFYING DATA

At the start of the evaluation the clinician needs a general orientation that provides a broad view of the context of the patient's life. The age of the patient, for example, identifies what developmental challenges are currently at issue. The struggles for autonomy and identity of the adolescent, the conflict between career and childbirth of a 30-year-old single woman, and the psychological and physiologic consequences of illness and infirmity in a senior may be salient and contributing to the insomnia. The adolescent has an increased sleep need and often weekend late-to-bed and late-to-rise sleep habits that may need to be assessed and managed to address morning sleepiness and trouble falling asleep.[10–12] The 30-year-old career woman may be bringing work stress home, thus preventing an adequate wind-down period before bed. Increased health concerns, psychosocial stressors, depression, pain, and discomfort are more common in seniors and interfere with sleep.[13–15] In addition, a variety of primary sleep disorders, such as periodic limb movement disorder, restless legs syndrome, and a variety of sleep-disordered breathing conditions, are more prevalent in seniors.[16]

In addition to age, other standard descriptive features of an individual's life may be noteworthy. What a patient does for a living, the stress involved, and the work schedule are factors that commonly play a role in sleep disturbance. In one case, the changing sleep schedule of the shift worker may be relevant, whereas in another case, a patient's over-concern with performance on the job may adversely

**Table 24-1.** Insomnia Complaints

Not enough sleep
Trouble falling asleep
Difficulty staying asleep
Early morning awakening
Light or unrefreshing sleep
Cannot sleep without sleeping pills
Sleep is unpredictable
Unable to sleep when work schedule permits

Source: Adapted from AJ Spielman, J Nunes, PB Glovinsky. Insomnia. In M Aldrich (ed), Neurologic Clinics (Vol. 14, no. 3). Philadelphia: Saunders, 1996;513.

affect sleep. Similarly, changes in marital status and family concerns are sources of stress. This type of background information sets the stage for understanding the patient's sleep problems within the overall context of their lives.

## COMPLAINT

### The Patient's Presentation of Unsatisfactory Sleep

The patient's description of the sleep problem is key in directing the clinician's attention toward particular domains (Table 24-1). The time of night that is most problematic is a major clue for the assessment and treatment of insomnia. Over time, chronic insomnia may change, for example, from being exclusively a difficulty with sleep onset to a problem that includes trouble staying asleep.[17,18] Although the temporal pattern of the sleep disturbance is not immutable, this does not diminish the value of knowing when in the night sleep is currently disturbed.

In patients with exclusively sleep-onset problems, there is little need to consider conditions that interrupt sleep, such as periodic limb movements, frequent urination, and alcohol consumption. Difficulty initiating sleep suggests particular problems, such as arousing activities too close to bedtime, maladaptive conditioning, ruminative anxiety, or the lack of coordination between the retiring time and the biological rhythm of sleep propensity.

Awakenings from sleep are common in all individuals. People without sleep disturbance only remember a few of these interruptions of sleep because they are brief. Awakenings that occur in the second half of sleep are potentially long and disruptive because the homeostatic need for sleep has been substantially discharged.[19] In older individuals, the second half of the night can be particularly problematic because of age-related changes in sleep architecture and the altered phase relationship between circadian rhythms.[20] The well-documented reductions in stages III and IV sleep produce a "lighter," more easily disrupted sleep. Furthermore, the timing of sleep tends to be earlier in older individuals and this shift results in the second half of the sleep period occurring at a time when the circadian rhythm of body temperature is rising. Work in time-free environments has shown that in individuals of all ages, the rising limb of the body temperature curve is the predominant time when subjects awake from sleep.[21] Therefore, for a variety of reasons, maintaining sleep in the later part of the night is particularly problematic.

The evaluation of sleep maintenance insomnia begins with a thorough description of the experience of the awakenings. Although there is no formula for translating individual features of the awakening back to the instigating factor, the details of the experience may suggest areas to be explored. Awakenings with epigastric pain or the need to void, for example, indicate specific conditions that require intervention. The solution to the problem is more complex with cases in which patients awaken abruptly and the only worry on their mind is how poorly they will perform the next day if they do not get back to sleep quickly.

Identifying the portion of the night that is most disturbed allows the clinician to prescribe a sleep schedule at the start of treatment that promotes sleep regardless of the specific mechanisms that are responsible for the problem. Consolidation of sleep is often one goal of treatment and can be accomplished by reducing time in bed.[22] In general, if the sleep disturbance is more prominent in the first half of the night, a later bedtime is scheduled. Conversely, poor sleep in the second half of the sleep period suggests establishing an earlier wake-up schedule. These new sleep schedules have the effect of reducing wakefulness at the time of the night when it is most problematic. The result is more compact, less fragmented sleep.

Similarly, the choice of sedative-hypnotic is also guided by the time of the night when sleep is disturbed. A patient with exclusively sleep-onset difficulties, for example, requires proper timing of drug administration so that therapeutic blood levels are present at the time of retiring. Because there is no need to sustain sleep, in this type of case, the medication should have a short or intermediate plasma elimination half-life if administered on a chronic basis. The time of the night that is disturbed will also determine the proper timing of exposure to bright light or exogenous melatonin administration to shift circadian rhythms to help ameliorate the insomnia.[23–26]

The frequency of poor sleep is a measure of severity and may suggest a structure to the inquiry. In cases of intermittent insomnia, for example, the inquiry will naturally focus on the different circumstances surrounding good and bad periods.

The patient's complaint of disturbed sleep is to be understood as a symptom that needs to be placed within a larger diagnostic context. The symptom of trouble falling asleep, for example, may be due to a dysthymic disorder with prominent ruminative features, a circadian rhythm disorder such as jet lag, or a learned psychophysiologic condition. If the clinician does not delve beneath the presentation to ascertain the meaning of the complaint, a symptom-relief approach to treatment may be prescribed by default.

### Date of Onset of Insomnia

Knowing when the insomnia began is crucial to discovering what produced the sleep disturbance. The circumstances of the patient's life at the time the sleep problem started may provide clues to the instigating factors. Job stress, for example, may have overwhelmed coping capacity and the insomnia that has resulted may be alleviated by emotional support, a strategic plan to address the problem, or reduced expectations of how good sleep will be given the challenges of the moment. Health and family concerns are also common stressors that trigger insomnia. The prevalence of psychopathology in patients with insomnia necessitates a thorough inquiry into psychological symptoms, thematic conflicts, and coping capacity at the time the sleep problem began.

Determining the date of the onset of the problem permits a comprehensive historical account of changes over time. It can also be valuable to include a survey of the premorbid conditions such as sleep schedule, practices of everyday living, drug regimen, and general sleep hygiene.

### Sleep-Wake Pattern

A thorough description of how the patient sleeps at night is at the center of the evaluation. All of the aspects of the case must be understood in their relationship to the disturbed sleep. It is therefore essential that the clinician gets a clear picture of the sleep-wake pattern early in the evaluation process. In addition, many of the descriptive features of how the patient sleeps are also potential etiologic factors in the insomnia. Prolonged tossing, turning, and ruminating in bed while trying to fall asleep, for example, are an indication of both the severity of the insomnia, as well as the possible pathogenic role of hyperarousal, excessive worrying, and too much time spent in bed.

An exclusive focus early in the evaluation on the numerous features of the sleep schedule, presleep habits, and nocturnal behavior, however, runs the risk of overemphasizing these features. For a more balanced investigation, we recommend that the clinician limit the scope of the inquiry at the beginning of the assessment to the key aspects of the sleep pattern described in this section. After other areas have been explored, we suggest a systematic survey of the remaining practices associated with the sleep pattern, described in Inadequate Sleep Hygiene later in this chapter.

How the patient sleeps at night provides a quantification of the severity of the problem. The report of the frequency of bad nights, the length of time to fall asleep, and the number and duration of nocturnal awakenings gives the clinician a measure of the seriousness of the sleep disturbance. Although the amount of sleep obtained is one important determinant of sleep adequacy, other features, such as the continuity and depth of sleep, also contribute to the value of sleep. In addition, nightly variability in the timing of sleep supplies information on the relative synchronization of sleep with other rhythmic biological functions.

The clinician needs to be alert to any changes that produce improvements or impairments in sleep. Changes in the sleep pattern, for example, on different nights of the week and when the patient sleeps away from home, offer clues to the mechanisms responsible for the sleep disturbance. Going to bed later on the weekend makes it easier for individuals with delayed sleep phase syndrome to fall asleep.[11] In contrast, a later bedtime exacerbates sleep-onset difficulties in individuals who worry so much about sleep loss that they believe starting out with less available sleep time is a strike against them.

Patients' reports of how they sleep may lack details that are important. Although sleep is the focus of the complaint in insomnia, nuances may not be recounted because of failures of memory. It is not unusual, for example, for patients to be unaware of how frequently they doze briefly in the evening while reading and watching television. In other cases, the patients may be more aware of a recent period during which sleep problems have been exacerbated than the more distantly experienced but more typical pattern of good nights mixed in with bad nights.

In addition to failures of memory, a faithful representation of the sleep problem may be compromised by a patient's desire to emphasize bad nights when asked for a portrayal of sleep. When asked how much sleep they get on average or on a typical night, patients may neglect to take into account the good nights. This biased presentation may be due to insomniacs' previous experience with clinicians who did not take their complaint seriously.

The use of a sleep log, prospectively filled out, helps avoid these and other problems of the retrospective history. We recommend that the patient fill out a simple diary that is easy to use and enables the clinician to grasp the pattern and details of the problem via a graphic format. Alongside each of the stacked 24-hour grids is a set of questions about sleep, alcohol, and medication use, as well as the quality of sleep and daytime fatigue. The reader is referred to Spielman et al.[8] for a detailed discussion and illustration of the use of the sleep log in clinical practice. We will present one case here, as an example. For clarity, we have omitted the questions that accompany each day's entry from the illustration (Figure 24-1).

A young computer programmer complained, "I can't fall asleep, no matter how tired I am." Sleep latencies of 1–3 hours during the week result in inadequate amounts of sleep because he "should get to work by 9 AM." Struggling to wake up in the morning, he often turns off his alarm, falls back to sleep, and is late for work. An analysis of the sleep log reveals the following items:

## SLEEP LOG:  Use these symbols

● Lights out or in bed trying to sleep    ⊢─┤ Asleep    ○ Lights on or out of bed for the night    C  Caffeinated coffee or soda

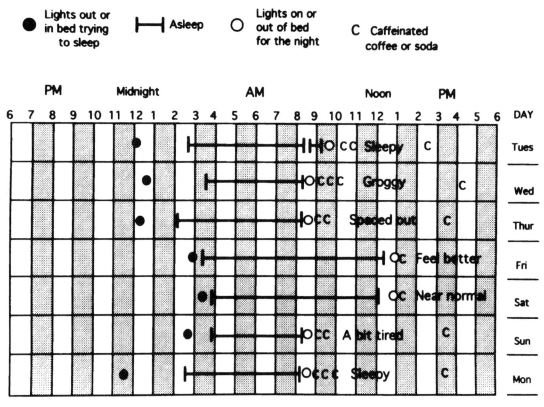

**Figure 24-1.** An illustration of the use of a sleep log in the evaluation of a case of a man with difficulty falling asleep at night and trouble waking and "getting going" in the morning.

- The problem is exclusively at the beginning of the night; once asleep, he sleeps well.
- Trouble waking in the morning is evident.
- The problem resolves on the weekends, when he goes to sleep later and sleeps into the afternoon.

This case can be understood as a mismatch between the patient's internal clock and his work schedule. The features of delayed sleep phase syndrome[11,27] are well-illustrated by the sleep log.

Details of the sleep schedule and sleep pattern are easily appreciated from the sleep log and provide information on both the problem that needs to be treated and the sleep hygiene practices that may be contributing to the sleep disturbance. To reduce redundancy, we systematically review all sleep hygiene practices and limit ourselves in this section to a description of the basic parameters of the sleep pattern. We suggest that the interview of the patient proceed in a chronologic order from events in the evening, such as medication use and sleep latency, to features present in the morning, such as the variability of the wake-up time and the patient's estimate of sleep duration.

*Sleep Medication*

The type and amount of sedative-hypnotics, as well as the time of administration and frequency with which they are used, are essential pieces of information. In addition, the efficacy, side effects, withdrawal effects on discontinuation, and the degree of drug tolerance that has developed to the sleeping medication are important to understand. This information helps the clinician to determine if the patient has a hypnotic-dependent sleep disorder.[27]

A more subtle source of valuable clinical material is the way in which patients decide whether to use sleeping medication on a particular night. Many patients will start the night by trying to fall asleep without a sleeping pill. On nights when they have difficulty they may wait an hour or more before they resort to the sleep medicine. The onset of action of the medicine will then be delayed until an adequate blood concentration is reached. In this case, the strategy of attempting to do without the pill did not work and resulted in the patient having spent a considerable portion of the night in distress and not sleeping. Furthermore, patients waiting to see if they can fall asleep on their own often leads to an arousing internal monologue. The patient may be preoccupied with the question of, "Should I throw in the towel and take the pill or tough it out?" This kind of internal monologue is counterproductive.

### Time at Which Patient Goes to Bed

Many patients get into bed well before trying to get to sleep. This affords them the chance to rest, watch television, and feel comforted. Although getting into bed before turning the lights out may be part of the presleep ritual that is conducive for sleep, it may also permit counterproductive dozing, negative conditioning, and variability in the time of falling asleep. Therefore, if there is substantial time spent in bed awake before attempting to go to sleep, the details of the patient's activities and experience need to be explored.

### Time for "Lights Out"

The variability of the time of retiring or lights out is one gauge of the regularity of sleep-wake habits that may have an impact on sleep. In addition, the reason for the irregular retiring time may provide clues to other contributions to the sleep problem. Patients who are pushed to stay at work late or pulled by social opportunities may be too keyed up to sleep well. Furthermore, widely varying lights-out times may be an indication of poor internal self-regulation or lack of mastery of life's challenges. Therefore, in addition to documenting the pattern of lights-out time, an exploration of the meaning of this parameter is also important.

Some individuals do not turn the lights off and begin to try to go to sleep, but set a timer that automatically switches off the television or radio. This may work, because it allows them to drift gradually into sleep. This is a strategy chosen by people who get aroused by preparations for sleep as minor as reaching up to turn off the bedside lamp.

### Sleep Latency

The time it takes to fall asleep is one measure of the severity of insomnia. The duration of sleep latency also gives an indication of the time the patient tosses and turns in bed struggling for sleep. The time of sleep onset, which can be calculated from the time of lights out and sleep latency, provides information on the phase of circadian rhythms. Individuals with delayed sleep phase syndrome, for example, may have a late but stable time of falling asleep, regardless of the time of lights out.

As discussed earlier, individuals who use a sleep timer on the television may have a sleep latency that is indeterminate. Because they do not decide to start trying to sleep, the only measure available that approximates the sleep latency is the time from getting into bed to the time of sleep onset.

### Awakenings

The number, timing, and duration of awakenings are important features of the pattern of insomnia. The experience of the awakening and how an individual copes during the night offer clues to the mechanisms responsible for the sleep disturbance.

### Wake-Up Time

A variable wake-up time has many origins, whereas an unvarying wake-up time suggests a circadian rhythm–timed arousal, a sleep stage–cued awakening, or environmental disturbance. It has been shown that in time-free conditions, waking up occurs as body temperature rises.[21] Although the circadian wakefulness stimulus becomes stronger as the endogenous circadian body temperature rhythm rises in the morning, studies suggest that in the real world of entrained conditions, the habitual time of spontaneous awakening is predominantly determined by the amount of sleep.[28] It has been demonstrated that the ability to awaken at a predetermined time is possible and may be a function of sleep stage.[29] Another source of arousal is the regular occurrence of environmental disturbances, such as sunrise, birds chirping, and the sounds associated with traffic, that may disturb the sleeper and produce a set wake-up time.

*Out-of-Bed Time*

The time that the sleep period ends supplies information on the variability of sleep-wake habits and the amount of time in bed, which are key features of sleep hygiene. Individuals who linger in bed long after they wake up may occasionally fall asleep again. Getting more sleep in the morning adds variability to the sleep-wake cycle. In some cases, the extra sleep obtained will delay sleep onset or reduce the amount or depth of sleep on the subsequent night.[30]

*Total Sleep Time*

The patient's estimate of the amount of sleep obtained is another index of the severity of the sleep disturbance and a predictor of the impact one can expect on daytime functioning. In addition, a log of the fluctuations in sleep duration from night to night is an opportunity for the clinician to discover the factors responsible for the insomnia. A patient able to fall asleep faster or stay asleep longer on the weekends suggests that the stresses present during the work week may play a role in the sleep problem in this individual. Alternatively, it may be easier to sleep on the weekends because the absence of a required, early wake-up time reduces anticipatory anxiety. The individual is less worried about a bad night's sleep, because there is ample time to sleep in.

*Total Time in Bed*

It is common knowledge that sleep during the day may interfere with sleep at night. Just as it is easy to forget to return borrowed book, failure to report a momentary nod is understandable. Therefore, the clinician is advised to use multiple terms in the inquiry, such as *nap, doze, nod,* and "zone out" to help record all instances of daytime sleep. Similarly, if the clinician asks only about daytime sleep episodes, the patient may exclude evening napping.

The sleep period, or time in bed, is calculated from the time of lights out to the time the subject gets out of bed. This feature of the sleep pattern needs to be considered, because insomniacs may cope with their sleeping difficulty by increasing the duration of this potential sleep period to maximize their opportunity to sleep.

The limited selection of features of the sleep-wake pattern discussed here include the essential informa-

tion for understanding a patient's insomnia. We will consider how these and other features contribute to the insomnia in the section Inadequate Sleep Hygiene.

It is also helpful to get the same information about the sleep-wake pattern from a time period before the sleep disturbance began. The perspective of the premorbid picture should help generate a reasonable set of goals for treatment. If the patient has always been a light sleeper but is now having trouble falling asleep, it may be useful for the patient and clinician to agree that the aim of treatment is explicitly focused on the circumscribed problem of sleep onset. Moreover, simple changes in sleep habits may have contributed to the problem. Patients may be unaware, for example, of how their recently adopted coping strategy of sleeping later on weekends to compensate for sleep loss during the week has reduced the stability of sleep.

## HISTORY OF THE PROBLEM

We have discussed the usefulness of a simple schema to classify historical material into predisposing, precipitating, and perpetuating factors that contribute to insomnia.[6-8,31,32] Assessing and addressing these different factors results in a comprehensive treatment plan.

Some individuals are predisposed to develop insomnia because of personality traits or concurrent conditions. People inclined to obsess and ruminate over past defeats or worry about anticipated failures, for example, are vulnerable to insomnia. They may be able to sleep well when their life is routine (Figure 24-2, premorbid), but when they make a mistake or face an upcoming challenge, intrusive cognitions may disrupt the sleeping process (Figure 24-2, acute). Similarly, an individual who has a lifelong pattern of being alert and active at night may have no sleeping problem until a time of increased stress. Dampening arousal at night to fall asleep may then become quite difficult for this "night-owl." The high degree of association between psychopathology such as depressive and anxiety disorders with insomnia are other examples of the link between predisposing conditions and chronic or recurrent sleep disturbance (Figure 24-3).

In addition to characteristics of the individual, the precipitating event that initiates an episode of insomnia is an important focus of the inquiry. Identification of the instigating factor allows therapy to target

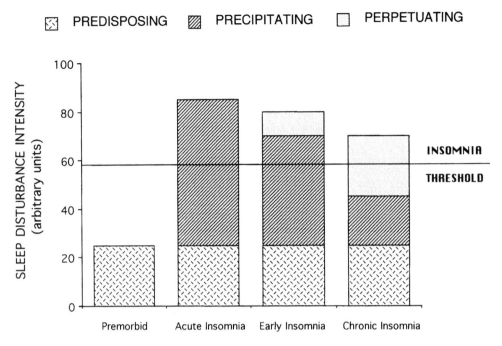

**Figure 24-2.** A schematic model of the development of an unspecified type of chronic insomnia and the changing factors that play a role over the course of the disorder. (Adapted with permission from AJ Spielman, L Caruso, PB Glovinsky. A Behavioral Perspective on Insomnia. In M Erman [ed], Psychiatric Clinics of North America. Philadelphia: Saunders, 1987.)

this cause of the problem. Insomnia secondary to retirement, for example, may suggest counseling the patient regarding loss of self-esteem, continuing to set the alarm clock in the morning, and avoiding the temptation to nap when there is nothing to do.

It is not always the case that triggering factors are relevant to the current insomnia, however, especially as time passes and the sleep disturbance has become chronic (see Figure 24-2, chronic). As insomnia becomes persistent, the patient may become so worried in anticipation of a bad night's sleep that the worry itself inhibits sleep. In other cases, patients change their habits to cope with the insomnia. Increased time spent in bed, for example, may sustain insomnia by weakening the self-sustaining properties of a regular sleep-wake schedule. Perpetuating factors may be of secondary importance or may become the principal determinants of the current sleep disturbance (see Figure 24-3, Table 24-2). We emphasize the importance of these sustaining factors because they are common and need to be addressed for successful treatment.

The role of predisposing, precipitating, and perpetuating factors is most convincingly seen in patients with recurrent insomnia. A log of the alter-

nating periods of adequate and troubled sleep provides the clinician with an opportunity to look for similarities in both the precipitating factors and the changes or interventions that produced remission. In cases in which the triggering event is similar, the clinician is in a strong position to help the patient examine himself or herself to discover the meaning of this vulnerability. In other individuals, the similarity between episodes that is striking is the intense worry over the consequences of poor sleep or the altered sleep schedule that they adopt to cope with the problem. These responses to the insomnia, referred to as *perpetuating factors*, may be the salient features that sustain the sleep problem.

In taking a history and when working with an insomnia patient over a protracted period, the clinician keeps an eye out for fluctuations in the severity of the sleep problem and any corresponding change in the patient, habits of daily living, or life circumstances. A determination needs to be made between features that covary with the sleep disturbance and may be contributing to the problem and features that are merely coincident. Although it has clinical value to discover that an insomniac, for example, suffers from untreated daytime panic attacks, whether anxi-

**Figure 24-3.** The development of chronic insomnia. Illustration of how predisposing and perpetuating factors may play either a separate or combined role in pathways leading to insomnia. (Adapted from AJ Spielman, J Nunes, PB Glovinsky. Insomnia. Neurol Clin 1996;14:513.)

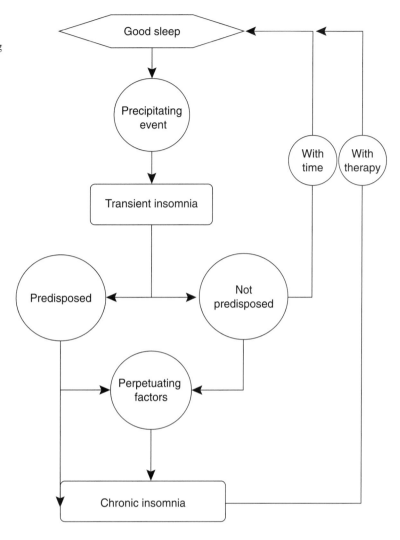

ety has any role in the insomnia must be ascertained and not assumed. If insomnia occurs only at times when panic has been present, then the covariation of these two problems suggests, but does not prove, causality. On the other hand, if it is clear that the two conditions do not occur at the same time, comorbidity rather than causality is suggested.

In many patients, there is partial covariation of poor sleep and a sleep disturber. There may be poor nights and good nights after both days with and without alcohol ingestion, for example. Although this suggests independence, it is only when insomnia and alcohol ingestion do not occur together that the clinician can discount any connection. Because insomnia is multidetermined, alcohol may contribute to sleeplessness but not be sufficient to produce sleep inter-

**Table 24-2.** Factors That Commonly Perpetuate Insomnia

Too much time in bed
Variable retiring and arising times
Unpredictability of sleep
Concern about daytime deficits
Napping, dozing, and nodding
Fragmentation of sleep
Maladaptive conditioning
Caffeine consumption
Hypnotic and alcohol ingestion

Source: Adapted from AJ Spielman, PB Glovinsky. The Evaluation and Differential Diagnosis of Insomnia. In M Pressman, W Orr (eds), Sleep and Biological Rhythms in Health and Sickness, Washington, DC: American Psychological Association, 1997.

ruption. In this and other cases of partial covariation, the alcohol should be considered a putative contributor to the insomnia until proven otherwise. The critical importance of covariation in identifying features that contribute to the insomnia is repeatedly represented in the CCNY Insomnia Interview by providing a place for the clinician to rate covariation on a scale.

The patient's answer to "What makes your sleep better or worse?" may uncover areas to explore, underscores the fact that the adequacy of sleep varies, and implicitly instructs the patient to be on the lookout for patterns that offer clues to the mechanisms responsible for the sleep disturbance.

### Daytime Consequences

In the final analysis, it is not the time to sleep onset, number of awakenings, depth of sleep, or amount of sleep obtained that matters, but how the experiences of the night affect the day. In general, the consequences of insomnia fall into the following broad categories: fatigue, sleepiness, impaired performance, mood disturbance, decreased motivation, and anxiety in anticipation of a bad night's sleep. Experimental studies that induce sleep loss or interrupt sleep continuity in noncomplaining subjects produce this set of effects with the exception of the anticipatory anxiety of sleeplessness.

In most cases, the patient's description of the severity of the nocturnal sleep disturbance corresponds to the depiction of the daytime functional impairment. In other cases, the daytime consequences appear to be substantially more or less severe than one would expect from the degree of nighttime disturbance.

In the extreme, there are patients who report that totally sleepless nights are common and yet they present with only moderate daytime problems. However, studies of normals have shown that profound decrements in alertness, performance, and motivation, as well as change in mood, are a reliable consequence of complete deprivation of sleep.[33] Thus, it is unlikely that these patients are getting as little sleep as they report. Typically, when patients who complain of obtaining no sleep at all are studied in the laboratory, their sleep is found to be relatively normal.[34]

Patients who have relatively normal sleep but report no sleep at all represent the extreme of sleep state misperception disorder.[27] It is well-known that patients with chronic insomnia generally overestimate nocturnal sleep latency and underestimate total sleep time when their subjective estimates are compared to polygraphically recorded sleep.[35-37] Nonetheless, it is important to remember that even in insomnia patients, there is a significant and strong positive relationship between subjective and objective sleep latency and subjective and objective total sleep time.[36] Thus, the patient's subjective report of the severity of the sleep disturbance does correspond to the results of the polygraph.

Patients diagnosed with sleep state misperception often have impaired daytime vigilance and, paradoxically, are mildly sleepier than patients with objective insomnia.[38] Our group found similar results in a group of middle-aged and elderly insomniacs.[39]

Sleep state misperception is not well-understood. Suggested explanations for the misperception include sleep continuity disturbances, subtle micro awakenings, and complaining due to psychological response style.[40-42] Some work has suggested that hypnotics are effective in treating insomnia not by improving sleep, but by changing the sleeping subject's perception of it.[43]

A similar mismatch is seen in the patient who complains of daytime impairments but reports only minor sleep disturbance. This combination of symptoms reminds us that the typical daytime problems of insomnia may be a product of psychopathology. The fatigue, depressive mood, irritability, anxiety, flagging motivation, and performance decrements seen in insomniacs are also the symptoms associated with depressive and anxiety conditions. Thus, the evaluation of insomnia will invariably include an assessment of psychological state.

An unexpected mismatch is the complaint of insufficient sleep without daytime sleepiness as a consequence. As a group, insomniacs have been shown to be no more sleepy than matched normal control subjects, despite lack of sleep.[44-48] The absence of measurable daytime sleepiness in some patients with insomnia, despite their complaints of poor or shortened nocturnal sleep, is consistent with the hyperarousal theory of insomnia (see Hyperarousal in this chapter). To make sense of these data, investigators have suggested that a generalized increase in physiologic arousal may be responsible for both the insomniac's nocturnal sleeplessness and lack of sleepiness during the day.[49]

Although insomniacs as a group are no sleepier during the day than normal control subjects, some data suggest borderline and pathologic sleepiness in a portion of patients with sleep disturbance. A number of studies have found Multiple Sleep Latency Test sleep latencies of fewer than 10 minutes in a substantial proportion of insomniacs,[38,44,45,50] and fewer than 6 minutes in a subset of these patients.[44,51] The hyperarousal theory of insomnia does not appear to account for this group of individuals.

It is important to recognize that although many individuals with insomnia may suffer from a form of central nervous system hyperarousal, others may be carrying around a moderate to severe level of daytime sleepiness. An assessment of daytime sleepiness in insomnia is important, because some standard behavioral treatments seek to increase sleep drive through mild, partial sleep deprivation.[22] These therapies may further reduce daytime alertness in compromised individuals. A thorough understanding of the daytime functioning in insomnia may provide us with more reliable diagnostic categories and better information on which to base our treatment decisions.

### Sleep-Related Cognition: Cognitive Hyperarousal and the Vicious Circle of Dysfunctional Reasoning and Worrying

The patient's opinion about the cause of the insomnia should be explicitly elicited. In addition to the potential validity of this understanding, the patient is also directing the clinician's attention to problematic areas of his or her life. The patient's hypothesis of what is provoking the sleep disturbance also informs the clinician of the individual's preferred mode of explanation. The idea, for example, that a "chemical imbalance in the brain" is responsible for the sleep disturbance in a rigid individual who is prone to somatizing serves as a caution that if psychogenic explanations are relevant, they must be offered with considerable tact.

As insomniacs know too well, an act of will is not sufficient to produce sleep. It is easy to arrange the external conditions that facilitate sleep, such as darkness, quiet, and an appropriate time for sleep onset. Similarly, the behavioral prerequisites for sleep, including recumbency, stillness, and closed eyes, are readily performed. It is the quiet mind that is often elusive, and without it, the insomniac is unprepared

for sleep. When the mind is churning, anticipating dangers and rewards, surveying losses, and planning for the future, the path to sleep is blocked.

Origins of the unquiet mind are diverse. A state of cognitive hyperarousal may be produced by events during the day that keep the individual keyed up at night. The worrying, racing, ruminative mind may be a more enduring trait or cognitive style in individuals with psychological conflicts that keep the mind scanning for trouble ahead and appraising the damage done. Another common cause of the overactive ideation is the sleep disturbance itself. As a result of repeated experiences of poor sleep, the expectation of a bad night produces worry and anxiety that exacerbate the problem.[52] This vicious circle is frustrating and causes many insomniacs to plead that, if they could just stop worrying about their sleep, the problem would be solved. Learning counterproductive cognitive associations is considered part of the pathogenesis of psychophysiologic insomnia.[27,53]

Dysfunctional sleep-related thinking processes have been proposed as contributors to insomnia.[54,55] This cognitive perspective suggests that it is the insomniac's way of framing his or her sleep experience that becomes problematic. Many insomniacs, for example, conclude that their insomnia is due to a loss of personal control rather than external circumstances. The individual may therefore believe that he or she no longer has mastery over the sleeping process and this threatening prospect may make sleeping more difficult. Similarly, the insomniac's inference that the cause of the sleep problem is chronic and unavoidable fuels worries about sleep. Another way that insomniacs' thinking affects their sleep is the overemphasis or exclusive focus on poor sleep as the root cause of all of their problems. The importance thus placed on getting a good night's sleep may be counterproductive.

The patient with psychophysiologic insomnia can devote extraordinary amounts of time during the day worrying about their sleep and tend to "catastrophize" or exaggerate the consequences of even modestly impaired nighttime sleep.[56] They often compare their own sleep quantity and quality to an unrealistic ideal that further increases their anxiety. They may view all of the day's misfortunes, mood swings, and angry outbursts as a direct and exclusive result of their poor sleep at night. The increased anxiety about their sleep pattern is often a major barrier to falling asleep for these patients.

A personality characteristic that is associated with individuals who are prone to chronic and recurrent insomnia is a high degree of reactivity to bad sleep. Individuals predisposed to insomnia cannot tolerate a brief period of poor sleep without reaching out for some relief, such as sleeping pills, compensatory naps, or spending extra time in bed trying to catch up on lost sleep. These vulnerable individuals feel like they are caught in a vicious circle. Their overconcern or excessive reaction to a bad night's sleep is, in part, responsible for the entrenched nature of the sleep problem.

It is worth noting that a period of poor sleep is essentially a universal human experience. Most individuals weather this sleeplessness with the expectation that this stormy period will be transient. They posit circumscribed and specific reasons for the trouble sleeping and they do not blame themselves. They put up with the problem and allow self-correcting processes to take hold. Thus, the enhanced sleep propensity due to sleep loss together with the central nervous system's periodic programming of sleep are relied on to re-establish a regular sleep regimen.

In contrast, the insomniac worries or expects that the sleep disturbance will be stable and long-lived. They may have a limited understanding of the cause of the poor sleep or assume that the factors responsible are ubiquitous, unavoidable, and part of who they are. They identify themselves as insomniacs, thus completing the circle and establishing a self-fulfilling prophesy. Individuals who are unable to tolerate a period of bad sleep may take some action to correct the problem that does more harm than good.

In general, the clinical evaluation needs to examine how and what the patient thinks about their sleep and consequent daytime functioning. This material will enable the clinician to understand what insomniacs make of their sleep problem, to analyze the implicit meanings, misperceptions, selective recall, catastrophizing, and covert reasoning that characterize the individual's cognitive processing and contribute to the insomnia. Understanding and addressing the sleep-related concerns of the patient that are a part of the self-perpetuating vicious circle of insomnia are fundamental for successful treatment of chronic insomnia.

To assist the clinician in discovering these sleep-related cognitions, the patients may be asked to fill out a questionnaire or systematically monitor themselves for ideas, beliefs, and expectations about their sleep problem.[55] An ongoing, open-ended discussion of the validity and personal meaning of the sleep problem enables the clinician to point out that the way the sleep problem is construed is part of "who you are and what you make of it," not merely "how things are." This enlarges the patient's perspective and helps foster optimism for treatment.

## Psychological and Social Determinants of Insomnia

### Psychopathology

The two most frequent types of diagnoses of insomnia are insomnia associated with an affective disorder and insomnia associated with an anxiety disorder.[57,58] Therefore, the role of psychological and psychiatric problems in the patient complaining of insomnia needs to be thoroughly examined.

**Depression.**    Sleep disturbance is so commonly a part of the symptom complex of major depressive disorder that it is one of the diagnostic criteria of the disorder.[59] In addition to this categorical connection, there is a parallel temporal connection. It has been shown that changes in the frequency of depressed affect over a 3-year period in older individuals correspond to changes in reported sleep difficulties.[60] Not only is insomnia contemporaneous with depression but it can be considered a risk factor that predates the mood disorder.[2] In a prospective study, nondepressed individuals in whom insomnia persisted were more likely to become depressed 1 year later.

Altered neurophysiology, neuroendocrine and neurochemical features of sleep, and biological rhythms are part of the depressive profile and suggest pathophysiologic mechanisms. These features include a short time from sleep onset to the first rapid eye movement (REM) sleep episode, a shift to an earlier time (called a *phase advance*) of a number of circadian rhythms, nonsuppressed cortisol in the first half of the night, and a potentiated cholinergic system.[61] In addition, the role of sleep in major depression is suggested by different studies showing that several weeks of REM sleep deprivation and one night of total sleep deprivation are antidepressant.[62]

A conundrum often arises with cases in which it is not clear that there is a depressive disorder independent of the insomnia. The question that needs to be answered is, "Do the sleep loss and resulting daytime deficits produce the depressive features or is there a depressive disorder that produces insomnia as one of its symptoms?" The clinician may conclude that the insomnia is primary if the depressive features vary with fluctuations in the severity of the insomnia. However, it is often quite difficult to tease apart cause and effect. Consider, for example, the individual who lacks the motivation to complete occupational tasks and either worries about the job while going to sleep or tries to compensate for lack of productivity by working late into the night. The nocturnal activation interferes with sleep and the next day the patient's mood is distinctly depressed. The clinician will have a hard time deciding if it is simply the sleep loss that is producing the depressive state or if the lack of motivation as a symptom of depression is setting the process of insomnia in motion.

In such difficult cases it is important that the patient understand that both the sleep problem and the depression may need to be addressed for a satisfactory outcome. It is generally the case that a modest improvement in sleep is more readily obtained than a change in the depressive state. We have found that the encouragement gained from even marginally improved sleep often motivates patients to be more hopeful and more engaged with the clinician for the difficult task of addressing the depressive process. Treatment of the sleep disturbance exclusively may, in some cases, be sufficient to improve the entire symptom complex. It is often the case that there are grounds to suspect underlying psychological problems, however, and the clinician needs to help the patient to focus therapeutic attention on these issues.

**Anxiety.**    A substantial proportion of insomniacs are suffering from anxiety disorders.[1,18,57] The mechanisms that produce the arousal in these conditions is unclear. Some investigators have concluded that the personality of insomniacs results in internalization rather than an outward expression of conflicts.[52] The result is emotional and physiologic arousal interfering with sleep.

Awakening with a jolt is seen in hypervigilant individuals who consciously or unconsciously feel threatened. Interestingly, the content of the nocturnal rumination after such abrupt awakenings is often not related to the active psychological conflict. It is the suddenness of the awakening that encourages the clinician to find the psychological threat. The pressure to produce on the job, mourning, jealousy, and humiliation are some of the psychological themes in the lives of patients with startling awakenings. Another clinical example of this mechanism is the distinct subgroup of patients who have recently heard of the illness or death of a friend or relative and begin to awaken suddenly with a rapid and pounding heartbeat or with the feeling that they cannot catch their breath. Although a sleep-disordered breathing problem like sleep apnea needs to be considered in these cases, a psychological mechanism may also be responsible.

**Other Psychopathology and Subsyndromal Conditions.**    Insomniacs often complain that they cannot sleep because they cannot control their "racing" mind.[63] This lack of cognitive control at night is often part of more generalized anxious worrying, frank obsessive, compulsive, or phobic symptoms. In other cases, the content of the thoughts is self-deprecatory or guilt-ridden, and a sense of hopelessness pervades this characteristic depressive thinking. Whether this intrusive ideation is part of a psychopathologic syndrome or exclusively sleep related, the disruption of sleep needs to be addressed.

*Stress*

The tight temporal coincidence of stress and sleep disturbance may be striking. This is more often the case when the sleep problem is of recent origin and the circumstances are fresh in the patient's mind. Studies of diverse groups of chronic insomniacs such as older individuals and holocaust survivors, for example, have confirmed the association of stress and sleep disturbance.[64,65] Diagnoses appropriate to these conditions are adjustment sleep disorder and insomnia associated with post-traumatic stress disorder.[27]

In addition to correlative studies, experimental studies have shown that inducing stress by the anticipation of public speaking, for example, interferes with sleep. Another study examined the pattern of neuroendocrine response to the nighttime preparations before morning surgery.[66] It is not surprising that a major release of cortisol occurred during the body shave prepping for surgery that was not typical of this time of day. This study suggests one possible mechanism by which stress affects sleep.

Although it is common knowledge that excessive demands, difficult decisions, the problems of family and work, and illness interfere with sleep, it is often difficult for individuals to gauge their own level of chronic stress. It appears that people adapt to stress and then lose perspective on the cost to their health and sense of well-being. Circumstances that remove the person from the context of their lives, such as weekends, holidays, and illness, can provide a valuable perspective on the pressures of everyday living. A look at the adequacy of sleep during these relatively stress-free periods may suggest the impact of stress in the more typical life circumstances.

*Inadequate Sleep Hygiene*

The collective habits and practices of everyday living that promote good sleep and optimal daytime functioning have been called *sleep hygiene*. It is clear that some daytime activities, such as evening caffeine consumption or a long nap close to bedtime, may adversely affect sleep. However, most individuals do not appreciate the wide range of habits and actions that may have an impact on sleep. In part, this is because sleep is sufficiently robust in good sleepers to withstand some degree of perturbation. Therefore, conforming to good sleep hygiene practices is not necessary to sleep well.[67,68] If an individual's sleep is trouble-free and daytime mood and functioning are therefore uncompromised, little attention need be given to sleep hygiene. Insomnia sufferers, however, will be well-served by abiding by good sleep hygiene.

In general, sleep hygiene practices (e.g., establishing regular bedtimes) are in agreement with common sense and established principles of sleep regulation. Some practices that appear to be common sense to the insomniac trying to cope with poor sleep, however, may be ill-advised. Sleeping in on the weekends to catch up on lost sleep, for example, is a tried and true strategy for many hardworking individuals. Drinking alcohol in the evening helps many people unwind and relieve the stress of the day. Resting and relaxing in bed watching television for the better part of the evening is a great comfort to many individuals. It is a paradox that these activities, salutary in the good sleeper, are pathogenic in the insomniac.

The clinician should survey the patient's sleep hygiene practices thoroughly, regardless of the etiology of the sleep problem. Even cases in which the cause of the sleep disturbance is clear and circumscribed, habits and practices of everyday living often play a subsidiary role in the problem. Addressing these minor contributions may be easier at the start of treatment than tackling ingrained depressive personality characteristics or the stress of the patient's job. Even minor success in improving sleep by waking up the same time on weekends as the weekdays, for example, may encourage the patient to begin the long process of changing aspects of character, outlook, and work habits.

The following discussion of sleep hygiene practices is organized according to the order in which the patient is asked to describe a typical day in the interview. We review daytime, evening, nighttime, and morning activities by eliciting a description of an ordinary day for the patient in sequence, probing for pertinent information with specific questions. This sequential organization gives structure to the inquiry and yields a detailed picture of the habits of the individual's life.

Collectively, the patient's habits may produce trouble falling or staying asleep. However, it is possible for a single habit of poor sleep hygiene to produce a specific problem. A very brief doze late in the evening, for example, may alert the individual sufficiently to cause falling asleep to become difficult. Nodding for a few seconds does not discharge the need for sleep, however, and once the individual gets to sleep, the continuity of sleep will likely be unaffected.

**Daytime: Caffeine and Napping.**   The benefits of limiting caffeine consumption and not indulging in a nap are intuitively understood by most individuals. Due to the stress of increasing occupational and family demands, however, or as a result of a few poor nights of sleep, we may eschew our typical habits. For example, we may attempt to increase our work speed and efficiency with extra coffee and take a nap to counter drowsiness and boost performance. These strategies may help us keep up with increasing demands but they do not promote good sleep.

It is common knowledge that caffeine's stimulant properties can interfere with falling asleep. It is less well-known, however, that caffeine can produce arousals and sleep fragmentation during the night. Thus, some patients with exclusively sleep maintenance problems drink coffee in the evening because they have no trouble falling sleep. This is a counterproductive habit. Caffeine has a half-life of approximately 3–7 hours in young individuals.[69] With increasing age there is a reduced capacity to metabolize and eliminate caffeine. This results in an increased plasma half-life that reaches 10 hours in some older individuals. Patients and doctors are little aware of the adverse impact of even low doses of caffeine consumed early in the day on sleep continuity. Studies have shown that a dose of caffeine equivalent to 2 cups of strong coffee has an objective impact on electroencephalography (EEG) 24 hours after ingestion.[70] Furthermore, studies have shown that individuals may not be able to tell if they have been given caffeine or a placebo. Thus, it is often difficult for the individual to make a connection between caffeine consumption and trouble falling or staying asleep.

Napping improves alertness and performance but discharges the need for sleep and thus reduces the ability to sleep at night. A vicious circle may then become established if insufficient nocturnal sleep due to the nap produces daytime sleepiness and the need for further napping. Napping at different times of day and for different durations may be particularly disruptive. Lying down to relax or meditate promotes napping.[71] Just as the perception of being asleep at night is not straightforward,[35–37] some individuals may not be aware that they are asleep during a rest period.

Daytime sleep does not invariably produce insomnia. When napping is consistent, the routine can be accommodated. Although there is less total nocturnal sleep, no sleep disturbance is produced. However, this routine does create the need for the daytime sleep episode. Without the regular nap, deficits in performance and daytime alertness will occur. Similarly, it may be unreasonable to expect older individuals who have difficulty sustaining nocturnal sleep to obtain a night's sleep sufficient to permit optimal daytime functioning. A case can be made for scheduled naps with these individuals.

Some worried individuals believe a daytime nap will lead to better sleep at night. In this case, the individual may be frightened that too little sleep will be obtained at night. A daytime nap may ease these worries and thereby foster nocturnal sleep.[72]

**Evening: Presleep Thinking, Consumption, and Habits.**    Creating the calm necessary for sleep requires some interval of time. Arriving home late in the evening because of a long day at work or socializing into the night may therefore interfere with sleep. Settling down may call for the rituals of reading the newspaper, watching television, reestablishing the bond with one's spouse, or the libations of the bathroom.

A wind-down period in the evening before bedtime allows us to decompress from the excitements and woes of the day. Those individuals who work into the night and hold onto the cares of the day until the last moment often suffer continued rumination and tension well into the night. Like the new mother at home with her newborn[7] or the physician who goes to sleep in the hospital while on call, the psychological vigilance continues while these individuals' sleep and the quality and continuity of sleep suffer as a result.[73] Good sleep is promoted when an individual can leave work at the office and feel confident about the amount and quality of work completed. Insecurity, a perfectionist need to review the details of an assignment, and the stress that comes with an impending deadline can all keep the individual keyed up before and during sleep.

As bedtime approaches and the individual anticipates struggling to go to sleep, apprehension increases. This increased worrying is counterproductive and has been discussed earlier (see Sleep-Related Cognition: Cognitive Hyperarousal and the Vicious Circle of Dysfunctional Reasoning and Worrying).

Many insomnia patients do not create a safe haven for sleep. The time before bedtime may be filled with action plans for work. Late evenings during the week may be the only opportunity parents have to discuss family problems. The evening may be the time the patient pursues fitness with intense exercise. The bedroom itself may be a battleground of marital discord or the hub of activities such as late-night telephone calls and work to meet deadlines. The expectation that a flurry of intense and arousing activity at night can be abruptly stopped and sleep should ensue promptly thereafter is unrealistic for many individuals.

In addition to allowing a wind-down period to facilitate sleep, patients with insomnia must not allow the habits of smoking, drinking alcohol, and eating to interfere with sleep. Although the physiologic stimulation produced by caffeine is widely known, the activation resulting from nicotine is less well-appreciated.[74] Alcohol is a mixed blessing for sleep. Relief of the stresses of the day and the sleep-inducing property of alcohol will help individuals fall asleep. However, the continuity of sleep is often interrupted by alcohol. It is unclear what characteristics of alcohol produce the sleep fragmentation but the disruption in the second half of the night is a reliable phenomenon. In a similar vein, eating in the evening may have both sleep-promoting and disruptive effects.[75–79] There is a distinct diurnal rhythm of gastric acid secretion with peak levels occurring around midnight.[80] Eating in the late evening stimulates acid production and will therefore add to this already high level of acidity. As a result, heartburn or acid reflux may occur, which can interfere with falling asleep or wake the individual in the early part of the night. Individuals with this sensitivity should avoid eating late in the evening.

In addition to the potential disruption caused by food consumption, fluid consumption may exacerbate the need to void during the night. Urination during the night interferes with sleep in some individuals, especially in women after childbirth and in older men. It is not clear if the urge to void provokes the awakening or if awareness of the need to urinate becomes evident during an awakening. All of us wake, albeit briefly, numerous times each night, although we remember few of these interruptions from sleep. If during one of these many normal awakenings the need to urinate comes into consciousness, the awakening is prolonged. Going to the bathroom may be sufficiently arousing to prevent a rapid return to sleep.

Intense physical exercise late at night also disrupts sleep.[81] The increase in body temperature and heart rate as a result of exertion are purported mechanisms that produce an arousal that interferes with sleep.

Dozing (even very briefly) or watching television in a trancelike state in the evening can lead to trouble falling asleep that is out of proportion to the brevity of the sleep episode or altered state of consciousness. This may be the origin of some patients' reports that if they do not fall asleep within a narrow window of opportunity at night, they become aroused and sleep will elude them for hours. It appears that just becoming sedentary or "spacing out" may be sufficient to relieve some drowsiness and increase arousal. In other cases, patients are relaxed until the decision to go to sleep propels them to engage in presleep preparations that are arousing. To understand these patterns of paradoxical alertness, the clinician must get the details of the patient's evening.

If the bed becomes the hub of nonsleep activities at night, the demarcation between the waking day and the sleeping night will become blurred. Seemingly innocuous activities performed in bed such as talking on the phone, preparing assignments for work, and just relaxing can become associated with the bed and anticipated as part of the in-bed experience. The bed no longer serves as a cue that evokes the sleep response; rather, it may produce arousal by association with these waking activities (see Maladaptive Conditioning).

**Night: In-Bed Schedule and Behavior.**    The burgeoning field of chronobiology is elucidating the mechanisms and processes of sleep and adding to the understanding of the value of a regular sleep-wake cycle in promoting good sleep. When sleep and wakefulness occur at nearly the same time day after day, these behaviors coordinate and regulate a set of physiologic rhythms as well as establish external time cues, such as the light-dark cycle, to synchronize physiologic rhythms. The result is stable and synchronized phase relationships between a host of rhythms. This coupling of rhythms is self-sustaining and results in the regular timing of sleep propensity that is the foundation of good sleep. For example, the habit of arising in the morning at a set time results in exposure to light, a major synchronizer of circadian rhythms, at the same time each day.

The insomniac's practice of occasionally spending extra time in bed is a double-edged sword. On one hand, there are potential long-term negative effects of permitting sleep to occur at a wide range of times. Sleeping late on weekends, for example, precludes the regular timing of exposure to external time cues and thus forfeits the synchronizing cadence of light. In addition, extending time in bed will result in shallow sleep that is vulnerable to arousal. Too much time in bed, therefore, promotes fragmentation of sleep and increased wakefulness during the night. On the other hand, getting into bed early or staying in bed late may allow for more sleep, especially in those insomniacs who have accumulated significant sleep loss. The beneficial effects of this compensatory sleep will manifest immediately.

There are individuals who cope with difficulty falling asleep by going to sleep with the television or radio on. This practice may produce an awakening when the sleep timer shuts off the device. More insidious is the association that develops as this experience is repeated night after night. The habit will establish the television or radio as necessary cues to elicit sleep during the night, as arousals occur. If the patient has already obtained a substantial amount of sleep, he or she might be alert enough to become interested and aroused by the television program in the middle of the night.

Although the solution to the stimulation of night-time television is clear and easy to implement, the provocative behavior of a bed partner, such as snoring and tossing and turning, may be more difficult to control. Snoring, more prevalent in men and with increasing age, is common. Typical strategies include going to sleep before the snorer, wearing ear plugs, masking the snoring sounds with "white noise," and sleeping elsewhere. Although adaptation to regular mild snoring is often reported, it is more difficult to avoid the disruptive effects of the changing patterns of loud snoring. Although many couples are reluctant to sleep apart, this is a viable solution, along with weight loss or uvulopalatopharyngeal surgery for the snorer.

The practice of checking the clock after an awakening may lead to frustration, worry, and increased arousal. The patient may run through a series of calculations, including how much time has been spent sleeping, how long he or she has been awake, and how much time is left to sleep. The night becomes filled with anxious predictions about the next day's fatigue, poor performance, and irritability. These worries lead to increased efforts at falling asleep, which are often self-defeating.

Awake during the night, the insomniac is faced with the dilemma of whether to stay in bed or temporarily give up and get out of bed. Either way, there are costs and benefits. If the individual stays in bed, there is the possibility of falling asleep shortly. Thus, hope springs eternal in many insomniacs. If sleep does not ensue quickly, however, the tossing, turning, and thinking will foster associations between the bed and the agitation that is detrimental to sleep. On the other hand, getting out of bed during the night may be stimulating and preclude falling asleep. From the perspective of sleep hygiene, getting out of bed is the preferred strategy. Although arising sacrifices the potential for a rapid return to sleep on that night, it will improve sleep in the long term.

**Morning: Clangs and Cues.**    The environment can be the source of disruptive noise, such as a snoring or restless bed partner and barking dogs demanding to be walked. Similarly, light streaming into the bedroom may awaken the sleeper. These disruptions should not be ignored, even if they are intermittent and play only a minor role in the insomnia.

Individuals who linger in bed for long periods of time after they wake up may drift in and out of sleep. This habit creates irregularity in the wake-up time, which weakens the time cues in the morning that reset and synchronize circadian rhythms. Ignoring the regular wake-up time on the weekend and sleeping in may result in the shift of rhythmic processes to a later time. Although the extra sleep on the weekend may help the individual recover from sleep lost during the week by paying the sleep debt, it may also make it more difficult to get to sleep on Sunday night.

A different type of problem may be produced in individuals who go outdoors for an extended period of time shortly after waking in the morning. Light exposure soon after waking shifts circadian rhythms to an earlier time. This will produce both sleepiness earlier in the evening and arousal from sleep earlier in the morning. These effects depend on bright light and will thus be most pronounced when sunrise is earlier in the day. Therefore, spring and summer are the times of year when individuals are most susceptible to this early-morning light influence.

**Maladaptive Conditioning.**    In good sleepers, the rituals before bedtime and the bedroom environment are associated with falling asleep rapidly. Bedtime rituals establish the presleep behaviors and environment as cues that facilitate falling asleep. This learning process can go awry in two ways. The distinctiveness of the cues can be diminished and an association with difficulty falling asleep can be established.

Individuals who go into their bedroom early in the evening and spend hours in bed engaged in reading, watching television, and doing paper work are weakening the distinctive association between presleep cues and sleep. The environmental cues have become signals for a variety of behaviors and no longer help prepare the individual for sleep.

Even regular presleep rituals and going into the bedroom and getting into bed just before turning the lights out do not ensure that these cues will facilitate sleep. Staying in bed for hours and struggling to fall asleep establishes an association between the bed and sleeplessness. As this experience is repeated over time, the individual learns that the presleep cues and the bed are forerunners of agitation. Thus, it is not surprising that as bedtime approaches the insomniac dreads getting into bed. This process of maladaptive conditioning in combination with increased physiologic arousal are the mechanisms responsible for psychophysiologic insomnia.[27,53]

Insomniacs commonly use coping strategies to deal with interrupted sleep that make sense to them but in fact are ill-advised. Hoping to get back to sleep quickly and fearing that getting out of bed will increase arousal lead many insomniacs to stay in bed during long nocturnal waking episodes. In other cases, patients believe that it is good for their health to get rest by staying in bed if they are awake during the night. Spending time in bed awake forges an association between the bed and wakefulness, so that the bed becomes an arousing cue that interferes with falling asleep.

Many parents know the frustration and exhaustion of trying to put an infant or toddler back to sleep during the night. These youngsters wake and begin to cry and will not settle down unless held, rocked, and cared for by the parent. The child's sleep maintenance insomnia results from the child's having learned that at the beginning of the night the parent stays with them, ministering to their needs until they fall asleep. The child has been trained that the necessary conditions for falling asleep include parental presence and attention. The child protests if the parent leaves the room before he or she has fallen

asleep. This association can be unlearned by conditioning the child to fall asleep with the parent absent at both bedtime and during the night.

Similarly, adults who have established a fixed bedtime ritual may have great difficulty falling back to sleep if they shun this same routine during a nighttime awakening. In one scenario, the struggle to fall asleep during the night is the result of not engaging in the same set of behaviors and not repeating the environmental cues that promote sleep at the beginning of the night. There are some individuals, for example, who go to sleep at night by first watching the news on television while sitting up in bed and then lying down to go to sleep. These individuals may have trouble falling back asleep during the night when they remain lying down and the television is not on.

A thorough assessment of the role of maladaptive conditioning in insomnia requires a systematic review of sleep-wake habits and practices. One telltale indication of a learned aspect of insomnia is the report of better sleep out of the habitual sleeping environment, such as on vacation, in other people's houses, in hotels, or on the couch.

### Physiologic Determinants of Insomnia

#### Hyperarousal

High levels of physiologic arousal are incompatible with sleep. Measures of hyperarousal shown to be present in insomnia include elevated core body temperature and lower skin temperatures, increased muscle tone, lower auditory arousal threshold, decreased skin resistance, and higher respiratory and heart rate.[82–84] These indices of increased activation, in some contexts referred to as *somatized tension*, are consistent with the diagnosis of psychophysiologic insomnia, which, in a multisite sleep disorder center study, was the second most common primary diagnosis.[57] Because of bias in sampling methods, however, many sleep specialists believe that this type of insomnia may be as common as insomnia associated with psychiatric disorders.[85]

Although their sleep may not be as disturbed as they insist, objective polygraphic sleep recordings have consistently demonstrated that the sleep of insomniacs is worse than that of matched normal controls.[35-37,86] They have longer sleep latencies, reduced sleep continuity or efficiency, and an increase in the frequency of both brief and long awakenings. Although psychophysiologic patients also complain of "light sleep," there have been few reliable reports that show meaningful differences in sleep architecture between groups of insomnia sufferers and normal controls.[87]

It is well-known that stress produces a transient sleep disturbance. In most individuals, sleep returns to normal when the stressors are effectively neutralized. In patients with psychophysiologic insomnia, however, their sleep does not return to baseline so readily. In these susceptible individuals, the rituals of going to bed have come to function not as triggers for sleep, but as cues for cognitive and physiologic arousal.[88] This arousal delays sleep onset and perpetuates the cycle of sleeplessness. The harder these individuals try to fall asleep, the more anxious and tense they become, in turn resulting in redoubled efforts to try to sleep. All of this effort serves to increase the intensity of the insomnia, further strengthening the negative cues for sleep.

In the clinical setting, it is difficult to determine if an individual's physiologic arousal level is high. There is no standard objective and practical measure sufficiently sensitive to gauge the degree of hyperarousal of insomniacs. Therefore, assessment of this parameter is currently based on clinical phenomena such as high activity level, muscle tension, cold hands and feet, rapid speech, reactivity to stress, and the inability to nap.

In addition to the correlative association between physiologic level of arousal and sleep disturbance in psychophysiologic insomnia, manipulations that produce elevations in physiologic state adversely affect sleep. For example, intense physical exercise shortly before bedtime and activating agents, such as caffeine, interfere with sleep.[79,89]

*Circadian Rhythm Disturbances*

The physiologic level of arousal does not have to be tonically elevated to interfere with sleep. Alterations in the timing of the normal fluctuation in arousal may produce activation that interferes with sleep. For example, the core body temperature rhythm can be considered a summary measure of the level of physiologic arousal and the peak of the rhythm can be thought of as the time of greatest activation. The trough of the body temperature rhythm is well-established as the time of the greatest propensity for sleep.[28,90] It is well-known that body temperature, driven by the endogenous circadian oscillator, fluctuates by more than 1°F over the course of the day.[91]

The peak of the rhythm of core body temperature, as an index of the greatest physiologic activation, may be delayed or advanced resulting in higher than normal temperatures occurring at a later or earlier hour, respectively. It has been demonstrated that some individuals with chronic difficulties falling asleep have a delayed phase of their body temperature rhythm with respect to the sleep cycle.[92,93] Thus, these individuals have a higher body temperature compared to noncomplaining individuals at the time of retiring. Conversely, individuals with an early morning awakening type of sleep disturbance have a phase advance in the temperature rhythm. Body temperature starts to rise earlier in the morning in these individuals compared to normal controls. These differences in body temperature at different times of day are due to shifts in the entire rhythm, although there may be no difference in mean body temperature over the day. This chronobiological perspective has lead to effective treatments of sleep onset and early morning awakening insomnia based on an understanding of the regulation of circadian rhythmicity.

**"Night-Owl" Pattern.**    Some individuals become more alert in the evening and just do not feel like heading for bed at a time when going to sleep would enable them to get sufficient sleep. When they delay bedtime by a few hours, as on the weekends or holidays, they have no difficulty falling asleep. Furthermore, once asleep, they have no trouble staying asleep and may on occasion have long sleep episodes. Individuals with this "night-owl" propensity often have trouble waking in the morning. They may be in a daze in the morning or be frankly sleepy. This pattern suggests that the rhythm of sleep propensity is delayed to a later clock hour. In some individuals this pattern is clinically significant and is called *delayed sleep phase syndrome*.[27] The problems with falling asleep and waking in the morning are more severe in these patients, with consequences such as insufficient sleep, sleeping through the alarm and not meeting morning obligations, and poor functioning in the morning.

Investigators examining the 24-hour pattern of sleep propensity in normal individuals have described a time in the evening when individuals are least likely to choose to go to sleep. This time of day has been called the *maintenance of wakefulness zone*, suggesting that the sleep gate is closed. Even when asked to sleep after total sleep deprivation, this time of day, approximately 2–5 hours before the habitual bedtime, appears to be unfavorable for sleep.[90,92,94] It has been proposed that in individuals with delayed sleep phase syndrome, difficulty falling asleep at a desirable clock hour is due to the maintenance of wakefulness zone coinciding with the desired bedtime.

**"Morning-Lark" Pattern.**   Birds of a different feather have difficulty staying alert and awake in the evening and fall asleep readily. Early risers feel best in the morning. This pattern suggests that the rhythm of sleep propensity is advanced to an earlier clock hour. Individuals for whom this pattern of early-evening sleepiness and early-morning awakening becomes a problem have a condition called *advanced sleep phase syndrome*.[27] Trouble extending their sleep in the morning makes it difficult for these individuals to recover from sleep loss. This pattern is present in many older individuals and may result from either a shortening of the endogenous period length or a phase-advance of rhythms.

The change in phase-angle between clock time and the underlying circadian temperature rhythm may be responsible for the early morning awakenings. In patients with advanced sleep phase syndrome, a significant portion of the sleep episode occurs on the rising limb of the temperature curve, a time when it is known that sleep is difficult to sustain.[28,90] A phase-advance shift in the sleep-wake and other biological rhythms to an earlier clock time can be produced if an individual receives light exposure in the early morning hours. We are not referring to a morning awakening produced by the disturbing effect of a beam of light streaming into the bedroom window. The shift is due to light as a time cue being transduced by the nervous system and producing changes in the output of the endogenous circadian oscillator. The mechanisms responsible for these shifts include the stimulus parameters that produce the changes in the direction and magnitude of the shift, the neuroanatomic pathways involved, and the biochemical processes at the level of gene expression.

**Desynchronosis**

SHIFT WORK SLEEP DISORDER.   Complaints of insomnia are common in individuals who work permanent nights, work nights irregularly, or rotate consistently onto the night shift. Not only do shift workers complain of poor and unrefreshing sleep, but they also experience significant sleepiness during their work hours, with as many as 20% admitting that they regularly fall asleep while on the job.[95] Because shift workers frequently are forced to attempt sleep outside their normal circadian sleep phase, sleep episodes tend to be short, fragmented, and unrefreshing. It has been shown that shift workers have increased risk for gastrointestinal disorders, heart disease, and marital and family discord.[96] Although the consequences of disturbed sleep are unambiguous and readily understood on the basis of normal circadian sleep-wake physiology, whether workers' sleep problems can be classified as a sleep disorder or if they are better understood as predictable problems that arise from a choice to work certain work schedules is debated.[97]

TIME ZONE CHANGE (JET LAG) SYNDROME.   Rapid travel across multiple time zones can result in a complaint of insomnia that may vary in intensity and specific features. Depending on the direction and length of travel, sleep onset, sleep maintenance, or early morning awakening insomnia may be experienced.[98] The symptoms of jet lag are not trivial. In addition to poor sleep, individuals frequently complain of performance deficits, irritability and depression, and sleepiness at inopportune times. Jet lag insomnia is due to the inability of our biological timing system to adjust to rapid time zone changes that are a consequence of transmeridian travel. Under normal conditions, an individual's circadian timing system or body clock can only adjust by approximately 1 hour a day. Thus, it might take an individual 7 days to fully adjust to jet travel across seven time zones. Middle-aged and older individuals take longer to recover from jet lag compared to younger individuals.[99]

NON–24-HOUR SLEEP-WAKE SYNDROME.   A sleep-wake pattern that resembles normal subjects living in laboratory conditions without the benefit of time cues is present in some individuals in normal conditions. This circadian rhythm sleep disorder, called *non–24-hour sleep-wake syndrome*, can present as either sleep-onset or sleep maintenance insomnia. It is extremely rare, but it is more common in blind individuals.[100] Because they cannot entrain or synchronize to the 24-hour day, they adhere to a sleep-wake schedule that is consistent with their own internal clock. Thus, the individual typically chooses to go to bed 1–2 hours later each day.

In blind individuals, non–24-hour sleep-wake syndrome is probably due to the inability of light to influence or synchronize the circadian pacemaker to the 24-hour day. Consistent with this theory is one report in which 0.5 mg of exogenous melatonin administration at 2100 hours successfully treated a sighted person with non–24-hour sleep-wake syndrome.[101] Subsequently, this patient was found to be subsensitive to bright light, suggesting that although the optical system governing sight was functional, the system translating light information to the circadian system, which governs the timing of sleep and wakefulness, was inoperative.

IRREGULAR SLEEP-WAKE PATTERN.    The essential feature of irregular sleep-wake pattern disorder is the presence of a markedly irregular sleep-wake pattern to the extent that few observable regularities in sleep behavior can be discerned. Bouts of sleep are irregular in duration. Sleep may occur at any time during the day or night, although an analysis of sleep log data usually reveals that the total amount of sleep in the average day is within normal limits for age. This sleep-wake pattern is most likely to appear in the nursing home resident and in various patients with moderate-to-severe developmental or acquired neurologic dysfunction. A few cases may appear in non-neurologic patients, whose significant personality idiosyncrasies lead them to ignore shared social time.[102]

*Sleep-Related Disorders*

**Restless Legs Syndrome.**    Patients with restless legs syndrome[27] complain of an uncomfortable sensation of restlessness in their calf muscles (less frequently in their thighs or arms), which is sometimes described as a "burning," "tingling," "pulling," or "drawing" sensation (see Chapter 26). A relatively common condition in individuals older than 50 years of age with sleep complaints, restless legs syndrome is not commonly confirmed through laboratory testing procedures and therefore the diagnosis is made from the clinical history alone. Movement provides temporary relief, but the

unpleasant and highly distracting sensations often return soon after the movement stops. The symptoms of restless legs are worse when patients are relaxed and lying down and are usually confined to the late evening, they may contribute to sleep-onset problems in affected patients. A genetic mode of inheritance of the disorder has been described in some families.[103]

Although the syndrome is idiopathic in most cases, restless legs appears to be common in patients with peripheral neuropathy, anemia, and kidney failure. In other cases, substances such as tricyclic antidepressants, caffeine, and antihistamines may be implicated. The mechanism that produces the predominantly evening occurrence of restless legs is not clear, but circadian rhythm processes and fatigue due to prolonged wakefulness are under investigation. Up to 90% of patients who experience restless legs have periodic limb movement disorder.[27]

**Periodic Limb Movement Disorder.**    Although patients may be aware of events, conditions, and treatments that disturb sleep, it is rare for an individual to be aware of periodic leg movements that commonly arouse or fully awaken the sleeper. These movements are slow writhing retractions of the foot and leg that are often brief, lasting a second or two. The signature feature of these movements is the relatively equal intervals of approximately 20–40 seconds between successive movements, primarily occurring during non-REM stages I and II sleep.[104] This condition is diagnosed by overnight polysomnography. Standard scoring rules have been developed with attention to whether the muscle movement or limb twitch is associated with EEG arousal.[105] In patients with a complaint of insomnia, five limb movements per hour with an associated EEG arousal is considered to be the minimum requirement to make a diagnosis of periodic limb movement disorder.[27]

The sleep disturbance or fragmentation immediately after the limb movement is thought to be responsible for the complaint of insomnia in affected individuals. One study found that up to one-third of the stereotypic limb movements were preceded by signs of an EEG arousal, such as a K complex followed by the alpha rhythm. This finding suggests that both the limb movements and EEG arousals may be the result of some common underlying CNS pathology rather than the limb movement causing the arousal.[106]

Regardless of how clearly causative other factors may be, until a sleep maintenance insomnia is successfully treated, the clinician must keep in mind the possibility that periodic limb movement disorder is playing a role.

**Insomnia Associated with Sleep Apnea.**    Central sleep apnea syndrome, characterized by repetitive episodes of diminished or absent airflow plus an absence of ventilatory effort, may result in complaints of insomnia.[107] Individuals with central sleep apnea experience marked difficulties maintaining sleep with associated complaints of nonrestorative sleep, daytime fatigue, and daytime sleepiness.[27,108] This condition is often observed in patients with congestive heart failure, neuromuscular disorders, and poststroke syndrome.

Clinicians also need to be aware that some patients presenting with a complaint of insomnia may have obstructive sleep apnea syndrome[27] or upper airway resistance syndrome.[109] Patients complaining of insomnia, nonrestorative sleep, or fatigue should be questioned vigorously about a history of snoring, observed apneas, or restless sleep during the night. One report found that 15% of patients complaining of insomnia evaluated at a sleep disorders clinic were found to have significant obstructive sleep apnea-hypopnea syndrome.[110] It has been shown that women with mild craniofacial abnormalities who complain of tiredness, fatigue, and nocturnal sleep disruption may have underlying sleep apnea syndrome or upper airway resistance syndrome.[111] For cases in which sleep-disordered breathing is suspected, a full polysomnogram may be revealing. For cases in which the insomnia could be plausibly linked to occult sleep-disordered breathing, hypnotics are contraindicated and behavioral treatment is likely to be ineffective.

## BACKGROUND INFORMATION

A wide range of patient background information can be obtained in the clinical evaluation, including a survey of other sleep disorders, psychosocial history, history of psychopathology, and general medical history. This history can uncover important information and provides a broad view of the patient. It is not uncommon for patients with chronic medical conditions to complain of insomnia. The insomnia may be secondary to the disease process itself, arise from medications used to treat the illness, or the underlying disease process may be exacerbated by the sleeping state. Although insomnia stemming from the development of an acute medical condition will likely resolve and be self-limiting, patients with chronic medical conditions may experience bouts of insomnia that fluctuate with the symptoms of the underlying disease. A review of the medical conditions that produce insomnia is beyond the scope of this chapter. We will only comment briefly and unsystematically on this broad area.

Common central nervous system disorders such as headache, infection, trauma, or peripheral neuropathy are often associated with complaints of poor sleep and daytime tiredness. The sleep of patients with Alzheimer's or Parkinson's disease is characterized by increased sleep fragmentation, reduced total sleep time at night, increased napping during the day, and an increased incidence of primary sleep disorders such as periodic limb movement disorder and REM sleep behavior disorder.[27]

Other medical disorders that frequently lead to complaints of disturbed sleep are endocrine disorders, renal failure, rheumatologic disorders, gastrointestinal disorders, congestive heart failure, and chronic obstructive pulmonary disease. Patients with renal failure often have frequent periodic limb movements in sleep and patients with congestive heart failure may demonstrate Cheyne-Stokes respiration during sleep, resulting in sleep fragmentation, insomnia, and daytime sleepiness. Patients with pulmonary disorders have a higher incidence of insomnia compared to those without breathing problems and the sleeplessness covaries with nocturnal cough, wheezing, and dyspnea.[112] Intermittent activity such as cardiac arrhythmias and gastroesophageal reflux may be sudden enough to produce awakenings.

The need to urinate during the night may contribute to sleep maintenance difficulty. An intense urge to void is rarely so salient that it wakes the individual. During any awakening, however, an individual may become aware of the need to void and get up to use the bathroom. Just walking to the

**Table 24-3.** Clinical Indications for Polysomnography in the Evaluation of Insomnia

| |
|---|
| When clinical diagnosis suggests |
|    Sleep-related breathing disorders |
|    Periodic limb movement disorder |
| When clinical diagnosis is uncertain and |
|    Treatment is unsuccessful |
|    Precipitous arousals or violent behavior interrupts sleep |
|    Persistent circadian rhythm disorder is present |

Source: Adapted from Standards of Practice Committee of the American Sleep Disorders Association. Practice parameters for the use of polysomnography in the evaluation of insomnia. Sleep 1995;18:155.

bathroom and urinating may be sufficiently arousing to produce a long awakening.

The utility of polysomnography in insomnia has recently been reviewed and recommendations offered.[113] In general, the consensus is that polysomnographic evaluation of insomnia in the clinical setting is useful in a limited number of circumstances (Table 24-3). However, a number of investigators in clinical practice have shown that the use of polysomnography has resulted in additional diagnoses, revision of diagnosis, and altered treatment planning in a substantial proportion of patients.[114,115]

## IMPRESSION

The diagnostic formulation and differential diagnosis properly belongs at the end of the clinical evaluation. To suit our didactic purpose, we have integrated our diagnostic formulations within the context of the clinical evaluation as presented in this chapter.

## PLAN

Treatment of insomnia within the context of the doctor-patient relationship is recommended. Insomnia is complex and multidetermined and often requires both specific and general interventions to be dealt with adequately.[31,32] The clinician is concerned with the entire person, not just the disorder. Therefore, stress management, improved coping skills, and helping establish more satisfactory interpersonal relationships are commonly a part of the therapeutic relationship that benefits the patient globally and

the insomnia in particular. Furthermore, the counseling, support, and understanding that is part of the doctor-patient relationship is indicated because of the common comorbidity of psychopathology with insomnia and the need for encouragement and monitoring necessary to change lifestyle habits that interfere with sleep.

The means by which treatments of insomnia work fall into four categories: (1) enabling sleep by addressing disorders and conditions that interfere with sleep, such as depression, pain, hyperarousal, and excessive napping; (2) training the individual to sleep by conditioning; (3) enhancing sleep by promoting central mechanisms of sleep induction and maintenance and sleep-wake rhythmicity; and (4) mitigating the consequences of insomnia and thereby reducing excessive sleep-related worrying. Currently available treatments work primarily by a combination of these mechanisms of action. Stimulus control instructions, for example, are purported to help patients learn to associate the appropriate cues with rapid sleep onset.[88] However, the mild sleep deprivation and the regularity of bedtimes that this treatment produces may also enhance central mechanisms by increasing sleep propensity and synchronizing sleep with circadian rhythms. Similarly, hypnotic medications may enhance central mechanisms of sleep generation and the simple knowledge that a sleeping pill is available can relieve the anticipatory anxiety of a bad night's sleep.

In addition to the lack of specificity of insomnia treatments, there is limited information available to suggest which treatment is most effective for a particular insomnia disorder.[116] If we take insomnia secondary to an anxiety disorder as an example, a case can be made for any of the following interventions: enabling sleep by targeting the anxiety with behavioral techniques; reducing the maladaptive conditioning resulting from the association of anxiety and lying awake in bed for long periods of time; scheduling less time in bed to produce mild sleep loss, which will enhance sleep propensity; and taking a daytime nap to alleviate the physiologic and mental consequences of insomnia.

Studies and clinical experience have demonstrated that both behavioral and drug treatment alone or in combination are capable of reducing sleep latency and reducing nocturnal awakenings. Although the state of the field has not matured sufficiently for a comprehensive and scientifically based rationale for therapeutics, general principles can be identified that guide the choice of treatment.

As a general guideline in therapeutics, it is preferable to address the pathogenic mechanism responsible for the condition rather than symptomatic treatment. For example, this is clearly the case in the treatment of medical conditions that produce pain and discomfort or that interfere with sleep. A symptomatic treatment consisting of sedative-hypnotics would help the patient stay asleep by raising the threshold for the perception of pain. Notwithstanding the merits of this approach, it is preferable to treat the underlying condition. Another example of addressing the mechanism of the disorder instead of the symptom of sleeplessness is the treatment of periodic limb movement disorder, in which at least some of the fragmentation of sleep is secondary to the arousal produced by the movements. Current practice recommends drug treatments, such as dopaminergic agents, which reduce or eliminate the sleep-related movements. The alternative symptomatic approach is sedative-hypnotic treatment, which is effective in suppressing the arousal from sleep but does not reduce the movements. Again, the symptom-relief approach of using the hypnotic, although not the first line of treatment, is not without merit in certain clinical circumstances.

The clinical state of the patient may suggest treatment choice, as in the case of an individual in an acute state of agitation. When rapid amelioration of the sleep disturbance is clinically indicated, pharmacologic agents are more likely to bring immediate relief compared to behavioral techniques. In addition, the patient's preference for treatment needs to be considered when choosing a treatment modality. For example, as a group, insomnia patients prefer nondrug approaches.[117]

Trouble falling asleep may be understood as the result of a number of conditions as diverse as restless legs syndrome and generalized anxiety disorder. The isolated complaint of waking too early in the morning may be due to major depressive disorder or inadequate sleep hygiene. An alternative to this diagnostic viewpoint is a chronobiological perspective that sees these complaints as problems in the timing of sleep onset and sleep offset. Relatively new approaches that address the timing of sleep as the purported pathogenic mechanism use phase-shifting strategies, such as bright light exposure and melatonin administration, to reset or entrain the biological clock.

If sleep-disordered breathing is present, such as central sleep apnea, medical and drug treatment may be appropriate. Obstructive sleep apnea, although almost invariably producing the complaint of sleepiness, may be occasionally seen in an insomnic and a variety of treatments are available to prevent occlusive sleep-related apneas. In these cases, sedative-hypnotic drug therapy is contraindicated because of the respiratory suppression, reduction in nasopharyngeal and oropharyngeal muscle tone, and reduction of the arousal response that is a concomitant of this type of treatment.

We first briefly review the major treatment modalities and purported mechanism of action. The clinician should not forget that education of the patient regarding basic principles of sleep regulation helps reduce the mystery of sleep and addresses false beliefs the patient may have about sleep.

### Stimulus Control Instructions

Individuals with insomnia repeatedly experience the frustration of restless tossing and turning while trying to go to sleep. Eventually, an association is formed between (1) presleep behavior and the bedroom environment with (2) the inability to fall asleep. The bedtime rituals and the bed itself become cues for arousal rather than the threshold for sleep.

Stimulus control instructions help re-establish the connection between bedtime cues and rapid sleep onset and have demonstrated efficacy in insomnia.[88] Patients are told to stay out of bed except for sex and sleep. They are to go to sleep only when sleepy. If not asleep within approximately 20 minutes, they are to get out of bed. When drowsy, they are to return to bed. These procedures result in, on occasion, the experience of getting into bed and falling asleep rapidly, which begins to rebuild the association between the bed and bedtime rituals with unencumbered sleep. Additional instructions—to get up at the same time every morning and to forego napping—are in line with sleep hygiene principles.

Stimulus control instructions are generally effective in treatment for trouble falling asleep, and there is some evidence that it is also useful for patients with trouble maintaining sleep. It is specifically indicated when conditioning appears to be playing a role, for example, in patients who report sleeping better away from home or those who spend hours in bed engaged in nonsleep activities. As in all of the behavioral techniques, patient compliance is necessary for success. Providing support and encouragement, for example, to get out of bed in the middle of the night instead of struggling for sleep, is an ongoing function of the therapeutic relationship.

### Sleep Restriction Therapy

Curtailing time in bed, although paradoxical to patients who are trying to get more sleep, sets in motion a number of processes that promote sleep.[22] Patients are prescribed a time in bed that is equal in duration to their subjective report of sleep time. The patient reporting 7.5 hours in bed and sleeping 5 hours, for example, is prescribed a specific 5 hours in bed at the start of treatment. The result is mild sleep loss, reduced time to fall asleep, reduced wakefulness during the night, consolidated sleep and more stable sleep from night to night. As treatment proceeds and the patient is sleeping more consistently, the amount of time allowed in bed is increased by 15 or 30 minutes. The decision to increase the time in bed can be based on a 5-day average sleep efficiency [(total sleep time ÷ time in bed) × 100%] of more than 85–90%.[22,118] Alternatively, increases in bedtime can be scheduled each week.[119] When further increases of time in bed produce small changes in sleep and increased wakefulness, the point of diminishing returns has been reached and no additional changes in sleep schedule are warranted. Sleep restriction is thought to work by enhancing central sleep mechanisms and has been shown to be effective by itself[22,39,118–121] and when used in conjunction with other treatments.[122–125]

Patients should be put on notice that besides the improved depth and consolidation of sleep, it is expected that mild sleep loss will occur at first, and they will likely feel more tired, irritable, sleepy, and less able to cope. These side effects are short-lived and disappear as time in bed is systematically increased. In very sleepy individuals, this treatment may be contraindicated. In addition, sleep restriction is not appropriate when the patient complains of an insufficient amount of sleep in the context of a compact, unfragmented sleep period.

An effective strategy for a wide range of insomnia disorders, not just for patients who spend too much time in bed, sleep restriction therapy is use-

ful alone, in multimodal interventions, and to assist withdrawal from sleeping medication.

### Relaxation Training and Biofeedback Techniques

Many insomniacs fail to fall asleep because they are anxious or tense, and various relaxation techniques have been tested and shown to be effective for sleep onset insomnia.[54] Biofeedback modalities have been used to enhance relaxation training, including muscle tension and EEG frequencies in the alpha and theta bandwidths.[126–128] Patients with high anxiety, high frontalis muscle tension, or long sleep latencies benefit from EMG or EMG plus theta-EEG biofeedback. A different biofeedback technique is effective for patients who wake up frequently during the night, are tired in the morning, or have difficult-to-score polysomnograms with poorly formed sleep spindles. In these patients, daytime biofeedback to reward increases in the 12- to 15-Hz activity over the sensorimotor cortex has been shown to increase nighttime spindle activity and reduce the number and length of nighttime awakenings.

The purpose of relaxation and EMG biofeedback techniques is to reduce physiologic arousal so that the normal mechanisms of sleep induction can take effect. In contrast, sensorimotor rhythm biofeedback is designed to enhance central sleep mechanisms.

Biofeedback or relaxation training may require anywhere from two or three to 50 or 60 sessions, depending on individual differences in learning capacity. Because there is no simple way to predict how easily a particular patient will learn these techniques, an empiric trial is necessary to determine suitability. Furthermore, not all clinicians are skilled in these modalities and specialized equipment is sometimes necessary.

### Cognitive Control Procedures and Psychotherapy

A host of treatments have been developed to address cognitive hyperarousal and sleep-related worries that contribute to the vicious circle of insomnia.[54,55] The techniques of guided imagery, meditation, deep breathing, and thought stopping are strategies that are designed to directly control excessive ideation. In guided imagery, the individual practices an internal monologue in which a scenario is imagined, with a time line having a beginning, middle, and end. The individual focuses on details and sensations that help conjure up the scene. The goal is to "make it real" and try to be in the scene, as if having the experience. To the extent that the patient can imagine the scene as real and salient, thoughts and worries that are extraneous to the imagery are excluded and the mind settles down. Keeping personally meaningful, intrusive ideation out of the mind for a time by various techniques removes the cognitive obstacles to sleep. In addition to excluding particular thought content, these techniques change a disjointed thinking process or racing mind into a smoother, more well-regulated flow of consciousness.

Guided imagery and similar tasks prevent the patient from engaging in the counterproductive struggle of "trying to sleep." When engaged in the task, the patients cannot worry that they have "lost control" over sleep. Capturing the individual's attention, these techniques preclude frustration and self-criticism.[129] When first attempted, guided imagery and other techniques may be arousing rather than relaxing. A training period of daytime practice for a few weeks is usually necessary to develop sufficient proficiency before the technique can be used with success at night.

A different approach is taken by strategies that direct therapeutic attention to the mental schemas underlying the cognitive hyperarousal. Many of these broadly conceived techniques can be understood as aiming for cognitive restructuring or modification of cognitive distortions of the patient's views of the causes and consequences of the sleep disturbance. After identification of the personal meaning of the sleep problem, such as loss of personal control and mastery, overgeneralizing and magnifying the consequences of the insomnia, and rigid and unrealistic expectation of how well we can expect to sleep, cognitive therapy helps patients re-evaluate the validity of their explanations and reasoning. The aim is to help patients gain a more realistic view of their insomnia.

An insomniac who complains that his or her life is ruined by poor performance due to sleeplessness, for example, may be helped by putting things in perspective. The sensitive clinician attempts to appreciate the patient's distress and does not deny the impact of sleep loss on functioning. Helping the patient accept less than stellar work and settle for merely adequate performance at this time, however, has considerable value. Directing attention away from the view that life is measured only by productivity may help this patient appreciate other aspects of life, such as interpersonal, family, and community relationships. This altered focus or reassessment may reduce the perceived impact of the insomnia.

This type of work with patients is essentially psychotherapy within a circumscribed domain. Less formulaic and more creative for the clinician than other therapeutic approaches to insomnia, it requires a rapport and working relationship that allows for trying out approaches and perspectives. The potential success of a line of reasoning or challenge to a patient's beliefs depends at least as much on who the patient is and the quality of the relationship with the clinician as it does on the logic of the argument or persuasive power of the clinician.

Cognitive therapy's appeal to logic and the view that the patient's distorted thinking and irrational beliefs need to be corrected have limited the success of this valuable perspective. That the cognitive approach may go awry is easily seen in those cases in which the clinician's attempt to persuade the patient to abandon the "incorrect" or "irrational" position leads to confrontation, argument, and intransigence, rather than consideration, reframing, and transformation. It is a more subtle and avoidable limitation of the cognitive approach, however, that we want to point out. Some clinicians start with the assumption that what is necessary is the identification of dysfunctional thinking processes, followed by various means to modify them. As pointed out in a different but highly relevant context, this approach is like "hypothesis testing."[130] The clinician knows he or she will find dysfunctional cognitions and when they are identified, therapy requires coming up with ways to "correct" these ways of thinking. This approach may be seen by the patient as "The doctor knows what's right and I don't." Although promoting this attitude may be helpful in particular patients, we present a different way of proceeding that has its own merits.

An alternative approach to the patient's beliefs and reasoning (labeled "incorrect" and "irrational" in the standard cognitive approach) is to appreciate that this thinking makes sense to the patient. The clinician's first step is to help the patient see this thinking process as one possible way of construing experience. From this perspective, the next step would not be "correction" but rather an exploration of the origins and implications of such a personal perspective. Helping the individual interpret his or her experience from a different perspective encourages the patient to appreciate the subjective nature of his or her point of view. The clinician promotes the view that the patient's articulation of the causes and consequences of the sleep problem is not the only faithful rendering of reality but one *personally relevant* rendering of reality. This approach incorporates the cognitive perspective and has been described as *hypothesis generation*.[130] If the patient can become detached from his or her experience in this manner, the grip of the dysfunctional thinking is loosened.

In our view, the cognitive perspective is fundamental, in that the patient's internal world of experience and meanings is a central focus of the psychotherapeutic process. What particular ways are most helpful in addressing the patient's inner world is an ongoing challenge to clinicians.

### Timed Bright Light Exposure

It has been demonstrated that bright light is a time cue in humans and the timing and duration of light exposure results in shifts in the endogenous circadian phase that are predictable in direction and magnitude.[23,131,132] This information has led to the use of timed bright light exposure to treat conditions in which the primary difficulty is trouble falling asleep, such as delayed sleep phase syndrome, or problems waking too early, such as advanced sleep phase syndrome.

To shift circadian rhythms to an earlier clock time in an effort to help patients fall asleep faster and earlier, bright light exposure should occur some time between the time of the trough of the endogenous circadian phase (often indexed by the low point of the core body temperature rhythm) and for a number of hours later. The determination of the endogenous circadian phase is difficult, however; in clinical practice, therefore, it is assumed that the time the patient habitually wakes up is a time of day when the circadian system is sensitive to phase advancing effects by bright light. Light treatment of delayed sleep phase syndrome, for example, is therefore scheduled immediately after the habitual arising time.[25] Although the longer the exposure the greater the phase shift of the rhythm, duration of exposure is often between 15 minutes and 2 hours, based on practical considerations. In addition, bright light exposure is avoided in the evening because this tends to shift the rhythms in the opposite, undesired, direction.

Treatment for patients with sleepiness too early in the evening and difficulty maintaining sleep in the morning requires bright light exposure in the evening shortly before the desired bedtime. Studies have shown that in older individuals, 2 hours of bright indoor light from approximately 8–10 PM is capable of increasing evening alertness, delaying wake-up time, and increasing total sleep time.[26]

Bright light therapy requires motivation to keep to a sleep schedule and spend considerable time receiving the light treatment. This technique is a reliable way to shift the timing of sleep, however, and it is applicable to a wide range of insomnia disorders in which the primary complaint is either difficulty initiating sleep or waking too early.

### Sleep Hygiene

Treatment of patients with inadequate sleep hygiene requires the rectification of the specific practice that is contributing to the sleep disturbance. Therefore, if it is suspected that alcohol in the evening is one of the factors responsible for trouble maintaining sleep, then the patient should be encouraged to taper and then discontinue evening alcohol consumption. We have described inadequate sleep hygiene practices in detail. We do not systematically review the interventions that are required to address these problems because they are straightforward. We suggest, however, that the clinician not be dissuaded from proscribing any habit due to the fact that the patient may have already discontinued this particular habit for a period of time in the past with no relief from the insomnia. It is usually the case that a set of habits, practices, or conditions are contributing to the sleep problem. Although the elimination of one contributing cause alone may be insufficient to improve the condition, failure to discontinue that particular contribution in combination with others may delay or prevent improvement.

Not yet mentioned are practices of everyday living that promote sleep. Hot baths, for example, increase the depth of sleep by enhancing slow-wave sleep.[133,134] The water temperature needs to be approximately 106°F to achieve this effect. The time of night the bath is taken and its duration need to be explored to see what works for a particular patient. In general, the bath should last between 30 and 90 minutes and should begin between 1 and 5 hours before going to bed. This approach is not indicated for children, and the clinician should be aware that there are rare individuals in whom seizures are induced by hot baths. Standing up slowly and taking precautions to avoid falls when exiting the bath are recommended.

Another proactive approach to improving sleep is to engage in physical exercise. There is evidence that both aerobic and resistance training are efficacious for sleep problems.[135–140] It is hypothesized that the increase in body temperature resulting from intense exercise may be responsible for an increase in slow-wave sleep and the perceived improvement in sleep. However, not all findings are consistent with this view.[141,142] As in the use of a hot bath, the timing of the exercise may be an important parameter and individuals may differ in how close to bedtime the exercise needs to take place to be effective.

Setting aside time early in the evening to review the day, plan for the future, and worry is a useful discipline to help prepare for sleep. The goal is to create a boundary between the cares and concerns of the waking day and the rest and repose that are conducive for sleep. When this scheduled worry time is over, the individual should feel like he or she has completed work for the day and the rest of the evening can be carefree.

In addition to restricting fluids in the evening to help limit the need to void at night, bladder training during the day may also be of benefit.[143] The patient exerts willpower by progressively increasing the time between the urge to urinate and the act of voiding. An initial delay of 10–15 minutes before urinating is lengthened in steps over a 6-week period.

### Sedative-Hypnotics

A number of compounds are now available that are safe and effective for the symptomatic relief of insomnia. The benzodiazepine and imidazopyridine sedative-hypnotics have been shown to be rapidly and reliably effective over the course of short-term use. Although less well-studied, the benzodiazepine

**Table 24-4.** Principles of Rational Pharmacotherapy of Insomnia

| |
| --- |
| Prescribe the lowest effective dose |
| Use intermittent dosing |
| Do not extend regular use beyond 4 weeks |
| Discontinuation should be gradual |
| Manage rebound insomnia during withdrawal |
| Minimize daytime drug hangover by using lower dosage or drugs with shorter elimination half-lives |

Source: Adapted from D Kupfer, C Reynolds. Management of insomnia. N Engl J Med 1997;336:341.

anxiolytics and sedating antidepressants are commonly prescribed for their sleep-promoting effects. The guidelines for prudent drug treatment of insomnia have been reviewed and follow from a set of fundamental principles (Table 24-4).[144,145]

### Importance of Dose After a Single Administration

The clinical effects of the benzodiazepine-hypnotics include sedation; sleep; performance and memory impairment; and anxiolytic, myorelaxant, and anticonvulsant effects. Studies have shown that factors such as dose and the closely related measure of plasma concentration of the compound are significant determinants of these clinical effects, especially with a single dose or short-term use.[146,147] Similarly, the time to onset of action as well as the maximum effect and duration of action are functions of dose and corresponding drug plasma levels. Therefore, we use the agents' plasma concentration as the metric to represent both the pharmacokinetic and pharmacodynamic effects.

### Time to Onset of Action: Dissolution, Absorption, and Lipophilicity

The time from drug ingestion to its first appearance in the systemic circulation and the time to reach a plasma concentration that is sufficient to produce a clinical effect depend on a number of factors. Although the speed of the drug's dissolution in the stomach and the transit time to the small intestine play a role, it is the rate of absorption through the gastrointestinal tract and finally into the systemic circulation that is a major determinant of the timing of the drug's initial action. In addition, the degree of lipid solubility of the compound will affect how

**Figure 24-4.** The hypothetical function plasma concentration (C) by time for an unspecified benzodiazepine hypnotic. The role of time of administration on onset of action is illustrated. (Adapted from DJ Greenblatt. Benzodiazepine hypnotics: sorting the pharmacokinetics facts. J Clin Psychiatry 1991;52:S4.)

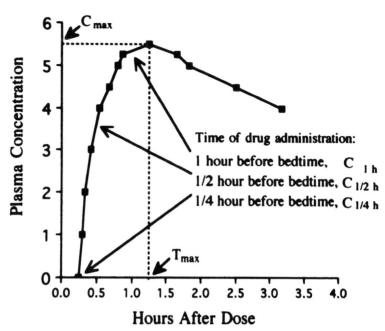

fast the drug moves from the systemic circulation into the brain. However, of all the factors affecting speed of onset of action, absorption is the rate-limiting step.

The benzodiazepine and imidazopyridine compounds used as hypnotics generally have a rapid onset of action. Time to initial clinical effects ranges between 15 and 45 minutes in different compounds and will determine how effectively sleep latency is reduced.

*Timing of Drug Administration: A Strategy to Optimize Drug Efficacy at the Lowest Effective Dose*

An area of pharmacotherapy of sedative-hypnotics that has received scant attention is the timing of drug administration. Perhaps little has been said because, as a class, the benzodiazepine and imidazopyridine hypnotics have a rapid onset of action due to rapid absorption and high lipophilicity. We have developed a strategy for optimizing drug efficacy based on the pharmacodynamic and pharmacokinetic features of the agent and the temporal pattern of the sleep disturbance of the individual.

The time to peak plasma concentration for the parent compound of the sedative-hypnotics cur-

rently marketed in the United States is between approximately 0.75 and 1.25 hours. Agents such as flurazepam and quazepam have, in addition to the parent compound, an active metabolite with a delay to peak plasma concentration of approximately 8 hours. As can be seen in Figure 24-4, the plasma concentration of this hypothetical sedative-hypnotic with no active metabolite is zero at 0.25 hours after ingestion ($C_{1/4\ h}$), due to the "lag time" associated with dissolution, transit to the small bowel, absorption, and travel through the hepatic to the systemic circulation.[147] Furthermore, the plasma concentration is lower at 0.5 hours after ingestion ($C_{1/2\ h}$) compared with 1 hour after ingestion ($C_{1\ h}$). The direct relationship between plasma concentration levels and therapeutic effects suggests that the time of drug ingestion should be scheduled so that the peak plasma levels are achieved at the time of the night when sleep is disturbed.

The strategy we suggest for optimizing drug efficacy starts by categorizing each case into one of two classic temporal patterns of insomnia: trouble falling asleep or trouble remaining asleep. In cases of sleep maintenance insomnia, for example, there is no need to establish therapeutic plasma levels at the beginning of the night. Therefore, in this type of insomnia, the sedative-hypnotic should be ingested immediately before turning the lights off to go to sleep. Peak blood levels will then occur approximately 0.75–1.25 hours later, depending on the agent chosen. The positively skewed tail of the typical plasma concentration curve (corresponding to the distribution and elimination phases) will provide effective hypnotic action when it is needed in the middle of the night. To further delay the onset of action for cases in which sleep is disturbed near the end of the night, absorption can be delayed by eating a snack along with the pill ingestion just before retiring. In contrast, patients with sleep onset insomnia need to take the drug some time before going to sleep, so that peak plasma levels are reached at around the time of retiring. In most cases, drug ingestion 1 hour before bedtime will satisfy this requirement.

These guidelines are presented not as a substitute for recommendations based on dosage and choice of drug based on length of elimination half-life. Clearly, higher plasma concentration at the beginning and end of the night can be produced by either increasing the dose or with chronic administration of compounds that have an intermediate or long elimination half-life. The import of our recommendations regarding the time of drug administration is that it allows the lowest possible dose to be administered with optimization of efficacy. To take a clear-cut example, sleep latency will be facilitated by either a high dose of a sedative-hypnotic ingested 15–30 minutes before bedtime or a lower dose of the same compound administered 60 minutes before bedtime. These same guidelines can be applied to other sedating compounds, such as anxiolytics and sedating antidepressants, based on their time to peak plasma concentration.

*Duration of Action: Elimination Rate, Distribution into Peripheral Tissue and Enzymatic Inactivation*

In general, discussions of which sedating agent to use have focused on the elimination half-life of the different compounds, which is a characteristic that varies widely within the benzodiazepine class. Drugs with an ultrashort and short elimination half-life have been recommended for patients with problems falling asleep, whereas drugs with an intermediate and long elimination half-life are sug-

gested for problems staying asleep.[144,145] These guidelines are most relevant when drug usage is chronic. With repeated dosing, the duration of action becomes markedly different in short versus long half-life compounds. This is due to the differences in drug accumulation. Although the compounds with an ultra-short and short elimination half-life produce no accrual of plasma concentration with daily dosing, there is substantial accumulation in plasma for the drugs with an intermediate and long half-life. The increased duration of action with the chronic administration of longer half-life drugs is desirable in patients with difficulty maintaining sleep or early morning awakening.

An additional characteristic of the compound that will determine duration of action in certain circumstances is the volume of drug distribution.[148] The distribution of the compound from the systemic circulation to peripheral tissues, other than the brain, may reduce the plasma concentration sufficiently to terminate the clinical effects. The extent of distribution is especially relevant to the termination of effects when the dose is low and little drug accumulation has occurred.

The enzymatic inactivation of a subset of the benzodiazepines by microsomal oxidation is affected by patient characteristics and the concurrent use of other drugs.[144] Age, liver disease, and use of certain drugs (e.g., cimetidine, erythromycin, estrogens, some of the selective serotonin-reuptake inhibitors) compromise the drug's degradation by the microsomal enzymes. The resulting reduced clearance capacity produces higher plasma concentrations and increased duration of action and drug hangover effects. A different subset of benzodiazepines, exclusively inactivated by hepatic glucuronide conjugation (e.g., lorazepam and temazepam), is not affected by age, liver disease, and competing drug effects. Therefore, the clinician may need to consider these metabolic factors in addition to dose and elimination half-life if prolonged duration of action is to be avoided.

*Undesirable Effects: Dose, Duration of Action, and Patient Age*

The size of the dose is a major determinant of the occurrence and intensity of side effects and withdrawal effects (Table 24-5). Drug-induced sedation, slowed cognitive performance, compromised infor-

**Table 24-5.** Side Effects Associated with the Use and Discontinuation of Sedative Hypnotics

---

Associated with intermediate and long half-life compounds
    Daytime sedation or drug hangover
    Impaired information acquisition and anterograde amnesia
    Depressed mood
Associated with short half-life compounds
    Daytime anxiety
    Early morning insomnia
    Impaired information acquisition and anterograde amnesia
    Depressed mood
    Withdrawal effects, including rebound insomnia and
      anxiety

---

mation acquisition and recall, and impairment in performance on tasks involving memory and visual-motor speed show a direct dose-response relationship.[149–153] These same undesirable drug effects will be more likely after administration of drugs with long compared to short elimination half-life. This is due to the extended duration of action (mentioned earlier) when drugs with intermediate and long elimination half-life are used chronically because of drug accumulation. The reduced metabolic clearance rate in older individuals also results in extended duration of action and this has been shown to be associated with an increased risk of drug hangover and falls in the morning.[154–160] Therefore, chronic administration of drugs with long elimination half-life is contraindicated in the elderly individuals.

A somewhat different profile of unwanted effects is associated with the use or abrupt withdrawal of rapidly eliminated hypnotic drugs (see Table 24-5). Although the risk of anterograde amnesia may be greater with the short half-life compared with the longer acting compounds the sedation produced by drug hangover is much less problematic.[154–159,161] Drugs which differ in their elimination half-lives have different effects on anxiety. Chronic use or abrupt withdrawal of short half-life hypnotics may produce daytime anxiety, whereas chronic use of drugs with a long half-life may reduce daytime anxiety.[162,163]

The abrupt discontinuation of short half-life drugs produces a withdrawal sleep disturbance called *rebound insomnia*. In contrast, a benefit of the prolonged duration of action of chronically administered compounds with long elimination half-lives is that rebound insomnia and rebound anxiety are unlikely after discontinuation. This is due to the gradual reduction of plasma levels after termination of drug use, which can be viewed as "self-tapering."

An important caution is that hypnotic drugs should be used with great care or not at all in individuals with sleep apnea conditions. The pauses in respiration during sleep in these common disorders are more frequent and longer in duration when sedating compounds are used. This increases the potential for cardiopulmonary dysfunction.

The current recommendations for short-term and intermittent use are in part attempts to prevent the development of tolerance and drug dependence. Because tolerance develops at a slower rate for some side effects compared with desirable clinical effects, increasing dosage as tolerance develops increases the risk for unwanted effects.

Melatonin,[164] a non–FDA-approved hormone available over the counter as a sleeping aid, has shown promise for several types of sleep disturbances. It has been used in doses (0.1–0.5 mg) that produce blood levels in the physiologic range and doses (1–10 mg and higher) that produce supraphysiologic levels. There is substantial evidence that exogenous melatonin administration at specific times of day is capable of shifting circadian rhythms.[23] To shift the endogenous circadian rhythm to an earlier time, melatonin is ingested in the late afternoon to early evening. Conversely, melatonin ingestion in the morning produces a shift of rhythms to a later time. This phase-shifting effect provides the rationale for the use of melatonin to treat jet lag syndrome, delayed sleep phase syndrome, and the non–24-hour sleep-wake disorder of blind individuals.

The evidence that exogenous melatonin produces sleepiness and promotes sleep is mounting. The facts that melatonin is a naturally occurring hormone, has few side effects, and has been reported to have efficacy by some controlled studies have peaked the interest of insomniacs and scientists alike. There is no consensus on the recommended dosage, time of administration, indications, and contraindications.

Many sedating antidepressants are commonly used to treat insomnia.[165] Although not yet established, the possible advantages of using these compounds is that tolerance to the sleep-promoting effects may not develop and these drugs may be safer than standard hypnotics in individuals with concurrent sleep-disordered breathing.

Accompanying the physiologic effects of drugs for insomnia is the psychological meaning that using sleep medications has for the patient. Many patients take solace in the knowledge that a pill is at hand to help get them through the night if necessary. In contrast, there are patients who feel dependent and vulnerable because of their reliance on sedative-hypnotics. In some cases, physicians and patients collaborate in a sequence of futile attempts to achieve satisfactory sleep. In this scenario an escalation in dosage is the first step, followed by a switch to different medications and ending in multiple drug use. When drug-assisted sleep remains unsatisfactory or daytime functioning is impaired as a drug side effect, the meaning to the patients is clear. They are not in control. The clinician should be alert to this potential downside of sleep medication use. Patients prescribed sedative-hypnotics should understand that these compounds are sleep aids, not sleep cures. They improve sleep but may not eliminate the problem entirely. Thus, limiting expectations and engaging the patient in additional therapeutic interventions are ways to avoid the psychological vulnerability that dependence on sleep medications may foster.

## CONCLUSION

This chapter presents the clinical phenomena, diagnostic reasoning, and treatment modalities that are part of the clinical decision-making process for insomnia disorders. The organization of the material corresponds to the sequence we recommend the clinician follow in the diagnostic interview. A semistructured interview based on this chapter is offered as an aid to assessment (the chapter appendix). A systematic evaluation consisting of an inquiry into the domains covered in the CCNY Insomnia Interview and a sleep log filled out for 1 week is suggested for the routine assessment of insomnia. This comprehensive approach is necessary because insomnia disorders are often caused or perpetuated by multiple factors. They usually require multiple treatment modalities, therefore, to adequately address the condition. Effective behavioral, cognitive, and biological treatments are available to help this under-served patient population.

*Acknowledgements*

We thank our colleagues who have contributed to this work in various ways. The following include our teachers, collaborators, and reviewers: Richard R. Bootzin, Lauren Broch, Scott S. Campbell, Charles A. Czeisler, Colin A. Espie, Paul B. Glovinsky, Peter J. Hauri, Charles M. Morin, Charles P. Pollack, Howard P. Roffwarg, Michael J. Thorpy, Daniel R. Wagner, and the late Eliott D, Weitzman.

## REFERENCES

1. Mellinger GD, Balter MB, Uhlenhuth EH. Insomnia and its treatment. Prevalence and correlates. Arch Gen Psychiatry 1985;42:225.
2. Ford D, Kamerow D. Epidemiologic study of sleep disturbances and psychiatric disorders. JAMA 1989;262:1479.
3. Ganguli M, Reynolds CF, Gilby JE. Prevalence and persistence of sleep complaints in a rural older community sample: the movies project. J Am Geriatr Soc 1996;44:778.
4. Gallup Organization. Sleep in America. Princeton, NJ: Gallup Organization, 1995.
5. Everitt DE, Avoran J. Clinical decision-making in the evaluation and treatment of insomnia. Am J Med 1990;89:357.
6. Spielman AJ. Assessment of insomnia. Clin Psychol Rev 1986;6:11.
7. Spielman AJ, Glovinsky PB. The Varied Nature of Insomnia. In P Hauri (ed), Case Studies in Insomnia. New York: Plenum, 1991;1.
8. Spielman AJ, Nunes J, Glovinsky PB. Insomnia. In M Aldrich (ed), Neurologic Clinics (vol 14, no 3). Philadelphia: Saunders, 1996;513.
9. Lacks P, Morin CM. Recent advances in the assessment and the treatment of insomnia. J Consult Clin Psychol 1992;60:586.
10. Carskadon MA, Harvey K, Duke P, et al. Pubertal changes in daytime sleepiness. Sleep 1980;2:453.
11. Weitzman ED, Czeisler CA, Coleman R, et al. Delayed sleep phase syndrome: a chronobiological disorder with sleep onset insomnia. Arch Gen Psychiatry 1981;38:737.
12. Thorpy MJ, Korman E, Spielman AJ, Glovinsky PB. Delayed sleep phase syndrome in adolescents. J Adolesc Health Care 1988;9:22.
13. Reynolds CF, Buysse DJ, Kupfer DJ. Disordered Sleep: Developmental and Biopsychosocial Perspectives on the Diagnosis and Treatment of Persistent Insomnia. In FE Bloom, DJ Kupfer (eds), Psychopharmacology: The Fourth Generation of Progress. New York: Raven, 1995;1617.
14. Dew M, Reynolds C, Monk T, et al. Psychosocial correlates and sequelae of electroencephalographic sleep in healthy elders. J Gerontol 1994;49:8.

15. Reynolds CF, Kupfer DJ. Sleep research in affective illness: state of the art. Sleep 1987;10:199.

16. Bliwise DL. Normal Aging. In M Kryger, T Roth, WC Dement (eds), Principles and Practices of Sleep Medicine (2nd ed). Philadelphia: Saunders, 1994;26.

17. Angst J, Koch R. The Zurich Study. Eur Arch Psychiatry Neurol Sci 1989;238:285.

18. Vollrath M, Wicki W, Angst J. The Zurich Study. VIII. Insomnia: association with depression, anxiety, somantic syndromes, and course of insomnia. Eur Arch Psychiatry Neurol Sci 1989;239:113.

19. Borbely AA. A two-process model of sleep regulation. Human Neurobiol 1982;1:195.

20. Kales A, Bixler EO, Vela-Bueno A, et al. Biopsychobehavioral correlates of insomnia. III: Polygraphic findings of sleep difficulty and their relationship to psychopathology. Int J Neurosci 1984;23:43.

21. Strogatz SH. The Mathematical Structure of the Human Sleep-Wake Cycle. Berlin: Springer, 1986.

22. Spielman AJ, Saskin P, Thorpy MJ. Treatment of chronic insomnia by restriction of time spent in bed. Sleep 1987;10:45.

23. Czeisler CA, Kronauer RE, Allan JS, et al. Bright light induction of strong (type 0) resetting of the human circadian pacemaker. Science 1989;244:1328.

24. Lewy AJ, Ahmed S, Jackson JM, Sack RL. Melatonin shifts human circadian rhythms according to a phase-response curve. Chronobiol Int 1992;9:380.

25. Rosenthal NE, Joseph-Vanderpool JR, Levendosky AA, et al. Phase-shifting effects of bright morning light as treatment for delayed sleep phase syndrome. Sleep 1990;13:354.

26. Campbell SS, Dawson D, Anderson MW. Alleviation of sleep maintenance insomnia with timed exposure to bright light. J Am Geriatr Soc 1993;41:829.

27. American Sleep Disorders Association. International Classification of Sleep Disorders (rev). Diagnostic and Coding Manual. Rochester, MN: American Sleep Disorders Association, 1997.

28. Dijk D, Czeisler CA. Contribution of the circadian pacemaker and the sleep hemostat to sleep propensity, sleep structure, electroencephalographic slow waves, and sleep spindle activity in humans. J Neurosci 1995;15:3526.

29. Moorcroft WH, Kayser KH, Griggs AJ. Subjective and objective confirmation of the ability to self-awaken at a predetermined time without using external means. Sleep 1997;20:40.

30. Feinberg I, Maloney T, March JD. Precise conservation of NREM period 1 (NREMP1) delta across naps and nocturnal sleep: implications for REM latency and NREM/REM alternation. Sleep 1992;15:400.

31. Spielman AJ, Caruso L, Glovinsky PB. A Behavioral Perspective on Insomnia. In M Erman (ed), Psychiatric Clinics of North America. Philadelphia: Saunders, 1987.

32. Spielman AJ, Glovinsky PB. The Evaluation and Differential Diagnosis of Insomnia. In M Pressman, W Orr (eds), Sleep and Biological Rhythms in Health and Sickness. Washington, DC: American Psychological Association, 1997.

33. Bonnet MH. Sleep Deprivation. In M Kryger, T Roth, WC Dement (eds), Principles and Practices of Sleep Medicine (2nd ed). Philadelphia: Saunders, 1994;50.

34. McCall WV, Edinger JD. Subjective total insomnia: an example of sleep state misperception. Sleep 1992;15:71.

35. Baekeland F, Hoy P. Reported vs recorded sleep characteristics. Arch Gen Psychiatry 1971;24:548.

36. Carskadon MA, Dement WC, Mitler MM, et al. Self-reports versus sleep laboratory findings in 122 drug-free subjects with complaints of chronic insomnia. Am J Psychiatry 1976;133:1382.

37. Frankel BL, Coursey RD, Buchbinder R, Snyder F. Recorded and reported sleep in chronic primary insomnia. Arch Gen Psychiatry 1976;33:615.

38. Sugerman JL, Stern JA, Walsh JK. Daytime alertness in subjective and objective insomnia. Biol Psychiatry 1985;20:741.

39. Anderson MW, Zendell SM, Rosa DP, et al. Comparison of sleep restriction therapy and stimulus control in older insomniacs: an update. Sleep Res 1988;17:141.

40. Sewitch DE. NREM sleep continuity and the sense of having slept in normal sleepers. Sleep 1984;7:147.

41. Dement WC, Seidel WF, Carskadon MA. Daytime alertness, insomnia, and benzodiazepines. Sleep 1982;5:S28.

42. Beutler LE, Thornby JI. Psychological Variables in the Diagnosis of Insomnia. In Williams RL, Karacan I (eds), Sleep Disorders: Diagnosis and Treatment. New York: Wiley, 1978;61.

43. Mendelson WB, Martin JV, Shepher H, et al. Effects of flurazepam on sleep, arousal threshold, and the perception of being asleep. Psychopharmacology 1988;95:258.

44. Seidel WF, Ball S, Cohen S, et al. Daytime alertness in relation to mood, performance, and nocturnal sleep in chronic insomniacs and noncomplaining sleepers. Sleep 1984;7:230.

45. Stepanski EJ, Zorick F, Roehrs TA, et al. Daytime alertness in patients with chronic insomnia compared to asymptomatic control subjects. Sleep 1988;11:54.

46. Mendelson WB, Garnett D, Gillin JC, Weingartner H. The experience of insomnia and daytime and nighttime functioning. Psychiatry Res 1984;12:235.

47. Lichstein KL, Wilson NM, Noe SL, et al. Daytime sleepiness in insomnia: behavioral, biological and subjective indices. Sleep 1994;17:693.

48. Seidel WF, Dement WC. Sleepiness in insomnia: evaluation and treatment. Sleep 1982;5:S182.

49. Bonnet MH, Arand DL. 24-hour metabolic rate in insomniacs and matched normal sleepers. Sleep 1995;19:581.

50. Hauri P, Wisby J. The MSLT in insomnia. Sleep Res 1990;19:141.

51. Anderson MW, Rubinstein ML, Rothenberg SA, Spielman AJ, et al. Relationships between total sleep time and the MSLT in insomnia. Sleep Res 1991;20:203.

52. Kales A, Caldwell AB, Preston TA, et al. Personality patterns in insomnia. Arch Gen Psychiatry 1976;33:1128.

53. Association of Sleep Disorders Centers, Howard Roffwarg, Chairman. Diagnostic classification of sleep and arousal disorders. Sleep 1979;2:1.

54. Espie CA. The Psychological Treatment of Insomnia. New York: Wiley, 1991.

55. Morin CM. Insomnia: Psychological Assessment and Management. New York: Guilford, 1993.

56. Marchini EJ, Coates TJ, Magistad JG, Waldum SJ. What do insomniacs do, think, and feel during the day? A preliminary study. Sleep 1983;6:147.

57. Coleman RM, Roffwarg HP, Kennedy SV, et al. Sleep-wake disorders based on a polysomnographic diagnosis: a national cooperative study. JAMA 1982;247:997.

58. Kales A, Kales JD. Evaluation and Treatment of Insomnia. New York: Oxford University Press, 1984.

59. American Psychiatric Association. Diagnostic and Statistical Manual of Mental Disorders (4th ed). Washington, DC: American Psychiatric Association, 1994.

60. Rodin J, McAvay G, Timko C. A longitudinal study of depressed mood and sleep disturbances in the elderly. J Gerontol B Psychol Sci Soc Sci 1984;43:45.

61. Benca RM. Mood Disorders. In M Kryger, T Roth, WC Dement (eds), Principles and Practices of Sleep Medicine (2nd ed). Philadelphia: Saunders, 1994;899.

62. Wu JC, Bunney WE. The biological basis of an antidepressant response to sleep deprivation and relapse: review and hypothesis. Am J Psychiatry 1990;147:14.

63. Lichstein KL, Rosenthal TL. Insomniacs' perceptions of cognitive versus somatic determinants of sleep disturbances. J Abnorm Psychol 1980;89:105.

64. Rosen J, Reynolds CF, Yeager AL, et al. Sleep disturbance in survivors of the Nazi holocaust. Am J Psychiatry 1991;148:62.

65. Ross RJ, Ball WA, Sullivan KA, Caroff SN. Sleep disturbance as the hallmark of posttraumatic stress disorder. Am J Psychiatry 1989;146:697.

66. Czeisler CA, Moore-Ede MC, Regestein QR, et al. Episodic 24-hour cortisol secretory patterns in patients awaiting elective cardiac surgery. J Clin Endocrinol Metab 1976;42:273.

67. Lacks P, Rotert M. Knowledge and practice of sleep hygiene techniques in insomniacs and good sleepers. Behav Res Ther 1986;24:365.

68. Schoicket SL, Bertelson AD, Lacks P. Is sleep hygiene a sufficient treatment for sleep-maintenance insomnia? Behav Ther 1988;19:183.

69. Curatolo PW, Robertson D. The health consequences of caffeine. Ann Intern Med 1983;5:641.

70. Landolt HP, Werth E, Borbely AA, Dijk DJ. Caffeine intake (200 mg) in the morning affects human sleep and EEG power spectra at night. Brain Res 1995; 675:67.

71. Pagano RR, Rose RM, Stivers RM, Warrenburg S. Sleep during transcendental meditation. Science 1976; 191:308.

72. Hauri PJ. Sleep Hygiene, Relaxation Therapy, and Cognitive Interventions. In P Hauri (ed), Case Studies in Insomnia. New York: Plenum, 1991;65.

73. Torsvall L, Akerstedt T. Disturbed sleep while being on call: an EEG study of ship's engineers. Sleep 1988;11:35.

74. Soldatos CR, Kales J, Scharf MB, et al. Cigarette smoking associated with sleep difficulty. Science 1980;207:551.

75. Porter JM, Horne JA. Bed-time food supplements and sleep: effects of different carbohydrate levels. Electroencephalogr Clin Neurophysiol 1981;51:426.

76. Lacey JH, Stanley P, Hartmann M, et al. The immediate effect of intravenous specific nutrients on EEG sleep. Electroencephalogr Clin Neurophysiol 1978; 44:275.

77. Phillips F, Chen CN, Crisp AH, et al. Isocaloric diet changes and electroencephalographic sleep. Lancet 1975;2:723.

78. Stahl ML, Orr WC, Bollinger C. Postprandial sleepiness: objective documentation via polysomnography. Sleep 1983;6:29.

79. Orr W. Gastrointestinal Disorders. In M Kryger, T Roth, WC Dement (eds), Principles and Practices of Sleep Medicine (2nd ed). Philadelphia: Saunders, 1994;861.

80. Moore JG, Englert E. Circadian rhythm of gastric acid secretion in man. Nature 1970;226:1261.

81. Browman CP, Tepas DI. The effects of presleep activity on all-night sleep. Psychophysiology 1976;13:536.

82. Monroe LJ. Psychological and physiological differences between good and poor sleepers. J Abnorm Psychol 1967;72:255.

83. Haynes SN, Fitzgerald SG, Shute G, O'Meary M. Responses of psychophysiologic and subjective insomniacs to auditory stimuli during sleep: a replication and extension. J Abnorm Psychol 1985;94:338.

84. Freedman RR, Sattler HL. Physiological and psychological factors in sleep-onset insomnia. J Abnorm Psychol 1982;91:380.

85. Stepanski E, Koshorek AS, Zorick F, et al. Characteristics of individuals who do or do not seek treatment for chronic insomnia. Psychosomatics 1989;30:421.

86. Coates TJ, Killen JD, Marchini E, et al. Discriminating good sleepers from insomniacs using all-night polysomnograms conducted at home. J Nerv Ment Dis 1982;170:224.

87. Hauri P, Fisher J. Persistent psychophysiologic (learned) insomnia. Sleep 1986;9:38.

88. Bootzin RR, Nicassio PM. Behavioral Treatments for Insomnia. In M Hersen, RE Eisler, PM Miller (eds), Progress in Behavior Modification (vol 6). New York: Academic, 1978;1.

89. Karacan I, Thornby JI, Anch AM, et al. Dose-related sleep disturbances induced by coffee and caffeine. Clin Pharmacol Ther 1977;20:682.

90. Czeisler CA, Weitzman ED, Moore-Ede MC, et al. Human sleep: its duration and organization depend on its circadian phase. Science 1980;210:1264.

91. Glotzbach SF, Heller HC. Temperature Regulation. In M Kryger, T Roth, WC Dement (eds), Principles and

Practices of Sleep Medicine (2nd ed). Philadelphia: Saunders, 1994;260.

92. Strogatz SH, Kronauer RE, Czeisler CA. Circadian pacemaker interferes with sleep onset at specific times each day: role in insomnia. Am J Physiol 1987;253:R172.

93. Morris M, Lack L, Dawson D. Sleep-onset insomniacs have delayed temperature rhythms. Sleep 1990;13:1.

94. Lavie P. Ultradian rhythms in human sleep. III. Gates and 'forbidden zones' for sleep. Electroencephalogr Clin Neurophysiol 1986;63:414.

95. Akerstedt T. Sleepiness as a consequence of shiftwork. Sleep 1988;11:17.

96. Moore-Ede MC, Sulzman FM, Fuller CA. The Clocks that Time Us. Cambridge: Harvard University Press, 1982.

97. Regestein QR, Monk TM. Is the poor sleep of shift workers a disorder? Am J Psychiatry 1991;148:1487.

98. Monk TH, Moline ML, Graeber RC. Inducing jet lag in the laboratory: patterns of adjustment to an acute shift in routine. Aviat Space Environ Med 1988;59:703.

99. Moline ML, Pollak CP, Monk TH, et al. Age-related differences in recovery from simulated jet-lag. Sleep 1991;14:42.

100. Sack RL, Lewy AJ, Blood ML, et al. Circadian rhythm abnormalities in totally blind people: incidence and clinical significance. J Clin Endocrinol Metab 1992;75:127.

101. McArthur AJ, Lewy AJ, Sack RL. Non-24-hour sleep-wake syndrome in a sighted man: circadian rhythm studies and efficacy of melatonin treatment. Sleep 1996;19:544.

102. Wagner DR. Disorders of the Circadian Sleep-Wake Cycle. In M Aldrich (ed), Neurologic Clinics. Philadelphia: Saunders, 1996;14:651.

103. Montplaisir J, Godbout R, Boghen MD, et al. Familial restless legs with periodic movements in sleep: electrophysiological, biochemical, and pharmacological study. Neurology 1985;35:130.

104. Coleman RM, Pollak CP, Weitzman ED. Periodic limb movements in sleep (nocturnal myoclonus): relation to sleep disorders. Ann Neurol 1980;8:416.

105. American Sleep Disorders Association. Recording and scoring leg movements. Sleep 1993;16:749.

106. Montplaisir J, Boucher S, Gosselin A, et al. Persistence of repetitive EEG arousals (K-alpha complexes) in RLS patients treated with L-dopa. Sleep 1996;19:196.

107. Guilleminault C, Eldridge FL, Dement WC. Insomniacs with sleep apnea. Science 1973;181:856.

108. Guilleminault C, Robinson A. Central Sleep Apnea. In M Aldrich (ed), Neurologic Clinics. Philadelphia: Saunders, 1996;14:611.

109. Guilleminault C, Stoohs R, Clerk A, et al. A cause of excessive daytime sleepiness: the upper airway resistance syndrome. Chest 1993;104:781.

110. Lund S, Zammit GK, Feldman J, et al. Occurrence of respiratory disturbance in patients presenting with insomnia [abstract]. Sleep Res 1993;22:230.

111. Guilleminault C, Stoohs R, Yound-do K, et al. Upper airway sleep-disordered breathing in women. Ann Intern Med 1995;122:493.

112. Klink ME, Dodge R, Quan SF. The relation of sleep complaints to respiratory symptoms in a general population. Chest 1994;105:151.

113. Standards of Practice Committee of the American Sleep Disorders Association. Practice parameters for the use of polysomnography in the evaluation of insomnia. Sleep 1995;18:155.

114. Jacobs E, Reyonlds C, Kumpfer D, et al. The role of polysomnography in the differential diagnosis of chronic insomnia. Am J Psychiatry 1988;145:346.

115. Edinger JD, Hoelscher TJ, Webb MD, et al. Polysomnographic assessment of DIMS: empirical evaluation of its diagnostic value. Sleep 1989; 12:315.

116. Nowell P, Buysse D, Morin C, et al. Effective Treatments for Selected DSM-IV Sleep Disorders. In PE Nathan, J Gorman (eds), A Guide to Treatments that Work. New York: Oxford University Press, 1996.

117. Morin CM, Gaulier B, Barry T, Kowatch RA. Patients' acceptance of psychological and pharmacological therapies for insomnia. Sleep 1992;15:302.

118. Glovinsky PB, Spielman AJ. Sleep Restriction Therapy. In P Hauri (ed), Case Studies in Insomnia. New York: Plenum, 1991;49.

119. Rubinstein ML, Rothenberg SA, Maheswaran S, et al. Modified sleep restriction therapy in middle-aged and elderly chronic insomniacs. Sleep Res 1990;19:276.

120. Morin CM, Kowatch RA, O'Shanick G. Sleep restriction for the inpatient treatment of insomnia. Sleep 1990;13:183.

121. Friedman L, Bliwise DL, Yesavage JA, Salom SR. A preliminary study comparing sleep restriction and relaxation treatments for insomnia in older adults. J Gerontol 1991;46:P1.

122. Hoelscher T, Edinger J. Treatment of sleep-maintenance insomnia in older adults: sleep period reduction, sleep education, and modified stimulus control. Psychol Aging 1988;3:258.

123. Morin CM, Kowatch RA, Barry T, Walton E. Cognitive-behavior therapy for late-life insomnia. J Consult Clin Psychol 1993;61:137.

124. Jacobs GD, Benson H, Friedman R. Home-based central nervous system assessment of a multifactor behavioral intervention for chronic sleep-onset insomnia. Behav Ther 1993;24:159.

125. Espie C. Conference on "Behavioral Methods in the Evaluation and Treatment of Insomnia." Rome, Italy: Universita di Roma "La Sapienza," 1996.

126. Haynes SN, Sides H, Lockwood G. Relaxation instructions and electromyographic biofeedback intervention with insomnia. Behav Ther 1977;4:644.

127. Hauri P. Treating psychophysiologic insomnia with biofeedback. Arch Gen Psychiatry 1981;38:752.

128. Hauri P, Percy L, Hellekson C, et al. The treatment of psychophysiologic insomnia with biofeedback: a replication study. Biofeedback Self Regul 1982; 7:223.

129. Gallwey WT. The Inner Game of Tennis. New York: Random House, 1974.

130. Wachtel PL. Psychoanalysis, Behavior Therapy, and the Relational World. Washington, DC: American Psychological Association, 1997.

131. Honma K, Honma S, Wada T. Entrainment of human circadian rhythms by artificial bright light cycles. Experientia 1987;43:572.

132. Boivin DB, Duffy JF, Kronauer RE, Czeisler CA. Dose-response relationships for resetting of human circadian clock by light. Nature 1996;379:540.

133. Horne JA, Reid J. Nighttime sleep EEG changes following body heating in a warm bath. Electroencephalogr Clin Neurophysiol 1985;60:154.

134. Bunnell DE, Agnew JA, Horvath SM, et al. Passive body heating and sleep: influence of proximity to sleep. Sleep 1988;11:210.

135. Horne JA, Porter JM. Time of day effects with standardized exercise upon subsequent sleep. Electroencephalogr Clin Neurophysiol 1976;40:178.

136. Horne JA. The effects of exercise upon sleep: a critical review. Biol Psychol 1981;12:241.

137. Shapiro CM, Bortz R, Mitchell D. Slow-wave sleep: a recovery period after exercise. Science 1981;214:1253.

138. Horne JA, Staff LH. Exercise and sleep: body-heating effects. Sleep 1983;6:36.

139. King AC, Oman RF, Brassington GS, et al. Moderate-intensity exercise and self-rated quality of sleep in older adults: a randomized controlled trial. JAMA 1997; 277:32.

140. Singh NA, Clements KM, Flatarone MA. A randomized controlled trial of the effect of exercise on sleep. Sleep 1997;20:95.

141. Trinder J, Paxton SJ, Montgomery I, Fraser G. Endurance as opposed to power training: their effect on sleep. Psychophysiology 1985;22:668.

142. Kupfer DJ, Sewitch DE, Epstein LH, et al. Exercise and subsequent sleep in male runners: failure to support the slow wave sleep-mood-exercise hypothesis. Neuropsychobiology 1985;14:5.

143. Espie CA. Treatment of excessive urinary urgency and frequency by retention control training and desensitization: three case studies. Behav Res Ther 1985;23:205.

144. Gillin JC, Byerley WF. The diagnosis and management of insomnia. N Engl J Med 1990;322:239.

145. Kupfer D, Reynolds C. Management of insomnia. N Engl J Med 1997;336:341.

146. Greenblatt DJ. Pharmacology of benzodiazephine hypnotics. J Clin Psychiatry 1992;53:7.

147. Greenblatt DJ. Benzodiazepine hypnotics: sorting the pharmacokinetics facts. J Clin Psychiatry 1991;52:S4.

148. Greenblatt DJ, Ehrenberg BL, Gunderman J, et al. Kinetic and dynamic study of intravenous lorazepam: comparison with intravenous diazepam. J Pharmacol Exp Ther 1989;250:130.

149. Greenblatt DJ, Harmatz JS, Shapiro L, et al. Sensitivity to triazolam in the elderly. N Engl J Med 1991;324:1691.

150. Locniskar A, Greenblatt DJ. Oxidative versus conjugative biotransformation of temazepam. Biopharm Drug Dispos 1990;11:499.

151. Morris HH, Estes ML. Traveler's amnesia: transient global amnesia secondary to triazolam. JAMA 1987; 258:945.

152. Johnson LC, Chernik DA. Sedative-hypnotics and human performance. Psychopharmacology (Berl) 1982;76:101.

153. Salkind MR, Silverstone TA. Clinical and psychometric evaluation of flurazepam. Br J Clin Pharmacol 1975; 2:223.

154. Ogura C, Nakazawa K, Majima K, et al. Residual effects of hypnotics: triazolam, flurazepam, and nitrazepam. Psychopharmacology 1980;68:61.

155. Bliwise D, Seidel W, Karacan I, et al. Daytime sleepiness as a criterion in hypnotic medication trials: comparison of triazolam and flurazepam. Sleep 1983;6:156.

156. Carskadon MA, Seidel WF, Greenblatt DJ, et al. Daytime carryover of triazolam and flurazepam in elderly insomniacs. Sleep 1982;5:361.

157. Mitler MM, Seidel WF, Van Den Hoed J, et al. Comparative hypnotic effects of flurazepam, triazolam, and placebo: a long-term simultaneous nighttime and daytime study. J Clin Psychopharmacol 1984;4:2.

158. Bliwise D, Seidel W, Greenblatt DJ, et al. Nighttime and daytime efficacy of flurazepam and oxazepam in chronic insomnia. Am J Psychiatry 1984;141:191.

159. Roehrs T, Kribbs N, Zorick F, et al. Hypnotic residual effects of benzodiazepines with repeated administration. Sleep 1986;9:309.

160. Ray WA, Griffin MR, Schaffner W, et al. Psychotrophic drug use and the risk of hip fracture. N Engl J Med 1987;316:363.

161. Spinweber CL, Johnson LC. Effects of triazolam (0.5 mg) on sleep, performances, memory, and arousal threshold. Psychopharmacology (Berl) 1982;76:5.

162. Kales A, Soldatos CR, Bixler EO, Kales JD. Rebound insomnia and rebound anxiety: a review. Pharmacology 1983;26:121.

163. Adams K, Oswald I. Can a rapidly-eliminated hypnotic cause daytime anxiety? Pharmacopsychiatry 1989;22:115.

164. Brezinski A. Melatonin in humans. N Engl J Med 1997;336:186.

165. Ware JC. Tricyclic antidepressants in the treatment of insomnia. J Clin Psychiatry 1983;44:25.

# Chapter 24 Appendix

## CCNY Semistructured Interview for Insomnia

I. IDENTIFYING DATA _____ _____ M F _____ ___/___/___
name          age     ethnicity     date

Sin Mar Sep Div Wid _____ _____ _____ _____
date      children      occupation      referral

II. COMPLAINT
  A. PRESENTATION

| | primary | secondary |
|---|---|---|
| trouble falling asleep | O | O |
| trouble staying asleep | O | O |
| waking too early | O | O |
| not enough sleep | O | O |
| light sleep | O | O |
| sleep is unpredictable | O | O |
| work schedule interferes | O | O |
| need drugs to sleep | O | O |
| unrefreshing sleep | O | O |

frequency _____

  B. DATE OF ONSET _____

  C. SLEEP-WAKE PATTERN
  Based on sleep log O or
  retrospective report O      Weekday      Weekend      prior to problem-      yr

  1. Sleep medication _____
  type, amount, time, carryover

  2. Time into bed _____

  3. 'Lights-out' time _____

  4. Sleep latency _____

  _____

  5. Awakenings _____

  _____

  6. Wake-up time _____

  7. Time out of bed _____

  8. Total sleep time _____

  _____

  9. Calculated sleep period - _____     _____     _____
    time in bed, 2. to 7.
  10. Napping, _____
     nodding,
     dozing _____

❏ *Hypnotic-dependent sleep disorder**

❏ *Inadequate sleep hygiene*

\* All items in italics are from, International classification of sleep disorders, revised:
Diagnostic and coding manual. Rochester, Minnesota: American Sleep Disorders Association. 1997.     © 1997, A. **Spielman**

III. HISTORY OF THE PROBLEM - The course of insomnia - changing patterns over time. Duration and circumstances
of good nights/asymptomatic periods. What makes it better, worse? Past bouts of insomnia. Response to treatment
Predisposing, precipitating and perpetuating factors.

A. DAYTIME CONSEQUENCES
tired, fatigue, sleepiness, irritable, wired, depressed
↓ thinking, performance, motivation

Clinician rates    severity        co-varies with poor sleep
          1  2  3  4  5        1  2  3  4  5
     not at all      alot    not at all     hi correlation

❐ *Sleep state misperception*

B. SLEEP-RELATED COGNITIONS - What do you think is causing your insomnia?
Cognitive hyperarousal and the vicious circle of dysfunctional reasoning and worrying.
Pessimism: 'loss of the ability to sleep', 'can't change life to help sleep'
Overconcerned about sleeplessness: health fears, ruining life,
   can't function, blames all problems on poor sleep, 'sleep always bad'

       severity        co-varies with poor sleep
          1  2  3  4  5        1  2  3  4  5
     not at all      alot    not at all     hi correlation

❐ *Psychophysiologic insomnia*

C. PSYCHOLOGICAL AND SOCIAL DETERMINANTS OF INSOMNIA

1. Psychopathology
a) Depression
biological - ↓ ↑ appetite, ↑ fatigue, ↓ sex drive
     ↑ depression in am, ↓ ↑ motoric activity
cognitive - worthless, hopeless, guilty, ↓ concentration
    catastrophizing, self-deprecatory
mood - distinct sadness, crying,
    ↓ capacity for pleasure
other - depressed facies, social withdrawal
    suicidal thoughts/actions

       severity        co-varies with poor sleep
          1  2  3  4  5        1  2  3  4  5
 not at all      alot    not at all     hi correlation

❐ *Insomnia associated with an affective disorder*

b) Anxiety -- anxious, phobic, obsessive, compulsive

       severity        co-varies with poor sleep
          1  2  3  4  5        1  2  3  4  5
 not at all      alot    not at all     hi correlation

❐ *Insomnia associated with an anxiety disorder*

c) Other psychopathology and subsyndromal conditions
racing mind, worrier, cognitive hyperarousal, over-reactive, alcohol/substance abuse ...

       severity        co-varies with poor sleep
          1  2  3  4  5        1  2  3  4  5
 not at all      alot    not at all     hi correlation

2. <u>Stress</u> -- work, social support, family, financial, illness, duration

```
              severity               co-varies with poor sleep
         1  2  3  4  5               1  2  3  4  5
     not at all      alot        not at all      hi correlation
```

☐ *Adjustment sleep disorder*
☐ *Insomnia associated with post-traumatic stress disorder*

3. <u>Sleep hygiene</u>: Sleep-wake habits and life style that interfere with sleep

### a) Daytime, and b) evening habits

[ ]  problem for both falling and staying asleep
    ○  problem for falling asleep
        ◇  problem for staying asleep

↓   ↓   ↓

[ ]  naps, nods, dozes -
    times/week <1 1 2 3 4 5 6 7 10 14+   [ ]
    avg duration, min <5 15 30 45 60 120+   [ ]
[ ]  lies down to relax, meditate
[ ]  caffeine
[ ]  cigarettes
[ ]  in bed before lights out
    ○  exercise late pm
    ○  get home late
    ○  insufficient wind-down in evening
    ○  evening apprehension of sleep
    ○  distressing pillow talk
    ○  in a trance, semi-awake in evening
    ○  preparations for bed are arousing
    ○  no regular pre-sleep ritual
        ◇  alcohol
        ◇  food, fluid after ~9 pm
        ◇  frequent urination

### c) Nighttime habits

[ ]  problem for both falling and staying asleep
    ◇  problem for staying asleep

↓   ↓

[ ]  lights out time varies
time patient gets out of bed varies
too much time in bed
[ ]  falls asleep with TV/radio left on
[ ]  bedpartner snores, or . . .
[ ]  clock watching
[ ]  trying too hard to sleep
[ ]  stays in bed during awakenings

### d) Morning habits

[ ]  lingering in bed awake in am
[ ]  extra sleep weekends
    ◇  noise, light, pet
    ◇  outdoor light exposure in am

---

---

---

---

☐ *Inadequate sleep hygiene*
☐ *Environmental sleep disorder*
☐ *Alcohol-dependent sleep disorder*

### e) Maladaptive conditioning

sleeps better away from home/bedroom Yes ___ No ___, anticipates sleep with dread
no pre-sleep ritual, in bed before lights out, irregular sleep-wake schedule,
stays in bed during awakenings, lingers in bed in am, falls asleep when not trying

☐ *Psychophysiologic insomnia*

B. PHYSIOLOGICAL DETERMINANTS OF INSOMNIA                                                4

    1. <u>Hyperarousal</u> - agitation, tension, cold extremities, rapid speech, rapid/pounding heart rate, hypervigilant, unable to nap, racing mind

|  | severity |  |  | co-varies with poor sleep |  |
|---|---|---|---|---|---|
|  | 1  2  3  4  5 |  |  | 1  2  3  4  5 |  |
|  | not at all | alot |  | not at all | hi correlation |

    ❏ *Psychophysiologic insomnia*

    2. <u>Circadian rhythm disturbance</u>

        a) "Night-owl" - trouble falling asleep, difficulty waking in am less of a problem on weekends and vacation

|  | severity |  |
|---|---|---|
|  | 1  2  3  4  5 |  |
|  | not at all | alot |

        ❏ *Delayed sleep phase syndrome*

        b) "Morning-lark" - waking too early, easy to get up, alert in morning, fatigued and sleepy in pm, rapid sleep onset

|  | severity |  |
|---|---|---|
|  | 1  2  3  4  5 |  |
|  | not at all | alot |

        ❏ *Advanced sleep phase syndrome*

        c) 'Desynchronosis'
        ❏ *Time zone change (jet lag) syndrome*
        ❏ *Shift work sleep disorder*
        ❏ *Irregular sleep-wake pattern*
        ❏ *Non-24 hour sleep-wake disorder*

    3. <u>Sleep-related disorders</u>

        a) Restless legs - restless legs in evening, when at rest, relieved by movement

|  | severity |  |  | co-varies with poor sleep |  |
|---|---|---|---|---|---|
|  | 1  2  3  4  5 |  |  | 1  2  3  4  5 |  |
|  | not at all | alot |  | not at all | hi correlation |

        b) Periodic limb movements in sleep
        ◯ substances - caffeine, antidepressants, antihistamines
        ◯ disorders - anemia, peripheral neuropathy or vascular insufficiency, renal, diabetes
        ◯ bedpartner reports patient kicks/restless sleeper, bedsheets in disarray

        ❏ *Restless legs syndrome*
        ❏ *Periodic limb movement disorder*

        c) Insomnia associated with sleep apnea
        ◯ heavy snoring, respiratory pauses, gasps, choking, resuscitative breathing, sleepiness
        ◯ obese, thick neck, retro-placed mandible, overbite
        ◯ central apnea:  neurological, neuromuscular or lung disease or taking respiratory suppressant agent

        ❏ *Insomnia associated with sleep apnea*

C. SURVEY OF OTHER SLEEP DISORDERS

    sleep walking, REM behavior disorder, enuresis, bruxism
    night terrors, nightmares, somniloquy, sleep starts

D. PSYCHOSOCIAL BACKGROUND                                          5

    family history
    personality growing up
    relatives with sleep problems
    family medical history

E. HISTORY OF PSYCHOPATHOLOGY

    condition
    substance abuse
    treatment

F. PAST MEDICAL HISTORY

medications:
<u>name</u>                          <u>dosage</u>                          <u>regimen</u>

    ❑ *Insomnia associated with medical and/or neurologic disorders*

IV. FINDINGS
    A. PHYSICAL EXAM

    B. POLYSOMNOGRAPHY
    C. OTHER

V. IMPRESSION

VI. PLAN

_____
    signature

# Chapter 25
# Narcolepsy

## Anstella Robinson and Christian Guilleminault

## A HISTORICAL VIEW

The term *narcolepsy* was first coined by Gelineau[1] in 1880 to designate a pathologic condition characterized by irresistible episodes of sleep of short duration recurring at close intervals. In the same report, he wrote that attacks were sometimes accompanied by falls or "astasias," a condition later referred to as *cataplexy*.[2] In the 1930s, Daniels[3] emphasized the association of daytime sleepiness, cataplexy, sleep paralysis, and hypnagogic hallucination. Calling these symptoms the *clinical tetrad*, Yoss and Daly[4] and Vogel[5] reported a nocturnal period of sleep-onset rapid eye movement (REM) in narcoleptic patients, a finding confirmed in subsequent years.[6–9] In 1975, participants in the First International Symposium on Narcolepsy defined the syndrome as follows:

> The word narcolepsy refers to a syndrome of unknown origin that is characterized by abnormal sleep tendencies, including excessive daytime sleepiness (EDS) and, often, disturbed nocturnal sleep and pathologic manifestations of REM sleep. The REM sleep abnormalities include sleep-onset REM periods and the dissociated REM sleep inhibitory processes cataplexy and sleep paralysis. EDS, cataplexy, and, less often, sleep paralysis and hypnagogic hallucinations, are the major symptoms of the disease.[10]

This definition highlighted the need for further research, as many unanswered questions remained about the causes of narcolepsy. In 1980, a Japanese group described a weak but significant association of this condition with HLA-Bw35. This finding was fol-lowed 3 years later by the discovery by Honda and colleagues[11,12] that virtually all Japanese narcoleptics tested carried the specific antigen DR2. The consensus in 1975, therefore, was that the syndrome involved deranged REM-sleep mechanisms. Yet pathophysiologically, narcolepsy is the loss of boundaries between wakefulness, non-REM (NREM) sleep, and REM sleep.

Honda and Juji[13] criticized this definition for being too broad and for overemphasizing the importance of polygraphic studies. They proposed the following two diagnostic criteria: recurrent daytime naps and lapses into sleep occurring almost every day for a period of at least 6 months as well as clinical confirmation of cataplexy in the patient's history concurrent with the history of napping.

These criteria are based on strict findings as follows:

### Daytime sleep
- The duration of each episode of daytime sleep is usually less than 1 hour. Sleep can be easily terminated by external stimulation.
- The patient usually feels refreshed after sleeping.
- Central nervous system (CNS) stimulants such as methylphenidate, pemoline, and amphetamine are effective against the somnolence.
- The condition lasts at least 6 months and usually many years.

### Cataplexy
- Consciousness and memory are not impaired during cataplexy.

- The duration of cataplexy is usually short, from seconds to a few minutes.
- Clomipramine and imipramine are effective in markedly reducing cataplexy.

With these clinical criteria, presence of HLA-DR2 (DR2 changed in 1990 under the new World Health Organization HLA nosology to DRw15, Dw2, DQw6) and sleep-onset REM periods on polysomnography (PSG) confirm the diagnosis.[13]

Although there is some controversy over this definition, at present the *International Classification of Sleep Disorders Diagnostic and Coding Manual* does not require HLA-DQw6 (specificity DQB1-0602) for the definition of narcolepsy, nor is this HLA type sufficient for the diagnosis of narcolepsy.[12] The requirement for clear investigation of clinical findings has the advantage of avoiding vagueness and of obtaining a good sleep history from patients.

## CLINICAL FEATURES

Narcolepsy is characterized by a set of clinical symptoms, including abnormal sleep features, overwhelming episodes of sleep, EDS, hypnagogic hallucinations, disturbed nocturnal sleep, and manifestations of paroxysmal muscle weakness, cataplexy, and sleep paralysis.

### Daytime Naps and Excessive Daytime Sleepiness

Unwanted episodes of sleep recur several times a day, not only under favorable circumstances such as monotonous sedentary activity or a heavy meal but also in situations when the subject is fully involved in a task. The duration of the episode may vary from a few minutes if the subject is in an uncomfortable position to more than an hour if the subject is reclining. Narcoleptics characteristically wake up refreshed, and there is a refractory period of 1 to several hours before the next episode occurs.

Apart from sleep episodes, patients may feel abnormally drowsy, spending the day at an unpleasantly low level of alertness that is responsible for poor performance at work, memory lapses, and even gestural, deambulatory, or speech automatisms.

### Cataplexy

Cataplexy is an abrupt and reversible decrease or loss of muscle tone most frequently elicited by emotion. It may involve a limited (commonly postural) number of muscles or the entire voluntary musculature. Most typically, the jaw sags, the head falls forward, the arms drop to the side, and the knees unlock. The duration of a cataplectic attack, partial or total, is highly variable but is commonly from a few seconds to 30 minutes. Attacks may be elicited by emotion, stress, fatigue, or heavy meals. Laughter and anger seem to be the most common triggers, but the attacks can also be induced by feeling elation while listening to music, reading a book, or watching a movie. Cataplexy can also occur without clear precipitating acts or emotions.

The severity and extent of a cataplexy attack can vary from a state of absolute powerlessness that seems to involve the entire voluntary musculature, to limited involvement of certain muscle groups, to no more than a fleeting sensation of weakness throughout the body. Although the extraocular muscles are probably not involved, eye weakness can occur, and the patient may complain of blurred vision. Although complete paralysis of extraocular muscles has never been reported, the palpebral muscle may be affected. Speech may be impaired and respiration may become irregular during an attack—symptoms that may be related to weakness of the abdominal muscles. Long diaphragmatic pauses have never been recorded, but short diaphragmatic pauses similar to those seen during nocturnal REM sleep have been noted. Complete loss of muscle tone may be experienced during a cataplectic attack, resulting in total collapse with risk of serious injuries, including skull and other fractures. Commonly, however, the attacks are not so dramatic, and they may even be unnoticed by nearby individuals. An attack may consist only of a slight buckling of the knees. Patients may perceive this abrupt and very short-lived weakness and stop moving or stand against a wall. The condition may be slightly more obvious when there is a combination of sagging jaw and inclined head. Speech may be broken because of intermittent weakness affecting the arytenoid muscles. As seen during nocturnal REM sleep, the abrupt muscle inhibition is interrupted by sudden bursts of returning muscle tone, which at times even seems enhanced. If the weakness involves only the jaw or speech, the subject may exhibit masticatory movement or an attack of stuttering. If it involves the upper limbs, the patient complains of clumsiness, reporting episodes such as dropping cups or spilling liquids when surprised, laughing, and so forth.

Because these attacks of partial flaccidity are short and may not resemble a classic full-blown attack of cataplexy, they are often ignored by physicians, even though this is by far the most common way these attacks present. Without an electromyographic (EMG) recording, their transience may make them easy to miss, even by a skilled observer.

Cataplexy is associated with inhibition of the monosynaptic H and muscle stretch reflexes. Physiologically, H reflex activity is fully suppressed only during REM sleep, which points to the relationship between the motor inhibitory components of REM sleep and the sudden atonia and areflexia seen during a cataplectic attack.

### Sleep Paralysis and Hypnagogic Hallucinations

Sleep paralysis is a terrifying experience that occurs when a narcoleptic falls asleep or awakens. Patients find themselves suddenly unable to move their extremities, speak, open their eyes, or even breathe deeply, although they are fully aware of their condition and able to recall the experience afterward. In many episodes of sleep paralysis, especially the first occurrence, the patient may be prey to extreme anxiety associated with the fear of dying. This anxiety is often greatly intensified by the hallucinations that can accompany the sleep paralysis. The narcoleptic's hypnagogic hallucinations often involve vision, and the manifestations usually consist of simple forms (colored circles, parts of objects) that may be constant in size or changing. The image of an animal or a person may present itself abruptly in black and white or, more often, in color. Auditory hallucinations are also common, but other senses are seldom involved. The auditory hallucinations can range from a collection of sounds to an elaborate melody. The patient may also be menaced by threatening sentences or harsh invective. With more experience of the phenomenon, the patient usually learns that episodes are brief and benign, rarely lasting longer than 20 minutes and always ending spontaneously. Although sleep paralysis may occur at sleep onset

or termination, it is more common at sleep onset in narcoleptics.

A common and interesting type of hallucination reported at sleep onset involves elementary cenesthopathic (abnormal) sensations (e.g., picking, rubbing, light touching), changes in location of body parts, or feelings of levitation or extracorporeal experiences, which may be quite elaborate. For example, the patient may say, "I am above my bed and I can also see my body below," or, "I am a few feet up and people jump over my body." The association of sleep paralysis has led researchers to postulate gamma loop involvement in some of these hallucinations. The abrupt motor inhibition that involves the spinal cord motor neurons may lead to a significant decrease in feedback of information normally used by the CNS to gauge the position of the body and the relation of the limb segments to each other. The night sleep of the narcoleptic is often interrupted by repeated awakenings and is sometimes interspersed with terrifying dreams.

## ONSET OF CLINICAL SYMPTOMS

The first symptoms of narcolepsy often develop near puberty. The peak age of reported symptoms is between 15 and 25 years in women, but narcolepsy and other symptoms have been noted at 3–6 years and a second, smaller peak of onset between 35 and 45 years, near menopause.

EDS and irresistible sleep episodes usually occur as the first symptoms, either independently or associated with one or more other symptoms. They are enhanced by high temperature, indoor activity, and idleness. Symptoms may abate with time but they never phase out completely. Attacks of cataplexy generally appear in conjunction with abnormal episodes of sleep but they may occur as much as 20 years later. Occasionally, but seldom, they occur before the abnormal sleep episodes, in which case they are a major source of difficulty in diagnosis. They can vary in frequency from a few episodes during the subject's entire lifetime to one or several episodes per day.

Hypnagogic hallucinations and sleep paralysis do not affect all subjects and often are transitory. Disturbed nocturnal sleep seldom occurs in the first stages and generally increases with age.[14]

## DIAGNOSTIC PROCEDURES: EVALUATION OF SLEEPINESS

The six-point Stanford Sleepiness Scale[15] was developed to quantify the subjective sleepiness of patients, but its reliability for chronically sleepy patients is questionable. Several tests have been designed to evaluate sleepiness objectively. Yoss and coworkers[16] described the electronic pupillogram (EPG) as a method of measuring increased levels of sleepiness. Schmidt and Fortin[17] reviewed the advantages and limitations of EPG in arousal disorders. The use of EPG as a test is based on the facts that peripheral autonomic manifestations are associated with states of arousal or excitation as well as sleep and the pupil is an index of autonomic (vagal) activity. Berlucchi and colleagues[18] clearly demonstrated the pupil's constriction during sleep. A normal, alert person sitting quietly in total darkness can maintain a stable pupil diameter, usually well above 7 mm, for at least 10 minutes without subjective difficulty or pupillary oscillation. The pupillary diameter in excessively sleepy patients, however, is unstable when they are adapting to the dark. The EPG technique is often performed with a series of light stimuli. (Schmidt and Fortin[17] recommend 15 foot-candle intensity attenuated by a 4.0-log neutral-density filter.)

There are problems and limitations with this technique.[17] Patients with ocular problems or autonomic (CNS) lesions must be identified and excluded. A patient's ability and willingness to cooperate are critical. Excessively sleepy subjects have trouble avoiding lid drooping or closure. Small initial pupil diameter, dark irises, and excessive eye makeup all pose problems. Finally, the data may be difficult to interpret, particularly if recording conditions are not standardized. Although at one time experts did attempt to use EPG to diagnose narcolepsy, it essentially diagnoses only sleepiness. The test does not indicate the underlying causes of EDS.

The Multiple Sleep Latency Test (MSLT) was designed by Carskadon and Dement[19] to measure physiologic sleep tendencies in the absence of alerting factors. It consists of four or five scheduled naps, usually at 10:00 AM and 12:00, 2:00, 4:00, and 6:00 PM, during which the subject is polygraphically monitored in a comfortable, soundproof, dark bedroom. The latency between lights-out time and sleep onset is calculated for each nap. The criteria for sleep onset are those outlined in Rechtschaffen and Kales' international manual.[20] The type of sleep, REM or NREM, is also noted. After each 20-minute monitoring period, patients stay awake until the next scheduled nap. The MSLT records the latency for each nap, the mean sleep latency, and the presence or absence of REM sleep in any of the naps. Based on polygraphic recording, REM sleep that occurs within 15 minutes of sleep onset is considered a sleep-onset REM period. Guidelines for performance of the MSLT have been published by the American Sleep Disorders Association (ASDA).[21]

In normal populations, MSLT scores vary with age. Puberty is the critical landmark; prepubertal children between ages 6 and 11 years appear to be hyperalert. Mean MSLT scores under 8 minutes are generally considered to be in the pathologic range, whereas those over 10 minutes are considered normal. When the range is between 8 and 10 minutes, the test should be interpreted with greater care and in light of factors associated with age. Mean scores of 9–10 minutes are in the gray zone.[22]

An MSLT performed alone has the same drawbacks as EPG (i.e., it measures sleepiness regardless of its cause, which may simply be sleep deprivation). The MSLT also ignores repetitive microsleeps that can lead, in borderline cases, to daytime impairment not scored by conventional analysis. To be clinically relevant, the MSLT must be conducted under specific conditions. Subjects must be off medication for a sufficient period (usually 15 days) to avoid drug interaction. A subject's sleep-wake schedule must be stabilized on the basis of a sleep diary. The night preceding the MSLT, patients must undergo nocturnal PSG (i.e., polygraphic recording of variables defining wakefulness and sleep states or stages, using electroencephalography [EEG]; electro-oculogram [EOG]; chin EMG; and other biological variables, including cardiac, pulmonary, and gastrointestinal). Esophageal manometry increases the sensitivity of the overnight PSG for subtle breathing disorders such as upper airway resistance syndrome. Throughout the total nocturnal sleep period, any sleep-related biological abnormalities responsible for sleep fragmentation and sleep deprivation should be recorded.

Further evidence of the limitation of the MSLT was demonstrated by the prospective evaluation at Stanford University of 72 patients with isolated EDS. This study revealed upper airway resistance syndrome in 16 of the 72. Three of these patients (all women) had pathologic sleep latencies on MSLT and more than one sleep-onset REM period. These individuals were indistinguishable from other patients by their clinical histories or nocturnal polysomnograms. Sleep-wake schedules, professional activities, body mass index, and demographics were also not predictive of the findings. Although two patients improved with continuous positive airway pressure therapy, the third did not. The importance of a thorough evaluation for sleep-disordered breathing, before committing the patient to a lifetime of stimulant medication, cannot be overstated.

The nocturnal PSG indicates the underlying cause for the complaint of sleepiness; the MSLT indicates the severity of the problem. Once the nocturnal sleep recording has eliminated specific diseases and demonstrated that a patient is sleeping normally through the night, the MSLT confirms the presence of narcolepsy if there are two or more sleep-onset REM periods.

Browman and associates[23] proposed adding a test for the maintenance of wakefulness to the MSLT. The patient is to remain awake in a comfortable sitting position in a dark room for five 20-minute trials given at 10:00 AM and 12:00, 2:00, 4:00, and 6:00 PM. The test may be helpful in specific pharmacologic trials, but it has proved unsatisfactory as a diagnostic procedure.[23]

Another procedure is a continuous 24- or 36-hour PSG monitoring that provides information about the actual number, duration, times, and types of daytime sleep episodes and about disrupted night-time sleep. In addition, this long polygraphic recording may identify the dissociated REM sleep inhibitory process that characterizes cataplexy. This dissociated REM process combines an awake EEG and EOG recording associated with complete absence of chin EMG recording and bursts of muscle twitches also typical of REM sleep. This may allow monitoring of microsleeps and microarousals. Microarousals, or transient alpha arousals, are short bursts of alpha EEG activity lasting 3–14 seconds (usually 5–10 seconds), which interrupt any eye movements. The ASDA Task Force on Terminology, Techniques, and Scoring System[24] preliminary report indicates that a sleep EEG must last at least 10 seconds to be called a *transient alpha arousal*. Microsleeps, by analogy with transient alpha arousals, are changes

in EEG to stage I NREM sleep or a REM-sleep pattern lasting 3–14 seconds.

Broughton and colleagues[25] proposed using auditory evoked potentials to evaluate sleepiness. Once again, however, this test, which may be very helpful in evaluating pharmacologic agents, has not been sufficiently discriminatory to be used as a diagnostic tool. All of these tests must be performed in association with a urine drug test to ascertain the presence or absence of stimulants or drugs that have an impact on the sleep-wake cycle.

The positive diagnosis of narcolepsy requires a minimum of two major symptoms: EDS and sleep attacks or attacks of cataplexy associated with objectively documented sleep-onset REM episodes. The clinical association of daytime sleepiness and cataplexy, when observed by a physician, is pathognomonic of the narcolepsy syndrome.

If EDS and cataplectic attacks are sufficient to confirm narcolepsy, why require PSG in cases in which one or both are absent? The history of cataplexy can be difficult to affirm. Absolute cataplexy, which causes the patient to collapse on the floor, is uncommon. Often, subjects have time to reach a chair or wall to prevent a complete collapse. Most commonly, cataplexy is only partial, involving the head and neck, upper limbs, mandibular and upper airway muscles, or weak knees. This partial cataplexy is often difficult to interpret, especially in cases when the subject has only a positive history of cataplexy without current symptoms. It is in these cases that polygraphic monitoring with positive MSLT findings can confirm the diagnosis.

### Can a Subject with Excessive Daytime Sleepiness and a History of Cataplexy Have a Negative Multiple Sleep Latency Test?

Van den Hoed and coworkers[22] and Moscovitch and colleagues[26] reviewed the issue of whether subjects who meet the criteria of having EDS and a history of cataplexy can receive a negative score (fewer than two sleep-onset REM periods) on the MSLT. Both groups analyzed patients seen at the Stanford University Sleep Disorders Clinic. Moscovitch's group had a larger population (306 narcoleptics). Seventy-seven percent of these patients had been seen by the same physician, who had a great deal of experience with narcolepsy. Based on clinical data, all were believed to have cataplexy, but only 84% of them presented with two or more sleep-onset REM periods at one PSG-MSLT period. Four successive days of MSLTs were necessary to observe two or more sleep-onset REM periods in every subject in the population.

### Can Someone Be Diagnosed as Narcoleptic Who Has No Cataplexy but Has Sleep-Onset REM Periods?

Considering the need for strict criteria in epidemiologic studies and the gloomy prognosis linked to the diagnosis of narcolepsy (a lifelong illness), it is strongly recommended that physicians avoid using the term *narcolepsy* and, rather, describe the findings (i.e., excessive daytime somnolence with *X* number of sleep-onset REM periods). The subject may be developing narcolepsy and may not yet have developed cataplexy. Seven young individuals followed by the Stanford Sleep Clinic had EDS and two or more sleep-onset REM periods at MSLT approximately 5–24 months before they exhibited cataplexy. (Some other teenagers exhibited cataplexy before they had two or more sleep-onset REM periods at 1-day MSLT.) Thus, a subject with two or more sleep-onset REM periods may be narcoleptic. In addition, family members of narcoleptics have presented with EDS and two sleep-onset REM periods (five subjects older than 30 years in the Stanford Sleep Clinic database). However, 54 of 306 EDS subjects in the Stanford database aged 32 years and older presented no cataplexy and two or more sleep-onset REM periods, and had no family history of narcolepsy. Investigations performed on a large group of sleepy patients indicates that a small number of narcoleptics never develop cataplexy.[14]

### Can Human Leukocyte Antigen Aid in Diagnosis?

As indicated by Guilleminault and colleagues,[27] the HLA-DR2 DQw6 DQB1-0602 haplotype is neither sufficient nor necessary for narcolepsy. As stated previously, the World Health Organization nomenclature[28] labels the HLA haplotype most commonly associated with narcolepsy DRwl5 Dw2 DQw6 (DQw6 was formerly DQwl). Although it is frequently noted, this haplotype may not be associated with independent and familial cases of narcolepsy. Conversely, at least 10% of narcoleptics with cataplexy do not present with DQB1-0602.[29]

### Can Multiple Sleep Latency Test Scores for Excessive Daytime Sleepiness in Narcoleptics Be Outside the Range Usually Reported?

Once again drawing from the Stanford University database, of 500 narcoleptics with clear cataplexy and complaints of mild sleepiness, two presented a mean MSLT score of 11 at two repeated investigations. Each of them had two sleep-onset REM periods at the MSLT; however, 85% of the narcoleptics in van den Hoed's[22] and Moscovitch's[26] groups had a mean sleep latency on MSLT of less than 5 minutes.

In summary, cataplexy is a key feature for the diagnosis of narcolepsy. A PSG evaluation followed by an MSLT the next day demonstrates two or more sleep-onset REM periods in 84% of the cases. Descriptive language is recommended in questionable cases.

## EPIDEMIOLOGY AND GENETICS

Narcolepsy is not a rare condition. Its prevalence has been reported at as little as 0.0002% in Israel to 0.16% in Japan.[30] It's been calculated at 0.05% in the San Francisco Bay area[31] and 0.067% in the Los Angeles area.[32] There has been strong criticism of some of these surveys because of their methodology (i.e., some of the studies did not involve an appropriate sample of the population of the considered country). More recently, the prevalence has been calculated at between 0.03% and 0.05% in Europe and North America. There is no sex predominance in this disorder. The former reports of increased male to female affect ratios were probably due to the higher numbers of men in the studies as well as cases of sleep apnea, which affects predominantly men, mistaken for narcolepsy. Age at onset varies from childhood to the fifth decade and peaks in the second decade. A special circumstance such as an abrupt change of sleep-wake schedule or a severe psychological stress—death of a relative, divorce—precedes the occurrence of the first symptom in half of the cases.[14]

The genetic aspect of narcolepsy has been investigated by several groups. Among the first-degree relatives of 50 narcoleptic probands, Kessler and coworkers[33] found nine narcoleptic patients (18%) and 17 subjects with EDS (34%). Among the parents and siblings of 232 narcoleptic probands, Honda and associates[34] found 14 narcoleptic patients (6%) and 56 subjects with EDS (24%). These findings led these two groups of authors to suggest a two-threshold, multifactorial model of inheritance, with EDS being the more prevalent and less severe manifestation and narcolepsy the less prevalent and more severe manifestation of the same genetic predisposition.[33,34]

The discovery by Japanese researchers of a link between a class II antigen of the major histocompatibility complex then known as DR2 DQw1 and narcolepsy led to a new investigation of the genetic basis of this disorder.[35] Honda and his team[35] have discovered that 100% of the Japanese narcoleptic patients studied to date express the haplotype now known as DR15 DQw6. British, French, Canadian, and U.S. investigators have confirmed the findings that, with few initial exceptions,[36–44] the great majority of white and black narcoleptics studied also express HLA-DR15 DQw6. This clear association strongly supports a genetic basis for the susceptibility to the illness. It has been demonstrated across racial groups in a transethnic study, and is the best current genetic marker for this disease. Matsuki et al.[45] and Mignot et al.[46] have shown that DQw6 is a better marker than DRw15. For example, only 70% of black American narcoleptics carry DRw15, although nearly all carry the DQw6 subtype.[45,46] Oligotyping demonstrated further that DQB1-0602 is the most common haplotype associated with narcolepsy. More recent family studies of narcoleptic index cases performed by our team and others, however, have provided challenging data.

In a survey (interviews and questionnaires) published in 1988, Montplaisir and Poirier[47] found that 23% of index cases had a family history of the disease and that 44% had at least one other relative who suffered from daytime sleepiness. In 1988, we pooled 334 probands who exhibited sleep attacks and cataplexy and abnormal sleep-onset REM periods at polygraphic recordings.[27] All of these patients would have met the strictest criteria for the definition of narcolepsy, including those of Honda and Juji.[13] Direct patient interviews, rather than questionnaires sent to patients, assured us that questions were well understood. It became clear that the family history was often inaccurate and more vague than had been suspected. Deceased subjects were

reported to have presented a higher rate of symptoms of daytime sleepiness or sleep attacks and cataplexy than living subjects, which obviously could not be verified. After interviewing these well-documented probands, we obtained the following results: 176 patients (53%) had no known family history of sleep attacks and cataplexy; 18 patients (5%) reported a history of sleep attacks and cataplexy in a family member; and 132 patients (40%) reported EDS in another family member.[27]

We compared our results with our previous investigation[33] in 1972 and 1973. The 1972 study involved only 50 probands; at that time we had found a low rate of narcolepsy and cataplexy (5.5%) in the surveyed population but a family history of EDS in 34%. To complete our new study, we asked 20 sleepy family members to be evaluated using objective criteria for sleepiness. One family member had an abnormal sleep-wake schedule and only two would have qualified for the diagnosis of isolated idiopathic sleepiness. Although it is difficult to generalize from these findings, we believe that the published number of isolated EDS cases that can appropriately be related to narcolepsy (in questionnaire studies covering family members of narcoleptics) has been inflated. Determining the relationship between narcolepsy syndrome and EDS in family members requires systematic monitoring of all family members suspected of having EDS. This could be very expensive and difficult; in our population, most relatives lived outside the area.

Thus, the first finding from these data was that a relationship did not necessarily exist between narcolepsy and EDS in other family members. Our second finding, echoed by the Japanese, Canadian, French, and German researchers, was that familial occurrence of narcolepsy is not a very frequent phenomenon.[48] Investigation of published pedigrees of families with several affected members has further complicated the issue. It must be emphasized that families with at least three living narcoleptic members who have all had HLA typing are rare in the literature.

Several noteworthy findings have been obtained from a group of approximately 50 families with several affected members that have been sent to Stanford from all over the world. In two families, one proband was HLA-DR2 DQw6 DQB1-0602 homozygous. In the German family studied by Mueller-Eckhardt and associates,[44] three siblings and one parent presented narcolepsy. One affected sibling did not share the same HLA haplotype (coming from the affected parent) with the two other affected siblings. This made the interpretation that the genetic transmission of the illness is purely through HLA-DR2 DQw6 unlikely. To explain the discrepancy, it has been suggested that there is a recombinant haplotype.[44-48] This notion is credible, but at best it is only one of many possibilities. Probably the most damaging evidence against the genetic transmission of narcolepsy only through DQB1-0602 or a closely located gene is our report of a family in which six members presented all the clinical symptoms of narcolepsy and PSG-documented sleep-onset REM periods but had negative tests for HLA-DR15 DQw6 DQB1-0602. Not only were all family members DR15-DQw6–negative, but three-fourths of the patients with cataplexy did not share similar haplotypes. There was, however, a high familial incidence of both daytime sleepiness and cataplexy through several generations. The existence of a genetic element was therefore strongly supported. The first proband had two affected daughters born of two different fathers, eliminating a recessive gene hypothesis for this family. The transmission of narcolepsy in this family can in some respects be compared with the canine model of narcolepsy, in which genetic transmission has been shown to be different from the dog leukocyte antigen complex and is consistent with the classic mendelian mode of inheritance. A similar family was reported by Singh and colleagues.[49] The percentage of narcoleptics who are positive for HLA-DQB1-0602 is estimated at 90–93%. Well-documented cases of non–HLA-DR2 DQw6 DQB1-0602 narcoleptics prove that it is not necessary to be HLA-DR2 DQw6 DQB1-0602–positive to be narcoleptic. Moreover, family studies throughout the world have shown that many family members have shared the HLA haplotype for disease susceptibility with the proband and have never developed narcolepsy. For example, in one Japanese investigation of 17 families, 22 subjects had the same haplotype for disease susceptibility as the proband, but 13 subjects had no symptoms whatsoever, eight presented EDS in non-PSG studies, and only one suffered from narcolepsy.[44,47] Our investigation showed similar results in the 18 families studied.[27]

A final critical observation has been made by Montplaisir and Poirier[47] and our group at Stanford: We have observed monozygotic twin pairs who are discordant for narcolepsy. Twin studies are always important in genetic investigations, and cases of monozygotic twins in which narcolepsy was diagnosed are often cited as evidence for a genetic etiology of the disease. Many of the older cases, however, are unconvincing when judged by present standards. Before 1985, HLA typing was not widespread, and MSLTs often were not performed in the course of clinical evaluations of narcolepsy. Montplaisir and Poirier[47] (two pairs) and our team[27] (one pair) have now investigated in depth three pairs of monozygotic twins discordant for narcolepsy. The two pairs of Canadian twins are over 50 years of age, and their monozygocity was established by HLA typing. The pair we are studying are 42 years old, and monozygocity was established by HLA typing and DNA fingerprinting. In each case, the affected twin developed symptoms during the teenage years. Both express DR2 DQw6. The existence of discordant monozygotic twins indicates that nongenetic factors participate in the development of narcolepsy. We reiterate, however, that although up to 4% of patients may not express HLA-DR2, the major association between HLA-DR2 DQw6 DQB1-0602 and narcolepsy cannot be dismissed. We conclude that an association frequently exists between narcolepsy and the presence of HLA-DQB1-0602 but that the association is neither sufficient nor necessary for the development of narcolepsy.

The association between HLA-DR2 DQw6 DQB1-0602 and narcolepsy is of particular interest because of the link between the HLA antigen and autoimmune disease. Although there is very little evidence at this date to implicate the immune system in the pathogenesis of narcolepsy, the very strong association between this haplotype and the disease makes a compelling argument for immune system involvement. Investigations in Doberman pinschers have shown that, in this dog breed, narcolepsy is transmitted through a single autosomal recessive gene called *canarc1*. Gene markers for *canarc1* have indicated that it is not linked to the canine major histocompatibility complex but is tightly linked to a mu-like gene. Mu is the switch region of the immunoglobulin heavy chain gene. This last finding in canine narcolepsy also suggests involvement of the immune system in the pathophysiology of the disease. One could propose a model in which a combination of several factors would be necessary for the development of narcolepsy in most cases: (1) a genetic factor not linked to the HLA system, which would be a susceptibility gene; (2) the presence of HLA-DRwl5 DQlw6 (the key element is a locus near DQB1-0602); and (3) the involvement of at least one environmental factor, possibly a viral infection. This model would not explain the non–DQB1-0602 cases, which are much less common than the non-DRwl5 cases, but until the susceptibility gene is identified, non–DQB1-0602 cases cannot be clearly explained.

### *Is There Any Support for Possible Immune System or Viral Involvement in the Development of Narcolepsy?*

In a study involving 52 narcoleptics, Billiard and coworkers[50] reported that elevated antibody to streptolysin O (ABO titers) was found in 22 patients (compared with one in 49 controls), and elevated antibody to DNase B titers was observed in 13 patients and none of the controls. However, Montplaisir (personal communication, 1990) was unable to replicate the ABO findings in his patient population.

One must conclude that some combination of genetic and environmental factors is probably involved in the development of human narcolepsy. The sequencing of DR in two narcoleptic patients (in England and the United States) has not shown any difference between these patients and an unaffected subject. Further investigation of canine narcolepsy, which allows one to obtain back-crosses and several affected litters, may be of further help.

## ETIOLOGIC AND PHARMACOLOGIC STUDIES AND THE ANIMAL MODEL

Over the past 10 years, an animal model of the narcolepsy-cataplexy syndrome has been developed at Stanford University. Several breeds of dogs have been collected that exhibit symptoms closely resembling those of human narcolepsy. The usefulness of studying a naturally occurring disorder in an animal model depends on its similarity to the human form of the disorder. Of the four major symptoms of human narcolepsy, two—EDS and cataplexy—are present in most human patients and in dogs afflicted with narcolepsy. Excessive sleepiness may be documented in these animals using the canine version of the MSLT and PSG recordings of the narcoleptic and control animals.[51]

Cataplexy is a brief episode of generalized non-reciprocal motor inhibition that is entirely reversible. It is essentially identical in humans and dogs.[52,53] In canine cataplexy, the episode is often induced by a clear emotional component such as feeding, chewing, playing, or appetitive behaviors such as gnawing on a package of food or attempting sexual intercourse. Because canine cataplexy is elicited by emotional excitement, the Stanford Sleep Laboratory has developed the food elicited cataplexy test. This is a biological assay for quantifying cataplexy in narcoleptic canines. This study is performed by placing 12 pieces of food (1 cm$^3$ in size) 30 cm apart in a circle on the floor, and dogs that have been previously trained to eat all the pieces of food in serial order are introduced to the testing room. The number and duration of cataplectic attacks are recorded, as is the time required for the dogs to complete the test.[54] As in humans, there is no loss of alertness during the briefer cataplectic attacks or during the initial stage of longer attacks in dogs. The waking state sensorium remains intact, and the dog visually tracks objects if its eyes are open. Tendon reflexes are inactive during a cataplectic attack, but they return once cataplexy is terminated and there are no residual neurologic abnormalities. Electrographic variables resemble those of wakefulness during the initial stage of cataplexy, whereas the later stage is indistinguishable from REM sleep. Finally, cataplexy in dogs is suppressed by the same REM-suppressant drugs that are used to treat human cataplexy.[55–59] In addition, narcoleptic dogs consistently have short sleep latency, typically less than 5 minutes on all tests, whereas normal dogs show much longer latencies.[48] Investigations in Dobermans and Labrador retrievers have shown transmission via an identical autosomal recessive mode[58,59]; the recessive gene has full penetrance. Not all dog breeds exhibit genetic transmission of narcolepsy, as evidenced by unsuccessful efforts to breed affected poodles and beagles. These findings suggest that there may be different causes for the canine narcolepsy syndrome: (1) inheritance via a single autosomal recessive gene with complete penetrance; (2) nongenetic mechanisms such as developmental accidents or CNS trauma; and (3) more complex polygenic mechanisms that produce unaffected offspring from narcoleptic parents. The Doberman and Labrador models have allowed the performance of pharmacologic studies searching for specific receptor defects.

## CURRENT TREATMENT

The drugs most widely used against EDS are the CNS stimulants. Amphetamines were first proposed by Prinzmetal and Bloomberg[60] in 1935. The alerting effect of a single oral dose of amphetamine is at its maximum 2–4 hours after administration, and many patients require daily or twice-daily dosing. A number of side effects, including irritability, tachycardia, nocturnal sleep disturbances, and sometimes tolerance and drug dependence may arise. The use of methylphenidate was later encouraged[61] because of faster action and lower incidence of side effects. Pemoline, an oxazolidine derivative with a longer half-life and slower onset of action, is less efficient but well tolerated.[62] Modafinil is a medication with a less defined mode of action that has been described as like that of $\alpha_1$ stimulants. It is used in Europe and Canada and currently under investigation in the United States. A French study found that it caused substantial improvement.[63] The new monoamine oxidase B inhibitor selegiline has none of the tyramine-related side effects and appears to be helpful in the treatment of EDS.[64] The pharmacologic activity of the drug on sleepiness may be related to a levoamphetamine metabolite.

Mazindol, an imidazoline derivative, has been shown to reduce the number of daytime sleep episodes in narcoleptics in a dose range of 3–8 mg. Side effects are minor.[65] γ-Hydroxybutyrate (GHB) (available in France and Canada and under investigation in the United States), which is given orally at bedtime and at the time of a night awakening, has been shown to be of definite value even though its efficiency varies among patients.[66] This substance has been shown to increase slow-wave and REM sleep in normal individuals.

The treatment of cataplexy, sleep paralysis, and hypnagogic hallucinations calls for tricyclic medications and the new serotonin antagonists. Both protriptyline in North America and clomipramine in Europe have been widely used, often with good results. Other tricyclic medications, such as imipramine and desipramine hydrochloride (Norpramin), are also effective; however, the atropine-like side effects—particularly impotence in men—

have prompted a search for other drugs. Selective serotonin-reuptake inhibitors have been added to the pharmacologic armamentarium for the relief of daytime sleepiness as well as the control of cataplexy.[67] The advantage of improving nocturnal sleep is significant not only for daytime sleepiness but also for cataplexy, though stimulant medications are often necessary with GHB. Patients who present the full clinical tetrad frequently need a combination of drugs, particularly stimulants and tricyclics; GHB, antiserotonergic drugs, or a benzodiazepine may be needed at night.

To better understand the efficacy of the different available drugs, Mitler and Hajdukovic[68] compared the efficacy of putative therapeutic agents on daytime sleepiness results from MSLT and maintenance of wakefulness test published in the literature. The authors normalized the data, obtained on 179 narcoleptics, and reported the results as percentages of normal values obtained on a control group. The drugs tested were dextroamphetamine, methylphenidate, pemoline, modafinil, protriptyline, viloxazine, ritanserin, codeine, and GHB.

The study shows that even with the largest recommended doses, no drug brings narcoleptics to normal alertness. Dexedrine (dextroamphetamine) and methylphenidate most improved patients' alertness. GHB, protriptyline, and ritanserin had an insignificant impact. Viloxazine, modafinil, and pemoline had mild to moderate effect. Codeine is the least investigated of these drugs, but it actually shows more promise than viloxazine, modafinil, or pemoline.

Drugs that stimulate norepinephrine release (amphetamines and methylphenidate) seem to have the greatest impact on sleepiness. This seems to be true also in the dog model of narcolepsy. As $\alpha_{1b}$ agonists appear to significantly improve canine narcolepsy, it is possible that such agents will prove beneficial to humans. Modafinil does not have a direct effect on the $\alpha_{1b}$, which may explain its limited activity. More specific compounds may give better results.

Two other therapeutic approaches must be emphasized: short daytime naps and support groups. A 15- to 20-minute nap taken three times daily helps maintain a satisfactory level of vigilance. It has never been demonstrated that stimulant medications improve alertness more effectively. Naps have to be repeated throughout the day, as the "refractory" sleep period after a nap varies between 90 and 120 minutes. Narcolepsy is a disabling disorder, leading in many instances to loss of gainful employment because of daytime sleepiness and automatic behavior. It is also often ill-understood by patients, family members, and peers. It can result in rejection from family and other social groups, in divorce, loss of self-esteem, and depressive reactions. For these reasons, as well as the young age at onset of the syndrome, it is important to put narcolepsy patients in contact with support groups and to help create regional narcolepsy associations and patient groups. Tables 25-1 and A25-1 (see the chapter appendix) summarize the drugs and other treatments currently available for narcolepsy.

## CLINICAL VARIANTS AND ASSOCIATED ILLNESSES

There are some rare but clearly documented forms of "secondary" narcolepsy, with EDS and cataplexy, that appear coincident to head trauma or as a result of brain lesions. In most reported instances, the lesion invaded the floor of the third ventricle and upper brain stem. A paper presenting a series of case reports and a review of the literature on this subject detailed 16 cases, seven of whom had tissue typing performed.[69] Three of the six were HLA-DR2 DQw6–positive. This reinforces the concept that a particular genetic background is important to the expression of this disease. Four, nonetheless, were not HLA-DR2 DQw6–positive, indicating that the CNS lesion played a primary role in those cases.[69] Lankford and colleagues[70] evaluated nine patients with EDS after closed head injury. Five of these patients also exhibited cataplexy. These researchers concluded that the location of the head injury was unrelated to symptoms or the sleep parameters.[70]

The subject of narcolepsy (with or without cataplexy) and its possible association with multiple sclerosis is interesting. Both disorders have been postulated to be disorders of immunoreactivity, and the frequency of DQw6 DQB1-0602 is also increased among multiple sclerosis patients, but a preliminary study has not demonstrated a significant difference in sleepiness complaints between MS patients who express this allele and those who do not. Similarly, if rheumatoid arthritis, another DR2-linked disorder, occurs with narcolepsy, the association is far from frequent. Because DQw6 may be more important than DRw15, the lack of association may not be surprising.

**Table 25-1.** Currently Available Narcolepsy Drugs

| Drugs | Maximum Dosage* (mg/day) |
|---|---|
| **Treatment of excessive daytime sleepiness** | |
| Stimulants | |
|     Amphetamine | 40 |
|     Methylphenidate | 60 (in divided doses) |
|     Mazindol | 5 |
|     Pemoline | 150 |
| Adjunctive effect drugs (i.e., improve EDS if associated with stimulant) | |
|     Protriptyline | 10 |
|     Viloxazine | 200 |
| **Treatment of auxiliary effects** | |
| Tricyclic antidepressants with atropine-like side effects | |
|     Protriptyline | 20 |
|     Imipramine | 200 |
|     Clomipramine | 200 |
|     Desipramine | 200 |
| Tricyclic antidepressants without atropine-like side effects: viloxazine | 200 |
| **Experimental drugs or drugs available in very few countries** | |
| Stimulant | |
|     CRL 40476 | |
|     Codeine (given as stimulant) | |
| Cataplexy antagonist and mild stimulant: γ-hydroxybutyrate | |

EDS = excessive daytime sleepiness
*All drugs are taken orally.

Sleep apnea may be seen more frequently with narcolepsy. As obstructive sleep apnea may lead to significant sleep fragmentation, the association of sleep-onset REM periods and daytime sleepiness at MSLT is insufficient to consider a disorder's association. A study of 100 sleep apnea patients found that 24% of them had two or more sleep-onset REM periods at MSLT (personal observation). The association of daytime sleepiness, cataplexy, and sleep apnea, however, can undoubtedly be noted, with cataplexy affirming the presence of the narcolepsy syndrome.[71] The association between periodic leg movement syndrome (PLMS) and narcolepsy has been mentioned, although one must remember that imipramine, clomipramine, and protriptyline increase the number of PLMS during sleep, an increase that also is associated with aging. PLMS seems to be more common in narcoleptic patients than in the general population,[72] though Montplaisir and Godbout[73] do not believe, from their own analysis, that PMLS is an important factor in nocturnal sleep disturbance in narcolepsy.

## DIFFERENTIAL DIAGNOSIS

The major items in the differential diagnosis of narcolepsy are idiopathic hypersomnia and the syndromes associating EDS with the presence of one or several sleep-onset REM periods, as discussed in the Diagnostic Procedures section. Idiopathic hypersomnia, which is characterized by EDS, should be considered a possible diagnosis only when obstructive sleep apnea syndrome and upper airway resistance syndrome have been ruled out. Unlike narcolepsy, the daytime somnolence associated with idiopathic hypersomnia is rarely relieved by short naps. In fact, naps may lead to sleep drunkenness and complaints of increased tiredness. Frequently reported with this syndrome are mild symptoms of autonomic nervous system dysfunction such as cold hands, cold feet (Raynaud's-type phenomena), lightheadedness (rarely associated with a drop in systolic blood pressure sufficient to be called *orthostatic hypotension*), and frequent dull headaches that may have a typical migraine presentation. In some instances the syndrome develops immediately after mononucleosis, Guillain-Barré syndrome, viral hepatitis, or atypical pneumonia, particularly that involving echoviruses, which suggests that a virus might participate in the appearance of idiopathic hypersomnia. PSG and MSLT show lack of sleep-onset REM periods and a mean sleep latency of approximately 6 minutes. Tables A25-2 and A25-3 summarize the pertinent features for diagnosis and differential diagnosis of narcolepsy.

In conclusion, despite the many studies and publications on narcolepsy during the past 90 years, a complete understanding of the narcolepsy syndrome eludes us. Narcolepsy remains a disabling neurologic illness that is poorly or incompletely controlled by treatment. It leads to a variety of complications when it goes undiagnosed, such as traffic and industrial accidents. Narcolepsy is a major employment problem for its victims, owing to many employers' unwillingness to allow short (15-minute) naps two or three times during the day. The disorder is often the source of job discrimination, job dismissal, early retirement, and depression secondary to these circumstances.[74]

The question of whether EDS slowly worsens with age is unresolved at this time. As aging is often associated with more disturbed nocturnal sleep, it is possible that the nocturnal sleep disturbances noted with aging worsen the EDS of narcoleptics. A survey performed on the Stanford Sleep Disorders Clinic narcoleptic population showed that 62% of narcoleptics older than 47 years of age had no recourse other than to apply for Social Security disability benefits.

## REFERENCES

1. Gelineau J. De la narcolepsie. Gaz Hop (Paris) 1880; 53:626, 54:635.
2. Henneberg R. Uber genuine Narkolepsie. Neurol Zb1 1916;30:282.
3. Daniels L. Narcolepsy. Medicine 1934;13:1.
4. Yoss RE, Daly DD. Criteria for the diagnosis of the narcoleptic syndrome. Proc Staff Meet Mayo Clin 1957; 32:320.
5. Vogel G. Studies in the psychophysiology of dreams. III. The dream of narcolepsy. Arch Gen Psychiatry 1960; 3:421.
6. Rechtschaffen A, Wolpert E, Dement WC, et al. Nocturnal sleep of narcoleptics. Electroencephalogr Clin Neurophysiol 1963;15:599.
7. Takahashi Y, Jimbo M. Polygraphic study of narcoleptic syndrome with special reference to hypnagogic hallucinations and cataplexy. Folia Psychiatr Neurol (Jap) 1963;7:S343.
8. Passouant P, Schwab RS, Cadilhac J, et al. Narcolepsie-cataplexie. Étude du sommeil de nuit et du sommeil de jour. Rev Neurol (Paris) 1964;3:415.
9. Hishikawa Y, Kaneko Z. Electroencephalographic study on narcolepsy. Electroencephalogr Clin Neurophysiol 1965;18:249.
10. Guilleminault C, Dement WC, Passouant P (eds). Narcolepsy. New York: Spectrum, 1975;1.
11. Honda Y, Asaka A, Tanaka Y, Juji T. Discrimination of narcolepsy by using genetic markers and HLA. Sleep Res 1983;12:254.
12. Diagnostic Classification Steering Committee. International Classification of Sleep Disorders: Diagnostic and Coding Manual. Rochester, MN: American Sleep Disorders Association, 1990.
13. Honda Y, Juji T (eds). HLA in Narcolepsy. Berlin: Springer, 1988;208.
14. Billiard M, Besset A, Cadilhac J. The Clinical and Polygraphic Development of Narcolepsy. In C Guillem-

inault, E Lugaresi (eds), Sleep/Wake Disorders: Natural History, Epidemiology, and Long-Term Evolution. New York: Raven, 1983;187.

15. Hoddes E, Dement WC, Zarcone V. The development and use of the Stanford Sleepiness Scale (SSS). Psychophysiology 1972;9:150.

16. Yoss RE, Mayer NJ, Ogle KN. The pupillogram and narcolepsy. Neurology 1969;19:921.

17. Schmidt HS, Fortin LD. Electronic Pupillography in Disorders of Arousal. In C Guilleminault (ed), Sleep and Waking Disorders: Indications and Techniques. Menlo Park, CA: Addison-Wesley, 1981;127.

18. Berlucchi G, Moruzzi G, Salva G, et al. Pupil behavior and ocular movements during synchronized and desynchronized sleep. Arch Ital Biol 1964;102:230.

19. Carskadon MA, Dement WC. The multiple sleep latency test: what does it measure? Sleep 1982;5:67.

20. Rechtschaffen A, Kales AD. A Manual of Standardized Terminology, Techniques and Scoring System for Sleep Stages of Human Subjects. Los Angeles: Brain Information Service/Brain Research Institute, UCLA, 1968.

21. Association of Professional Sleep Societies Guidelines Committee. Guidelines for the Multiple Sleep Latency Test (MSLT): a standard measure of sleepiness. Sleep 1986;9:519.

22. Van den Hoed J, Kraemer H, Guilleminault C, et al. Disorders of excessive daytime somnolence: polygraphic and clinical data for 100 patients. Sleep 1981;4:23.

23. Browman CP, Gujavarty KS, Sampson MG, et al. REM sleep episodes during the maintenance of wakefulness tests in patients with sleep apnea syndrome and patients with narcolepsy. Sleep 1983;6:23.

24. Sleep Disorders Atlas Task Force of the American Sleep Disorders Association. EEG arousals: scoring rules and examples: a preliminary report. Sleep 1992;15:174.

25. Broughton R, Low R, Valley V, et al. Auditory evoked potentials compared to EEG and performance measures of impaired vigilance in narcolepsy-cataplexy. Sleep Res 1981;10:184.

26. Moscovitch A, Partinen M, Patterson-Rhoads N, et al. Cataplexy in differentiation of excessive daytime somnolence. Sleep Res 1991;20:303.

27. Guilleminault C, Mignot E, Grumet C. Family study of narcolepsy. Lancet 1989;11:1376.

28. World Health Organization (WHO) Nomenclature Committee for Factors of the HLA System. Nomenclature for factors of the HLA system, 1989. Immunogenetics 1990;31:131.

29. Mignot E, Hayduk R, Black J, et al. HLA DQB1*0602 is associated with cataplexy in 509 narcoleptic patients. Sleep 1997;20:2012.

30. Aldrich MS. The neurobiology of narcolepsy-cataplexy. Prog Neurobiol 1993;41:533.

31. Dement WC, Zarcone V, Varner V, et al. The prevalence of narcolepsy. Sleep 1972;1:148.

32. Dement WC, Carskadon MA, Ley R. The prevalence of narcolepsy. Sleep Res 1973;2:147.

33. Kessler S, Guilleminault C, Dement WC. A family study of 50 REM narceptics. Arch Neurol Scand 1974;50:503.

34. Honda Y, Asaka A, Tanimura M, et al. A Genetic Study of Narcolepsy and Excessive Daytime Sleepiness in 308 Families with a Narcolepsy of Hypersomnia Proband. In C Guilleminault, E Lugaresi (eds), Sleep/Wake Disorders: Natural History, Epidemiology and Long-Term Evolution. New York: Raven, 1983; 187.

35. Honda Y, Asaka A, Tanaka Y, et al. Discrimination of narcoleptic patients by using genetic markers and HLA [abstract]. Sleep Res 1983;12:254.

36. Langdon N, Welch KI, Dam MV, et al. Genetic markers in narcolepsy. Lancet 1984;2:1178.

37. Guilleminault C, Grumet C. HLA-DR2 and narcolepsy: not all narcoleptic cataplectic patients are DR2. Hum Immunol 1986;17:1.

38. Juji T, Satake M, Honda Y, et al. HLA antigens in Japanese patients with narcolepsy—all the patients were DR2 positive. Tissue Antigens 1984;24:316.

39. Seignalet J, Billiard M. Possible associations between HLA-B7 and narcolepsy. Tissue Antigens 1984;23:188.

40. Billiard M, Seignalet J. Extraordinary association between HLA-DR2 and narcolepsy. Lancet 1985;2:226.

41. Poirier G, Montplaisir J, Decary F, et al. HLA antigens in narcolepsy and idiopathic central nervous system hypersomnolence. Sleep 1986;9:153.

42. Langdon N, Lock C, Welsh K, et al. Immune factors in narcolepsy. Sleep 1986;9:143.

43. Neely SE, Rosenberg AS, Spire JP, et al. HLA antigens in narcolepsy. Neurology 1987;37:1858.

44. Mueller-Eckhardt G, Meier-Ewert K, Schendel DJ, et al. HLA and narcolepsy in a German population. Tissue Antigens 1986;28:163.

45. Matsuki K, Grumet FC, Lin X, et al. HLA DQB1-0602 rather than HLA DRw15 (DR2) is the disease susceptibility gene in black narcolepsy. Lancet 1992;339:1052.

46. Mignot E, Lin X, Arrigoni J, et al. DQB1*0602 and DQA*0102 (DQ1) are better markers than DR2 for narcolepsy in caucasian and black Americans. Sleep 1994;17:S60.

47. Montplaisir J, Poirier G. HLA in Narcolepsy in Canada. In Y Honda, T Juji (eds), HLA in Narcolepsy. Berlin: Springer, 1988;97.

48. Matsuki K, Honda Y, Satake M, et al. HLA in Narcolepsy in Japan. In Y Honda, T Juji (eds), HLA in Narcolepsy. Berlin: Springer, 1988;58.

49. Singh S, George CFP, Kryger MH, et al. Genetic heterogeneity in narcolepsy. Lancet 1990;21:726.

50. Billiard M, Laaberki MF, Reygrobillet C, et al. Elevated antibody to streptolysin O and antibody to DNase B titers in narcoleptic subjects. Sleep Res 1989;18:201.

51. Lucas EA, Foutz AS, Mitler MM, et al. Multiple sleep latency test in normal and narcoleptic canines [abstract]. Soc Neurosci 1978;4:541.

52. Mitler MM, Boysen BG, Campbell L, et al. Narcolepsy-cataplexy in a female dog. Exp Neurol 1974;45:332.

53. Mitler MM, Dement WC. Sleep studies on canine narcolepsy: pattern and cycle comparisons between affected and normal dogs. Electroencephalogr Clin Neurophysiol 1977;43:691.

54. Nishino S, Reiid MS, Dement WC, Mignot E. Neuropharmacology and neurochemistry of canine narcolepsy. Sleep 1994;17:S84.

55. Delashaw J, Foutz Z, Guilleminault C, et al. Cholinergic mechanisms and cataplexy in dogs. Exp Neurol 1978;66:745.

56. Foutz AS, Delashaw JB Jr, Guilleminault C, et al. Monoaminergic mechanisms and experimental cataplexy. Neurology 1981;10:369.

57. Lucas EA. A study of the daily sleep and waking patterns of the laboratory cat and dog. Sleep Res 1978;7:142.

58. Foutz AS, Mitler MM, Cavalli-Sforza LL, et al. Genetic factors in canine narcolepsy. Sleep 1979;1:413.

59. Baker TL, Narver EL, Dement WC, et al. Effects of imipramine, chlorimipramine, and fluoxetine on cataplexy in dogs. Pharmacol Biochem Behav 1976;5:599.

60. Prinzmetal M, Bloomberg W. The use of benzedrine for treatment of narcolepsy. JAMA 1935;105:2051.

61. Yoss RE, Daly DD. Treatment of narcolepsy with Ritalin. Neurology 1952;9:171.

62. Honda Y, Hishikawa Y. Effectiveness of pemoline in narcolepsy. Sleep Res 1970;8:192.

63. Farma L, Galland Y. Treatment of Narcoleptics with CRL-40476, an Alpha Stimulant Medication [abstract]. Munich, FRG: Seventh European Sleep Congress, 1984.

64. Roselaar SE, Langdon N, Lock CB, et al. Selegiline in narcolepsy. Sleep 1987;10;491.

65. Parkes JD, Schacter M. Mazindol in the treatment of narcolepsy. Acta Neurol Scand 1979;60:250.

66. Broughton R, Mamelak M. Effects of nocturnal gamma-hydroxybutyrate on sleep/waking patterns in narcolepsy-cataplexy. Can J Neurol Sci 1980;7:23.

67. Nishino S, Arrigoni J, Shelton J, et al. Desmethyl metabolites of serotonergic uptake inhibitors are more potent for suppressing canine cataplexy than their parent compounds. Sleep 1993;16:706.

68. Mitler M, Hajdukovic R. Relative efficacy of drugs for the treatment of sleepiness in narcolepsy. Sleep 1991;14:218.

69. Clavelou P, Tournilhac M, Vidal C, et al. Narcolepsy associated with arteriovenous malformation of the diencephalon. Sleep 1995;18:202.

70. Lankford DA, Wellman JJ, O'Hara C. Posttraumatic narcolepsy in mild to moderate closed head injury. Sleep 1994;17:S25.

71. Guilleminault C, Van den Hoed J, Mitler MM. Clinical Overview of the Sleep Apnea Syndromes. In C Guilleminault, Dement WC (eds), Sleep Apnea Syndromes. New York: Liss, 1978;1.

72. Baker TL, Guilleminault C, Nino-Murcia G, et al. Comparative polysomnographic study of narcolepsy and idiopathic central nervous system hypersomnia. Sleep 1986;9:232.

73. Montplaisir J, Godbout R. Nocturnal sleep of narcoleptic patients: revisited. Sleep 1986;9:159.

74. Broughton R, Ghanem Q, Hishikawa Y, et al. Life effects of narcolepsy in 180 patients from North America, Asia, and Europe compared to matched controls. Can J Sci 1981;8:299.

# Chapter 25 Appendix

**Table A25-1.** Treatment for Narcolepsy

I. Treatment for cataplexy and sleep paralysis, with or without hypnagogic hallucinations or panic reaction to sleep paralysis, is tricyclic antidepressants. Best medications are nonatropinic tricyclics, as they have fewer side effects.

    Viloxazine HCl (50-mg tablets) PO; normal dose, 150–200 mg daily.

    Fluoxetine HCl (20-mg tablets) PO; normal dose (in the morning).

    Clomipramine (25- or 50-mg tablets) PO; normal dose, 75–125 mg daily (at bedtime).

  Other tricyclics with atropine-like side effects:

    Protriptyline (5-mg tablets) PO; normal dose, 10–15 mg (in the morning or divided). Impotence is common with 15–20 mg.

    Imipramine (25- or 30-mg tablets) PO; normal dose, 75–125 mg daily (divided or in the evening).

II. Treatment for sleepiness

  A. Behavioral treatment

    Scheduled short 15-minute daytime naps

    Best times: 10:30 AM, 1:00 PM, 4:00 PM

    Schedules most frequently used by patients: 1:00–2:00 PM and 4:30–6:00 PM

  B. Nutrition: Avoid heavy lunches, alcohol, and foods or beverages that have paradoxical effects, such as chocolate.

  C. Medication: No medication completely alleviates daytime sleepiness, but some help to improve performance.

  Best medications:

    For children and adolescents: pemoline (18.75- and 37.5-mg tablets). Efficacy increases progressively over 1 week. Dosage varies with age (weight) between 37 and 150 mg/day.

    For adults:

    1. Methylphenidate (5-mg tablets) PO, taken at least 30–45 minutes before or after a meal. Repeat dose throughout the day and avoid one large dose (short half-life).

      Advantages: can be taken when needed; rapid action

      Usual dosage: 20–40 mg/day; avoid more than 50 mg/day—no clinical gain

      The slow-release (SR) form of this drug is available and may be used in the morning by U.S. Medicaid patients, whose only authorized dose is 20-mg tablets.

    2. Pemoline (37.5-mg tablets) PO; 1 or 2 daily doses (morning, noon). Normal dosage is 100–150 mg/day.

    3. Dexedrine (5-mg tablets) PO. Normal dosage is 10–40 mg/day. Divided doses or SR formula recommended to avoid side effects. New patients should first be treated with other drugs.

    4. Mazindol (2-mg tablets) PO. Normal dosage is 4–8 mg/day in 2 doses.

    5. Modafinil is available in several European countries on a restricted basis, presented as a nonamphetamine stimulant.

**Table A25-1.** *continued.*

III. Examples of treatment packages
  A. Prepubertal children
    1. For sleepiness
        Contact school to alert teachers
        Nap at lunchtime
        Nap at 4:00–5:00 PM
        Medication: pemoline, one to three 18.75-mg tablets daily
    2. For cataplexy: clomipramine, 25–50 mg at bedtime
  B. Pubertal children: for sleepiness
        Contact school to alert teachers
        Emphasize need for regular nocturnal sleep schedule
        Try to obtain 9 hours nocturnal sleep
        Nap at lunch time and at 4:00 or 5:00 PM
        Medications: pemoline, one to three 37.5-mg tablets daily
  C. Adults
        Avoid shifting sleep schedule
        Avoid heavy meals and alcohol
        Regular timing of nocturnal sleep: 10:30 PM to 7:00 AM
        Naps: 15 minutes at lunch time and at 5:30 PM
    1. For daytime sleepiness:
        Methylphenidate, 5 mg × 3/4 or 20 mg SR morning, on empty stomach
        If difficulties persist:

|  |  |
|---|---|
| Methylphenidate (SR): | 20 mg in the morning |
|  | 5 mg after noon nap |
|  | 5 mg at 4:00 PM |

        If no response:

|  |  |
|---|---|
| Dexedrine spansule (SR): | 15 mg at awakening |
|  | 5 mg after noon nap |
|  | 5 mg at 3:30 or 4:00 PM |
|  | 15 mg at awakening |
|  | 15 mg after noon nap |

    2. For cataplexy:
        Clomipramine, 75–125 mg, *or*
        Vivactil, 150–200 mg, *or*
        Imipramine, 75–125 mg

**Table A25-2.** How to Diagnose Narcolepsy

| | | |
|---|---|---|
| A. Patient reports partial or complete cataplectic attacks, daytime sleepiness, and napping. | Patient is narcoleptic. | Confirm by nocturnal PSG and MSLT on the following day. MSLT shows short sleep latencies. PSG shows presence or absence of sleep apnea, presence or absence of PLMs. Risk of MSLT being negative with 1-day test is 3%. |
| B. Patient reports a history of partial or complete cataplectic attacks and current daytime sleepiness and napping. | | |
| C. Patient reports partial or complete cataplectic attacks and intermittent daytime drowsiness several times a week. | | |
| D. Patient reports isolated cataplexy; no reports of EDS or napping. | Patient has isolated cataplexy, is not narcoleptic, but . . . | 1. Confirm absence of EDS by PSG and MSLT.<br>2. Investigate family history for narcolepsy.<br>3. Perform HLA typing to search for DR2 DQw6. |
| E. Patient reports isolated EDS and daytime napping. | | |
| F. Patient reports EDS, daytime napping, hypnagogic hallucinations, sleep paralysis. | Patient is not narcoleptic. See Table A25-3. | Patient may be developing narcolepsy. Follow patient. |

PSG = polysomnography; MSLT = Multiple Sleep Latency Test; EDS = excessive daytime sleep; PLMs = periodic limb movements.

**Table A25-3.** What to Do When Patient is Not a Bona Fide Narcoleptic*

| IF, | THEN |
|---|---|
| Patient presents with EDS, daytime napping, hypnagogic hallucinations, and sleep paralysis | 1. Perform polygraphic recordings and daytime MSLT; <br> 2. investigate first-degree relatives for narcolepsy; and <br> 3. consider patient's age. |
| 1. Patient is young; <br> 2. sleep latencies in MSLT are short; <br> 3. there is more than one sleep-onset REM period; <br> 4. PSG shows no cause for EDS; *and* <br> 5. there is family (first-degree relative) of narcolepsy | Patient is probably developing narcolepsy. Follow and treat as a narcoleptic. Do HLA typing and determine whether DR2 DQw6 is expressed. |
| Patient presents with isolated EDS and daytime napping | 1. Obtain good sleep disorders history; <br> 2. perform nocturnal PSG and daytime MSLT; <br> 3. investigate family history for causes of EDS; and <br> 4. consider patient's age. |
| 1. Patient has no clinical symptoms for other causes of EDS; <br> 2. tests produce a good, undisrupted nocturnal PSG without evidence of sleep-related problems; <br> 3. MSLT produces short latencies but ≤1 sleep-onset REM period; <br> 4. the family history includes narcolepsy; *and* <br> 5. patient is young | Patient may be developing narcolepsy. Follow and treat as a narcoleptic. Perform HLA typing. |
| 1. Findings are identical to 1–4 above; and <br> 2. patient is middle-aged or older, with several years' history of sleepiness | Patient is considered to have a disorder of daytime sleepiness (probably related to narcolepsy, but unproved to date). HLA typing is of scientific interest for better definition of the syndrome. Treat as a narcoleptic. |
| 1. Patient has no clinical symptoms for other causes of EDS; <br> 2. tests produce good, undisrupted nocturnal PSG without evidence of sleep-related problems; <br> 3. MSLT produces short sleep latencies and ≥2 sleep-onset periods; <br> 4. there is no family history of narcolepsy; *and* <br> 5. patient is young, middle-aged, or older with several years' history of sleepiness | Patient may be developing narcolepsy and must be followed. Condition is considered a disorder of isolated sleepiness (possibly a disorder of REM sleep; the relation to narcolepsy is unknown). HLA typing is of scientific interest for better understanding of the syndrome. Treat with stimulants. |
| 1. Patient has no clinical symptoms for other causes of EDS; <br> 2. tests produce good, undisrupted nocturnal PSG without evidence of sleep-related problems; <br> 3. MSLT produces short sleep latencies with ≤1 sleep-onset REM period; and <br> 4. and there is no family history of narcolepsy | Patient of any age is considered to have CNS hypersomnia (relation to narcolepsy unknown). Investigate for viral infection concomitant with syndrome onset, and possibly perform serologic studies for positive history. Investigate family for history of isolated daytime sleepiness. HLA typing is of scientific interest for better definition of the syndrome (most commonly subjects express HLA-DR2 DQw6). Treat with stimulants. |

EDS = excessive daytime sleepiness; MSLT = multiple sleep latency test; PSG = polysomnography; CNS = central nervous system.
*That is, if cataplexy is not currently and never has been, present.

# Chapter 26
# Motor Functions and Dysfunctions of Sleep

Wayne A. Hening, Richard Allen, Arthur S. Walters,
and Sudhansu Chokroverty

The motor system is highly modulated by the changes in state from wake to drowsiness to slow-wave sleep (SWS) and then to rapid eye movement (REM) sleep. Indeed, so significant are the changes in motor activity depending on state that various researchers have used quantitative recordings of motor activity, known as *actigraphy*, as a basis for determining sleep and wake states.[1] The importance of measuring such activity is growing and reflected in a new section of this chapter that deals with the use of actigraphy in assessing sleep disorders.

This chapter is divided into three sections. The first briefly reviews normal motor activity and its changes during sleep, whereas the next two sections examine motor disturbances associated with sleep. These two sections are informally divided into two categories. On the one hand, there are motor disturbances present during the day (diurnal movement disorders) that may impact sleep, either directly through their motor effects or indirectly through a variety of other mechanisms. These are *movement disorders* that are seen by a neurologist or movement disorder specialist. On the other hand, there are the motor disturbances that are predominantly associated with sleep. They may be motor activity similar to what is normally found during waking hours that intrudes on sleep (some parasomnias, such as sleep walking, are of this type) or abnormal motor activity that does not occur during the wake state, but is aroused by sleep. These are generally classified as *sleep dis-*

*orders* and typically treated by a sleep disorder specialist. These two main categories are by no means completely unique, however, and it is not unusual for a patient with a disorder in one category to be seen by a specialist in the other category. It is, therefore, useful to consider these two categories of sleep disturbances together in this chapter.

This chapter has two major purposes: to describe and compare the various motor disturbances of sleep and to demonstrate a usable approach to the diagnosis and treatment of motor disturbances of sleep. Although this chapter touches briefly on the distinctions between the various movement disorders, it does not pretend to be a general review of movement disorders. Those in the sleep field who wish to refer to a general discussion of movement disorders can find a number of reviews that deal extensively with a wide spectrum of movement disorders.[2–5] There are also a number of excellent, more abbreviated treatments of this field in medical and neurologic textbooks.[6,7] The remaining chapters in this volume provide a suitable background for sleep-related issues for the neurologist or other individual whose primary field is movement disorders. Where issues have overlapped—such as those parasomnias that cause motor disturbances—we have referred to other chapters in this volume so as not to unnecessarily increase the length of this one.

## THE MOTOR SYSTEM
## IN RELATION TO SLEEP

Before discussing specific motor disturbances of sleep, we review the normal physiology of the motor system during sleep and the patterns of normal motor activity that vary with the circadian rhythm, the different sleep stages, and human development and aging. Abnormal activity, in different cases, may follow this same background activity pattern or deviate from it in striking ways.

### *The Normal Motor System and Sleep*

The normal motor system shows marked variations in activity and responsiveness as a function both of time of day (based on circadian rhythm as well as sleep history) and of sleep-wake state. Age is also an important factor, as the relation of the motor system to sleep changes throughout the life span. Another important factor is laterality: the nondominant hand moves considerably more often during sleep than the dominant hand.[8]

### *Circadian Activity Cycles*

In many, if not most, animal species, the motor system's level of activity is dependent on the time of day. Even in the absence of a day-night light cycle (i.e., under constant conditions), such activity cycling persists in a *free running state* with a circadian period. As discussed in Chapter 30 on chronobiology, many other important physiologic variables, such as temperature, also show circadian periods. Although there are currently believed to be at least two important circadian "clocks" generating these rhythms,[9] the suprachiasmatic nucleus is thought to be the center responsible for the circadian variation of motor activity. In humans, sleep is usually at night, so that activity is concentrated during the day. This basic pattern, however, can be disturbed in a number of different settings, including shift work or other unusual schedules and a variety of sleep disorders or degenerative neurologic conditions.

### *The Motor System and Sleep Stages*

Changes in motor activity are dependent on the sleep state (i.e., wake, REM, non-REM [NREM]

sleep stages). One frequently used monitor of the sleep-wake state, the chin electromyogram (EMG), is an indicator of branchial (brain stem) muscle tone. During the wake state, chin muscle tone is high and a tonically active chin EMG is interrupted by phasic contractions (facial expressions, tension, chewing, etc.). With relaxation and drowsiness, the level of EMG activity decreases. It further decreases as NREM sleep is achieved and deepens to SWS levels. During REM sleep, EMG activity becomes minimal or even inapparent, although it may be occasionally interrupted with brief, irregular bursts of activity. These changes mirror, to a fair degree, the changes undergone by much of the motor system during sleep. As explained later, much of this variability can be understood on the basis of the altered activity of different levels of the motor system, as well as their interaction, during different sleep stages.

It is important to note that the relationship between motor activities and sleep stages may need to be qualified in various contexts: (1) It should be remembered that at a technical level, sleep scoring may not adequately reflect the underlying brain processes at the time of a given event such as a movement. Sleep is generally scored as arbitrary epochs of fixed length, usually 30 seconds, whereas physiologic processes may occur on a variety of time scales. This has led some investigators to examine microepochs of a few seconds for momentary state.[10] (2) It may not be possible to adequately score some sleep according to the current rules. This has led to various proposals for revising the scoring system or even to use very different methods of scoring. McGregor and colleagues, for example, have proposed the use of transitional (or T sleep) epochs, in which, because of disruptive events such as sleep apnea, there is an alternation of some sleep stage with arousal.[11] Terzano and colleagues have defined a pattern seen in NREM sleep, the cyclic alternating pattern, showing alternation between active and quiet sleep phases.[12] This pattern is often associated in a time-locked fashion with sleep disorders such as sleep apnea or periodic limb movements in sleep (PLMS).[13] (3) The sleep stages themselves are not fully discrete or comprehensive. Fragments of a stage, such as REM-related atonia, may occur during other states, even in fully normal individuals. For example, Mahowald and Schenck[14] reported on six patients with marked admixture of features from the different sleep-wake states (i.e., wake, NREM sleep, REM sleep). These patients showed abnormal distribution of motor activity with relation to sleep features. (4) Motor events, although typical of one sleep stage or state, may less commonly occur in other stages. Although PLMS occur primarily in NREM sleep, they may occur in REM sleep.[15] In our experience, similar movements may occur during arousals or periods of wakefulness after sleep onset, usually as part of a periodic sequence of movements that span the sleep-wake divide. (5) Many conditions are not completely pure but contain a combination of disorders related to different sleep stages. For example, narcolepsy is highly associated with PLMS[16] and patients with somnambulism, which typically occurs in NREM sleep, may show REM sleep motor abnormalities suggestive of REM sleep behavior disorder (RBD).[17]

Table 26-1 summarizes the frequency of normal and abnormal motor activities that occur during the various phases of sleep and wake. Because many of these movements have not been exhaustively studied, this table is a preliminary guide rather than a definitive pronouncement.

**Drowsiness, Sleep Onset, and Arousals.** In the period before sleep begins, humans, as well as other animals, enter a period of relative repose. The transition to sleep is signaled by a variety of behavioral and electroencephalographic (EEG) features.[18] Even before sleep onset, the motor system reduces its level of activity. It is during this period that the symptoms of restless legs syndrome (RLS) become prominent. RLS is relatively distinctive in that, unlike almost all other movement disorders, it is activated by relaxation.

The transition to sleep is often marked by a sleep-related movement, the sleep start or hypnic jerk.[19] This is an abrupt, often asymmetric myoclonic flexion movement, generalized or partial, which may be accompanied by a sensation or an illusion of falling. Unless it occurs very frequently (which is rare[20]), this is a benign movement that has little effect on sleep and carries no negative prognosis. It probably occurs in the majority of people. It is typically a single event, causing a brief arousal. EMG records show relatively brief EMG complexes (<250 msec in duration) that may be simultaneous or sequential in various muscles.

Arousals, brief periods of interrupted, lighter sleep that may lead to full awakening, are often associated with movements. Arousals may both follow and lead movements such as body shifts. Abnormal movements, such as parkinsonian tremor, may recur during arousals. Sleep-related movements, such as PLMS, may provoke frequent arousals or even awakenings, and may also continue during periods of arousal from sleep.

Transitions into and out of sleep may also be associated with sleep paralysis. In this condition, an individual is unable to move, although awake. Breathing and eye movements are usually preserved. This condition is thought to represent a variety of REM sleep tonic motor inhibition, as recordings of the state can show REMs together with an electrophysiologic pattern consistent with REM sleep.[21] The state transition may be associated with arousal from a REM period or, less commonly except in narcolepsy, progress into REM sleep from wake. Although most frequent in narcolepsy, sleep paralysis also occurs in many non-narcoleptic individuals, sometimes with a familial pattern. Some studies suggest that, at least in some populations, sleep paralysis may be common.[22,23] It has been suggested that sleep paralysis may occur when there is an early-onset REM period, such as after an awakening from NREM.[24] Sleep paralysis may be infrequent in normal individuals, but may cause significant anxiety, especially the first episode. In the absence of other narcoleptic phenomena or abnormal neurologic findings, someone with occasional sleep paralysis may be reassured that it is almost certainly benign. A similar condition, nocturnal alternating hemiplegia, involves paralysis limited to one side while awakening from sleep.[25] This may be a variant of hemiplegic migraine, a complicated headache disorder with paralysis due to suppressed activity in certain brain regions.

**Non–Rapid Eye Movement Sleep.** In NREM sleep, motor activity is less than in the wake or resting state. Postural shifts, which may signal stage changes (into or from wake or REM), occur. There are also small flickering movements called *sleep myoclonus*, which may cause no apparent movement and are associated with very brief, highly localized EMG potentials.[26,27] In some cases, the amplitude and frequency of these movements increase, at which point they are called *fragmentary*

**Table 26-1.** Persistence of Motor Activity of Sleep

| Motor Activity | Awake/ Active | Drowsiness/ Sleep Onset | Arousal/ Awakening | Stage I NREM | Stage II NREM | Stage III NREM | REM Sleep |
|---|---|---|---|---|---|---|---|
| **Normal motor activity** | | | | | | | |
| Postural shifts | Very frequent | Frequent | Frequent | Common | Occasional | Rare | Occasional |
| Sleep myoclonus | Unreported | Rare | Rare | Common | Occasional | Rare | Frequent |
| Hypnic jerk | Unreported | Frequent | Occasional | Occasional | Rare | Rare | Unreported |
| Sleep paralysis | Unreported* | Common | Common | Rare | Unreported | Unreported | Usual |
| **Movement disorders** | | | | | | | |
| Bobble-headed doll syndrome | Frequent | Diminished | Diminished | None? | None? | None? | None? |
| Chorea | Very frequent | Frequent | Common | Occasional | Rare | Very rare | Rare |
| Dystonia | Very frequent | Common | Common | Occasional | Rare | Very rare | Rare |
| Fasciculations | Present | Present | Present | Present | Present | Present | Present |
| Hemiballismus | Very frequent | Common | Common | Occasional? | Occasional? | Very rare | Occasional? |
| Hemifacial spasm | Very frequent | Frequent | Frequent | Common | Common | Occasional? | Common |
| Hiccups (chronic) | Frequent | Frequent | Frequent | Common | Common | Common | Common |
| Myoclonus: cortical/sub- cortical | Very frequent | Common? | Occasional? | Occasional? | Occasional? | Rare | Rare |
| Myoclonus: spinal | Very frequent | Frequent | Common | Common? | Common? | Occasional | Common? |
| Palatal tremor | Constant | Frequent | Frequent | Frequent | Frequent | Common? | Common? |
| Parkinsonian tremor | Very frequent | Common | Common | Occasional | Rare | Very rare | Occasional |
| Tics | Very frequent | Common | Common | Occasional | Occasional | Rare | Common |
| **Sleep disorders** | | | | | | | |
| Benign infantile myoclonus | ? | Unreported | Unreported | Common | Common | Common | Common |
| Bruxism | Common | Occasional? | Occasional? | Frequent | Frequent | Occasional | Frequent |
| Fragmentary myoclonus | Unreported | Unreported | Unreported | Frequent | Frequent | Common | Occasional |
| Nocturnal parox- ysmal dys- tonia | — | Unreported | Common? | Frequent | Frequent | Occasional | Rare |
| PLMS: isolated or with RLS | Rare | Occasional | Occasional | Frequent | Common | Occasional | Occasional |
| PLMS: narco- lepsy, RBD | Rare | Occasional? | Occasional? | Frequent | Common | Rare | Common |
| Propriospinal myoclonus at rest | — | Frequent | Occasional | Rare | None | None | None |
| REM sleep behavior disorder | — | Unreported | Occasional? | Rare | Rare | Rare | Frequent |
| Rhythmic move- ment disorder | Common | Very frequent | Common? | Common | Common | Rare | Occasional? |
| RLS: restlessness | Rare | Very frequent | Frequent | Occasional | — | — | — |
| Somnambulism | — | Unreported | Common? | Occasional | Common | Frequent | Occasional |

*In narcolepsy, presents as cataplexy in wake state.

? = limited information; REM = rapid eye movement; NREM = non-REM sleep; PLMS = periodic limb movement in sleep; RLS = restless legs syndrome; RBD = REM sleep behavior disorder.

*myoclonus*, a possible sleep disorder.[28] The frequency of all movements decreases with depth of sleep, being least in SWS (NREM stages III and IV).[29,30] Postural shifts rarely occur before SWS. This reduced activity is consistent with the quiescent state of the nervous system documented by physiologic studies (discussed later).

A number of abnormal motor activities (discussed later), such as somnambulism or PLMS, occur predominantly during NREM sleep.

**Rapid Eye Movement Sleep.**   REM is dramatically different from NREM sleep. The motor system is dominated by central activation and peripheral inhibition, so that muscle tone is tonically reduced even below that of SWS. However, bursts of small movements (sleep myoclonus) similar to those seen in NREM sleep, but more clustered, occur phasically in association with REMs.

As discussed later under Motor Physiology, during REM sleep there is increased nervous system activity and a close balance between strong upper motor center excitation and inhibition at the level of the motor effector. When the inhibitory influences break down, significant motor activity may be released. This results from lesions in the brain stem of animals that destroy the inhibitory centers[31] and, it is believed, in human sleep disorders such as RBD. The resulting movements may represent an "acting out" of dreams, which characteristically have a motoric component.[32]

*Ontogeny of the Motor System During Sleep*

In addition to sleep stage, normal sleep movements are also affected by age: The number of movements during sleep is greatest in infants, then decreases with age.[29] For example, De Koninck and colleagues found that position shifts during sleep decreased from 4.7 per hour in sleepers of 8–12 years to 2.1 per hour in those 65–80 years old.[33] Children are also thought to lack a fully "mature" sleep regulatory system. For instance, Kohyama[34] found that younger infants appear to lack the profound motor inhibition during phasic REM that is seen in older children and adults. Perhaps as a result of such immaturity, parasomnias such as bruxism, somnambulism, or soliloquy are present with a greater prevalence during childhood, tending to decrease with age from early childhood on. Toward the end of life,

however, as neural and other bodily systems age or deteriorate, some forms of excessive motor activity may emerge again, including PLMS or RBD. In at least one study, movements were increased in the elderly compared to younger adults.[35]

*Physiology of the Motor System in Relation to Sleep*

The motor system can be very roughly considered to have three main units or levels: higher centers, segmental centers, and the motor unit (motor neuron and related muscle fibers). The higher centers are located within the brain and brain stem where they receive diverse information from other brain regions including those involved with the senses. These centers include the motor, premotor, and supplementary motor cortices; the basal ganglia and cerebellum; and various brain stem nuclei including the reticular nuclei of the pons and medulla. They provide descending control to segmental motor centers located at the brain stem and spinal cord level, as well as some direct connections in the human to motor neurons. The segmental centers, in turn, channel and moderate descending and afferent inputs from somatosensory organs so as to control the "final common path," the motor neuron. In addition to serving as way or integrating stations, the segmental centers may generate their own activity. Many studies have shown that the brain stem and spinal cord, even in complete isolation, can produce patterned motor activity such as locomotion.[36-38] This indicates that they have endogenous oscillators that are based on organized neural networks. The motor neuron, with its associated set of muscle fibers within a specific muscle, collectively known as the *motor unit*, is the ultimate effector responsible for motor activity. Between the levels, there is continuous two-way communication. In addition, the motor system receives a continuous flow of inputs from the various afferent systems, including the different sensory systems. In later sections of the chapter, as we discuss different normal and abnormal sleep-related motor activity, we refer to this model of the motor system to suggest the levels likely to be involved or disturbed in a particular condition. Most motor disturbances of sleep originate at the level of the higher motor centers, although some arise at the segmental level and a few motor phenomena derive from the level of the motor unit.

Our understanding of the phenomena of normal and abnormal movements in sleep depends on our understanding of how the motor system functions and is controlled. In higher animals, like humans, our understanding does not approach the precise mapping of identified, unique neurons and their subsequent manipulation that is possible in a lower animal such as the pleurobranch mollusk *Aplysia* or the nematode worm *Caenorhabditis elegans*.[39] Several techniques, however, do allow us to begin to assemble a model of how the motor system changes during different states such as drowsiness, NREM, and REM sleep: (1) It is possible to record the activity and, with intracellular recordings, the underlying membrane events in single neurons. Most of these studies are performed in animals, including rats, cats, and monkeys, but such techniques can occasionally be used on humans in the course of surgery for cerebral disorders. This technique has been used to record a wide range of neurons during sleep. Most relevant for the motor system are studies of brain stem neurons, which control sleep states and their motoric concomitants, and the motor neurons themselves. This technique is the only one that allows us to uncover the role of specific neural elements in state-dependent function, although each study usually deals with only a limited set of neural elements. Lacking the full picture, the investigator must usually guess about the significance of any individual finding. With time and increasingly better techniques and analysis, it will be possible to put together a more complete picture of state-dependent motor behavior. (2) It is possible to determine the motor output of the sleeping subject through the application of a variety of stimuli to elicit reflex responses or evoked potentials. By relating response to stimulus, this technique probes some of the lumped properties of the sensorimotor system. The information obtained is usually restricted to some measure of overall excitability, however, and the elucidation of what controls these excitability changes must be pursued by other techniques, such as single-neuron recording. (3) Information about the behavior of specific brain regions can be obtained by a variety of techniques that measure aggregate neural activity. Some of the most interesting results of probing human brain activity has come from the development of a variety of imaging techniques

including positron emission tomography (PET) and single-photon emission computed tomography (SPECT) scanning and functional magnetic resonance imaging (MRI). Although never as precise as single-unit recording, imaging offers the possibility of noninvasively mapping the activity of many brain regions at once and re-examining them in a number of different sleep-wake states. In the following sections, some of the most important directions and findings that have been obtained with these techniques are summarized.

*Studies of Activity in Individual Neurons*

Two major kinds of studies have been done in individual neurons: (1) Patterns of activity in various brain centers have been studied, usually without clear knowledge of the function of the recorded neurons. These studies have indicated overall patterns of activity during different sleep stages. (2) Extracellular and intracellular studies have been performed on identified motor neurons located in the brain stem and spinal cord. These studies have been able to identify some of the specific mechanisms for altered motor neuron function during sleep.

During the wake state, most brain cells tend to fire irregularly, at different frequencies in different brain regions. The general change during NREM sleep, and especially SWS, is for cells to fire more slowly (at a lower frequency) but with more of a tendency to fire bursts.[40] During SWS, for example, thalamic cells fire slowly and are less responsive to afferent activity. These changes are related to the greater synchronization of surface electrical activity (EEG) during sleep. In REM sleep, by contrast, cellular activity is increased in many regions. Motor areas of the brain often show these activity increases, such as the primary motor cortex,[41] motor thalamus, red nucleus, and cerebellum.[40] This increased firing in the motor centers of the brain is thought to be related to the increased descending drive that occurs during REM sleep. Because single-unit studies have, in the main, merely examined rates of firing, however, it is not possible to say whether the neuronal activity in brain centers during REM sleep has the same pattern and organization as in the wake state.

More focused studies have examined motor neurons in the brain stem and spinal cord and traced backward some of the descending influences that modulate them, depending on state. As Chapter 3 indicates, studies have begun to establish the brain stem centers whose altered activity is related to the various stages of sleep and wake and associated alterations in motor activity. Particular information has been obtained about the control of REM sleep. Neurons located near the border between the pons and midbrain appear to release acetylcholine into the more central reticular formation of the pons and medulla. Various (poorly defined) centers or cell groups in the reticular formation are then stimulated[42] to exert descending influences that act on motor neurons. Recordings from the motor neurons themselves, however, have shown distinct sleep-dependent changes in their physiology. In relaxation and NREM sleep, motor neurons are slightly hyperpolarized (moved electrically away from their firing threshold) and less excitable.[43,44] This is due to inhibitory inputs, inhibitory postsynaptic potentials (IPSPs). In REM sleep, the motor neurons are further hyperpolarized due to an increased frequency of small IPSPs as well as large IPSPs that occur only during phasic REMs.[45] At least the larger and perhaps both classes of IPSPs can be suppressed by perfusion of strychnine, suggesting that they are mediated by the neurotransmitter glycine.[44] Some of these IPSPs are likely to arise from the gigantocellular reticular nucleus of the medulla. IPSPs blocked by strychnine can be evoked by stimulating this nucleus, but only during a state similar to REM sleep (induced by carbachol stimulation of the pons in an animal model).[46] Moreover, the same descending inhibitory input depresses the Ia monosynaptic reflex, thereby decreasing the excitation of motor neurons by reflex input.[47] As a result of this inhibition of the motor neurons, the increased activity of the central motor system in REM sleep is generally not reflected in increased motor activity. Rather, muscles such as the mentalis show atonia, whereas limb movements, either centrally or reflexly generated, are rare. The bursts of myoclonic movements that sometimes accompany REMs apparently arise from a superimposed phasic excitation via excitatory postsynaptic potentials (EPSPs). This excitation does not depend on the major voluntary motor pathways, such as the corticospinal or rubrospinal tract, but presumably originates in the brain stem.[48] Pharmacologic studies suggest that these EPSPs are mediated by non–$N$-methyl-D-aspartate excitatory synapses.[49] Neuronal state has also been probed by measuring the level of c-*fos* in cells; this protein is associated with active nuclear transcription and protein synthesis. Whereas many interneuronal regions of the brain stem show increased activity in REM sleep, motor nuclei (masseter, facial, and hypoglossal nuclei) show depressed activity.[50]

*Studies of Reflex Activity and Evoked Responses*

Because much of motor behavior is generated in part by reflexes, the study of reflexes can be relevant to examining changes of the motor system with state. The most commonly studied reflex has been the tendon reflex or its electrical counterpart, the H reflex. Constant stimuli are applied and the resulting motor response, monitored as force, movement, or EMG, is measured to determine the reflex gain (output per unit input). The tendon reflex is called a *monosynaptic* reflex because it is driven primarily by action across a single synapse, the excitatory connection from the afferent Ia muscle tendon fiber to the alpha motor neuron. The complete reflex can be elicited at the segmental level, although it is clearly modulated by descending influences from higher centers. This reflex is diminished in NREM sleep, especially SWS, and then almost completely abolished in REM sleep, especially during REMs.[48,51] Polysynaptic spinal reflexes, which cross many synapses (e.g., cutaneous reflexes), are similarly depressed in NREM and REM sleep.[48] A somewhat related bulbar reflex, the response of the genioglossus muscle to negative pressure in the airway, is decreased in NREM sleep.[52] This reduced response has significant consequences, because reduced reflex gain may contribute to airway collapse and respiratory difficulties in sleep, especially obstructive sleep apnea (OSA). It has been noted that some brain stem reflexes, such as vestibular reflexes and the blink reflex, show decreased gain in NREM sleep but may then recover partially in REM sleep.[53–55] This recovery of brain stem reflexes during REM sleep parallels the relatively greater activity of the eye muscles, compared with trunk and limb muscles at that time, and reinforces the mixed picture of excitation and inhibition characteristic of REM. Even drowsiness can attenuate some reflexes, including the vestibulo-ocular reflex, which has two outputs: quick restorative jerks to head rotation and slower smooth compensatory eye deviations.[56] The more polysynaptic quick jerks are more easily suppressed by even modest drowsiness. Although all these various changes in reflex gain indicate altered excitability, they do not indicate where in the reflex arc the changes occur.

The basis for much of the reduced reflex gain during sleep is most likely inhibition of motor output. In one supportive study, Morrison and colleagues[57] placed pontine tegmental lesions in cats that caused REM sleep without atonia. They found that orienting to both tone stimuli and acoustic startle responses was evident in REM sleep in the lesioned cats, but rare or absent throughout sleep in intact cats. Because the same tones elicited brain stem–generated ponto-geniculo-occipital waves in both normal and lesioned cats, it seems likely that the block to the further responses of orienting and startle reflexes is on the motor side of the reflex arc. On the other hand, sensory transmission may itself be altered by sleep. A number of studies have indicated that in primary afferent neurons located both in the spinal cord[58] and the brain stem,[59] there is a significant, presynaptic decrease in responsiveness during REM sleep, but not NREM sleep. Sensory transmission can be more directly studied by examining evoked responses, synchronized electrical activity that arises as a result of sensory input (or electrical shocks to selected nerves) and indicates the nervous system's response to the input.[60] Responses are described as *short, medium,* and *long latency,* depending on how long after the sensory stimulus they occur: earlier responses travel faster pathways, with fewer synaptic relays, than do later responses and are, thus, more purely "sensory" in nature. The general rule has been that medium- and long-latency components of evoked responses may be altered by NREM sleep, whereas the short-latency components remain relatively stable.[61,62] Even short-latency somatosensory evoked potentials, however, may show diminished responsiveness with increased latency in stage II sleep.[63,64] Some studies have supported the idea that even output of primary sensory nuclei is decreased by NREM and (more powerfully) by the REM sleep state.[65] Visual evoked responses, of course, are profoundly altered, even by drowsiness. During REM sleep, some later responses make at least a partial recovery. For example, the midlatency P1 potential of the brain stem auditory evoked response (BAER) returns to its waking configuration.[61] But some late components, such as the N300 component of the auditory evoked response, are further suppressed in REM sleep and may even show reduction in the transition to REM sleep.[47] In general, it would appear that those effects (i.e., potentials and responses) that manifest the simplest and most direct pathways (e.g., monosynaptic) are best preserved in sleep. For instance, in a study comparing the rat's P13 response to auditory stimuli (equivalent to the human P1 component of BAER) to the associated startle response, Miyazato and colleagues[66] found that the more complex startle response was both more easily habituated in waking and more easily abolished by sleep.

To more directly examine the impact of sleep on the motor system, motor evoked potentials (MEPs) can be studied. These potentials are muscle responses, usually measured by surface EMG, that are elicited by stimulating motor nerves in the periphery or the central nervous system. They are therefore largely restricted to activity in the motor pathways. In one study of MEPs evoked by stimulating the motor cortex with a strong magnetic stimulus during sleep, it was noted that the MEPs decreased during NREM sleep.[67] Results during REM sleep have shown a much greater degree of variability in amplitude of evoked responses. Hess and colleagues[67] found that responses were of normal or increased amplitude, whereas Fish and coworkers[68] found that average amplitude was decreased in three normal subjects, despite some responses of higher amplitude than normal in relaxed waking. The latter group also noted prolonged latencies of the MEPs, consistent with inhibitory processes. In a group of narcoleptic patients, stimulation during cataplexy resulted in apparently normal MEPs.[69] Although these results remain to be harmonized, the variability is consistent with the fluctuating balance between inhibitory and excitatory processes in REM. A finding of decreased mean amplitude, however, is more consistent with the general inhibitory balance of REM sleep in normals.

It should be noted that sleep, although dulling higher coordinated or voluntary motor activity, does not completely abolish it. Complex responses such as scratching can occur during sleep and human subjects can respond selectively to different sounds.[70] Such complex responses are most active in stage I sleep, least active in SWS, with responsiveness in REM being intermediate in level. In one study, normal subjects were required to respond to infrequent moderate amplitude auditory stimuli with a key press.[71] They were able to do this only when the stimuli were presented in the lighter phases of stage I polysomnographic (PSG) sleep. A cortical potential related to specific events in the wake state (event related potential P300), however, was found in deeper stage I NREM and in REM sleep, indicating that some of the cerebral activity underlying voluntary behavior remained despite the absence of the behavior itself. Such findings suggest that various phases of information processing are present during light NREM sleep or REM sleep.[72] Consistent with the presence of such processing, elementary forms of learning, such as classical conditioning, may occur during sleep.[73] Such abilities to adapt and alter cortical connectivity and function are consistent with the proposed role of the sleeping brain, especially during REM sleep, in further processing and consolidating learning that occurs while awake.[74,75] Indeed, some studies have suggested that the amount of REM sleep increases after learning to carry out this function.[76]

Reflexes can also change their characteristic motor output in sleep,[77] indicating that sleep is not merely a general change in activity levels but a rearranged organization of responsiveness. In addition, certain reflexes that would be abnormal while awake, such as the Babinski sign, may be elicited in sleep.[78,79]

*Imaging Studies*

The development of new imaging techniques that permit assessment of activity in the waking brain provides an additional method of studying regional contributions to state-dependent motor activity. Studies of cerebral blood flow and metabolism have largely paralleled those of cellular activity. Blood flow and metabolism may be greater during REM sleep than in waking, but are widely depressed during NREM sleep, especially SWS.[80–83] More recent studies have been able to differentiate among brain regions, revealing selective changes that accompany the sleep states. The picture that emerges is both preliminary, coarse, and complex, but already intriguing and suggestive. In one study, Hofle and colleagues[84] correlated activity in different brain regions with power in different EEG frequency domains (e.g., delta, here 1.5–4.0 Hz). The greatest decrement associated with increased delta power (characteristic of SWS) was in the thalamus, con-

sistent with the depressed thalamic activity of sleep. During REM sleep, in contrast, there is activation of the brain stem core and thalamus as well as limbic areas of the brain and primary and secondary sensory areas.[83,85] Hong and colleagues[86] examined the association between REMs and blood flow and found associations both with the midline attentional system active in REM sleep and areas involved in generating waking saccadic eye movements and subserving visual attention. Higher cortical areas, including prefrontal cortex and multimodal sensory and associative cortex, remain suppressed during all sleep stages.[83,87] Two additional studies have shown that the basal ganglia are suppressed in SWS, but very strongly activated in REM sleep.[81–83] The significance of these basal ganglia changes for the motor system and for movement disorders in sleep remains unclear, but is of great potential interest. These preliminary results in imaging studies suggest further studies may give a much clearer picture of sleep states in terms of the involved brain structures. So far, the studies bear only indirectly on the motor system, but they should clarify how motor activity is modulated during sleep by revealing the controlling or suppressed brain regions involved.

*Summary of Physiologic Studies*

The relatively consistent picture that has developed is that NREM sleep is a quiescent period, with decreased activity and reduced responsiveness at all levels of the motor system in comparison to the wake state. REM sleep, in contrast, is a more unstable state in which excitatory and inhibitory influences are balanced. Although the brain centers show increased activity, the motor unit is bombarded with both excitation and inhibition with, in the normal state, a functional preponderance of inhibitory tone. This result is precarious and, in some cases such as reflexes, there may be increased activity during REM sleep.

## MOVEMENT DISORDERS IN RELATION TO SLEEP

The relation between the diurnal movement disorders and sleep has become better known over the past several decades, in large part because of the major increase in the study of sleep. It has become more evident that movement disorders, even if most of their symptoms are appreciated during the day, also have significant impact on sleep. It has also become clear that many movement disorders do persist to some extent during sleep. In some conditions, the level of symptoms may vary systematically with the sleep-wake cycle. For example, in dopa-responsive dystonia (DRD), the patient feels best in the early morning (after a night of sleep) and deteriorates throughout the day. In addition, movement disorder specialists have become more aware of certain conditions primarily categorized as sleep disorders, such as RLS or nocturnal paroxysmal dystonia (NPD), that are more active during the night or during sleep.

### Diurnal Movement Disorders

Most diurnal movement disorders are present during the day and it is the resultant impairment of function during the day that leads patients to seek medical care. It has become increasingly apparent, however, that movement disorders are not absent during sleep and they may cause or be associated with a variety of sleep disturbances. Surveys of patients with Parkinson's disease (PD) have shown that the majority believe they have difficulty with sleep. Large numbers of patients complain of difficulty getting to sleep, inadequate time asleep, disrupted sleep, and daytime sleepiness. It has therefore become important for clinicians involved with movement disorders to be aware of the impact of these conditions on sleep and be ready to assist patients in dealing with sleep problems. Sleep disorder specialists should also be sensitive to the increased sleep dysfunction of patients with movement disorders.

### Persistence of Movement Disorders During Sleep

Different diurnal movement disorders show various degrees of persistence during sleep (see Table 26-1). Until fairly recently, it was almost universally believed that most movement disorders are abolished by sleep, such as the increased tonic spasms of dystonia and essential or parkinsonian tremor. However, careful studies generally find that there are remnants of abnormal activity that persist during sleep or occur during brief transitions to light sleep or waking. As a rule, movement disorders are most likely to be present at transitions into and out of sleep or during the lighter stages of NREM sleep. Occasionally, they will be reactivated during REM sleep as well.

Some movement disorders have been reported to occur fairly commonly during sleep. Tics, especially in children, have been noted to occur during sleep. In children, this may reflect a relative immaturity of the mechanisms for suppressing unwanted movement during sleep.

In a thorough and careful study using EMG, accelerometry, and split-screen video recording, Fish and colleagues[10] examined the relation of motor activity not only to conventional sleep staging, but also to epochs with transitions (to lighter or deeper sleep stages or waking). They also monitored the 2-second periods before onset of dyskinesias in patients with PD, Huntington's disease (HD), Tourette's syndrome, and torsion dystonia (both primary generalized and secondary) and scored them for presence of arousals, REM, sleep spindles, and slow waves. They compared these dyskinesias to normal movements both in patients and in normal subjects. Of 43 patients, 41 had characteristic movements that persisted in sleep. Both normal movements and dyskinesias for every disorder followed the same general pattern: movements and dyskinesias were most common in awakening epochs, then lightened during stage I, REM, and stage II sleep; there was no movement in pure stages III, IV, and deepening sleep. Only Tourette's patients had dyskinesias during transition from wake to sleep. Arousals were most common in the 2-second period before both normal and abnormal movements, REM was second most common, and spindles and slow waves were extremely unlikely to occur. These results support previous speculation[88] that both dyskinesias and normal movements are likely to be modulated by sleep in a similar fashion. The authors suggest this may be due either to the general suppression of centers for both normal and dyskinetic movements or suppression of some common descending path, such as the pyramidal tract. It should be noted that all of these abnormal motor activities are thought to be generated in what we have called the *higher motor centers*, most of them from centers above the brain stem.

Movement disorders associated with abnormalities of the lower motor centers persist most commonly during sleep. Most typical are the palatal myoclonus or palatal tremor family in which there is low-frequency (typically, 1.5–2.5 Hz) oscillatory activity associated with brain stem damage within Mollaret's triangle (dentatorubro-olivary pathways, with damage most common in the central tegmental tract that runs from the region of the red nucleus to the ipsilateral olive).[89] In addition, spinal myoclonus will often persist during sleep. These conditions can, in a general sense, be lumped together as segmental myoclonias. Similar persistence may be seen in hemifacial spasm, which is thought to involve damage either in the brain stem facial nucleus or in the peripheral nerve (cross-talk due to ephaptic transmission) or both. In addition, fasciculations due to damage to the lower motor neuron may persist in sleep.

It has been said that psychogenic movement disorders subside during sleep or anesthesia. Although this is generally true, there may be violations of this rule in rare cases. Patients with psychogenic movement disorders have not been studied systematically enough to reach a conclusion, but it can be expected that they would be most likely to show persistent abnormalities at sleep onset, during very light sleep stages, and in the course of arousals, and least likely to show persistent abnormalities in deep SWS.

*Sleep Dysfunctions Associated with Diurnal Movement Disorders*

A basic problem occurs when movement disorders prevent sleep or arouse patients from sleep. However, such direct effects of movement disorders are not the only effects on sleep. Additional problems arise because the movement disorder, or its treatment, may bring about disturbed sleep. Movement disorder patients may also be at risk for sleep disturbances such as sleep apnea or parasomnias. Moreover, many movement disorder patients are elderly or demented and may have the impaired sleep often seen with aging and degenerative disease. Before discussing the sleep problems of individual movement disorders, we first review the general kinds of sleep problems that may occur in these patients.

**Respiratory Disturbances.** A major problem for movement disorder patients is the prevalence of respiratory disturbances during sleep. Respiratory disturbances are common in the motor disorders that involve neuronal degeneration. Especially vulnerable are those patients with degenerative diseases such as PD that involve brain stem loci. In the more widespread degenerative diseases such as olivopontocerebellar atrophy (OPCA) or multisystem atrophy (MSA), there may be respiratory disturbances based on disturbed central regulation of breathing, problems with neuromuscular function leading to obstruction or laryngeal stridor, or impaired feedback control of respiration. These difficulties and the situation of patients with MSA are also discussed in Chapter 27.

**Sleep Fragmentation.** A primary concomitant of a degenerative movement disorder is disrupted sleep—increased awakenings, more stage transitions, and partial and complete arousals. The result is usually a sleep characterized by more time awake, less SWS, and, perhaps, less REM sleep. This sleep fragmentation has been reported as a complication of many movement abnormalities. It should be remembered, however, that many of these movement disorders occur primarily in older patients and that sleep quality declines even in the relatively healthy elderly. Sleep may improve once effective therapy is found for the underlying condition.[90] Therapy for movement disorders may also interfere with sleep and this must be considered in assessments of sleep problems. Because both the primary disease and its therapy may cause sleep disruption, completely successful management may not be possible.

**Dyssomnias and Parasomnias.** Parasomnias or other motor disturbances of sleep are more likely to occur in patients with a number of movement disorders than in the general population. Children with tics are reported to have an increased incidence of parasomnias such as somnambulism and somniloquy. Increased prevalence of PLMS or RLS has been reported with a variety of movement disorders such as Huntington's chorea[15] or PD.[91–93] A number of movement disorders, especially PD and related syndromes, may be associated with RBD.[94,95]

The degree to which additional motor abnormalities are seen in patients with diurnal movement disorders is not yet clear. Although good epidemiologic studies have not been done, it seems increasingly likely that they may be common. The frequency of associations reported indicates that additional motor abnormalities during sleep must be considered in patients who report a movement disorder.

**Circadian Rhythm Disturbances.** Circadian rhythm disturbances, especially changes in sleep phase or chaotic sleep rhythms, are often seen in patients with degenerative conditions. Many of these patients are elderly, incapacitated, or demented, all features that may weaken the circadian regulation of activity. Patients may have multiple factors that upset the circadian rhythm, including their medication. Nocturnal confusion or "sundowning" often occurs in this setting.

Circadian rhythm disturbances are difficult to treat, especially in patients with cognitive compromise. Careful adjustment of medication, attempts to maintain wakefulness during the day, and good sleep hygiene may help. Sleeping medications may be counterproductive, leading to additional difficulties such as confusion. Because these patients are often homebound or institutionalized, they may lack adequate bright light exposure to reset their circadian rhythms. A trial of bright light therapy should be considered in suitable patients.

Patients with PD are prone to endogenous and reactive depression.[96,97] They may show a classic pattern of sleep phase advance with increased and early-onset REM periods. In this situation, they may respond to judicious use of antidepressants.

**Excessive Daytime Somnolence.** Because of the varied difficulties associated with movement disorders—such as inadequate sleep, sleep fragmentation, sleep apnea, and circadian rhythm disturbances—excessive daytime somnolence (EDS) may be a major problem for patients. This problem can be aggravated by medications such as L-dopa, which can induce sleepiness at peak blood concentration.

*Sleep and Sleep Disturbances
in Specific Movement Disorders*

Movement disorders have traditionally been categorized according to their appearance or phenomenology. Two major categories of movement disorders have been identified: (1) the akinetic or hypokinetic disorders, predominantly PD and related entities, in which the most salient feature is a paucity or deficiency of movement, and (2) the hyperkinetic disorders, such as chorea or myoclonus, in which the most salient features are excessive movements superimposed on normal motor behavior. These two classes are by no means exclu-sive, because akinetic syndromes will exhibit hyperkinetic features, even without treatment (e.g., dystonia in PD). Indeed, in juvenile-onset cases of dystonia-parkinsonism, it has been difficult to differentiate one from another or to decide which is the primary motor disorder. These classes are also applied primarily to the more classic basal ganglia or "extrapyramidal" disorders. Other motor problems of central origin, such as cerebellar ataxia or paresis due to stroke, are often not categorized along with the basal ganglia disorders.

**Akinetic-Hypokinetic Disorders.** The paradigmatic akinetic-hypokinetic disorder is PD. However, many other conditions have some of the same symptoms as a part of their clinical picture. Patients with these conditions may be said to show parkinsonism.[98] When many other systems are involved, as in multisystem atrophy, the clinical picture can become far more complicated. Such syndromes are discussed in Chapter 27. In this chapter, we focus primarily on PD, which has been investigated to a fair degree from the point of view of sleep, with a lesser focus on related conditions.

As well as being a common movement disorder, parkinsonism is associated with a variety of sleep complaints. This association is sufficiently important to be recognized in the new international sleep classification. Sleep problems of parkinsonism are given their own coding category as a medical/psychiatric sleep disorder associated with neurologic disorders.[99]

PARKINSON'S DISEASE. PD is defined by the following: resting tremor, rigidity (resistance to passive movement of the limbs), poverty of movement (slow movement, bradykinesia, and reduced spontaneous movement or akinesia), and poor postural reflexes leading to falls.[98] Classically, PD has been associated with the presence of Lewy bodies in the brain stem nuclei and depigmentation of the substantia nigra, the major nucleus providing dopaminergic innervation to the basal ganglia. Recently, it has become clear that PD can be caused by a genetic defect in the gene for α-synuclein, a protein involved in presynaptic function. The gene is mutated in some families (most prominently the extensive Italian Contursi kindred), who display a dominant inheritance for PD.[99a] Although a mutation in this gene is not responsible for the bulk of PD, including most familial PD,[99b] the gene product α-synuclein may be important in the development of Lewy bodies.[99c] It has become clear that this Lewy body pathology is not specific to PD, but may present with other features, such as dementia. In most patients with PD, dementia is seen only late in the course of the disease or in old age. Although juvenile cases of PD have been reported, most patients present older than the age of 40 with incidence increasing at least through the 80s. A typical course is progressive, although many patients achieve plateaus that last for years and developments in therapy have succeeded in maintaining some degree of function in many patients for decades.

Pathologically, PD affects not only the substantia nigra, but also other brain stem nuclei, such as the locus coeruleus and raphe nuclei,[100,101] that directly impact on sleep (see Chapters 3 and 4). It is, therefore, reasonable to expect that patients with PD or pathologically related disorders will have sleep disturbances. One interesting physiologic observation has been that parkinsonian patients have diminished amplitude and frequency of sleep spindles,[102] which may be reversed by therapy.[103] The explanation for this phenomenon is not yet clear, but some patients with hyperkinetic disorders such as dystonia have been found to have increased spindles. These alterations may derive from interaction between the basal ganglia and the thalamus, where spindles originate, because the thalamus is a major target for basal ganglia output.

Overall movement during sleep is sometimes been found to be altered in PD. Although some investigators found normal large body movements such as position shifts decreased in patients,[104,105] more recent studies using actigraphy have found that there may be increased movements associated with disrupted sleep,[106] especially in more advanced patients[107] with response fluctuations and dyskinesias. A final conclusion on this matter will require resolution of differences in technique, which may reflect different kinds of motor activity.

The characteristic motor abnormalities of parkinsonism, tremor, and rigidity were once thought to disappear in sleep. This was first pointed out by Parkinson himself, who also noted exceptions in very severe cases. More recently, some authors have pointed out that tremor can persist during sleep, usually occurring during lighter sleep stages and often associated with arousals.[108–110] April[109] found that tremor could also appear in undisturbed SWS; in contrast, Fish and colleagues[10] have discovered that tremor is associated with awakenings or lightenings, rarely or never with deep SWS. Fish and colleagues[10] also found that, in two cases, tremor

was precipitated in PD patients by PLMS. In summary, this work appears to show that tremor may occur during the night, but that it is almost invariably associated with those intermediate states of sleep between sleep and waking and rarely occurs either in REM sleep or SWS.

Other motor activity during sleep may be abnormal in PD. A number of investigators examining sleep in PD have reported complex, unusual motor activity[90,111]; PLMS, involving arms as well as legs[90,111]; REM-onset blepharospasm[112]; and brain stem myoclonus.[113] The association of reduced REM atonia with PD was first reported as increased chin muscle tone in sleep.[112] More recently, it has become clear that RBD occurs with increased frequency in PD. This may be present late in the course of the disease in advanced patients[114] or may occur as a prodrome, noted before any diurnal motor difficulties.[115] Schenck and colleagues,[95] who have followed a large series of such patients, note that 11 of 29 (38%) RBD patients first diagnosed as having an idiopathic disorder were subsequently diagnosed with PD. The lag from beginning of RBD to diagnosis of PD averaged 12.3 years in this group. The authors speculate that the RBD is related to degeneration of the enteropeduncular nucleus, which is known to be affected in PD. In some patients, it has been noted that RBD is worse at the onset and early in the course of PD, but may be less of a problem later. In other patients, it may be precipitated by particular therapies (e.g., selegiline[116]).

Treatment of PD itself may alleviate abnormal motor activity during sleep[90,111] or it may require separate treatment. Clonazepam has been highly successful in treatment of RBD, with or without PD.[95] It may well be that the various motor abnormalities of sleep depend on duration or stage of the PD, response to therapy, kind of therapy and dosage, and any dyskinetic complications of therapy. Therefore, these motor abnormalities cannot be neatly categorized or resolved.

Sleep difficulties have been found to be common in patients with PD.[117] Indeed, survey studies have found that patients have numerous and frequent sleep complaints. Some of these complaints may be explained by the age of the patients, however, as age-matched controls may have almost as many, if not more, general sleep complaints.[118–120] In a study by Lees and colleagues[117] of 220 patients contacted through support groups, at least 32% of the respondents complained about each of the following sleep-related problems: excessive nocturia, inability to turn over during the night or on waking, inability to get out of bed unaided, leg cramps and jerks, dystonic spasms of the limbs or face, and back pain during the night. In this population, 44% felt their sleep was good, but 18% rated it as poor. Only 4% of the patients had no sleep-related complaint. In a study by Factor et al.,[118] parkinsonian subjects had more sleep problems, but the difference from controls was not significant, except for spontaneous episodes of falling asleep during the day. Nocturnal vocalizations only occurred in the parkinsonians. van Hilten and colleagues[107] found recurrent parkinsonian symptoms (stiffness and difficulty turning over) as well as abnormal dreams increased in parkinsonian patients. Hening and colleagues[121] reported increased sleep complaints in 71 parkinsonian patients with significant increases in daytime sleepiness, troubling dreams, and a variety of motor complaints (including falls out of bed, leg discomfort, disturbing movements, vocalizations). In summary, it appears that parkinsonian patients are troubled by a number of different problems in sleep, with motor difficulties, abnormal movements and vocalizations, and disturbing dreams emphasized in several studies.

Polysomnographic studies, usually uncontrolled, have identified poor sleep as common in PD,[102,122–124] usually worsening with duration of the disease.[125] The most frequently found abnormal features of sleep include decreased sleep efficiency and increased time awake,[105] after a basic pattern of sleep fragmentation. There is no single cause of poor sleep in patients with parkinsonism; rather, a series of associated sleep problems may impair sleep, including the following:

- Patients may have a variety of abnormal movements such as persistent tremor, noted earlier, or dyskinesias or disease-related dystonia. Akathisia, and possibly restless legs, can occur in the evening and disrupt sleep initiation.
- There may be awakening with reactivation of symptoms such as difficulty changing position or getting out of bed or inability to initiate movement.[126]
- Other abnormal movements such as increased chin EMG during REM sleep (REM motor dysfunction), RBD, PLMS, or REM-onset blinking may also disrupt sleep. These may occur with increased frequency in PD.
- There may be an increase in sleep-fragmenting respiratory disorders, such as sleep apnea or

upper airway resistance syndrome, which may be more common in PD. Although respiratory problems are not prominent in PD, a number do occur and can have an impact on sleep.[127,128] Patients have been noted to have a restrictive type of lung defect, due to an intrinsic defect in breathing control, impaired respiratory muscle function due to rigidity, and faulty autonomic control of the lungs.[129] Patients may also have an obstructive respiratory defect,[130] stridor or laryngeal spasm associated with off-states or dystonic episodes,[131,132] diaphragmatic dyskinesias,[127,133] L-dopa–induced respiratory arrhythmia and dyspnea,[134] and upper airway dysfunction with tremor-like oscillations.[135] The incidence of respiratory difficulties is likely to be higher in patients with additional autonomic dysfunction.[124] Unlike patients with multisystem atrophy, however, PD patients do not usually have vocal cord abductor paralysis that is worsened during sleep.[136]

Given that these respiratory difficulties may be detected when patients are awake, it is not surprising that respiratory dysfunction has been reported to be increased in the sleep of parkinsonian patients. Obstructive, central, and mixed apneas can occur,[127,137] although not all authors have found them to be present.[124] Some authors have speculated that respiratory-related sleep disorders in parkinsonism may cause the increased early morning mortality noted in these patients.[138]

- Patients with PD, as in patients with degenerative diseases generally, may suffer a loss of central nervous system sleep regulation, leading to weakened circadian rhythmicity and poor sleep maintenance. On the other hand, they may have an onset of confusion during the nocturnal hours (sundowning) that leads to disruptive behavior and disturbed sleep.[139]
- Patients with PD are prone to depression, which in itself may cause sleep abnormalities such as reduced REM sleep latency.[140] Depression may aggravate the response to other parkinsonian symptoms, such as pain, and magnify their impact on sleep.[96,97] One study, however, did not confirm a generally adverse impact of depression in PD on overall sleep quality.[141]
- Medication effects can cause sleep disruption through varied mechanisms, including myoclonus or vivid and frightening nightmares.[142]

Klawans and colleagues[125,142] have studied parkinsonian patients treated over long periods with L-dopa who develop a progressive sleep disturbance that includes impaired sleep maintenance, EDS with frequent naps, sleep talking, sleepwalking, frightening dreams, and myoclonic jerks. The condition may progress to hallucinosis and frank psychosis.[143] Because it is presumed to be due to L-dopa therapy, it may be alleviated by reducing medications or switching in part or entirely to other agents. Like many of the late complications of treated PD, this may require careful balancing of medications. Patients with hallucinations have been shown on PSG to have more sleep problems than those without hallucinations.[114,144] Hallucinations are also not rare: Sanchez-Ramos and colleagues[145] found them present in 55 of 214 patients (26%) in one large series study.

Treatment of PD has not been found to consistently improve sleep, with some authors reporting parallel benefits to sleep and movement,[90,126] whereas others have shown persistent abnormalities in sleep.[122,124] A difficulty of interpreting these studies, however, has been the failure to fully examine the different sources of sleep abnormalities (see earlier) in parkinsonism. It may be that, in undermedicated patients, sleep will improve in parallel with PD when medication is increased but that, over time, the patient may be caught between the need for medication to maintain function and side effects of the medication that impact on sleep. In patients with reactivation of parkinsonian symptoms during the night, adjustments in the timing and kind of medication taken may help. Patients who are taking medications only early in the day may benefit from evening or bedtime doses. Longer-acting preparations of L-dopa may also help,[146–148] especially when taken near bedtime. The catechol O-methyltransferase (COMT) inhibitor tolcapone, which can prolong the action of L-dopa, is now available.[149–151] Dopamine agonists (bromocriptine, pergolide, pramipexole, ropinirole) also have sustained action and may provide better nocturnal coverage. Anticholinergics may assist with sleep in some patients, but can also cause vivid nightmares and awakenings. Other patients may require judicious balancing of their medication schedule or switching to a different combination of agents.[152] Antihistamines, such as diphenhydramine,

may be the most reasonable sleep medications, particularly because they may also produce some antiparkinsonian benefit. Specific motor disorders of sleep may be treated with appropriate medications: clonazepam for RBD or PLMS, opioids for RLS, and clozapine for nocturnal akathisia.[116] Similarly, respiratory disorders should be treated with appropriate modalities (continuous positive airway pressure, bilevel positive airway pressure).

Although typical PD may occur at least as early as young adult life, some patients with early onset have distinct conditions.[153] These patients often show marked diurnal fluctuations in their symptoms.[154–156] On initial presentation, these patients may overlap clinically with those who have the Segawa variant of DRD,[157,158] although they can usually be differentiated by testing for the known genetic abnormality in DRD. Whereas the DRD patients generally maintain a good response to L-dopa for prolonged periods,[159] the juvenile Parkinson's patients, although L-dopa–responsive, quickly develop dyskinetic side effects. Pathologic studies in one series indicated that the pathology of juvenile PD is unlike that of the ordinary adult-onset idiopathic disorder. Juvenile-onset patients had neuronal loss in the substantia nigra and locus ceruleus without any Lewy bodies.[155]

Improvement after sleep has also been reported to be common in PD with onset at a later age,[160,161] although not all patients experience this benefit. The literature, which has generally relied on patient report, does not show a consistent subgroup of patients who benefit most. Factor et al.[118] found that roughly equal groups of patients reported improvement, worsening, or no change after sleeping, with the group reporting improvement having relatively mild disease. Currie and colleagues[162] reported that 33% of patients claimed sleep benefit, with those who had younger onset, longer duration, higher L-dopa doses, and better mental and physical function most likely to claim benefit. Merello[163] reported that 55% of 312 patients experienced a sleep benefit lasting an average of 85 minutes, allowing many patients to delay their initial dose of medication. Benefit was more likely in men, older patients, and those with more long-standing disease, but did not depend on sleep quality. In contrast with these findings, in one controlled study, sleep deprivation also led to an improvement in parkinsonian symptoms.[164]

NEUROLOGIC DISORDERS RELATED TO PARKINSON'S DISEASE.   A number of degenerative diseases are similar to PD but have a different pathology and, typically, additional features. The multisystem atrophies and olivopontocerebellar atrophies are discussed in Chapter 27. Here, we discuss two specific conditions whose relationship to sleep have been studied as well as a particular syndrome of parkinsonism described earlier.

Postencephalitic parkinsonism is a condition due to infectious damage to the central nervous system, typically as a result of the encephalitis lethargica epidemics of the 1920s (see Kleitman[78] for a discussion of encephalitis lethargica). Although not studied extensively, respiratory problems appear to be more common in this syndrome than in patients with PD, perhaps due to the more widespread brain stem pathology in these patients.[127] These patients have been found to have poor voluntary respiratory control[165] as well as hypoventilation,[166] even while awake, which has been linked to a decreased sensitivity of central chemoreceptors regulating breathing.[166,167] These patients may also have greater sleep problems than idiopathic PD patients, including greater respiratory compromise in sleep.[138]

Progressive supranuclear palsy (PSP) is a condition with parkinsonism related to early gait disturbance and dystonia, especially of the neck and face, and progressive, eventually marked impairment of eye movements.[168–170] The condition involves cell loss and overgrowth of glial cells in a number of brain stem nuclei, including the locus coeruleus. It is not surprising, therefore, that sleep is affected in this condition. There have been a number of studies of sleep in this condition. These patients have been reported to have severe sleep disruption with reduced total sleep, marked diminution in sleep spindles, reduced REM sleep time with abnormal REM, disordered sleep architecture, and frequent awakenings.[171–177] Patients may develop RBD, which, in one case, was presaged by the development of somniloquy.[178] Sleep disruption was noted to increase with severity of the motor abnormalities in three studies,[173,175,179] but not to be related in a fourth.[174] The greater sleep abnormalities of PSP compared to PD may be due to the greater brain stem pathology, especially that in the pedunculopontine tegmentum, a region linked to control of REM sleep.[177]

Therapy for PSP generally follows that for PD, but is often relatively unavailing. For daytime symptoms, a combination of L-dopa (with carbidopa) and a dopamine agonist may work better than either medication alone. Little is known about treatment of the sleep dysfunctions in this condition.

There have been two reports of a familial syndrome of parkinsonism with alveolar hypoventilation. Purdy and colleagues[180] described identical twins who experienced ataxia of breathing with episodes of apnea that were more severe during sleep. These patients sustained breathing only by voluntary efforts, so their condition could be described as *Ondine's curse*, the failure of automatic breathing resulting in severe apnea during sleep. On autopsy, the twins had extensive damage to brain stem regions related to control of breathing, as well as pathology typical of PD. Roy and colleagues[181] described a family in which six members were affected with parkinsonism, depression, and central hypoventilation. Three died suddenly of suspected respiratory arrest.

**Hyperkinetic Disorders.** The hyperkinetic disorders are a diverse group characterized by excessive involuntary movement, often coupled with a deficiency of voluntary movement such as bradykinesia. In some cases, the conditions are known to have a very specific etiology, such as HD, which is presumed to be due always to a single genetic defect.

CHOREA.    Chorea consists of movements that occur in a flowing or irregular pattern and appear to migrate from one part of the body to another.[182] They may be increased with action and typically are seen in the face and distal limbs.

The best known cause of chorea is HD, a dominant disease with a known mutation of the *IT15* gene located on the short arm of chromosome 4.[183] The mutation in HD is the expansion of a CAG repeat in the DNA that leads to increased length of a polyglutamine tract in the protein product, now called *huntingtin*. Currently, research is directed at finding the function of huntingtin in the normal brain and the elucidation of the toxic effect of the mutated protein. Although huntingtin is widely distributed in the brain,[184] the pathology of HD is more restricted. Patients also have prominent psychological symptoms, including depression, psychosis, and character disorders. Onset is typically between the ages of 25 and 50, although it may occur even in the first decade or in late adult life. Progression is slow but relentless, with eventual debility, dementia, and inanition occurring in those with onset before old age.

Sleep has been studied by a number of investigators in HD. These investigators have shown a variable persistence of chorea during sleep, with most chorea present in the lighter stages of NREM sleep (stages I and II).[108,111,185] Fish and colleagues[10] found that most choreiform movements occurred during awakening, lightening of sleep stages, or in stage I sleep, similar to other dyskinesias. One study reported an increase in overall sleep movements in HD.[104] Alterations in sleep spindles in HD have been inconsistent. Whereas one study found sleep spindles to be largely absent,[186] other studies have found that their frequency increased.[102,187]

Sleep has been found to be variably impaired in HD, although only some studies have used matched control groups. The general finding has been that sleep is disturbed, and especially fragmented, particularly in those patients with more advanced disease. Deficits include prolonged sleep latency, excessive waking, decreased SWS and REM sleep, and decreased sleep efficiency.[185–188] In one study, these sleep abnormalities were specifically correlated with caudate atrophy.[189] Some studies have reported that many patients have essentially normal sleep architecture and stages.[102] Unlike patients with parkinsonism, HD patients have not been found to have a significant number of sleep apneas contributing to impaired sleep.[187,188,190]

Sleep has not been well-studied in other conditions with predominant chorea. Broughton et al.[191] reported that four patients with Sydenham's chorea, which follows a streptococcal infection, had reactivation of their movements during REM sleep.

Because sleep complaints are not prominent in HD, little is known about the response to therapy or the effects of treatment for the motor manifestations of HD on sleep features.

DYSTONIA.  Dystonia[192] is a condition characterized by sustained distorting or twisting postures, often mixed with a variety of more jerklike or oscillatory movements (see Fahn et al.[193] for a general discussion). Dystonia can be primary or secondary and can be of variable extent, either focal, segmental, or generalized, depending on the area of involvement. Dystonia includes a number of different conditions, some of which, like early onset torsion dystonia, have a single-gene basis.[194,195] The protein for early-onset torsion dystonia, torsin A, has been found to bind adenosine triphosphate,[196] but how it causes dystonia itself remains unresolved

as of 1997. Not all idiopathic dystonia patients have been shown to have a genetic mutation, however, and there are many cases of secondary dystonia that do not appear to depend on common dystonia genes.[197] One problem in evaluating sleep studies in dystonia is that the studies have often examined a fairly heterogeneous collection of patients with different distributions of dystonia and different etiologies. This will change, however, because patients can be selected for studies on a genetic basis.

Although they usually subside significantly, dystonic movements may persist during sleep at a reduced frequency and amplitude. They are maximally reduced during SWS and may be partially reactivated during REM sleep episodes.[111,198] In the study by Fish et al.[10] of dyskinetic movements, both primary and secondary dystonic patients followed the general pattern of more frequent dyskinetic movements during awakening or lightening epochs; fewer movements in stage I sleep; only infrequent movements in stage II, REM, and SWS; and no movements during epochs of deepening sleep. In a study including focal and segmental dystonias, Silvestri and colleagues[199] found that Meige's syndrome (oromandibular dystonia), blepharospasm, and tonic foot syndrome all showed persistent abnormal activity during sleep, with reduced amplitude, duration, and frequency of EMG bursts. The greatest suppression was in SWS and REM sleep.

A number of studies have reported the presence of exaggerated sleep spindles in dystonia.[111,198,200] One study, however, found that this was, at best, a variable finding in a carefully studied group with primary and secondary dystonia.[201]

It has been suggested that inhibitory mechanisms are defective in dystonia.[202] This prompted Fish and colleagues[68] to study whether REM inhibition is intact in both primary and secondary dystonics. They found that primary dystonics had normal chin EMG atonia, whereas secondary dystonics showed significantly decreased chin EMG activity. No patients had complex abnormal activity during REM sleep. In an attempt to analyze motor excitability, the authors successfully stimulated three normals and four dystonics with a magnetic coil over the vertex to evoke a motor response in the fifth finger abductor, the abductor digiti minimi. Whereas response amplitudes were highly variable, dystonics, like controls, showed a decrease in the mean response relative to responses obtained before and after the sleep study in relaxed wakefulness. Latencies were prolonged on average in all groups. The findings of decreased amplitude and prolonged latency were consistent with REM motor inhibition. Occasional high-amplitude responses may have corresponded to periods of phasic excitation. These results indicate that, whatever the decreased inhibitory processes in dystonia, they do not involve the descending inhibitory pathways of REM sleep.

Studies of sleep in dystonia have not been systematic; studies have involved small numbers of patients on diverse medications, some of whom had prior thalamic surgery. In these studies, sleep has been found to be inconsistently disrupted,[111,200] with more severe fragmentation seen in more advanced cases.[203] The major therapeutic effort in these patients is the attempt to reduce the dystonic movements (for review of therapy, see Fahn et al.[192,193]). Successful therapy of the movements should also improve sleep.[204]

It is not known to what degree different forms of dystonia—early- versus late-onset, focal versus generalized—have different relationships to sleep, although one striking form of dystonia, variably called *hereditary progressive dystonia with marked diurnal fluctuations* (HPD), DRD, and the *Segawa variant*, often shows distinct circadian variability.[157,205] These patients typically present at a young age, often in the middle of the first decade, with postural dystonia, usually affecting one leg and sparing the trunk and neck. Thereafter, the dystonia spreads and parkinsonian signs, which are present at onset in a minority of patients, become more prominent. The condition is usually inherited in an autosomal dominant mode with a mutation in *GTP cyclohydrolase I (GCHI)*.[206] A number of different mutations in *GCHI* have been described,[195,207] but, less commonly, it seems that the condition can be inherited recessively with a mutation in *tyrosine hydroxylase*.[194] Some studies have found that even patients thought to have more typical idiopathic torsion dystonia may harbor a mutation in the *GCHI* gene.[208] These patients may obtain significant symptomatic relief from sleep and therefore are minimally impaired early in the day,[157] although this is not true of all patients (57 of 86, in one review[209]), and some dystonic patients unresponsive to L-dopa may have similar benefit from sleep.[158,210] Patients with PD may also show sleep benefit.[118,160] Whether only REM sleep[157] or NREM sleep or even rest can improve symptoms remains controversial.[158]

Patients do show abnormal sleep motility. Segawa and colleagues[157,211] obtained movement counts from PSG with multiple EMG channels (8–12 surface recordings on trunk and limbs) and found that in DRD, there is a decrease in gross body movements in stage I sleep, an increase in stage II sleep, and a decrease in REM sleep. In contrast, localized twitch movements were depressed in all sleep stages, but followed the normal relative distribution between stages.[157,211]

Patients with diurnal dystonia or the nocturnal sleep abnormalities of DRD are responsive to low doses of L-dopa,[157] often as little as 50–200 mg per day with decarboxylase inhibitor. Some patients can maintain a stable therapeutic effect with doses every other day. Patients with long-standing disease (24–45 years before treatment) may benefit as well as those with recent onset.[209,212,213] DRD patients can use L-dopa without the development of the dyskinetic side effects that are so prominent in juvenile parkinsonism.[158,159,213] A few patients may develop "wearing off" phenomena, the re-emergence of symptoms several hours after an oral dose of L-dopa.[213] Older family members may present with a "parkinsonian picture," but still show the same persistent, positive response to L-dopa.[158,159,214] This finding is consistent with the idea that a single underlying disease has different manifestations that vary with age, dystonia being prominent early and parkinsonism late.[214]

With fluorodopa PET scanning, it has been shown in a number of families that patients with DRD have normal to modestly reduced striatal uptake of fluorodopa,[215] including those who present with parkinsonian features later in life.[214] Because of this finding, it can be concluded that these patients have relatively intact dopamine uptake, decarboxylation, and storage systems in the striatum. The genetic abnormalities so far uncovered are involved with the dopamine synthetic system. Some authors have speculated that the diurnal fluctuations that characterize DRD may be due to the circadian variation in dopamine production, with greater synthetic activity possible at night.[212]

One study found that acute dystonia secondary to neuroleptic medication also shows a circadian pattern,[216] with maximal dystonia present between 12:00 noon and 11:00 PM. This could not be accounted for by sleep, fatigue, or time since the last dose of medication (in this case, injections twice daily).

Some of this circadian variability may be accounted for by circadian variations in the dopamine system, which seem to show the least activity in the evening hours with maximal activity in the morning.[217]

MYOCLONUS.    The myoclonias (for a general discussion, see Fahn et al.[218]) are a diverse group of conditions with abnormal movements generated at various levels of the neuraxis, from cortex (cortical reflex or epileptic myoclonus) to spinal cord (spinal or segmental myoclonus). The basic abnormal movement is a single, repeated, or periodic jerk, most typically abrupt and "lightning-like." The categorization of these disorders is in a state of flux and some conditions (e.g., nocturnal myoclonus, now known as *periodic limb movement disorder* [PLMD]), are likely to be removed from the overall myoclonus category, primarily because they lack the lightning-like quality of the movements in "true" myoclonus. The most typical myoclonus arises from higher motor centers, whereas more rhythmical movements, less truly myoclonic, appear to arise from segmental motor centers.

Most of the studies of myoclonus and sleep have focused on the persistence of myoclonic movements during sleep. Some of these dyskinesias are highly persistent. Lugaresi and colleagues[219] studied a range of patients with myoclonus and found that persistence of the movements during sleep depended on the source of the abnormal discharge: myoclonus with a cortical source showed suppressed movements during sleep while (as in epilepsy) cortical discharges persisted, myoclonus of presumed subcortical origin was rapidly suppressed during sleep, and myoclonus of lower-level origins (spinal cord or secondary to peripheral damage) persisted during sleep. Myoclonic jerks associated with startle disease also persist during sleep, although with diminished intensity.[220]

Among persistent myoclonic conditions, palatal myoclonus, sometimes called *palatal tremor*, has been found to persist in sleep and even during anesthesia.[89] Electrophysiologic studies in a small number of patients with palatal and associated eye and sometimes limb movements[221,222] have demonstrated that palatal contractions persist during sleep, albeit with shifts in amplitude and frequency or even altered rhythmicity. The eye or limb movements show a greater decrease during sleep. One study found that patients with symptomatic palatal myoclonus (caused by a recognized disorder) were more likely to show sleep persistence than patients with essential palatal myoclonus.[223] The range of such cyclic motor dyskinesias may be broader than currently known: A similar tongue movement was reported to persist largely unchanged in sleep.[224] The finding of persistent rhythmicity suggests a relatively autonomous oscillator consistent with the idea that these segmental myoclonias may represent release of a primitive rhythmic center.[89] In contrast to other forms of myoclonus, these dyskinesias appear to arise at a segmental level and to be associated with decreased motor control from higher centers. This dissociation may explain their resistance to modulation by descending inhibitory influences during sleep. The dyskinesias are not completely removed from higher motor centers or the periphery, however, because they may disappear in sleep, change with state, and be influenced by attention.[225,226] In one interesting case, palatal myoclonus was associated with time-locked respiration, suggesting a coupling of these two rhythms.[227] Spinal myoclonus, another segmental myoclonus, although more likely to disappear in sleep,[228,229] can also persist (see Walters et al.[230]). A similar observation was one of auricular myoclonus that persisted in sleep.[231] One patient was also reported with generalized, repetitive disabling myoclonus throughout the ocular and branchial musculature (including the eyes, face, pharynx, larynx, and diaphragm) associated with inhibition of limb muscles (negative myoclonus).[232] This apparently brain stem–mediated myoclonus persisted during sleep. The variable persistence of different segmental myoclonias is consistent with the suggestion of Lugaresi et al.[219] that these myoclonias should persist during sleep.

A conclusion to be drawn from these findings is that, when the sleep system is intact, dyskinesias arising from dysfunction of the higher motor centers are blocked from expression by the normal inhibitory controls of sleep. Dyskinesias from lower centers, segmental- and effector-level (e.g., fasciculations), may be associated with damage to descending control systems and, therefore, be less regulated by the sleep-wake cycle.

Little is known about sleep in the myoclonic conditions. When movements persist, they are likely to disrupt sleep to some extent,[233] although the movements of palatal myoclonus are usually too modest and continuous to be a source of arousals. Standard therapy for myoclonus may improve any sleep disruption related to the movements themselves.[234]

TICS.   Tics are typically brisk, stereotyped, complex, often repetitive movements.[235,236] Usually, any given patient has a somewhat limited repertoire of movements that may change over a period of months to years. The prototypical tic disorder is Gilles de la Tourette's syndrome, a condition involving multiple motor tics with vocalizations that usually begins in childhood or adolescence, but may subside in later adult life. Tics may be associated with a sensory penumbra and an urge to move.[237] Tourette's patients also have a number of commonly associated behavioral abnormalities, especially obsessive-compulsive disorder. Most sleep studies have been done in Tourette's patients.

Typically, younger Tourette's patients, who are the more severely affected in most cases, have been studied with PSG or sleep monitoring.[238–240] Tics in Tourette's syndrome have been found to persist during sleep in most cases, mostly in stages I and II of NREM sleep, with fewer during SWS or REM sleep.[240,241] In addition, bodily movements in general may be increased in tics. Hashimoto and colleagues[239] found that both twitchlike and gross body movements were increased over controls during all stages of sleep, with total movements in tic patients markedly increased during REM sleep. Those authors did not attempt to analyze such movements in detail, so it is not clear what fraction of them were actual tics.

Sleep has been reported to be impaired in patients with tics.[241] Various investigators have reported increased sleep disruption, an elevated prevalence of parasomnias, and respiratory disturbances during sleep in Tourette's patients.[240] In one study, 22 of 50 (44%) patients were reported to have disturbed sleep based on patient and family report.[238] One large study ($N = 57$ in each group) that found increased parasomnias used two control groups, one of children with learning disorders and another of children with seizures[242]: somnambulism occurred in 17.5% of tic patients, significantly more than either of the two control groups. Sleepwalking is a frequently noted problem by younger Tourette's patients.[243]

In one study, patients were monitored after successful treatment of their movements with tetrabenazine and it was found that sleep was also improved.[244]

**Other Movement Disorders.**   There are scattered reports of sleep studies in a variety of other motor conditions that can be considered movement disorders. These have been studied less than the conditions discussed earlier and a systematic picture of their relation to sleep is not yet possible.

In athetoid cerebral palsy, abnormalities of REM sleep have been noted. Hayashi and colleagues[245] reported on a group of severe adolescent and young adult patients. The significant motor abnormalities were associated with REM sleep: three patients had decreased numbers of REM, two had increased chin muscle tone, and seven had reduced numbers of muscular twitches. The authors suggest this may be related to brain stem pathology in these birth-injured patients. It has also been noted that this patient group is commonly affected by childhood OSA and may benefit from surgical management.[246]

Neuroacanthocytosis is an often inherited movement disorder with tics, chorea, vocalizations, and self-mutilation together with frequent seizures, associated with elevated acanthocytes (spiked red cells) in blood smears.[247] Silvestri and colleagues[199] reported that abnormal movements persisted during sleep, but with decreased amplitude, duration, and frequency. Patients frequently vocalized during REM sleep. Sleep was fragmented and of poor quality.[248] Two siblings with neuroacanthocytosis showed EEG slowing (predominantly delta) both while awake and during REM sleep,[249] indicating abnormal cerebral function.

In hemiballism, there are proximal flinging movements of one side of the body, which may be of a violent nature, associated with damage to the contralateral subthalamic nucleus.[250] It was initially thought that the movements totally subsided in sleep. Askenasy,[111] however, reported a patient whose movements persisted in sleep and Silvestri and colleagues[199] found that the movements were present during stages I and II NREM sleep as well as during REM sleep, although diminished in intensity and frequency. Puca and colleagues[251] reported one case in which spindle density and amplitude were greater ipsilateral to the damaged subthalamic nucleus. There was also disrupted sleep, with prolonged latency and an absence of both SWS and REM sleep. Successful treatment with haloperidol improved the sleep and decreased the spindling. In most cases, hemiballism is a transient phenomenon after local injury to the subthalamus, usually ischemic, although it may be transformed into a chronic choreiform disorder.

Hemifacial spasm is a synchronous contraction of one side of the face, which is usually repetitive and jerklike, but may sometimes be sustained.[252,253] It is thought to arise from damage to the facial nerve or nucleus. EMG recording shows highly synchronous discharges in upper and lower facial muscles. Montagna and colleagues[254] studied 16 patients, recording from upper and lower facial muscles during sleep studies. In most patients, the dyskinesias decreased during sleep, being approximately 80% less frequent in SWS and REM sleep. One patient showed almost no change in the prevalence of spasms. Current therapy for hemifacial spasm includes medications such as carbamazepine and botulinum toxin injection into the affected muscles. We are aware of no reports of sleep studies after successful therapy, but it seems likely that the dyskinesias are relieved.

One family with five generations affected by paroxysmal dystonic choreoathetosis with dominant transmission was found to show substantial benefit from even brief periods of sleep.[255]

*Therapy*

Specific therapies for different sleep disturbances in the movement disorders have been discussed earlier within the text dealing with those disorders, but a number of specific suggestions can be made about how to proceed.

The first step in tailoring therapy is to determine whether the sleep problem is a direct consequence of the movement disorder itself or due to a coexisting sleep disorder, which may be primary (e.g., sleep apnea) or secondary (e.g., insomnia due to depression). Therapy should then be appropriately addressed to the movement disorder, the coexisting sleep disorder, or its underlying cause. Most sleep disorders coexisting with movement disorders would be treated in the usual fashion (e.g., with continuous positive airway pressure for OSA or antidepressants for insomnia due to depression).

A second consideration is to consider whether behavioral measures, such as good sleep hygiene, can help with the sleep problem. Even demented patients with highly disrupted circadian rhythms may benefit from some imposed temporal order on their daily activity. Bright light therapy can regularize circadian rhythms[256] and improve sleep-maintenance insomnia[257,258] and some work suggests that extraocular receptors may be stimulated, for instance, through light applied behind the knee,[259] making such therapy less uncomfortable and cumbersome. Such therapy may then be applied even to those in whom degeneration has damaged the sleep and circadian regulatory circuits of the brain.[260] Exercise may also improve sleep and circadian cycling.[261]

The third step is to begin therapy with low doses and only gradually build up to full dose schedules, especially in the elderly or those with degenerative neurologic disease. This caution may avoid many side effects. In some cases, however, slow buildup may be too discouraging to the patient, who may be looking for a more rapid effect; in this case, the process of building up to a therapeutic dose may need to be modified.

The fourth consideration for providing therapy is the avoidance of regular, protracted use of hypnotic medications. In some cases, they may be used for a short time to regularize sleep or on an occasional basis to avoid particularly difficult nights. Antihistamines such as diphenhydramine or anticholinergic antidepressants such as amitriptyline may substitute for benzodiazepines.

### Movement Disorders Evoked by Sleep

Movement disorders evoked by sleep or rest fall into two primary categories in the *International Classification of Sleep Disorders*.[99] RLS and PLMD are considered to be *intrinsic sleep disorders*, whereas other movement abnormalities are classified as *parasomnias*. At least one condition, fragmentary myoclonus, is categorized as a tentative disorder.

The motor parasomnias are extensively reviewed in Chapter 31. Therefore, we restrict our discussion of these conditions, including some commentary on two of the more important motor parasomnias, NPD and RBD. We review RLS and PLMD more extensively.

*Restless Legs Syndrome and Periodic Limb Movements in Sleep*

RLS, first described in a comprehensive manner by Ekbom[262] and more recently reviewed a number of

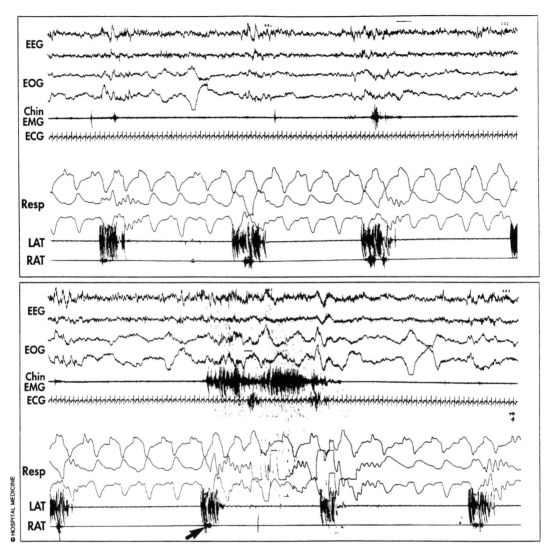

**Figure 26-1.** Continuous 2-minute sequence of sleep study with periodic leg movements in sleep (PLMS) in patient with severe restless legs syndrome. Channels indicated include electroencephalography (EEG, derivations: C3-A2 above, O1-A2 below); electro-oculography (EOG, derivations: LOC-A2 above, ROC-A2 below); chin EMG (on mentalis muscle); electrocardiography (ECG); respiratory monitoring (Resp, top line, airflow from nose and mouth combined; middle, chest excursion; bottom, abdominal excursion); left anterior tibialis muscle EMG (LAT); and right anterior tibialis muscle EMG (RAT). Arrow indicates sustained arousal caused by PLMS. Except for arousal, the patient is in stage II non-REM sleep. (Reprinted from Hospital Medicine, November 1997, by permission of Quadrant Healthcom Inc.)

times,[263–267] is an intrinsic sleep disorder in which leg symptoms lead to difficulties with sleep initiation and may disrupt sleep. The cardinal symptoms are leg dysesthesias, provoked by rest, that are associated with an urge to move and relieved by movement such as walking. Most patients with RLS (approximately 70–80%[15,268,269]) studied by PSG have PLMS (Figure 26-1). PLMS, however, are common in patients without RLS. In this case, they form a separate intrinsic sleep disorder, PLMD. It has been estimated that approximately one-third of patients with PLMS will be found to have RLS. In many older and possibly some newer studies, specific questions were not asked to determine if

**Table 26-2.** Characteristics of Periodic Limb Movements

**Movement character:** flexion of hip and knee and dorsiflexion of foot and great toe, as in triple withdrawal reflex; varies from minimal in toe to rapid and forceful and may involve arms or whole body

**Movement speed:** typically of moderate speed similar to voluntary movement, but may be rapid (myoclonic) or sustained (dystonic)

**Movement distribution:** may be in one or both legs, switch sides, or involve distant parts; generally, all involved parts move with the same period as complex but rarely see desynchrony and different period in two limbs

**Movement association:** may be related to periodic apneas with respiratory disorder or to cyclic electroencephalography changes during sleep

**Duration of electromyography burst:** 1- to 5-second complex; may have more brief, high-amplitude components (50–200 msec)

**Period of movements:** by definition, may range from 4 to 120 seconds (by different standards); typical period is 10–60 seconds, most commonly 15–40 seconds

**Severity index:** count per hour of sleep (periodic limb movement index [PLMI]) or with associated arousals per hour of sleep (periodic limb movement arousal index [PLMAI]); by definition, periodic limb movement disorder requires a PLMI of ≥5; a moderate disorder requires a PLMI of ≥25; a severe disorder requires a PLMI of ≥50 or a PLMAI of ≥25

---

patients also had RLS. In these studies, mixed groups of patients were therefore studied. The importance of this distinction is unknown. Although the response of the two conditions to medications is quite similar, some differences may exist: One study reported that carbamazepine benefited RLS, but had no effect on PLMS, suggesting they have distinguishable pathophysiologies.[268] This section of the chapter begins with a discussion of the clinical features, diagnosis, and epidemiology of these disorders. Because PLMS form a component of RLS, they are described first. The pathophysiology and treatment of the two conditions subsequently are discussed together.

**Periodic Limb Movements in Sleep.** These movements are repetitive, often stereotyped movements that typically recur at intervals of 15–40 seconds during NREM sleep (Table 26-2). They usually involve the legs, where they may consist of extension of the great toe associated with flexion at the ankle, knee, and hip. Because of their occasional jerklike character and the initial lumping together of several different motor disorders, these movements were first called *nocturnal myoclonus*[270] and may still be so labeled in some papers. Later, the term *periodic movements in sleep* was introduced to emphasize their periodicity and de-emphasize their myoclonic nature, because they are not usually myoclonic in speed.[271] Subsequently, when the abbreviation for the condition, PMS, was confused with premenstrual syndrome, the name began to

shift to periodic *leg* movements in sleep or periodic *limb* movements in sleep (PLMS). The latter is preferable because, although less common, the arms or trunk may be involved. In the 1990 classification of sleep disorders, the disorder associated with PLMS is known as *PLMD*.[99]

The individual leg movements of PLMS have been described as resembling a Babinski reflex (extension of the great toe with fanning of the other toes)[272] or a triple flexion reflex.[273] However, a fairly wide variety of movements have been described and the arms, as well as trunk, may be less commonly involved.[274] Most movements are too slow to be called *myoclonus* and they typically last a few seconds. However, the movements may begin with one or more brief, myoclonic jerks which then blend into a more tonic phase[15,230,273,275] or a more sustained movement may terminate in a jerk.[275] Movements are often bilateral, involving both legs, but may be predominant in one leg during a bout or alternate between legs. In most patients, both legs show some involvement in the course of a night's recording, but one leg may be much more involved than the other. In a minority of patients, the arms may also be involved.[276] Their most characteristic feature is their repetitive, often strikingly periodic nature. In the typical moderate to severely affected patient, PLMS occur in bouts of dozens to a 100 or more movements that last for many minutes. At a typical period (20 seconds), a patient could have 180 PLMS in an hour. Although most movements occur in the lighter stages of NREM sleep (stages I and II), some movements may occur in SWS and REM sleep as well as during the wake state, especially when it occurs in the middle of a sleep episode.[277] Bouts of PLMS often end with a shift in body position, which may have occurred in response to the movements.[278] Because PLMS movements may occur while awake, a broader term, periodic limb movements (PLMs) has been used to designate these movements independent of the state in which they occur.

PLMS is generally diagnosed by PSG recording or ambulatory sleep monitoring (for PSG standards, see Atlas Task Force of the American Sleep Disorders Association[279]). Although the precise categorization of leg movement activity varies, most investigators use a definition that includes EMG burst duration length, period between movements, and number of movements in a series. A typical scheme, such as that proposed in the current version of the *International Classification of Sleep Disorders*,[99] will count movements if they occur in series of 4 or more movements during any sleep stage (wake excluded) at intervals of 5–90 seconds (in other publications, intervals as short as 4 seconds or as long as 120 seconds have been accepted). EMG bursts must last 0.5–5.0 seconds. The number of movements associated with arousals may also be counted.[280] Criteria for diagnosis or severity typically use an index determined by dividing the total number of movements (PLMS index [PLMI]) or movements associated with arousals (PLMS arousal index [PLMAI]) by total sleep time. A PLMI greater than 5 is considered abnormal. The *International Classification* defines PLMD as mild, moderate, or severe: Mild PLMD has a PLMI of 5 but less than 25 associated with mild insomnia or sleepiness; moderate PLMS has a PLMI of 25 but less than 50 associated with moderate insomnia or sleepiness; and severe PLMS has a PLMI of 50 or more or a PLMAI greater than 25 associated with severe sleepiness or insomnia. One criticism of this scheme is that it only counts movements that occur during sleep, although many PLMD patients may also have movements while awake.[277]

Patients with PLMS may be asymptomatic, but severely affected patients may have complaints of difficulty maintaining sleep or EDS. Bed partners may actually complain more about the movements than the patients and are often an excellent source of information about the condition and its severity.

The importance of PLMS has been questioned by some authors and in some contexts,[271,281] but many sleep specialists believe that severe cases do cause significant sleep disturbance and warrant therapy. This may be particularly true in patients with RLS whose PLMS can be quite severe.[282] As noted earlier, the *International Classification* requires that the PLMS impact on either sleep continuity (insomnia) or daytime functioning (sleepiness) for a diagnosis of PLMD.[99]

In RBD, LaPierre and Montplaisir[283] found that PLMS occurred as often in REM as NREM sleep. They concluded from this that the center driving these movements continues to be active during REM sleep, but that, in otherwise normal patients, the movements are suppressed during REM sleep by the descending inhibition. Because the RBD patients lack the normal REM inhibition, they have PLMS during REM sleep. Patients with narcolepsy also have PLMS during REM sleep,[284] which may be consistent with their having a degree of decreased REM inhibition. It may not be surprising then that Schenck and Mahowald have reported that patients with narcolepsy have an increased incidence of REM without atonia, including RBD,[16] further supporting the contention that deficient REM inhibitory control can disclose the continued operation of a PLMS pacemaker. In normal patients, when PLMs occur in REM, their period is increased and their amplitude and tendency to cause arousals are decreased,[277] suggesting that REM inhibitory influences can act directly on the PLMS pacemakers (higher or segmental level) as well as on the individual movements (motor unit level).

PLMS may begin at any age, but prevalence increases markedly in later life until more than 30% of individuals older than 65 may have a significant number of PLMS.[285] Indeed, because of night-to-night variability,[285] it is possible that as many as 80% of elderly individuals have more than five PLMs per hour relatively frequently. In one large-scale study, Dickel and Mosko[286] examined 100 healthy, community-dwelling seniors with few sleep complaints (only 18% expressed complaints), and found that 71% had some PLMS on two nights of PSG (after one adaptation night), with 58% having a PLMI greater than 5. Because PLMS are so common in the elderly, merely finding some PLMs may not reveal much about underlying sleep problems. Some studies have found no association between

PLMs and either objective measures of sleep or symptomatic reports in the elderly or only very weak associations.[285] Dickel and Mosko using a threshold PLMI of 5, 20, or 40 could not find significant associations between PLMS and sleep complaints, although sleep was objectively more disrupted in those with greater PLMIs. Interestingly, for the 71 subjects with PLMS, a mean of only 25% of sleep time was dominated by epochs of PLMS. Because of these findings, elderly patients with PLMS on PSG or ambulatory recording should only be treated when the PLMS can be linked to their sleep complaints, which usually means excluding other sources of sleep dysfunction. One longitudinal study found that, although PLMs are, in general, common in the elderly, their frequency and severity may not progressively increase with additional aging.[287]

One home study of DIMS patients with previously documented PLMS found that their night-to-night variability, although significant in some individual cases, only rarely resulted in major changes in clinical classification.[288] Patients who were blindly rated as severe by sleep clinicians based on home ambulatory sleep monitoring were usually (five of seven patients) rated as severe on each of the three night studies in which they participated. The initial night study was rated as severe in each of these patients.

PLMS may occur as an isolated condition or may be associated with a large number of other medical, neurologic, or sleep disorders or with medications and other pharmacologic agents (Table 26-3). Unfortunately, few studies are controlled and it is often not possible to say whether an association is more than a matter of chance. Now that it has become clear that large numbers of older individuals have PLMS, the significance of a modest percentage of affected subjects in association with some other condition must be more closely scrutinized. For instance, PLMS is common in patients with OSA and RBD, but these patients are elderly. Some comparative studies have shown similar prevalence of PLMS among normals and insomniacs.[289] Patients with sleep disorders may have a similar prevalence of PLMS.[271] Among sleep disorders, the more striking associations are with narcolepsy[16,290,291] and RLS, because PLMS is common in these patients even if they are relatively young. OSA patients may actually have more PLMs, sometimes with significant sleep fragmentation,

after successful treatment of their apnea and PLMs may cause residual sleep difficulty in otherwise successfully treated patients with sleep apnea.[292] Among medical conditions, the association between PLMS and uremia is likely to be an important one. In some conditions, PLMS may be of great significance for sleep: In one actigraphic and PSG study of 13 patients with rheumatoid arthritis, sleep efficiency was more highly negatively linked to PLMs than to measures of disease activity, suggesting that the PLMs were a major factor for sleep fragmentation in these patients.[293] In some cases, especially that of medications, it may be that PLMs are aggravated, rather than precipitated, by the condition or medication. In general, a full understanding of which conditions increase PLMs may need to await more sweeping and thorough epidemiologic studies. Until such studies are undertaken, however, it is probably worth keeping in mind the associations already suggested, with their general notion that altered nervous system function may often be expressed as PLMs, if patients with other disorders present with complaints of poor sleep maintenance or EDS.

**Restless Legs Syndrome.** Table 26-4 indicates the features of RLS. The most distinctive characteristic of RLS is that the sensory and motor symptoms are evoked by rest, either quiet wakefulness or attempts to sleep. Patients typically describe their symptoms as worst when lying or sitting. Patients almost always describe uncomfortable sensations, most common in the legs, especially in the region of the calves, that may be variably described as tingling, burning, like water moving or insects crawling, aching, grabbing, or painful, although a wide variety of other descriptions may be offered[294] and a significant number of patients cannot describe the sensations at all. Although the symptoms are most commonly experienced in the legs, a significant minority of patients have symptoms in the arms.[294] Associated discomfort of the trunk or genitals is also known, but distinctly less common, and associated head symptoms have not been reported. These sensations are usually associated with an urge to move, although some patients report such an urge or inner feeling of restlessness without any clear precipitating sensation. In response to the urge to move, patients typically walk around, although a wide variety of movements such as rocking, shak-

**Table 26-3.** Conditions Associated with Restless Legs Syndrome (RLS) and Periodic Limb Movement Syndrome (PLMS)

| Underlying Condition | Associated with RLS | Associated with PLMS |
|---|:---:|:---:|
| **Sleep disorders** | | |
| Obstructive sleep apnea | X | X |
| Narcolepsy | | X |
| Rapid eye movement behavior disorder | | X |
| Sleep-related breathing disorder | X | |
| **Neurologic and psychiatric disorders** | | |
| Attention-deficit disorder, attention-deficit hyperactivity disorder | X | X |
| Akathisia | | X |
| Amyotrophic lateral sclerosis | X | X |
| Huntington's disease | | X |
| Isaacs' syndrome | | X |
| Multiple sclerosis | X | X |
| Myelopathies | X | X |
| Parkinson's disease | X | X |
| Peripheral neuropathies | X | X |
| Poliomyelitis | X | |
| Post-traumatic stress disorder | | X |
| Radiculopathies | X | X |
| Seizure disorders | | X |
| Spinal cord lesions | | X |
| Startle disease | | X |
| Stiff-man syndrome | | X |
| Tic disorders | X | |
| **Medical disorders** | | |
| Amyloidosis | X | |
| Anemia | X | |
| Cancer | X | |
| Chronic fatigue syndrome | | X |
| Congestive heart failure | | X |
| Chronic obstructive pulmonary disease | X | X |
| Diabetes | X | X |
| Ferritin deficiency | X | |
| Fibromyalgia | X | |
| Fibrositis syndrome | | X |
| Folate deficiency | X | |
| Gastrectomy | X | |
| Impotence | | X |
| Iron deficiency | X | |
| Leukemia | | X |
| Rheumatoid arthritis | X | |
| Sjögren's syndrome | X | |
| Telangiectasia | X | |
| Uremia | X | |
| Varicose veins | X | |
| Vascular insufficiency | X | |

| Underlying Condition | Associated with RLS | Associated with PLMS |
|---|---|---|
| **Exogenous chemicals** | | |
| Caffeine | X | |
| Ethanol | | X |
| L-Dopa | | X |
| Lithium | X | |
| Neuroleptics | X | |
| Serotonin-reuptake blockers | X | X |
| Tricyclic antidepressants | | X |
| Withdrawal | X | |

**Table 26-4.** Key Features of Idiopathic Restless Legs Syndrome

**Critical diagnostic features**
Desire to move the limbs usually associated with paresthesias/dysesthesias
Motor restlessness
Exacerbation of sensorimotor features with repose, relief with activity
Circadian variability with symptoms worst in the evening and early in the night

**Additional clinical features**
Sleep disturbance, especially difficulty in sleep initiation
Involuntary movements (periodic limb movements) that can occur asleep or awake while at rest
Absence of associated abnormalities on neurologic examination
Onset at any age; most severely affected individuals are middle aged or older; frequent onset or aggravation during pregnancy
Typical course chronic and progressive; occasional remissions
Exacerbation by caffeine and dopamine blockers common
Suggestive family history consistent with dominant inheritance often present

Source: Adapted from The International Restless Legs Syndrome Study Group; AS Walters, Group Organizer and Correspondent. Towards a better definition of the restless legs syndrome. Mov Disord 1995;10:634.

ing, stretching, marching in place, or bending may be tried for relief.[295] These varied movements that patients select to reduce their symptoms are under voluntary control and can be suppressed by the patient on command. Suppression, however, may greatly increase patient discomfort and few severely affected patients are willing to suppress their restless movements for more than a brief period when they are symptomatic. Many patients report that they use also a variety of sensory stimuli such as massage, applying oils or other materials, hot baths, or cold showers to bring at least temporary relief.

While awake, patients may also have involuntary movements that they cannot suppress by will alone. These are typically jerklike movements with an appearance and distribution similar to that of PLMS, but with greater intensity and speed, which have been also called *dyskinesias while awake* (DWAs).[295] Although the movements may take a variable form, like those of PLMS, they are most characteristically a flexion jerk, with flexion at hip, knee, and ankle. In the flexed leg, the movements may appear primarily extensor in direction, consis-

tent with our EMG observation (unpublished studies) that there is usually co-contraction in flexor and extensor muscles during the dyskinesias. Although they may have a wide range of speeds, DWAs are often myoclonic in speed. Because these jerks are influenced by ongoing voluntary activity—such as movement or position (flexion may suppress the jerks)—they are less periodic than PLMs and may appear to be either aperiodic or clustered into bursts. In many patients, these movements will merge with PLMs at sleep onset or termination. It has been noted that the jerks while awake have a shorter period than PLMs.[230,277,296] A published videotape illustrates the different voluntary and involuntary movements that patients experience.[295]

Most commonly, the various symptoms occur during the evening or early part of the night (between approximately 6 PM and 4 AM). Patients are less bothered by symptoms during the day and, even if severely affected, often obtain some relief near dawn. The increase in the number of hours when patients have RLS is often a good measure of severity. The Hopkins group has used the hour at which RLS symptoms begin as a marker for severity.[297] In general, patients experience the abnormal sensations, involuntary movements, and urge to move or restlessness under the same conditions. Indeed, these different symptoms tend to respond to the same medications.[298–300] The underlying variation in symptom intensity appears to follow a definite circadian rhythm. In two studies completed in a total of 16 RLS patients,[301,302] the patients were periodically immobilized while awake and monitored for PLMS during sleep in a 72-hour laboratory study. While awake and immobile (a modified suggested immobilization test[303] [mSIT]), they rated their sensory symptoms and were either told to remain immobile, allowing clear EMG detection of PLMS, or to move around to relieve their symptoms, allowing actigraphic assessment of restlessness. The frequency of PLMS, subjective discomfort, and restlessness all peaked between midnight and 4 AM (awake or asleep), whereas the same RLS features reached a minimum between 9 AM and 3 PM. Because activity during the mSIT was held constant, this finding indicated a time-of-day pattern independent of level of activity. Moreover, because RLS features decreased the day after a night's sleep deprivation, without intervening sleep, these features did not merely reflect time since last sleep. In 12 patients with adequate recordings, rectally measured core body temperatures showed a relatively normal nadir for age (between 2 and 6 AM). By comparing RLS features to the circadian temperature curve, it could be shown that all RLS features were maximal during the latter part of the falling phase of the temperature curve.[304]

Patients with RLS have sleep disturbance because of their symptoms and their PLMS. They have a primary difficulty getting to sleep because lying down and trying to relax activates their symptoms, which may only be relieved by activity. In severe cases, patients may have frequent nights where sleep is delayed for several hours because of their symptoms. In addition to a prolonged sleep latency, patients may have difficulty maintaining sleep. An important contribution to this may be their PLMs, which can arouse and awaken them. Approximately 70–80% of patients with RLS have associated PLMs.[269] In severe cases, this disturbance can be quite significant.[305] As a result of these difficulties in achieving sleep, patients may, in severe cases, have a total sleep

time of only 3 or 4 hours a night. In such cases, EDS can occur and may be severe and significant. However, it has been noted, although not formally studied, that RLS patients are less likely to complain of EDS than patients with similarly sleep-disruptive OSA, patients with equivalent sleep reduction, or patients with narcolepsy. Although RLS is a condition that impairs quality of life, it has not been thought to carry an adverse prognosis. However, in one study, Pollak and colleagues found that, in women, RLS was a significant predictor of mortality.[306] The significance of that association remains to be further defined. On the other hand, there have been various anecdotal reports of patients who have contemplated suicide and at least one case report of suicide in a patient with RLS.[307] It seems clear, then, that for some patients the impact of RLS is very severe.

Prevalence estimates for RLS have generally ranged from 1% to 15%. Two studies in general medical populations using clinical diagnosis led to estimates between 3.2% and 5%.[262,308] Questionnaire studies of clinical populations have given the most widely varying results, from 2.0% in a group of headache patients[309] to 29% in a group of VA outpatients.[310] One study in a control group of diabetes patients found a prevalence of 7%.[311] In one large-scale study performed in Canada,[312] Montplaisir and colleagues used two questions about bedtime restless and unpleasant leg sensations on waking to determine prevalence of RLS. In the total population surveyed (age-stratified sample of those 18 or older), 15% answered yes to the first question and 10% answered yes to the second. Prevalence, as estimated from these two questions, increased with age and was higher among women, those who lived in Eastern Canada (Quebec and the Atlantic provinces), and those who were Catholic or French speaking. This may suggest an underlying ethnic difference in prevalence. A number of investigators have noted that African-Americans are relatively rarely diagnosed with RLS. For instance, in a clinical study by Ondo and Jankovic,[294] 53 of 54 patients were noted to be Caucasian. Two additional large-scale questionnaire studies, in the United States generally and in Kentucky, have led to similar conclusions about overall prevalence as the Canadian survey.[313,314] Approximately 10% of adults say they often have symptoms suggestive of RLS. None of these population-based studies did

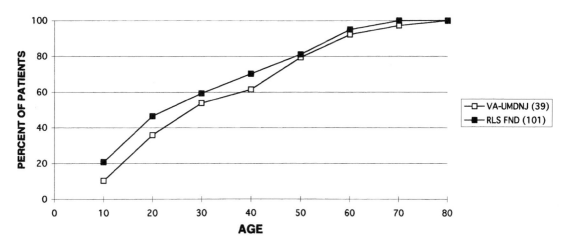

**Figure 26-2.** Cumulative prevalence of restless legs syndrome before a given age (*x* axis) gauged from date of onset of symptoms in two case series: 39 patients studied by Dr. Walters and colleagues at the UMDNJ-Robert Wood Johnson Medical School and at Lyons, New Jersey, Department of Veterans Affairs Medical Center, and 101 patients interviewed by a team directed by Dr. Walters who were initially contacted through the RLS Foundation by Virginia Walker, secretary. (Modified from AS Walters, K Hickey, J Maltzman, et al. A questionnaire study of 138 patients with restless legs syndrome: the 'Night-Walkers' survey. Neurology 1996;46:92.)

follow-ups to determine how many patients with RLS might have been missed and what proportion of those who answered positively to RLS questions actually had RLS. The likelihood is that these population studies overestimate the prevalence of RLS. Clinically significant RLS probably occurs in 1–5% of the population, and the total prevalence may be as high as 3–8%.

Although often considered a disorder of older persons, it has been known since Ekbom's pioneering studies in the 1940s that RLS can occur in children.[262] Some studies have emphasized that RLS symptoms frequently appear in childhood and adolescence,[315,316] although they typically are more severe in older patients, indicating that the disease is often progressive.[99,294,316,317] Symptoms, however, may remit for periods, even later in the course of the disorder[99,294,316,317] but in most cases, RLS is a chronic condition, whether treated or not.[318] A summary of the age of onset derived from a study performed by Walters and colleagues[316] is plotted in Figure 26-2 as a cumulative prevalence, demonstrating graphically the increase in prevalence that occurs with increasing age. Similar results, indicating a widely distributed age of onset from childhood on and a chronic course leading to increased prevalence in older groups, have been reported by Ondo and Jankovic[294] and Montplaisir's group.[319]

Pregnancy is a known precipitant of the condition,[320,321] which may first appear, usually later in pregnancy, and then subsequently remit, only to reappear in a more chronic form in later years. Since Ekbom,[262] it has been noted that RLS can be found in first-degree relatives. One factor that has made the familial clustering less obvious is that probands are often uninformed about the presence of the condition even in close relatives. However, efforts to find familial clustering have been quite successful, including seven large pedigrees with many affected members used by members of the International RLS Study Group in genetic studies.[296,317,318,322–324] Informal inspection of these pedigrees indicates that they are consistent with an autosomal dominant form of inheritance.[15,317] In older family members, the proportion of those who have RLS approaches the expected Mendelian proportion[325] for a single autosomal dominant gene (50% of those at risk affected). Therefore, gene penetrance may be high, although full expression may not occur until near the end of the life span. Another finding, the possible presence of anticipation in one large kindred,[325] raises the question of whether RLS might be another triplet repeat disorder.[326] Current studies aimed at determining a linkage for RLS have not been successful, however, suggesting either genetic heterogeneity, a more complex genetic model than a major gene autosomal dominant inheritance, or difficulties with exact diagnosis. The relatively high frequency expected for a gene (on the order of 2–10%) and the possibility of environmental phenocopies may also be important in complicating the linkage studies. Finding a testable genetic factor (linkage or gene) would, of course, provide a substantial benefit for a full range of studies (epidemiologic, pathophysiologic, therapeutic) in RLS.

One factor supporting a genetic or at least familial basis in idiopathic RLS is the relatively increased percentage of individuals with family members positive for RLS when the proband's RLS seems idiopathic, without antecedent cause. A study by Ondo and Jankovic[294] found a very high familial incidence of RLS in idiopathic cases (92%), but a much lower familial association (13%) in RLS possibly secondary to neuropathy.[294] A similar difference was found by Stautner and colleagues who compared idiopathic to uremic RLS[327]: 54% of the idiopathic patients had a positive family history compared to 12% of the uremic patients. Another support for a genetic factor in RLS is the finding of a significantly elevated prevalence of RLS in first-degree relatives (4- to 8-fold increase) of RLS patients seen at sleep centers compared to unaffected controls.[328] Although our impression is that the majority of cases of RLS are idiopathic (although no studies have been done to establish this epidemiologic point), there have been many different reports that linked RLS to other medical, neurologic, or sleep disorders (see Table 26-3). The most important associations with pathologic conditions are with iron deficiency (with or without frank anemia),[329] uremia,[327,330,331] rheumatoid arthritis,[332] and diabetes.[311] In each of these conditions, the true prevalence of RLS almost certainly exceeds 10%. Iron deficiency, with or without anemias, is a very important provocative factor for RLS.[329] Treating iron deficiency, best measured by the ferritin level, can alleviate RLS or improve the patient's response to other medications. It has been suggested that ferritin levels as high as 45, which is well within the normal range, may benefit from iron supplementation. RLS is only one of a spectrum of motor abnormalities that occur in uremia and may need to be distinguished from action myoclonus, asterixis, tremor, or akathisia. Some studies indicate that RLS in uremic RLS is quite similar to that seen in idiopathic patients, although the number of PLMs may be greater. In one study, uremic dialysis patients with RLS (40% of 55 dialysis patients) were more likely to be anemic than other dialysis patients, but had no more neuropathy than those without RLS.[333] Correcting the anemia in an open-label, long-term trial led to significantly decreased subjective complaints. Another study found that 23% of 136 dialysis patients had RLS,[331] but they did not differ from the other patients in anemia or iron levels. The one difference between the groups was lower parathormone levels in the RLS patient.

Although peripheral neuropathy has long been associated with RLS,[334–336] clear evidence for increased prevalence in neuropathy of mixed etiology has not yet been presented. However, there are clearly cases that develop in the same time frame as peripheral neuropathy or radiculopathy.[294,316,337] so that the association is important to remember.

One intriguing suggestion is that there may be an association between childhood RLS and attention-deficit hyperactivity disorder (ADHD).[338] The two disorders share restlessness and may respond to the same medications, including both stimulants and dopaminergic agents. There may also be a relationship in childhood between tic syndromes and RLS.[339] Perhaps these conditions share some pathogenetic features.

Diagnosis of RLS is based on clinical features, mostly the clinical interview. It is important to establish, first, that the four diagnostic features for RLS are present in a more than incidental way (general degrees of severity are specified in the *International Classification*[99]). There are currently no widely accepted diagnostic or evaluative questionnaire instruments, although a number of groups are currently developing and standardizing such instruments. Evaluation of RLS involves a general medical history and physical examination to rule out possible secondary causes of the syndrome. In idiopathic RLS, the neurologic examination is normal unless some additional neurologic disorder is present. Blood tests should be performed to exclude anemia (including iron, ferritin, and probably folate levels), uremia, and diabetes, if recent previous results are not available. In long-standing cases with no findings on history or examination, that may end the work-up for cause. With sensory findings or a complaint suggestive of root damage, an EMG and nerve conduction study should be performed. Eval-

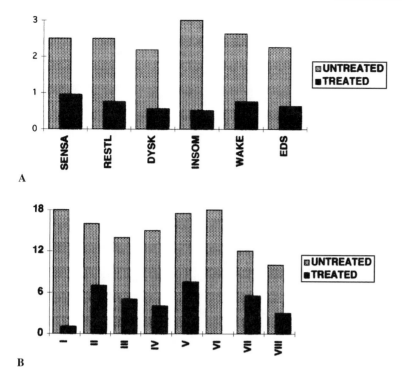

A

B

**Figure 26-3.** Effects of opioid therapy in eight patients with restless legs syndrome. Patients rated six symptoms on a 0–3 scale before therapy (untreated) and on opioid therapy (treated; in five patients, treatment included additional medications). (A) Mean rating per symptom across eight patients (all differences significant, $p < .05$, paired $t$ test). (B) The sum of the six ratings for each individual patient, I–VIII (sum ranges from 0 to 18). (SENSA = uncomfortable sensations; RESTL = degree of motor restlessness or urge to move; DYSK = dyskinesias while awake; INSOM = difficulty in getting to sleep; WAKE = waking after sleep onset; EDS = excessive daytime somnolence.)

uation of RLS should include sleep logs, as part of the general evaluation of the sleep complaint, and specific questions about RLS. Although there is no standardized instrument to assess the severity of RLS, we have rated subjective discomfort on a scale of 0–3 points, where 0 is asymptomatic and 1–3 represent mild, moderate, or severe symptoms. Patients assess their leg discomfort, restlessness, jerks while awake, difficulty getting asleep, difficulty staying asleep, and daytime somnolence, so that a maximally affected patient would have an RLS score of 18. This scale has been helpful in assessing subjective response to therapy[300] (Figure 26-3). Although PSG is not indicated to diagnose RLS,[340] it may be necessary to rule out other sleep disorders or assess the contribution of PLMS to sleep disruption.

It may often be important to distinguish RLS from akathisia, which has at times been called *restless legs*. Akathisia, most typically due to neuroleptic medications (neuroleptic-induced akathisia [NIA]), is a similar motor restlessness which may have sleep abnormalities and PLMS.[341,342] In one study, however, Lipinski and colleagues did not find PLMS, but rather a distinctive rhythmic activity at sleep onset and during arousals that may represent a rhythmic manifestation of the akathisia.[343] Akathisia can be distinguished from RLS by history and examination of the patient.[341,344] We have noted, based on patient interviews and observation, that there are several telling historical distinctions between RLS and NIA[341]: (1) RLS patients complain most about uncomfortable sensations as a source of restlessness (19 of 20), whereas this is less common in NIA patients (5 of 20) who have a more primary sense of inner restlessness (15 of 20); (2) RLS patients more commonly complain about nighttime aggravation of their symptoms (18 of 20 vs. 6 of 20 NIA patients), whereas NIA patients have continuous symptoms or symptoms related to the timing of neuroleptic doses; (3) RLS patients more frequently report they are worst lying down (16 of 20 vs. 3 of 20 NIA patients); and (4) NIA patients tend to have persistent, repetitive, cyclic movements like body rocking and marching in place, whereas RLS patients less commonly and then only in association with nighttime symptoms and restlessness have similar kinds of movements. Akathisia is associated with a number of disorders, such as PD, as well as medications, but is almost always secondary. Idiopathic or essential akathisia is rare.

**Pathophysiology of Restless Legs Syndrome and Periodic Limb Movements in Sleep.**    Despite the suggestion that idiopathic RLS may have a genetic basis, there is no known and clearly established pathology associated with the syndrome. The only exceptions to this observation are secondary cases where pathology appropriate to the primary disorder may be present. However, various clinical observations and studies have shed some light on the pathophysiology of RLS and PLMS and the location of its abnormal centers.

Electrophysiology has been used to determine whether there is some abnormal level of function within the nervous system in RLS, either increased reflexes or damaged peripheral nerves, to assess involvement of the cortex in PLMS, and to map muscle activation as a means of finding some clue as to how the nervous system coordinates the different muscles active during PLMS. In general, these studies have followed suggestions that proved useful in the study of myoclonus, because PLMS were once called "nocturnal myoclonus." Several studies have examined patients with RLS or PLMS (usually not clearly distinguished) and found inconsistent support for the presence of some hyperexcitable brain stem or transcortical reflexes.[345,346] Two studies have re-examined the question: One found enhanced excitability of the blink reflex (persistent R2 component) in sleep apnea patients with PLMS compared to apneic controls[347]; whereas the other, examining unmedicated patients with RLS, found no abnormalities of the blink reflex or the H reflex in these patients.[348] Because of the continuing reports of inconsistent results, it is not possible to determine whether there is abnormal excitability in RLS and PLMS. The further question of whether abnormal function might be present only when patients are symptomatic also remains to be addressed.

Again, pursuing a research theme that has yielded results in myoclonus, several groups have looked for cortical prepotentials before the waking and sleeping PLMS. This result could indicate a cortical source or involvement in the generation of PLMS. However, the researchers either found no prepoten-

tial[15] or one that was unlike other known pathologic prepotentials[349] and, to some degree, resembled the normal prepotential occurring before voluntary movement.[350] In the most thorough study reported to date, Trenkwalder and colleagues[351] examined the cortical potential before waking PLMS in 13 RLS patients. They found no prepotential before the PLMS, but normal premovement potentials when the RLS patients simulated their movements. There was no difference between the latter prepotentials and those made by control subjects moving their legs. As a result, it now appears unlikely that the cortex is the generator for the PLMS. Even those investigators who found a movement prepotential[350] noted that it might well represent activity projected upward from subcortical sites.

PLMs have also been studied to see whether there is a distinctive pattern of muscular activation. Trenkwalder and colleagues[352] found consistent descending or ascending patterns in 7 of 18 patients demonstrating progressive activation within the L3–S1 levels. The rate of spinal conduction appeared to be slow, suggesting transmission by some secondary pathways as suggested for propriospinal myoclonus. This is consistent with a potential spinal location for a generator for PLMS, perhaps a segmental oscillator. To support this localization, several groups have now reported the presence of PLMS in patients with lesions of the spinal cord including seemingly complete thoracic cord transection.[273,353] It is now clear that such generators exist in the isolated spinal cord for a number of different cyclical motor behaviors,[36] although in many cases the movements produced by the isolated cord are reduced in amplitude, frequency, or complexity. Such a finding does not exclude, however, the possibility that these spinal generators might be elements in a more complex generator circuit or controlled by descending influences. In addition, some small series and case reports have now shown that there can be different periods for PLMS simultaneously present in different limbs, including arm and leg,[276,354] two legs,[355] or two arms.[354] These preliminary observations thus support the presence of individual limb oscillators capable of producing PLMS.

In the absence of a known pathologic lesion in RLS, attempts have been made to determine whether there might be some detectable abnormality using a variety of imaging techniques. Imaging studies have also been undertaken to find a locus for RLS and

PLMS pathology. Neither structural MRI studies[348] nor fluorodeoxyglucose PET studies[356] revealed any consistent abnormalities of cerebral structure or blood flow in RLS patients. One study used functional MRI to examine patients when they were symptomatic.[357] Nineteen patients were studied when they had sensory symptoms alone ($N = 7$) and when they had, in addition, PLMs ($N = 12$). Either condition was associated with bilateral cerebellar activation and thalamic activation contralateral to the affected leg. When PLMs were also present, there was additional activation of the red nuclei and of brain stem sites in the region of the reticular formation (11 of 12 patients with PLMs). Mimicking of PLMs by either patients or controls led to more attenuated activation of thalamic, cerebellar, and red nuclei sites, but no appreciable brain stem activation. In addition, mimicking led to activation of the pallidum and motor cortex not seen with PLMs. This study, therefore, shows that PLMs have a pattern of activation that differs from voluntary movement. The lack of motor cortex activation is consistent with the absence of a clear-cut cortical prepotential for PLMs. It remains a possibility, however, that all or much of the activated regions are largely reflecting activity projected upward from the spinal cord.

In a series of studies, Staedt and colleagues examined patients with PLMS, some of whom also had RLS, and found decreased striatal binding of IBZM, an iodinated ligand that selectively binds to $D_2$ receptors.[358] After treatment, four patients treated with dopaminergic agents showed an increased IBZM binding, suggesting that there were then more $D_2$ receptors in the striatum.[359] These results are somewhat puzzling, because the efficacy of dopaminergic agents in RLS suggests that any dopamine deficiency should be presynaptic. Moreover, the area involved, the striatum, would primarily relate to the nigrostriatal pathways. Presynaptic degeneration in those pathways produces PD, but parkinsonism is not present in most patients with RLS (although patients with PD are at increased risk for both RLS and PLMS[92,141]). In another study, four patients with RLS were examined when asymptomatic using fluorodopa PET scanning to examine the presynaptic dopamine system: No abnormalities were detected compared to age-matched controls (Eidelberg, personal communication, 1997).

Because they often occur without RLS and are so common in the elderly, PLMs must have some relatively separate or independent pathophysiology. Lugaresi and colleagues have suggested that the oscillation may be linked to autonomic periodicities generated primarily within the brain stem.[360] This would couple the oscillator to apparently normal rhythms within the central nervous system. Further support for this proposal is found in the shifts in heart rate and respiratory rate reported in some patients in phase with the PLMS.[361] Some studies in RBD, which show persistent PLMs during REM sleep, suggest that the oscillator may be active throughout all sleep stages, but that its manifestations, the leg movements, are suppressed selectively during REM sleep.[283] The same may apply during SWS. Alternatively, the oscillator may be itself inhibited by the REM-generating mechanism in patients without RBD, whereas RBD patients have a parallel failure of atonia and suppression of the PLMS oscillator.

Several other findings have important potential pathophysiologic implications for RLS and PLMS. The efficacy of dopaminergic and opioid medications suggests the likelihood that the dopaminergic and endogenous opioid systems are involved in the pathogenesis of RLS and PLMS. The influence of a circadian factor and of activity factors on RLS suggests that there must be circadian and activity-dependent physiologic changes that are important for pathogenesis. The association of RLS with pregnancy, and perhaps with other hormonally changing states in women (e.g., the menstrual cycle, surgical menopause), suggests there may also be some hormonal influence on RLS.

**Therapy of Restless Legs Syndrome and Periodic Limb Movement Disorder.**    Therapy for RLS (Table 26-5) has been developed over the last 15–20 years, and there are now a large number of different treatments whose effectiveness has been more or less rigorously established (for a general discussion, consult reviews of RLS[15,263,265–267,295,317,362–365]). The history of treatment for RLS goes back several centuries to Willis' use of laudanum, an opioid.[366] However, only recently have developments led to a revolution in the therapeutic attitude toward RLS and PLMD, from despair over the lack of treatment[367] to a more cautious optimism and concern for finding the most effective and least potentially dangerous therapy.[267,269,368–370] Two points should be made about interpreting this material. First,

**Table 26-5.** Medications Useful in Restless Legs Syndrome (RLS) and Periodic Limb Movement Disorder (PLMD)

**Primary therapy**
Dopaminergic agents
    Dopamine precursors: levodopa combined with car-
      bidopa or benserazide, in regular or sustained-
      released preparations
    Dopamine agonists
      Established: pergolide, bromocriptine
      Potential: pramipexole, ropinirole
    Other dopaminergic agents: selegiline, amantadine
Benzodiazepines
    Most often used: clonazepam, temazepam, triazolam
    Also used: nitrazepam, alprazolam, diazepam, lorazepam
Opioids
    Short half-life: propoxyphene, codeine, oxycodone,
      hydrocodone, pentazocine
    Long half-life: methadone, levorphanol, sustained-
      release morphine

**Secondary therapy**
Anticonvulsants: gabapentin, carbamazepine, valproate
Others relatively well studied: clonidine, baclofen
Only suggestive reports: tramadol, lamotrigine, barbitu-
    rates, beta blockers, 5-hydroxytryptophan, phenoxyben-
    zamine, orphenadrine citrate, γ-hydroxybutyrate,
    amitriptyline, fluoxetine, alcohol

**Symptomatic therapy**
Iron
Vasodilators
Vitamins and minerals: folate; vitamins $B_{12}$, C, and E;
    magnesium

**Ancillary therapy**
Good sleep hygiene and moderate activity
Nonpharmacologic therapies
    Increasing blood flow to feet (?)
    Electrical stimulation
    Behavioral modification
    Sclerotherapy
Avoiding foods or drugs that may aggravate RLS
    Caffeine
    Antidepressant medications, especially tricyclics, but
      perhaps also serotonin-reuptake blockers (mixed
      reports)
    Dopamine-blocking agents: neuroleptics, antiemetic and
      antigastric dumping medications (e.g., prochlorper-
      azine, metoclopramide)

Note: This table includes some agents that are suggested for RLS or PLMD but not well studied and are not dealt with in the text. Note that in some cases the literature is either contradictory, containing both beneficial and harmful reports, or minimal.

because effective therapies are multiple and only recently developed, there is no fixed consensus on treatment and recommended treatment paradigms have been evolving rapidly. Second, therapeutic choices today must be based on an evaluation of the literature and expert practice, because RLS is not an approved indication for any medication in the United States.

Since the mid-1980s, there have been controlled clinical trials of therapeutic agents in RLS which have involved double-blind drug and placebo studies. These have established the usefulness to some degree of a number of medications for RLS and PLMS including benzodiazepines,[371–373] opioids,[374] dopamine precursors,[303] dopamine agonists,[299] baclofen,[375] carbamazepine,[376] clonidine,[377] and γ-hydroxybutyrate.[378] Many of these trials and others have used a variety of measures for improvement including subjective report of symptom severity, PSG variables such as sleep latency and sleep efficiency, quantitation of PLMS or of PLMS associated with arousals and awakenings, actigraphic recordings of movement, and provoked waking symptoms (e.g., the Suggested Immobilization Test [SIT] which requests the patient to sit still for 30 minutes or more).[303]

Treatment for RLS and PLMS can be broken down into several categories. Primary treatment is that best established to reduce the subjective complaints of patients and their objective findings. Symptomatic treatment is directed at an underlying cause. Secondary treatment is that whose efficacy is not as well-established or whose usefulness is restricted or more modest. Ancillary treatments may assist pharmacologic therapy. These include lifestyle changes that can often be used for mild or more stoic patients. Most severe patients with RLS will need pharmacotherapy to adequately manage their symptoms.

Primary treatment is with medications selected from the three primary classes whose effectiveness in RLS has been best established: dopaminergic agents, opioids, and benzodiazepines.

The dopaminergic agents are useful for treatment of both RLS and PLMD. They improve all cardinal features of RLS including subjective discomfort, dyskinesias while awake, PLMS, and sleep quality. Dopamine precursors were first used, either regular carbidopa/L-dopa or sustained-release compounds. Typical doses have been 25/100 to 100/400 (carbidopa/L-dopa) taken in divided doses before bed-time or before bedtime and during the night. Two major problems have been noted: (1) *rebound*, the tendency of symptoms to recur late in the night lead-ing to poor sleep quality near morning, and (2) *aug-mentation*, the tendency for symptoms to develop earlier in the day (e.g., late afternoon[379] instead of midevening) and to be more severe than before treat-ment. Side effects include gastrointestinal discom-fort, nausea and vomiting, light-headedness, or headache. The degree to which sustained-release preparations overcome this problem is not clear. Long-term treatment has only rarely led to the kinds of dyskinetic movements that follow treatment of PD.[263,380] The major alternative dopaminergic treat-ment uses dopamine agonists that act directly on the dopamine receptor. Both bromocriptine and per-golide have been tried successfully in patients with RLS and PLMS. Typical doses for therapy have been 5–20 mg of bromocriptine or 0.10–0.60 mg of pergolide, either drug taken in divided doses before bedtime. These dopamine agonists do not seem to show to the same degree the problems of rebound and augmentation seen with L-dopa–based com-pounds. Nasal stuffiness, gastrointestinal discomfort, and hypotension have occurred as side effects. Par-ticularly with pergolide, the dose must be carefully increased (from 0.05 mg per day) to avoid symp-tomatic hypotension. If possible, domperidone, a peripheral blocker, can be obtained from Canada to prevent the frequent gastrointestinal symptoms and nasal congestion that occur early during pergolide therapy. One report demonstrated excellent results with bromocriptine,[299] whereas pergolide has been more widely used and has now been tried in a num-ber of variously designed trials with notable suc-cess.[297,381,382] Initial reports also suggest that newly approved dopamine agonists, pramipexole[382a] and ropinirole, are useful in RLS. Dosages remain to be established, but the initial indication is that, as with bromocriptine and pergolide, the optimal doses will be lower than those used in PD (less than 1 mg per day for pramipexole in most cases). In one open-label study, the mean dose was 0.3 mg per day.[382a]

Some now regard pergolide as the best agent for chronic therapy of RLS, especially for patients with moderate to severe disease who have daily symp-toms and require continuous therapy. If hypotension is a major problem, some patients can be managed with blood pressure supporting agents such as flu-drocortisone acetate. Other side effects can often also be managed by additional medications—for example, decongestants for nasal stuffiness. Side effects often seen in PD patients treated with L-dopa or other agents, including dopa-induced dyskinesias and mental changes such as hallucinations, are rarely seen in RLS, but may be a worry for those on high doses for long periods, especially the elderly. Worries that L-dopa might induce degeneration of the endogenous dopamine system have been calmed to some degree by an autopsy series that showed no degeneration of the main dopaminergic nucleus, the substantia nigra, in nonparkinsonian patients treated with high doses of L-dopa.[383] In selected cases, sig-nificantly higher doses of the dopaminergic agents than those mentioned here have been used. A final point is that the COMT blockers, tolcapone and entacapone (entacapone not approved), may help extend the effects of L-dopa therapy.[151,384]

The opioid medications are clearly useful for treating RLS and are also effective for some cases of PLMD. Many different opioids have been tried infor-mally, including codeine, propoxyphene, oxycodone, pentazocine, levorphanol, and methadone. Doses have been quite variable, but typical doses used for patients have been codeine, 15–120 mg per day; propoxyphene, 130–520 mg per day; oxycodone, 2.5–20.0 mg per day; pentazocine, 50–200 mg per day; and methadone, 5–30 mg per day. In one double-blind controlled trial, subjective symptoms, sleep measures, and PLMs were all significantly improved with oxycodone at a mean dose of 15.9 mg per day.[374] In contrast, two double-blind studies of propoxyphene napsylate (up to 300 mg per night) found benefits to subjective symptoms and total motor activity, but no significant reduction in PLMs.[385,386] One study of patients with PLMD alone found that some responded quite well to the opioid medications.[387] Stronger opioids are reserved for more severely affected or resistant patients. Problems have included constipation and addictive behavior, in a few patients. Moderate tolerance has been noted, although we have some patients who remain on constant doses for many years with per-ceived continued efficacy[300] and recurrence of symptoms when the medication is tapered. A major problem for prescribing these medications is the physician's imagined or real fear of social or regu-latory disapproval. Recently, an opioid active med-ication, tramadol, which is not classified like an opioid for regulatory purposes, has become available. There have been some scattered clinical reports of benefit, but clarifying the benefits of this agent, which is also active as a serotonin-reuptake blocker, will require formal study.

The benzodiazepines are useful for treatment of both RLS and PLMD. Their strong point is in improving the quality of sleep and reducing its fragmentation. They may also benefit waking symptoms in RLS, but their degree of benefit is less well-established. The number of PLMs has not always been significantly decreased, although some studies have shown significant decreases.[372,388] Clonazepam, 0.5–4.0 mg; temazepam, 15–30 mg[373]; and triazolam,[389] 0.125–0.500 mg, are taken at bedtime. Doses for daytime treatment of RLS are less well-established. Diazepam has also been used for daytime symptoms; a typical dose might be 5 mg twice a day. Drawbacks include the potential for confusion or daytime sleepiness, especially in older patients. One additional benefit of clonazepam is that it may treat related motor sleep disorders such as RBD that are more common in older patients and may coexist with RLS or PLMD. Some experts have found that patients can do well for years on low-dose benzodiazepines.[390]

The most promising of the secondary therapies currently are the anticonvulsants. In the last few years, gabapentin has been reported in open trials to be a successful medication for RLS.[391–394] It appears to be most useful in cases of RLS whose disturbing sensations seem truly painful. It seems to work best in mild to moderate cases. Carbamazepine has been shown in a double-blind trial with only clinical monitoring to benefit RLS.[376] In a PSG study, it was found to benefit subjective symptoms, sleep latency and sleep efficiency, but not PLMs.[268] There is, however, one report of a dramatic response of PLMS to carbamazepine,[395] so it should not be completely disregarded. Other anticonvulsants such as valproic acid[396] or lamotrigine[397] have also been reported to be effective in some cases. Patients may respond to doses lower than those commonly used to treat seizures; as is generally true in RLS, it is helpful to increase doses slowly so as not to miss a therapeutic window.

Adrenergic agents have also been found to benefit RLS. Clonidine, a centrally active α-adrenergic blocker, has been reported to be effective in both idiopathic[398] and uremic patients.[399] One double-blind study reported that clonidine had a significant benefit, especially on waking symptoms and sleep latency.[377] Another well-studied drug is baclofen, which was found in one double-blind study to reduce arousal related to PLMS, primarily by decreasing the response to movements. It appeared to decrease the intensity, but not the frequency of movements.[375] Its effect on RLS waking symptoms is not clear. γ-Hydroxybutyrate was suggested in an initial report of another double-blind study to have a similar effect at doses of 37.5 mg/kg.[378]

Other agents have been mentioned incidentally as useful for RLS or PLMD, but the evidence is not yet well developed.

When RLS or PLMD is due to some underlying disorder, treatment of the underlying condition may alleviate RLS or PLMD. This has not been generally well studied. An alternative is to use standard RLS therapy, as has been studied in uremia, which has been reported to respond to benzodiazepines,[400] dopaminergic agents,[401,402] opioids, and clonidine.[403] Deficiency states might be corrected. The most important deficiency state is probably iron deficiency. Low iron levels, best measured as serum ferritin, can bring out RLS, aggravate known RLS, and cause resistance to therapy. Iron supplementation has been shown to improve RLS in uncontrolled studies.[329] Women are particularly liable to have low iron levels. Low iron may contribute to RLS symptoms in pregnancy. Transfusion has sometimes helped RLS in anemia.[404] One group has linked folate deficiency to RLS and found improvement of RLS along with other symptoms with treatment,[405,406] whereas another has suggested magnesium treatment for magnesium deficiency.[233] Other treatments, including a number of different vitamins, such as vitamin C,[404] vitamin E,[407] or vitamin $B_{12}$,[405] are more speculatively linked to a deficiency. I am aware of no controlled trials demonstrating that these therapies are effective, although there are suggestive clinical reports.

Some disorders can be cured with consequent resolution of RLS: For instance, kidney transplantation may alleviate uremia and associated RLS,[402] whereas surgical decompression may alleviate spinal cord compression and associated PLMS.[408]

In addition to standard medications, a number of nonpharmacologic therapies have been suggested for RLS. These have generally been proposed after case studies or series of open trials. Such reports have dealt with the use of thermal feedback for PLMS[409] or the use of transdermal stimulation regimes.[410] A basis for the thermal feedback is the observation that PLMS may be associated with decreased blood flow to the feet and cold feet.[409] However, in one case report, adequate training for increased blood flow did not result in improved RLS.[411] So more study must be done to see whether this potentially attractive procedure will be of any real use. Edinger and colleagues have reported that behavioral therapies aimed at normalizing sleep may also benefit PLMD patients,[412] although PLMs do not decrease significantly. It has also been reported that varicose veins may be associated with RLS and relieved by sclerotherapy.[413]

Some substances should be avoided. Among the dietary substances and medications that have been suggested to increase RLS or PLMS are caffeine,[414] neuroleptics, and tricyclic antidepressants.[415,416] Patients taking more modern antidepressants, such as the serotonin-reuptake blockers, may also have RLS symptoms aggravated.[417] One small study showed increased PLMs in nine depressed patients treated with fluoxetine compared to six depressed controls.[418] Paradoxically, some patients apparently respond favorably to tricyclics[419] or to serotonin-reuptake blockers.[420,421]

The following comments suggest a general approach to treatment of different patient presentations in RLS. These recommendations are a composite derived by the first author from the literature, discussions with others treating RLS and PLMD, and the author's own clinical experience. A suggested algorithm for RLS and PLMD treatment is shown in Figure 26-4.

RLS patients should be treated when their symptoms are bothersome and cannot be managed by the tricks or routines that patients often use to ameliorate their condition, including hot baths, massages, avoiding caffeine or other problematic medications, or a bit of appropriately timed exercise. Before trying significant medications (e.g., benzodiazepines, opioids, or dopaminergic agents), lifestyle management including good sleep hygiene and avoidance of provocative circumstances or substances (caffeine, cigarettes, alcohol), appropriately timed exercise, or varied stratagems to relax. A trial of vitamins, vitamin E or folate, is also worthwhile, although they have not been established to be reliably helpful. PLMD patients should be treated when their movements appear to be the sole or a clearly major cause of disrupted sleep that is related to significant subjective complaints.

Where a treatable potential cause for RLS is known, it is best, when feasible, to initiate therapy with agents designed to eliminate or palliate that cause. As a general rule, treatment should be only as much as needed—for example, give medications that can be taken only when needed for sporadic symptoms. Build up doses slowly and try to limit final doses. Remember that some medicines—dopaminergic agents or beta blockers, for example—should not be discontinued abruptly. In general, patients who stop an RLS medication may feel transiently worse than before therapy.

If the patient has primarily complaints of sleep dysfunction and daytime somnolence, the first author's initial choice for therapy is a benzodiazepine, such as clonazepam or temazepam. This would be the case if the patient had PLMD alone. The initial dose of clonazepam would be 0.5 mg, increased as necessary to 2 mg; of temazepam, 15 mg increased to 30 mg, if necessary. If those failed, a dopaminergic agent can be added. Therapy needs to be tailored to the duration of daily symptoms. PLMs that persist throughout the night may indicate the need for a longer-acting agent. If the patient has primarily waking complaints, the first author would consider either a mild opioid such as propoxyphene or a dopaminergic agent. Carbidopa/L-dopa combinations, like the opioids, are useful when given as a single dose for symptoms that occur at specific times (e.g., during travel or public functions). The L-dopa dose should be kept low to avoid problems with augmentation. A maximum of 300–400 mg per day is probably a good limit, whereas no more than 200 mg per day of L-dopa is probably optimal for sustaining efficacy without augmentation. Dopamine agonists can be used for patients who do not respond to L-dopa. Typical doses are bromocriptine, 5–20 mg per day; pergolide, 0.1–1.0 mg per day; and pramipexole, 0.125–1.250 mg per day. Doses for ropinirole have not yet been established but are expected to be lower than typical doses used for treating PD. Patients who have severe RLS when first seen, especially those with symptoms throughout the night or during the daytime, will almost inevitably require multiple doses of L-dopa combined with carbidopa and high-dose levels. It is, therefore, best to begin dopaminergic therapy for such patients with an agonist, skipping L-dopa. Pergolide should almost always be initiated slowly (0.05 mg per day with dose increases only every few days) and coverage with domperidone provided, if feasible. Optimally, the domperidone is started a few days before the pergolide. An alternate medication for patients with waking complaints is clonidine.

**Starting treatment**

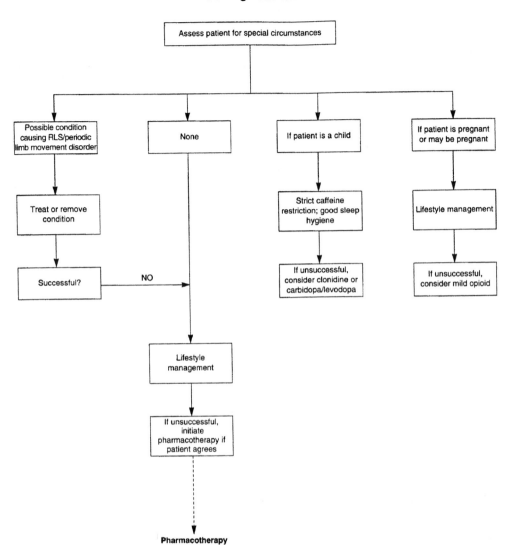

**Figure 26-4.** Flowchart for therapy in restless legs syndrome (RLS). This schematized flowchart shows how therapy can be initialized and tailored to individual patient needs. It represents the first author's viewpoint based on his own experience and the current literature on treatment of RLS and periodic limb movement disorder. Medication doses, dosing schedules and titrations, and side effects are discussed in the text. (Reprinted from Hospital Medicine, November 1997, by permission of Quadrant Healthcom Inc.)

Dose levels are tailored to the patients' needs, as is the timing of the individual doses. It is best to use as little medication as possible. It is to be expected that, over time, doses may need to increase. It is probably poor management to use L-dopa/carbidopa around the clock, as has happened to some patients whose symptoms shifted from evening and night to all hours. Instead, it is preferable to switch to a dopamine agonist or an opioid. Refractory cases have to be judiciously managed by increasing doses, switching primary medications, or using combination therapy. Patients often do well on a combination of a dopaminergic agent or opioid for daytime symptoms with a benzodiazepine at night. The worst cases may require triple therapy of opioid, dopaminergic agent, and benzodiazepine. Truly

**Pharmacotherapy**

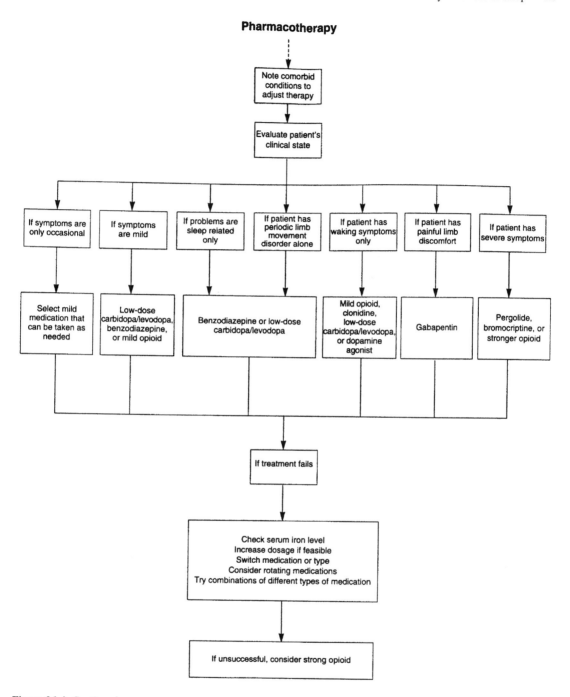

**Figure 26-4.** *Continued.*

refractory cases have responded to a long-acting opioid such as methadone or levorphanol.

Patients who complain of pain associated with RLS may do very well on gabapentin, at doses ranging from 300 to 1,800 mg per day. It is possible that other anticonvulsants (carbamazepine, valproate, lamotrigine) will be similarly useful in this context.

Some RLS or PLMD patients will have other medical or psychiatric disorders or be taking additional medications. These must be taken into account in planning RLS and PLMD therapy. For example, propranolol needs to be used very cautiously in patients with lung disease or diabetes and may cause excessively low blood pressure or hypotension in patients taking other medicines for high blood pressure. On the other hand, an RLS medication may also sometimes be beneficial for another condition. For example, clonidine or propranolol can benefit both RLS and high blood pressure. It may be possible to coordinate pharmacotherapy so that one medicine adequately treats two disorders.

Special care is required in treating children and pregnant women. In children, it is best to avoid pharmacotherapy if possible, concentrating on good sleep hygiene (regular bedtime and bedtime habits, cooling down period before bedtime, regular exercise) and perhaps avoidance of all caffeinated beverages, foods, and medications (including colas, chocolates, etc.).[422] If these procedures are inadequate, treatment with clonidine, L-dopa/carbidopa, or pergolide has been helpful (Picchietti, personal communication, 1997). In children with diagnoses of both RLS or PLMD and ADHD, both these agents have sometimes cured the sleep and the attention problems.[338,423] One study tested pergolide in children with tics and found pergolide was well tolerated and provided relief especially in children with RLS.[339] In pregnant women, most agents pose potential problems and possible teratogenicity. Therefore, medications should be avoided. RLS tends to get worse as pregnancy proceeds, so it may be possible to avoid medications at least until the third trimester, when they should do the least harm. Iron levels should be measured and corrected if at all low. If pharmacologic treatment is necessary, for the mother's sake (and perhaps her unborn child's), opioids are probably the first choice, because they seem not to be dangerous in this setting (Earley, personal communication, 1997).

## Other Motor Disturbances of Sleep

Most of the other motor disturbances of sleep are covered in other chapters, especially the chapter on parasomnias (Chapter 31). This section largely supplements that chapter by emphasizing some of the motoric aspects of the motor disturbances of sleep. What is crucial is that the motor disorders, in general, require a specific diagnostic approach and often share a differential diagnosis. After touching on some of the motoric aspects of these disorders, the chapter concludes with a discussion of general aspects of diagnosis and evaluation.

**Nocturnal Paroxysmal Dystonia and Related Conditions.** NPD was first described by Lugaresi's group as a condition that might be considered analogous to diurnal paroxysmal movement disorders.[424] NPD with short duration (seconds to minutes) attacks together with two other conditions, paroxysmal arousals[425,426] and episodic nocturnal wanderings,[427,428] have since been found to represent a spectrum of related disorders. They share the main features of sudden arousals or awakenings from NREM sleep and dyskinetic or semipurposive movements and vocalizations.

Short attacks of NPD begin with arousal, including an abrupt autonomic activation that can include substantial tachycardia, followed by dystonic movements and large-scale semipurposive movements of all limbs. Vocalizations are common. The attacks are quite diverse if considered between patients, but appear to be stereotyped in a single patient. Attacks last about 1 minute (range, 15 seconds to 2 minutes for typical attacks) and may be vaguely remembered. Neither tongue biting nor urinary incontinence is common. In some patients, the attacks are decidedly unilateral.[429] Other patients have been described with paroxysmal dystonic movements both during the day and night, both types of attacks thought to be epileptic.[430] Paroxysmal arousals[426] are brief attacks lasting several seconds in which patients awake abruptly from NREM sleep, perhaps with a start or cry, and have fleeting dyskinetic movements, then fall back to sleep. Episodic nocturnal wanderings[428,431] are attacks of sudden motor activity, including violent ambulation, loud vocalizations, and a variety of forceful gestures that can cause significant injury. The attacks commonly occur in stage II NREM sleep.

It has become increasingly clear that these represent a form of sleep-activated focal epilepsy.[426,428,432–434] Consistent with this etiology, there is an increased prevalence of seizures in patients, interictal EEG abnormalities, and the response of many patients to anticonvulsants (especially carbamazepine). Meierkord and colleagues demonstrated that the episodes of NPD overlap substantially in character with nocturnal attacks of patients with an established diagnosis of epilepsy.[433] It is also possible that there is some overlap in the pathophysiology of epileptic motor attacks and nonepileptic dystonia. Both are largely dependent on motor tracts descending from cortex to cause abnormal muscle activation and, in certain conditions, there may be a common basis.[430]

However, there may still remain a residual group of disorders that may not be of epileptic origin. In the original description, two cases had longer duration (2–50 minutes) attacks, with no epileptic associations.[435] In one case, a patient afflicted with such attacks for 20 years developed HD. There are a number of more recently described disorders of at least uncertain etiology. Lugaresi's group described a periodic form of NPD[436] that recurs every 30 seconds to 2 minutes with usually quite brief attacks (2–13 seconds' duration) and associated arousals that they called *atypical periodic movements in sleep*. While showing overlap with the short-lasting NPD, this condition was unresponsive to seizure medications, although one patient in the original series had a vascular orbital frontal tumor on CT and spikes on depth recording. Other such disorders include dystonic attacks provoked both by sleep and exercise,[437] apnea-associated paroxysmal dyskinetic movements,[438] and post-traumatic paroxysmal nocturnal hemidystonia.[439]

NPD events must be studied, best with video PSG and multichannel EEG, to determine whether they are consistent with epilepsy. They must also be distinguished from other eruptive motor events of sleep such as PLMS, RBD, nightmares, sleep terrors, and other parasomnias. In the absence of clear-cut evidence for an epileptic focus, the main distinction between NPD and RBD often hinges on the clear association of the latter with REM and the response of NPD to anticonvulsants. Although treatment of the epilepsy-like attacks with anticonvulsants, especially carbamazepine, is usually successful, treatment of the various nonepileptic attacks remains uncertain.

**Rapid Eye Movement Sleep Behavior Disorder.** Patients with RBD (see also Chapter 31) typically present with a history of vivid dreams and excessive movements in sleep, sometimes violent and causing injury to the patient or bed partner.[440–442] Such violent actions can also interfere with medical treatment, for example, newly emerging or becoming troublesome in the intensive care unit.[443] The condition may begin insidiously and progress over many years, with a so-called prodrome consisting primarily of vocalizations and limb jerks, reported in 17 of 70 patients in a large series described by Schenck and Mahowald.[444] Violent behavior may be specifically related to dream content, which is often repetitive and stereotyped and commonly involves the patient's engaging with some form of threat. For example, the patient may dream that he is rescuing his wife from attackers, although, at that time, he is actually striking her.[442]

Although RBD may occur at all ages, including childhood, it is far more common in the elderly. Men are more commonly afflicted than women, and there may be a familial tendency in some patients.[442] It has been suggested that the male predominance is related not to REM control, but to the different dream content of men and women.[445] Women with RBD do not have such violent dreams and therefore are not at the same risk for injury or so disturbing to the bed partner. Although it can clearly occur in otherwise healthy and neurologically intact individuals, RBD appears to have a significantly increased prevalence in those with neurodegenerative disorders or vascular lesions involving the brain stem.[446] It has been reported to occur in PD,[444] diffuse Lewy body disease,[447] OPCA,[448] MSA or Shy-Drager syndrome,[94] and corticobasal degeneration.[449] Either full-blown RBD or a subclinical variant, REM-sleep motor dysfunction, was found in 20 of 21 patients with MSA studied by PSG.[450] None had a complaint of RBD before study, suggesting that some degree of dysfunction, primarily vocalizations and REM without atonia, is an almost universal concomitant of MSA, which heavily involves the brain stem nuclei. In another series of 39 MSA patients, 27 voiced complaints consistent with RBD and 90% had REM-sleep motor dysfunction on PSG.[451] Similar transient conditions may occur in situations of drug toxicity or withdrawal as well as other conditions of acute brain insult.[442] Fluoxetine, which increases motor activity during various sleep stages,[452] may also be a cause of RBD at nontoxic levels.

It has become apparent that RBD may herald the onset of neurodegenerative diseases involving the brain stem. For instance, in a series of MSA cases collected by the Bologna group, 12 of 39 patients (44%) had RBD predating evident MSA by more than 1 year.[451] As discussed earlier, a prodrome of RBD has been noted in PD and a substantial fraction of patients with idiopathic RBD may go on to develop PD.[95]

Contrary to the usual predilection for the elderly, Schenck and Mahowald have reported RBD to be common in narcolepsy (more than 10% of PSG studied patients).[16] Narcolepsy, of course, involves various abnormalities of REM organization. This group is exceptional in the youthful age of onset of RBD (mean age of onset in Schenck and Mahowald's study was 28.4 years). These patients also had an elevated incidence of PLMS (in 10 of 17), another condition more typically associated with advanced years. Another younger group with evidence of REM motor dysfunction are RBD patients with post-traumatic stress disorder,[342] who also have disturbing dreams and waking visual intrusions, or "flashbacks."

Patients with this condition show increased EMG tone in the mentalis on PSG during REM sleep together with excessive phasic movement outbursts. Patients also have other sleep motor disturbances, with many having both PLMD and excessive fragmentary myoclonus in NREM sleep or other NREM periodic movements.[441,446] In a series reported by Schenck and Mahowald, 44 of 70 patients had PLMD and 28 of 70 had aperiodic NREM movements.[444] LaPierre and Montplaisir found in a small controlled series that the PLMS of RBD occurred as often in REM as NREM sleep.[283] They conclude that this occurs because the RBD patients lack a normal atonia that would mask the PLMS. One subgroup of relatively young patients has additional parasomnias, including somnambulism and sleep terrors, either as an essential disorder or secondary to other brain dysfunction.[453] Schenck and colleagues have called this condition *parasomnia overlap disorder* and note that, like RBD alone, it responds well to clonazepam (65% of 20 patients), alprazolam, carbamazepine, or, in one case, self-hypnosis.

Other than the motor disturbances, sleep architecture is usually normal in RBD patients, although patients may have greater than expected SWS and REM sleep for their age. In the Schenck and Mahowald series, 28 of 65 evaluable patients had increased REM percent (>25% of total sleep time) and 42 of 50 patients older than the age of 57 had increased SWS (>15% of total sleep time).[444] In another study of seven otherwise healthy elderly patients, Tachibana and colleagues[454] found normal sleep architecture. The patients had increases in both tonic REM sleep EMG and in phasic EMG increases, as measured in chin EMG. Their only other abnormality was an increase in REM density (number of REMs per minute of REM sleep).

Diagnosis relies on a mixture of clinical and PSG features. On PSG, the patients must have at least some tonic or phasic abnormality in muscle tone during REM (and usually will have both— LaPierre and Montplaisir have proposed that both should be required[283]). Violent, dream-related behaviors must be documented either by excessive, complex, or violent behaviors during PSG recorded REM sleep or a significant history of abrupt, dangerous, or sleep-disrupting behaviors. In addition, seizures must be excluded by suitable EEG recording.[442] The differential diagnosis includes those sleep disorders that cause disrupted movements and sleep, as well as awakenings, and would include somnambulism, night terrors, and NPD, as well as some cases of sleep apnea or PLMD. Dissociated states can also be confused with RBD. All of these can generally be discriminated by a combination of a careful sleep history, including interviewing of the bed partner, and adequate PSG (with video or observational monitoring, EMG leads on legs, and suitable EEG montage for seizure study).

Pathophysiologically, RBD appears to be a human analogue of REM sleep without atonia—a breakdown of the normal REM inhibition of the lower motor neuron with resulting translation of cortical impulses into motor behavior. It is, therefore, likely an abnormality of the higher regulatory centers. Animal models of this condition have been available for several decades, caused by specific lesions within the brain stem: Different lesions may cause different forms of behavioral abnormality.[31] The disruption may be specific to atonia, with normal descending drive intact, because, in one controlled study, patients had the same number of REMs as normal subjects.[283] Various pathologies that involve the brain stem may, therefore, cause RBD. One publication has suggested that the key pathology should be found in the pedunculopontine nucleus, which is involved in sleep regulation and damaged in PD.[455] One possible pathogenetic relationship between PD and RBD is suggested by the finding of Lewy bodies, the pathologic hallmark of PD, in the degenerated locus coeruleus of a nonparkinsonian patient with RBD.[456] Lewy body disease, therefore, may be another route to damaging the brain stem centers responsible for REM atonia.

Another potential route to RBD may be immunologic. In one report, it was noted that RBD patients had an increased frequency of the HLA class II antigen DQw1.[457] Attempts to find circulating antibodies to the locus coeruleus, a possible substrate for an immunologic pathophysiology, were unavailing, however,[458] so the significance of the HLA association remains uncertain.

Most patients respond well to clonazepam, which may be particularly effective in suppressing the dangerous, violent sleep behavior.[442] However, occasional breakthrough behaviors may occur, such that the patient's environment should be rendered safe even if treatment appears to be working. Other medications that may be effective include L-dopa (combined with carbidopa), clonidine,[444] and carbamazepine.[459] In one case report, a 64-year-old man appeared to be substantially benefited by melatonin.[460]

**Other Sleep-Related Movement Disorders.** Benign neonatal myoclonus, also a parasomnia, is a transient, sometimes familial condition that begins soon after birth and resolves within months.[461] The myoclonic jerks are brief, asynchronous, and repetitive, involving primarily the distal limbs, but also the trunk. The jerks occur during all stages of sleep, with most occurring in NREM sleep, and typically do not arouse or wake the infant.[462,463] The pathophysiology of this disorder is unknown. It is not typically associated with other nervous system disease and the EEG is not epileptogenic, distinguishing this condition from a seizure disorder.[464] It may be an exaggeration of the normally greater sleep-related movements in infants.[465]

Fragmentary myoclonus is considered a possible sleep disorder.[99] The abnormal movements of this condition are brief, asymmetric, focal jerks of the face and limbs that occur primarily during NREM sleep,[28] although they may occur in REM.[466] They are least common in SWS.[466] The associated EMG shows brief bursts (<150 msec) of variable amplitude, the larger bursts associated with visible movements. Fragmentary myoclonus may be associated with a variety of sleep disorders or occur in isolation.[28] Because the myoclonus is similar to the jerks of sleep starts or hypnic myoclonus, it may represent an exaggeration of normal sleep movements.

This condition may be another in which inadequate inhibitory drive fails to block descending activation from higher centers or it may represent a condition of excessive activation of higher centers during sleep.

Fatal familial insomnia (FFI)[467,468] is a prion disorder that involves progressive insomnia with derangement of sleep states,[469] loss of circadian rhythm and associated endocrine cycles,[470,471] autonomic abnormalities,[472] and abnormal motor signs, especially ataxia (loss of coordination) and myoclonus. It is classified as a medical/psychiatric sleep disorder associated with a neurologic disorder in the current sleep classification.[99] In some patients, the motor symptoms are the first to be noted.[467] The condition appears to be inherited in an autosomal dominant pattern (with parent to children of both sex transmission). Genetic linkage studies have established that the disease is related to a mutation in the prion protein that also causes Creutzfeldt-Jakob disease (CJD), a rapidly progressive dementia often accompanied by myoclonus. Indeed, the mutation in FFI is identical to that of one familial form of CJD (asparagine substituted for aspartic acid at locus 178 of the prion protein).[473] Familial manifestation as either FFI or CJD apparently depends on which common polymorphism occurs in the mutant allele at locus 129: Methionine results in FFI, whereas valine yields CJD. The primary pathology is a degeneration of the thalamic nuclei.[474] Although the disorder appears to be inexorably fatal, one report has suggested some relief from insomnia may be obtained with γ-hydroxybutyrate.[475]

A number of the more classic parasomnias, dealt with in Chapter 31, such as somnambulism, rhythmic movement disorder (formerly known as *head banging* or *jactatio capitis nocturna* for the paradigmatic form of this disorder), or bruxism, contain a prominent motor component. Therefore, they may be in the differential diagnosis for the other sleep-related motor disorders and, thus, must be kept in mind by the investigator who is studying an unknown sleep-related motor disturbance.

Somnambulism, for instance, might be considered in the differential diagnosis of RBD or NPD, conditions that may involve similar motor activity in sleep, or RLS, in which patients may wake up and seek relief in walking. Somnambulism in adults, like RBD, may be a frequent cause of injury.[17] Like RBD, which it may resemble, somnambulism responds well to clonazepam.

Rhythmic movement disorder may need to be distinguished from tremor or segmental myoclonias, as well as RBD or NPD, whereas bruxism may need to be distinguished from oromandibular dystonia. Bruxism declines in prevalence with age,[312] whereas rhythmic movement disorder is most common in prepubertal children. However, there are older children[476] and also adults[477,478] who will show persistent rhythmic movement. These disorders can also cause significant injury. Most rhythmic movements occur at sleep onset or in NREM sleep, but rarely a case may show a REM predominance.[479] It is also to be remembered that in some patients, such as children with tics, such parasomnias may be more common. This may also be true in patients with diurnal movement disorders, especially elderly patients suffering from a degenerative process. In evaluating the significance of parasomnias found in a patient with another motor disturbance of sleep, however, it should be remembered that parasomnias are quite common in children, especially if they are only occasional, and also of increased occurrence in the elderly. Therefore, their association with another motor disturbance of sleep may be a benign coincidence.

## SOME REMARKS ABOUT SPECIAL CONSIDERATIONS FOR EVALUATING AND TREATING DISORDERS OF THE MOTOR SYSTEM IN SLEEP

### *History and Examination*

As in all sleep disorders, a detailed sleep history is important in evaluating these patients. A sleep diary and specific questions about sleep symptoms will prove useful, as in the general sleep patient. Frequency and timing of the movements are also important to note, because these may provide diagnostic clues or indicate how likely studies are to uncover the nature of the movements. In women, the relation of the disorder to pregnancy or the menstrual cycle should be ascertained. The history should also include all associated medical conditions, whether neurologic or referable to other organ systems, because a motor sleep disturbance may be secondary to an antecedent medical condition. All medications should also be ascertained, because they may cause secondary motor

and sleep disturbances, aggravate pre-existing conditions, or even mask some sleep problems serendipitously (as pain medications can ameliorate RLS).

In patients with movement disorders, it is important to elucidate the relation and timing of the sleep complaint relative to the motor disease and its treatment. It is important to consider whether the sleep problem is due to the movement disorder itself (in which case management may be directed at the symptoms of the movement disorder as a first approach), a secondary consequence of the movement disorder, independent of the movement disorder (as a pre-existing condition or one only coincidentally present, which may be then best addressed by the specific therapy for the sleep problem), or a consequence of the treatment of the movement disorder (in which case therapy might be adjusted, if feasible). This categorization will provide some guidance as to which way therapy should be directed. The sleep specialist may need to become somewhat familiar, through reading or consultation, with the features of the movement disorder. Obtaining a clear picture from a referring neurologist or movement disorder specialist, through discussion or review of notes and summaries, of the evaluation and treatment of the patient's movement disorder is often critical to rational advice and therapy. Ideally, there will be an active collaboration, when needed, between a sleep medicine specialist and a specialist capable of handling the movement disorder itself.

Because motor sleep disturbances are not generally evident in the physician's office, and may provide little that could assist diagnosis on physical examination, it is important to probe more deeply into the patient's symptoms than is usually the case. The bed partner may provide a wealth of information about movements; their timing during the night; patient drowsiness during the daytime; and the frequency of motor disturbances, noises, confusion, and hallucinations. As appropriate, all of these should be discussed because the patient may be unaware of these phenomena. We have found it helpful to probe waking movements by asking the patient to re-enact them in the office, discussing whether they can be suppressed, finding details of how the patient handles the movements or uncomfortable sensations (as in RLS), and eliciting provocative factors, such as time of day or night, position, and so forth. When patients do not freely provide information on their own, we have sometimes modeled potential movements for them, to show them what might have occurred.

It is important to probe specific features of the patients' histories when particular diagnoses are under consideration. For example, in considering whether epilepsy might figure in the clinical picture, it is important to ask about such sequelae of epileptic attacks as incontinence, tongue biting, or muscle soreness. In considering the possibility of RBD, it is important to determine the character of the movements, whether they can injure the patient or whether the patient actually leaves the bed in the course of the attack.

Some motor conditions, such as RLS, may have a familial clustering. It is important, therefore, to attempt to obtain a thorough family history. In cases of RLS, this may require independent interviewing of other family members because, we have found, the symptoms of RLS are often not communicated to other family members, even those who might be expected to be quite close. For example, we interviewed two sisters, both single and in weekly contact with each other, each of whom was severely affected by RLS and unaware that the other sister was also affected. Although this concern may be diminishing as RLS becomes better known in the press, it still remains a concern when a familial pattern is important to establish.

As a final consideration, in this day of the personal videocameras, many patients may own home videotaping equipment and may be willing to take some videos of the patient's movements awake or asleep. These can provide unique invaluable insights into the patient's situation.

In sleep-related motor disturbances, as in sleep disturbances generally, a variety of paper instruments—symptom checklists, lists of sleep complaints, sleep logs, or questionnaires aimed at specific sleep symptoms (e.g., EDS[480])—can be helpful in delineating the clinical picture. In using such instruments, it is important to review them with regard to relevant motor complaints. It is also important to use bed partners or others close to the patient as additional sources of information. These individuals may provide better information about the nature, severity, and frequency of the sleep problem than patients do. They may have unique insights into what causes awakenings in patients and can describe the extent and characteristics of abnormal movements.

## Sleep Studies

Standard sleep studies have been held to be of established worth in evaluating motor disturbances of sleep.[481] A standard polysomnogram, with at least one EMG lead for the legs, provides a fair amount of information about motor disturbances. This should be supplemented by technician observations, wherever feasible, to explain motor events on the record. Where motor disturbances are the primary concern and seizures are in the differential diagnosis, it is helpful to perform video PSG. In an optimal set-up, this may include multiple EEG channels, as for a regular EEG study (8–12 channels in a montage that can span the head and provide information about frontal and temporal activity), split screen recording, and a facility for playing back the EEG record at the conventional daytime paper speed of 30 mm per second.

The following sections include a number of suggestions about the use of different modalities for studying motor phenomenon in sleep, then comment on alternate schemes from the regular polysomnogram for assessing sleep-related motor disturbances. PSG, together with the Multiple Sleep Latency Test (MSLT), has been accepted as having established value for studies of PLMD as well as for studies of movements that can provoke violence in sleep (which includes RBD, seizures, somnambulism, and related conditions).[340,481,482]

### Polysomnography

In deciding how to proceed with PSG, it is important to think about what conditions are being studied. Because the differential of unknown motor disorders of sleep is relatively broad, it is usually important to monitor breathing as well as to obtain extensive EEG and EMG recordings. Accurate technician observation and videotaping may be extremely helpful in conducting studies that yield accurate diagnoses.

**Electroencephalography Montages.**    The standard sleep study may use only two EEG leads—a central lead (C3-A2 or C4-A1) together with an occipital lead (O1, O2, or Oz linked to an ear electrode). However, in cases where seizures may be in the differential, as in unknown motor disorders of sleep, more elaborate montages may be necessary to adequately rule out seizure activity. Special electrodes may be required (see Chapter 34 on sleep and epilepsy as well as Chapter 6 on PSG techniques).

**Electromyography Recording.** Standard sleep recording uses the chin EMG and leads on one or both legs for evaluation of possible PLMS. Where a specific motor complaint is noted that involves movement of other body parts—arms, trunk, abdomen, neck, or face—additional leads can be applied. Most laboratories perform EMGs with a standard EEG filter setting (bandpass of 5–70 Hz), but the first and last authors have found that more artifact-free recording can be obtained if a higher bandpass (e.g., 50–1,500 Hz) is used. These frequencies better match the frequency of actual muscle potentials. It is also useful to set the amplitude before the study so that a maximal voluntary contraction is near or slightly above the full pen excursion for a polygraphic recorder.

**Videotaping.** Videotape studies can be extremely helpful in sorting out various abnormal movements or gaining some insight into their severity.[483] This can permit correlation of paper records of movement or EMG potentials with actual movements and allow, in some cases, distinguishing further the character of the movements. Split screen studies, with polygraphic montages correlated directly with videotaping of the associated behavior, are especially helpful in this regard. Patients may also have different categories of movements that may be distinguished by the videotape record, but not the PSG. To provide best natural conditions, infrared cameras are optimal, although many modern color video cameras can perform under relatively low light conditions. If possible, subjects should sleep with minimal covers, because this makes visualization of movements much easier. To do this, carefully temperature-controlled rooms, especially warmer ones, are helpful. Time bases, including those added by special effects generators or an on-screen clock, can facilitate search and retrieval of movements.

In one study of the utility of video PSG, Aldrich and Jahnke[484] found that, in 86 patients without known epilepsy who had reported abnormal motor activity in sleep, these studies provided useful diagnostic information for 52 patients. Fully 69% of those with prominent motor activity received such information. In 36 patients with known epilepsy, the studies provided useful diagnostic information about unclear motor phenomena in 28 (78%). For both groups of patients, the diagnostic outcomes included both seizure and nonseizure disorders. The authors emphasize that ability to play back the record at slower speed, afforded by some digital EEG systems, improves the ability to discriminate seizure activity from other motor phenomena. They also emphasize, as is generally true of PSGs to evaluate motor abnormalities, that yield increases with the frequency of the disturbance. Conditions that manifest every night can usually be usefully evaluated.

*Home-Based Polysomnography*

A variety of systems are available for home or ambulatory monitoring of sleep, with capacity that can now include 16 or more channels. Most of the customary sleep monitors can be used in the ambulatory setting. Generally, technicians prepare the patient for study either in the laboratory or at home. The various channels are recorded on tape for later display and analysis with computer systems. The advantage of these systems is that they reduce the personnel required and can reduce cost. This may permit analysis of less-frequent phenomena than those profitably studied in the laboratory or permit repeated studies to guide therapeutic options. In addition, the patient is studied under his or her normal conditions in the more relevant home environment. However, because these systems lack supervision, clear identification of abnormal events may not be feasible. Therefore, for diagnostic purposes, they may best be used as screening procedures, rather than a full substitute for laboratory-based PSG.[485] Once a clear question is available (How well is the patient sleeping? How many typical events occur?) they may provide more exact answers to questions.

*Other Recording Systems*

The static charge sensitive bed is a device,[486] suitable for adult and pediatric[487] recordings, that is highly sensitive to movements, including such physiologic movements as those associated with breathing or the heart beat. Different kinds of movement, such as body movements or respiratory pauses, can be differentiated by selective filtration of the potentials transmitted by the bed.[488] This can allow for quantification of sleep states[489] or for counting of movements. Because the bed itself is rather simple and not particularly expensive, it may offer an alternative to some PSG in the future, although, like other simplified recording systems, it is not as yet as accurate as PSG in detailing sleep states and associated movements.[490] It has been reported to have good accuracy in quantifying PLMS.[491]

*Automatic Scoring of Sleep Studies*

One of the more interesting and challenging current developments in the sleep field is the development of technologies based on digitized PSGs that are processed by computer and stored on electronic media. This leads, in some cases, to "paperless" records. As a corollary of the computerized processing of studies, it becomes possible to perform automatic sleep analysis. This can offer the advantage of decreased scorer time; more consistent scoring criteria; and the ability to readily redisplay, reformat, and rescore records. Quantitation of normal and abnormal sleep phenomena becomes substantially easier. As a result, cost may decrease, although this has not yet happened. All current digital systems are still in a state of development. An experienced scorer can extract more information from a record and can respond far more flexibly to altered recording conditions.[492] The long-term prospect, nevertheless, is that digital systems with automatic scoring will continue to play an ever-increasing role in the field of sleep studies. We believe that these systems are becoming the predominant ones used for sleep studies, whether in a sleep laboratory or in the ambulatory setting. New techniques using frequency decomposition,[493,494] neural network algorithms,[495,496] or both[497] are among the currently promising techniques for advancing this field.

In the area of motor disturbances, the greatest promise of automatic scoring is the ability to score PLMS, whose stereotyped form allows for relatively simple discrimination of PLMS from non-PLMS. A number of systems for such scoring are currently available, with reasonable reliability with respect to human scorers. Kayed and colleagues reported one system that matched human performance, but on occasion disregarded PLMS not meeting exact criteria that were accepted by the human scorers.[498] In scoring PLMS, one distinct advantage of these systems is the ability to readily prepare graphic displays of the movements and to analyze them quantitatively. Other possible functions of automated scoring in the area of motor function may be the quantification of muscle activity (such as chin EMG), as by rectification and integration, and automatic scoring of movement time epochs. It should also be possible to relate various motor activities to other sleep events, such as arousals, awakenings, or K complexes.

In the more distant future, the combination of expert systems with digital PSG may lead to scoring and record analysis that far exceeds the capacity of even the most experienced scorer.

*Activity Monitoring*

Activity monitoring or actigraphy is the technique of quantifying and recording movements. A value for movement is determined and assigned to a sample period that can range from a few milliseconds up to many hours. Actigraphy can be used for various purposes: to measure the degree of movement, to demonstrate circadian or other cyclical patterns of movement, and to discriminate wake from sleep.[1]

Activity monitoring has a number of advantages over sleep-laboratory PSG or even ambulatory PSG monitoring. First, it can be efficiently and inexpensively used for extended periods. Depending on the equipment and technique used, recordings can be made for many days or even months. In assessing sleep disorders, this extended recording can allow for the capture of rare events, overcoming the problem of variability, which can limit the accuracy of more abbreviated studies, and permit repeated measurement of sleep in different conditions (disease progression or remission, therapeutic responses). One of the major problems with the movement disorders in sleep is the large night-to-night variation in expression of the disorder. Sleepwalking may occur only once a week or even less often. PLMs in sleep correlate across three consecutive nights at significant but at relatively low levels ($r^2 = 0.36$–$0.64$). The correlations for amount of wake time appear to be even lower and not consistently significant ($r^2 = 0.30$–$0.62$).[499] Thus, although a one-night PSG may suffice for diagnosis for severe cases, it is less satisfactory for determining severity. Even for diagnostic purposes, the one-night PSG is likely to miss some significant cases. Indeed a three-night study of 46 healthy seniors (28 with PLMs) included one who had no PLMs on one night and 37 per hour on another night.[500] Moreover, the night-to-night variation in PLM rate for the elderly is estimated to be four times larger than that for sleep-related breathing disorders.[501] Although adequate for evaluating sleep-related breathing disorders, the one-night PSG is probably not satisfactory for PLMD. This instability in PLM rate seriously hampers both clinical treatments and research studies. For example, the degree of morbidity due to PLMD has been controversial. Clinical studies in the elderly indicate that PLMD is a major cause of insomnia in the elderly[502] but surveys have been inconsistent in finding relations between PLMs and subjective symptoms.[285,286,503] It appears individuals differ greatly in the degree to which these movements disturb their functioning. The clinical presentation of RLS syndrome similarly shows marked night-to-night variation. Patients with a mild degree of symptoms report they may occur only about once every week or so. Thus, given the large variability between individuals and across nights and in some cases the unpredictable nature of a significant but rare event, the study of many movement disorders of sleep needs to involve fairly large sample sizes and multiple night recordings. The inconvenience and expense of the PSG currently makes this technique impractical for such extended or repeated studies. The usual ambulatory PSG alternatives (such as the Vitalog or Oxford Medilog systems) are also both expensive and inconvenient because they still require staff intervention (e.g., for applying EMG electrodes). Second, because the activity monitors are usually small, light weight, and self-contained, activity monitoring can occur in multiple settings, including the home, and in varied activity states. The activity monitors can be taken out of the laboratory, self-applied, and even transmitted by mail. They may be useful in uncooperative patient groups with degenerative disease who would not tolerate a laboratory sleep study[504,505] and may simplify large studies of therapeutic interventions in insomnia or other sleep disturbances. Third, some PSG channels, such as EMG, may indicate activity that is not, in fact, significant for the patient. Activity monitoring can discriminate actual movement from EMG potentials, which may occur without any significant displacement of a limb.

The limitations on activity monitoring result from the relatively nonspecific results and the limited information monitored. The results are generally nonspecific because all movement, even transmitted movement, is recorded. Certain nonspecific movements, such as gravity or almost constant velocity

movement (e.g., as in a car on a highway), can be largely eliminated by filtering, but activity monitors may not discriminate between normal or abnormal movements or even active and passive movements. As discussed later, this limitation is being overcome to some extent by additional processing of activity recordings. The information obtained by activity monitoring is limited because there may be no information about cerebral state (EEG), eye movements (too small to be reflected in a limb monitor), or breathing. Therefore, they do not provide much useful information about physiologic state and crucial information about exact sleep stages.

Typically, activity-monitoring devices use accelerometry to quantify movement. Several small self-contained devices currently available provide a direct assessment of the amount of activity or body movement at the point of the body where they are attached. These are all derived from the work of Coleman and Smith, who produced the first of these meters and documented the methods for others to use.[506] Virtually all of these use a piezoelectric sensor (usually a ceramic bender unit). The ceramic bender generates its own electric current that is directly proportional to the amount of acceleration. The activity devices usually include a volatile memory chip and a small computer or micro-controller chip. They are programmed to determine the amount of activity in a unit time and record that amount at a determined storage frequency. The activity accepted by these devices is usually filtered so that they cover the dominant frequency ranges for human movement of approximately 0.5 to 10.0–15.0 Hz.[507] Later the data are downloaded to a computer, typically a desktop or laptop PC, usually through a special interface device. Various manipulations can then be performed on the downloaded data for further quantification or illustration. The activity data are maintained with a time-date code so that the activity can be analyzed by the time of each day recorded. The self-contained units are battery powered; current models provide batteries capable of actively recording for from 14 days to 4 years. Although shorter battery life does limit the maximum duration of the recording, battery life should increase as this technology develops. Another limitation on the duration of monitoring is the amount of computer memory available to retain the stored values. Currently, the memory size available for these monitors is 32–1,024 Kb. Duration of monitoring is inversely proportional to the rate at which values are stored. For low storage frequencies (e.g., once every minute), these capacities translate into a total monitoring period of 22–720 days. However, at high storage rates useful for examining individual movements (e.g., 10 per second), total monitoring would only be from about 50 minutes up to 28 hours.

These devices all use internal circuitry to sample the output voltage at a certain frequency (sample frequency or rate). The amount of activity can be determined by checking the number of times the voltage reaches or exceeds a minimum criteria (threshold crossing) or by some integration or summation of the total voltage from the individual samples. Integration provides the more sensitive approach, especially for examining individual movements as opposed to total activity. After a certain number of samples, the result in total threshold crosses or integrated voltage is stored. The storage frequency or rate limits the time resolution of this technique. For assessing total activity occurring in spans of a few seconds to minutes, the digital sampling can be at relatively low rates (e.g., 4–8 Hz) and still provide an adequate measurement. But for higher storage frequencies designed to examine individual movements, a sampling frequency of 10–40 Hz is probably necessary. Storage rates of 10 Hz or more would be ideal although slower movements can be analyzed with storage rates perhaps as low as 1 Hz.

One main use of activity monitoring has been in the multiday assessment of sleep and wake. Whereas the determination of circadian activity patterns through activity monitoring is well worked out,[508] the assessment of sleep has been less clear. Sleep as determined by activity monitoring, with monitors typically placed on the nondominant wrist, has been compared to that indicated on PSG and shows both random and systematic errors.[509] In one study, three-fourths of 36 patients with insomnia assessed for 3 days with both actigraphy and PSG showed a mean discrepancy of less than 1 hour per night, but one-fourth showed a larger discrepancy.[510] This has led to recommendations by the American Sleep Disorders Association (ASDA) that actigraphy be used primarily as an adjunct to detailed history and other examinations to reveal multiday rest-activity patterns with implications for the diagnosis, severity grading, and treatment response of sleep disorders.[511] Some efforts have

been made to increase the accuracy of sleep detection by further processing the activity measures.[512–515] One of the authors (Allen) and colleagues have shown that activity during the night's sleep has a small hysteresis effect for state changes between sleep and waking so that the duration of inactivity preceding sleep onset after a period of wakefulness depends on the prior state as defined by length of the preceding awakening.[516] Using this finding and comparing results to a PSG standard, 90% of the 30-second epochs were correctly identified as sleep or wake in 10 normals and 77% of epochs in 10 insomniacs.[517] This would yield a substantial improvement in summed sleep states over the whole night.

For movement disorders, the activity monitor is placed at the site of the movement. In general, the goal of such recording is to count and quantify such movements, not merely to indicate when movement occurs. Various earlier studies showed that abnormal movements associated with hyperkinetic disorders could be quantified using actigraphy,[518,519] if appropriate filtering was used to select for frequencies associated with the movements. Early studies attempted such a quantitation in PLMS. The total movement activity during sleep for patients was determined from activity monitors worn on the ankle of the affected leg, but the correlations between overall activity and the number of PLM were not high ($r$ values of about 0.6).[520] This method is not adequate except possibly for evaluating treatment response.

The solution to this problem of weak correlation between total activity and specific abnormal movements may be a finer-grain analysis, which has now been attempted.[521] Such an analysis may challenge the capacities of most monitors. Recognizing the distinctive profile of individual movements requires matching the descriptive powers of an EMG record. To detect the onset and end of a specific movement requires sensitivity to higher-frequency components of the movement, necessitating sampling rates in the range of 10 to 40 Hz. Moreover, there are major data-storage problems for this condition. Abnormal PLMs are, by definition, greater than 0.5 seconds in duration (ASDA nosology[99]). Activity measurements of them must have storage frequencies of at least 4 Hz and preferably 8–10 Hz to enhance measurement accuracy. A fine-grain analysis with 40-Hz sampling and storage at 10 Hz available from one of these monitors (Individual Monitoring Services, Baltimore, MD) provides a description closely matching the EMG recordings for these movements. The recording time is, however, still limited to one night (14 hours).

An alternative has been developed by one of the authors (Allen) and colleagues that uses a computerized program in the monitor itself to detect the periodic movements and measure the duration and intensity of the movement as well as the interval between movements. These detections are based on sampling at 40 Hz. Storing the descriptive information about the movement along with total activity per second permits a review of machine scoring to determine if criteria are met for abnormal periodic movements of sleep or waking. This "two-pass" approach allows recording for 5–10 days using a monitor that has a 512-Kb memory. It provides an excellent agreement with the nocturnal PSG for number of leg movements with a correlation of 0.997 and an average error for rates per hour of less than 1.0.[522] Similar excellent agreement for periodic movement while lying awake has also been shown. These monitors may in the future permit determination of the abnormal patterns of periodic movement during the waking day providing for the first time a complete 24-hour picture of the involuntary movement characteristics of RLS.

The use of the new ambulatory monitors that provide this fine-grain analyses of movements might be further extended to assess other movement disorders in sleep, such as RBD or rhythmic movement disorder. But even such a development would fail to provide relevant information about the patient's sleep-wake state. This can be approached by adding illumination[504,523] or position information. To detect body position, a system developed by one of the coauthors (Allen) and colleagues requires wearing small monitors on the trunk and also on the leg just above the knee. Each monitor records position in three-dimensional space for each epoch (30 seconds to 1 minute), and the combination of the two provides a description of the overall body position as standing, sitting, reclining, supine, prone, or lying on the right or left side. These monitors, when compared to direct observation of a subject's body position, show an excellent overall agreement (contingency coefficients C = 0.85–0.91, maximum value of C for these data = 0.913).[524] Activity data collected at the same time as position data permits differentiating abnormal movements that occur while the patient is lying down from those while standing or sitting. It also permits the detection of events during the sleep time when the patient sits or stands up, such as occurs for sleepwalking.

### Daytime and Evening Evaluation

Patients with sleep motor disturbances can be evaluated with MSLT for EDS, as can sleep patients generally. The American Academy of Neurology now accepts these studies as useful for patients with a variety of sleep disorders who complain of EDS.[481]

Daytime sleep studies, sometimes done with sleep deprivation for the night before, can occasionally be useful in disclosing sleep motor disturbances, such as RLS or PLMS or may assist in the evaluation of a patient with possible epilepsy. However, negative studies under these conditions are not helpful and the limited yield of daytime studies makes full nighttime monitoring far more desirable.

There is a great need for developing a test for the waking movements and discomfort of RLS. A number of investigators have proposed preliminary tests that allow for quantification of movements through EMG, videotapes, or actigraphy, together with subjective indicators of abnormal sensations.[524a] In our studies, we have asked patients to lie quietly for up to 90 minutes. Patients rated the severity of uncomfortable sensations every 10 or 15 minutes; involuntary movements were counted by EMG, and restlessness by actigraphy[525] (Figure 26-5). Other forms of an immobilization test, such as the Forced Immobilization Test (FIT),[526] in which patients' legs are restrained in bed in an extended position for 1 hour, or the SIT,[303] may be used to elicit sensory complaints and involuntary movements. Patients press a button at the onset of every abnormal sensation, while movements are quantified by EMG. The first and third authors and colleagues have modified this test through instructions and with activity monitoring to measure either the involuntary[301] or restless voluntary movements[302] of RLS.

## SUMMARY

The past quarter century has witnessed a great increase in knowledge about the motor disorders

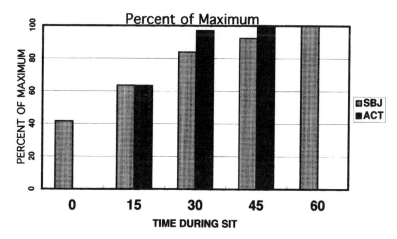

**Figure 26-5.** Restless legs syndrome discomfort (SBJ) ($N = 7$) and summed actigraphic measures of restlessness (ACT) ($N = 6$) during modified Subjective Immobilization Tests (SITs). During the test, patients sat with their legs maintained in an extended position for 1 hour. This was repeated at different times for a total of 14–17 SITs per subject; the values from individual SITs were then averaged for each patient and the final value obtained by averaging across the subjects. Subjective measures were obtained with a 10-point visual analogue scale related to leg discomfort administered every 15 minutes from the beginning of the test (time = 0); actigraphic measures were obtained by summing the movement counts from an activity meter (Minimitter, Inc.) for 15-minute intervals that included the second through fourth subjective assessment. To compare values, the data are presented as a percent of maximum averaged value, which was the last subjective assessment (time = 60 minutes) and the last actigraphic sum (interval spanning time = 45 minutes). The first 5 minutes and last 10 minutes of the SIT were not counted in the actigraphic assessment to avoid including counts associated with the start and end of the SIT.

and sleep. New disorders—such as RBD and NPD—have been described, and other disorders, such as RLS, have been clarified. The importance of sleep dysfunction in the diurnal movement disorders, especially PD and related conditions, has been established. From the viewpoint of treatment, new therapies, both for long-known and recently described disorders, have been developed.

Newly developed techniques such as brain imaging and genetic analysis promise that an explosion of knowledge about brain function will also lead to much better answers about why sleep is needed and how it is regulated. We may also gain a much better understanding of how motor disturbances of sleep intrude on normal function. These answers should help provide guides for more specific therapy. Advances in understanding the genetics of a number of conditions, both diurnal movement disorders and sleep disorders such as RLS, may provide specific clues as to how the sleep-regulating system is disordered.

Currently, we are beginning to develop a sharper picture of how both normal and abnormal move-

ments are controlled during sleep. In the normal or "ideal" case, there are three discrete states: waking, NREM sleep, and REM sleep.[14] Both sleep states act to provide two key functions: a relative dissociation of higher sleep centers from the external world and from lower levels of the nervous system and a partial suppression of overt motor activity. The waking state, in contrast, attempts to optimize association between higher centers, lower centers, and the world, and to facilitate motor expression. The two sleep states differ in the autonomous activity of higher centers, which appears to be much greater in REM sleep. Both normal movements and most abnormal movements due to diurnal movement disorders show a characteristic pattern in sleep. They are most likely to occur during the lightest stages of sleep (stage I NREM), often in association with lightenings or arousals. They are less likely to occur in stage II NREM or REM sleep and least likely to occur in SWS or during deepening sleep. This pattern seems to be followed by those movement disorders whose presumed generator is in a higher motor center, either cortical or subcortical. In contrast, movements generated at the segmental level or at the level of the motor neuron are relatively resistant to modulation by sleep, perhaps because their mere presence is evidence for a reduced degree of higher control.

NREM and REM sleep disorders involve separate but interrelated sensorimotor dysfunctions. NREM disorders, such as many parasomnias, RLS, and PLMD, are activated by repose and sleep. In the case of RLS, the activation may begin in the predormital phase, as relaxation and drowsiness overshadow awake alertness. Presumably, these conditions arise, especially RLS and PLMD, because of some changing control from higher centers that allows the expression of a more primitive motor rhythmicity. In case of parasomnias that are similar to normal motor behavior, such as somnambulism or somniloquy, the major defect may be an excessive activity of higher centers or a relative failure of the NREM motor inhibitory system. NREM disorders probably would occur during REM sleep as well, as seen with PLMD in the RBD[283] and narcolepsy,[284] but the additional inhibition that occurs during REM sleep suppresses them. REM disorders, by contrast, involve some shift in the critical REM sleep balance between excitation and inhibition. Although the exact changes are not clear, it seems most likely that this is a change in higher influence and most likely a deficiency in inhibitory systems in the brain stem, as analogous to the animal lesion models of REM sleep without atonia.[31] A unifying thesis for both NREM and REM disorders is that they can involve a failure of descending inhibition. The different conditions are likely to involve partially distinct, but related inhibitory processes.

NREM and REM disorders, then, are likely to be activated by processes that impinge on the inhibitory systems of the brain stem. Because the balance between excitation and inhibition is fairly exacting, a variety of different influences, such as neurodegenerative disorders or even normal aging, may result in the emergence of disorders. Conditions, such as narcolepsy, that are associated with poor state regulation, are very likely to be associated with additional NREM and REM disorders— hence the report that narcoleptics at a young age may have both PLMD and RBD.[16] The overall inter-relatedness of failures of sleep inhibitory control can be seen in two further facts. First, that REM and NREM disorders often overlap. For example,

there is a high incidence of PLMD and fragmentary myoclonus in RBD.[444] Second, that certain medications, such as the benzodiazepines and dopaminergic agents, may be useful in a number of the NREM and REM motor disturbances, as well as in state dyscontrol conditions such as narcolepsy.

The further resolution of the pathophysiology of motor disturbances of sleep will now await a more exact understanding of the sleep regulatory systems of the brain, especially those responsible for the descending inhibition of the segmental and effector levels of the motor system.

## REFERENCES

1. Tryon WW. Activity Measurement in Psychology and Medicine. New York: Plenum, 1991.
2. Weiner WJ, Lang AE. Movement Disorders: A Comprehensive Survey. Mt. Kisco, NY: Futura, 1989.
3. Chokroverty S. Movement Disorders. Costa Mesa, CA: PMA, 1990.
4. Marsden CD, Fahn S. Movement Disorders 3. Boston: Butterworth–Heinemann, 1994.
5. Watts RL, Koller WC. Movement Disorders: Neurologic Principles and Practice. New York: McGraw-Hill, 1997.
6. Fauct A, Braunwald E, Isselbacher KJ, et al. Harrison's Principles of Internal Medicine (14th ed). New York: McGraw-Hill, 1997.
7. Rowland LP. Merritt's Textbook of Neurology (9th ed). Philadelphia: Lea & Febiger, 1995.
8. Lauerma H, Lehtinen I, Lehtinen P, et al. Laterality of motor activity during normal and disturbed sleep. Biol Psychiatry 1992;32:191.
9. Minors DS, Waterhouse JM. Circadian rhythms and their mechanisms. Experientia 1986;42:1.
10. Fish DR, Sawyers D, Allen PJ, et al. The effect of sleep on the dyskinetic movements of Parkinson's disease, Gilles de la Tourette syndrome, Huntington's disease, and torsion dystonia. Arch Neurol 1991;48:210.
11. McGregor P, Thorpy MJ, Schmidt-Nowara WW, et al. T-sleep: an improved method for scoring breathing-disordered sleep. Sleep 1992;15:359.
12. Terzano MG, Mancia D, Salati MR, et al. The cyclic alternating pattern as a physiological component of normal NREM sleep. Sleep 1985;8:137.
13. Terzano MG, Parrino L. Clinical applications of cyclic alternating pattern. Physiol Behav 1993;54:807. (Published erratum appears in Physiol Behav 1994;55:199.)
14. Mahowald MW, Schenck CH. Status dissociatus—a perspective on states of being. Sleep 1991;14:69.
15. Lugaresi E, Cirignotta F, Coccagna G, Montagna P. Nocturnal Myoclonus and Restless Legs Syndrome. In S Fahn, CD Marsden, M Van Woert (eds), Myoclonus. New York: Raven, 1986;295.

16. Schenck CH, Mahowald MW. Motor dyscontrol in narcolepsy: rapid-eye-movement (REM) sleep without atonia and REM sleep behavior disorder. Ann Neurol 1992;32:3.

17. Schenck CH, Milner DM, Hurwitz TD, et al. A polysomnographic and clinical report on sleep-related injury in 100 adult patients. Am J Psychiatry 1989;146:1166.

18. Santamaria J, Chiappa KH. The EEG of drowsiness in normal adults. J Clin Neurophysiol 1987;4:327.

19. Oswald I. Sudden bodily jerks on falling asleep. Brain 1959;82:92.

20. Broughton R. Pathological Fragmentary Myoclonus, Intensified Sleep Starts and Hypnagogic Foot Tremor: Three Unusual Sleep Related Disorders. In WP Koella (ed), Sleep 1986. New York: Fischer, 1988;240.

21. Dyken ME, Yamada T, Lin-Dyken DC, et al. Diagnosing narcolepsy through the simultaneous clinical and electrophysiologic analysis of cataplexy. Arch Neurol 1996;53:456.

22. Bell CC, Dixie-Bell DD, Thompson B. Further studies on the prevalence of isolated sleep paralysis in black subjects. J Natl Med Assoc 1986;78:649.

23. Fukuda K, Miyasita A, Inugami M, Ishihara K. High prevalence of isolated sleep paralysis: *kanashibari* phenomenon in Japan. Sleep 1987;10:279.

24. Takeuchi T, Miyasita A, Sasaki Y, et al. Isolated sleep paralysis elicited by sleep interruption. Sleep 1992;15:217.

25. Andermann E, Andermann F, Silver K, et al. Benign familial nocturnal alternating hemiplegia of childhood. Neurology 1994;44:1812.

26. Dagnino N, Loeb C, Massazza G, Sacco G. Hypnic physiological myoclonus in man: an EEG-EMG study in normals and neurological patients. Eur Neurol 1969;2:47.

27. Montagna P, Liguori R, Zucconi M, et al. Physiological hypnic myoclonus. Electroencephalogr Clin Neurophysiol 1988;70:172.

28. Broughton R, Tolentino MA, Krelina M. Excessive fragmentary myoclonus in NREM sleep: a report of 38 cases. Electroencephalogr Clin Neurophysiol 1985;61:121.

29. Gardner R Jr, Grossman WI. Normal Motor Patterns in Sleep in Man. In E Weitzman (ed), Advances in Sleep Research (Vol 2). New York: Spectrum, 1975;67.

30. Wilde-Frenz J, Schulz H. Rate and distribution of body movements during sleep in humans. Percept Mot Skills 1983;56:275.

31. Hendricks JC, Morrison AR, Mann GL. Different behaviors during paradoxical sleep without atonia depend on pontine lesion site. Brain Res 1982;239:81.

32. McCarley RW. Dreams and the Biology of Sleep. In MH Kryger, T Roth, WC Dement (eds), Principles and Practice of Sleep Medicine (2nd ed). Philadelphia: Saunders, 1994;373.

33. De Koninck J, Lorrain D, Gagnon P. Sleep positions and position shifts in five age groups: an ontogenetic picture. Sleep 1992;15:143.

34. Kohyama J. A quantitative assessment of the maturation of phasic motor inhibition during REM sleep. J Neurol Sci 1996;143:150.

35. Ohnaka T, Tochihara Y, Kanda K. Body movements of the elderly during sleep and thermal conditions in bedrooms in summer. Appl Human Sci 1995;14:89.

36. Grillner S. Neurobiological bases of rhythmic motor acts in vertebrates. Science 1985;228:143.

37. Grillner S, Dubuc R. Control of locomotion in vertebrates: spinal and supraspinal mechanisms. Adv Neurol 1988;47:425.

38. Mortin LI, Stein PS. Spinal cord segments containing key elements of the central pattern generators for three forms of scratch reflex in the turtle. J Neurosci 1989;9:2285.

39. Kandel ER, Schwartz JH, Jessell TM. Principles of Neural Science. New York: Elsevier, 1991.

40. Steriade M, Hobson JA. Neuronal activity during the sleep-waking cycle. Prog Neurobiol 1976;6:155.

41. Evarts EV. Temporal patterns of discharge of pyramidal tract neurons during sleep and waking in the monkey. J Neurophysiol 1964;27:152.

42. Imon H, Ito K, Dauphin L, McCarley RW. Electrical stimulation of the cholinergic laterodorsal tegmental nucleus elicits scopolamine-sensitive excitatory postsynaptic potentials in medial pontine reticular formation neurons. Neuroscience 1996;74:393.

43. Chase MH, Morales FR. The Control of Motoneurons During Sleep. In MH Kryger, T Roth, WC Dement (eds), Principles and Practice of Sleep Medicine (2nd ed). Philadelphia: Saunders, 1994;163.

44. Chase MH, Morales FR. The atonia and myoclonia of active (REM) sleep. Annu Rev Psychol 1990;41:557.

45. Morales FR, Boxer P, Chase MH. Behavioral state-specific inhibitory postsynaptic potentials impinge on cat lumbar motoneurons during active sleep. Exp Neurol 1987;98:418.

46. Yamuy J, Jimenez I, Morales F, et al. Population synaptic potentials evoked in lumbar motoneurons following stimulation of the nucleus reticularis gigantocellularis during carbachol-induced atonia. Brain Res 1994;639:313.

47. Pereda AE, Morales FR, Chase MH. Medullary control of lumbar motoneurons during carbachol-induced motor inhibition. Brain Res 1990;514:175.

48. Pompeiano O. The Neurophysiological Mechanisms of the Postural and Motor Events During Desynchronized Sleep. In SS Kety, EV Evarts, HL Williams (eds), Sleep and Altered States of Consciousness. Baltimore: Williams & Wilkins, 1967;351.

49. Soja PJ, Lopez-Rodriguez F, Morales FR, Chase MH. Effects of excitatory amino acid antagonists on the phasic depolarizing events that occur in lumbar motoneurons during REM periods of active sleep. J Neurosci 1995;15:4068.

50. Yamuy J, Mancillas JR, Morales FR, Chase MH. C-fos expression in the pons and medulla of the cat during carbachol-induced active sleep. J Neurosci 1993;13:2703.

51. Hodes R, Dement WC. Depression of electrically induced reflexes ("H-reflexes") in man during low voltage EEG "sleep." Electroencephalogr Clin Neurophysiol 1964;17:617.

52. Horner RL, Innes JA, Morrell MJ, et al. The effect of sleep on reflex genioglossus muscle activation by stimuli of negative airway pressure in humans. J Physiol (Lond) 1994;476:141.

53. Kimura J, Harada O. Excitability of the orbicularis oculi reflex in all night sleep: its suppression in non-rapid eye movement and recovery in rapid eye movement sleep. Electroencephalogr Clin Neurophysiol 1972;33:369.

54. Reding GR, Fernandez C. Effects of vestibular stimulation during sleep. Electroencephalogr Clin Neurophysiol 1968;24:75.

55. Hoshina Y, Sakuma Y. Changes in photically evoked blink reflex during sleep and wakefulness. Jpn J Ophthalmol 1991;35:182.

56. Kasper J, Diefenhardt A, Mackert A, Thoden U. The vestibulo-ocular response during transient arousal shifts in man. Acta Otolaryngol (Stockh) 1992;112:1.

57. Morrison AR, Sanford LD, Ball WA, et al. Stimulus-elicited behavior in rapid eye movement sleep without atonia. Behav Neurosci 1995;109:972.

58. Soja PJ, Oka JI, Fragoso M. Synaptic transmission through cat lumbar ascending sensory pathways is suppressed during active sleep. J Neurophysiol 1993;70:1708.

59. Cairns BE, Fragoso MC, Soja PJ. Active-sleep-related suppression of feline trigeminal sensory neurons: evidence implicating presynaptic inhibition via a process of primary afferent depolarization. J Neurophysiol 1996;75:1152.

60. Chiappa KH. Evoked Potentials in Clinical Medicine. (3rd ed). Philadelphia: Lippincott–Raven, 1997.

61. Erwin R, Buchwald JS. Midlatency auditory evoked responses: differential effects of sleep in human. Electroencephalogr Clin Neurophysiol 1986;65:383.

62. Litscher G. Continuous brainstem auditory evoked potential monitoring during nocturnal sleep. Int J Neurosci 1995;82:135.

63. Emerson RG, Sgro JA, Pedley TA, Hauser WA. State-dependent changes in the N20 component of the median nerve somatosensory evoked potential. Neurology 1988;38:64.

64. Nakano S, Tsuji S, Matsunaga K, Murai Y. Effect of sleep stage on somatosensory evoked potentials by median nerve stimulation. Electroencephalogr Clin Neurophysiol 1995;96:385.

65. Cairns BE, Fragoso MC, Soja PJ. Activity of rostral trigeminal sensory neurons in the cat during wakefulness and sleep. J Neurophysiol 1995;73:2486.

66. Miyazato H, Skinner RD, Reese NB, et al. Midlatency auditory evoked potentials and the startle response in the rat. Neuroscience 1996;75:289.

67. Hess CW, Mills KR, Murray NMF, Schriefer TN. Excitability of the human cortex is enhanced during REM sleep. Neurosci Lett 1987;82:47.

68. Fish DR, Sawyers D, Smith SJM, et al. Motor inhibition from the brainstem is normal in torsion dystonia during REM sleep. J Neurol Neurosurg Psychiatry 1991;54:140.

69. Rosler KM, Nirkko AC, Rihs F, Hess CW. Motor-evoked responses to transcranial brain stimulation persist during cataplexy: a case report. Sleep 1994;17:168.

70. Williams HL, Morlock HC Jr, Morlock JV. Instrumental behavior during sleep. Psychophysiology 1966;2:208.

71. Niiyama Y, Fujiwara R, Satoh N, Hishikawa Y. Endogenous components of event-related potential appearing during NREM stage 1 and REM sleep in man. Int J Psychophysiol 1994;17:165.

72. Hamon JF, Gauthier P, Gottesmann C. Event-related potentials in humans as indices of access to stored information during sleep. Acta Physiol Hung 1994;82:87.

73. Ikeda K, Morotomi T. Classical conditioning during human NREM sleep and response transfer to wakefulness. Sleep 1996;19:72.

74. Hennevin E, Hars B, Maho C, Bloch V. Processing of learned information in paradoxical sleep: relevance for memory. Behav Brain Res 1995;69:125.

75. Smith C. Sleep states, memory processes and synaptic plasticity. Behav Brain Res 1996;78:49.

76. De Koninck J, Christ G, Hebert G, Rinfret N. Language learning efficiency, dreams and REM sleep. Psychiatr J Univ Ott 1990;15:91.

77. Cirignotta F, Montagna P, Lugaresi E. Reversal of Motor Excitation to Motor Inhibition Induced by Sleep in Man. In M Chase, ED Weitzman (eds), Sleep Disorders: Basic and Clinical Research. New York: Spectrum, 1983;129.

78. Kleitman N. Sleep and Wakefulness. Chicago: University of Chicago Press, 1963.

79. Fujiki A, Shimizu A, Yamada Y, et al. The Babinski reflex during sleep and wakefulness. Electroencephalogr Clin Neurophysiol 1971;31:610.

80. Balkin TJ, Wesensten NJ, Braun AR, et al. Sleep-mediated changes in regional cerebral blood flow in humans. J Sleep Res 1992;1:S14.

81. Maquet P. Positron emission tomography studies of sleep and sleep disorders. J Neurol 1997;244:S23.

82. Maquet P, Degueldre C, Delfiore G, et al. Functional neuroanatomy of human slow wave sleep. J Neurosci 1997;17:2807.

83. Braun AR, Balkin TJ, Wesenten NJ, et al. Regional cerebral blood flow throughout the sleep-wake cycle. An H2(15)O PET study. Brain 1997;120:1173.

84. Hofle N, Paus T, Reutens D, et al. Regional cerebral blood flow changes as a function of delta and spindle activity during slow wave sleep in humans. J Neurosci 1997;17:4800.

85. Maquet P, Peters J, Aerts J, et al. Functional neuroanatomy of human rapid-eye-movement sleep and dreaming. Nature 1996;383:163.

86. Hong CC, Gillin JC, Dow BM, et al. Localized and lateralized cerebral glucose metabolism associated with eye movements during REM sleep and wakefulness: a positron emission tomography (PET) study. Sleep 1995;18:570.

87. Hetta J, Onoe H, Andersson J, et al. Cerebral blood flow during sleep—a positron emission tomographic (PET) study of regional changes. Sleep Res 1995;24:A87.

88. Hening WA, Walters AS, Chokroverty S. Movement Disorders and Sleep. In S Chokroverty (ed), Movement Disorders. Costa Mesa, CA: PMA, 1990;127.

89. Lapresle J. Palatal Myoclonus. In S Fahn, CD Marsden, MH Van Woert (eds), Myoclonus. New York: Lippincott–Raven. 1986;265.

90. Askenasy JJM, Yahr MD. Reversal of sleep disturbance in Parkinson's disease by antiparkinsonian therapy: a preliminary study. Neurology 1985;35:527.

91. Askenasy JJM. Sleep in Parkinson's disease. Acta Neurol Scand 1993;87:167.

92. Vanderheyden JE. Restless legs syndrome and nocturnal myoclonus in Parkinson's disease. Mov Disord 1996;11:S101.

93. Wetter TC, Seidel VC, Scheidtmann K, Trenkwalder C. A comparative polysomnographic study of patients with Parkinson's disease and multiple system atrophy. Sleep Res 1997;26:604.

94. Shimizu T, Inami Y, Sugita Y, et al. REM sleep without muscle atonia (stage 1-REM) and its relation to delirious behavior during sleep in patients with degenerative diseases involving the brainstem. Jpn J Psychiatr Neurol 1990;44:681.

95. Schenck CH, Bundlie SR, Mahowald MW. Delayed emergence of a parkinsonian disorder in 38% of 29 older men initially diagnosed with idiopathic rapid eye movement sleep behaviour disorder. Neurology 1996; 46:388. (Published erratum appears in Neurology 1996; 46:1787.)

96. Goetz CG, Wilson RS, Tanner CM, Garron DC. Relationships Among Pain, Depression, and Sleep Alteration in Parkinson's Disease. In MD Yahr, KJ Bergmann (eds), Parkinson's Disease. New York: Raven, 1986;345.

97. Starkstein SE, Preziosi TJ, Robinson RG. Sleep disorders, pain, and depression in Parkinson's disease. Eur Neurol 1991;31:352.

98. Duvoisin RC, Sage JI. The Spectrum of Parkinsonism. In S Chokroverty (ed), Movement Disorders. Costa Mesa, CA: PMA, 1990;159.

99. Diagnostic Classification Steering Committee of the American Sleep Disorders Association, MJ Thorpy, Chairperson. The International Classification of Sleep Disorders: Diagnostic and Coding Manual. Rochester, MN: American Sleep Disorders Association, 1990.

99a. Polymeropoulos MH, Lavedan C, Leroy E, et al. Mutation in the alpha-synuclein gene identified in families with Parkinson's disease. Science 1997;276:2045.

99b. Chan P, Tanner CM, Jiang X, Langston JW. Failure to find the alpha-synuclein gene missense mutation (G209A) in 100 patients with younger onset Parkinson's disease. Neurology 1998;50:513.

99c. Irizarry MC, Growdon W, Goméz-Isla T, et al. Nigral and cortical Lewy bodies and dystrophic nigral neurites in Parkinson's disease and cortical Lewy body disease contain alpha-synuclein immunoreactivity. J Neuropathol Exp Neurol 1998;57:334.

100. Jellinger K. Overview of Morphological Changes in Parkinson's Disease. In MD Yahr, KJ Bergmann (eds), Parkinson's Disease, Advanced Neurology 45. New York: Raven, 1987;1.

101. German DC, Manaye KF, White CL III, et al. Disease-specific patterns of locus coeruleus cell loss. Ann Neurol 1992;32:667.

102. Emser W, Brenner M, Stober T, Schimrigk K. Changes in nocturnal sleep in Huntington's and Parkinson's disease. J Neurol 1988;235:177.

103. Puca FM, Bricolo A, Turella G. Effect of L-dopa or amantadine therapy on sleep spindles in parkinsonism. Electroencephalogr Clin Neurophysiol 1973; 35:327.

104. Shima F, Imai H, Segawa M. Polygraphic study on body movements during sleep in cases with involuntary movement. Clin Electroencephalogr 1974;16:229.

105. Laihinen A, Alihanka J, Raitasuo S, Rinne UK. Sleep movements and associated autonomic nervous activities in patients with Parkinson's disease. Acta Neurol Scand 1987;76:64.

106. van Hilten B, Hoff JI, Middelkoop HA, et al. Sleep disruption in Parkinson's disease. Assessment by continuous activity monitoring. Arch Neurol 1994;51:922.

107. van Hilten JJ, Weggeman M, van der Velde EA, et al. Sleep, excessive daytime sleepiness and fatigue in Parkinson's disease. J Neural Transm Park Dis Dement Sect 1993;5:235.

108. Tassinari CA, Broughton R, Poire R, et al. Sur l' Evolution des Mouvements Anormaux au Cours du Sommeil. In H Fischgold (ed), Le Sommeil de Nuit Normal et Pathologique. Paris: Masson, 1965;314.

109. April R. Observations on parkinsonian tremor in all-night sleep. Neurology 1966;16:720.

110. Stern M, Roffwarg H, Duvoisin R. The parkinsonian tremor in sleep. J Nerv Ment Dis 1968;147:202.

111. Askenasy JJM. Sleep patterns in extrapyramidal disorders. Int J Neurol 1981;15:62.

112. Mouret J. Differences in sleep in patients with Parkinson's disease. Electroencephalogr Clin Neurophysiol 1975;38:653.

113. Clouston PD, Lim CL, Fung V, et al. Brainstem myoclonus in a patient with non-dopa-responsive parkinsonism. Mov Disord 1996;11:404.

114. Comella CL, Tanner CM, Ristanovic RK. Polysomnographic sleep measures in Parkinson's disease patients with treatment-induced hallucinations. Ann Neurol 1993;34:710.

115. Tan A, Salgado M, Fahn S. Rapid eye movement sleep behavior disorder preceding Parkinson's disease with therapeutic response to levodopa. Mov Disord 1996; 11:214.

116. Louden MB, Morehead MA, Schmidt HS. Activation by selegiline (Eldepryle) of REM sleep behavior disorder in parkinsonism. W V Med J 1995;91:101.

117. Lees AJ, Blackburn NA, Campbell VL. The nighttime problems of Parkinson's disease. Clin Neuropharmacol 1988;11:512.

118. Factor SA, McAlarney T, Sanchez-Ramos JR, Weiner WJ. Sleep disorders and sleep effect in Parkinson's disease. Mov Disord 1990;5:280.

119. Rubio P, Burgeura JA, Sobrino R, et al. Trastornos del sueño y enfermedad de Parkinson: estudio de una casuísta. Rev Neurol (Barc) 1995;23:265.

120. Smith MC, Ellgring H, Oertel WH. Sleep disturbances in Parkinson's disease patients and spouses. J Am Geriatr Soc 1997;45:194.

121. Hening W, Rolleri M, Chokroverty S. Parkinson's disease patients have impaired sleep quality and frequent sleep complaints. Sleep Res 1996;25:418.

122. Kales A, Ansel RD, Markham CH, et al. Sleep in patients with Parkinson's disease and normal subjects prior to and following levodopa administration. Clin Pharmacol Ther 1971;12:397.

123. Bergonzi P, Chiurulla C, Cianchetti C, Tempesta E. Clinical pharmacology as an approach to the study of biochemical sleep mechanisms: the action of L-dopa. Confin Neurol 1974;36:5.

124. Apps MCP, Sheaff PC, Ingram DA, et al. Respiration and sleep in Parkinson's disease. J Neurol Neurosurg Psychiatry 1985;48:1240.

125. Nausieda PA, Weiner WJ, Kaplan LR, et al. Sleep disruption in the course of chronic levodopa therapy: an early feature of the levodopa psychosis. Clin Neuropharmacol 1982;5:183.

126. Bergonzi P, Chiurulla C, Gambi D, et al. L-Dopa plus decarboxylase inhibitor: sleep organization in Parkinson's syndrome before and after treatment. Acta Neurol Belg 1975;75:5.

127. Chokroverty S. The Spectrum of Ventilatory Disturbances in Movement Disorders. In S Chokroverty (ed), Movement Disorders. Costa Mesa, CA: PMA, 1990;365.

128. Hovestadt A, Bogaard JM, Meerwaldt JD, et al. Pulmonary function in Parkinson's disease. J Neurol Neurosurg Psychiatry 1989;52:329.

129. Lilker ES, Woolf CR. Pulmonary functions in Parkinson syndrome. Can Med Assoc J 1968;99:752.

130. Obenour WH, Stevens PM, Cohen AA, McCutchen JJ. The causes of abnormal pulmonary function in Parkinson's disease. Am Rev Respir Dis 1972;105:382.

131. Vas CJ, Parsonage M, Lord OC. Parkinsonism associated with laryngeal spasm. J Neurol Neurosurg Psychiatry 1965;28:401.

132. Corbin DO, Williams AC. Stridor during dystonic phases of Parkinson's disease (Letter). J Neurol Neurosurg Psychiatry 1987;50:821.

133. Weiner WJ, Goetz G, Nausieda PA, Klawans HL. Respiratory dyskinesias: extrapyramidal dysfunction and dyspnea. Ann Intern Med 1978;88:327.

134. De Keyser J, Vincken W. L-Dopa–induced respiratory disturbance in Parkinson's disease suppressed by tiapride. Neurology 1985;35:235.

135. Vincken WG, Gauthier SG, Dollfuss RE, et al. Involvement of upper airway muscles in extrapyramidal disorders. N Engl J Med 1984;311:438.

136. Isozaki E, Shimizu T, Takamoto K, et al. Vocal cord abductor paralysis (VCAP) in Parkinson's disease: difference from VCAP in multiple system atrophy. J Neurol Sci 1995;130:197.

137. Hardie RJ, Efthimiou J, Stern GM. Respiration and sleep in Parkinson's disease. J Neurol Neurosurg Psychiatry 1986;50:1326.

138. Efthimiou J, Ellis SJ, Hardie RJ, Stern GM. Sleep Apnea in Idiopathic and Postencephalitic Parkinsonism. In MD Yahr, KJ Bergmann (eds), Parkinson's Disease, Advanced Neurology 45. New York: Raven, 1986;275.

139. Bliwise DL, Watts RL, Watts N, et al. Disruptive nocturnal behavior in Parkinson's disease and Alzheimer's disease (see comments). J Geriatr Psychiatry Neurol 1995;8:107.

140. Kostic VS, Susic V, Covickovic-Sternic N, et al. Reduced rapid eye movement sleep latency in patients with Parkinson's disease. J Neurol 1989;236:421.

141. Menza MA, Rosen RC. Sleep in Parkinson's disease. The role of depression and anxiety. Psychosomatics 1995;36:262.

142. Sharf B, Moskovitz C, Lupton MD, Klawans HL. Dream phenomena induced by chronic levodopa therapy. J Neural Transm 1978;43:143.

143. Factor SA, Molho ES, Podskalny GD, Brown D. Parkinson's disease: drug-induced psychiatric states. Adv Neurol 1995;65:115.

144. Klein C, Kompf D, Pulkowski U, et al. A study of visual hallucinations in patients with Parkinson's disease. J Neurol 1997;244:371.

145. Sanchez-Ramos JR, Ortoll R, Paulson GW. Visual hallucinations associated with Parkinson's disease (see comments). Arch Neurol 1996;53:1265.

146. Van den Kerchove M, Jacquy J, Gonce M, De Deyn PP. Sustained-release levodopa in parkinsonian patients with nocturnal disabilities. Acta Neurol Belg 1993;93:32.

147. Pahwa R, Busenbark K, Huber SJ, et al. Clinical experience with controlled-release carbidopa/levodopa in Parkinson's disease (see comments). Neurology 1993;43:677.

148. Garcia de Yebenes J, Mateo D, Pino MA, et al. The effect of controlled release of DOPA and carbidopa on clinical response and plasma pharmacokinetics of DOPA in parkinsonian patients. Neurologia 1997;12:145.

149. Ruottinen HM, Rinne UK. Entacapone prolongs levodopa response in a one month double blind study in parkinsonian patients with levodopa related fluctuations. J Neurol Neurosurg Psychiatry 1996;60:36.

150. Rajput AH, Martin W, Saint-Hilaire MH, et al. Tolcapone improves motor function in parkinsonian patients with the "wearing-off" phenomenon: a double-blind, placebo-controlled, multicenter trial. Neurology 1997;49:1066.

151. LeWitt PA. New options for treatment of Parkinson's disease. Baillieres Clin Neurol 1997;6:109.

152. Stocchi F, Nordera G, Marsden CD. Strategies for treating patients with advanced Parkinson's disease with

disastrous fluctuations and dyskinesias. Clin Neuropharmacol 1997;20:95.

153. Quinn N, Critchley P, Marsden CD. Young onset Parkinson's disease. Mov Disord 1987;2:73.

154. Yamamura Y, Sobue I, Ando K, et al. Paralysis agitans of early onset with marked diurnal fluctuations of symptoms. Neurology 1973;23:239.

155. Takahashi H, Ohama E, Suzuki S, et al. Familial juvenile parkinsonism: clinical and pathologic study in a family. Neurology 1994;44:437.

156. Ishikawa A, Tsuji S. Clinical analysis of 17 patients in 12 Japanese families with autosomal-recessive type juvenile parkinsonism. Neurology 1996;47:160.

157. Segawa M, Hosaka A, Miyagawa F, et al. Hereditary progressive dystonia with marked diurnal fluctuations. Adv Neurol 1976;14:215.

158. Nygaard TG. Dopa-Responsive Dystonia: 20 Years into the L-Dopa Era. In NP Quinn, PG Jenner (eds), Disorders of Movement: Clinical, Pharmacological, and Physiological Aspects. New York: Academic, 1989;323.

159. Segawa M, Nomura Y, Yamashita S, et al. Long-Term Effects of L-Dopa on Hereditary Progressive Dystonia with Marked Diurnal Fluctuation. In A Berardelli, R Benecke, M Manfredi, CD Marsden (eds), Motor Disturbances II. New York: Academic, 1990;305.

160. Marsden CD, Parkes JD, Quinn N. Fluctuations of Disability in Parkinson's Disease—Clinical Aspects. In CD Marsden, S Fahn (eds), Movement Disorders. Boston: Butterworth Scientific, 1982;96.

161. Comella CL, Bohmer J, Stebbins GT. Sleep benefit in Parkinson's disease. Neurology 1995;45(Suppl 4):A286.

162. Currie LJ, Bennett JP Jr, Harrison MB, et al. Clinical correlates of sleep benefit in Parkinson's disease. Neurology 1997;48:1115.

163. Merello M, Hughes A, Colosimo C, et al. Sleep benefit in Parkinson's disease. Mov Disord 1997;12:506.

164. Reist C, Sokolski KN, Chen CC, et al. The effect of sleep deprivation on motor impairment and retinal adaptation in Parkinson's disease. Prog Neuropsychopharmacol Biol Psychiatry 1995;19:445.

165. Kim R. The chronic residual respiratory disorder in post encephalitic Parkinsonism. J Neurol Neurosurg Psychiatry 1968;31:393.

166. Garland T, Linderholm H. Hypoventilation syndrome in a case of chronic epidemic encephalitis. Acta Med Scand 1958;162:333.

167. DaCosta JL. Chronic hypoventilation due to diminished sensitivity of the respiratory centre associated with Parkinsonism. Med J Aust 1972;1:373.

168. Steele JC, Richardson JC, Olszewski J. Progressive supranuclear palsy. Arch Neurol 1964;10:333.

169. Golbe LI, Davis PH, Schoenberg BS, Duvoisin RC. Prevalence and natural history of progressive supranuclear palsy. Neurology 1988;38:1031.

170. Jankovic J, Van der Linden C. Progressive Supranuclear Palsy (Steel-Richardson-Olszewski Syndrome). In S Chokroverty (ed), Movement Disorders. Costa Mesa, CA: PMA, 1990;267.

171. Gross RA, Spehlmann R, Daniels JC. Sleep disturbances in progressive supranuclear palsy. Electroencephalogr Clin Neurophysiol 1978;45:16.

172. Laffont F, Autret A, Minz M, et al. Étude polygraphique du sommeil dans 9 cas de maladie de Steele-Richardson. Rev Neurol 1979;135:127.

173. Massetani R, Arena R, Bonuccelli U, et al. Sleep in progressive supranuclear palsy. Riv Patol Nerv Ment 1982;103:215.

174. Laffont F, Leger JM, Penicaud A, et al. Sleep abnormalities and evoked potentials (VEP-BAER-SEP) in progressive supranuclear palsy. Neurophysiol Clin 1988;18:255.

175. Aldrich MS, Foster NL, White RF, et al. Sleep abnormalities in progressive supranuclear palsy. Ann Neurol 1989;25:577.

176. De Bruin VS, Machado C, Howard RS, et al. Nocturnal and respiratory disturbances in Steele-Richardson-Olszewski syndrome (progressive supranuclear palsy). Postgrad Med J 1996;72:293.

177. Montplaisir J, Petit D, Decary A, et al. Sleep and quantitative EEG in patients with progressive supranuclear palsy. Neurology 1997;49:999.

178. Pareja JA, Caminero AB, Masa JF, Dobato JL. A first case of progressive supranuclear palsy and pre-clinical REM sleep behavior disorder presenting as inhibition of speech during wakefulness and somniloquy with phasic muscle twitching during REM sleep. Neurologia 1996;11:304.

179. Perret JL, Jouvet M. Étude du sommeil dans la paralyse supra-nucléaire progressive. Electroencephalogr Clin Neurophysiol 1980;49:323.

180. Purdy A, Hahn A, Barnett JM, et al. Familial fatal Parkinsonism with alveolar hypoventilation and mental depression. Ann Neurol 1979;6:523.

181. Roy EP, Riggs JE, Martin JD, et al. Familial parkinsonism, apathy, weight loss, and central hypoventilation: successful long-term management. Neurology 1988;38:637.

182. Thompson PD. Chorea. In NP Quinn, PG Jenner (eds), Disorders of Movement: Clinical, Pharmacological and Physiological Aspects. New York: Academic, 1989;455.

183. The Huntington's Disease Collaborative Research Group. A novel gene containing a trinucleotide repeat that is expanded and unstable on Huntington's disease chromosomes. Cell 1993;72:971.

184. Gourfinkel-An I, Cancel G, Trottier Y, et al. Differential distribution of the normal and mutated forms of huntingtin in the human brain. Ann Neurol 1997;42:712.

185. Spire JP, Bliwise DL, Noronha ABC, Roos RP. Sleep profiles in Huntington disease. Neurology 1981;31:151.

186. Sishta SK, Troupe A, Marszalek KS, Kremer LM. Huntington's chorea: an electroencephalographic and psychometric study. Electroencephalogr Clin Neurophysiol 1974;36:387.

187. Wiegand M, Moller AA, Lauer CJ, et al. Nocturnal sleep in Huntington's disease. J Neurol 1991;238:203.

188. Hansotia P, Wall R, Berendes J. Sleep disturbances and severity of Huntington's disease. Neurology 1985;35:1672.

189. Wiegand M, Moller AA, Schreiber W, et al. Brain morphology and sleep EEG in patients with Huntington's disease. Eur Arch Psychiatry Clin Neurosci 1991;240:148.

190. Bollen EL, Den Heijer JC, Ponsioen C, et al. Respiration during sleep in Huntington's chorea. J Neurol Sci 1988;84:63.

191. Broughton R, Tassinari CA, Gastaut JR, et al. A polygraphic study of abnormal movements during different stages of sleep. Can Med Assoc J 1967;97:243.

192. Fahn S. Recent Concepts in the Diagnosis and Treatment of Dystonias. In S Chokroverty (ed), Movement Disorders. Costa Mesa, CA: PMA, 1990;237.

193. Fahn S, Marsden CD, Calne DB. New York: Raven, 1988;705.

194. Knappskog PM, Flatmark T, Mallet J, et al. Recessively inherited L-DOPA-responsive dystonia caused by a point mutation (Q381K) in the tyrosine hydroxylase gene. Hum Mol Genet 1995;4:1209.

195. Bandmann O, Nygaard TG, Surtees R, et al. Dopa-responsive dystonia in British patients: new mutations of the GTP-cyclohydrolase I gene and evidence for genetic heterogeneity. Hum Mol Genet 1996;5:403.

196. Ozelius LJ, Hewett JW, Page CE, et al. The early-onset torsion dystonia gene (DYT1) encodes an ATP-binding protein. Nat Genet 1997;17:40.

197. Bressman SB, de Leon D, Raymond D, et al. Secondary dystonia and the DYTI gene. Neurology 1997;48:1571.

198. Shiozawa Z, Mano T, Sobue I. Polygraphic studies on involuntary movements during sleep in cases of dystonia, choreo-athetosis, and ballism. Rinsho Shinkeigaku 1978;18:547.

199. Silvestri R, De Domenico P, Di Rosa AE, et al. The effect of nocturnal physiological sleep on various movement disorders. Mov Disord 1990;5:8.

200. Jankel WR, Allen RP, Niedermeyer E, Kalsher MJ. Polysomnographic findings in dystonia musculorum deformans. Sleep 1983;6:281.

201. Fish DR, Allen PJ, Sawyers D, Marsden CD. Sleep spindles in torsion dystonia. Arch Neurol 1990;47:216.

202. Berardelli A. The Pathophysiology of Dystonia. In NP Quinn, PG Jenner (eds), Disorders of Movement: Clinical, Pharmacological, and Physiological Aspects. New York: Academic, 1989;251.

203. Wein A, Golubev V. Polygraphic analysis of sleep in dystonia musculorum deformans. Waking Sleeping 1979;3:41.

204. Jankel WR, Niedermeyer E, Graf M, Kalsher MJ. Case report: polysomnographic effects of thalamotomy for torsion dystonia. Neurosurgery 1984;14:495.

205. Segawa M, Nomura Y. Hereditary Progressive Dystonia with Marked Diurnal Fluctuations. In T Nagatsu, H Narabayashi, M Yoshida (eds), Parkinson's Disease. From Clinical Aspects to Molecular Basis. New York: Springer, 1991;167.

206. Ichinose H, Ohye T, Takahashi E, et al. Hereditary progressive dystonia with marked diurnal fluctuation caused by mutations in the GTP cyclohydrolase I gene (see comments). Nat Genet 1994;8:236.

207. Imaiso Y, Taniwaki T, Yamada T, et al. A novel mutation of the GTP-cyclohydrolase I gene in a patient with hereditary progressive dystonia/dopa-responsive dystonia. Neurology 1998;50:517.

208. Jarman PR, Bandmann O, Marsden CD, Wood NW. GTP cyclohydrolase I mutations in patients with dystonia responsive to anticholinergic drugs. J Neurol Neurosurg Psychiatry 1997;63:304.

209. Nygaard TG, Marsden CD, Duvoisin RC. Dopa-Responsive Dystonia. In Fahn S, Marsden CD, Calne DB (eds), Dystonia 2, Advanced Neurology 50. New York: Raven, 1988;377.

210. Montagna P, Procaccianti G, Lugaresi A, et al. Diurnal variability in cranial dystonia. Mov Disord 1990;5:44.

211. Segawa M, Nomura Y, Tanaka S, et al. Hereditary Progressive Dystonia with Marked Diurnal Fluctuations—Consideration on Its Pathophysiology Based on the Characteristics of Clinical and Polysomnographical Findings. In S Fahn, CD Marsden, DB Calne (eds), Dystonia 2, Advanced Neurology 50. New York: Raven, 1988;367.

212. de Yebenes JG, Moskowitz C, Fahn S, Saint-Hilaire MH. Long-Term Treatment with Levodopa in a Family with Autosomal Dominant Torsion Dystonia. In S Fahn, CD Marsden, DB Calne (eds), Dystonia 2. New York: Raven, 1988;101.

213. Nygaard TG, Marsden CD, Fahn S. Dopa-responsive dystonia: long-term treatment response and prognosis. Neurology 1991;41:174.

214. Nygaard TG, Takahashi H, Heiman GA, et al. Long-term treatment response and fluorodopa positron emission tomographic scanning of parkinsonism in a family with dopa-responsive dystonia. Ann Neurol 1992;32:603.

215. Sawle GV, Leenders KL, Brooks DJ, et al. Dopa-responsive dystonia: [$^{18}$F] dopa positron emission tomography. Ann Neurol 1991;30:24.

216. Mazurek MF, Rosebush PI. Circadian pattern of acute, neuroleptic-induced dystonic reactions. Am J Psychiatry 1996;153:708.

217. Davila R, Zumarraga M, Andia I, Friedhoff AJ. Persistence of cyclicity of the plasma dopamine metabolite, homovanillic acid, in neuroleptic treated schizophrenic patients. Life Sci 1989;44:1117.

218. Fahn S, Marsden CD, Van Woert M. Myoclonus. New York: Raven, 1986;730.

219. Lugaresi E, Coccagna G, Mantovani M, et al. The evolution of different types of myoclonus during sleep. A polygraphic study. Eur Neurol 1970;4:321.

220. Lugaresi E, Cirignotta F, Montagna P, Coccagna G. Myoclonus and Related Phenomena During Sleep. In M Chase, ED Weitzman (eds), Sleep Disorders: Basic and Clinical Research. New York: Spectrum, 1983;123.

221. Chokroverty S, Barron KD. Palatal myoclonus and rhythmic ocular movements: a polygraphic study. Neurology 1969;19:975.

222. Tahmoush AJ, Brooks JE, Keltner JL. Palatal myoclonus associated with abnormal ocular and extremity movements: a polygraphic study. Arch Neurol 1972;27:431.

223. Deuschl G, Toro C, Valls-Sole J, et al. Symptomatic and essential palatal tremor. 1. Clinical, physiological and MRI analysis. Brain 1994;117:775.

224. Postert T, Amoiridis G, Pohlau D, et al. Episodic undulating hyperkinesias of the tongue associated with brainstem ischemia. Mov Disord 1997;12:619.

225. Jacobs L, Newman RP, Bozian D. Disappearing palatal myoclonus. Neurology 1981;31:748.

226. Kayed K, Sjaastad O, Magnussen I, Mårvik R. Palatal myoclonus during sleep. Sleep 1983;6:130.

227. Sakurai N, Koike Y, Kaneoke Y, et al. Sleep apnea and palatal myoclonus in a patient with neuro-Behçet syndrome. Intern Med 1993;32:336.

228. Hoehn MM, Cherington M. Spinal myoclonus. Neurology 1977;27:942.

229. Bauleo S, De Mitri P, Coccagna G. Evolution of segmental myoclonus during sleep: polygraphic study of two cases. Ital J Neurol Sci 1996;17:227.

230. Walters A, Hening W, Côte L, Fahn S. Dominantly Inherited Restless Legs with Myoclonus and Periodic Movements of Sleep: A Syndrome Related to the Endogenous Opiates? In S Fahn, CD Marsden, M Van Woert (eds), Myoclonus, Advanced Neurology 43. New York: Raven, 1986;309.

231. Kirk A, Heilman KM. Auricular myoclonus. Can J Neurol Sci 1991;18:503.

232. Palmer JB, Tippett DC, Wolf JS. Synchronous positive and negative myoclonus due to pontine hemorrhage. Muscle Nerve 1991;14:124.

233. Popoviciu L, Asgian B, Delast-Popoviciu D, et al. Clinical, EEG, electromyographic and polysomnographic studies in restless legs syndrome caused by magnesium deficiency. Rom J Neurol Psychiatry 1993;31:55.

234. Ikeda A, Shibasaki H, Tashiro K, et al. Clinical trial of piracetam in patients with myoclonus: nationwide multiinstitution study in Japan. The Myoclonus/Piracetam Study Group. Mov Disord 1996;11:691.

235. Jankovic J. The Neurology of Tics. In CD Marsden, S Fahn (eds), Movement Disorders 2. Boston: Butterworth, 1987;383.

236. Van Woert MH. Gilles de la Tourette Syndrome. In S Chokroverty (ed), Movement Disorders. Costa Mesa, CA: PMA, 1990;309.

237. Jankovic J. Tourette syndrome. Phenomenology and classification of tics. Neurol Clin 1997;15:267.

238. Nee LE, Caine ED, Polinsky RJ, et al. Gilles de la Tourette syndrome: clinical and family study of 50 cases. Ann Neurol 1980;7:41.

239. Hashimoto T, Endo S, Fukuda K, et al. Increased body movements during sleep in Gilles de la Tourette syndrome. Brain Dev 1981;3:31.

240. Glaze DG, Frost JD Jr, Jankovic J. Sleep in Gilles de la Tourette syndrome: disorder of arousal. Neurology 1983;33:586.

241. Drake ME Jr, Hietter SA, Bogner JE, Andrews JM. Cassette EEG sleep recordings in Gilles de la Tourette syndrome. Clin Electroencephalogr 1992;23:142.

242. Barabas G, Matthews WS, Ferrari M. Somnambulism in children with Tourette syndrome. Dev Med 1984;26:457.

243. Wand RR, Matazow GS, Shady GA, et al. Tourette syndrome: associated symptoms and most disabling features. Neurosci Biobehav Rev 1993;17:271.

244. Jankovic J, Glaze DG, Frost JD Jr. Effect of tetrabenazine on tics and sleep of Gilles de la Tourette's syndrome. Neurology 1984;34:688.

245. Hayashi M, Inoue Y, Iwakawa Y, Sasaki H. REM sleep abnormalities in severe athetoid cerebral palsy. Brain Dev 1990;12:494.

246. Cohen SR, Lefaivre JF, Burstein FD, et al. Surgical treatment of obstructive sleep apnea in neurologically compromised patients. Plast Reconstr Surg 1997;99:638.

247. Yamamoto T, Hirose G, Shimazaki K, et al. Movement disorders of familial neuroacanthocytosis syndrome. Arch Neurol 1982;39:298.

248. Silvestri R, Raffaele M, De Domenico P, et al. Sleep features in Tourette's syndrome, neuroacanthocytosis and Huntington's chorea. Neurophysiol Clin 1995;25:66.

249. Hori A, Kazukawa S, Nakamura I, Endo M. Electroencephalographic findings in neuroacanthocytosis. Electroencephalogr Clin Neurophysiol 1985;61:342.

250. Shannon KM, Klawans HL. Hemiballismus. In S Chokroverty (ed), Movement Disorders. Costa Mesa, CA: PMA, 1990;353.

251. Puca FM, Minervini MG, Savarese M, et al. Evoluzione del sonno in un caso di emiballismo. Boll Soc Ital Biol Sper 1984;60:981.

252. Auger RG. Hemifacial spasm: clinical and electrophysiologic observations. Neurology 1979;29:1261.

253. Digre KB, Corbett JJ. Hemifacial Spasm: Differential Diagnosis, Mechanism and Treatment. In J Jankovic, E Tolosa (eds), Facial Dyskinesias. New York: Raven, 1988;151.

254. Montagna P, Imbriaco A, Zucconi M, et al. Hemifacial spasm in sleep. Neurology 1986;36:270.

255. Byrne E, White O, Cook M. Familial dystonic choreoathetosis with myokymia: a sleep responsive disorder. J Neurol Neurosurg Psychiatry 1991;54:1090.

256. Terman M, Lewy AJ, Dijk DJ, et al. Light treatment for sleep disorders: consensus report. IV. Sleep phase and duration disturbances. J Biol Rhythms 1995;10:135.

257. Campbell SS, Dawson D, Anderson MW. Alleviation of sleep maintenance insomnia with timed exposure to bright light. J Am Geriatr Soc 1993;41:829.

258. Campbell SS, Terman M, Lewy AJ, et al. Light treatment for sleep disorders: consensus report. V. Age-related disturbances. J Biol Rhythms 1995;10:151.

259. Campbell SS, Murphy PJ. Extraocular circadian phototransduction in humans (see comments). Science 1998; 279:396.

260. Satlin A, Volicer L, Ross V, et al. Bright light treatment of behavioral and sleep disturbances in patients with Alzheimer's disease. Am J Psychiatry 1992;149:1028.

261. Van Someren EJ, Lijzenga C, Mirmiran M, Swaab DF. Long-term fitness training improves the circadian rest-activity rhythm in healthy elderly males. J Biol Rhythms 1997;12:146.

262. Ekbom KA. Restless legs: a clinical study. Acta Med Scand Suppl 1945;158:1.

263. Montplaisir J, Godbout R, Pelletier G, Warnes H. Restless Legs Syndrome and Periodic Movements During Sleep. In MH Kryger, T Roth, WC Dement (eds), Principles and Practice of Sleep Medicine. Philadelphia: Saunders, 1994;589.

264. O'Keeffe ST. Restless legs syndrome. A review (see comments). Arch Intern Med 1996;156:243.

265. Trenkwalder C, Walters AS, Hening W. Periodic limb movements and restless legs syndrome. Neurol Clin 1996;14:629.

266. Silber MH. Restless legs syndrome. Mayo Clin Proc 1997;72:261.

267. Hening WA. Restless legs syndrome: diagnosis and treatment. Hosp Med 1997;33:54,61,68,73,75.

268. Zucconi M, Coccagna G, Petronelli R, et al. Nocturnal myoclonus in restless legs syndrome: effect of carbamazepine treatment. Funct Neurol 1989;4:263.

269. Montplaisir J, Lapierre O, Warnes H, Pelletier G. The treatment of the restless legs syndrome with or without periodic leg movements in sleep. Sleep 1992;15:391.

270. Symonds CP. Nocturnal myoclonus. J Neurol Neurosurg Psychiatry 1953;16:166.

271. Coleman RM, Pollak CP, Weitzman ED. Periodic movements in sleep (nocturnal myoclonus): relation to sleep disorders. Ann Neurol 1980;8:416.

272. Smith RC. Relationship of periodic movements in sleep (nocturnal myoclonus) and the Babinski sign. Sleep 1985;8:239.

273. Yokota T, Hirose K, Tanabe H, Tsukagoshi H. Sleep-related periodic leg movements (nocturnal myoclonus) due to spinal cord lesion. J Neurol Sci 1991;104:13.

274. Walters A, Hening W, Kavey N, et al. Restless Legs Syndrome: a pleomorphic sensorimotor disorder. Neurology 1984;34:S129.

275. Coccagna G. Restless Legs Syndrome/Periodic Leg Movements in Sleep. In MJ Thorpy (ed), Handbook of Sleep Disorders. New York: Marcel Dekker, 1990;457.

276. Hening WA, Walters AS, Chokroverty S, Truong D. Are there dual oscillators producing dyskinesias of the arms and legs in the restless legs syndrome (RLS)? Muscle Nerve 1989;12:751.

277. Pollmacher T, Schulz H. Periodic leg movements (PLM): their relationship to sleep stages. Sleep 1993;16:572.

278. Dzvonik ML, Kripke DF, Klauber M, Ancoli-Israel S. Body position changes and periodic movements in sleep. Sleep 1986;9:484.

279. Atlas Task Force of the American Sleep Disorders Association. Recording and scoring leg movements. Sleep 1993;16:748.

280. Atlas Task Force—ASDA Report. EEG arousals: scoring rules and examples. Sleep 1992;15:173.

281. Mendelson WB. Are periodic leg movements associated with clinical sleep disturbance? (see comments). Sleep 1996;19:219.

282. Kwan PC, Hening WA, Chokroverty S, Walters AS. Periodic limb movements in sleep may cause signifi-cant sleep disruption in patients with the restless legs syndrome. Sleep Res 1992;21:222.

283. Lapierre O, Montplaisir J. Polysomnographic features of REM sleep behavior disorder: development of a scoring method. Neurology 1992;42:1371.

284. Godbout R, Montplaisir J, Poirier G, Bédard MA. Distinctive electrographic manifestations of periodic leg movements during sleep in narcoleptic vs insomniac patients. Sleep Res 1988;17:182.

285. Ancoli-Israel S, Kripke DF, Klauber MR, et al. Periodic limb movements in sleep in community-dwelling elderly. Sleep 1991;14:496.

286. Dickel MJ, Mosko SS. Morbidity cut-offs for sleep apnea and periodic leg movements in predicting subjective complaints in seniors. Sleep 1990;13:155.

287. Phoha RL, Dickel MJ, Mosko SS. Preliminary longitudinal assessment of sleep in the elderly. Sleep 1990;13:425.

288. Edinger JD, McCall WV, Marsh GR, et al. Periodic limb movement variability in older DIMS patients across consecutive nights of home monitoring. Sleep 1992;15:156.

289. Kales A, Bixler EO, Soldatos CR, et al. Biopsychobehavioral correlates of insomnia. Part 1: Role of sleep apnea and nocturnal myoclonus. Psychosomatics 1982;23:589.

290. Wittig R, Zorick F, Piccione P, et al. Narcolepsy and disturbed nocturnal sleep. Clin Electroencephalogr 1983;14:130.

291. Baker TL, Guilleminault C, Nino-Murcia G, Dement WC. Comparative polysomnographic study of narcolepsy and idiopathic central nervous system hypersomnia. Sleep 1986;9:232.

292. Guilleminault C, Philip P. Tiredness and somnolence despite initial treatment of obstructive sleep apnea syndrome (what to do when an OSAS patient stays hypersomnolent despite treatment). Sleep 1996;19:S117.

293. Lavie P, Epstein R, Tzischinsky O, et al. Actigraphic measurements of sleep in rheumatoid arthritis: comparison of patients with low back pain and healthy controls. J Rheumatol 1992;19:362.

294. Ondo W, Jankovic J. Restless legs syndrome: clinicoetiologic correlates. Neurology 1996;47:1435.

295. Walters AS, Hening WA, Chokroverty S. Review and videotape recognition of idiopathic restless legs syndrome. Mov Disord 1991;6:105 & videotape.

296. Montplaisir J, Godbout R, Boghen D. Familial restless legs with periodic movements in sleep: electrophysiologic, biochemical and pharmacologic study. Neurology 1985;35:130.

297. Earley CJ, Allen RP. Pergolide and carbidopa/levodopa treatment of the restless legs syndrome and periodic leg movements in sleep in a consecutive series of patients. Sleep 1996;19:801.

298. Montplaisir J, Godbout R, Poirier G, Bédard MA. Restless legs syndrome and periodic movements in sleep: physiopathology and treatment with L-dopa. Clin Neuropharmacol 1986;9:456.

299. Walters AS, Hening WA, Kavey N, et al. A double-blind randomized cross-over trial of bromocriptine and placebo in the restless legs syndrome. Ann Neurol 1988;24:455.

300. Hening WA, Walters AS. Successful long-term therapy of the restless legs syndrome with opioid medications. Sleep Res 1989;18:241.

301. Trenkwalder C, Walters AS, Hening W, et al. Circadian rhythm of patients with the idiopathic restless legs syndrome. Sleep Res 1995;24:360.

302. Hening W, Walters A, Wagner M, et al. Motor restlessness follows a circadian pattern in the restless legs syndrome. Sleep Res 1997;26:375.

303. Brodeur C, Montplaisir J, Godbout R, Marinier R. Treatment of restless legs syndrome and periodic movements during sleep with L-dopa: a double-blind controlled study. Neurology 1988;38:1845.

304. Hening WA, Walters AS, Campbell S, et al. Circadian rhythm of the restless legs syndrome: subjective complaint and restless movements peak on the falling phase of the core temperature cycle. Sleep 1998; 21(suppl):143.

305. Kwan PC, Hening WA, Chokroverty S, Walters AS. Periodic limb movements in sleep may cause significant sleep disruption in patients with the restless legs syndrome. Sleep Res 1992;21:222.

306. Pollak CP, Perlick D, Linsner JP, et al. Sleep problems in the community elderly as predictors of death and nursing home placement. J Community Health 1990;15:123.

307. Akpinar S. Restless legs syndrome treatment with dopaminergic drugs. Clin Neuropharmacol 1987;10:69.

308. Strang RR. The symptoms of restless legs. Med J Aust 1967;1:1211.

309. Banerji N, Hurwitz L. Restless legs syndrome, with particular reference to its occurrence after gastric surgery. BMJ 1970;4:774.

310. Oboler SK, Prochazka AV, Meyer TJ. Leg symptoms in outpatient veterans. West J Med 1991;155:256.

311. O'Hare JA, Abuaisha F, Geoghegan M. Prevalence and forms of neuropathic morbidity in 800 diabetics. Ir J Med Sci 1994;163:132.

312. Lavigne GJ, Montplaisir JY. Restless legs syndrome and sleep bruxism: prevalence and association among Canadians. Sleep 1994;17:739.

313. Goldberg J. New Gallup Findings: Americans Know They're Sleep-Deprived, but Do Not Seek Effective Relief. New York: National Sleep Foundation, 1995.

314. Purvis C, Phillips B, Asher K, et al. Self reports of restless legs syndrome: 1996 Kentucky behavior risk factor surveillance survey. Sleep Res 1997;26:474.

315. Walters AS, Picchietti DL, Ehrenberg BL, Wagner ML. Restless legs syndrome in childhood and adolescence. Pediatr Neurol 1994;11:241.

316. Walters AS, Hickey K, Maltzman J, et al. A questionnaire study of 138 patients with restless legs syndrome: the 'Night-Walkers' survey. Neurology 1996;46:92.

317. The International Restless Legs Syndrome Study Group; Walters AS, Group Organizer and Correspondent. Towards a better definition of the restless legs syndrome. Mov Disord 1995;10:634.

318. Montagna P, Coccagna G, Cirignotta F, Lugaresi E. Familial Restless Legs Syndrome: Long-Term Follow-Up. In C Guilleminault, E Lugaresi (eds), Sleep/Wake Disorders: Natural History, Epidemiology, and Long-Term Evolution. New York: Raven, 1983;231.

319. Montplaisir J, Boucher S, Poirier G, et al. Clinical, polysomnographic, and genetic characteristics of restless legs syndrome: a study of 133 patients diagnosed with new standard criteria. Mov Disord 1997;12:61.

320. Ekbom KA. Restless legs syndrome. Neurology 1960; 10:868.

321. McParland P, Pearce JM. Restless legs syndrome in pregnancy. Case reports. Clin Exp Obstet Gynecol 1990;17:5.

322. Boghen D, Peyronnard JM. Myoclonus in familial restless legs syndrome. Arch Neurol 1976;33:368.

323. Godbout R, Montplaisir J, Poirier G. Epidemiological data in familial restless legs syndrome. Sleep Res 1987;16:338.

324. Walters A, Johnson W, Hening W, et al. Preliminary evidence for possible genetic linkage in the restless legs syndrome. J Sleep Res 1992;1:S248.

325. Trenkwalder C, Seidel VC, Gasser T, Oertel WH. Clinical symptoms and possible anticipation in a large kindred of familial restless legs syndrome. Mov Disord 1996;11:389.

326. Paulson HL, Fischbeck KH. Trinucleotide repeats in neurogenetic disorders. Annu Rev Neurosci 1996;19:79.

327. Stautner A, Stiasny K, Collado-Seidel V, et al. Comparison of idiopathic and uremic restless legs syndrome: results of a database of 134 patients. Mov Disord 1996;11:S98.

328. Allen RP, LaBuda MC, Becker PM, Earley CJ. Family history study of RLS patients from two clinical populations. Sleep Res 1997;26:309.

329. O'Keeffe ST, Gavin K, Lavan JN. Iron status and restless legs syndrome in the elderly. Age Ageing 1994;23:200.

330. Callaghan N. Restless legs syndrome in uremic neuropathy. Neurology 1966;16:359.

331. Collado-Seidel V, Kohnen R, Samtleben W, et al. Clinical and biochemical findings in uremic patients with and without restless legs syndrome. Am J Kidney Dis 1998;31:324.

332. Salih AM, Gray RE, Mills KR, Webley M. A clinical, serological and neurophysiological study of restless legs syndrome in rheumatoid arthritis. Br J Rheumatol 1994;33:60.

333. Roger SD, Harris DCH, Stewart JH. Possible relation between restless legs and anaemia in renal dialysis patients. Lancet 1991;337:1551.

334. Gorman CA, Dyck PJ, Pearson JS. Symptoms of restless legs. Arch Intern Med 1965;115:155.

335. Rutkove SB, Matheson JK, Logigian EL. Restless legs syndrome in patients with polyneuropathy. Muscle Nerve 1996;19:670.

336. Gemignani F, Marbini A, Di Giovanni G, et al. Cryoglobulinaemic neuropathy manifesting with restless legs syndrome. J Neurol Sci 1997;152:218.

337. Walters AS, Wagner M, Hening WA. Periodic limb movements as the initial manifestation of restless legs syndrome triggered by lumbosacral radiculopathy [letter]. Sleep 1996;19:825.

338. Picchietti DL, Walters AS. Restless Legs Syndrome and Periodic Limb Movement Disorder in Children and Adolescents: Comorbidity with Attention-Deficit Hyperactivity Disorder. In RE Dahl (ed), Child and Adolescent Psychiatric Clinics of North America: Sleep Disorders. Philadelphia: Saunders, 1996;729.

339. Lipinski JF, Sallee FR, Jackson C, Sethuraman G. Dopamine agonist treatment of Tourette disorder in children: results of an open-label trial of pergolide. Mov Disord 1997;12:402.

340. Polysomnography Task Force, American Sleep Disorders Association Standards of Practice Committee. Practice parameters for the indications for polysomnography and related procedures. Sleep 1997;20:406.

341. Walters AS, Hening W, Rubinstein M, Chokroverty S. A clinical and polysomnographic comparison of neuroleptic-induced akathisia and the idiopathic restless legs syndrome. Sleep 1991;14:339.

342. Ross RJ, Ball WA, Dinges DF, et al. Motor dysfunction during sleep in posttraumatic stress disorder. Sleep 1994;17:723.

343. Lipinski JF, Hudson JI, Cunningham SL, et al. Polysomnographic characteristics of neuroleptic-induced akathisia. Clin Neuropharmacol 1991;14:413.

344. Walters AS, Hening WA, Chokroverty S. Frequent occurrence of myoclonus while awake and at rest, body rocking and marching in place in a subpopulation of patients with restless legs syndrome. Acta Neurol Scand 1988;77:418.

345. Wechsler LR, Stakes JW, Shahani BT, Busis NA. Periodic leg movements of sleep (nocturnal myoclonus): an electrophysiological study. Ann Neurol 1986; 19:168.

346. Mosko SS, Nudleman KL. Somatosensory and brainstem auditory evoked responses in sleep-related periodic leg movements. Sleep 1986;9:399.

347. Briellmann RS, Rosler KM, Hess CW. Blink reflex excitability is abnormal in patients with periodic leg movements in sleep. Mov Disord 1996;11:710.

348. Bucher SF, Trenkwalder C, Oertel WH. Reflex studies and MRI in the restless legs syndrome. Acta Neurol Scand 1996;94:145.

349. Hening WA, Chokroverty S, Walters AS. Presence of a biphasic cortical potential before leg jerks in the restless legs syndrome. Sleep Res 1990;19:235.

350. Hening W, Chokroverty S, Rolleri M, Walters A. The cortical premovement potential of restless legs syndrome jerks: differences in potentials before simulated versus symptomatic jerks. Sleep Res 1991; 20:355.

351. Trenkwalder C, Bucher SF, Oertel WH, et al. Bereitschaftspotential in idiopathic and symptomatic restless legs syndrome. Electroencephalogr Clin Neurophysiol 1993;89:95.

352. Trenkwalder C, Bucher SF, Oertel WH. Electrophysiological pattern of involuntary limb movements in the restless legs syndrome. Muscle Nerve 1996;19:155.

353. de Mello MT, Lauro FA, Silva AC, Tufik S. Incidence of periodic leg movements and of the restless legs syndrome during sleep following acute physical activity in spinal cord injury subjects. Spinal Cord 1996;34:294.

354. Yokota T, Shiojiri T, Hirashima F. Sleep-related periodic arm movement [letter]. Sleep 1995;18:707.

355. Gupta P, Hening W, Rahman K, et al. Periodic limb movements (PLMs) in a patient with multiple sclerosis and central sleep apnea: independent right and left leg movement periods suggest lateralized PLM oscillators. Sleep Res 1996;25:417.

356. Walters AS, Trenkwalder C, Hening WA, et al. Fluorodeoxyglucose PET scanning in 5 patients with the restless legs syndrome. Sleep Res 1995;24:365.

357. Bucher SF, Seelos KC, Oertel WH, et al. Cerebral generators involved in the pathogenesis of the restless legs syndrome. Ann Neurol 1997;41:639.

358. Staedt J, Stoppe G, Kogler A, et al. Nocturnal myoclonus syndrome (periodic movements in sleep) related to central dopamine $D_2$-receptor alteration. Eur Arch Psychiatry Clin Neurosci 1995;245:8.

359. Staedt J, Stoppe G, Kogler A, et al. Single photon emission tomography (SPET) imaging of dopamine $D_2$ receptors in the course of dopamine replacement therapy in patients with nocturnal myoclonus syndrome (NMS). J Neural Transm Gen Sect 1995;99:187.

360. Lugaresi E, Coccagna G, Montovani M, Lebrun R. Some periodic phenomena arising during drowsiness and sleep in man. Electroencephalogr Clin Neurophysiol 1972;32:701.

361. Ali NJ, Davies RJO, Fleetham JA, Stradling JR. Periodic movements of the legs during sleep associated with rises in systemic blood pressure. Sleep 1991;14:163.

362. Hening WA, Walters AS, Chokroverty S. Motor Functions and Dysfunctions of Sleep. In S Chokroverty (ed), Sleep Disorders Medicine (1st ed). Boston: Butterworth–Heinemann, 1994;255.

363. Hening WA. The diagnosis and clinical features of the restless legs syndrome. ASDA News 1995;2(2):6.

364. Sachdev P. Akathisia and Restless Legs. New York: Cambridge University Press, 1995.

365. Wilson V. Sleep Thief: Restless Legs Syndrome. Orange Park, FL: Galaxy Books, 1996.

366. Willis T. De Animae Brutorum. London: Wells & Scott, 1672.

367. Coleman RM. Periodic Movements in Sleep (Nocturnal Myoclonus) and Restless Legs Syndrome. In C Guilleminault (ed), Sleeping and Waking Disorders: Indications and Techniques. Menlo Park, CA: Addison Wesley, 1982;265.

368. Walters AS, Hening W. Review of the clinical presentation and neuropharmacology of restless legs syndrome. Clin Neuropharmacol 1987;10:225. Erratum 482.

369. Krueger BR. Restless legs syndrome and periodic movements of sleep. Mayo Clin Proc 1990;65:999.

370. Silber MH. Restless legs syndrome. Mayo Clin Proc 1997;72:261.

371. Montagna P, de Bianchi LS, Zucconi M, et al. Clonazepam and vibration in restless leg syndrome. Acta Neurol Scand 1984;69:428.

372. Ohanna N, Peled R, Rubin AHE. Periodic leg movements in sleep: effect of clonazepam treatment. Neurology 1985;35:408.

373. Mitler MM, Browman CP, Menh SJ, et al. Nocturnal myoclonus: treatment efficacy of clonazepam and temazepam. Sleep 1986;9:385.

374. Walters AS, Wagner ML, Hening WA, et al. Successful treatment of the idiopathic restless legs syndrome in a randomized double-blind trial of oxycodone versus placebo. Sleep 1993;16:327.

375. Guilleminault C, Flagg W. Effect of baclofen on sleep-related periodic leg movements. Ann Neurol 1984;15:234.

376. Telstad W, Sørensen O, Larsen S, et al. Treatment of the restless legs syndrome with carbamazepine: a double blind study. BMJ 1984;288:444.

377. Wagner ML, Walters AS, Coleman RG, et al. Randomized, double-blind, placebo-controlled study of clonidine in restless legs syndrome. Sleep 1996;19:52.

378. Scrima L, Johnson FH Jr, Thomas EE, et al. Gamma-hydroxybutyrate effect on nocturnal myoclonus: a double-blind study. Sleep Res 1990;19:289.

379. Allen RP, Earley CJ. Augmentation of the restless legs syndrome with carbidopa/levodopa. Sleep 1996;19:205.

380. Von Scheele C, Kempi V. Long-term effect of dopaminergic drugs in restless legs: a 2 year follow-up. Arch Neurol 1990;47:1223.

381. Staedt J, Wassmuth F, Ziemann U, et al. Pergolide: treatment of choice in restless legs syndrome (RLS) and nocturnal myoclonus syndrome (NMS). A double-blind randomized crossover trial of pergolide versus L-dopa. J Neural Transm 1997;104:461.

382. Silber MH, Shepard JW Jr, Wisbey JA. Pergolide in the management of restless legs syndrome: an extended study [in process citation]. Sleep 1997;20:878.

382a. Lin SC, Kaplan J, Burger CD, Frederickson PA. Effect of pramipexole in treatment of resistant restless legs syndrome. Mayo Clin Proc 1998;73:497.

383. Rajput AH, Fenton M, Birdi S, Macaulay R. Is levodopa toxic to human substantia nigra? Mov Disord 1997;12:634.

384. Gottwald MD, Bainbridge JL, Dowling GA, et al. New pharmacotherapy for Parkinson's disease. Ann Pharmacother 1997;31:1205.

385. Allen RP, Kaplan PW, Buchholz DW, et al. Double-blinded, placebo controlled comparison of high dose propoxyphene and moderate dose carbidopa/levodopa for treatment of periodic limb movements in sleep. Sleep Res 1992;21:166.

386. Allen RP, Kaplan PW, Buchholz DW, Walters JK. A double-blind, placebo controlled study of the treatment of periodic limb movements in sleep using carbidopa/levodopa and propoxyphene. Sleep 1993;16:717.

387. Kavey N, Walters AS, Hening W, Gidro-Frank S. Opioid treatment of periodic movements in sleep in patients without restless legs. Neuropeptides 1988;11:181.

388. Horiguchi J, Inami Y, Sasaki A, et al. Periodic leg movements in sleep with restless legs syndrome: effect of clonazepam treatment. Jpn J Psychol Neurol 1992;46:727.

389. Bonnet MH, Arand DL. The use of triazolam in older patients with periodic leg movements, fragmented sleep, and daytime sleepiness. J Gerontol Med Sci 1990;45:139.

390. Schenck CH, Mahowald MW. Long-term, nightly benzodiazepine treatment of injurious parasomnias and other disorders of disrupted nocturnal sleep in 170 adults. Am J Med 1996;100:333.

391. Mellick GA, Mellick LB. Management of restless legs syndrome with gabapentin (Neurontin) [letter]. Sleep 1996;19:224.

392. Allen RP, Earley CJ. An open label clinical trial with structured subjective reports and objective leg activity measures comparing gabapentin with alternative treatment in the restless legs syndrome. Sleep Res 1996; 25:184.

393. Adler CH. Treatment of restless legs syndrome with gabapentin. Clin Neuropharmacol 1997;20:148.

394. Ehrenberg BL, Muller-Schwarze A, Frankel F. Open-label trial of gabapentin for periodic limb movement disorder of sleep. Neurology 1997;48:A278.

395. Laschewski F, Sanner B, Konermann M, et al. Pronounced hypersomnia in a 13-year-old patient with periodic leg movements. Pneumologie 1997;51(Suppl 3):725.

396. Ehrenberg B, Eisensehr I, Walters A. Influence of valproate on sleep and periodic limb movement disorder. Sleep Res 1995;24:227.

397. Staedt J, Stoppe G, Riemann H, et al. Lamotrigine in the treatment of nocturnal myoclonus syndrome (NMS): two case reports. J Neural Transm 1996;103:355.

398. Handwerker JV, Palmer RF. Clonidine in the treatment of restless legs syndrome. N Engl J Med 1985;313:1228.

399. Cavatorta F, Vagge R, Solari P, Queirolo C. Risultati preliminari con clonidina nella sindrome delle gambe senza riposo in due pazienti uremici emodializzati. Min Urol Nefrol 1987;39:93.

400. Read D, Feest T, Nassim M. Clonazepam: effective treatment for restless legs syndrome in uremia. BMJ 1981;283:885.

401. Walker SL, Fine A, Kryger MH. L-DOPA/carbidopa for nocturnal movement disorders in uremia. Sleep 1996;19:214.

402. Trenkwalder C, Stiasny K, Pollmacher T, et al. L-DOPA therapy of uremic and idiopathic restless legs syndrome: a double-blind crossover trial. Sleep 1995;18:681.

403. Ausserwinkler M, Schmidt P. Successful clonidine treatment of restless legs syndrome in chronic kidney insufficiency. Schweiz Med Wochenschr 1989;119:184.

404. Nordlander NB. Therapy in restless legs. Acta Med Scand 1953;145:453.

405. Botez MI, Cadotte M, Beaulieu R, et al. Neurologic disorders responsive to folic acid therapy. Can Med Assoc J 1976;115:217.

406. Botez MI, Fontaine F, Botez T, Bachevalier J. Folate-responsive neurological and mental disorders: report of 16 cases. Eur Neurol 1977;15:230.

407. Ayres S, Mihan R. Nocturnal leg cramps (systremma): a progress report on response to vitamin E. South Med J 1974;67:1308.

408. Lee MS, Choi YC, Lee SH, Lee SB. Sleep-related periodic leg movements associated with spinal cord lesions. Mov Disord 1996;11:719.

409. Ancoli-Israel S, Seifert AR, Lemon M. Thermal biofeedback and periodic movements in sleep: patients' subjective report and a case study. Biofeedback Self Regul 1986;11:177.

410. Kovacevic-Ristanovic R, Cartwright RD, Lloyd S. Non-pharmacologic treatment of periodic leg movements in sleep. Arch Phys Med Rehabil 1991;72:385.

411. Knowles J, Ancoli-Israel S, Gevirtz R, Poceta JS. The evaluation of thermal biofeedback in the treatment of periodic limb movement disorder. Sleep Res 1996;25:265.

412. Edinger JD, Fins AI, Sullivan RJ, et al. Comparison of pharmacologic and nonpharmacologic treatments of periodic limb movement disorder. Sleep Res 1995;24:224.

413. Kanter AH. The effect of sclerotherapy on restless legs syndrome. Dermatol Surg 1995;21:328.

414. Lutz EG. Restless legs, anxiety, and caffeinism. J Clin Psychiatry 1978;39:693.

415. Ware JC, Brown FW, Moorad PJ, et al. Nocturnal myoclonus and tricyclic antidepressants. Sleep Res 1984;13:72.

416. Garvey MJ, Tollefson GD. Occurrence of myoclonus in patients treated with tricyclic antidepressants. Arch Gen Psychiatry 1987;44:269.

417. Bakshi R. Fluoxetine and restless legs syndrome. J Neurol Sci 1996;142:151.

418. Dorsey CM, Lukas SE, Cunningham SL. Fluoxetine-induced sleep disturbance in depressed patients. Neuropsychopharmacology 1996;14:437.

419. Sandyk R, Iacono RP, Bamford CR. Spinal cord mechanisms in amitriptyline responsive restless legs syndrome in Parkinson's disease. Int J Neurosci 1988;38:121.

420. Fleming J. The effect of trazodone hydrochloride on periodic leg movements. Sleep Res 1988;17:39.

421. Shaffer JI, Tallman JB, Boecker MR, et al. A report on the PLM suppressing properties of serotonin reuptake inhibitors. Sleep Res 1995;24:347.

422. Picchietti D. Growing Pains: RLS in Children. In V Wilson, A Walters (eds), Sleep Thief: Restless Legs Syndrome. Orange Park, FL: Galaxy Books, 1996;82.

423. Picchietti DL, Walters AS. Restless legs syndrome: parent-child pairs. Sleep Res 1995;24:319.

424. Lugaresi E, Cirignotta F, Montagna P. Nocturnal paroxysmal dystonia. J Neurol Neurosurg Psychiatry 1986;49:375.

425. Peled R, Lavie P. Paroxysmal awakenings from sleep associated with excessive daytime somnolence: a form of nocturnal epilepsy. Neurology 1986;36:95.

426. Zucconi M, Oldani A, Ferini-Strambi L, et al. Nocturnal paroxysmal arousals with motor behaviors during sleep: frontal lobe epilepsy or parasomnia? J Clin Neurophysiol 1997;14:513.

427. Pedley TA, Guilleminault C. Episodic nocturnal wanderings responsive to anticonvulsant drug therapy. Ann Neurol 1977;2:30.

428. Plazzi G, Tinuper P, Montagna P, et al. Epileptic nocturnal wanderings. Sleep 1995;18:749.

429. Oguni M, Oguni H, Kozasa M, Fukuyama Y. A case with nocturnal paroxysmal unilateral dystonia and interictal right frontal epileptic EEG focus: a lateralized variant of nocturnal paroxysmal dystonia? Brain Dev 1992;14:412.

430. de Saint-Martin A, Badinand N, Picard F, et al. Diurnal and nocturnal paroxysmal dyskinesia in young children: a new entity? Rev Neurol (Paris) 1997;153:262.

431. Montagna P. Nocturnal paroxysmal dystonia and nocturnal wandering. Neurology 1992;42:61.

432. Tinuper P, Cerullo A, Cirignotta F, et al. Nocturnal paroxysmal dystonia with short-lasting attacks: three cases with evidence for an epileptic frontal lobe origin of seizures. Epilepsia 1990;31:549.

433. Meierkord H, Fish DR, Smith SJM, et al. Is nocturnal paroxysmal dystonia a form of frontal lobe epilepsy? Mov Disord 1992;7:38.

434. Scheffer IE, Bhatia KP, Lopes-Cendes I, et al. Autosomal dominant frontal epilepsy misdiagnosed as sleep disorder (see comments). Lancet 1994;343:515.

435. Montagna P. Nocturnal paroxysmal dystonia and nocturnal wandering. Neurology 1992;42:61.

436. Lugaresi E, Montagna P, Sforza E. Nocturnal Paroxysmal Dystonia. In MG Terzano, P Halasz, AC Declerck (eds), Phasic Events and Dynamic Organization of Sleep. New York: Raven, 1991;1.

437. Montagna P, Cirignotta F, Giovanardi Rossi P, Lugaresi E. Dystonic attacks related to sleep and exercise. Eur Neurol 1992;32:185.

438. van Sweden B, Kemp B, van Dijk JG, Kamphuisen HA. Ambulatory monitoring in sleep apnoea presenting with nocturnal episodic phenomena. Int J Psychophysiol 1990;10:181.

439. Biary N, Singh B, Bahou Y, et al. Posttraumatic paroxysmal nocturnal hemidystonia. Mov Disord 1994;9:98.

440. Schenck CH, Bundlie SR, Ettinger MG, Mahowald MW. Chronic behavioral disorders of human REM sleep: a new category of parasomnia. Sleep 1986;293.

441. Schenck CH, Bundlie SR, Patterson AL, Mahowald MW. Rapid eye movement sleep behavior disorder. JAMA 1987;257:1786.

442. Mahowald MW, Schenck CH. REM Sleep Behavior Disorder. In MH Kryger, T Roth, WC Dement (eds),

Principles and Practice of Sleep Medicine (2nd ed). Philadelphia: Saunders, 1994;574.

443. Schenck CH, Mahowald MW. Injurious sleep behavior disorders (parasomnias) affecting patients on intensive care units. Intensive Care Med 1991;17:219.

444. Schenck CH, Mahowald MW. Polysomnographic, neurologic, psychiatric, and clinical outcome report on 70 consecutive cases with REM sleep behavior disorder (RBD): sustained clonazepam efficacy in 89.5% of 57 cases. Cleve Clin J Med 1990;57:S9.

445. Tatman JE, Sind JM. REM behavior disorder manifests differently in women and men. Sleep Res 1996; 25:380.

446. Culebras A, Moore JT. Magnetic resonance findings in REM sleep behavior disorder. Neurology 1989; 39:1519.

447. Turner RS, Chervin RD, Frey KA, et al. Probable diffuse Lewy body disease presenting as REM sleep behavior disorder. Neurology 1997;49:523.

448. Septien L, Didi-Roy R, Marin A, Giroud M. REM-sleep behavior disorder and olivo-ponto-cerebellar atrophy: a case report. Neurophysiol Clin 1992;22:459.

449. Kimura K, Tachibana N, Aso T, et al. Subclinical REM sleep behavior disorder in a patient with corticobasal degeneration. Sleep 1997;20:891.

450. Tachibana N, Kimura K, Kitajima K, et al. REM sleep motor dysfunction in multiple system atrophy: with special emphasis on sleep talk as its early clinical manifestation. J Neurol Neurosurg Psychiatry 1997;63:678.

451. Plazzi G, Corsini R, Provini F, et al. REM sleep behavior disorders in multiple system atrophy. Neurology 1997;48:1094.

452. Armitage R, Trivedi M, Rush AJ. Fluoxetine and oculomotor activity during sleep in depressed patients. Neuropsychopharmacology 1995;12:159.

453. Schenck CH, Boyd JL, Mahowald MW. A parasomnia overlap disorder involving sleepwalking, sleep terrors, and REM sleep behavior disorder in 33 polysomnographically confirmed cases. Sleep 1997;20:972.

454. Tachibana N, Sugita Y, Terashima K, et al. Polysomnographic characteristics of healthy elderly subjects with somnambulism-like behaviors. Biol Psychiatry 1991;30:4.

455. Sforza E, Krieger J, Petiau C. REM sleep behavior disorder: clinical and physiopathological findings. Sleep Med Rev 1997;1:57.

456. Uchiyama M, Isse K, Tanaka K, et al. Incidental Lewy body disease in a patient with REM sleep behavior disorder (see comments). Neurology 1995;45:709.

457. Schenck CH, Garcia-Rill E, Segall M, et al. HLA class II genes associated with REM sleep behavior disorder. Ann Neurol 1996;39:261.

458. Schenck CH, Ullevig CM, Mahowald MW, et al. A controlled study of serum anti-locus ceruleus antibodies in REM sleep behavior disorder. Sleep 1997;20:349.

459. Bamford CR. Carbamazepine in REM sleep behavior disorder. Sleep 1993;16:33.

460. Kunz D, Bes F. Melatonin effects in a patient with severe REM sleep behavior disorder: case report and theoretical considerations. Neuropsychobiology 1997;36:211.

461. Coulter DL, Allen RJ. Benign neonatal sleep myoclonus. Arch Neurol 1982;39:191.

462. Resnick TJ, Moshe SL, Perotta L, Chambers HJ. Benign neonatal sleep myoclonus. Relationship to sleep states. Arch Neurol 1986;43:266.

463. Di Capua M, Fusco L, Ricci S, Vigevano F. Benign neonatal sleep myoclonus: clinical features and videopolygraphic recordings. Mov Disord 1993;8:191.

464. Daoust-Roy J, Seshia SS. Benign neonatal sleep myoclonus. A differential diagnosis of neonatal seizures. Am J Dis Child 1992;146:1236.

465. Fukumoto M, Mochizuki N, Takeishi M, et al. Studies of body movements during night sleep in infancy. Brain Dev 1981;3:37.

466. Lins O, Castonguay M, Dunham W, et al. Excessive fragmentary myoclonus: time of night and sleep stage distributions. Can J Neurol Sci 1993;20:142.

467. Manetto V, Medori R, Cortelli P, et al. Fatal familial insomnia: clinical and pathological study of five new cases. Neurology 1992;42:312.

468. Fiorino AS. Sleep, genes and death: fatal familial insomnia. Brain Res Brain Res Rev 1996;22:258.

469. Sforza E, Montagna P, Tinuper P, et al. Sleep-wake cycle abnormalities in fatal familial insomnia. Evidence of the role of the thalamus in sleep regulation. Electroencephalogr Clin Neurophysiol 1995;94:398.

470. Portaluppi F, Cortelli P, Avoni P, et al. Progressive disruption of the circadian rhythm of melatonin in fatal familial insomnia. J Clin Endocrinol Metab 1994;78:1075.

471. Portaluppi F, Cortelli P, Avoni P, et al. Dissociated 24-hour patterns of somatotropin and prolactin in fatal familial insomnia. Neuroendocrinology 1995;61:731.

472. Portaluppi F, Cortelli P, Avoni P, et al. Diurnal blood pressure variation and hormonal correlates in fatal familial insomnia. Hypertension 1994;23:569.

473. Goldfarb LG, Petersen RB, Tabaton M, et al. Fatal familial insomnia and familial Creutzfeldt-Jakob disease: disease phenotype determined by a DNA polymorphism. Science 1992;258:806.

474. Macchi G, Rossi G, Abbamondi AL, et al. Diffuse thalamic degeneration in fatal familial insomnia. A morphometric study. Brain Res 1997;771:154.

475. Reder AT, Mednick AS, Brown P, et al. Clinical and genetic studies of fatal familial insomnia. Neurology 1995;45:1068.

476. Bramble D. Two cases of severe head-banging parasomnias in peripubertal males resulting from otitis media in toddlerhood. Child Care Health Dev 1995; 21:247.

477. Bastuji H. Rhythms of falling asleep persisting in adults. Two cases without mental deficiency. Neurophysiol Clin 1994;24:160.

478. Chisholm T, Morehouse RL. Adult headbanging: sleep studies and treatment. Sleep 1996;19:343.

479. Kempenaers C, Bouillon E, Mendlewicz J. A rhythmic movement disorder in REM sleep: a case report. Sleep 1994;17:274.

480. Johns MW. A new method for measuring daytime sleepiness: the Epworth Sleepiness scale. Sleep 1991;14:540.

481. Therapeutic and Technology Assessment Subcommittee of the American Academy of Neurology. Assessment: techniques associated with the diagnosis and management of sleep disorders. Neurology 1992; 42:269.

482. Chesson AL Jr, Ferber RA, Fry JM, et al. The indications for polysomnography and related procedures. Sleep 1997;20:423.

483. Dyken ME, Lin-Dyken DC, Yamada T. Diagnosing rhythmic movement disorder with video-polysomnography. Pediatr Neurol 1997;16:37.

484. Aldrich MS, Jahnke B. Diagnostic value of video-EEG polysomnography. Neurology 1991;41:1060.

485. Broughton RJ, Fleming JA, Fleetham J. Home assessment of sleep disorders by portable monitoring. J Clin Neurophysiol 1996;13:272.

486. Alihanka J, Vaahtoranta K, Saarikivi J. A new method of long-term monitoring of the ballistocardiogram, heart rate and respiration. Am J Physiol 1981;240:384.

487. Erkinjuntti M, Vaahtoranta K, Alihanka J, Kero P. Use of the SCSB method for monitoring of the respiration, body movements, and ballistocardiogram in infants. Early Hum Dev 1984;9:119.

488. Salmi T, Leinonen L. Automatic analysis of sleep records with static charge sensitive bed. Electroencephalogr Clin Neurophysiol 1986;64:84.

489. Erkinjuntti M, Kero P, Halonen JP, et al. SCSB method compared to EEG-based polygraphy in sleep state scoring of newborn infants. Acta Paediatr Scand 1990;79:274.

490. Salmi T, Telakivi T, Partinen M. Evaluation of automatic analysis of SCSB airflow and oxygen saturation signals in patients with sleep related apneas. Chest 1989;96:255.

491. Rauhala E, Erkinjuntti M, Polo O. Detection of periodic leg movements with a static-charge-sensitive bed. J Sleep Res 1996;5:246.

492. Sforza E, Vandi S. Automatic Oxford-Medilog 9200 sleep staging scoring: comparison with visual analysis. J Clin Neurophysiol 1996;13:227.

493. Jobert M, Schulz H, Jahnig P, et al. A computerized method for detecting episodes of wakefulness during sleep based on the alpha slow-wave index (ASI). Sleep 1994;17:37.

494. Jobert M, Escola H, Poiseau E, Gaillard P. Automatic analysis of sleep using two parameters based on principal component analysis of electroencephalography spectral data. Biol Cybern 1994;71:197.

495. Schaltenbrand N, Lengelle R, Toussaint M, et al. Sleep stage scoring using the neural network model: comparison between visual and automatic analysis in normal subjects and patients. Sleep 1996;19:26.

496. Baumgart-Schmitt R, Herrmann WM, Eilers R, Bes F. On the use of neural network techniques to analyse sleep EEG data. First communication: application of evolutionary and genetic algorithms to reduce the feature space and to develop classification rules. Neuropsychobiology 1997;36:194.

497. Schaltenbrand N, Lengelle R, Macher JP. Neural network model: application to automatic analysis of human sleep. Comput Biomed Res 1993;26:157.

498. Kayed K, Roberts S, Davies WL. Computer detection and analysis of periodic movements in sleep. Sleep 1990;13:253.

499. Coleman RM, Bliwise DL, Sajben N, et al. Epidemiology of Periodic Movements During Sleep. In C Guilleminault, E Lugaresi (eds), Sleep/Wake Disorders: Natural History, Epidemiology, and Long-Term Evolution. New York: Raven, 1983;217.

500. Dickel M, Mosko S. Sleep apnea and sleep-related periodic leg movements in the elderly: night-to-night variability. Sleep Res 1988;17:168.

501. Bliwise DL, Carskadon MA, Dement WC. Nightly variation of periodic leg movements in sleep in middle aged and elderly individuals. Arch Gerontol Geriatr 1988;7:273.

502. Roehrs T, Zorick F, Sicklesteel J, et al. Age-related sleep-wake disorders at a sleep disorders center. J Am Geriatr Soc 1983;31:364.

503. Mosko SS, Dickel MJ, Paul T, et al. Sleep apnea and sleep-related periodic leg movements in community resident seniors. J Am Geriatr Soc 1988;36:502.

504. Ancoli-Israel S, Clopton P, Klauber MR, et al. Use of wrist activity for monitoring sleep/wake in demented nursing-home patients. Sleep 1997;20:24.

505. Van Someren EJ. Actigraphic monitoring of movement and rest-activity rhythms in aging, Alzheimer's disease, and Parkinson's disease. IEEE Trans Rehabil Eng 1997;5:394.

506. Colburn T, Smith B, Guarini J, Simmons N. An ambulatory activity monitor with solid state memory. ISA Trans 1976;15:149.

507. Redmond DP, Hegge FW. Observations on the design and specification of a wrist-worn activity monitor. Behav Res Meth Instr Comput 1985;17:639.

508. Brown AC, Smolensky MH, D'Alonzo GE, Redman DP. Actigraphy: a means of assessing circadian patterns in human activity. Chronobiol Int 1990;7:125.

509. Sadeh A, Hauri PJ, Kripke DF, Lavie P. The role of actigraphy in the evaluation of sleep disorders. Sleep 1995;18:288.

510. Hauri PJ, Wisbey J. Wrist actigraphy in insomnia (see comments). Sleep 1992;15:293.

511. American Sleep Disorders Association. Practice parameters for the use of actigraphy in the clinical assessment of sleep disorders. Sleep 1995;18:285.

512. Cole RJ, Kripke DF, Gruen W, et al. Automatic sleep/wake identification from wrist activity. Sleep 1992;15:461.

513. Jean-Louis G, von Gizycki H, Zizi F, et al. Determination of sleep and wakefulness with the actigraph data analysis software (ADAS). Sleep 1996;19:739.

514. Jean-Louis G, von Gizycki H, Zizi F, et al. The actigraph data analysis software: I. A novel approach to scoring and interpreting sleep-wake activity. Percept Mot Skills 1997;85:207.

515. Jean-Louis G, von Gizycki H, Zizi F, et al. The actigraph data analysis software: II. A novel approach to scoring and interpreting sleep-wake activity. Percept Mot Skills 1997;85:219.

516. Allen RP, Gorny SW, Krausman DT, Earley CJ. Activity and eye blink rates prior to initial sleep onset and return to sleep as a function of prior wake time and time since initial sleep onset for normals and insomnia patients. Sleep Res 1996;25:91.

517. Gorny S, Allen RP, Karausman D, et al. A parametric and sleep hysteresis approach to assessing sleep and wake from a wrist activity meter with enhanced frequency range. Sleep Res 1997;26:662.

518. Caligiuri MP, Lohr JB, Bracha HS, Jeste DV. Clinical and instrumental assessment of neuroleptic-induced parkinsonism in patients with tardive dyskinesia. Biol Psychiatry 1991;29:139.

519. Caligiuri MP, Lohr JB, Rotrosen J, et al. Reliability of an instrumental assessment of tardive dyskinesia: results from VA Cooperative Study #394. Psychopharmacology (Berl) 1997;132:61.

520. Allen RP, Kaplan PW, Buchholz DW, et al. Accuracy of a physical activity monitor (PAM) worn on the ankle for assessment of treatment response for periodic limb movements in sleep. Sleep Res 1992;21:329.

521. Kazenwadel J, Pollmacher T, Trenkwalder C, et al. New actigraphic assessment method for periodic leg movements (PLM). Sleep 1995;18:689.

522. Allen RP. Activity Monitoring to Diagnose and Evaluate Motor Abnormalities of Sleep. In W Hening, S Chokroverty (eds), Topics in Movement Disorders of Sleep (Course Syllabus: ASDA Annual Meeting, San Francisco). Rochester, MN: American Sleep Disorders Association, 1997.

523. Ancoli-Israel S, Klauber MR, Jones DW, et al. Variations in circadian rhythms of activity, sleep, and light exposure related to dementia in nursing-home patients. Sleep 1997;20:18.

524. Allen RP, Gorny S, Krausman DT, et al. Ambulatory 3-D body position monitor for patients with sleep walking or the restless legs syndrome. Sleep Res 1997; 26:639.

524a. Montplaisir J, Boucher S, Nicolas A, et al. Immobilization tests and periodic leg movements in sleep for the diagnosis of restless leg syndrome. Mov Disor 1998;13:324.

525. Hening WA, Walters AS, Chokroverty S. A test for monitoring symptom severity in the restless legs syndrome. Neurosci Abstr 1988;14:908.

526. Pelletier G, Lorrain D, Montplaisir J. Sensory and motor components of the restless legs syndrome. Neurology 1992;42:1663.

# Chapter 27
# Sleep, Breathing, and Neurologic Disorders

## Sudhansu Chokroverty

To understand the effects of neurologic lesions on sleep-wake cycles and sleep states, and to understand the normal interactions of sleep and breathing, it is important to have a clear understanding of the functional anatomy of sleep and breathing. In the first section of the chapter, therefore, a brief overview of the anatomy and physiology of sleep is presented. The section of the functional anatomy of sleep is followed by a short discussion of the control of breathing during sleep. For details readers are referred to some excellent reviews[1–10] and monographs, and to Chapters 3, 4, and 6 in this volume.

Most of the anatomic structures that control sleep and breathing are located in the central nervous systems (CNS). These regions are influenced not only by other CNS structures but also by inputs from the peripheral neuromuscular system and other body systems. It is very common to encounter in practice a variety of neurologic disorders that affect sleep and breathing. It is important to understand not only that the neurologic illnesses may affect sleep and breathing but also that alterations of sleep and breathing may adversely affect the natural history of a neurologic disorder. A number of excellent sources provide systematic descriptions of the effects of neurologic lesions on the pattern and control of breathing.[11–21] The effect of acute and chronic neurologic disorders on the state of sleep and the resulting interaction on breathing have received scant attention. An understanding of such an interaction is essential for treatment and prognostic purposes in various neurologic disorders. In

neurologic illnesses, breathing disorders may manifest as hypopnea, apnea, irregular or periodic breathing, or cessation of breathing. Similarly, sleep disturbances may manifest as hypersomnia, hyposomnia (insomnia), parasomnia, or circadian rhythm sleep disorders. The sections after those on functional anatomy and physiology of sleep and breathing deal with the clinical manifestations, laboratory assessment, and treatment of sleep and breathing disorders that accompany neurologic illnesses. The discussion is grouped into two major sections: (1) sleep and breathing disorders secondary to somatic neurologic illness and (2) sleep and breathing disorders secondary to autonomic failure. The somatic neurologic disorders are subdivided into CNS disorders and peripheral neuromuscular disorders.

## FUNCTIONAL ANATOMY OF SLEEP

Neurophysiologic studies of sleep really began after astute clinicopathologic observers examined patients with encephalitis lethargica at the beginning of the twentieth century.[22] It was noted that lesions of encephalitis lethargica, which severely affected the posterior hypothalamic area, were associated with the clinical manifestation of extreme somnolence whereas morphologic alterations in the anterior hypothalamic region were associated with sleeplessness. These observations led scientists to believe in the existence of the so-called sleep-wake centers.[22–25]

Before the middle of the century, the emphasis of sleep physiologists was on the passive[25–27] theories of sleep. Beginning in the late 1950s thought shifted toward active sleep theories.[3,5,28–37] The passive theory postulates that sleep results from withdrawal of both specific and nonspecific afferent stimuli to the brain stem and the cerebral hemisphere. Proponents of active sleep theories suggest that activity of sleep-promoting neurons or the fibers of these so-called centers determine the onset of sleep. Most likely, proponents of both active and passive theories are partially correct, as far as the physiology and anatomy of sleep are concerned. These conclusions are based on stimulation, ablation, or lesion experiments. Later, these studies were extended to include extracellular as well as intracellular recordings, and pharmacologic injections of chemicals into discrete areas to induce different states of sleep or to inhibit sleep.[38]

The passive theory originated with two classic preparations in cats by Bremer,[26,39] *cerveau isolé* and *encéphale isolé*. Bremer found that midcollicular transection (*cerveau isolé*) produced somnolence in the acute stage and that transection at C1 vertebral level, to disconnect the entire brain from the spinal cord (*encéphale isolé*), caused electroencephalographic (EEG) recordings to fluctuate between wakefulness and sleep. From these experiments Bremer concluded that in *cerveau isolé* preparations all the specific sensory afferent stimuli were withdrawn and thus sleep was facilitated, whereas such stimuli maintained the activation of the brain in *encéphale isolé* preparation. These conclusions, however, have been modified since the discovery by Moruzzi and Magoun[27] in 1949 of the existence of nonspecific groups of neurons and fibers in the center of the brain stem called the *reticular formation*. Moruzzi and Magoun[27] stated that the ascending reticular activating brain stem system energized the forebrain and that withdrawal of this influence in *cerveau isolé* preparation resulted in somnolence or coma. The observations of Moruzzi and Magoun[27] that EEG desynchronization results from activation of the midbrain reticular neurons, which directly excite the thalamocortical projections, have been confirmed by more recent intracellular studies.[40,41] It was thought that wakefulness resulted from activation of the ascending reticular activating system and diffuse thalamocortical projections.[1] After stimulation of these structures, EEG shows diffuse desynchronization, whereas lesions

in these structures produce EEG synchronization or the EEG non–rapid eye movement (NREM) sleep pattern. This also supports the suggestion of Steriade et al.[42] that, at the onset of NREM sleep, there is deafferentation of the brain due to blockage of afferent information first at the thalamic level, causing the waking open brain to be converted into a closed brain resulting from thalamocortical inhibition. It has been demonstrated that the origin of the sleep spindles are related to the reticular nucleus of the thalamus.[1] Stimulation of this nucleus produces spindlelike activity, whereas destruction of it abolishes the spindles unilaterally and bilateral destruction abolishes the spindles on both sides.

The passive sleep theories were challenged by findings that came in the wake of midpontine pretrigeminal brain stem transection in cats performed by Batini and coworkers.[29,30] This preparation is only a few millimeters below the section that produces *cerveau isolé* preparation. In contrast to the somnolence produced by *cerveau isolé* preparation, the midpontine pretrigeminal section produced persistent EEG and behavioral signs of alertness. These observations imply that structures located in the brain stem regions between these two preparations (*cerveau isolé* and midpontine pretrigeminal preparations) are responsible for wakefulness. Data demonstrate cholinergic neurons in the pedunculopontine tegmental (PPT) nucleus and in the laterodorsal tegmental nucleus in the region of the midbrain-pontine junction.[1] These groups of cholinergic neurons have been shown to have thalamic and basal forebrain projections as well as projections toward the medial pontine reticular formation. The neurons are likely responsible for activation and for generation of REM sleep (see Chapter 3). The forebrain cholinergic neurons from the basal nucleus of Meynert project to the cerebral hemisphere, particularly to the sensory-motor cortex, and lesions in these neurons disrupt the EEG waves and elicit diffuse slow waves.[1] The finding of cholinergic neurons at the mesopontine junction confirms the conclusions drawn by Batini and colleagues[29,30] after midpontine pretrigeminal transections. Transection experiments by Jouvet[43] through different regions of the midbrain, pons, and medulla of cats clearly show the existence of REM sleep–generating neurons in the pontine cat brain (see Chapter 3).

The active hypnogenic neurons for NREM sleep are thought to be located in two regions[1]:

(1) the region of the nucleus tractus solitarius (NTS) in the medulla and (2) the preoptic area of the hypothalamus and the basal forebrain area (see Chapter 4). The evidence is based on stimulation, lesion, and ablation studies, as well as extracellular and intercellular recordings.[1] The active inhibitory role of the lower brain stem hypnogenic neurons on the upper brain stem ascending reticular activating systems has been clearly demonstrated by Batini's[29,30] experiment of midpontine pretrigeminal section. Similarly, electrical[34] stimulation of the preoptic area, which produced EEG synchronization and behavioral state of sleep, supported the idea of the existence of active hypnogenic neurons in the preoptic area.[1] Nauta's[25] experiments in 1946 that showed insomnia after lesions of the preoptic region also supported the hypothesis of active hypnogenic neurons in the forebrain preoptic area. Later experiments by McGinty and Sterman[36] in 1968 confirmed Nauta's observations. More recently, ibotenic lesions in the preoptic region have been found to produce insomnia, and these results support the active hypnogenic role of preoptic area.[1,44] In the same experiments, however, injections of muscimol (a $\gamma$-aminobutyric acid [GABA] agonist) in the posterior hypothalamus transiently recovered sleep, suggesting that the sleep-promoting role of the anterior hypothalamus is dependent on inhibition of posterior hypothalamic histaminergic awakening neurons.

Intracellular studies by Szymusiak and McGinty[45] again challenged the concept of active hypnogenic neurons in the preoptic area. In these experiments, only a small number of neurons showed discharge rates that were higher during EEG synchronization than in REM sleep or wakefulness; therefore, the majority of these forebrain neurons are found to be state-indifferent or waking-active.[1,45] On the other hand, experiments in cats by Detari et al.[46] and Buzsaki et al.[47] have clearly shown increased firing rates for basal forebrain neurons during EEG desynchronization associated with appropriate behavioral state. Thus, Steriade and McCarley[1] concluded that the idea of an active hypnogenic center or group of neurons still awaits confirmation at the cellular level. They suggested that the search for the active hypnogenic neurons should be conducted in the region of the basal forebrain rather than any other brain region, however, because cholinergic pathways that descend from the basal forebrain to the PPT nucleus in the mesopontine junction have been found.[1,48,49] In summary, the active and passive theories of sleep may be viewed as complementary rather than mutually exclusive mechanisms.[1] The role of postulated humoral sleep factors (e.g., prostaglandin $D_2$, growth hormone–releasing factor, muramyl peptides) remains undetermined in the absence of experiments to test their role at the cellular level in critical brain areas.

It has been suggested that adenosine, a neuromodulator, may act as a physiologic sleep factor modulating the somnogenic effects of prolonged wakefulness.[50] This has been postulated after experiments in cats have shown that adenosine extracellular concentration in the basal forebrain cholinergic region increased progressively during prolonged spontaneous wakefulness.

For additional discussion on the functional anatomy of sleep, the reader is referred to Chapters 3 and 4.

## FUNCTIONAL ANATOMY OF RESPIRATION IN SLEEP AND WAKEFULNESS

The neuroanatomy of respiration, its control, and physiologic changes during sleep in healthy individuals are described in detail in Chapter 6. Briefly, respiration is controlled by the automatic or metabolic and behavioral systems.[11–14,51–54] The two systems are complemented by a third system known as the *arousal system*, which may also be called the *system for wakefulness stimulus*.[54,55] These respiratory systems work in concert with the various peripheral and central inputs to maintain acid-base regulation and respiratory homeostasis.[9] The location of the respiratory neurons makes them easily vulnerable to a variety of central and peripheral neurologic disorders, particularly central neurologic disorders involving the brain stem. Many acute and chronic neurologic illnesses may affect central or peripheral respiratory pathways, giving rise to acute respiratory failure in wakefulness and sleep. Some conditions may affect control of breathing only during sleep. Such a condition may cause undesirable, often catastrophic, results, including cardiorespiratory failure and even sudden death.

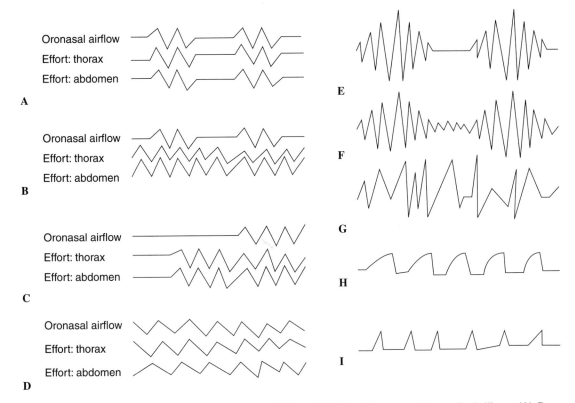

**Figure 27-1.** Schematic diagram to show different types of sleep-related breathing patterns in neurologic illness. **(A)** Central apnea. **(B)** Upper airway obstructive apnea. **(C)** Mixed apnea (initial central followed by obstructive). **(D)** Paradoxical breathing. **(E)** Cheyne-Stokes respiration. **(F)** Cheyne-Stokes variant pattern. **(G)** Dysrhythmic breathing. **(H)** Apneustic breathing. **(I)** Inspiratory gasp. (Reproduced with permission from S Chokroverty. Sleep Apnea and Respiratory Disturbances in Multiple System Atrophy with Progressive Autonomic Failure [Shy-Drager Syndrome]. In R Bannister [ed], Autonomic Failure [2nd ed]. London: Oxford University Press, 1988;432.)

## SLEEP-RELATED RESPIRATORY DYSRHYTHMIA IN NEUROLOGIC DISORDERS

Many types of sleep-related respiratory dysrhythmia have been noted in association with neurologic illnesses[54,56,57] (Figure 27-1). The most common type is sleep apnea or sleep hypopnea.

### Sleep Apnea

Three types of sleep apnea have been noted[58]: central, upper airway obstructive, and mixed. Normal individuals may experience a few episodes of sleep apnea, particularly central apnea, at the onset of NREM sleep and during REM sleep. To be of pathologic significance, the sleep apnea should last at least 10 seconds, apnea index (number of apneas per hour of sleep) should be at least 5, and the patient should have at least 30 periods of apneas during 7 hours of all-night sleep.[59]

Cessation of airflow with no respiratory effort constitutes central apnea. During this period there is no diaphragmatic and intercostal muscle activity or air exchange through the nose or mouth. Upper airway obstructive sleep apnea (OSA) is manifested by absence of air exchange through the nose or mouth but persistence of the diaphragmatic and intercostal muscle activity.

During mixed apnea, initially airflow ceases, as does respiratory effort (central apnea); this is followed by a period of upper airway OSA. On rare occasions this pattern may be reversed, resulting in an initial period of OSA followed by central apnea (Figure 27-2).

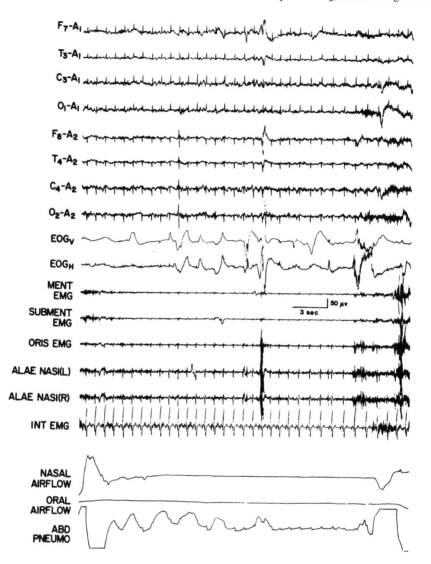

**Figure 27-2.** Polysomnography recording in a patient with narcolepsy and sleep apnea showing EEG (top eight channels); vertical (EOG$_V$) and horizontal (EOG$_H$) electro-oculograms; mentalis (MENT), submental (SUBMENT), orbicularis oris (ORIS), left (L) and right (R) alae nasi, and intercostal (INT) electromyogram (EMG); nasal and oral airflow; and abdominal pneumogram (ABD PNEUMO). Note unusual type of mixed apnea (initial obstructive apnea for a period of 14 seconds followed by central apnea for a period of 8 seconds) during REM sleep.

### Sleep-Related Hypopnea

Sleep-related hypopnea is manifested by a decrease in airflow at the mouth and nose and decreased chest movement, which causes a reduction in tidal volume and a reduction of the amplitude of the oronasal thermistor or the pneumographic signal to half the volume measured during the preceding or following respiratory cycles.[60] Some investigators consider a reduction of one-third of the tidal volume associated with 4% reduction of oxygen ($O_2$) desaturation to be consistent with a diagnosis of hypopnea. There is, at present, no precise standardized definition of hypopnea.[61,62,63] Respiratory disturbance index (RDI), or apnea-hypopnea index (AHI), is defined as the number of apneas plus hypopneas per hour of sleep. A normal index is less than 5. However, most investigators consider an AHI or RDI of 10 or more to be significant.

Sleep-related apneas and hypopneas in neurologic diseases are secondary sleep apnea syndromes, in contrast to primary OSA syndrome, in which no cause is found except for minor upper airway anatomic configuration in some cases to account for the appearance of apnea. The neurologic illness may be aggravated by the secondary sleep apnea because of the adverse effects of sleep-induced hypoxemia and hypercapnia and repeated sleep arousals with sleep fragmentation. In long-standing cases there may be pulmonary hypertension, congestive cardiac failure, and other manifestations of chronic sleep deprivation.

## Paradoxical Breathing

The thorax and abdomen move in opposite directions during paradoxical breathing, indicating increased upper airway resistance. In upper airway resistance syndrome, this may be noted without any change in oronasal airflow; in OSA, however, paradoxical breathing is accompanied by reduction or absence of oronasal airflow.

## Cheyne-Stokes and Cheyne-Stokes Variant Pattern of Breathing

Cheyne-Stokes breathing is a special type of central apnea manifested as cyclic changes in breathing with crescendo-decrescendo sequence separated by central apneas.[60,64,65] The Cheyne-Stokes *variant pattern* of breathing is distinguished by the substitution of hypopneas for apneas.[19,21] In neurologic disorders, Cheyne-Stokes type of breathing is mostly noted in bilateral cerebral hemispheric lesions[12,13] and it worsens during sleep, whereas Cheyne-Stokes variant patterns of breathing may also be noted in brain stem lesions, in addition to bilateral cerebral hemisphere disease.

## Dysrhythmic Breathing

Dysrhythmic breathing[60,66] is characterized by nonrhythmic respiration of irregular rate, rhythm, and amplitude during wakefulness with or without $O_2$ desaturation that becomes worse during sleep. Dysrhythmic breathing may result from an abnormality in the automatic respiratory pattern generator in the brain stem.

## Apneustic Breathing

Apneustic breathing is characterized by prolonged inspiration with an increase in the ratio of inspiratory to expiratory time.[64] This type of breathing may result from a neurologic lesion in the caudal pons that disconnects the so-called apneustic center in the lower pons from the pneumotaxic center (parabrachial and Kolliker-Fuse nuclei) in the upper pons in association with vagotomy.[67,68]

## Inspiratory Gasp

Inspiratory gasp is characterized by a short inspiration time and a relatively prolonged expiration (reduced inspiratory-expiratory time ratio).[69] Gasping or irregular breathing has been noted after lesion in the medulla.[16,64]

## Other Abnormal Breathing Patterns

The following abnormal breathing patterns have also been noted in neurologic disorders, particularly in patients with Shy-Drager syndrome[54,57]:

- Nocturnal stridor causing severe inspiratory breathing difficulty
- Periodic central apnea in the erect position accompanied by postural fall of blood pressure in Shy-Drager syndrome[70a]
- Prolonged periods of central apnea accompanied by mild $O_2$ desaturation in relaxed wakefulness, as if the respiratory centers "forgot" to breathe[60,66]
- Transient occlusion of the upper airway or transient uncoupling of intercostal and diaphragmatic muscle activity[66]
- Transient sudden respiratory arrest

## MECHANISM OF RESPIRATORY DYSRHYTHMIAS IN NEUROLOGIC DISEASE

Several mechanisms may be responsible for the respiratory abnormalities in sleep associated with neurologic disorders.[54,60]

1. Direct involvement causing structural alterations of the medullary respiratory neurons (automatic or metabolic respiratory controlling system) may result in apnea or hypopnea during NREM and REM sleep. During REM sleep, this problem may be aggravated because of the additional complicating factor of oropharyngeal or other upper airway muscle hypotonia contributing to upper airway OSA.

2. Involvement of the voluntary respiratory control system causes respiratory dysfunction during wakefulness and may give rise to respiratory apraxia.

3. Functional or neurochemical alteration of the respiratory neurons, causing respiratory dysrhythmia.

4. Interference with the afferent inputs to the medullary respiratory neurons (e.g., compromise of the peripheral chemoreceptors located in the vagal and glossopharyngeal nerve endings), supramedullary pathways, and central chemoreceptors in the ventrolateral medulla, causing abnormal breathing.

5. Direct involvement of the efferent mechanism through respiratory muscle weakness may result from either direct involvement of the muscles, as in myopathies, or involvement of the lower motor neurons to the respiratory muscles. In patients with weakness of the principal respiratory and the accessory respiratory muscles, the central respiratory neurons may increase their rate of firing or recruit additional respiratory neurons during wakefulness to maintain ventilation at a level adequate to drive the weak respiratory muscles. Because of the normal vulnerability of the respiratory neurons during sleep, the central respiratory neurons may not be able to participate in such compensatory mechanisms in patients with respiratory muscle weakness. Ventilatory problems may thus be aggravated, causing more severe hypoventilation and even apnea during sleep. In addition, weakness of the upper airway muscles, which in fact are respiratory muscles and receive phasic inspiratory drive from the respiratory neurons in the brain stem, may cause obstructive apnea.

## SLEEP DISTURBANCES IN NEUROLOGIC DISORDERS

Sleep disorders in neurologic illnesses may be divided broadly into two groups: (1) *dyssomnias*, which include insomnia, hypersomnia, and circadian rhythm sleep disorders; and (2) *parasomnias*, which are not primary disorders of sleep but disorders of arousal and sleep stage transition associated with abnormal movements and behavior that disrupt sleep but do not alter sleep architecture.

Insomnia may be manifested as difficulty in initiating or maintaining sleep, and hypersomnia as excessive daytime somnolence (EDS) and other symptoms. Most of the neurologic disorders cause hypersomnia, but sometimes insomnia is the presenting complaint.[70b] An important but rare example, fatal familial insomnia (FFI), is described later in this chapter.

Hypersomnia is generally noted in patients with sleep-related respiratory dysrhythmias. In acute neurologic disorders, the clinical features of neurologic dysfunction may overshadow the sleep and sleep-related respiratory problems.[60] Furthermore, many patients with acute neurologic disorders are actually in stupor or coma. Neurologic lesions may disrupt the sleep architecture, for example, altering the percentage of different sleep stages, increasing awakenings, or causing sleep stage shifts. In addition, sleep apnea, which may occur in various neurologic diseases; intrusion of abnormal movements in sleep; and repeated seizures may disrupt the morphology of sleep and sleep stages. Sleep disturbances may impair memory, cognition, or behavior, or cause cardiopulmonary changes secondary to repeated hypoxemia. These effects, secondary to sleep disturbance, can aggravate the primary neurologic condition.

### Clinical Manifestations

The general symptoms of insomnia and hypersomnia have been described in Chapters 18 and 24.

The clinical manifestations of sleep and breathing disorders in chronic neurologic illnesses may be divided into specific and general features.[54,60] The specific manifestations depend on the nature of the neurologic deficit. The general features that are relevant to the diagnosis of sleep-related hypoventilation and apnea include EDS, fatigue, early morning headache, disturbed nocturnal sleep, intellectual deterioration, personality changes, and in men, impotence. Breathlessness is generally not an important feature of CNS disorders except those illnesses that affect the lower motor neurons to the respiratory muscles. The general symptoms of daytime fatigue, somnolence, and morning headache may be related to frequent arousals at night secondary to repeated apnea or hypopnea and carbon dioxide retention.[71] In patients with neurologic disorders it is very important to recognize alveolar hypoventilation during sleep because assisted ventilation at night improves the symptoms and protects patients from fatal apnea during sleep. Furthermore, such treatment may prevent the development of serious complications resulting from episodic or prolonged hypoxemia, hypercapnia, and respiratory acidosis in sleep, complications that may include pulmonary hypertension, cor pulmonale, congestive cardiac failure, and occasionally cardiac arrhythmias. Occasionally, neurologic disorders may cause an inversion of the sleep-wake rhythm that is manifested by excessive somnolence during the day and insomnia with agitation during the night.[72]

To make a clinical diagnosis of sleep disorders or sleep-related breathing disorders, a careful history—from the patient and the caregiver—and a physical examination are essential.

## Mechanisms of Sleep Disturbances in Neurologic Disorders

Neurologic disorders can be metabolic or structural (e.g., head injury, tumor, infection, toxic-metabolic brain dysfunction, vascular and degenerative CNS disease, headache from any cause, painful peripheral neuropathy, or other neuromuscular disorder). The following are the suggested mechanisms of the sleep disturbances associated with neurologic disorders[54,60,73]:

1. Direct involvement of the hypnogenic neurons; hypofunction of the hypothalamic preoptic nuclei or the lower brain stem hypnogenic neurons, for example, alters the balance between the waking and the sleeping brain, causing wakefulness or sleeplessness. Similarly, a disorder of the posterior hypothalamic, the ascending reticular activating system, or other brain regions responsible for waking and alertness causes hypersomnolence.
2. Indirect mechanisms associated with the disorder, such as pain, confusional episodes, changes in the sensorimotor system, and movement disorders, can interfere with sleep.

3. Medications used to treat neurologic illnesses (e.g., anticonvulsants, antidepressants, dopamine agonists, anticholinergics, hypnotics, sedatives) may have a direct effect on sleep and breathing.
4. Neurologic diseases (e.g., hyperkinetic movement disorders, Rett syndrome) may change the neurochemical environment of the sleep-generating and sleep-promoting neurons.[74]
5. Associated depression or anxiety, which may be a secondary manifestation of neurologic disease, can disrupt sleep.
6. Sleep-wake schedule disturbances can interfere with sleep.
7. Sleep-related respiratory dysrhythmias may result in sleep fragmentation.

## SLEEP AND BREATHING DYSFUNCTION

### Cerebral Hemispheric and Diencephalic Diseases

Sleep disturbances in neurologic diseases affecting the cerebral hemispheres and the diencephalon have been noted in two groups of patients: those with sleep-related breathing disorders and those without sleep-disordered breathing. Plum and coworkers noted[11–13,17,75] that the major effects of cerebral hemispheric disease on respiration in sleep consisted of the following: (1) Cheyne-Stokes respiration or long-cycle Cheyne-Stokes breathing associated with hypocapnia; this was associated with brain damage deep in both cerebral hemispheres. In unilateral cerebral infarction this may be due to the phenomenon of diaschisis.* (2) Posthyperventilation apnea was noted in 70% of patients with bilateral and 6% with unilateral cerebral dysfunction, and the apnea became more marked during sleep. On the other hand, Lee and coworkers[21] found Cheyne-Stokes and Cheyne-Stokes variant pattern breathing in patients with extensive bilateral pontine lesions. Plum and coworkers[11–13,17,75] rarely found Cheyne-Stokes respiration in lesions located as low as the upper pons but mostly noted it with bilateral cerebral hemispheric or diencephalic lesions. It must be remembered that many patients with cerebral hemispheric and diencephalic lesions

---

*Diaschisis implies physiologic dysfunction of the contralateral homologous area without anatomic disconnection.

remain in stupor and coma; these patients' sleep and respiration during sleep cannot be assessed.

Sleep disturbances in cerebral hemispheric and diencephalic diseases may result from cerebral vascular diseases, brain tumors, degenerative dementia (e.g., Alzheimer's disease [AD]), head trauma, encephalitis, or toxic-metabolic encephalopathy or any diffuse cerebral dysfunction that could directly or indirectly affect the diffuse thalamocortical projection system and thalamic-hypothalamic regions.

### Sleep and Breathing Disturbances in Alzheimer's Disease

AD, or senile dementia of the Alzheimer's type, is characterized by progressive intellectual deterioration occurring in middle or later life associated with characteristic neuropathologic findings, including cerebral cortical atrophy and neuronal loss in the nucleus basalis of Meynert. There is also evidence of alterations in the forebrain cholinergic, and in many cases also in the noradrenergic, system.[76] For the diagnosis of probable, possible, and definite AD, readers are referred to the clinical criteria developed by NINCDS-ADRDA (National Institute of Neurological and Communicative Disorders and Stroke–Alzheimer's Disease and Related Diseases Association) work (Table 27-1).[77] Sleep disturbances in AD may be related partly to the severity of the loss of the cholinergic neurons in the basal forebrain regions, as well as to changes in the brain stem aminergic systems.

Sleep disorders in AD may increase cognitive and behavioral dysfunction. Such sleep disorders may arise directly from the disease itself, as a consequence of the degeneration of the brain stem and other centers that regulate sleep,[78] or indirectly from changes in sleep associated with aging (see Chapter 32). Sleep disorders can have a number of undesirable consequences, including increasing cardiovascular and even cerebrovascular morbidity as well as impairing daytime alertness and functioning.[58,59,79]

A number of studies have examined the differences between demented patients and normal elderly individuals and have demonstrated higher prevalence for sleep apnea and for poorer sleep quality when patients are compared to age-matched controls.[78–80] Although the results vary somewhat from study to study, these investigations have shown deterioration of sleep parameters, including reduced total length of sleep, decreased REM and stage IV NREM sleep, loss of phasic components (spindles and K complexes) of NREM sleep, and sleep-wake rhythm disturbances in demented patients.[80–85] Montplaisir et al.[85] documented EEG slowing during both wakefulness and REM sleep in AD patients. The authors suggested that degeneration of nucleus basalis of Meynert, which is the main source of cholinergic input to the cerebral cortex, may be responsible for EEG slowing and REM sleep changes. This pattern of disorder is different from that of depressed elderly patients, who most clearly show poor sleep maintenance, often with increased REM sleep.[81] Most of the studies, however, have not used current diagnostic criteria for dementia and have lumped together patients with different forms of it. When more accurate diagnostic groupings were made, similar results were found for AD patients usually defined by clinical course. Some studies have shown a clear association between greater sleep disturbance and impaired mental functioning or severity of dementia.[78,86–88]

Some of the inconsistencies noted in the sleep architecture in AD patients[89,90] may be related to the fact that in many studies, mild, moderate, and severe AD patients were grouped together and not necessarily analyzed separately. Another point to remember is that it is often difficult to separate the effects of the disease on sleep from the effects of medication and periodic limb movements in sleep (PLMS) or sleep apneas, both of which are common in elderly patients. Additionally, sleep architectural alterations noted during overnight sleep studies in the laboratory may be partly environmentally determined, as AD patients may become confused, displaying features of "sun-downing," in the artificial and foreign environment of the laboratory.

Sleep apnea has been observed in approximately 33–53% of demented patients with probable AD.[78,87,88,91] Although sleep apnea may be associated with disease severity, no longitudinal studies have been conducted to determine whether sleep apnea increases the severity of disease in individual patients and whether sleep apnea may be associated with more rapid progression of the disease. Such a deleterious effect of sleep apnea is to be expected, as it is thought to increase the intellectual deficit of demented patients.[81,91] Because sleep apnea may be treated by a number of modalities, it is possible that therapy may improve behavior and cognitive function, although

**Table 27-1.** Criteria for the Clinical Diagnosis of Alzheimer's Disease

---

I. The criteria for the clinical diagnosis of probable Alzheimer's disease include

Dementia established by clinical examination and documented by the Mini-Mental Status Examination, Blessed Dementia Scale, or some similar examination, and confirmed by neuropsychologic tests;

Deficits in two or more areas of cognition;

Progressive worsening of memory and other cognitive functions;

No disturbance of consciousness;

Onset between ages of 40 and 90 years, most often older than age 65; and

Absence of systemic disorders or other brain diseases that could account for the progressive deficits in memory and cognition.

II. The diagnosis of probable Alzheimer's disease is supported by

Progressive deterioration of specific cognitive functions such as language (aphasia), motor skills (apraxia), and perception (agnosia);

Impaired activities of daily living and altered patterns of behavior;

Family history of similar disorders, particularly if confirmed neuropathologically; and

Laboratory results as follows:

Normal lumbar puncture as evaluated by standard techniques;

Normal pattern or nonspecific changes in EEG, such as increased slow-wave activity; and

Evidence of cerebral atrophy on computed tomography with progression documented by serial observations.

III. Other clinical features consistent with the diagnosis of probable Alzheimer's disease, after exclusion of causes of dementia other than Alzheimer's disease, include

Plateaus in the course of progression of the illness;

Associated symptoms of depression; insomnia; incontinence; delusions; illusions; hallucinations; catastrophic verbal, emotional, or physical outbursts; sexual disorders; and weight loss. Other neurologic abnormalities seen in some patients, especially those with more advanced disease, include motor signs such as increased muscle tone, myoclonus, and gait disorder;

Seizures in advanced disease; and

Computed tomography normal for age.

IV. Features that make the diagnosis of probable Alzheimer's disease uncertain or unlikely include

Sudden, apoplectic onset;

Focal neurologic findings such as hemiparesis, sensory loss, visual field deficits, and lack of coordination early in the course of the illness; and

Seizures or gait disturbances at the onset or very early in the course of the illness.

V. Clinical diagnosis of possible Alzheimer's disease

May be made on the basis of the dementia syndrome in the absence of other neurologic, psychiatric, or systemic disorders sufficient to cause dementia, and in the presence of variations in the onset, presentation, or clinical course;

May be made in the presence of a second systemic or brain disorder sufficient to produce dementia but not considered to be the cause of the dementia; and

Should be used in research studies when a single, gradually progressive, severe cognitive deficit is identified in the absence of other identifiable cause.

VI. Criteria for the diagnosis of definite Alzheimer's disease include the clinical criteria for probable Alzheimer's disease and histopathologic evidence obtained from a biopsy or autopsy.

VII. Classification of Alzheimer's disease for research purposes should specify features that may differentiate subtypes of the disorder, such as

Familial occurrence;

Onset before age 65 years;

Presence of trisomy 21; and

Coexistence of other relevant conditions, such as Parkinson's disease.

---

Source: Reprinted with permission from G McKhann, D Drachman, M Folstein, et al. Clinical diagnosis of Alzheimer's disease: report of the NINCDS-ADRDA work under the auspices of Department of Health and Human Services Task Force on Alzheimer's Disease. Neurology 1984;34:939.

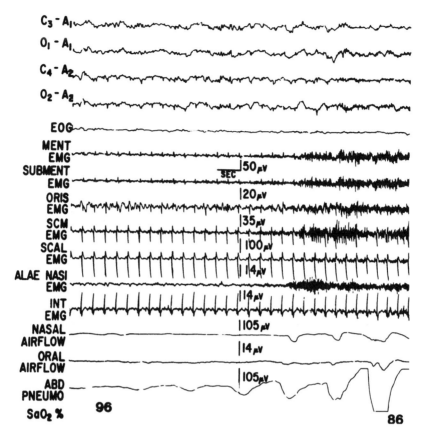

**Figure 27-3.** Polysomnography recording of a patient in an advanced stage of Alzheimer's disease shows a portion of mixed apnea during stage II non-REM sleep accompanied by oxygen desaturation. Top four channels represent EEG (Key: international electrode placement system). Electromyograms (EMG) of mentalis (MENT), submental (SUBMENT), orbicularis (ORIS), sternocleidomastoid (SCM), scalenus anticus (SCAL), alae nasi, and intercostal (INT) muscles are shown. Also shown are nasal and oral airflow, abdominal pneumogram (ABD PNEUMO) and oxygen saturation (Sao$_2$%). (EOG = electro-oculogram.) (Reproduced with permission from S Chokroverty. Sleep and Breathing in Neurological Disorders. In NH Edelman, TV Santiago [eds], Breathing Disorders of Sleep. New York: Churchill Livingstone, 1986;225.)

as yet there are no reports of the effects of treatment of sleep apnea in AD or dementia.

According to Smallwood and colleagues,[88] the incidence of sleep apnea in male AD patients is similar to that of healthy elderly subjects. Reynolds and coworkers[92] reported a higher prevalence of sleep apnea in female AD patients during the later stage of the illness than in controls. These findings have been confirmed by Vitiello[93] and Mant[94] and their associates.

PLMS is common in the elderly, and there is no significant difference in incidence between AD patients and healthy elderly subjects.[95] The incidence and severity of sleep apnea and PLMS did not significantly differ in elderly subjects and AD

patients.[95] Figure 27-3 shows mixed sleep apnea associated with significant O$_2$ desaturation in a 68-year-old man with advanced AD who was studied with polysomnography (PSG). In view of the documentation by Carskadon and associates (summarized by Miles and Dement[96]) of a high prevalence of apnea in asymptomatic ambulatory elderly volunteers, and the findings of Smallwood's group,[88] it is difficult to estimate the true incidence of sleep apnea in AD patients.

Sleep-wake rhythm disturbances are common in AD.[97] The inability of patients to follow a normal schedule can present a significant management problem; sun-downing, an inversion of sleep schedule (wakefulness at night and somnolence in the daytime) is particularly troublesome. It may be that the suprachiasmatic nucleus of the hypothalamus, a well-established regulator of circadian activity rhythm in lower animals, likely plays a similar role in humans[98] and is involved in AD. Decreased REM sleep could also result from degeneration of brain stem neurons, such as noradrenergic neurons of the locus coeruleus, which are affected in AD,[99] and the cholinergic neurons of the brain stem. These neurons have been strongly implicated in the control of sleep-wake rhythm.[4,100]

Vitiello and coworkers[93,97] and others[80,81,84,101–104] reported sleep disturbances in AD associated with a decrease in slow-wave sleep and an increase in nighttime awakenings. In a study of 45 control subjects and 44 mild AD patients Vitiello's group[105] confirmed their previous findings of disturbed sleep-wake patterns in AD patients, but the phenomenon of sleep disturbances was not diagnostically useful for discriminating between those with a mild stage of AD and control subjects.

In summary, it is known that sleep dysfunction is common in AD. It is unclear, however, whether a specific set of sleep abnormalities will be found to be associated with AD that are different from those observed in other dementias. It has been shown that the abnormalities in dementia are significantly different from those of depressive pseudodementia.[81] Reynolds and coworkers[81] suggested that sleep dysfunction in AD may be related to progression of the disease and may cause ongoing deterioration of alertness, orientation, and cognitive function.

### Sleep, Breathing, and Hemispheric-Diencephalic Stroke

Stroke is an acute neurologic deficit resulting from vascular injury to the brain. Vascular injury could be ischemic (thrombotic or embolic) or hemorrhagic. In this section, sleep and breathing disorders in cerebral hemispheric and thalamic strokes are described. Those resulting from brain stem stroke are discussed in a later section.

There are a few scattered reports of sleep complaints after stroke and several reports of sleep-related breathing disorders after cerebral infarction, but there is a dearth of well-controlled studies of the relationship between sleep disorders and cerebral vascular disease. Such studies are important from prognostic and therapeutic points of view.

### Hemispheric Stroke

Sleep disruption and sleep complaints resulting from sleep-related breathing dysrhythmias have been reported in many patients with cerebral hemispheric stroke. Sleep apnea, snoring, and stroke are intimately related. Sleep apnea may predispose to stroke and stroke may predispose to sleep apnea. There is increasing evidence based on case-control, epidemiologic, and laboratory studies that snoring and sleep apnea are risk factors for stroke. Confounding variables that are common risk factors for snoring, sleep apnea, and stroke (e.g., hypertension, cardiac disease, age, body mass index, smoking, and alcohol consumption) should be considered when attempting to establish relationships among snoring, sleep apnea, and stroke. A history of habitual snoring (established through questionnaire studies and interviews with a bed partner or other family members) is a clear risk factor for stroke. There is an increased frequency of sleep apnea in both the infratentorial and supratentorial strokes. Sleep apnea may adversely affect the short-term and long-term outcomes in patients with stroke both in terms of morbidity and mortality. It is important to make the diagnosis of sleep apnea in stroke patients, as there is effective treatment for sleep apnea that can decrease the risk of future stroke.

Dyken et al.[106] prospectively performed overnight PSG studies in 24 patients who had experienced a recent stroke with a mean age of approximately 65 (13 men and 11 women) and 27 control subjects with a mean age of approximately 62 (13 men and 14 women). The authors concluded that patients with stroke had a high incidence of significant OSAs compared to the normal age- and sex-matched control subjects. Similarly, Good et al.[107] used computerized overnight oximetric study in 47 patients with recent ischemic stroke and performed a PSG in 19 of these patients. These authors found that 18 of 19 subjects who had a PSG study had an AHI of more than 10 per hour of sleep. They also observed that the sleep-disordered breathing was associated with higher mortality at 1 year and a lower Barthel index at follow-up. This study, however, suffers from the serious drawbacks of having no control group and failing to exclude other causes of hypoxemia.

Bassetti et al.[108] prospectively obtained PSG in 36 of 59 subjects within 12 days of acute hemispheric stroke or transient ischemic episodes (TIAs) and in 19 age- and sex-matched control subjects. The PSG study showed an AHI of 10 or more in 25 of 36 subjects (69%). The proportion of subjects with sleep apnea was similar in the TIA and stroke groups. The authors concluded that sleep apnea has a high frequency in patients in the acute phase of TIA or stroke. In addition, although they could not reliably predict sleep apnea on clinical grounds alone, it was more likely in patients with habitual snoring, severe stroke, or a high score on a sleep disorder questionnaire. Spriggs et al.[109] found that in addition to increasing the risk for stroke, snoring adversely affected the prognosis after a stroke. Mohsenin and Valor[110] noted that stroke can cause sleep apnea.

Case-control and epidemiologic studies have established an association between hypertension and habitual snoring[111–114] and between habitual snoring and stroke.[114–119] Sleep apnea is noted more frequently in patients with multiple cerebral infarction than in patients with AD or normal elderly individuals.[120,121] The prospective study by Koskenvuo et al.[114] adjusted for other risk factors and found that habitual snorers had a significantly increased risk of new ischemic heart disease or new stroke. Neau et al.[122] also found a significantly increased adjusted risk of stroke in habitual snorers. In contrast, in a community-based study of snoring and sleep-disordered breathing, Olson and colleagues[123] found that the adjusted odds ratio for subjects with sleep-disordered breathing was elevated but not statistically significant for stroke. In a more recent review, Wright et al.[124] questioned the validity of a causal relationship between sleep apnea and the range of poor health outcomes, including stroke. There is, however, compelling evidence that stroke, sleep disorders, and sleep apnea are strongly associated, as discussed earlier in this section.

Cerebral hemispheric strokes can cause a decrease in NREM and REM sleep that may be correlated with clinical outcomes.[125,126] Korner and colleagues[127] made an important PSG study in a group of patients with infarction in the territory of the middle cerebral artery. They found marked attenuation of REM sleep after right cerebral hemispheric stroke and a reduction of slow-wave sleep after left hemispheric stroke; however, the numbers

are too few to be statistically significant and further studies are needed to confirm this conclusion.

In a previous brief report, Kapen and coworkers[128] reported a high incidence of OSA in hemispheric stroke patients. Because of associated risk factors such as obesity and hypertension in most of these patients, however, a definite causal relationship between OSA and stroke cannot be claimed. In a later study[129] of 53 stroke patients, these authors confirmed their previous reports of peak prevalence for the onset of stroke in the morning during a 6-hour period after awakening from sleep. This is similar to the peak incidence in the morning hours for myocardial infarction and sudden cardiac death. All of these conditions may be aggravated by a combination of circadian increase of corticosteroids and catecholamines, increased blood pressure and heart rate in the morning, and increased platelet "aggregability." (Normal subjects exhibit increased platelet aggregability in the early morning.[130]) In several other studies, the incidence of stroke was highest during sleep at night[131] or during early morning hours after awakening from nocturnal sleep.[115,132–134]

Stroke may predispose to a number of sleep disorders. Kleine-Levin syndrome can occur after multiple cerebral infarction.[135] Narcolepsy-cataplexy has been reported to follow cerebral hypoxic-ischemia.[136] Insomnia is commonly noted after cerebral infarction, but this may be partly due to the depression that typically follows stroke.[137]

### Diencephalic Stroke

Thalamic stroke may cause ipsilateral loss of sleep spindles,[138] and bilateral paramedian thalamic infarcts may be associated with hypersomnia.[139,140] Bassetti et al.[140] evaluated 12 patients with magnetic resonance imaging (MRI)-proven isolated paramedian thalamic stroke and hypersomnia. The patients were evenly divided between groups of severe and mild hypersomnia. Nocturnal PSG findings included increased stage I NREM sleep, reduced stage II NREM sleep, and a reduced number of sleep spindles. Bassetti et al.[140] found intact REM sleep as well as circadian, ultradian, and homeostatic sleep regulation, however, in their patients. The authors concluded that hypersomnia after paramedian thalamic stroke is accompanied by deficient arousal during the day and insufficient spindling and slow-wave sleep production at night. Their observation supported the hypothesis of a dual role of the paramedian thalamus for the maintenance of sleep-wake regulation. In contrast, Guilleminault et al.[141] reported three patients with pseudohypersomnia and presleep behavior with bilateral paramedian thalamic lesions. These authors used long-term monitoring with an infrared video camera and polygraphic study to document that their patients did not develop the normal NREM cycling during the day; rather, the EEG indicated a mixture of low-amplitude theta and alpha frequency waves during the day, with "sleep-like behavior." The patients exhibited the behavioral aspects of sleep during the day, suggesting to Guilleminault et al.[141] that these subjects did not present hypersomnia but a "de-arousal" and are left in the transition between wakefulness and sleep. These authors[141] cited a report by Catsman-Berrevoets and von Harskamp,[142] who reported a similar patient with compulsive presleep behavior and apathy due to bilateral thalamic stroke who responded to bromocriptine.

### Basal Ganglia Disorders

Sleep disturbances and sleep-related respiratory dysrhythmias are noted in many patients with basal ganglia disorders, but a systematic study to evaluate such dysfunction has not been undertaken in a large number of patients. A review of sleep and movement disorders is given in Chapter 26.

### Disorders of Cerebellum and Brain Stem

Olivopontocerebellar atrophy (OPCA) defines chronic progressive hereditary (usually dominant, occasionally recessive, rarely sporadic) cerebellar degeneration manifested by cerebellar-parkinsonian or parkinsonian-cerebellar syndrome and associated with atrophy of the pontine nuclei and cerebellar cortex and degenerative lesions of the olivopontocerebellar regions.[143-145] There have been a few reports on sleep disturbances and sleep-related respiratory dysrhythmias in OPCA.

Cerebellar influence on the sleep-wakefulness mechanism has been clearly demonstrated in experimental animal studies.[146] The role of the cerebel-

lum, however, on the respiratory control mechanism in sleep is not known. Brain stem neurons, which are known to be degenerated in OPCA,[144,145] lie close to the hypnogenic[39] and respiratory neurons.[52] Thus, dysfunction of the respiratory control, in parallel with the somatic structural dysfunction in OPCA, may be expected. The known morphologic changes of OPCA[144,145] are adequate to explain the sleep disturbances and sleep apnea in this condition. Several authors[147-150] described EEG sleep alterations in degenerative cerebellar atrophy. Reduced or absent REM sleep, reduced slow-wave sleep, and increased awakenings are the essential PSG findings. In several cases of OPCA, REM sleep without muscle atonia accompanied by the typical features of REM behavior disorder (RBD) has been described.[151-153] Jouvet and Delorme[154] produced REM sleep without atonia in cats by bilateral pontine tegmental lesions. A similar lesion in OPCA may be also responsible for RBD in this condition. OPCA has also been associated with hyposomnia.[155]

Sleep apnea has been described in several cases of OPCA.[150,155-158] It should be noted that patients with sporadic OPCA associated with prominent autonomic failure are now classified under the term *multiple-system atrophy* (MSA) or *Shy-Drager syndrome* (see Assessment of Sleep and Sleep-Related Breathing Disorders in Autonomic Failure, later in this chapter). Chokroverty and colleagues[156] described five patients with OPCA and sleep apnea. PSG study showed repeated episodes of central, upper airway obstructive, and mixed apneas (Figure 27-4) during sleep; the apneic episodes lasted from 10 to 62 seconds and the apnea index was 30–55. Pure central apnea was noted in three patients, but all three types of apnea were seen in two, and most of the apneic episodes occurred during NREM sleep stage II. Thus, these findings suggested central neuronal dysfunction in an area where respiratory and sleep-waking systems are closely interrelated, such as the NTS and the pontomedullary reticular formation. Salazar-Grueso and associates[150] described a 37-year-old man with a 19-year history of autosomal dominant OPCA and EDS whose PSG demonstrated episodes of mixed and central (predominantly central) sleep apnea and no sleep spindles or REM sleep. Trazodone treatment normalized the sleep architecture and reduced the apneic episodes.

Occasionally, sleep disturbances are associated with other types of cerebellar lesions, although

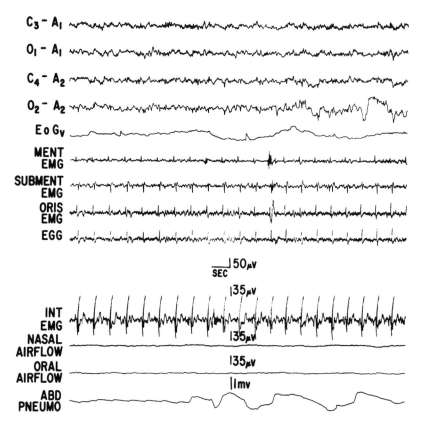

$C_3 - A_1$

$O_1 - A_1$

$C_4 - A_2$

$O_2 - A_2$

$EoG_V$

MENT EMG

SUBMENT EMG

ORIS EMG

EGG

$\overline{SEC}$ |50µv

|35µv

INT EMG

NASAL AIRFLOW    |35µv

ORAL AIRFLOW    |35µv

ABD PNEUMO    ||mv

**Figure 27-4.** Polysomnography recording in a patient with olivopontocerebellar atrophy showing a portion of an episode of mixed apnea (central followed by upper airway obstructive apnea) during stage II NREM sleep. EEGs are shown in the top four channels. ($EOG_V$ = vertical electro-oculogram; MENT = mentalis; EMG = electromyography; SUBMENT = submental; ORIS = orbicularis; INT = intercostal muscles; ABD PNEUMO = abdominal pneumogram; EGG = electroglossogram.) (Reproduced with permission from S Chokroverty, R Sachdeo, J Masdeu. Autonomic dysfunction and sleep apnea in olivopontocerebellar degeneration. Arch Neurol 1984;41:509.)

systematic studies are lacking. Bergamasco and colleagues[159] made a polygraphic study of a 13-year-old girl with a diagnosis of dyssynergia cerebellaris myoclonica (Ramsey-Hunt syndrome). All-night sleep study showed no REM sleep and increased slow-wave sleep. The EEG showed multiple spike-wave discharges accompanied by myoclonic generalized seizures, and on other occasions desynchronized EEG was noted during tonic seizure.

### Brain Stem Lesions

The metabolic and autonomic respiratory neurons and the lower brain stem hypnogenic neurons are located in the medulla. These neurons are influ-enced by the supramedullary respiration-controlling inputs and hypothalamic preoptic nuclei, as well as by the peripheral afferent inputs to the respiratory centers (see Chapter 6). Therefore, sleep and respiratory disturbances should be common manifestations of lesions in the brain stem, and many such cases have been described. Such disorders have included brain stem vascular lesions, tumors, traumatic lesions, multiple sclerosis (MS), bulbar poliomyelitis and postpolio syndrome, brain stem encephalitis, motor neuron disease affecting the bulbar nuclei, syringobulbia, and Arnold-Chiari malformation.[60] In addition, several cases in which brain stem lesions caused symptomatic or secondary narcolepsy have been described.[139,160–165] Generally, all the characteristic features of narcolepsy are not seen in the secondary syndrome.

The causes have included infarction,[139] trauma, tumors[160] (including third ventricle tumor[161]), and arteriovenous malformation invading the third ventricle and affecting the hypothalamus,[162] and some cases have been associated with MS.[163–165]

*Brain Stem Vascular Lesions*

Brain stem vascular lesions include infarction, hemorrhage, arterial compression, and localized brain stem ischemia. Sleep disturbances have been described in brain stem infarction by Markand and Dyken[166] and several other authors.[19,21,167,168] PSG findings generally consisted of increased wakefulness after sleep onset and decreased REM and slow-wave sleep. Several reports of EEG or PSG studies to document sleep disturbances have been described in patients with locked-in syndrome (LIS), which is characterized by quadriplegia associated with deafferentation and results from ventral pontine infarction. Patients are generally aware of the surroundings and are conscious. They cannot speak because of facial muscle paralysis but can respond by moving the eyes, whose control is spared. Sleep EEG recordings of LIS patients have been reported by Feldman,[169] Freemon and coworkers,[170] Markand and Dyken,[166] Cummings and Greenberg,[171] Oxenberg and colleagues,[172] and Nordgren et al.[173] The EEG findings in these reports generally showed reduced or absent REM sleep and variable changes in NREM sleep including reduction of slow-wave sleep and total sleep time. Oxenberg's group,[172] however, described only minor alterations in the initial recording in contrast to the more marked alterations noted in the other reports. The authors thought that the difference could be related to the extent of the lesion. Feldman[169] found in his patient reduced REM, stage IV NREM and total sleep time. Markand and Dyken[166] noted in five of seven LIS patients total absence of REM sleep and variable changes in NREM sleep. Cummings and Greenberg[171] described that one patient had reduced slow-wave sleep and the other reduced NREM sleep and no REM sleep. Autret and coworkers[174] also found a reduction of REM and NREM sleep in four patients after medial pontine tegmental stroke.

Kushida and associates[175] described marked asymmetry in the EEG of REM sleep in a 24-year-old woman with a left pontine hematoma, suggesting to the authors that a unilateral pontine lesion may cause disruption of the normal REM sleep EEG in the ipsilateral hemisphere. The lesion did not affect the other characteristics of REM sleep, such as REMs and muscle atonia.

The term *Ondine's curse*, or the *syndrome of primary failure of automatic respiration*, was coined by Severinghaus and Mitchell[176] to describe three patients who experienced long periods of apnea even when awake but could breathe on command. They became apneic after surgery involving the brain stem and high cervical spinal cord and required artificial ventilation while asleep. When their consciousness was altered by nitrous oxide or thiopental, they became apneic. Carbon dioxide response to breathing showed low sensitivity. One patient died in apnea and the two others improved in 1 week. The authors suggested that Ondine's curse resulted from damage to the medullary carbon dioxide chemoreceptors. It is notable that the term *Ondine's curse* was derived from the sea nymph in German mythology, whose curse rendered her unfaithful lover incapable of automatic respiratory function and caused his death. This eponymic syndrome generated considerable controversy and confusion.[177] The syndrome of the Ondine's curse is usually caused by bilateral lesions anywhere caudal to the fifth cranial nerve in the pons down to the upper cervical spinal cord in the ventrolateral region. Levin and Margolis[168] described a 52-year-old man with unilateral medullary infarction, however, who lost automatic respiratory control. At autopsy the lesion was found to extend from the left lower pons through the left lateral medullary tegmentum to the upper cervical spinal cord and to involve the left paramedian pontine reticular formation. Thus, in some patients, automatic respiratory control can reside unilaterally in the pontomedullary tegmentum.

A case of the inverse Ondine's curse syndrome in whom there was selective paralysis of voluntary respiration but preservation of automatic respiration was described by Munschauer et al.[178] This was a 36-year-old man with sudden onset of quadriparesis and bulbar dysfunction in whom the MRI demonstrated a well-demarcated lesion restricted to the ventral basis pontis. His hypercapnic ventilatory response and breathing during sleep were normal. Emotional stimuli producing laughter, crying, or anxiety appropriately modulated automatic respiration but the patient could not voluntarily modify any respiratory parameters. The findings in this case suggested that descending limbic influences on automatic respiration are anatomically and functionally independent of the voluntary respiratory systems.

Bogousslavsky et al.[179] reported a clinical pathologic correlation in two patients who had central hypoventilation and unilateral infarct in the caudal brain stem. The authors suggested that unilateral involvement of pontomedullary reticular formation and nucleus ambiguus is sufficient for generating a loss of automatic respiration, whereas associated lesion of the NTS may lead to more severe respiratory failure involving both automatic and voluntary responses.[179]

Respiratory rate and pattern were studied by Lee and colleagues[19] by impedance pneumography in 14 patients with acute brain stem or cerebral infarction, and in a subsequent study they reported on another 23 patients with acute brain stem infarction.[21] They found frequent abnormalities of respiratory pattern and rate in such patients, and these abnormalities became worse during sleep. The abnormal pattern included Cheyne-Stokes and Cheyne-Stokes variant types of breathing, in addition to tachypnea and cluster breathing in some. In contrast to the observations of Plum and coworkers[11–13,75] that such breathing patterns are associated with bilateral cerebral hemispheric and diencephalic lesions but rarely with lesions in the upper pons, Lee's group[21] observed Cheyne-Stokes respiration in patients with extensive bilateral pontine lesions. They suggested that the size and the bilaterality of the lesions determined the types of respiratory pattern abnormalities.

Devereaux and coworkers[167] reported sleep apnea that required ventilatory support in two women who breathed normally while awake. Aged 36 and 59 years, they had bilateral infarctions limited to the lateral medullary tegmentum. One of these patient's carbon dioxide response was markedly depressed. Although the authors stated that acute automatic respiratory failure did not generally evolve into a chronic alveolar hypoventilation syndrome, their second patient continued to have sleep-induced apnea after many months.

Sleep apnea after bulbar stroke was also described by Askenasy and Goldhammer.[180] Their patient had a left-sided Wallenberg's syndrome (lateral medullary syndrome) and two nights' PSG recordings documented mostly obstructive or mixed apneas and hypopneas. This was a clinical diagno-

sis, and neuroimaging did not define the exact anatomy of the lesion. Their report, however, should direct attention to the possibility that unilateral brain stem lesions can cause sleep apnea syndrome. In such patients it is important to diagnose and promptly treat ventilatory dysfunction during sleep.

Miyazaki and associates[181] described a 5-year-old boy with central sleep apnea (CSA) (documented by PSG recording) associated with compression of the ventral medulla by abnormal looping of the vertebral artery as documented by MRI. The authors suggested that the aberrant vertebral artery might have compressed the respiratory center, although the hypercapnic ventilatory response, which reflects central chemoreceptor function, was normal during sleep in this case.

Periodic breathing, apnea, and cyanosis were described in a 57-year-old woman after carotid endarterectomy.[182] The authors suggested that respiratory depression resulted from midbrain hypoxia and edema.

Brain stem ischemic damage may also cause respiratory dysfunction. Beal and colleagues[183] described a 19-year-old man who had failure of automatic respiration and other signs of brain stem dysfunction after nearly drowning. He had sleep apneas, and PSG study confirmed the presence of CSAs. During wakefulness, his breathing was normal. Hypercapnic ventilatory response was markedly impaired, but hypoxic ventilatory response appeared to be normal. Autopsy findings 8 months later, after sudden death, documented marked bilateral neuron loss in the tractus solitarius, ambiguus, and retroambigualis nuclei. These most likely resulted from anoxia or ischemia.

### Brain Stem Tumor

Brain stem glioma with automatic respiratory failure was mentioned by Plum.[13] Ito et al.[184] described two children with brain stem gliomas and sleep apnea. A patient of mine with a medullary tumor that caused severe hypoventilation during sleep, required tracheostomy (unpublished observation). The central apneic episodes in the same patient became prolonged when the tracheostomy tube was occluded. Brain stem tumor may cause disorganization of the tonic and the phasic events of REM sleep, as described in a patient whose pontine tumor caused a marked decrease in the atonia of REM sleep.[185] Lee et al.[186] reported a 74-year-old woman with recurrent acoustic neuroma at the cerebello-pontine angle presenting as central alveolar hypoventilation. The patient had shallow breathing during sleep and had hypersomnolence during the daytime. Arterial blood gases showed increased $PaCO_2$ and decreased $PaO_2$. Tumor resection eliminated hypersomnolence and respiratory failure.

*Brain Stem Trauma*

Traumatic brain injuries (TBIs) include concussion, contusion, laceration, hemorrhage, and cerebral edema. After a severe TBI, the brain stem function is severely compromised and the patient becomes comatose. There have been many EEG studies in patients with coma and some patients may demonstrate sleep patterns such as spindles and K complexes. Such patterns are designated as *spindle coma*.[187] It is often stated that the presence of EEG sleep patterns means a favorable prognosis[188] but this may not be necessarily true. On recovering from the coma during this stage of rehabilitation, many patients may have sleep-wake disturbances. However, there have been no adequate studies addressing the sleep-wake abnormalities in such patients. It is surprising, considering that one editorial labeled TBI as a silent epidemic.[189] There is a dearth of studies addressing sleep-wake abnormalities after minor brain injuries that did not result in coma but caused a transient loss of consciousness. Many of these patients experience so-called postconcussion syndrome, characterized by a variety of behavioral disturbances, headache, and sleep-wake abnormalities.[190] A few reports[190–193] list subjective complaints of sleep disturbances but do not include formal sleep studies. In one report by Prigatano et al.,[194] PSG studies in patients with post-traumatic insomnia documented sleep maintenance insomnia with an increased number of awakenings and decreased night sleep in closed-head injury patients. The mechanism of these sleep abnormalities is unknown. All-night studies of 105 cases of brain-damaged patients after TBI were performed by Harada et al.,[195] showing a normalization of sleep organization and a parallel improvement of REM sleep recovery and cognition.

Insomnia, hypersomnia, and circadian sleep disturbances may occur after TBI but objective sleep studies rather than anecdotal reports or single case reports are necessary to determine this.[190] Post-traumatic hyper-somnolence has been listed in the *International Classification of Sleep Disorders* (*ICSD*).[196] Guilleminault et al.[197] evaluated 20 patients with post-traumatic hypersomnia using PSG and the Multiple Sleep Latency Test (MSLT). The causes were multiple, including cases secondary to sleep apnea syndrome. TBI may cause central and upper airway OSA by inflicting functional or structural alterations of the brain stem respiratory control system. It is important to remember, however, that many patients may have sleep apnea syndrome before sustaining TBI.

North and Jennett[18] recorded irregular breathing patterns in patients with traumatic lesions of the medulla and pons. However, they did not discuss the changes in the breathing patterns during sleep in these patients. In contrast to the findings of Plum and Posner,[75] they did not find that long- or short-cycle Cheyne-Stokes respirations helped localize the site of brain damage.

Okawa et al.[198] described disturbance of circadian rhythms in severely brain-damaged patients. Patten and Lauderdale[199] reported a case of delayed sleep phase syndrome in a 13-year-old boy after a minor head injury sustained in a motorcycle accident (5 minutes' loss of consciousness followed by headache and drowsiness without other objective neurologic findings). Billiard et al.[200] reported a reversal of the normal circadian rhythmicity in seven of nine severely head-injured patients. Quinto et al.[200a] briefly reported a case of a delayed sleep phase syndrome in a 48-year-old man after TBI.

*Demyelinating Lesion in the Brain Stem*

In individuals with MS, a demyelinating plaque may involve the hypnogenic and respiratory neurons in the brain stem, giving rise to sleep and to sleep-related breathing disorders. A few such cases have been described in MS patients. An interesting patient, a 38-year-old man, was described by Newsom Davis.[201] The patient had a clinical diagnosis of acute demyelinating lesion in the cervicomedullary junction. He had an autonomous breathing pattern, but he could neither take a voluntary breath nor stop breathing, thus illustrating the apparent independence of the mechanisms controlling metabolic and behavioral respiratory control systems. The patient of Rizvi and coworkers[202] whose brain stem dysfunction was consistent with MS, became apneic when asleep but was able to breathe when awake. His hypercapnic and hypoxic ventilatory responses were normal. Boor and associates[203] described a 40-year-old patient with paralysis of automatic respiration. During relaxation, the patient had recurrent apnea, but the breathing was stable when the patient was alert. The discovery at postmortem examination of a large, demyelinating lesion in the central medulla involving the medullary respiratory neurons explained the respiratory failure.

In addition to sleep-related breathing abnormalities, other sleep difficulties have been commonly reported in MS patients, including insomnia, EDS, and depression.[204–208] Sleep disturbances in MS may result from immobility, spasticity, urinary bladder sphincter disturbances, and sleep-related respiratory dysrhythmias due to respiratory muscle affection or impaired central control of breathing. Tachibana et al.[207] evaluated 28 consecutive patients with MS, 15 of whom had sleep problems that included difficulty initiating sleep, frequent awakenings, difficulty maintaining sleep, habitual snoring, and nocturia. All-night oximetric study showed sleep-related $O_2$ desaturation in three patients, and two of whom had sleep apnea on PSG investigations. The authors concluded that sleep disturbance in MS is common but poorly recognized and is usually due to leg spasms, pain, immobility, nocturia, or medication but not commonly associated with nocturnal respiratory dysfunction. Ferini-Strambi et al.[208] performed PSG studies in 25 MS patients and compared the results with 25 age- and sex-matched controls. They found reduced sleep efficiency with increased awakenings during sleep and an excess of PLMS in patients as compared with the controls.

### Bulbar Poliomyelitis and Postpolio Syndrome

In the acute and convalescent stages of poliomyelitis, respiratory disturbances commonly get worse during sleep. Some patients are left with the sequelae of respiratory dysrhythmia, particularly sleep-related apnea or hypoventilation requiring ventilatory support, especially at night. Another group of patients decades later developed symptoms that constitute *postpolio syndrome*. Sleep disturbances and sleep apnea or hypoventilation are also noted in postpolio syndrome. Medullary respiratory and hypnogenic neurons are involved directly by the poliovirus infection, and this explains the patients' symptoms.

Hypoventilation syndrome in bulbar poliomyelitis was first documented quantitatively by Sarnoff and colleagues.[209] They described four patients who could breathe voluntarily on command but hypoventilated during periods of sleep and quiescence. The authors described irregular rate and rhythm of respiration, incoordination of the muscles of respiration, and hypoventilation resulting from decreased sensitivity of the respiratory center to $Pco_2$ as a result of direct involvement of the respiratory center by the poliomyelitis virus. Two of their patients benefited from electrophrenic respiration.

An extensive report on the clinical and physiologic findings in 20 of 250 poliomyelitis patients with central respiratory disturbances was given by Plum and Swanson.[16] These patients' respiratory disturbances could not be explained by involvement of the spinal motor neurons or airway obstruction. In acute bulbar poliomyelitis, the disordered breathing progressed through three successive stages. Stage I was characterized by disorder of respiratory rhythm during sleep, when breathing became irregular in rate and depth with periods of apnea ranging from 4 to 12 seconds. During stage II, normal breathing required increasing effort and concentration, and strong auditory or painful stimuli were necessary to maintain respiratory rhythmicity. At this stage the patients had impaired chemosensitivity of the central respiratory centers as evidenced by a reduction in ventilation and carbon dioxide retention after $O_2$ inhalation. Sleep exacerbated the breathing difficulty, and there were longer periods of apnea. The respiratory homeostasis was lost entirely in stage III, and there was no ventilatory responsiveness to reflex, chemical, or other neuronal stimuli. The respiratory pattern was chaotic, with varying periods of apnea. The patients required ventilatory support to maintain respiratory homeostasis. Severe inflammatory changes and small areas of necrosis in the ventrolateral reticular formation of the medulla were noted in two patients on neuropathologic examination. The breathing abnormalities in this series rarely lasted more than 2 weeks, but two patients had sleep-related irregular respiration that persisted many months after acute poliomyelitis. These two patients also demonstrated impaired hypercapnic ventilatory response and hypoventilation during administration of 100% $O_2$.

The physiologic abnormalities suggested severe and permanent dysfunction of the medullary respiratory neurons. In several convalescent spinal poliomyelitis patients, the authors also observed subnormal ventilatory response to carbon dioxide with reduction of maximum breathing capacity or vital capacity to less than 50% of predicted normal values. These findings implied that peripheral mechanisms that cause restriction of chest movements may also contribute to impaired ventilatory response to carbon dioxide.

*Postpolio Syndrome*

Postpolio syndrome is manifested clinically by increasing weakness or wasting of the previously affected muscles and by involvement of previously unaffected regions of the body, fatigue, aches and pains, and sometimes symptoms secondary to sleep-related hypoventilation such as EDS and tiredness.[210,211] The exact mechanism of postpolio syndrome is not known.[212] Some of the symptoms (e.g., EDS and fatigue) could result from sleep-related hypoventilation or apnea and sleep disturbances.[213] Thus, it is important to be aware of sleep apnea in such patients. This syndrome has been described in patients who had poliomyelitis decades earlier. Guilleminault and Motta[214] reported on five such men who had a history of bulbar poliomyelitis 16 years earlier. All had EDS, and PSG study documented numerous episodes of apneas, which were predominantly central but also mixed and upper airway obstructive types associated with $O_2$ desaturation. Their longest apneas were seen during REM sleep. It is important to know that these patients resemble those with primary sleep apnea syndrome. Presumably, the lesions in these cases involved the medullary respiratory neurons and thus central lesions were responsible for all three types of apneas. The patients' symptoms improved and daytime somnolence decreased after ventilatory assistance at night. A 41-year-old woman with a history of bulbar poliomyelitis 20 years earlier was reported by Solliday and associates.[215] This patient had chronic hypoventilation with marked hypoxemia and hypercapnia during sleep. Hypercapnic ventilatory response was impaired, but the hypoxic ventilatory response was normal, suggesting that the patient had impaired central chemoreceptors but functioning peripheral chemoreceptors.

Steljes and coworkers[213] performed PSG examinations on 13 postpolio patients, five of whom used rocking beds for ventilatory assistance and eight of whom had no ventilatory assistance. Patients who required ventilatory assistance demonstrated severe sleep disturbances with decreased total sleep time; reduced sleep efficiency; decreased percentage of stage II, slow-wave sleep and REM sleep; but increased awakenings and percentage of stage I sleep. Respiratory abnormalities in these patients consisted of hypoventilation, apneas, and hypopneas associated with significant $O_2$ desaturation. These patients did not respond to continuous positive airway pressure (CPAP) treatment with the rocking bed, but they showed improvement in sleep structure and respiratory function after mechanical ventilation via nasal mask. Five of the eight patients who required no ventilatory assistance also showed impairment of sleep architecture similar to the other group's, but the findings were less severe. All but one patient from the second group had obstructive or mixed apneas, which were treated successfully with nasal CPAP. One patient with mixed apnea and marked hypoventilation improved after treatment with nasal ventilation by mask.

PSG and pulmonary function studies by Bye[216] and Ellis[217] and their coworkers documented respiratory failure and sleep hypoxemia, particularly during REM sleep, in patients with postpolio respiratory muscle weakness. Sleep studies by Ellis' group[217] under controlled conditions without respiratory support showed repeated arousals with disruption and fragmentation of REM-NREM cycle. Bye's group[216] and Howard's[218] found a direct relationship between forced vital capacity, sleep hypoxemia, and nocturnal hypoventilation in such patients.

In questionnaire studies, Cosgrove et al.[219] found sleep disturbances in 31% of postpolio patients. Van Kralingen et al.[220] reported sleep complaints (i.e., daytime sleepiness and fatigue, morning headache, and restless legs) in almost 50% of 43 postpolio patients.

*Syringobulbia-Myelia*

Some patients with syringobulbia-myelia may have alveolar hypoventilation and sleep-related apneas or irregular breathing and stridor. Haponik and colleagues[221] described such a case. The patient was a 35-year-old woman whose polygraphic examination showed 370 upper airway obstructive apneas lasting 10–170 seconds associated with hypoxemia during 7 hours of NREM stages I and II sleep. The patient died 9 months after the onset of the illness, and neuropathologic examination disclosed a syrinx that extended from the lower third of the medulla to the upper thoracic spinal cord.

## Western Equine Encephalitis

Cohn and Kuida[222] and White and coworkers[223] described alveolar hypoventilation, CSA, EDS, and subnormal hypercapnic ventilatory response after western equine encephalitis. The respiratory center was thought to have been damaged by the virus.

## Arnold-Chiari Malformation

CSA may result from Arnold-Chiari malformation.[224–226] On the basis of autopsy findings in their patient with Arnold-Chiari malformation, Papasozomenos and Roessman[224] suggested that CSA resulted from brain stem compression and ischemia with vascular stretching. In their report of Chiari I malformation in children, Dure and associates[225] did not have MRI or computed tomographic (CT) evidence of brain stem vascular compression. Upper airway OSA has also been described in Arnold-Chiari malformation.[227,228] Ely et al.[228] reported a patient with severe OSA associated with a unique combination of syringobulbia-myelia, Chiari malformation type I, absent hypoxic ventilatory drive, vocal cord paralysis, obesity, and acute respiratory failure requiring mechanical ventilation. Sleep apnea in this patient obviously resulted from multiple factors. Earlier, Campbell[229] described two patients with Arnold-Chiari malformation who had profound hypoventilation. Bokinsky and colleagues[230] described an 18-year-old patient with Arnold-Chiari malformation and syringomyelia accompanied by dysfunction of the ninth, tenth, and twelfth cranial nerves. They noted absent hypoxic ventilatory response but normal hypercapnic ventilatory response in their patient. These findings are consistent with bilateral ninth cranial nerve dysfunction.

## Diseases of the Spinal Cord

In spinal cord disorders, sleep disturbances occur as a result of sleep-related respiratory dysrhythmias

causing sleep apneas, hypopneas, or hypoventilation associated with hypoxemia and repeated arousals. The voluntary or the behavioral respiratory control system descends via the corticospinal tracts, and the metabolic or automatic respiratory controlling system descends via the reticulospinal tracts, and the two systems are integrated in the spinal cord (see also Chapter 6). The behavioral system is located in the dorsolateral quadrant of the cervical spinal cord[13,14] and the automatic respiratory system in the ventrolateral quadrant. These two systems control the final common respiratory pathways of the spinal respiratory motor neurons, which send impulses along the phrenic and intercostal nerves to the main respiratory muscles. The anterior horn cells in the third, fourth, and fifth cervical spinal cord segments give rise to phrenic nerves and the intercostal nerves originate from the ventral rami from the anterior horn cells in the thoracic spinal cord. It is known that transection of either the dorsolateral or the ventrolateral quadrant of the spinal cord may independently affect the voluntary and the automatic respiratory controlling systems.[53] Most of the reports, however, refer to transection of the ventrolateral tracts giving rise to dysfunction of the metabolic respiratory control system. Direct involvement of the lower motor respiratory pathways, either in the anterior horn or in the phrenic and intercostal nerves, may also give rise to respiratory dysfunction. Several patterns of respiratory dysfunction have been summarized by Krieger and Rosomoff[231]: (1) efferent motor impairment (e.g., phrenic nerve paralysis causing diaphragmatic weakness) associated with reduced vital capacity, (2) impaired hypercapnic ventilatory response without significant chest wall or diaphragmatic weakness and with normal vital capacity, and (3) a mixture of these two abnormalities. The lesions that cause such dysfunction in the spinal cord may include spinal surgery, spinal trauma, amyotrophic lateral sclerosis (ALS), syringomyelia, cervical spinal cord tumor, and cervical myelitis (demyelinating or nonspecific myelitis).

## Spinal Surgery

Several cases of sleep apnea have been described after spinal surgery.[231–234] Belmusto and colleagues[232] noted ineffective breathing during sleep that required assisted ventilation in a patient treated with bilateral high cervical cordotomy for intractable pain. Damage to the reticulospinal tracts was thought to be responsible for the breathing difficulty. Tenicela's group[233] and Krieger and Rosomoff[231] also described sleep apnea after high cervical cordotomy. Krieger and Rosomoff[231] observed respiratory dysfunction with 24–48 hours of bilateral percutaneous cervical cordotomy in 10 patients. Sleep apnea was associated with impaired hypercapnic ventilatory response, and the respiratory dysrhythmia lasted from 3 to 32 days in those who survived (two of the patients died in their sleep). The patients' breathing was normal during wakefulness but they had intermittent apnea and irregular rate and depth of breathing during sleep. Although the authors concluded that the ascending reticular fibers in the ventrolateral segment of the spinal cord that relay afferent impulses to the medullary respiratory center had been damaged in their patients, it is most likely that selective damage to the descending automatic respiratory controlling fibers in the ventrolateral quadrant of the spinal cord was the lesion responsible. In two other patients, Krieger and Rosomoff[234] described sleep apnea that required assisted ventilation at night for several days after anterior spinal surgery at C3–C4 interspace. Thus, these reports clearly document Ondine's curse as a sequela of high cervical spinal cord lesions.

*Spinal Trauma*

OSA has also been described in patients with cervical spine fractures[235] or high spinal cord injury.[236,237] Additionally, alterations of EEG sleep patterns after high cervical lesions have also been noted.[238] Guilleminault[59] described eight victims of neck trauma who showed sleep apnea, hypoxemia, and EDS. The long-term prognosis of these patients is variable, and some may require tracheostomy. Guilleminault[59] suggested that mild compression of the lower medulla and upper cervical spinal cord might cause respiratory disturbances during sleep after severe whiplash injury or odontoid fractures. Bach and Wang[239] evaluated 10 C4–C7 traumatic tetraplegic individuals at least 6 months postinjury and again 5 years later. Five patients had an increased number of transient nocturnal O$_2$ desaturations and eight of nine patients restudied by capnography were hypercapnic. However, the day-

time blood gases were normal. The authors concluded that in tetraplegic patients, this nocturnal O$_2$ desaturation and hypercapnia increased as a function of age.

There are a few scattered reports of PLMS associated with paraplegia due to spinal cord injury or other spinal cord lesions.[239–243] The authors of these papers concluded that the PLMS resulted from disinhibition of the spinal locomotor generator.[239–243] It should be noted that the question of the spinal cord as the generator for PLMS remains highly speculative and controversial.

*Amyotrophic Lateral Sclerosis,*
*or Motor Neuron Disease*

ALS is a degenerative CNS disease of the middle aged and elderly. The illness is characterized by progressive degeneration of the ventral horn cells of the spinal cord, motor neurons of the bulbar nuclei, and upper motor neurons (primarily cortical), which produces a combination of lower and upper motor neuron signs. The natural history of the disease shows a relentless progression without impairment of mental function or sensation. Patients with ALS often have sleep complaints and sleep-related respiratory dysrhythmias. Weaknesses of the upper airway, diaphragm, and intercostal muscles secondary to involvement of the bulbar, phrenic, and intercostal nerve nuclei are the main contributing factors for sleep-disordered breathing in this condition. There may also be degeneration of the central respiratory neurons, accounting for both CSAs and OSAs in this condition. Literature on sleep disorders in ALS is sparse.

Respiratory failure in ALS generally occurs late, but occasionally it is a presenting feature and requires mechanical ventilation.[244] Thorpy and colleagues[245] described a 52-year-old man with spinal muscular atrophy and diaphragmatic paralysis who complained of nocturnal respiratory difficulty and progressive daytime somnolence for 10 years. Sleep-related nonobstructive hypoventilation associated with O$_2$ desaturation was noted on PSG examination. The patient's symptoms of hypersomnolence and daytime ventilation improved after assisted respiration at night. Newsom Davis' group[246] described eight patients with diaphragmatic paralysis resulting from a variety of motor disorders. One of their

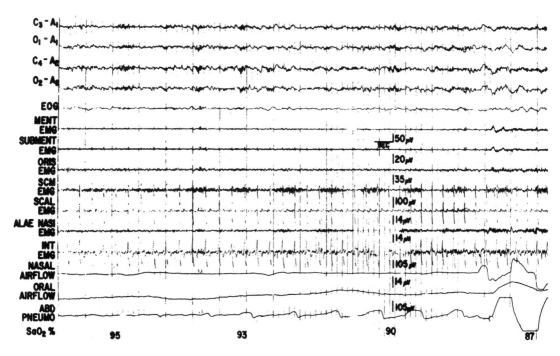

**Figure 27-5.** Polysomnography recording showing mixed apnea during stage II NREM sleep accompanied by oxygen desaturation in a patient with amyotrophic lateral sclerosis. Channel key as for Figure 27-3. (Reproduced with permission from S Chokroverty. Sleep and Breathing in Neurological Disorders. In NH Edelman, TV Santiago [eds], Breathing Disorders of Sleep. New York: Churchill Livingstone, 1986;225.)

patients had Kugelberg-Welander syndrome, which is considered a variant of juvenile type motor neuron disease. The following features may be helpful in the diagnosis of diaphragmatic paralysis[60,246]: (1) breathlessness and EDS suggesting alveolar hypoventilation; (2) paradoxical inward movement of the abdomen with epigastric retraction instead of protrusion during inspiration; (3) an elevated diaphragm on chest radiography and paradoxical movement or decreased excursion of the diaphragm on fluoroscopy; (4) documentation of a very sensitive measurement showing a lack of change in the transdiaphragmatic pressure during a maximum inspiration; (5) diaphragmatic electromyographic (EMG) findings; (6) respiratory function tests with evidence of a restrictive pattern; (7) blood gases showing hypoxemia and hypercapnia, suggesting alveolar hypoventilation; and (8) documentation of sleep-related breathing abnormalities on PSG.

Serpick and colleagues[247] described a patient with ALS who had hypersomnolence, periodic breathing, hypercapnia, and hypoxia. The authors suggested that medullary dysfunction was responsible for ventilatory impairment. Sleep-related respiratory dysrhythmia in two patients with ALS was described by the present writer,[248] who since has seen several other cases of sleep apnea associated with motor neuron disease (unpublished observations). Polygraphic study of one of these patients (Figure 27-5) documents both central and upper airway obstructive apnea.

Gay and coworkers[249] performed PSG studies of 18 patients with ALS. This study emphasized sleep-disordered breathing and pulmonary functions rather than detailed descriptions of sleep architecture. Ferguson and colleagues[250] studied 18 ALS patients with mild to severe bulbar muscle involvement and 10 age-matched control subjects. Most patients complained of difficulty initiating and maintaining sleep. All patients and controls had overnight PSG study and 13 ALS patients had a second night of PSG study. ALS patients had more arousals and stage changes per hour, more stage I NREM sleep, and shorter total sleep time than controls. ALS patients had mild sleep-disordered breathing with greater AHI than controls. It is notable that sleep-disordered breathing was similar in ALS patients with or without respiratory muscle weakness. The sleep-disordered breathing consisted of REM-related nonobstructive and central apneas, and none had significant sleep apnea. In an early study, Minz and colleagues[251] described PSG findings in 12 ALS patients, six men and six women. Four patients had both central and obstructive apneas. Sleep structure was normal in eight, but others had frequent awakenings. Bye's group[216] studied three patients with motor neuron disease using PSG and pulmonary function tests. They noted hypoventilation, particularly during REM sleep.

Howard and colleagues[252] described 14 patients with motor neuron disease associated with respiratory dysfunction. Eleven received respiratory support, with considerable benefit. Seven of eight with typical features of ALS had mainly diaphragmatic paralysis and one had generalized respiratory muscle weakness. Seven of these patients had negative pressure ventilation by cuirass, which improved the respiratory problem and the quality of sleep. Three with mainly bulbar type of ALS had sleep apnea or hypoventilation; one of these patients with additional diaphragmatic weakness was treated with a cuirass, CPAP, and later intermittent positive-pressure ventilation (IPPV) at night. Three patients with predominantly diaphragmatic paresis with sleep apnea were treated with nocturnal CPAP, cuirass, or IPPV with symptomatic relief. The series by Howard and coworkers[252] included three patients with sleep apnea (all had obstructive apnea and one also had central apnea) and four who suffered nocturnal hypoventilation. The authors concluded that sleep-related respiratory dysrhythmia is a significant complication of motor neuron disease and may contribute to daytime hypersomnolence.

Hetta and Jansson[253] reported that sleep disturbances in ALS patients can result from factors such as reduced mobility, muscle cramps, swallowing problems, anxiety, and respiratory problems. Based on interviews only, the authors reported insomnia in 25% of 24 patients with ALS. They mentioned sleep-onset and maintenance insomnia. They also stated that patients in the terminal stage of the disease had a higher frequency of sleep disturbance.

### Sleep and Sleep-Disordered Breathing in Polyneuropathies

The cardinal manifestations of polyneuropathies are bilaterally symmetric, distal sensory symptoms and signs and muscle weakness and wasting (affecting the legs more often than the arms). Peripheral neuropathies may be caused by a variety of heredofamilial and acquired lesions. Disorders of the phrenic, intercostal, and other nerves supplying the accessory muscles of respiration can cause weakness of the diaphragm, intercostal, and accessory respiratory muscles, giving rise to breathlessness on exertion, hypoxia, and hypercapnia. These respiratory dysrhythmias become worse during sleep. Sleep disturbances in polyneuropathies may result from painful neuropathies, partial immobility owing to a paralysis of the muscles, or sleep-related breathing disorders.

Trauma, inflammatory polyneuropathy, and infiltrative lesions (e.g., neoplasms) may cause phrenic neuropathy. The most common cause of respiratory dysfunction in polyneuropathy is acute inflammatory demyelinating polyradiculoneuropathy (Landry-Guillain-Barré-Strohl) syndrome. The characteristic clinical manifestations consist of predominantly motor deficits associated with rapidly progressive ascending paralysis beginning in the legs and manifesting maximally in 2–3 weeks. In approximately 20–25% of cases, severe respiratory involvement has been reported, and the critical period is usually the first 3–4 weeks of the illness. It is important to recognize and treat the ventilatory dysfunction. Even the mild respiratory dysrhythmia during wakefulness may worsen during sleep, causing sleep apnea and hypoventilation. Phrenic neuropathy may also be secondary to varicella-zoster virus infection or to the diphtheritic neuropathy.[254] Goldstein and colleagues[255] described a patient with peripheral neuropathy and severe involvement of the phrenic nerves who presented with hypoventilation.

Diaphragmatic dysfunction has also been described in siblings with hereditary motor and sensory neuropathy (Charcot-Marie-Tooth disease).[256] Bilateral glossopharyngeal and vagal neuropathy can also cause respiratory dysfunction.[230]

## Sleep and Breathing Disorders Associated with Primary Muscle Diseases

Myopathies are primary muscle disorders characterized by weakness and wasting of the muscles resulting from a defect in the muscle membrane or the contractile elements that is not secondary to a structural or functional derangement of the lower or upper motor neurons.[60] The characteristic clinical presentation consists of symmetric, proximal muscle weakness and wasting in the upper or lower limbs without sensory impairment or fasciculations. The causes include hereditary muscular dystrophies with or without myotonia; glycogen storage diseases; myoglobinuric myopathies; congenital nonprogressive myopathies with distinct morphologic characteristics; and various acquired metabolic, inflammatory, and noninflammatory myopathies. Some of these patients may report breathing disorders during sleep or worsening of the respiratory dysfunction during sleep. Generally, respiratory disorders show manifestations in the advanced stage, but a small number of them may present with respiratory failure at an early stage. In many such patients, the true incidence of the sleep disturbances and sleep-related respiratory dysrhythmias in these muscle disorders cannot be determined without a systematic PSG study. Factors responsible for breathing disorders associated with hypoventilation and sleep apnea in these patients may be summarized as follows[60]: impairment of chest bellows owing to weakness of the respiratory and chest wall muscles, increased work of breathing, and functional changes in the medullary respiratory neurons that could be due to hyporesponsive or unresponsive chemoreceptors acquired secondarily.[257] The other suggestion for carbon dioxide hyposensitivity is altered afferent input from the skeletal muscle receptors.[258] Sleep disturbances generally occur in muscle disorders secondary to sleep-related respiratory dysrhythmias. Alveolar hypoventilation, both during wakefulness and sleep, should be diagnosed early in these patients to prevent the fatal or dangerous hypoventilation during sleep or during administration of drugs, general anesthetic agents, and respiratory infections.[60] Complaints of daytime hypersomnolence and breathlessness should direct attention to the possibility of sleep-disordered breathing in these patients.

## Muscular Dystrophy

A few cases of muscular dystrophy with sleep complaints and sleep-related respiratory dysrhythmias have been described. Smith and associates[259] described 14 patients with Duchenne's muscular dystrophy who had sleep apneas or hypopneas associated with marked $O_2$ desaturation. These authors state that the severity of sleep-disordered breathing in Duchenne's muscular dystrophy could not reliably be ascertained from daytime pulmonary function studies and assert that sleep studies are essential.

Bye's[216] and Ellis's[217] groups also included patients with muscular dystrophy in their reports of patients with neuromuscular disorders who also had sleep-related breathing disorders. The REM sleep showed significant $O_2$ desaturation. Sleep study showed repeated arousals and sleep fragmentation.[217]

Gross and coworkers[260] described a 22-year-old patient with Duchenne's muscular dystrophy who was wheelchair bound and experienced breathlessness after meals. The blood gas studies showed hypercapnia and hypoxemia during wakefulness. A PSG study revealed nonapneic and hypopneic $O_2$ desaturation, which was more marked during REM than NREM sleep. After progressive inspiratory muscle training and administration of $O_2$ at a rate of 2 liters per minute via nasal prongs, the patient's subjective daytime symptoms of fatigue and breathlessness subsided.

Howard et al.[261] described nocturnal hypoventilation and respiratory failure in 84 patients with primary muscle disorders that included Duchenne's, Becker, limb-girdle, and facioscapulohumeral muscular dystrophies; adult-onset acid maltase deficiency; myotonic dystrophy; polymyositis; congenital myopathies; and rigid spine syndrome. All patients needed ventilatory support in the form of negative or positive pressure ventilation or tracheostomy.

Sleep-related respiratory dysrhythmias (both obstructive and central apneas) accompanied by $O_2$ desaturation and daytime hypersomnolence have been described in many patients with Duchenne's muscular dystrophy.[262–272] Although respiratory failure is most commonly noted in Duchenne's muscular dystrophy, sometimes it also occurs in the more advanced stages of Becker's, limb-girdle, and facioscapulohumeral muscular dystrophies.[272] In a pilot study, Kerr and Kohrman[262] described sleep apnea (obstructive and central) in five of 11 patients with Duchenne's muscular dystrophy. Khan and Heckmatt[264] studied 21 patients with Duchenne's muscular dystrophy aged 13–23 years using two consecutive nights of PSG and 12 age-matched controls. They noted apneas, 60% of which were obstructive in nature, with hypoxemia in 12 patients. Takasugi et al.[268] studied 42 patients with Duchenne's muscular dystrophy. PSG study documented three patterns of sleep-related respiratory disorders: obstructive apnea, central apnea, and paradoxical breathing without upper airway obstruction (nonobstructive paradoxical breathing). Obstructive apnea was the most common type. They concluded that sleep disorders are common in patients with Duchenne's muscular dystrophy. Obstructive apnea was the most common type of sleep disorder found, often accompanied by hypercapnia and central apnea in advanced cases, resulting from both respiratory muscle weakness and respiratory center abnormalities.

Khan et al.[273] described eight children 6–13 years old with congenital myopathy, congenital muscular dystrophy, and rigid spine syndromes with respiratory failure. PSG documented nocturnal hypoxemia and severe hypoventilation. Sleep disturbances included repeated awakenings.

*Myotonic Dystrophy*

*Dystrophica myotonica*, or myotonic dystrophy, is an adult-onset, dominantly inherited muscular dystrophy associated with myotonia. Benaim and Worster-Drought[274] were most probably the first to describe alveolar hypoventilation in myotonic dystrophy. Alveolar hypoventilation associated with hypoxemia, and impaired hypercapnic and hypoxic ventilatory responses may be present in both the early and late stages of the illness. A few authors[270–271,275–277] performed polygraphic studies that showed central, mixed, and upper airway OSAs, and sleep-onset REM was noted in some patients. The latter finding may have been due to sleep deprivation secondary to sleep-related respiratory disturbances. Two fundamental mechanisms account for the sleep-related breathing disorders in this illness: (1) weakness and myotonia of the respiratory and upper airway muscles and (2) an inherited abnormality of the central control of ventilation, most likely related to a common generalized membrane abnormality of the muscles and other tissues,

including brain stem neurons that regulate breathing and sleep.[276–279]

Sleep studies by Bye and colleagues[216] in four patients with myotonic dystrophy showed REM sleep–related $O_2$ desaturation and sleep disorganization. Several other authors have described alveolar hypoventilation, daytime somnolence, and periodic breathing in patients with myotonic dystrophy in single case reports and small and large series.[271,280–294]

Begin et al.[289] found a high prevalence of chronic alveolar hypoventilation in a series of 134 patients with myotonic dystrophy. The authors suggested that the central ventilatory control mechanism is abnormal in myotonic dystrophy patients, contributing to chronic alveolar hypoventilation. These authors concluded that the chronic alveolar hypoventilation resulted from a combination of inspiratory muscle weakness and loading. In addition, the presence of EDS suggested reduced central ventilatory drive or sleep apnea in these patients. The clinicopathologic study by Ono et al.[293,294] of one patient with myotonic dystrophy, alveolar-hypoventilation, and hypersomnia supported the hypothesis postulated by Begin et al.[289] On postmortem examination of this patient, Ono et al.[293,294] observed significant neuronal loss and gliosis in the midbrain and pontine raphe, as well as the pontomedullary reticular formation.

Park and Radtke[292] reviewed seven patients with myotonic dystrophy referred to their sleep disorders center. All patients had PSG. Five patients were subsequently given an MSLT. Each of the five who had an MSLT showed evidence of moderate hypersomnia. Three of these five patients had two sleep-onset REM episodes, only one of whom showed evidence of sleep apnea in the overnight PSG study. HLA typing was negative for DQW2 but DQW1 was present in two patients. The authors reviewed the literature available (they published their own paper in 1995) and found 86 patients, including their seven patients, with myotonic dystrophy who also had hypersomnolence. Ten percent of the reported patients with hypersomnolence had documented alveolar hypoventilation. Respiratory center hypoexcitability or myotonic muscle weakness is thought to be responsible for alveolar hypoventilation. Correction of hypoventilation does not always lead to improvement of EDS.[285] Sleep-disordered breathing events were noted in 57% of the reported patients with EDS and both central and obstructive sleep apneas were observed. The presence of sleep-onset REMs in these patients supported the hypothesis of a primary CNS abnormality as the cause of EDS.[292] EDS in myotonic dystrophy patients often occurs in absence of sleep apnea.[292] EDS in their patients[292] responded to methylphenidate treatment.

The danger of administering anesthetic agents to these patients is demonstrated by Kaufman[283]: Five of 25 myotonic patients in this series had marked respiratory depression during operation, and another four died in the postoperative period.

Guilleminault's group[276] described six adult myotonic patients with EDS, two of whom had obstructive, mixed, and central apneas associated with $O_2$ desaturation. Armagast and associates[288] described three women with myotonic dystrophy who complained of fatigue and daytime somnolence. All three had central apnea, but one also had obstructive and mixed apneas. The patients' symptoms and $O_2$ desaturation improved after treatment with dichlorphenamide, a carbonic anhydrase inhibitor and a respiratory stimulant.

Striano and coworkers[279] described predominantly OSA associated with daytime hypersomnolence in a patient with dominantly inherited myotonia congenita. Because the patient was obese and also had obstructive pulmonary disease, the relationship between sleep apnea and myotonia congenita remains inconclusive.

Proximal myotonic myopathy (PROMM) is a hereditary myotonic disorder that is differentiated from myotonic dystrophy by absence of the chromosome 19 C-T-G trinucleotide repeat that is associated with myotonic dystrophy.[295–298] In a brief report, we described sleep disturbances in two sisters, ages 51 and 53, with PROMM.[298] The patients had difficulty initiating sleep, EDS, snoring, and frequent awakenings and movements during sleep. Overnight PSG study in these two patients showed decreased sleep efficiency, increased number of arousals, and sleep architecture abnormalities. One patient had absent REM sleep and the other patient had dissociated REM sleep characterized by phasic REM bursts associated with EEG patterns showing sleep spindles and alpha intrusions. These sleep abnormalities in PROMM suggested involvement of the REM-NREM generating neurons as part of a multisystem membrane disorder. The MRI findings of white matter hyperintensity in T2-weighted images in six patients from three families with PROMM described by Hund et al.[297] suggested brain involvement in PROMM, but the relationship between the sleep disturbances and the MRI abnormalities remains to be determined.

### Acid Maltase Deficiency and Other Glycogen Storage Disorders

Alveolar hypoventilation has been described in several cases of mild to moderate myopathy associated with adult-onset acid maltase deficiency, a variant of glycogen storage disease.[246,257,261,299–301] In this condition, correct diagnosis can be established by performing respiratory function testing; EMG; and biochemical, histochemical, or morphologic examination of muscle biopsy samples. Hypoxemia, hypercapnia, and impaired hypercapnic ventilatory response may be seen in these patients. Diaphragmatic dysfunction may account for the alveolar hypoventilation. Rosenow and Engel[299] suggested that the hypoxemia in their patients was secondary to a combination of hypoventilation due to muscle weakness and an impairment of the ventilation-perfusion ratio resulting from compression atelectasis due to elevated diaphragm. The patient of Martin's group[301] on polygraphic study showed prolonged periods of hypopnea accompanied by $O_2$ desaturation. The patient improved considerably after inspiratory muscle training.

Bye and coworkers[216] also described REM sleep–related hypoxemia and sleep disorganization in a patient with acid maltase deficiency and another with Pompe's disease. An adult patient with acid maltase deficiency with severe OSA and respiratory failure was reported by Margolis et al.[302] The patient had mild daytime hypersomnolence, and the sleep study documented severe upper airway obstructive apnea with $O_2$ desaturation. Despite ventilatory support, the patient died. At postmortem examination, profound muscle replacement by fibrofatty tissue was noted in the tongue and diaphragm. The authors suggested that severe tongue weakness due to fatty metamorphosis associated with macroglossia contributed to the upper airway obstruction in this patient. The brain was not examined at the autopsy.

*Other Varieties of Congenital Myopathies*

Riley and coworkers[258] described alveolar hypoventilation in two patients with congenital myopathies (one with nemaline myopathy and the other with a myopathy of uncertain type). The patients' ventilatory response to carbon dioxide was absent, and the authors suggested that the alveolar hypoventilation may have been due to a primary defect in the central chemoreceptor control of breathing. Their other suggestion was that the sensory stimuli from skeletal muscle receptors (e.g., muscle spindles) may have played a role in the blunted hypercapnic ventilatory response by altering afferent input to the CNS.

Bye and colleagues[216] also studied a patient with central core myopathy who had sleep disruption and sleep hypoxemia. Kryger and colleagues[303] described two sisters with congenital muscular dystrophy who had CSA and blunted chemical drive to breathing in the index case. These abnormalities were thought to be out of proportion to the somatic and respiratory muscle weakness. The authors suggested that this patient's central control of breathing was defective. There are other reports of sleep hypoventilation in congenital myopathy.[273,304,305]

*Miscellaneous Myopathies*

Sleep-related hypoxemia and sleep disturbances have also been described in patients with polymyositis[216,261,271] and mitochondrial encephalomyopathy.[306,307]

*Neuromuscular Junction Disorders*

Myasthenia gravis, myasthenic syndrome, botulism, and tic paralysis are several neuromuscular junction disorders characterized by easy fatigability of the muscles, including the bulbar and other respiratory muscles, owing to failure of neuromuscular junctional transmission of the nerve impulses. The most important of these conditions is myasthenia gravis, an autoimmune disease characterized by a reduction in the number of functional acetylcholine receptors in the postjunctional region. Acute respiratory failure is often a dreaded complication of myasthenia gravis, and patients need immediate assisted ventilation for life support.[60,308] The respiratory failure, moreover, may be mild during wakefulness but may deteriorate considerably during sleep.

An important study by Quera-Salva and colleagues[309] reported the pulmonary function and PSG studies of 16 women and four men whose mean age was 40 years and who were diagnosed and treated for myasthenia gravis. PSG findings included moderately disturbed nocturnal sleep with an increase in stage I NREM and decreased slow-wave and REM sleep. Eleven patients had an RDI of 5 or higher. They had central, obstructive, and mixed apneas and hypopneas accompanied by decreased $O_2$ saturation. All patients with REM sleep–related apneas or hypopneas had disturbed nocturnal sleep with a sensation of breathlessness. Twelve patients had insufficient sleep owing to awakening in the middle of the night and early morning hours with a sensation of breathlessness. Four of the 12 patients also had daytime hypersomnolence. The authors suggested that those patients of advancing age, moderately increased body mass index, abnormal pulmonary function results, and daytime blood gas concentrations are at particular risk for sleep-disordered breathing. Before this report, brief reports of sleep disruptions and sleep apnea[310–312] appeared in the literature. Since this report, there have been a few other reports of upper airway obstruction and sleep apnea in patients with myasthenia gravis.[313–315]

Shintani et al.[312] studied 10 patients with myasthenia gravis using PSG and observed obstructive and central apneas in six of these 10 patients. Manni et al.[313] studied breathing patterns during sleep in 14 patients with mild generalized myasthenia gravis. PSG study documented infrequent central apneas, mainly during REM sleep in five patients associated with $O_2$ desaturation. Putman and Wise[314] described a 54-year-old woman with myasthenia gravis and episodes of shortness of breath, which were more severe at night. The flow-volume loops suggested extrathoracic airway obstruction. They surveyed a total of 61 myasthenia gravis patients referred to their pulmonary function laboratory during 42 months. They found a pattern of extrathoracic upper airway obstruction in seven of the 12 patients who had flow-volume loops. Stepansky et al.[315] performed overnight PSG study in 19 middle-aged myasthenia gravis patients and 10 age-matched controls. In 60% of the myasthenics, they observed mild CSAs with $O_2$ desaturation without any impairment of the sleep profile.

Myasthenic syndrome, or Lambert-Eaton syndrome, is a disorder of the neuromuscular junction in the presynaptic region and is often a paraneoplastic manifestation, mostly of oat cell carcinoma of the lungs. Patients complain of muscle weakness and fatigue involving the limbs accompanied by decreased or absent muscle stretch reflexes and characteristic electrodiagnostic findings that differentiate this from myasthenia gravis.

Botulism caused by *Clostridium botulinum* and tic paralysis caused by the female wood tic *Dermacentor andersoni* may also cause neuromuscular junctional transmission defects, which are due to released toxin.

In all of these conditions, respiratory muscles may be affected and patients may require assisted ventilation. They can exhibit sleep hypoventilation and sleep apnea.

### Assessment of Sleep and Sleep-Related Breathing Disorders in Autonomic Failure

Anatomically and functionally, sleep, breathing, and the autonomic nervous system (ANS) are closely interrelated.[60,316–321] To understand sleep and breathing disorders in autonomic failure it is important to understand the functional anatomy of sleep, control of breathing, and the central autonomic network. A brief review of the functional anatomy of sleep is given in the beginning of this chapter, and the neurophysiology of sleep is also described extensively in Chapters 3 and 4. Functional neuroanatomy of respiration, control of breathing during sleep and wakefulness, and the central autonomic network with its integration of sleep and breathing are reviewed briefly in Chapter 6.

Sleep has a profound effect on the functions of the ANS.[318,319] Sleep disorders and respiratory dysrhythmias during sleep in patients with autonomic failure are, therefore, logical expectations. Such sleep and breathing disorders have in fact been described in many patients with autonomic failure. It is also important to remember that the peripheral respiratory receptors, the central respiratory, and the hypnogenic neurons in the preoptic-hypothalamic area and the region of the NTS in the medulla are intimately linked by the ANS, making it easy to comprehend why sleep and breathing disorders should be associated with autonomic failure.

Autonomic failure may be grouped as primary and secondary types. Primary autonomic failure (without known cause) includes pure autonomic failure without any somatic neurologic deficits and MSA, or Shy-Drager syndrome. The most well-known condition with autonomic failure in which sleep and respiratory disturbances have been reported and well described is MSA with progressive autonomic failure, or Shy-Drager syndrome. In a consensus statement[322] sponsored by the American Autonomic Society and the American Academy of Neurology, *multiple-system atrophy* is the favored term, replacing *Shy-Drager syndrome*. MSA defines a sporadic, adult-onset progressive disorder characterized by autonomic dysfunction, parkinsonism, and ataxia in any combination. *Striatonigral degeneration* is the term used when the predominant feature is parkinsonism. The term *sporadic olivopontocerebellar atrophy* is used when cerebellar features are present. Finally, when autonomic failure is the predominant feature, the term *Shy-Drager syndrome* is often used. Familial dysautonomia, a recessively inherited primarily autonomic failure, is also known to be associated with disturbances of breathing and sleep. A large number of neurologic and general medical disorders are associated with prominent secondary autonomic failure. In many patients with diabetic autonomic neuropathies, amyloid neuropathy, and Guillain-Barré syndrome, sleep and sleep-related respiratory disturbances have been noted. In many neurologic conditions, sleep and respiratory disturbances are secondary to the structural lesions involving central hypnogenic or respiratory neurons.

### Multiple-System Atrophy with Progressive Autonomic Failure (Shy-Drager Syndrome)

In 1960, Shy and Drager[323] described a neurodegenerative disorder characterized by autonomic failure and MSA. Since their description, there have been many reports[54,55,143,318,324–333] of the condition, which has generally come to be known as *Shy-Drager syndrome* or *multiple-system atrophy with progressive autonomic failure*. Patients frequently manifest sleep and respiratory disturbances. Initially, they present with autonomic failure of both the sympathetic and parasympathetic systems. They may present with symptoms related to orthostatic hypotension (e.g., postural dizziness and faintness or even frank loss of consciousness in the erect posture), urinary sphincter dysfunction (e.g., frequency, urgency, hesitancy, dribbling, or overflow incontinence), hypohidrosis or anhidrosis, and impotence in men. After 2–6 years, patients lapse into the second stage, showing some combination of pyramidal, extrapyramidal, upper motor neuron, and lower motor neuron dysfunction, including bulbar deficits. Most patients manifest a parkinsonian-cerebellar syndrome. In some, atypical parkinsonian features (e.g., bradykinesia, rigidity, postural instability) predominate; in others, pancerebellar dysfunction predominates. In the later stages of the illness, a variety of respiratory and sleep disturbances add to the progressive disability. Occasionally, respiratory dysfunction, particularly dysrhythmic breathing in wakefulness that becomes worse during sleep, manifests in the initial stage of the illness. In the final stage, progressive autonomic and somatic dysfunction are compounded by respiratory failure. Ventilatory disturbances now may be present in both wakefulness and sleep. Pathologically, there are various combinations of striatonigral degeneration, OPCA, and degeneration of the autonomic neurons. A distinctive but not a specific neuropathologic alteration in MSA is thought to be the presence of argyrophilic oligodendroglial cytoplasmic inclusions in the cortical motor, premotor, and supplementary motor areas; extrapyramidal and corticocerebellar systems; brain stem reticular formation; and supraspinal autonomic systems and their targets.[332] This inclusion-bearing oligodendroglial degeneration may cause or contribute to the manifestations of clinical symptoms in MSA.

**Sleep Disturbances in Multiple-System Atrophy.** The most common sleep disorders in MSA result from a variety of sleep-related respiratory dysrhythmias similar to those described in other neurologic conditions (see Figure 27-1). The most common types of respiratory dysrhythmias consist of the sleep apnea and hypopnea associated with repeated arousals and hypoxemia,[54,66,334–345] dysrhythmic breathing,[54,66] and laryngeal stridor due to laryngeal abductor[324,325,336–341,346–348] paralysis. Less commonly, apneustic breathing[335] and inspiratory gasping[54,325,341] may occur. Hypersomnia often results from nocturnal sleep disruption. Sudden nocturnal death in patients with MSA in some cases probably is due to respiratory arrest and other cardiorespiratory abnormalities.

Laryngeal stridor and excessive snoring resulting from laryngeal abductor paralysis have been described in cases of MSA by groups led by Bannister,[324,326] Martin,[336] Israel,[337] Guilleminault,[338] Williams,[339] Kenyon,[340] Munschauer,[341] Sadaoka,[346] Isozaki,[347] and McBrien.[348] The nocturnal stridor can be inspiratory, expiratory, or both and cause upper airway obstruction during sleep. The stridor may result in a striking noise likened to a donkey's braying.[328] Williams's group[339] noted this abnormality in eight of 12 cases. The stridor can be relieved by tracheostomy. The group led by Guilleminault[342–344] described eight patients with predominantly upper airway OSA associated with $O_2$ desaturation.

McNicholas and coworkers[66] described two patients with MSA whose impaired hypoxic and hypercapnic ventilatory responses suggested a defect in the metabolic respiratory control system. Their pattern of breathing during sleep was highly irregular. They had approximately 61–79 apneic episodes in all during NREM stages I and II but without $O_2$ desaturation. The apneic episodes were mostly central, but occasionally they had transient occlusion of the upper airway or transient uncoupling of intercostal and diaphragmatic muscle activity. The most striking abnormality was an irregular pattern of breathing during sleep, as documented by overnight PSG study. These findings suggested a defective automatic respiratory rhythm generator in the brain stem.

In our early study of four patients with MSA,[70] we observed periodic central apnea in the erect position and Cheyne-Stokes type breathing in one patient during the last stage of the illness. In one patient, hypercapnic ventilatory response in the supine position was impaired and the neuropathologic findings in the same patient—neuronal loss and astrocytosis in the pontine tegmentum—suggested involvement of the respiratory neurons in the brain stem. In our later studies,[54] we described 10 other patients with MSA who showed central apnea, including Cheyne-Stokes or Cheyne-Stokes variant–type breathing and upper airway obstructive and mixed apneas accompanied by $O_2$ desaturation, predominantly during NREM sleep stages I and II and REM sleep (Figure 27-6). During sleep, seven patients had central apnea, two had upper airway OSA, and three had mixed apneas. The

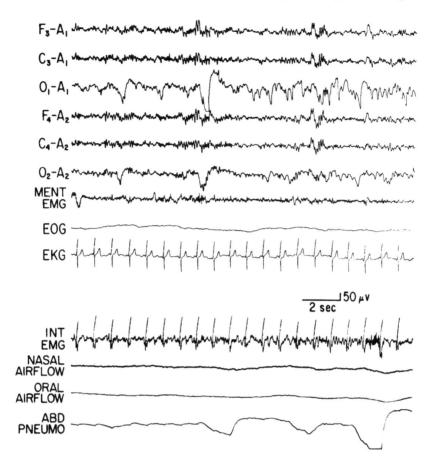

**Figure 27-6.** A portion of an episode of mixed apnea during stage II non-REM sleep associated with oxygen desaturation in a patient with multiple-system atrophy. EEGs are shown in the top six channels. Also shown are electromyography (EMG) of the mentalis (MENT) and intercostal (INT) muscles, electrocardiogram (EKG), nasal and oral airflow, and abdominal pneumogram (ABD PNEUMO). (Reproduced with permission from S Chokroverty. Sleep and Breathing in Neurological Disorders. In NH Edelman, TV Santiago [eds], Breathing Disorders of Sleep. New York: Churchill Livingstone, 1986;225.)

RDI varied from 20 to 80; the duration of apneas ranged from 10 to 65 seconds. The variation in the heart rate during apneic and eupneic cycles was not seen in these patients with evidence of cardiac autonomic denervation. This finding was in contrast to the bradyarrhythmias and tachyarrhythmias noted during apnea and immediately after resumption of normal breathing in patients with primary sleep apnea syndrome.[60] Four patients had several episodes of central apneas during relaxed wakefulness; it was as if the respiratory center "forgot" to breathe. Two patients had inspiratory gasps and two required tracheostomy for respiratory dysrhythmia. All-night PSG studies in two patients revealed the following sleep abnormalities in addition to recurrent episodes of sleep apneas accompanied by $O_2$ desaturation: marked reduction of NREM sleep stages III and IV and REM sleep, increased awakenings after sleep onset, snoring, and excessive body movements and frequent arousal responses in the EEG. Impaired hypercapnic ventilatory response and mouth occlusion pressure response in one patient suggested impairment of the metabolic respiratory system, whereas normal hypercapnic and hypoxic ventilatory responses in another patient (in the presence of an abnormal respiratory pattern resembling that noted by Lockwood[334]) suggested that the chemoreceptor control and respiratory pattern generator were probably subserved by different populations of neurons rendered selectively vulnerable in MSA. In eight of 10 patients, dysrhythmic breathing occurred mostly during sleep, although in four of the eight it was also present during wakefulness; this finding suggests that this type of respiratory dysrhythmia is very common in MSA. These observations are in agreement with the suggestion of McNicholas and colleagues[66] that such findings imply impaired respiratory pattern generator in these patients.

Some patients with MSA may complain of insomnia and many manifest RBD, which may occasionally be the presenting feature.[349–351]

It is important to recognize disturbed breathing events during sleep at night in these patients, so that appropriate treatment can be instituted to prevent sudden death from fatal sleep apnea. The clinical manifestations secondary to sleep-disordered breathing were described in the beginning of this chapter. Overnight PSG findings in MSA may be summarized as follows: reduction of total sleep time, decreased sleep efficiency, increased sleep latency in those with insomnia complaints, increased number of awakenings during sleep, reduction of slow-wave and REM sleep, absence of muscle atonia in REM sleep in those with RBD, and a variety of respiratory dysrhythmias.

**Mechanisms of Ventilatory Dysrhythmia in Multiple-System Atrophy.** There is ample evidence in the literature[143,323] of pathologic involvement of the pontine tegmentum, the reticular formation, NTS, nucleus ambiguus, hypoglossal nucleus, and, in some patients, anterior horn cells of the cervical and thoracic spinal cord. Lockwood[334] and Chokroverty and colleagues[70] correlated the physiologic and clinical findings of respiratory dysrhythmias with direct involvement of the regions of the brain stem that contain the respiratory neurons. In addition, physiologic studies of respiratory control[66] (also Chokroverty, unpublished data) showing impairment of hypercapnic and hypoxic ventilatory and mouth occlusion pressure responses indirectly suggested an impairment of the metabolic respiratory control system. Vagal and sympathetic denervation in these patients is firmly established.[143,323] The pathogenic mechanisms for the respiratory dysrhythmia include all that had been postulated in the beginning of this

chapter for the respiratory dysrhythmias in neurologic disorders.

Additional mechanisms for the respiratory dysrhythmia have been suggested[54]: interference with the forebrain, midbrain, and pontine inputs to the medullary respiratory neurons causing dysrhythmic and apneustic breathing; involvement of the direct projections from the hypothalamus and central nucleus of amygdala to the respiratory neurons in the NTS and nucleus ambiguus; involvement of the vagal afferents from the lower and upper airway receptors, which would reduce the input to the central respiratory neurons, causing respiratory dysrhythmia; sympathetic denervation of the nasal mucosa causing increased nasal resistance, thus promoting upper airway obstructive apnea; and discrete neurochemical alterations that may interfere with normal regulation of breathing. There is experimental evidence that noradrenaline, serotonin, and dopamine play distinct roles in the control of breathing.[352] Patients with MSA have been found to have low levels of dopamine and noradrenaline in the basal ganglia, the limbic-hypothalamic regions including the septal nuclei, and the locus coeruleus.[353] Furthermore, these patients may also have specific catecholamine enzyme deficits in the brain and sympathetic ganglia.[354]

*Familial Dysautonomia (Riley-Day Syndrome)*

Riley-Day syndrome is a recessively inherited disorder associated with autonomic failure. The condition usually presents in childhood and is peculiar to the Jewish population. The clinical features consist of a variety of autonomic and somatic manifestations[355]: autonomic, neuromuscular, cardiovascular, gastroesophageal, skeletal, renal, and respiratory abnormalities; absence of the fungiform papillae of the tongue; defective lacrimation and sweating; vasomotor instability and fluctuation of blood pressure (postural hypotension and paroxysmal hypertension); relative insensitivity to pain; and absent muscle stretch reflexes. Sleep dysfunction, associated with both CSAs and OSAs, has been described in most of these patients.[356] Sleep abnormalities consist of increased awakenings, delayed sleep onset, including prolonged REM-sleep onset (but reduced REM sleep time), and sleep apneas.

Patients with familial dysautonomia often have prolonged breath-holding spells, owing to defective responses of central respiratory neurons to changes in $Pa_{CO_2}$.

Gadoth and colleagues[356] performed PSG recordings of 13 patients (7 women and 6 men aged 5–31 years) with familial dysautonomia to investigate the role of ANS in sleep and breathing disorders in this condition. All had sleep apneas (an average of 73.5 per night), 11 had central apnea, and two had OSA. REM latency was prolonged, with decreased amount of REM in some patients, and adults also had increased sleep latency. All had orthostatic hypotension, and cardiac responses during apnea were absent, indicating cardiac autonomic denervation.

Guilleminault and colleagues[344] described two adolescent girls with familial dysautonomia who had respiratory irregularities. One also had esophageal reflux during sleep that gave rise to sleep disturbances due to frequent awakenings. McNicholas and coworkers[66] described dysrhythmic breathing in a patient with familial dysautonomia similar to the irregular breathing noted in patients with MSA. Maayan and associates[357] described a 42-year-old woman with familial dysautonomia who had several episodes of apnea during both wakefulness and sleep. The patient had megaesophagus associated with constriction in the lower esophageal region, which caused recurrent aspiration and apnea. After gastrostomy, no apneas were noted.

### Secondary Autonomic Failure

A group of patients experienced autonomic failure secondary to lesions in the central or peripheral nervous system, general medical disorders, drug effects, and other causes.[57,358]

An important example of an acquired nonprogressive dysautonomia syndrome was described by Frank and associates[359] in a 6-year-old girl who experienced subacute onset of hypoventilation and sleep apnea and gave evidence of dysautonomia. Frequent obstructive and central apneas were noted during all-night PSG study. The absence of variation in the heart rate suggested cardiac autonomic denervation. Postmortem findings 2 years after onset of the illness showed a ganglioneuroma of the lumbar sympathetic ganglia and neuron loss

with gliosis in the locus coeruleus, the reticular formation of the brain stem, and the Edinger-Westphal nuclei.

### Diabetic Neuropathy and Other Peripheral Autonomic Neuropathies

Many medical and neurologic conditions have associated autonomic neuropathies with peripheral neuropathies, but in most of these conditions, sleep and respiratory dysfunctions have not been adequately studied. However, there are many reports of such studies in diabetic polyneuropathies associated with autonomic neuropathy. This combination of somatic and autonomic neuropathies has been observed in some patients with acute inflammatory polyradiculoneuropathy (Guillain-Barré syndrome) and amyloidosis.

Rees and coworkers[360] observed 30 or more apneic episodes (in two patients mainly central and in one predominantly obstructive) during sleep at night in three of eight patients with diabetic autonomic neuropathy. In contrast, eight diabetes patients without autonomic neuropathy exhibited no sleep-related respiratory dysrhythmias. The authors speculate that sudden cardiorespiratory arrests that have been noted in some patients with diabetes may be related to autonomic failure and sleep apneas.

Guilleminault and coworkers[344] reported OSAs in two of four patients with juvenile diabetic autonomic neuropathy. One had central apnea and the other had irregular breathing associated with sleep-related esophageal reflux. Of the patients with primary sleep apnea syndrome described by Chokroverty and Sharp,[58] four had diabetes mellitus.

Mondini and Guilleminault[361] obtained PSG recordings for 12 type I and seven type II diabetics. They found obstructive and central apneas and an irregular pattern of breathing in five of 12 type I patients. They noted OSA in only one of seven type II diabetics. Autonomic neuropathy was present in all three type I patients with diabetes.

The findings of Catterall and coworkers[362] do not support the findings reported here of patients with diabetic autonomic neuropathy. They studied eight patients who had autonomic neuropathy and eight who did not and found no significant difference in frequency of apnea between the two groups.

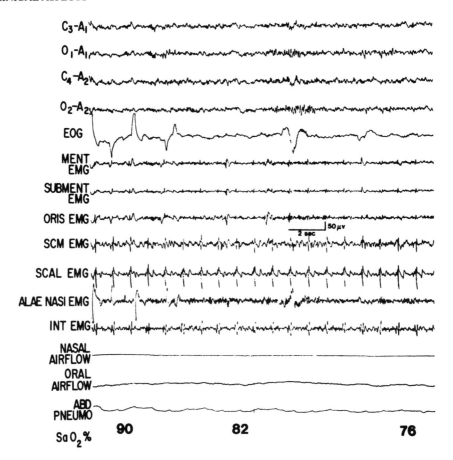

**Figure 27-7.** Polysomnography recording of a patient with narcolepsy showing four channels of EEG, vertical electro-oculogram (EOG), electromyograms (EMG) of mentalis (MENT), submental (SUBMENT), orbicularis oris (ORIS), sternocleidomastoid (SCM), scalenus anticus (SCAL), alae nasi, and intercostal (INT) muscles, nasal and oral airflow, abdominal pneumogram (ABD PNEUMO), and oxygen saturation ($Sao_2\%$) (ear oximeter). The patient has central apnea during REM sleep (only 18 of 30 seconds is shown). Note decrease of $Sao_2$ from 90% to 76% during apnea.

### Miscellaneous Neurologic Disorders

#### Sleep Apnea in Narcolepsy Syndrome

The narcolepsy syndrome is manifested by an irresistible desire to fall asleep at inappropriate times. Such attacks last a few seconds to as long as 20–30 minutes. They are often accompanied by cataplexy or other characteristic ancillary manifestations of narcolepsy (see Chapter 25). Sleep apnea is reported in some patients with narcolepsy syndrome.

Guilleminault's group[363] first reported CSA that lasted 20–90 seconds (during REM and NREM sleep) accompanied by $O_2$ desaturation in two patients with pure narcolepsy. In a later report, Guilleminault and colleagues[364] described 20 additional cases of narcolepsy with sleep apnea, which was predominantly central, although five also had mixed and obstructive apneas. The authors speculated that a dysfunction of the CNS structures that control the sleep and respiratory centers was responsible for the combined syndrome of sleep apnea and narcolepsy. Laffont and colleagues[365] also described central, obstructive, and mixed apneas in five of 18 narcolepsy patients. Chokroverty[366] made polygraphic observations in 16 patients with narcolepsy syndrome, 11 of whom showed central apneas and five upper airway OSAs during both REM and NREM sleep stages associated with $O_2$ desaturation (Figures 27-7 and 27-8).

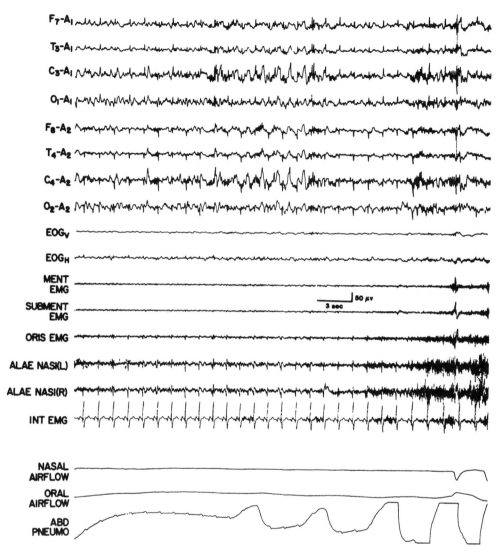

**Figure 27-8.** Polysomnography recording in a patient with narcolepsy and sleep apnea showing EEG (top eight channels); vertical ($EOG_V$) and horizontal ($EOG_H$) electro-oculograms; electromyography (EMG) of mentalis (MENT), submental (SUBMENT), orbicularis oris (ORIS), left (L) and right (R) alae nasi, and intercostal (INT) muscles; nasal and oral airflow, and abdominal pneumogram (ABD PNEUMO). Note mixed apnea (initial central apnea for a period of 13 seconds followed by obstructive apnea for a period of 19 seconds) during non-REM sleep stage II.

*Kleine-Levin Syndrome*

An episodic disorder occurring mostly in adolescent boys (but also described in girls[367]) and characterized by periodic hypersomnolence and bulimia was first described by Kleine[368] and later by Levin.[369] Critchley[370] gave a comprehensive description after analysis of 15 cases from the literature and 11 personal cases. The episodes usually occur three to four times per year, and each episode lasts days to weeks. During the sleep "attacks," patients sleep 16–18 hours a day or more, and on awakening they eat voraciously. Other behavior disturbances during the episode may include dull appearance, withdrawal, confusion, hallucinations, inattentiveness, memory impairment, and hypersexuality. In a later report, Billiard and Cadilhac[371] reviewed 123 cases collected from the literature. The condition is generally self-limited (although not always) and disappears by adulthood. PSG studies show normal sleep cycling and the MSLT shows pathologic sleepiness without sleep-onset REM. The cause of the condition remains undetermined, although a limbic-hypothalamic dysfunction has long been suspected but not proved. However, Gadoth et al.[372] described episodic hormone secretion during sleep in Kleine-Levin syndrome as evidence for hypothalamic dysfunction. The neuroendocrinologic assays by Chesson et al.[373] in a patient with Kleine-Levin syndrome during symptomatic and asymptomatic 24-hour periods also suggested a possible hypothalamic dysfunction. They found decreased growth hormone but increased thyroid stimulating hormone, prolactin, and cortisol during the symptomatic period, indicating a reduced hypothalamic dopaminergic tone. PSG study during the symptomatic period showed reduced slow-wave and REM sleep. In addition, the report by Gau et al.[374] of a 9-year-old Taiwanese boy with Prader-Willi syndrome associated with Kleine-Levin syndrome showing MRI evidence of a small hypothalamus further supports the hypothesis of a possible hypothalamic dysfunction in Kleine-Levin syndrome. Traditional treatment for this condition has been unsatisfactory but lithium treatment has been found to be effective.[375,376] In a letter to the editor, Crumley[377] mentioned valproic acid as a possible treatment for a 14-year-old boy with what the authors labeled Kleine-Levin syndrome. This boy had also been suffering from a bipolar disorder. Readers are referred to Orlosky[378] for a review of the Kleine-Levin syndrome.

*Idiopathic Recurrent Stupor*

Idiopathic recurrent stupor (IRS) is a condition of episodic loss of consciousness. A total of approximately 15 cases have appeared in the literature,[379] but the prevalence is probably higher than has been documented, as many patients admitted to intensive care units for stupor of unknown etiology remain undiagnosed.[379] In 1990, Cirignotta et al.[380] reported a patient with recurring coma and abnormal behavior in absence of toxic, metabolic, or vascular factors. In 1992, Tinuper et al.[381] described a similar patient, then described three more patients in 1994[382] in more detail. The clinical features are characterized by recurrent episodes of stupor in all of these patients, in whom no metabolic, toxic, or structural brain dysfunction was noted. Tinuper et al.[381] coined the term *idiopathic recurrent stupor* for this condition. These authors[382] described a characteristic EEG during an episode of stupor in these patients. The EEG showed

nonreactive, diffusely distributed fast rhythms (14–16 Hz). The frequency of the episodes of stupor varied between one to six to more than six per year; and the duration varied between 2 and 120 hours. A characteristic feature is that the patients were all briefly arousable from the stupor. In all three patients, AHI or RDI was higher than normal, somewhat complicating the issue. However, the characteristics of this disorder, including EEG and pharmacologic response, have not been described in patients with sleep apnea syndrome. Benzodiazepine-like activity identified as endozepine-4 in plasma and cerebrospinal fluid was markedly elevated in all patients. The clinical manifestations and the EEG abnormalities rapidly reversed to the normal state after administration of flumazenil (0.5–1.0 mg intravenously), a benzodiazepine-receptor antagonist. Lemesle et al.,[383] in a letter to the editor, confirmed the efficacy of flumazenil in IRS. Lotz et al.[384] described a somewhat similar patient with recurrent attacks of unconsciousness but with several differences from the patients described by Tinuper et al.[382] The patient described by Lotz et al.[384] had a characteristic EEG showing diffuse alphalike activity with frontal predominance and this patient was unarousable. The duration of each attack varied from 2 to 24 hours and the frequency of attacks was two to three per week. In addition, this patient had a family history with a similar illness in the father and two siblings. The patient responded to flumazenil treatment. Additional differences in the patient described by Lotz et al.[384] included prolonged I-V latency in brain stem auditory-evoked response, a nocturnal peak of melatonin secretion, and distal sensory-motor polyneuropathy. The description of these cases points to the role of benzodiazepine-like receptors in stupor and coma. Endozepines, benzodiazepine-like GABA$_a$ receptor modulators, are present in physiologically significant amounts in the brain.[385] It is notable that flumazenil injection also causes transient arousal in hepatic coma. It is possible that endozepines play a significant role in alterations of vigilance and mental status in various neurologic conditions.[386]

*Idiopathic Hypersomnia*

Idiopathic hypersomnia (IH), a condition of excessive somnolence, has no known cause. A disorder of the CNS has been suspected but not proved.[387,388] The syndrome has been described under a variety of labels, including *non–rapid eye movement narcolepsy*; *idiopathic central nervous system hypersomnia*; and *functional, mixed, or harmonious hypersomnia*. *Idiopathic hypersomnia* is the preferred term. The *ICSD*[196] defines IH as a disorder of presumed CNS cause that is associated with a normal or prolonged major sleep episode and excessive sleepiness consisting of prolonged (1–2 hours) sleep episodes of NREM sleep. The disease occurs insidiously and generally is manifested between ages 15 and 30 years. It closely resembles narcolepsy and sleep apnea. Although sometimes very difficult to distinguish from narcolepsy syndrome, the sleep pattern is different from that in narcolepsy or sleep apnea. The patient generally sleeps for hours, and the sleep is not refreshing. The patient does not give a history of snoring or repeated awakenings throughout the night. Sleep drunkenness is often seen in these patients, and they manifest automatic behavior with amnesia for the event. Physical examination shows no abnormal neurologic or other findings. The condition is disabling, and the patient is usually unemployable. It is generally a lifelong condition. PSG examination shows normal sleep structure and sleep cycling with prolonged NREM sleep accompanied by decreased stage I and increased stages III and IV NREM sleep. There is no sleep-onset REM. MSLT shows evidence of pathologic sleepiness without sleep-onset REM.

The differential diagnosis of the condition should include other causes of EDS such as classic narcolepsy with cataplexy, upper airway OSA syndrome, CSA syndrome, upper airway resistance syndrome, restless legs syndrome (RLS)-PLMS, insufficient sleep syndrome, drug-induced hypersomnia, and other medical or psychiatric disorders, particularly mood disorders. Post-traumatic hypersomnia, chronic fatigue syndrome, delayed sleep phase syndrome, and long sleepers should also be in the differential diagnostic considerations. Aldrich[389] suggested that IH is a heterogeneous syndrome. He based this suggestion on a retrospective review of clinical and PSG features, as well as questionnaire results derived from a database of 3,618 patients evaluated between 1985 and 1993 at a sleep disorders center. The study included patients with narcolepsy with cataplexy (39), narcolepsy without cataplexy (28), IH (26), EDS not otherwise specified (19), insufficient sleep syndrome (22), and patients with mild sleep-disordered breathing (21). In the same paper, the author directed our

attention to controversies and pitfalls in the diagnosis of IH. Aldrich[389] emphasized that patients with IH in his series did not exhibit prolonged night sleep, sleep drunkenness, nor frequent naps, and he questioned the validity of using prolonged or "deep" sleep as diagnostic criteria for IH. The author also did not find a significant difference in the proportion of subjects with sleep-related hallucinations and sleep paralysis between IH and those with narcolepsy without cataplexy. He suggested that clinical heterogeneity may reflect differences in etiology, such as the reports of preceding Epstein-Barr viral infection,[390] infectious mononucleosis or Guillain-Barré syndrome,[387,390] or HIV infection.[389] Finally, the author[389] argued for a re-evaluation of the diagnostic criteria for idiopathic disorders of sleepiness not associated with cataplexy. Some patients may have a positive family history[392,393] but the mode of inheritance is unknown. Montplaisir and Poirier[394] found an association with HLA-Cw2 and HLA-DR11 (a subtype of DR5) in a group of 18 subjects with IH. In contrast, Billiard[388] did not find this association in his population of 32 probands but he found a significant increase of DQ3. Harada et al.[395] found no significant difference in the distribution of HLAs in patients with essential hypersomnia and control subjects. Based on an analysis of the cerebrospinal fluid concentration of monoamine metabolites, a malfunction of the CNS norepinephrine system has been suggested in IH.[396] The treatment of IH is unsatisfactory and is somewhat similar to the stimulant treatment for narcolepsy. The behavioral approaches on sleep hygiene techniques have been advised but these do not have a significant impact on the disease. Compared with patients with classic narcolepsy with cataplexy, the stimulants are less effective in those with IH.

### Central Sleep Apnea Syndrome

CSA is defined as an apnea of at least 10 seconds' duration due to an absence of respiratory effort and airflow during sleep. Central hypopnea indicates the reduction in respiratory effort and airflow causing decreased tidal volume. CSA is a heterogeneous syndrome.[397–399] The condition can be classified into congenital central hypoventilation syndrome, acquired central hypoventilation syndrome, and acquired CSA syndrome. Congenital central hypoventilation syndrome causes alveolar hypoventilation with $CO_2$ retention and repetitive central apneas during sleep, and the condition manifests within the first few days of life.[400–403] There seems to be a congenital defect of the central chemoreceptors in the medulla. Based on the frequent association of congenital central hypoventilation syndrome with ganglioblastoma and Hirschsprung's disease, Guilleminault and Challamel[404] hypothesized that congenital central hypoventilation syndrome is a disorder of autonomic cell integration. Acquired CSA may result from neurologic, non-neurologic, or miscellaneous conditions. Neurologic causes of CSA and central alveolar hypoventilation syndrome include brain stem lesions, encephalitis, encephalopathy, neuromuscular and spinal cord disorders, and autonomic failure and have been described earlier in this section. Non-neurologic causes for CSA include left ventricle failure, nasal obstruction, acromegaly, myxedema, and chronic obstructive pulmonary disease. Most of these conditions have been described in Chapter 29. Under the miscellaneous category is high altitude. There is a decrease in the barometric pressure at high altitude associated with a decrease in $O_2$ tension causing reduced arterial $PaO_2$ and tissue oxygenation. Hypoxia stimulates ventilation, which in turn causes hypocapnia and reduced $PaCO_2$, thus lowering the $PaCO_2$ apnea threshold. (The level of arterial $CO_2$ tension at which an apnea occurs is called the *apnea threshold*.[405]) The lowering of the apnea threshold results in central apnea and periodic breathing (Cheyne-Stokes respiration) causing repeated awakenings and sleep fragmentation. Acetazolamide, a carbonic anhydrase inhibitor, will produce metabolic acidosis causing a shift in the $PaCO_2$ apnea threshold, and this has been used with success to treat central apnea at high altitude. This treatment may, however, cause OSA in such patients.[406] When all these conditions have been excluded, there remains a group of patients with CSA without any discernible cause. There are two subtypes, primary alveolar hypoventilation syndrome (PAH) and idiopathic CSA syndrome, that are thought to be associated with an occult or functional (chemical) neurologic lesion in the brain stem.

PAH is a syndrome of failure of automatic respiration without any recognizable disorder of the CNS or peripheral nervous system.[407] Central alveolar hypoventilation and central apnea syndrome associated with an organic neurologic disease should be differentiated from PAH.[407] The hallmark of PAH is a combination of arterial hypercapnia and hypoxemia during wakefulness that becomes worse during sleep.[408,409] Other manifestations include sleep apnea, congestive heart failure, pulmonary hypertension, and polycythemia. Central apnea is the usual type, but another feature of some cases is upper airway OSA. Impairment of hypercapnic ventilatory response is characteristic of this condition. The cause of the syndrome is unknown, and none of the reported cases of PAH showed evidence of CNS disease. Occasional postmortem reports showed no CNS structural lesions or nonspecific findings such as gliosis or mild loss of neurons in the medulla. A dysfunction of the medullary chemoreceptors is suspected, but no definite proof is available. Thus, the pathologic basis for PAH giving rise to the clinical manifestations of Ondine's curse remains undetermined. An important distinction from primary sleep apnea syndrome is that hypercapnic and hypoxic ventilatory responses during wakefulness are usually normal in primary sleep apnea syndrome.

Idiopathic CSA is not a common condition.[398,399,410,411] A common complaint in patients with CSA is insomnia[398,412] with frequent awakenings during sleep at night often accompanied by gasping for air or breathlessness. These patients may complain of EDS[397] but EDS is less common in CSA than in upper airway OSA patients. These patients are not generally obese. Depression is noted in many of these patients. These patients have recurrent episodes of CSA accompanied by $O_2$ desaturation, cardiac arrhythmias, and sleep fragmentation. The patients may develop pulmonary or systemic hypertension.[413] A later study by Podszus et al.,[414] however, found no change in pulmonary artery pressure during central apnea. In a large number of patients, the etiology of CSA remains unknown. CSA seems to result from a loss of ventilatory drive or respiratory rhythmicity but what causes this loss remains undetermined in many cases. In a subgroup of patients with EDS, nocturnal awakenings and sleep fragmentation, intermittent snoring and repeated CSAs, studied by Guilleminault et al.[399] and by Badr et al.[415] using fiberoptic scope and videoscope to visualize the upper airway, the authors found narrowing or occlusion of the upper airway during central apneas. Nasal CPAP reversed this CSA,[416–418] suggesting a role for the upper airway receptors in breathing during sleep.

### Sleep and Increased Intracranial Pressure

Increased intracranial pressure (ICP) may result from a variety of neurologic disorders (e.g., tumor, large infarction, intracranial hemorrhage, head trauma, focal abscess, diffuse encephalitis). Cooper and Hulme[419,420] found that the ICP of patients with intracranial lesions rose during REM and stage II NREM sleep. This was probably due to a combination of factors[421] (e.g., variations in cerebral blood flow, neurogenic reflex, cerebral vasoconstriction, enhanced brain metabolism). These observations have been confirmed by the findings of Munari and Calbucci[422] in 16 head trauma patients. In a study of children with craniosynostosis, Gonzalez et al.[423] observed both increased ICP and upper airway obstruction. They performed PSG studies along with continuous monitoring of ICP during sleep in 13 children with the syndrome of craniosynostosis and seven control patients with isolated unicoronal synostosis only. In 11 of 13 patients with this syndrome, they found upper airway obstruction, and eight of those 11 had frank OSAs. The other group of children showed no signs of upper airway obstruction during sleep. The causal relationship between upper airway obstruction and raised ICP in these children, however, remains undetermined.

### Headache Syndromes

Headaches and sleep complaints are common in day-to-day practice. Sleep disturbance (e.g., OSA syndrome) may cause headache and headache itself may cause sleep disturbances. The relationship between headache and sleep disorders is somewhat complex and remains ill understood. The *ICSD*[196] included cluster headache, chronic paroxysmal hemicrania (CPH), and migraine under the heading of sleep-related headaches. Migraine headache can, of course, occur both during the day and night. There are several reports showing a clear relationship between headache and sleep disorders but many of the reports are retrospective analysis and do not clearly eliminate the other confounding factors. Despite these limitations, there are clear indications from the various reports in the literature that there is a reciprocal interrelationship between headache and sleep disorders. Dexter and Weitzman[424] made the first PSG recording in patients with chronic migraine and cluster headaches and found a clear relationship between REM sleep and attacks of headache. Attacks occurred during REM or within 9 minutes after it terminated. In later studies,[425] Dexter also found a relationship between NREM stages III and IV and REM sleep and arousals with migraine headaches. Cluster headaches are thought to be REM related,[425–428] but cluster headaches may sometimes be triggered by NREM sleep.[429] CPH[430] is probably a variant of cluster headache. The attacks of CPH occur unilaterally and are briefer and more frequent than cluster headaches. CPH is most commonly associated with REM sleep[430] and it responds to indomethacin but in some cases may respond to calcium channel blockers.[431] Significant disruption of sleep architecture (decreased total and REM sleep time accompanied by increased number of awakenings during REM sleep) has been described in patients with CPH.[430] After a nocturnal polygraphic study, Conelli et al.[432] reported that CPH headache episodes were preceded by a sustained increase in blood pressure.

Kudrow and colleagues[427] found a high prevalence of CSA or OSA syndromes in patients who suffer cluster headaches, especially episodic cluster headaches.

Dexter[433] reported PSG-documented sleep apnea in 11 patients with chronic recurring headache syndrome. After surgical reconstruction in six patients with obstructive apneas, PSG demonstrated marked improvement in sleep apnea and considerable improvement in headache symptoms.

The relationship between chronic headache or early morning headache has remained somewhat controversial. Patients with upper airway OSA syndrome are thought to have an increasing incidence of morning headache as compared with controls,[433–435] and even improvement in morning headache has been reported after treatment of OSA syndrome.[436] In contrast, Aldrich and Chauncey[437] as well as Poceta and Dalessio,[438] after a survey, found that the complaint of morning headache was no different in patients with OSA syndrome than in those with other sleep disorders. The Copenhagen male study,[439] however, found that heavy snoring was an independent risk factor for headache. This study evaluated 3,323 men, aged 54–74 years. Ulfberg et al.[440] confirmed the association between heavy snoring, OSA, and headache in both men and women based on a questionnaire survey as well as sleep apnea screening that included 4 hours of sleep on the back of a static charge–sensitive bed and finger oximetry.

Paiva et al.[441] evaluated 49 subjects successfully seen in a headache clinic during a 6-month period with the predominant complaints of nocturnal or early morning headache. Based on the questionnaire and overnight sleep recordings, the authors found that headache was related to a specific sleep disorder (e.g., OSA syndrome, PLMS, sleep walking, sleep paralysis) in 55% of these subjects. They also found the treatment of these sleep disorders ameliorated the headaches. These findings confirmed the earlier observations of Paiva et al.[442] that morning or nocturnal headaches were frequent indicators of a sleep disturbance.

The hypnic headache syndrome (HHS) is a rare benign headache syndrome of the elderly that usually occurs after the age of 60 years and awakens the patient from sleep at a consistent time each night. Raskin[443] described six cases and Newman et al.[444] described two such cases who responded to lithium treatment. Raskin[443] suggested a relationship to REM sleep but no PSG study was performed to prove the hypothesis. HHS is differentiated from chronic cluster headache by its generalized distribution, age of onset and the lack of autonomic manifestations.

Another variety of unusual headache syndrome is "exploding head syndrome," which usually occurs in the transition from wake to sleep, abruptly arousing the patient with a feeling of an explosion of a sensation of bursting of the head.[445,446] The condition is benign and most likely represents a type of "sleep starts." PSG recordings[447,448] showed that the syndrome occurred both during wakefulness and REM sleep. In occasional cases, treatment with clomipramine may be effective.[447]

*Fatal Familial Insomnia*

FFI is a rare and rapidly progressive autosomal dominant prion disease with a mutation at codon 178 of the prion protein gene (*PrP*). Lugaresi and associates[449] originally described this entity in a family (14 affected members in three generations) with a progressive neurologic illness characterized by insomnia and dysautonomia that terminated in death. Age of onset of this illness is between 35 and 61 years and the clinical course runs from 7 to 48 months with an average of 12 months. Its clinical manifestations include impaired control of sleep-wake cycle including circadian rhythms; autonomic and neuroendocrine dysfunction; somatic neurologic, cognitive, and behavioral manifestations.[449–460]

Profound sleep disturbances and, in particular, severe insomnia are noted from the very beginning of the illness. PSG study[449,454,456,461,462] showed almost total absence of sleep patterns and only short episodes of REM sleep lasting for a few seconds or minutes, only without muscle atonia associated with dream-enacting behavior in the form of complex gestures and motions and myoclonus. As it progresses, there is progressive reduction of the total sleep time and reduced sleep cycles. The sleep cycle organization and stage shifts are lost from the very beginning. Sleep spindles and K complexes are markedly reduced and absent in the later stage of the illness, and slow-wave sleep is never recorded. The terminal stage of the illness is characterized by progressive slowing of the EEG and the patients remain in coma.

Autonomic function tests show evidence of sympathetic hyperactivity with preserved parasympathetic activity.[456,461–464] This unbalanced autonomic control results in persistent elevation of plasma catecholamines with further increase after upright tilt of the table.[461] There is increased heart rate response to atropine and diminished depressor effect after clonidine.[461] There is consistent elevation of blood pressure, heart rate, and core body temperature.[461,463] The nocturnal fall in blood pressure that occurs in normal individuals is lost from the early stages of the illness but nocturnal bradycardia still occurs.[461,463] Neuroendocrine functions[456,461,465,466] in FFI show a dysfunction of the pituitary-adrenal axis as manifested by striking elevation of serum cortisol but normal adrenocorticotrophic hormone (ACTH) indicating abnormal feedback suppression of ACTH.[461] Persistently elevated serum catecholamine levels associated with abnormal secretory patterns of growth hormones, prolactin, and melatonin are noted.[461,465,466] The nocturnal secretory peaks of growth hormone are absent but prolactin shows the expected nocturnal elevations except in the late stage. Plasma melatonin levels progressively decrease, but there is a complete obliteration of the melatonin rhythm in the most advanced stage of the illness.[461,465]

The somatic neurologic manifestations are present in all cases, particularly in the later stage of the illness and consist of ataxia, evidence of pyramidal tract dysfunction, myoclonus, tremor, and bizarre astasia-abasia. Neuropsychological studies reveal impairment of attention and vigilance, memory deficits involving data manipulation but leaving semantic, retrograde, and procedural memory intact, and relatively intact intellectual skills.[454,456,460] The disease progresses rapidly and in the final stage of the illness, the patients may also have breathing disturbances, mutism, and then end in coma and death.

Neuropathologically, the hallmark of FFI is severe atrophy of the thalamus, particularly the anterior ventral and dorsomedial thalamic nuclei associated with variable involvement of the inferior olive, striatum and cerebellum.[449,451,454,456,458–460] There are no spongiform changes, which are usually found in prion diseases, but a mild to moderate spongiform degeneration in the cerebral cortex has been noted in subjects with the longest duration of symptoms. A fluorodeoxyglucose positron emission tomographic (PET) study in seven FFI patients by Cortelli et al.[467] showed severe hypometabolism of the thalamus along with a mild hypometabolism of the cingulate cortex. Hypometabolism of other brain regions depends on the duration of symptoms, being more widespread in the heterozygotes (methionine-valine at codon 129) group. The data from Cortelli et al.[467] suggest that protease-resistant prion protein is the cause of neuronal dysfunction in FFI.

Based on the biochemical,[468] genetic,[469] and transmission[470,471] studies, it has been concluded that FFI is a transmissible prion disease resulting from a mutation at codon 178 of the prion protein gene associated with substitution of aspartic acid with asparagine along with the presence of methionine codon at position 129 of the mutant allele.[454,456,467] FFI subjects are divided into homozygotes (methionine/methionine 129) and heterozygotes (methionine/valine 129).[467] The heterozygotes pursue a longer course than the homozygotes. It should be noted that the same mutation at codon 178 of the prion protein gene is present in both FFI and familial Creutzfeldt-Jakob disease (CJD).[468,472,473,475] These two conditions, however, are separated by the methionine-valine polymorphism at codon 129 (CJD is invariably associated with valine).[474,475] All human prion diseases (CJD, Gerstmana-Straussler-Schenker syndrome)

should be considered in the differential diagnoses.[476–478] The other prion diseases that are known to exist consist of bovine spongiform encephalopathy (mad cow disease), scrapie (a disease of sheep), and kuru (described mostly in women and children in New Guinea in the past because of the practice of cannibalism).[476–478] The number of families of FFI sufferers included approximately 10 families, including one from Japan[459] and another from Australia.[458] The study of FFI has opened a new era in the molecular biology of the prion protein and its gene, and once again, rekindled the role of thalamus in sleep-wake regulating mechanisms.[451,456]

## LABORATORY INVESTIGATIONS

The laboratory tests should be directed at a diagnosis of the primary neurologic disorder and an assessment of sleep disturbances resulting from the neurologic illness.

### Laboratory Tests for the Primary Neurologic Disorders

It is beyond the scope of this chapter to delve into details of neurodiagnostic tests to assess the neurologic condition that gives rise to the sleep and sleep-related breathing disorders, so readers are referred to some excellent neurologic texts available.[479–481] Laboratory tests must subserve the findings of the history and physical examination, as discussed in Chapter 18. Laboratory tests are essential for diagnosis, prognosis, and treatment of the primary neurologic disorders. These investigations can be broadly divided into neurophysiologic tests, neuroimaging studies, examination of the cerebrospinal fluid, and general laboratory tests, including blood work and urinalysis. Special procedures such as tests to uncover autonomic deficits, neuroimmunologic, neurovirologic or neurourologic investigations, and brain biopsy are required to detect some neurologic disorders.

### Neurophysiologic Tests

Neurophysiologic tests include EEG, evoked potential and nerve conduction velocity studies, and EMG.

EEG, including 24-hour ambulatory and video-EEG examinations, is necessary to detect seizure disorder, metabolic-toxic-nutritional encephalopathies, and dementing illnesses (e.g., AD, CJD). Evoked potential studies include sensory (somatosensory, brain stem auditory, and visual evoked responses) and motor evoked potentials, and may be indicated in certain neurologic disorders, particularly demyelinating diseases such as MS. Nerve conduction measurements and EMG studies are necessary for diagnosis of various neuromuscular disorders, including neuromuscular junction diseases.

### Neuroimaging Studies

Cerebral angiography, including digital subtraction arteriography, may be necessary to investigate for strokes. CT and MRI are important studies for structural lesions of the CNS (e.g., tumors, infarctions, vascular malformations). CT and MRI are also helpful in patients with demyelinating and degenerative neurologic disorders that can be responsible for sleep and sleep-related breathing disturbances.

PET dynamically measures cerebral blood flow, $O_2$ uptake, and glucose utilization, and is helpful in diagnosis of dementing, degenerative (e.g., Parkinson's disease), and seizure disorders. It is very expensive, however, and is not available in most centers. Single-photon emission computed tomography (SPECT), which dynamically measures regional cerebral blood flow, may be useful for patients with cerebral vascular disease, AD, or seizure disorders. PET and SPECT studies can also be performed to investigate $D_2$-receptor alterations in RLS-PLMS and narcolepsy.[482–487] Functional MRI (fMRI) can be useful to study the generators and the areas of activation in RLS-PLMS.[488] Doppler ultrasonography is an important test for investigation of stroke due to extracranial vascular disease. Myelography other than CT and MRI is important for diagnosis of diseases of the spinal cord.

### Cerebrospinal Fluid Examination and Other Laboratory Tests

Cerebrospinal fluid examination is important for the diagnosis of meningoencephalitis, Lyme disease, and MS, all of which may give rise to sleep disturbances.

Hematologic tests and biochemical studies of blood and urine, as well as tests to assess endocrine, pulmonary, and cardiac disorders, are essential to undercover general medical disorders that may result in metabolic or toxic encephalopathies.

### Laboratory Tests to Investigate Sleep and Sleep-Related Breathing Disorders

#### Polysomnography

The importance of PSG in the diagnosis of sleep and sleep-related breathing disorders is discussed in Chapters 9 and 18. Sleep can adversely affect breathing, and, conversely, respiratory dysrhythmias can have deleterious effects on sleep (see Chapter 6). Both alterations can affect the severity and course of a neurologic illness, causing such sleep disturbances, and so the sleep architecture should be studied. The technique of PSG is described in detail in Chapter 9.

Multiple channels of EEG recordings are essential to document focal and diffuse neurologic lesions and to accurately localize epileptiform discharges in patients with seizure disorders (see Chapter 10). Multiple orofacial muscle EMGs, in addition to the standard chin EMG, may help assess upper airway muscle hypotonia (see Chapter 10). Multiple muscle EMGs, including tibialis anterior EMG, are essential for diagnosis of RLS, PLMS, some parasomnias (e.g., RBD), and paroxysmal nocturnal dystonia.

#### Multiple Sleep Latency Test

The MSLT is essential for objectively measuring daytime sleepiness. Sleep-onset latency of 5 minutes or less indicates pathologic sleepiness and may be seen in patients with narcolepsy, sleep apnea, idiopathic CNS hypersomnia, and other hypersomniac conditions. Additionally, sleep-onset REM during two of four or five recordings of MSLT is highly suggestive of narcolepsy. Further details about the recording technique and indications of MSLT are described in Chapter 13.

#### Maintenance of Wakefulness Test

The Maintenance of Wakefulness Test (MWT) measures the ability of the subject to remain awake. The test is similar to MSLT and is performed in a quiet, dark room with the patient in a semireclining position in a chair and instructed to resist sleep. The MWT really does not have a special advantage over MSLT but it may be useful for monitoring the effect of treatment in narcolepsy. For further details, see Chapter 14.

*Actigraphy*

Actigraphy is an activity monitor,[489] or a motion detector, designed to record activities during sleep and waking. This complements the sleep diary, or sleep log, data. It is a small device slightly larger than a wrist watch and is worn generally on the wrist but can also be worn at the ankle for 1–2 weeks. The actigraph stores the activity data in epoch-by-epoch samples in its internal memory until the end of the recording period, when it is downloaded to a computer to pool the data graphically and generate a report of the sleep-wake pattern. It is assumed that sleep is represented by long periods with very little to no movement. Actigraphy is a cost-effective method for assessment of sleep-wake pattern. It can assess sleep-wake schedules in normal and sleep-disordered patients. Actigraphy is very useful in the diagnosis of circadian rhythm sleep disorders, sleep state misperception, and other types of insomnia. It also can be used to detect and quantify PLMS and other sleep-related movements. However, it is not suitable for assessment of sleep-disordered breathing events. It is also not suitable for assessment in subjects who may feign a sleep problem. Several models are commercially available. Actigraphy and overnight PSG sleep measures are highly correlated in clinical studies. For additional information about actigraphy, see Chapter 26.

*Video-Polysomnography*

Video-PSG is important for monitoring patients suspected of having epilepsy or parasomnias that may be associated with certain neurologic disorders (see Chapters 18 and 27).

*Electroencephalography, Including 24-Hour Ambulatory EEG*

EEG, including 24-hour ambulatory EEG, is essential if epilepsy is suspected, as it can cause sleep disturbances that may sometimes be mistaken for parasomnias or sleep apneic episodes. For further details see Chapters 10 and 34.

*Pulmonary Function Tests*

Pulmonary function tests exclude intrinsic bronchopulmonary disease, which may affect sleep-related breathing disorders.[490] For additional detail on pulmonary function tests, see Chapter 12. The following is a brief list of pulmonary function tests:

- Ventilatory functions: forced expiratory volume in 1 second ($FEV_1$), forced vital capacity (FVC), $FEV_1$-FVC ratio, peak expiratory flow rate (PEFR), forced expiratory flow rate (FEF)
- Measurement of lung volumes: total lung capacity (TLC), residual volume (RV), functional residual capacity (FRC)
- Gas distribution and gas transfer: single-breath nitrogen test ($SBN_2$/L), diffusing capacity by the technique of single-breath apnea method using CO and helium ($DL_{CO}SB$)
- Arterial blood gases: $PaO_2$, $PaCO_2$

Other tests that may be performed in special situations include exercise tests and measurements of lung volumes and ventilatory functions before and after a bronchodilator is used.

The respiratory muscle function of individuals with neuromuscular disorders should be specifically assessed. According to Black and Hyatt,[491] it is important to measure the maximal static inspiratory and expiratory pressures, which are more important than the dynamic values. Such measurements, which require cooperation, may be difficult in many patients with neurologic disorders.

Chemical control of breathing may be impaired if neurologic disease causes dysfunction of the metabolic respiratory controllers.[9] Such impairment may be detected by hypercapnic ventilatory response ($\dot{V}E/PaCO_2$), hypoxic ventilatory response ($\dot{V}E/PaO_2$), and mouth occlusion pressure ($P_{0.1}$) response, with or without load.[9] Central respiratory drive and the inspiratory muscle strength independent of pulmonary mechanical factors are reflected in the $P_{0.1}$ response.

*Electrodiagnosis of the Respiratory Muscles*

EMG of the upper airway, diaphragmatic, and intercostal muscles (see Chapters 6 and 10) may detect affection of these muscles in neurologic diseases. In patients with MSA with laryngeal stridor, it is important to perform laryngeal EMG to detect laryngeal paresis.[492]

Phrenic nerve[493] and intercostal nerve conduction study[494] may detect phrenic and intercostal neuropathy, which may cause diaphragmatic and intercostal muscle affections in some patients with neurologic disorders.

## TREATMENT OF SLEEP AND RESPIRATORY DYSFUNCTION SECONDARY TO NEUROLOGIC DISORDERS

Treatment is discussed in two broad categories: (1) therapy for the primary neurologic illness and (2) therapy for the secondary sleep disturbance.

### Treatment of Primary Neurologic Illness

First and foremost is accurate diagnosis of the primary neurologic disorder. This is followed by vigorous treatment and monitoring of the neurologic illness. Such treatment may improve the sleep disturbances. It is beyond the scope of this volume to discuss the treatment of the primary neurologic disorders, and readers are referred to some excellent texts.[479–481]

### Treatment of Sleep Disturbances

Sleep disturbances in neurologic disorders include hypersomnia, insomnia, circadian rhythm sleep disturbances, and parasomnias. Treatment of these complaints is discussed in several chapters in this volume (see Chapters 22–26, 30–32, and 34). In this section, treatment of hypersomnia that results mainly from sleep-related respiratory dysrhythmias in neurologic disorders is discussed. In the final paragraph, general principles of treatment for sleep disturbances not related to the respiratory dysrhythmias in dementias are briefly reviewed.

### Treatment of Sleep-Related Breathing Disorders

The objective of treatment of sleep-related breathing disorders is twofold: (1) to improve the quality of life by improving the quality of sleep and (2) to prevent life-threatening cardiac arrhythmias, pulmonary hypertension, and congestive heart failure related to sleep-disordered breathing. The quality of sleep may be improved by eliminating repeated apneas during sleep and thus preventing repeated arousals, sleep fragmentation, nocturnal hypoxemia, and daytime hypersomnolence. The treatment modalities for sleep-related respiratory dysrhythmias resulting from neurologic illness may be divided into five categories: (1) general measures, (2) pharmacologic agents, (3) mechanical devices, (4) supplemental $O_2$ administration, and (5) surgical treatment.

### General Measures

General measures of treatment include reduction or elimination of risk factors that can aggravate sleep-related respiratory dysrhythmias. Avoidance of alcohol and sedative-hypnotic drugs[495] (e.g., benzodiazepines, barbiturates, narcotics) that can depress breathing during sleep is an important step in eliminating the risk factors. Alcohol is known to increase the frequency and duration of apneas, probably by two mechanisms[496–498]: (1) selective depression of the genioglossus and other upper airway muscles and (2) impairment of the arousal response by raising its threshold. For obese patients, weight loss is another important step in eliminating risk factors for sleep-related respiratory dysrhythmia.

### Drug Therapy

The three most important agents that have been tried with partial success for mild to moderate sleep apnea are protriptyline, medroxyprogesterone acetate, and acetazolamide. Protriptyline may be used in a dose of 5–20 mg at bedtime. Suppression of REM sleep, a specific alerting property; increased upper airway muscle tone; and conversion of apnea to hypopnea are cited as mechanisms of action of this drug.[495,499] Anticholinergic effects and cardiac arrhythmias are the limiting side effects of this drug.

Medroxyprogesterone acetate has been tried in many patients with sleep apnea, but the results have been disappointing.[500–505] It is thought to act by increasing ventilatory drive. Impotence in men is a limiting side effect. There are other side effects.[506]

Acetazolamide has been used with some success in central apnea, but development of obstructive apnea or aggravation of orthostatic hypotension owing to its diuretic and natriuretic effects should be kept in mind during treatment. Acetazolamide is a carbonic anhydrase inhibitor and will produce metabolic acidosis causing a shift in the $P_{CO_2}$ apnea threshold, and it has been used with some success to treat central apnea at high altitude.[398,399,507–510]

## Mechanical Devices

### Nasal Continuous Positive Airway Pressure

An important therapeutic advance in the treatment of OSA syndrome, CPAP is described in detail in Chapter 23. It should be given a trial in neurologic disease patients with upper airway OSAs associated with intermittent CSAs or with mixed apneas. Such treatment often improves the quality of sleep and reduces daytime symptoms by eliminating or reducing sleep-related obstructive or mixed apneas and $O_2$ desaturation. The role of nasal CPAP for CSA is highly controversial. A Stanford University group[511] found CPAP helpful for central apnea patients who had associated OSA or who showed sleep fragmentation and repeated sleep-wake changes. In a subgroup of patients with CSA with insomnia who may show narrowing or occlusion of the upper airway on fiberoptic scope, nasal CPAP reversed the CSA.[512–514] Instead of CPAP, some patients require BIPAP (see Chapter 23 for further details).

### Other Ventilatory Supports

Besides tracheostomy and diaphragmatic pacing, which is described under Surgical Treatment in this chapter, two types of ventilatory supports are available for patients with sleep-related apnea or hypoventilation (see also Chapter 23): (1) negative-pressure ventilators and (2) positive-pressure ventilators.[515–517] Many of these mechanical devices for ventilation were developed during the polio epidemics of the 1930s, 1940s, and 1950s.[517] There has been a resurgence for use of noninvasive positive pressure ventilation (NIPPV), however, for patients with respiratory failure with chronic hypoventilation associated with neuromuscular diseases. Negative pressure ventilators include "iron lung" or tank respirator, the "raincoat" or "Pneumo-Wrap ventilator," and the cuirass or "tortoise shell."[517–520] The tank respirator is the most effective negative pressure ventilator applying negative pressure to the entire body below the neck but it is bulky and limits the patient's acceptance.[517,518] Use of the negative pressure ventilator may be associated with upper airway OSA and $O_2$ desaturation, both in normal subjects[521] and in patients with neuromuscular diseases.[522]

The objectives of mechanical ventilation include improvement of pulmonary gas exchange, relief of respiratory muscle fatigue and respiratory distress, prevention of pulmonary atelectasis, and decrement of the work of breathing.[516] NIPPV can be used either with a face or nasal mask. Problems with the face mask include difficulty with swallowing saliva and aerophagia, and, therefore, the face mask has now been replaced by the nasal mask, which is more comfortable and acceptable to the patients.[517] Intermittent use of nasal NIPPV results in reduction of $Pa_{CO_2}$ and improvement of symptoms in various neuromuscular disorders[517]; patients with central hypoventilation and CSA may also respond.[517] NIPPV is, thus, an important therapeutic advance and current standard of care for chronic ventilatory failure is mainly NIPPV using nasal mask or prongs. Bach et al.[523] used these successfully through a mouthpiece in postpolio respiratory failure patients. Potential problems with the mouthpiece include air leaks and aspiration, and the patients need to have an adequate buccopharyngeal muscle strength.[515] Nasal route is, therefore, preferable but nasal IPPV requires intact bulbar function for protection of the upper airway.[515] Long-term NIPPV is not suitable for those with diffuse oropharyngeal muscle weakness who cannot ventilate on their own.[515] Nasal IPPV has similar complications as CPAP treatment for sleep apnea and may include dryness of the nose, nasal congestion, rhinorrhea, skin and eye irritation due to air leaks, and discomfort from inadequate mask fit and epistaxis[515,524] (see also Chapter 23). These complications can, however, be easily remediated.[525–527] Successful results using nocturnal NIPPV have been reported in case reports and in small and large series in patients with neuromuscular disorders and central ventilatory disorders.[217,269–271,515,524,525,528–535] Either pressure-cycled or volume-cycled ventilators may be used to deliver NIPPV. Bilevel positive airway pressure (BIPAP) with portable volume-cycled ventilators may be a useful alterative to NIPPV.[272,273,515,536–538] Using these methods, the group from Stanford[511] and others were able to avoid tracheostomy or diaphragmatic pacing and they were able to control sleep-related problems. It should be noted that the correct diagnosis of CSA syndrome (by modern methods) and identification of the causes of such apnea by sleep-wake studies are essential to correct treatment. NIPPV in appropriately selected patients with neuromuscular diseases associated with hypoventilation is useful to alleviate symptoms and improve the quality of life.[269–271,515]

In severe cases of poliomyelitis or postpolio syndrome, ventilatory support is required to maintain respiratory homeostasis. Some postpolio patients—those who have predominantly CSA—require a rocking bed[213] for ventilatory assistance. They do not respond to CPAP, but they do show improved sleep architecture and respiratory function after mechanical ventilation via nasal mask. Some patients may have obstructive or mixed apneas, and they improve with CPAP. Patients with hypoventilation improve after treatment with nasal ventilation via a mask.

For sleep apnea and hypoventilation in patients with ALS, ventilatory support is needed. Some of these patients may need the negative pressure ventilation by cuirass, which improves respiratory problems and sleep quality. Some with general respiratory muscle weakness, including diaphragmatic paresis, may require a combination of cuirass, CPAP, and, later, IPPV at night. Howard's group[252] treated patients with motor neuron disease with mechanical ventilation with considerable benefit. Some patients with mainly diaphragmatic muscle weakness were treated with negative pressure ventilation by cuirass, which improved their respiratory problems and the quality of sleep. Patients with sleep apnea or hypoventilation due to bulbar muscle weakness as well as diaphragmatic weakness were treated with cuirass, CPAP, and, later, with IPPV at night and had symptomatic relief.

## Oxygen

Supplemental $O_2$ therapy may decrease the severity of OSA in certain patients.[539] The recommended treatment of nocturnal hypoxemia is administration of $O_2$ at a low flow rate (1–2 liters per minute) via a nasal cannula (see Chapter 29). $O_2$ administration may not be safe for all patients with sleep apnea syndrome. Motta and Guilleminault[540] and Chokroverty and coworkers[541] observed prolongation of apneas after $O_2$ administration during sleep in patients with OSA syndrome. Gay and Edmonds[542] directed our attention to the possible exacerbation of hypercapnia after administration of low-flow $O_2$ in patients with neuromuscular disorders. In eight patients with neuromuscular disease and diaphragmatic dysfunction (patients with polymyositis, ALS, or inflammatory motor neuropathy), mean $Paco_2$ increased considerably after administration of low-flow supplemental $O_2$ (0.5–2.0 liters per minute). Four patients needed subsequent nocturnal assisted ventilation. The authors suggested that nocturnal assisted ventilation can be considered for patients with $O_2$-sensitive hypoventilation. In such patients, it may be possible to safely administer $O_2$ during the daytime.

## Surgical Treatment

### Diaphragmatic Pacing or Electrophrenic Respiration

Sarnoff and coworkers[543] first used electrophrenic stimulation in patients with poliomyelitis in 1951, but the technical difficulties at that time prevented its regular use for such treatment. Glenn and associates[544] improved the technique and studied extensively the electrophrenic respiration by diaphragm pacing (DP). This form of treatment is used successfully in patients with respiratory center involvement with CSA syndrome. Superimposed OSA may complicate the procedure, which may then require both electrophrenic respiration and tracheostomy for treating such patients. Glenn's group[544] used such treatment successfully in three groups of neurologic disease patients: those with respiratory center involvement, either direct or through interruption of the afferent or efferent neurons to the respiratory center; those with high cervical spinal cord lesions; and those with PAH. Chervin and Guilleminault[545] reviewed the topic of DP. The authors stated that the gold standard of treatment of hypoventilation due to neurologic including neuromuscular disorders is BIPAP or IPPV. For those who require ventilatory assistance during both day and night, however, DP is advantageous. The indications for DP include those patients with partial or total ventilatory failure, either during sleep or continuously. The causes for hypoventilation include neurologic disorders proximal to the phrenic motor neurons. The causes include both idiopathic CSA syndrome as well as congenital central hypoventilation syndrome in infants. Most of the patients on long-term DP require minimal or no additional ventilatory support, and most show improvement in the quality of life. Complications of DP include precipitation of upper airway OSA requiring CPAP or tracheostomy in many patients, damage to the phrenic nerve, diaphragmatic damage due to fatigue, equipment malfunction, surgical complications, neuromuscular junction failure, local infection, and interference with cardiac pacemakers. Finally, DP is an invasive procedure; despite the complications and disadvantages, DP is the preferred procedure for those requiring ventilatory assistance both during the day and night.

*Tracheostomy*

Tracheostomy remains the only effective measure for emergency treatment of patients with marked respiratory dysfunction with severe hypoxemia, patients with sudden respiratory arrest after resuscitation by intubation, and patients with severe laryngeal stridor due to laryngeal abductor paralysis. This used to be the definitive treatment for patients with severe OSA syndrome, but this has been largely replaced by CPAP or BIPAP since they became available. On improvement after emergency tracheostomy, patients may later be weaned from tracheostomy. Permanent tracheostomy may still be needed for patients with neuromuscular diseases; those with central respiratory drive abnormalities showing persistently elevated $Paco_2$ despite using NIPPV; those who are unable to handle oropharyngeal secretions and show continued deterioration of neuromuscular disorders with very brief periods of spontaneous ventilation; and those patients with sleep apnea who fail to improve after nasal CPAP and nasal ventilation.[515,517] In such patients, ventilatory assistance is provided at night with plugging of the tracheostomy tube during the daytime or the patient may use a commercially available portable

**Table 27-2.** Treatment of Sleep Disturbances in Alzheimer's Disease and Related Dementias

Reduce or eliminate medications that may contribute to sleep disturbance or sleep-related breathing disorders
Treat associated depression or anxiety
Eliminate alcohol and caffeine in the evening
Institute regular sleep schedule and sleep hygiene as much as possible
For insomnia, try an intermediate-acting benzodiazepine or zolpidem not more than three times per week
Use small doses of haloperidol (0.5–1.0 mg bid or tid) or thioridazine (25 mg tid)
Encourage the patient to avoid daytime naps
Encourage regular exercise

ventilator continuously if needed, using assist control mode.[517] Potential complications of tracheostomy and the care needed for maintenance of the tracheostomy should be discussed in detail with the patients and their families. Besides its invasiveness, the complications of tracheostomy include disfigurement, difficulty with speaking, tracheal stenosis, and tracheomalacia.[515,546]

### Treatment of Sleep Disturbances in Alzheimer's Disease and Related Dementias

Treatment of acute confusional states associated with dementia is described in Chapter 32. In this section, general principles of treatment of sleep disturbance in patients with dementia are outlined. Table 27-2 lists some certain general principles of treatment. Medications that could have an adverse effect on sleep and breathing should be reduced in dose or changed. Associated conditions that could interfere with sleep (e.g., pain due to arthritis and other causes) should be treated with analgesics. Depression is often an important feature in patients with AD, and a sedative antidepressant may be helpful. Frequency of urination in such patients may result from infection or enlarged prostate and may disturb sleep at night. Appropriate treatment should be directed toward such conditions. Patients should be encouraged to develop good sleep habits. They should be discouraged from taking daytime naps and should be encouraged to exercise (e.g., walking during the day). They should not drink caffeine before bedtime or in the evening. For sleeplessness, a trial with intermediate-acting benzodiazepines or zolpidem should be tried for a short period (see Chapter 24). For extreme agitation, patients should be treated with haloperidol, as for confusional episodes (see Chapter 32). In some patients, timed exposure to bright light may be helpful.[547–550] In limited studies, Satlin et al.[547] and Okawa et al.[548,549] reported improvement in nighttime sleep and a decrease in daytime sleepiness after bright light exposure in the evening. Further studies are needed to confirm these observations.

## CONCLUSION

The science of sleep is beginning to advance and probe even deeper into the significance and pathogenesis of sleep and its disorders. Dement[551] stated aptly that sleep medicine focuses on the sleeping brain and on all phenomena and pathologic effects that derive therefrom. This chapter summarizes how sleep, sleep disorders, and breathing interact in the brain and other neural structures, and how dysfunctions result in sleep and sleep-related breathing disturbances. Progress in research involving molecular neurobiology and neurophysiology of sleep, chronophysiology, chronobiology, and functional imaging of the brain (e.g., fMRI, PET scanning) holds great promise to unravel the mysteries of sleep even further and to direct our attention to finding more promising therapies for the unfortunate millions suffering from chronic disorders of sleep and wakefulness.

## REFERENCES

1. Steriade M, McCarley RW. Brainstem Control of Wakefulness and Sleep. New York: Plenum, 1990.
2. Vertes RP. Brainstem control of the events of REM sleep. Prog Neurobiol 1984;22:241.
3. Moruzzi G. The sleep waking cycle. Ergeb Physiol 1972;64:1.
4. Hobson JA, Lydic R, Baghdoyan HA. Evolving concepts of sleep cycle generation: from brain centers to neuronal populations. Behav Brain Sci 1986; 9:371.
5. Jouvet M. The role of monoamines and acetylcholine containing neurons in the regulation of the sleep-waking cycle. Ergeb Physiol 1972;64:166.
6. Bulow K. Respiration and wakefulness in man. Acta Physiol Scand Suppl 1963;59:1.
7. Phillipson EA. Control of breathing during sleep. Am Rev Respir Dis 1978;118:909.
8. Phillipson EA. Respiratory adaptations in sleep. Annu Rev Physiol 1978;40:133.
9. Phillipson EA, Bowes G. Control of Breathing During Sleep. In AF Fishman, NS Cherniack, JG Widdicombe (eds), Handbook of Physiology (Vol II, Part 2, Sect 3): The Respiratory System. Bethesda, MD: American Physiological Society, 1986;649.
10. McGinty DJ, Beahm EK. Neurobiology of Sleep. In NA Saunders, C Sullivan (eds), Sleep and Breathing. New York: Marcel Dekker, 1984;1.
11. Plum F, Brown HW. The effect on respiration of central nervous system disease. Ann N Y Acad Sci 1963;109:915.
12. Plum F. Breathlessness in Neurological Disease: The Effects of Neurological Disease on the Act of Breathing. In JBL Howell, EJM Campbell (eds), Breathlessness. Oxford: Blackwell, 1966;203.
13. Plum F. Neurological Integration of Behavioral and Metabolic Control of Breathing. In R Porter (ed), Ciba Foundation Symposium on Breathing. Herine-Breuer Centenary Symposium. London: Churchill, 1970;159.
14. Nathan PW. The descending respiratory pathway in man. J Neurol Neurosurg Psychiatry 1963;26:487.
15. Heyman A, Birchfield RI, Sieker HO. Effects of bilateral cerebral infarction on respiratory center sensitivity. Neurology 1958;8:694.
16. Plum F, Swanson AG. Abnormalities in central regulation of respiration in acute and convalescent poliomyelitis. Arch Neurol Psychiatry 1958;80:267.
17. Plum F, Brown HW, Snoep E. Neurologic significance of post-hyperventilation apnea. JAMA 1962;181:1050.
18. North JB, Jennett S. Impedance pneumography for the detection of abnormal breathing patterns associated with brain damage. Lancet 1972;2:212.
19. Lee MC, Klassen AC, Resch JA. Respiratory pattern disturbances in ischemic cerebral vascular disease. Stroke 1974;5:612.
20. North JB, Jennett S. Abnormal breathing patterns associated with acute brain damage. Arch Neurol 1974; 31:338.
21. Lee MC, Klassen AC, Heaney LM, et al. Respiratory rate and pattern disturbances in acute brain stem infarction. Stroke 1976;7:382.
22. Von Economo C. Die Pathologie des Schlafes. In A Bethe, G Bergmann, G Embden (eds), Handbuch der Normalen und Pathologischen Physiologie. Berlin: Springer, 1926;591.
23. Von Economo C. Encephalitis Lethargica. Its Sequelae and Treatment. London: Oxford University Press, 1931.
24. Hess WR. Le sommeil. C R Soc Biol (Paris) 1931; 107:1333.
25. Nauta WJH. Hypothalamic regulation of sleep in rats. An experimental study. J Neurophysiol 1946;9:285.
26. Bremer F. Cerveau "isolé" et physiologie due sommeil. C R Soc Biol (Paris) 1935;118:1235.
27. Moruzzi G, Magoun HW. Brain stem reticular formation and activation of the EEG. Electroencephalogr Clin Neurophysiol 1949;1:455.
28. Moruzzi G. Active processes in the brain stem during sleep. Harvey Lect 1963;58:233.

29. Batini C, Moruzzi G, Palestini M, et al. Persistent patterns of wakefulness in the pretrigeminal midpontine preparation. Science 1958;128:30–32.

30. Batini C, Moruzzi G, Palestini M, et al. Effect of complete pontine transections on the sleep-wakefulness rhythm: the mid-pontine pretrigeminal preparation. Arch Ital Biol 1959;97:1.

31. Jouvet M. Neurophysiology of the states of sleep. Physiol Rev 1967;47:117.

32. Magnes J, Moruzzi G, Pompeiano O. Synchronization of the EEG produced by low-frequency electrical stimulation of the region of the solitary tract. Arch Ital Biol 1961;99:33.

33. Sterman MB, Clemente CD. Forebrain inhibitory mechanisms: cortical synchronization induced by basal forebrain stimulation. Exp Neurol 1962;6:103.

34. Sterman MB, Clemente CD. Forebrain inhibitory mechanisms: sleep patterns induced by basal forebrain stimulation. Exp Neurol 1962;6:91.

35. Lucas EA, Sterman MB. Effect of a forebrain lesion on the polycyclic sleep-wake cycle and sleep-wake patterns in the cat. Exp Neurol 1975;46:368.

36. McGinty DJ, Sterman MB. Sleep suppression after basal forebrain lesions in the cat. Science 1968;160:1253.

37. Ricardo JA, Koh ET. Anatomical evidence of direct projections from the nucleus of the solitary tract to the hypothalamus, amygdala, and other forebrain structures in the rat. Brain Res 1978;153:1.

38. Jones BE. Mechanisms of Sleep-Wake States. In MH Kryger, T Roth, WC Dement (eds), Principles and Practice of Sleep Medicine (2nd ed). Philadelphia: Saunders, 1994;145.

39. Bremer F. Cerebral hypnogenic centers. Ann Neurol 1977;2:1.

40. Steriade M, Glenn LL. Neocortical and caudate projections of intralaminar thalamic neurons and their synaptic excitation from the midbrain reticular cord. J Neurophysiol 1982;48:352.

41. Steriade M, Oaskson G, Ropert N. Firing rates and patterns of midbrain reticular neurons during steady and transitional states of sleep-waking cycle. Exp Brain Res 1982;46:37.

42. Steriade M, McCormick DA, Sejnowski TJ. Thalamocortical oscillations in the sleeping and aroused brain. Science 1993;262:679.

43. Jouvet M. Recherches sur les structures nerveuses et les mecanismes responsables des differentes phases du sommeil physiologique. Arch Ital Biol 1962;100:125.

44. Sallanon M, Denoyer M, Kitahama K, et al. Long-lasting insomnia induced by preoptic neuron lesions and its transient reversal by muscimol injection into the posterior hypothalamus in the cat. Neuroscience 1989;32:669.

45. Szymusiak R, McGinty D. Sleep-related neuronal discharge in the basal forebrain of cats. Brain Res 1986;370:82.

46. Detari L, Juhasz G, Kukorelli T. Neuronal firing in the pallidal region: firing patterns during sleep-wakefulness cycle in cats. Electroencephalogr Clin Neurophysiol 1987;67:159.

47. Buzsaki G, Bickford RG, Ponomareff G, et al. Nucleus basalis and thalamic control of neocortical activity in the freely moving rat. J Neurosci 1988;8:4007.

48. Mesulam MM, Mufson EJ, Levey AI, et al. Atlas of cholinergic neurons in the forebrain and upper brainstem of the macaque based on monoclonal choline acetyltransferase immunohistochemistry and acetylcholinesterase histochemistry. Neuroscience 1984;12:669.

49. Swanson LW, Mogenson GJ, Simerly RB, et al. Anatomical and electrophysiological evidence for a projection from the medial preoptic area to the "mesencephalic and subthalamic locomotor regions" in the rat. Brain Res 1987;405:108.

50. Porkka-Hieskanen T, Strecker RE, Thakkar M, et al. Adenosine: a mediator of the sleep-inducing effects of prolonged wakefulness. Science 1997;276:1265.

51. Mitchell RA, Berger AJ. Neural regulation of respiration. Am Rev Respir Dis 1975;111:206.

52. Berger AJ, Mitchell RA, Severinghaus JW. Regulation of respiration. N Engl J Med 1977;297:92,138,194.

53. Mitchell RA. Neural regulation of respiration. Clin Chest Med 1980;1:3.

54. Chokroverty S. The Spectrum of Ventilatory Disturbances in Movement Disorders. In S Chokroverty (ed), Movement Disorders. Costa Mesa, CA: PMA, 1990;365.

55. Hugelin A, Cohen MI. The reticular activating system and respiratory regulation in the cat. Ann N Y Acad Sci 1963;109:586.

56. Chokroverty S. Sleep Apnea and Respiratory Disturbances in Multiple System Atrophy with Progressive Autonomic Failure (Shy-Drager Syndrome). In R Bannister (ed), Autonomic Failure (2nd ed). London: Oxford University Press, 1988;432.

57. Chokroverty S. The Shy-Drager syndrome. Neurol Neurosurg Update 1986;7:1.

58. Chokroverty S, Sharp JT. Primary sleep apnea syndrome. J Neurol Neurosurg Psychiatry 1981;44:970.

59. Guilleminault C. Sleep and Breathing. In C Guilleminault (ed), Sleeping and Waking Disorders: Indications and Techniques. Menlo Park, CA: Addison-Wesley, 1982;155.

60. Chokroverty S. Sleep and Breathing in Neurological Disorders. In NH Edelman, TV Santiago (eds), Breathing Disorders of Sleep. New York: Churchill Livingstone, 1986;225.

61. Gould GA, Whyte KF, Rhind GB, et al. The sleep hypopnea syndrome. Am Rev Respir Dis 1988;137:895.

62. Agency for Health Care Policy and Research. Polysomnography and Sleep Disorders Center: Health Technology Assessment Reports 1991, number 4. Public Health Service Publication No. 92-0027. Washington, DC: U.S. Department of Health and Human Services, 1992.

63. Moser NJ, Phillips BA, Berry DTR, Harbison L. What is hypopnea, anyway? Chest 1994;105:426.

64. Cherniack NS, Longobardo GA. Abnormalities in Respiratory Rhythm. In AF Fishman, NS Cherniack, JG Widdicombe (eds), Handbook of Physiology (Vol II, Part 2, Sect 3): The Respiratory System. Bethesda, MD: American Physiological Society, 1986;729.

65. Browne HW, Plum F. The neurologic basis of Cheyne-Stokes respiration. Am J Med 1961;30:849.

66. McNicholas WT, Rutherford R, Grossman R, et al. Abnormal respiratory pattern generation during sleep in patients with autonomic dysfunction. Am Rev Respir Dis 1983;128:429.

67. Lumsden T. Observations on the respiratory centers in the cat. J Physiol (Lond) 1923;57:153.

68. Wang SC, Ngai SH, Frumin MJ. Organization of central respiratory mechanisms in the brainstem of the cat: genesis of normal respiratory rhythmicity. Am J Physiol 1957;190:333.

69. Cohen MI. Neurogenesis of respiratory rhythm in the mammal. Physiol Rev 1979;59:1105.

70a. Chokroverty S, Sharp JT, Barron KD. Periodic respiration in erect posture in Shy-Drager syndrome. J Neurol Neurosurg Psychiatry 1978;41:980.

70b. Aldrich M. Insomnia in neurological diseases. J Psychosom Res 1993;37(Suppl 1):3.

71. Guilleminault C, Tilkian A, Dement WC. The sleep apnea syndromes. Annu Rev Med 1976;27:465.

72. Aldrich MS. Sleep and Degenerative Neurological Disorders Involving the Motor System. In MJ Thorpy (ed), Handbook of Sleep Disorders. New York: Marcel Dekker, 1990;673.

73. Tamura K, Karacan I, Williams R, Meyer JS. Disturbances of the sleep-waking cycle in patients with vascular brain stem lesions. Clin Electroencephalogr 1983;14:35.

74. Nomura Y, Segawa M. Anatomy of Rett syndrome. Am J Med Genet 1986;24:289.

75. Plum F, Posner JB. The Diagnosis of Stupor and Coma (3rd ed). Philadelphia: Davis, 1980.

76. Katzman R, Terry R. The Neurology of Aging. Philadelphia: Davis, 1983.

77. McKhann G, Drachman D, Folstein M, et al. Clinical diagnosis of Alzheimer's disease: report of the NINCDS-ADRDA work under the auspices of Department of Health and Human Services Task Force on Alzheimer's Disease. Neurology 1984;34:939.

78. Hoch CC, Reynolds CF III, Kupfer DJ, et al. Sleep-disordered breathing in normal and pathologic aging. J Clin Psychiatry 1986;47:499.

79. Erkinjuntti T, Partinen M, Sulkava R, et al. Sleep apnea in multi-infarct dementia and Alzheimer's disease. Sleep 1987;10:419.

80. Loewenstein RJ, Weingartner H, Gillin JC, et al. Disturbances of sleep and cognitive functioning in patients with dementia. Neurobiol Aging 1982;3:371.

81. Reynolds CF III, Kupfer DJ, Houck PR, et al. Reliable discrimination of elderly depressed and demented patients by electroencephalographic sleep data. Arch Gen Psychiatry 1988;45:358.

82. Allen SR, Seiler WO, Stahelin HB, et al. 72-Hour polygraphic and behavioral recordings of wakefulness and sleep in a hospital geriatric unit: comparison between demented and nondemented patients. Sleep 1987; 10:143.

83. Feinberg I, Koresko RL, Heller N. EEG sleep patterns as a function of normal and pathological aging in man. J Psychiatr Res 1967;5:107.

84. Prinz PN, Peskind ER, Vitaliano PP, et al. Changes in sleep and waking EEGs of non-demented and demented elderly subjects. J Am Geriatr Soc 1982;30:86.

85. Montplaisir J, Petit D, Lorrain D, et al. Sleep in Alzheimer's disease: further considerations on the role of brainstem and forebrain cholinergic populations in sleep-wake mechanisms. Sleep 1995;18:145.

86. Billiard M, Abboundi G, Dermenghem M, et al. Sleep apneas and mental deterioration in the elderly subjects. Rev Electroencephalogr Clin Neurophysiol 1981; 10:290.

87. Moldofsky H, Goldstein R, McNicholas WT, et al. Disordered Breathing During Sleep and Overnight Intellectual Deterioration in Patients with Pathological Aging. In C Guilleminault, E Lugaresi (eds), Sleep/Wake Disorders: Natural History, Epidemiology and Long-Term Evolution. New York: Raven, 1983;143.

88. Smallwood RG, Vitiello MV, Giblin EC, et al. Sleep apnea: relationship to age, sex and Alzheimer's dementia. Sleep 1983;6:16.

89. Benca RM, Obermeyer WH, Thisted RA, et al. Sleep and psychiatric disorders: a meta-analysis. Arch Gen Psychiatry 1992;49:651.

90. Bliwise DL. Dementia. In MH Kryger, T Roth, WC Dement (eds), Principles and Practice of Sleep Medicine. Philadelphia: Saunders, 1994;790.

91. Smirne S, Francschi M, Bareggi SR, et al. Sleep Apnea in Alzheimer's Disease. In Sleep 1980, 5th European Congress on Sleep Research, Amsterdam. Basel: Karger, 1981;442.

92. Reynolds CF, et al. Sleep apnea in Alzheimer's dementia: correlation with mental deterioration. J Clin Psychiatry 1985;46:7.

93. Vitiello M, Prinz P, Williams D, et al. Sleep related respiratory dysfunction in normal healthy aged individuals, Alzheimer's disease and major depressive disorder patients. Sleep Res 1987;16:453.

94. Mant A, Saunders NA, Eyland AE, et al. Sleep-related respiratory disturbance and dementia in elderly females. J Gerontol 1988;43:M140.

95. Ancoli-Israel S, Kripke DF, Mason W, et al. Sleep apnea and periodic movements in an aging sample. J Gerontol 1985;40:419.

96. Miles LE, Dement WC. Sleep and aging. Sleep 1980;3:119.

97. Vitiello MV, Prinz PN. Sleep/Wake Patterns and Sleep Disorders in Alzheimer's Disease. In MJ Thorpy (ed), Handbook of Sleep Disorders. New York: Marcel Dekker, 1990;703.

98. Moore-Ede MC. The circadian timing system in mammals: two pacemakers preside over many secondary oscillators. Fed Proc 1983;42:2802.

99. Tomlinson BE, Irving D, Blessed G. Cell loss in the locus coeruleus in senile dementia of the Alzheimer type. J Neurol Sci 1981;49:419.

100. Baghdoyan HA, McCarley RW, Hobson JA. Cholinergic Manipulation of Brainstem Reticular Systems: Effects on Desynchronized Sleep Generation. In A Waquier, J Monti, JP Gaillard, et al. (eds), Sleep: Neurotransmitters and Neuromodulators. New York: Raven, 1985;15.

101. Prinz P, Vitalianoi P, Vitiello M, et al. Sleep, EEG and mental functions changes in mild, moderate and severe senile dementia of the Alzheimer's type. Neurobiol Aging 1982;3:361.

102. Bliwise D. Sleep in normal aging and dementia. Review. Sleep 1993;16:40.

103. Reynolds C, Kupfer D, Taska L, et al. Slow wave sleep in elderly depressed, demented and healthy subjects. Sleep 1985;8:151.

104. Martin P, Loewenstein R, Kay W, et al. Sleep EEG in Korsakoff's psychosis and Alzheimer's disease. Neurology 1986;36:411.

105. Vitiello MV, Prinz PN, Williams DE, et al. Sleep disturbances in patients with mild stage Alzheimer's disease. J Gerontol 1990;45:M131.

106. Dyken ME, Somers VK, Yamada T, et al. Investigating the relationship between stroke and obstructive sleep apnea. Stroke 1996;27:401.

107. Good DC, Henkle JQ, Gelber D, et al. Sleep-disordered breathing and poor functional outcome after stroke. Stroke 1996;27:252.

108. Bassetti C, Aldrich M, Chervin R, Quinto D. Sleep apnea in the acute phase of TIA and stroke. Neurology 1996;47:1167.

109. Spriggs DA, French JM, Murdy JM, et al. Snoring increases the risk of stroke and adversely affects prognosis. QJM 1992;84:555.

110. Mohsenin V, Valor R. Sleep apnea in patients with hemispheric stroke. Arch Phys Med Rehabil 1995;76:71.

111. Lugaresi E, Cirignotta F, Coggagna G, et al. Some epidemiological data on snoring and cardiocirculatory disturbances. Sleep 1980;3:221.

112. Norton PG, Dunn EV. Snoring as a risk factor for disease: an epidemiological survey. Br Med J 1985;291:630.

113. Koskenvuo M, Kaprio J, Partinen M, et al. Snoring as a risk factor for hypertension and angina pectoris. Lancet 1985;1:893.

114. Koskenvuo M, Kaprio J, Telakivi T, et al. Snoring as a risk factor for ischaemic heart disease and stroke in men. BMJ 1987;294:16.

115. Palomaki H, Partinen M, Juvela S, et al. Snoring as a risk factor for sleep-related brain infarction. Stroke 1989;20:1311.

116. Partinen M, Palomaki H. Snoring and cerebral infarction. Lancet 1985;2:1325.

117. Palomaki H, Partinen M, Erkinjuntti T, et al. Snoring, sleep apnea syndrome and stroke. Neurology 1992;42(suppl 6):75.

118. Spriggs D, French JM, Murdy JM, et al. Historical risk factors for stroke: a case-control study. Age Ageing 1990;19:280.

119. Palomaki H. Snoring and risk of ischemic brain infarction. Stroke 1991;22:1021.

120. Erkinjuntti T, Partinen M, Sulkava R, et al. Are sleep apneas more common in vascular dementia than in Alzheimer's disease? Acta Neurol Scand 1984;69:S228.

121. Manni R, Marchioni E, Romani A, et al. Sleep-Apnea in Vascular and Primary Degenerative Dementia. In WP Koella, F Obal, H Schulz, et al. (eds), Sleep '86. Stuttgart: Gustav Fischer Verlag, 1988;427.

122. Neau JP, Meurice JC, Paquereau J, et al. Habitual snoring as a risk factor for brain infarction. Acta Neurol Scand 1995;92:63.

123. Olson LG, King MT, Hensley MJ, Saunders NA. A community study of snoring and sleep-disordered breathing. Health outcomes. Am J Respir Crit Care Med 1995;152:717.

124. Wright J, Johns R, Watt I, et al. Health effects of obstructive sleep apnoea and the effectiveness of continuous positive airway pressure: a systematic review of the research evidence. BMJ 1997;314:851.

125. Giubilei F, Iannilli M, Vitale A, et al. Sleep patterns in acute ischemic stroke. Acta Neurol Scand 1992;86:567.

126. Hachinski VC, Mamelak M, Norris JW. Clinical recovery and sleep architecture degradation. Can J Neurol Sci 1990;17:332.

127. Korner E, Flooh E, Reinhart B, et al. Sleep alterations in ischemic stroke. Eur Neurol 1986;25(suppl 2):104.

128. Kapen S, Park A, Goldberg J, et al. The incidence and severity of obstructive sleep apnea in ischemic cerebrovascular disease. Neurology 1991;41:S125.

129. Kapen S, Goldberg J, Diskin C, et al. The circadian rhythm of ischemic stroke and its relationship to obstructive sleep apnea. Sleep Res 1992;21:216.

130. Tofler GH, Brezinski D, Schafer AI, et al. Concurrent morning increase in platelet aggregability and the risk of myocardial infarction and sudden cardiac death. N Engl J Med 1987;316:1514.

131. Marshall J. Diurnal variation in occurrence of strokes. Stroke 1977;8:230.

132. Agnoli A, Manfredi M, Mossuto L, et al. Rapport entre les rythmes héméronyctaux de la tension artérielle et sa pathogenie de l'insuffance vasculaire cérébrale. Rev Neurol (Paris) 1975;131:597.

133. Tsementzis SA, Gilla JS, Hitchcock ER, et al. Diurnal variation of the activity during the onset of stroke. Neurosurgery 1985;17:901.

134. Mitler MM, Hajdukovic RM, Shafor R, et al. When people die? Cause of death versus time of death. Am J Med 1987;82:266.

135. Drake ME Jr. Kleine-Levin syndrome after multiple cerebral infarctions. Psychosomatics 1987;28:329.

136. Rivera VM, Meyer JS, Hata T, et al. Narcolepsy following cerebral hypoxic ischemia. Ann Neurol 1986; 19:505.

137. Partinen M. Cerebrovascular Disorders and Sleep. In MJ Thorpy (ed), Handbook of Sleep Disorders. New York: Marcel Dekker, 1990;693.

138. Chatrian GE, White LE Jr, Daly D. Electroencephalographic patterns resembling those of sleep in certain comatose states after injury to the head. Electroencephalogr Clin Neurophysiol 1963;15:272.

139. Castaigne P, Lhermitte F, Buge A, et al. Paramedian thalamic and midbrain infarcts. Clinical and neuropathological study. Ann Neurol 1981;10:127.

140. Bassetti C, Mathis J, Gugger M, et al. Hypersomnia following paramedian thalamic stroke: a report of 12 patients. Ann Neurol 1996;39:471.

141. Guilleminault C, Quera-Salva M, Goldberg MP. Pseudo-hypersomnia and pre-sleep behavior with bilateral paramedian thalamic lesions. Brain 1993;116:1549.

142. Catsman-Berrevoets CE, von Harskamp F. Compulsive pre-sleep behavior and apathy due to bilateral thalamic stroke: response to bromocriptine. Neurology 1988;38:647.

143. Chokroverty S. Autonomic Dysfunction in Olivopontocerebellar Atrophy. In RC Duvoisin, A Plaitakis (eds), The Olivopontocerebellar Atrophies. New York: Raven, 1984;105.

144. Eadie MJ. Olivopontocerebellar Atrophy. In Vinken PJ, Bruyn GW (eds), Handbook of Clinical Neurology. Amsterdam: Elsevier, 1975;21:415.

145. Oppenheimer DR. Disease of the Basal Ganglia, Cerebellum and Motor Neurons. In W Blackwood, JAN Corsellis (eds), Greenfield's Neuropathology (3rd ed). London: Edward Arnold, 1976;608.

146. Cunchillos JD, DeAndres I. Participation of the cerebellum in the regulation of the sleep-wakefulness cycle: results in cerebellectomized cats. Electroencephalogr Clin Neurophysiol 1982;53:549.

147. Neil JF, Holzer BC, Spiker DG, et al. EEG sleep alterations in olivopontocerebellar degeneration. Neurology 1980;30:660.

148. Osorio I, Daroff RB. Absence of REM and altered NREM sleep in patients with spinocerebellar degeneration and slow saccades. Ann Neurol 1980;7:277.

149. Cicirata F, Scrofani A, Biondi R. Spindle and EEG sleep alterations in subjects affected by cortical cerebellar atrophy. Eur Neurol 1987;26:120.

150. Salazar-Grueso EF, Rosenberg RS, Roos RP. Sleep apnea in olivopontocerebellar degeneration: treatment with trazodone. Ann Neurol 1988;23:399.

151. Quera-Salva MA, Guilleminault C. Olivopontocerebellar degeneration, abnormal sleep, and REM sleep without atonia. Neurology 1986;36:576.

152. Shimizu T, Sugita Y, Teshima Y, et al. Sleep Study in Patients with Spinocerebellar Degeneration and Related Disease. In WP Koella (ed), Sleep 1980. Basel: Karger, 1981;435.

153. Mahowald MW, Schenck CH. REM Sleep Behavior Disorder. In MH Kryger, T Roth, WC Dement (eds), Principles and Practice of Sleep Medicine. Philadelphia: Saunders, 1994.

154. Jouvet M, Delorme F. Locus coeruleus et sommeil paradoxal. C R Soc Biol 1965;159:895.

155. Bergonzi P, Gigli GL, Laudisio A, et al. Sleep and human cerebellar pathology. Int J Neurosci 1981;15:159.

156. Chokroverty S, Sachdeo R, Masdeu J. Autonomic dysfunction and sleep apnea in olivopontocerebellar degeneration. Arch Neurol 1984;41:926.

157. Adelman S, Dinner DS, Goren H, et al. Obstructive sleep apnea in association with posteria fossa neurologic diseases. Arch Neurol 1984;41:509.

158. Katayama S, Yokoyama S, Hirano Y, et al. TRH and Sleep Abnormalities in Spinocerebellar Degeneration (SCD). In I Sobue (ed), TRH and Spinocerebellar Degeneration. Amsterdam: Elsevier, 1986;227.

159. Bergamasco B, Bergamini L, Mutani R. Spontaneous sleep abnormalities in a case of dyssynergia cerebellaris myoclonica. Epilepsia 1967;8:271.

160. Stahl SM, Layzer RB, Aminoff MJ, et al. Continuous cataplexy in a patient with a midbrain tumor: the limp man syndrome. Neurology 1980;30:1115.

161. Anderson M, Salmon MV. Symptomatic cataplexy. J Neurol Neurosurg Psychiatry 1977;40:186.

162. Calvelou P, Tournilhse M, Vidal C, et al. Narcolepsy associated with arteriovenous malformation in the dienecephalo. Sleep 1995;18:202.

163. Berg O, Hanley J. Narcolepsy in two cases of multiple sclerosis. Acta Neurol Scand 1963;39:252.

164. Ekbom K. Familial multiple sclerosis associated with narcolepsy. Arch Neurol 1966;15:337.

165. Younger DS, Pedley TA, Thorpy MJ. Multiple sclerosis and narcolepsy: possible genetic susceptibility. Neurology 1991;41:447.

166. Markand ON, Dyken ML. Sleep abnormalities in patients with brainstem lesions. Neurology 1976;26:769.

167. Devereaux MW, Kleane JR, Davis RL. Automatic respiratory failure associated with infarction of the medulla. Arch Neurol 1973;29:46.

168. Levin B, Margolis G. Acute failure of autonomic respirations secondary to unilateral brain stem infarct. Ann Neurol 1977;1:583.

169. Feldman MH. Physiological observations in a chronic case of "locked-in" syndrome. Neurology 1971; 21:459.

170. Freemon FR, Salinas-Garcia RF, Ward JW. Sleep patterns in a patient with a brain stem infarction involving the raphe nucleus. Electroencephalogr Clin Neurophysiol 1974;36:657.

171. Cummings JL, Greenberg R. Sleep patterns in the "locked-in" syndrome. Electroencephalogr Clin Neurophysiol 1977;43:270.

172. Oxenberg A, Soroker N, Solzi P, Reider-Groswasser I. Polysomnography in locked-in syndrome. Electroencephalogr Clin Neurophysiol 1991;78:314.

173. Nordgren RE, Markesberry WR, Fukuda K, Reeves AG. Seven cases of cerebromedallospinal disconnection: the "locked-in" syndrome. Neurology 1971;21:1140.

174. Autret A, Laffont F, De Toofol B, et al. A syndrome of REM and non-REM sleep reduction and lateral gaze paresis after medial tegmental pontine stroke. Arch Neurol 1988;45:1236.

175. Kushida CA, Rye DB, Nummy D, et al. Cortical asymmetry of REM sleep EEG following unilateral pontine hemorrhage. Neurology 1991;41:5981.

176. Severinghaus JW, Mitchell RA. Ondine's curse—failure of respiratory center automaticity while awake. Clin Res 1962;10:122.

177. Comroe JH Jr. Frankenstein, Pickwick and Ondine. Am Rev Respir Dis 1975;111:689.

178. Munschauer FE, Madur MJ, Ahuja A, Jacobs L. Selective paralysis of voluntary but not limbically influenced automatic respiration. Arch Neurol 1991;48:1190.

179. Bogousslavsky J, Khurana R, Deruaz JP, et al. Respiratory failure and unilateral caudal brain stem infarction. Ann Neurol 1990;28:668.

180. Askenasy JJM, Goldhammer I. Sleep apnea as a feature of bulbar stroke. Stroke 1988;19:637.

181. Miyazaki M, Hashimoto T, Sakurama N, et al. Central sleep apnea and arterial compression of the medulla. Ann Neurol 1991;29:564.

182. Beamish D, Wildsmith JAW. Ondine's curse after carotid endarterectomy. BMJ 1978;2:1607.

183. Beal MF, Richardson EP Jr, Brandstetter R, et al. Localized brain stem ischemic damage and Ondine's curse after near-drowning. Neurology 1983;33:717.

184. Ito K, Murofushi T, Mizuno M, Semba T. Pediatric brain stem gliomas with the predominant symptom of sleep apnea. Int J Pediatr Otorhinolaryngol 1996;37:53.

185. de Barros-Ferreira M, Chodkiewicz JP, Lairy GC, et al. Disorganized relations of tonic and phasic events of REM sleep in a case of brain-stem tumour. Electroencephalogr Clin Neurophysiol 1975;38:203.

186. Lee DKP, Wahl GW, Swinburne AJ, Fedullo AJ. Recurrent acoustic neuroma presenting as central alveolar hypoventilation. Chest 1994;105:949.

187. Hansotia P, Gottschalk P, Greene P, Zis D. Spindle coma: incidence, clinical pathological correlates and prognostic value. Neurology 1981;31:83.

188. Chatrian GE, White LE Jr, Daly D. Electroencephalographic patterns resembling those of sleep in certain comatose states after injuries to the head. Electroencephalogr Clin Neurophysiol 1963;15:272.

189. Goldstein M. Traumatic brain injury: a silent epidemic. Ann Neurol 1990;27:327.

190. Mahowald M, Mahowald ML. Sleep Disorders. In M Rizzo, D Tranel (eds), Head Injury and Postconcussive Syndrome. New York: Churchill Livingstone, 1996;285.

191. Levine HS, Mattis S, Ruff RM, et al. Neurobehavior outcome following minor head injury: a 3-center study. J Neurosurgery 1987;66:234.

192. Parsons LC, Ver Beek D. Sleep-awake patterns following cerebral concussion. Nurs Res 1982;31:260.

193. Dikmen S, McLean A, Temkin N. Neuropsychological and psychosocial consequences of minor head injury. J Neurol Neurosurg Psychiatry 1986;49:1227.

194. Prigatano GP, Stahl ML, Orr WC, et al. Sleep and dreaming disturbances in closed head injury patients. J Neurol Neurosurg Psychiatry 1982;45:78.

195. Harada M, Minami R, Hattori E, et al. Sleep in brain damaged patients: an all night study of 105 cases. Kumamoto Med J 1976;29:110.

196. American Sleep Disorders Association. The International Classification of Sleep Disorders: Diagnostic and Coding Manual (rev ed). Rochester, MN: American Sleep Disorders Association, 1997.

197. Guilleminault C, Faull KF, Miles L, van den Hoed J. Post-traumatic excessive daytime sleepiness: review of 20 patients. Neurology 1983;33:1584.

198. Okawa M, Takahashi K, Sasaki H. Disturbance of circadian rhythms in severely brain-damaged patients correlated with CT findings. J Neurol 1986;233:274.

199. Patten SD, Lauderdale WM. Delayed sleep phase disorder after traumatic brain injury. J Am Acad Child Adolesc Psychiatry 1992;31:100.

200. Billiard M, Negri C, Baldy-Milliner M, et al. Organization du Sommeil Chez les Sujets atteints d'inconscience post-traumatique chronique. Rev Electroencephalogr Neurophysiol Clin 1979;9:149.

200a. Quinto C, Masleu J, Chokroverty S. Post-traumatic delayed sleep phase syndrome. Neurology 1998;50 (Suppl 4):A395.

201. Newsom Davis J. Autonomous breathing. Report of case. Arch Neurol 1974;30:480.

202. Rizvi SS, Ishikawa S, Faling LJ, et al. Defect in automatic respiration in a case of multiple sclerosis. Am J Med 1974;56;443.

203. Boor JW, Johnson RJ, Canales L, et al. Reversible paralysis of automatic respiration in multiple sclerosis. Arch Neurol 1977;34:686.

204. Clark CM, Fleming JA, Li D, et al. Sleep disturbance, depression and lesion site in patients with multiple sclerosis. Arch Neurol 1992;49:641.

205. Leo JG, Rao SM, Bernardin L. Sleep disturbances in multiple sclerosis. Neurology 1991;320;S727.

206. Saunders J, Whitham R, Schaumann B. Sleep disturbance, fatigue and depression in multiple sclerosis. Neurology 1991;41:S320,728.

207. Tachibana N, Howard RS, Hirsch NP, et al. Sleep problems in multiple sclerosis. Eur Neurol 1994;34:320.

208. Ferini-Strambi L, Filippi M, Martinelli V, et al. Nocturnal sleep study in multiple sclerosis: correlations with clinical and brain magnetic resonance imaging findings. J Neurol Sci 1994;125:194.

209. Sarnoff SJ, Whittenberger JL, Affeldt JE. Hypoventilation syndrome in bulbar poliomyelitis. JAMA 1951;147:30.

210. Speier JL, Owen RR, Knapp M, et al. Occurrence of Post-Polio Sequelae in an Epidemic Population. In LS

Halstead, DO Wiechers (eds), Research and Clinical Aspects of the Late Effects of Poliomyelitis. White Plains, NY: March of Dimes Birth Defects Foundation, 1987.

211. Codd MB, Mulder DW, Kurland LT, et al. Poliomyelitis in Rochester, Minnesota, 1935-1955: Epidemiology and Long-Term Sequelae: A Preliminary Report. Research and Clinical Aspects of the Late Effects of Poliomyelitis. White Plains, NY: March of Dimes Birth Defects Foundation, 1987.

212. Halsted LS, Rossi CD. New problems in old polio patients: results of a survey of 539 polio survivors. Orthopedics 1985;**8**:845.

213. Steljes DG, Kryger MH, Kirk BW, et al. Sleep in post-polio syndrome. Chest 1990;81:133.

214. Guilleminault C, Motta J. Sleep apnea syndrome as a long-term sequela of poliomyelitis. New York: Liss, 1978;309.

215. Solliday NH, Gaensler EA, Schwaber R, et al. Impaired central chemoreceptor function and chronic hypoventilation many years following poliomyelitis. Respiration 1974;31:177.

216. Bye PTP, Ellis ER, Issaq FG, et al. Respiratory failure and sleep in neuromuscular disease. Thorax 1990;45:241.

217. Ellis ER, Bye PTP, Bruderer JW, Sullivan CE. Treatment of respiratory failure during sleep in patients with neuromuscular disease: positive-pressure ventilation through a nose mask. Am Rev Respir Dis 1987;135:148.

218. Howard RS, Wiles CM, Spencer GT. The late sequelae of poliomyelitis. Q J Med 1988;66:219.

219. Cosgrove JL, Alexander MA, Kitts EL, et al. Late effects of poliomyelitis. Arch Phys Med Rehabil 1987;68:4.

220. Van Kralingen KW, Ivanyi B, Van Keimpema ARJ, et al. Sleep complaints in postpolio syndrome. Arch Phys Med Rehabil 1996;77:609.

221. Haponik EF, Givens D, Angelo J. Syringobulbia-myelia with obstructive sleep apnea. Neurology 1983;33:1046.

222. Cohn JE, Kuida H. Primary alveolar hypoventilation associated with western equine encephalitis. Ann Intern Med 1962;56:633.

223. White D, Miller F, Erickson R. Sleep apnea and nocturnal hypoventilation following western equine encephalitis. Am Rev Respir Dis 1983;127:132.

224. Papasozomenos S, Roessman U. Respiratory distress and Arnold-Chiari malformation. Neurology 1981; 91:97.

225. Dure LS, Percy AK, Cheek WR, et al. Chiari type I malformation in children. J Pediatr 1989;115:573.

226. Montserrat JM, Picado C, Agusti-Vidil A. Arnold-Chiari malformation and paralysis of the diaphragm. Respiration 1988;53:128.

227. Balk RA, Hiller FC, Lucas EA, et al. Sleep apnea and the Arnold-Chiari malformation. Am Rev Respir Dis 1985;132:929.

228. Ely ES, McCall WV, Haponik EF. Multifactorial obstructive sleep apnea in a patient with Chiari malformation. J Neurol Sci 1994;126:232.

229. Campbell EJM. Respiratory failure. BMJ 1965;1:1451.

230. Bokinsky GE, Hudson LD, Weil JV. Impaired peripheral chemosensitivity and acute respiratory failure in Arnold-Chiari malformation and syringomyelia. N Engl J Med 1973;288:947.

231. Krieger AJ, Rosomoff HL. Sleep-induced apnea. Part 1: A respiratory and autonomic dysfunction syndrome following bilateral percutaneous cervical cordotomy. J Neurosurg 1974;40:168.

232. Belmusto L, Woldring S, Owens G. Localization and patterns of potentials of the respiratory pathway in the cervical spinal cord in the dog. J Neurosurg 1965;22:277.

233. Tenicela R, Rosomoff HL, Feist J, et al. Pulmonary function following percutaneous cervical cordotomy. Anesthesiology 1968;29:7.

234. Krieger AJ, Rosomoff HL. Sleep-induced apnea. Part 2: Respiratory failure after anterior spinal surgery. J Neurosurg 1974;39:181.

235. Star AM, Osterman AL. Sleep apnea syndrome after spinal cord injury. Spine 1988;13:116.

236. Bonekat HW, Anderson G, Squires J. Obstructive disordered breathing during sleep in patients with spinal cord injury. Paraplegia 1990;28:292.

237. Short DJ, Stradling JR, Williams SJ. Prevalence of sleep apnea in patients over 40 years of age with spinal cord lesions. J Neurol Neurosurg Psychiatry 1992;55:1032.

238. Adey WR, Bors E, Porter RW. EEG sleep patterns after high cervical lesions in man. Arch Neurol 1968;19:377.

239. Bach JR, Wang T-J. Pulmonary function and sleep-disordered breathing in patients with traumatic tetroplegia: a longitudinal study. Arch Phys Med Rehabil 1994;75:279.

240. Yokata D, Hirosck T, Tsukagoshi H. Sleep-related periodic leg movements (nocturnal myoclonus) due to spinal cord lesions. J Neurol Sci 1991;104:13.

241. de Mello MT, Lauro FAA, Silva AC, Tufik S. Incidence of periodic leg movements and of the restless legs syndrome during sleep following acute physical activity in spinal cord injury subjects. Spinal Cord 1996;34:294.

242. Dickel MJ, Renfro WSD, Moore PT, Berry RB. Rapid eye movement sleep: periodic leg movements in patients with spinal cord injury. Sleep 1994;17:733.

243. Lee MS, Choy YC, Lee SH, Lee SB. Sleep-related periodic leg movements associated with spinal cord lesions. Mov Disord 1996;11:719.

244. Parhad IM, Clark AW, Barron KD, Staunton SB. Diaphragmatic paralysis in motor neuron disease. Report of two cases and a review of the literature. Neurology 1978;28:18.

245. Thorpy MJ, Schmidt-Nowara WW, Pollak C, Weitzman ED. Sleep-induced non-obstructive hypoventilation association with diaphragmatic paralysis. Ann Neurol 1982;12:308.

246. Newsom Davis J, Goldman M, Loh L, et al. Diaphragm function and alveolar hypoventilation. Q J Med 1976;45:87.

247. Serpick AA, Baker EL, Woodward TE. Motor system disease. Arch Intern Med 1965;115:192.

248. Chokroverty S. Sleep apnea in neurodegenerative diseases. Electroencephalogr Clin Neurophysiol 1982;53:22P.

249. Gay PC, Westbrook PR, Daube JR, et al. Effect of alterations in pulmonary function and sleep variables on survival in patients with amyotrophic lateral sclerosis. Mayo Clin Proc 1991;66:686.

250. Ferguson KA, Strong MJ, Ahmad D, George CSP. Sleep-disordered breathing in amyotrophic lateral sclerosis. Chest 1996;110:664.

251. Minz M, Autret A, Laffont F, et al. A study of sleep in amyotrophic lateral sclerosis. Biomedicine 1979;30:40.

252. Howard RS, Wiles CM, Loh L. Respiratory complications and their management in motor neuron disease. Brain 1989;112:1155.

253. Hetta J, Jansson I. Sleep in patients with amyotrophic lateral sclerosis. J Neurol 1997;244:S7.

254. Tanner CM. Respiratory Dysfunction and Peripheral Neuropathy. In WJ Weiner (ed), Respiratory Dysfunction in Neurologic Disease. Mount Kisco, NY: Futura, 1980;83.

255. Goldstein RFL, Hyde RW, Lapham LW, et al. Peripheral neuropathy presenting with respiratory insufficiency as the primary complaint. Am J Med 1974;56:443.

256. Chan CK, Mohsenin V, Loke J, et al. Diaphragmatic dysfunction in siblings with hereditary motor and sensory neuropathy (Charcot-Marie-Tooth disease). Chest 1987;91:567.

257. Bellamy D, Newsom Davis J, Hickey BP, et al. A case of primary alveolar hypoventilation associated with mild proximal myopathy. Am Rev Respir Dis 1975;112:867.

258. Riley DJ, Santiago TV, Danielle RP, et al. Blunted respiratory drive in congenital myopathy. Am J Med 1977;63:459.

259. Smith PEM, Calverley PMA, Edwards RHT. Hypoxemia during sleep in Duchenne muscular dystrophy. Am Rev Respir Dis 1988;137:884.

260. Gross D, Ladd HW, Riley EJ, et al. The effect of training on strength and endurance of the diaphragm in quadriplegia. Am J Med 1980;68:27.

261. Howard RS, Wiles CM, Hirsch NP, Spencer GT. Respiratory involvement in primary muscle disorders: assessment and management. Q J Med 1993;86:175.

262. Kerr SL, Kohrman MH. Polysomnographic abnormalities in Duchenne muscular dystrophy. J Child Neurol 1994;9:332.

263. Manni R, Ottolini A, Cerveri I, et al. Breathing patterns and HbSaO$_2$ changes during nocturnal sleep in patients with Duchenne muscular dystrophy. J Neurol 1989;236:391.

264. Khan Y, Heckmatt JZ. Obstructive apneas in Duchenne muscular dystrophy. Thorax 1994;49:157.

265. Barbe A, Quera-Salva MA, McCann C, et al. Sleep-related respiratory disturbances in patients with Duchenne muscular dystrophy. Eur Respir J 1994;7:1403.

266. Pradella M. Sleep polygraphic parameters in neuromuscular diseases. Arq Neuropsiquiatr 1994;52:476.

267. Khan Y, Heckmatt JZ. A double-blind cross-over trial of theophylline prophylaxis for sleep hypoxemia in Duchenne muscular dystrophy. Neuromuscul Disord 1997;7:75.

268. Takasugi T, Ishihera T, Kawamura J, et al. Respiratory disorders during sleep in Duchenne muscular dystrophy. Nippon Kyobu Shikkan Gakkai Zasshi 1995; 33:821.

269. Barbe A, Quera Salva MA, de Lattre J, et al. Long-term effects of nasal intermittent positive-pressure ventilation on pulmonary function and sleep architecture in patients with neuromuscular diseases. Chest 1996;110:1179.

270. Piper AJ, Sullivan CE. Effects of long-term nocturnal nasal ventilation on spontaneous breathing during sleep in neuromuscular and chest wall disorders. Eur Respir J 1996;9:1515.

271. Labanowski M, Schmidt-Nowara W, Guilleminault C. Sleep and neuromuscular disease: frequency of sleep-disordered breathing in a neuromuscular disease clinic population. Neurology 1996;47:1173.

272. Robertson PL, Roloff DW. Chronic respiratory failure in limb-girdle muscular dystrophy: successful long-term therapy with nasal bilevel positive airway pressure. Pediatr Neurol 1994;10:328.

273. Khan Y, Heckmatt JZ, Dubowitz V. Sleep studies and supportive ventilatory treatment in patients with congenital muscle disorders. Arch Dis Child 1996;74:195.

274. Benaim S, Worster-Drought C. Dystrophia myotonica with myotonia of diaphragm causing pulmonary hypoventilation with anoxaemia and secondary polycythaemia. Med Illus 1954;8:221.

275. Coccagna G, Mantovani M, Parchi C, et al. Alveolar hypoventilation and hypersomnia in myotonic dystrophy. J Neurol Neurosurg Psychiatry 1975;38:977.

276. Guilleminault C, Cummiskey J, Motta J, et al. Respiratory and hemodynamic study during wakefulness and sleep in myotonic dystrophy. Sleep 1978;1:19.

277. Hansotia P, Frens D. Hypersomnia associated with alveolar hypoventilation in myotonic dystrophy. Neurology 1981;31:1336.

278. Harper PS. Myotonic Dystrophy. Philadelphia: Saunders, 1979.

279. Striano S, Meo R, Bilo L, et al. Sleep apnea syndrome in Thomsen's disease. A case report. Electroencephalogr Clin Neurophysiol 1983;56:332.

280. Bashour F, Winchell P, Reddington J. Myotonia atrophica and cyanosis. N Engl J Med 1955;252:768.

281. Kilburn KH, Eagan JT, Heyman A. Cardiopulmonary insufficiency associated with myotonic dystrophy. Am J Med 1959;26:929.

282. Kohn NN, Faires JS, Rodman T. Unusual manifestations due to involvement of involuntary muscle in dystrophia myotonica. N Engl J Med 1964;271:1179.

283. Kaufman L. Anaesthesia in dystrophia myotonica. A review of the hazards of anesthesia. Proc R Soc Med 1966;53:183.

284. Gillam PMS, Heaf PJD, Kaufman L, et al. Respiration in dystrophia myotonica. Thorax 1964;19:112.

285. Coccagna G, Martinelli P, Lugaresi E. Sleep and alveolar hypoventilation in myotonic dystrophy. Acta Neurol Belg 1982;82:185.

286. Carroll JE, Zwillich CW, Weil JV. Ventilatory response in myotonic dystrophy. Neurology 1977;27:1125.

287. Begin R, Bureau MA, Lupien L, et al. Pathogenesis of respiratory insufficiency in myotonic dystrophy: the mechanical factors. Am Rev Respir Dis 1982; 125:312.

288. Armagast SJ, Ringel SP, Martin RJ. The effects of dichlorphenamide on sleep apnea in patients with myotonic dystrophy (abstract). Clin Res 1983;31:70.

289. Begin P, Mathieu J, Almirall J, Grassino A. Relationship between chronic hypercapnia and inspiratory muscle weakness in myotonic dystrophy. Am J Respir Crit Care Med 1997;156:133.

290. van der Mechefga FGA, Bogaard JM, van der Sluys JC, et al. Daytime sleep in myotonic dystrophy is not caused by sleep apnea. J Neurol Neurosurg Psychiatry 1994; 57:626.

291. Veale D, Cooper BJ, Gilmartin JJ, et al. Breathing pattern awake and asleep in patients with myotonic dystrophy. Eur Respir J 1995;8:815.

292. Park YD, Radtke RA. Hypersomnolence in myotonic dystrophy: demonstration of sleep onset REM sleep. J Neurol Neurosurg Psychiatry 1995;58:512.

293. Ono S, Kurisaki H, Sakuma A, Nagao K. Myotonic dystrophy with alveolar hypoventilation and hypersomnia: a clinical pathological study. J Neurol Psy 1995;128:225.

294. Ono S, Kanda F, Takashi K, et al. Neuronal loss in the medullary reticular formation in myotonic dystrophy: a clinical pathological study (abstract). Neurology 1996;46:171.

295. Ricker K, Koch MC, Lehmann-Horn F, et al. Proximal myotonic myopathy: a new dominant disorder with myotonia, muscle weakness and cataracts. Neurology 1994;44:1448.

296. Sander HW, Tavoulareas GP, Chokroverty S. Heat-sensitive myotonia in proximal myotonic myopathy. Neurology 1996;47:956.

297. Hund E, Jansen O, Koch MC, et al. Proximal myotonic myopathy with MRI white matter abnormalities of the brain. Neurology 1997;48:33.

298. Chokroverty S, Sander HW, Tavoulareas GP, Quinto C. Insomnia with absent or dissociated REM sleep in proximal myotonic myopathy (abstract). Neurology 1997;48:256.

299. Rosenow EC, Engel AG. Acid maltase deficiency in adults presenting as respiratory failure. Am J Med 1978;64:485.

300. Sivak ED, Salanga VD, Wilbourn AJ, et al. Adult-onset acid maltase deficiency presenting as diaphragmatic paralysis. Ann Neurol 1981;9:613.

301. Martin RJ, Sufit RL, Ringel SP, et al. Respiratory improvement by muscle training in adult-onset acid maltase deficiency. Muscle Nerve 1983;6:201.

302. Margolis ML, Howlett P, Goldberg R, et al. Obstructive sleep apnea syndrome in acid maltase deficiency. Chest 1994;105:947.

303. Kryger MH, Steljes DG, Yee W-C, et al. Central sleep apnoea in congenital muscular dystrophy. J Neurol Neurosurg Psychiatry 1991;54:710.

304. Maayan C, Springer C, Armon Y, et al. Nemaline myopathy as a cause of sleep hypoventilation. Pediatrics 1986;77:390.

305. Wilson DO, Sanders MH, Dauber JH. Abnormal ventilatory chemosensitivity and congenital myopathy. Arch Intern Med 1987;147:1773.

306. Tatsumi C, Takashashi M, Yorifugi S, et al. Mitochondrial encephalomyopathy with sleep apnea. Eur Neurol 1988;28:64.

307. Carroll JE, Zwillich C, Weil JV, et al. Depressed ventilatory response in oculocraniosomatic neuromuscular disease. Neurology 1976;26:146.

308. Mier-Jedrzejowicz A, Brophy C, Green M. Respiratory muscle function in myasthenia gravis. Am Rev Respir Dis 1988;138:867.

309. Quera-Salva MA, Guilleminault C, Chevret S, et al. Breathing disorders during sleep in myasthenia gravis. Ann Neurol 1992;31:86.

310. Mennumi G, Morante MT, Scoppeta, et al. Night sleep organization in myasthenic patients not undergoing therapy. Sleep Res 1983;12:84.

311. Shiozawa Z, Shintani S, Tsunoda S, et al. Sleep apnea in well-controlled myasthenia gravis. Sleep Res 1987;16:301.

312. Shintani S, Shiozawa Z, Shindo K, et al. Sleep apnea in well-controlled myasthenia gravis. Rinsho Shinkeigaku 1989;29:547.

313. Manni R, Piccolo G, Sartori I, et al. Breathing during sleep in myasthenia gravis. Ital J Neurol Sci 1995;16:589.

314. Putman MD, Wise RA. Myasthenia gravis and upper airway obstruction. Chest 1996;109:400.

315. Stepansky R, Weber G, Zeitlhofer J. Sleep apnea in myasthenia gravis. Wien Med Wochenschr 1996;146:209.

316. Chokroverty S. Functional Anatomy of the Autonomic Nervous System: Autonomic Dysfunction and Disorders of the CNS. In American Academy of Neurology Course No. 144. Boston: American Academy of Neurology, 1991;77.

317. Loewy AD, Spyer KM. Central Regulation of Autonomic Functions. New York: Oxford University Press, 1990.

318. Chokroverty S. Sleep Apnea and Autonomic Failure. In PA Low (ed), Clinical Autonomic Disorders (2nd ed). Boston: Little, Brown, 1997;633.

319. Parmeggiani PL, Morrison AR. Alterations of Autonomic Functions During Sleep. In AD Loewy, KM Spyer (eds), Central Regulation of Autonomic Functions. New York: Oxford University Press, 1990;367.

320. Loewy AD. Central Autonomic Pathways. In PA Low (ed), Clinical Autonomic Disorders. Boston: Little, Brown, 1993;88.

321. Barron KD, Chokroverty S. Anatomy of the Autonomic Nervous System: Brain and Brainstem. In PA Low (ed), Clinical Autonomic Disorders. Boston: Little, Brown, 1993;3.

322. Consensus statement on the definition of orthostatic hypotension, pure autonomic failure, and multiple system atrophy. Neurology 1996;46:1470.

323. Shy GM, Drager GA. A neurological syndrome associated with orthostatic hypotension. Arch Neurol 1960;2:511.

324. Bannister R, Ardill L, Fentem P. Defective autonomic control of blood vessels in idiopathic orthostatic hypotension. Brain 1967;90:725.

325. Bannister R, Oppenheimer DR. Degenerative disease of the nervous system associated with autonomic failure. Brain 1972;95:457.

326. Bannister R, Gibson W, Michaels L, Oppenheimer DR. Laryngeal abductor paralysis in multiple system atrophy. Brain 1981;104:351.

327. Chokroverty S, Barron KD, Katz FH, et al. The syndrome of primary orthostatic hypotension. Brain 1969;92:743.

328. Chokroverty S. The Assessment of Sleep Disturbances in Autonomic Failure. In R Bannister, C Mathias (eds), Autonomic Failure (3rd ed). Oxford: Oxford University Press, 1992;443.

329. Cohen J, Low P, Fealey R, et al. Somatic and autonomic function in progressive autonomic failure and multiple system atrophy. Ann Neurol 1987;22:692.

330. Quinn N. Multiple system atrophy: the nature of the beast. J Neurol Neurosurg Psychiatry 1989;52:S78.

331. Wenning GK, Shlomo YB, Magalhaes M, et al. The clinical features and natural history of multiple system atrophy: an analysis of 100 cases. Brain 1994; 117:835.

332. Papp MI, Lantos PL. The distribution of oligodendroglial inclusions in multiple system atrophy and its relevance to clinical symptomatology. Brain 1994; 117:235.

333. Wenning GK, Tison F, Ben Shlomo Y, et al. Multiple system atrophy: a review of 203 pathologically proven cases. Mov Disord 1997;12:133.

334. Lockwood AH. Shy-Drager syndrome with abnormal respirations and antidiuretic hormone release. Arch Neurol 1976;33:292.

335. Castaigne P, Laplane D, Autret A, et al. Syndrome de Shy et Drager avec troubles du rhythme respiratoire et de la vigilance. Rev Neurol (Paris) 1977;133:455.

336. Martin JB, Travis RH, Van Den Noort S. Centrally mediated orthostatic hypotension. Arch Neurol 1968; 19:163.

337. Israel RH, Marino JM. Upper airway obstruction in the Shy-Drager syndrome. Ann Neurol 1977;2:83.

338. Guilleminault C, Tilkian A, Lehrman K, et al. Sleep apnoea syndrome: states of sleep and autonomic dysfunction. J Neurol Neurosurg Psychiatry 1977;40:718.

339. Williams A, Hanson D, Calne DB. Vocal cord paralysis in the Shy-Drager syndrome. J Neurol Neurosurg Psychiatry 1979;42:151.

340. Kenyon GS, Apps MCP, Traub M. Stridor and obstructive sleep apnea in Shy-Drager syndrome treated by laryngofissure and cord lateralization. Laryngoscope 1984;94:1106.

341. Munschauer FE, Loh L, Bannister R, et al. Abnormal respiration and sudden death during sleep in multiple system atrophy with autonomic failure. Neurology 1990;40:677.

342. Lehrman KL, Guilleminault C, Schroeder JS, et al. Sleep apnea syndrome in a patient with Shy-Drager syndrome. Arch Intern Med 1978;138:206.

343. Briskin JG, Lehrman KL, Guilleminault C. Shy-Drager Syndrome and Sleep Apnea. In C Guilleminault, WC Dement (eds), Sleep Apnea Syndromes. New York: Liss, 1978;316.

344. Guilleminault C, Briskin JG, Greenfield MS, et al. The impact of autonomic nervous system dysfunction on breathing during sleep. Sleep 1981;4:263.

345. Harcourt J, Spraggs P, Mathias C, Brookes G. Sleep-related breathing disorders in the Shy-Drager syndrome. Observations on investigation and management. Eur J Neurol 1996;3:186.

346. Sadaoka T, Kakitsuba N, Fujiwara Y, et al. Sleep-related breathing disorders in patients with multiple system atrophy and vocal fold palsy. Sleep 1996;19:479.

347. Isozaki E, Naito A, Horiguchi S, et al. Early diagnosis and stage classification of vocal cord abductor paralysis in patients with multiple system atrophy. J Neurol Neurosurg Psychiatry 1996;60:399.

348. McBrien F, Spraggs PD, Harcourt JP, Croft CB. Abductor vocal fold palsy in the Shy-Drager syndrome presenting with snoring and sleep apnea. J Laryngol Otol 1996;110:681.

349. Shimizu T, Sugita Y, Iijima S, et al. Sleep study in Shy-Drager syndrome. Clin Neurol (Jpn) 1981;21:218.

350. Wright BA, Rosen JR, Buysse DJ, et al. Shy-Drager syndrome presenting as a REM behavioral disorder. J Geriatr Psychiatry Neurol 1990;3:110.

351. Tison F, Wenning GK, Quinn NP, et al. REM sleep behavior disorder as the presenting symptom of multiple system atrophy. J Neurol Neurosurg Psychiatry 1995;58:379.

352. Dempsey JA, Olson EB Jr, Skatrud JB. Hormones and Neurochemicals in the Regulation of Breathing. In AF Fishman, NS Cherniack, JG Widdicombe (eds), Handbook of Physiology (Vol II, Part I, Section 3): The Respiratory System. Bethesda, MD: American Physiological Society, 1986;181.

353. Spokes EG, Bannister R, Oppenheimer DR. Multiple system atrophy with autonomic failure: clinical, histological and neurochemical observations on 4 cases. J Neurol Sci 1979;43:59.

354. Black IB, Petito CK. Catecholamine enzymes in the degenerative neurological disease idiopathic orthostatic hypotension. Science 1976;192:910.

355. Brunt PW, McKusick V. Familial dysautonomia. Medicine 1970;49:343.

356. Gadoth N, Sokol J, Lavie P. Sleep structure and nocturnal disordered breathing in familial dysautonomia. J Neurol Sci 1983;60:117.

357. Maayan C, Oren A, Goldin E, et al. Megaesophagus and recurrent apnea in an adult patient with familial dysautonomia. Am J Gastroenterol 1990;85:729.

358. Chokroverty S. Functional Anatomy of the Autonomic Nervous System Correlated with Symptomatology of Neurologic Disease. In American Academy of Neurology Course No. 246. San Diego, CA: American Academy of Neurology, 1992;49.

359. Frank Y, Kravath RE, Inoue K, et al. Sleep apnea and hypoventilation syndrome associated with acquired nonprogressive dysautonomia: clinical and pathological studies in a child. Ann Neurol 1980;10:18.

360. Rees PJ, Prior JG, Cochrane GM, et al. Sleep apnoea in diabetic patients with autonomic neuropathy. J R Soc Med 1981;74:192.

361. Mondini S, Guilleminault C. Abnormal breathing patterns during sleep in diabetes. Ann Neurol 1985; 17:391.

362. Catterall JR, Calverley PMA, Ewing DJ, et al. Breathing, sleep and diabetic autonomic neuropathy. Diabetes 1984;33:1025.

363. Guilleminault C, Eldridge F, Dement WC. Insomnia, narcolepsy and sleep apneas. Bull Physiopathol Respir 1972;8:1127.

364. Guilleminault C, van den Hoed J, Mitler M. Clinical Overview of the Sleep Apnea Syndromes. In C Guilleminault, WC Dement (eds), Sleep Apnea Syndromes. New York: Liss, 1978;1.

365. Laffont F, Minz AM, Beillevaire T, et al. Sleep respiratory arrhythmias in control subjects, narcoleptics and non-cataplectic hypersomniacs. Electroencephalogr Clin Neurophysiol 1978;44:697.

366. Chokroverty S. Sleep apnea in narcolepsy. Sleep 1986;9:250.

367. Fukunishi I, Hosokwa K. A female case with the Kleine-Levin syndrome and its physiopathologic aspects. Jpn J Psychiatr Neurol 1989;43:45.

368. Kleine W. Periodische Schlafsucht. Mschr Psychiatr Neurol 1925;57:285.

369. Levin M. Periodic somnolence and morbid hunger: a new syndrome. Brain 1936;59:494.

370. Critchley M. Periodic hypersomnia and megaphagia in adolescent males. Brain 1962;85:627.

371. Billiard M, Cadilhac J. Les hypersomnies recurrentes. Rev Neurol (Paris) 1988;144:249.

372. Gadoth N, Dickerman Z, Becher M, et al. Episodic hormone secretion during sleep in Kleine-Levin syndrome: evidence for hypothalamic dysfunction. Brain Dev 1987;9:309.

373. Chesson AL Jr, Levine SN, Kong L-S, Lee SC. Neuroendocrine evaluation in Kleine-Levin syndrome: evidence of reduced dopaminergic tone during periods of hypersomnolence. Sleep 1991;14:226.

374. Gau S-F, Soong W-T, Liu H-M, et al. Kleine-Levin syndrome in a boy with Prader-Willi syndrome. Sleep 1996;19:13.

375. Pike M, Stores G. Kleine-Levin syndrome: a cause of diagnostic confusion. Arch Dis Child 1994;71:355.

376. Pfeiffer E. Kleine-Levin syndrome—diagnostic and therapeutic problems. Z Kinder Jugendpsychiatr 1997;25:117.

377. Crumley FE. Valproic acid for Kleine-Levin syndrome. J Am Acad Child Adolesc Psychiatry 1997;36:868.

378. Orlosky MJ. The Kleine-Levin syndrome: a review. Psychosomatics 1982;23:609.

379. Mahowald MW, Chokroverty S, Kader G, Shenck CH. Sleep disorders. Continuum [A program of the American Academy of Neurology]. 1997;3(4):46.

380. Cirignotta F, Baldini MI, Mondini S, et al. Recurring Coma and Abnormal Behavior. Case Report. In J Horne (ed), Sleep, 1990. Bochum: Pontenagel, 1990;1.

381. Tinuper P, Montagna P, Cortelli P, et al. Idiopathic recurring stupor: a case with possible involvement of the gamma-aminobutyric acid (GABAergic system). Ann Neurol 1992;31:503.

382. Tinuper P, Motgana P, Plazzi G, et al. Idiopathic recurring stupor. Neurology 1994;44:621.

383. Lemesle M, Aube H, Madinier G, et al. Idiopathic and recurrent stupor: efficacy of flumazenil (letter). Presse Med 1996;25:1847.

384. Lotz BP, Schutte CM, Bartel PR, Jacobs E. Recurrent attacks of unconsciousness with diffuse EEG alpha activity. Sleep 1993;16:671.

385. Rothstein JD, Guidotti A. Endozepines: Non-benzodiazepine Endogenous Allosteric Modulators of GABA Receptors. In I Izquierdo, J Medina (eds), Naturally Occurring Benzodiazepines: Structure, Distribution and Function. New York: Ellis Horwood, 1993;115.

386. Motagna P, Sforza E, Tinuper P, et al. Plasma endogenous benzodiazepine-like activity in sleep disorders with excessive daytime sleepiness. Neurology 1995; 45:1783.

387. Guilleminault C. Idiopathic Central Nervous System Hypersomnia. In MH Kryger, T Roth, WC Dement (eds), Principles and Practice of Sleep Medicine. Philadelphia: Saunders, 1994;562.

388. Billiard M. Idiopathic hypersomnia. Neurol Clin 1996;14:573.

389. Aldrich MS. The clinical spectrum of narcolepsy and idiopathic hypersomnia. Neurology 1996;46:393.

390. Guilleminault C, Mondini S. Mononucleosis and chronic daytime sleepiness: a long-term follow-up study. Arch Intern Med 1986;146:1333.

391. Aldrich MS, Rogers AE, Angell K. Excessive daytime sleepiness as a presenting manifestation of HIV infection (abstract). Sleep Res 1988;17:271.

392. Nevsimalovas-Bruhova S, Roth B. Heredofamilial aspects of narcolepsy and hypersomnia. Schweiz Arch Neurol Neurochir Psychiatr 1972;110:45.

393. Roth B. Narcolepsy and Hypersomnia. Basel: Karger, 1980.

394. Montplaisir J, Poirier G. HLA in Disorders of Excessive Daytime Sleepiness without Cataplexy in Canada. In Y Honda, T Juji (eds), HLA in Narcolepsy. Berlin: Springer, 1988;186.

395. Harada S, Matsuki K, Honda Y, et al. Disorders of Excessive Daytime Sleepiness without Cataplexy and their Relationship with HLA in Japan. In Y Honda, T Juji (eds), HLA in Narcolepsy. Berlin: Springer, 1988;172.

396. Faull KF, Thieman S, King RG, et al. Monoamine interactions in narcolepsy and hypersomnia: a preliminary report. Sleep 1986;9:246.

397. Bradley TD, McNicholas WT, Rutherford R, et al. Clinical and physiological heterogeneity of the central sleep apnea syndrome. Am Rev Respir Dis 1986; 134:217.

398. White DP. Central Sleep Apnea. In MH Kryger, T Roth, WC Dement (eds), Principles and Practice of Sleep Medicine (2nd ed). Philadelphia: Saunders, 1994;630.

399. Guilleminault C, Robinson A. Central sleep apnea. Neurol Clin 1996;14:611.

400. Fleming PJ, Cade D, Bryan MH, Bryan AC. Congenital central hypoventilation and sleep state. Pediatrics 1980;66:425.

401. Mellins RB, Balfour HH Jr, Turino GM, Winters RW. Failure of automatic control of ventilation (Ondine's curse). Report of an infant born with this syndrome and review of the literature. Medicine 1970;49:487.

402. Oren J, Kelly DH, Shannon DC. Long-term follow-up of children with congenital central hypoventilation syndrome. Pediatrics 1987;80:375.

403. Paton JY, Swaminathan S, Sargent CW, Keens TG. Hypoxic and hypercapnic ventilatory responses in awake children with congenital central hypoventilation syndrome. Am Rev Respir Dis 1989;140:368.

404. Guilleminault C, Challamel MJ. Congenital Central Hypoventilation Syndrome (CCHS): Independent Syndrome or Generalized Impairment of the Autonomic Nervous System? In C Guilleminault, R Korobkin (eds), Progress in Perinatal Neurology (Vol 1). Baltimore: Williams & Wilkins, 1981;107.

405. Dempsey JA, Skatrud JB. A sleep induced apneic threshold and its consequences. Am Rev Respir Dis 1986;133:1163.

406. Sharp J, Druz W, D'Souza V, et al. Effect of metabolic acidosis upon sleep apnea. Chest 1985;87:619.

407. Reichel J. Primary alveolar hypoventilation. Clin Chest Med 1980;1:119.

408. Fishman AP, Goldring RM, Turino GM. General alveolar hypoventilation: a syndrome of respiratory and cardiac failure in patients with normal lungs. Q J Med 1966;35:261.

409. Fishman AP. The syndrome of chronic alveolar hypoventilation. Bull Physiopathol Respir 1972;8:971.

410. Guilleminault C, van den Hoed J, Mitler M. Clinical Overview of the Sleep Apnea Syndromes. In C Guilleminault, W Dement (eds), Sleep Apnea Syndromes. New York: Liss, 1978;1.

411. Roehrs T, Conway W, Wittig R, et al. Sleep complaints in patients with sleep-related respiratory disturbances. Am Rev Respir Dis 1985;132:520.

412. Guilleminault C, Eldridge FL, Dement WC. Insomnia with sleep apnea: a new syndrome. Science 1973; 181: 856.

413. Schroeder J, Motta J, Guilleminault C. Hemodynamic Studies in Sleep Apnea. In C Guilleminault, W Dement (eds), Sleep Apnea Syndromes. New York: Liss, 1978;177.

414. Podszus T, Peter JH, Renke A, et al. Pulmonary artery pressure during central sleep apnea. Sleep Res 1988; 17:236.

415. Badr MS, Toiber F, Skatrud JB, et al. Pharyngeal narrowing/occlusion during central sleep apnea. J Appl Physiol 1995;78:1805.

416. Guilleminault C, Quera-Salva M, Nino-Murcia G, et al. Central sleep apnea and partial obstruction of the upper airway. Ann Neurol 1987;21:465.

417. Hoffstein V, Slutsky AS. Central apnea reversal by continuous positive airway pressure. Am Rev Respir Dis 1987;137:1210.

418. Issa FG, Sullivan CE. Reversal of central apnea using nasal CPAP. Chest 1986;90:165.

419. Cooper R, Hulme A. Intracranial pressure and related phenomena during sleep. J Neurol Neurosurg Psychiatry 1966;29:564.

420. Cooper R, Hulme A. Changes of the EEG, intracranial pressure and other variables during sleep in patients with intracranial lesions. Electroencephalogr Clin Neurophysiol 1969;27:12.

421. Martin RJ. Neuromuscular and Skeletal Abnormalities with Nocturnal Respiratory Disorders. In RJ Martin (ed), Cardiorespiratory Disorders during Sleep. Mount Kisco, NY: Futura, 1990;251.

422. Munari C, Calbucci F. Correlations between intracranial pressure and EEG during coma and sleep. Electroencephalogr Clin Neurophysiol 1981;51:170.

423. Gonzalez S, Hayward R, Jones B, Lane R. Upper airway obstruction and raised intracranial pressure in children with craniosynostosis. Eur Respir J 1997;10:367.

424. Dexter JD, Weitzman E. The relationship of nocturnal headaches to sleep stage patterns. Neurology 1970;20:513.

425. Dexter JD. The relationship between stage III[+], IV[+] REM sleep and arousals with migraine. Headache 1979;19:364.

426. Dexter JD, Riley TL. Studies in nocturnal migraine. Headache 1975;15:51.

427. Kudrow L, McGinty DJ, Phillips ER, Stevenson M. Sleep apnea in cluster headache. Cephalalgia 1984;4:33.

428. Pfaffenrath V, Pollmann W, Ruther E, et al. Onset of nocturnal attacks of chronic cluster headache in relation to sleep stages. Acta Neurol Scand 1986;73:403.

429. Sahota PK, Dexter JD. Reversible physiological insomnia associated with cluster headache. Sleep Res 1992;21:307.

430. Kayed K, Godtlibsen OB, Sjaastad O. Chronic paroxysmal hemicrania. IV. "REM sleep locked" nocturnal headache attacks. Sleep 1978;1:91.

431. Coria F, Claveria LE, et al. Episodic paroxysmal hemicrania responsive to calcium channel blockers. J Neurol Neurosurg Psychiatry 1992;55:166.

432. Conelli P, Plazzi G, Pierangeli G, et al. Cardiovascular Changes in Chronic Paroxysmal Hemicrania—A Nocturnal Polygraphic Study. In FC Rose (ed), New Advances in Headache Research. Great Britain: Smith-Gordon, 1994;225.

433. Dexter JD. Headache as a presenting complaint of sleep apnea syndrome. Headache 1984;24:171.

434. Guilleminault T. Clinical Features and Evaluation of Obstructive Sleep Apnea. In MH Kryger, T Roth, WC Dement (eds), Principles and Practice of Sleep Medicine (2nd ed). Philadelphia: Saunders, 1994;667.

435. Paiva T, Vasconcelos P, Leitao AN, Andrea M. Apneias obstrutivas do sono. Acta Med Port 1993;1:449.

436. Davis JA, Fine ED, Maniglia AJ. Uvulopalatopharyngoplasty for obstructive sleep apnea in adults: clinical correlation with polysomnographic results. Ear Nose Throat J 1993;72:63.

437. Aldrich MS, Chauncey JB. Are morning headaches part of obstructive sleep apnea syndrome? Arch Intern Med 1990;150:1265.

438. Poceta JS, Dalessio DJ. Identification and treatment of sleep apnea in patients with chronic headache. Headache 1995;35:586.

439. Jennum P, Hein HO, Suadicani D, Gyntelberg F. Headache and cognitive dysfunctions in snorers. A cross-sectional study of 3323 men, aged 54 to 74 years: the Copenhagen Male Study. Arch Neurol 1994; 51:937.

440. Ulfberg J, Carter N, Talbach M, Edling C. Headache, snoring and sleep apnea. J Neurol 1996;243:621.

441. Paiva T, Farinha A, Martins A, et al. Chronic headaches and sleep disorders. Arch Intern Med 1997;157:1701.

442. Paiva T, Batista A, Martins P, Martins A. The relationship between headaches and sleep disturbances. Headache 1995;35:590.

443. Raskin NH. The hypnic headache syndrome. Headache 1988;28:534.

444. Newman LC, Lipton RB, Solmon S. The hypnic headache syndrome: a benign headache disorder of the elderly. Neurology 1990;40:1904.

445. Pearce JMS. Clinical features of the exploding head syndrome. J Neurol Neurosurg Psychiatry 1989; 52:907.

446. Declerck AC, Arends JB. An exceptional case of parasomnia: the exploding head syndrome. Sleep-Wake Res Netherlands 1994;5:41.

447. Sachs C, Svanborg E. The exploding head syndrome: polysomnographic recordings and therapeutic suggestions. Sleep 1991;14:263.

448. Walsleben JA, O'Malley EB, et al. Polysomnographic and topographic mapping of EEG in the exploding head syndrome. Sleep Res 1993;22:284.

449. Lugaresi E, Medori R, Montagna P, et al. Fatal familial insomnia and dysautonomia with selective degeneration of thalamic nuclei. N Engl J Med 1986;315:997.

450. Manetto V, Medori R, Cortelli P, et al. Fatal familial insomnia and pathological study of five new cases. Neurology 1992;42:312.

451. Lugaresi E. The thalamus and insomnia. Neurology 1992;42(suppl 6):28.

452. Medori R, Montagna P, Tritschler HJ, et al. Fatal familial insomnia. A second kindred with mutation of prion protein gene at codon 178. Neurology 1992;42:669.

453. Gambetti P, Petersen R, Monari L, et al. Fatal familial insomnia and the widening spectrum of prion diseases. Br Med Bull 1993;49:980.

454. Fiorino AS. Sleep, genes and death: fatal familial insomnia. Brain Res Rev 1996;22:258.

455. Medori R, Tritschler HJ. Prion protein gene analysis in three kindreds with fatal familial insomnia (FFI): codon 178 mutation and codon 129 polymorphism. Am J Hum Genet 1993;53:822.

456. Montagna P, Cortelli P, Tinuper S, et al. Fatal Familial Insomnia. A Disease that Emphasizes the Role of the Thalamus in the Regulation of Sleep and Vegetative Functions. In C Guilleminualt, E Lugaresi, P Montagna, P Gambetti (eds), Fatal Familial Insomnia: Inherited Prion Diseases, Sleep and the Thalamus. New York: Raven, 1994;1.

457. Reder AT, Mednick AS, Brown P, et al. Clinical and genetic studies of fatal familial insomnia. Neurology 1995;45:1068.

458. McLean CAN, Storey E, Gardner RJ, et al. The D178N (cis-129M) "fatal familial insomnia" mutation associated with diverse clinicopathologic phenotypes in an Australian kindred. Neurology 1997;49:552.

459. Nagayama M, Shinohara Y, Furukawa H, Kitamoto T. Fatal familial insomnia with a mutation at codon 178 of the prion protein gene: first report from Japan. Neurology 1996;47:1313.

460. Gallassi R, Morreale A, Montagna P, et al. Fatal familial insomnia: behavioral and cognitive features. Neurology 1996;46:935.

461. Montagna P, Cortelli P, Gambetti P, Lugaresi E. Fatal familial insomnia: sleep, neuroendocrine and vegetative alterations. Adv Neuroimmunol 1995;5:13.

462. Sforza E, Montagna P, Tinuper P, et al. Sleep-wake cycle abnormalities in fatal familial insomnia. Evidence of the role of the thalamus in sleep regulation. Electroencephalogr Clin Neurophysiol 1995;94:398.

463. Portaluppi F, Cortelli P, Avoni P, et al. Diurnal blood pressure variation and hormonal correlates in fatal familial insomnia. Hypertension 1994;23:569.

464. Cortelli P, Parchi P, Contin M, et al. Cardiovascular dysautonomia in fatal familial insomnia. Clin Auton Res 1991;1:15.

465. Portaluppi F, Cortelli P, Avoni P, et al. Progressive disruption of the circadian rhythm of melatonin in fatal familial insomnia. J Clin Endocrinol Metab 1994;78:1075.

466. Portaluppi F, Cortelli P, Avoni P, et al. Dissociated 24-hour patterns of somatotropin and prolactin in fatal familial insomnia. Neuroendocrinology 1995;61:731.

467. Cortelli P, Perani D, Parchi P, et al. Cerebral metabolism in fatal familial insomnia: relation to duration, neuropathology, and distribution of protease-resistant prion protein. Neurology 1997;49:126.

468. Monari L, Chen SG, Brown P, et al. Fatal familial insomnia and familial Creutzfeldt-Jakob disease: different prion proteins determined by a DNA polymorphism. Proc Natl Acad Sci U S A 1994;91:28.

469. Medori R, Tritschler J, LeBlanc A, et al. Fatal familial prion protein gene. N Engl J Med 1992;326:444.

470. Tateishi J, Brown P, Kitamoto T, et al. First experimental transmission of fatal familial insomnia. Nature 1995;376:434.

471. Collinge J, Palmer MS, Sidle KCL, et al. Transmission of fatal familial insomnia to laboratory animals. Lancet 1995;346:569.

472. Collinge J, Palmer MS, Dryden AJ. Genetic predisposition to iatrogenic Creutzfeldt-Jakob disease. Lancet 1991;337:1441.

473. Goldfarb LG, Petersen RB, Tabaton M, et al. Fatal familial insomnia and familial Creutzfeldt-Jakob disease: disease phenotype determined by a DNA polymorphism. Science 1992;258:806.

474. Gambetti P. Fatal familial insomnia and familial Creutzfeldt-Jakob disease: a tale of two diseases with the same genetic mutation. Curr Top Microbiol Immunol 1996;207:19.

475. Gambetti P, Parchi P, Petersen RB, et al. Fatal familial insomnia and familial Creutzfeldt-Jakob disease: clinical, pathological and molecular features. Brain Pathol 1995;5:43.

476. Prusiner SB. Molecular biology and pathogenesis of prion diseases. Trends Biochem Sci 1996;21(12):482.

477. Ironside JW. Human prion diseases. J Neural Transm Suppl 1996;47:231.

478. Goldfarb LG, Brown P. The transmissible spongiform encephalopathies. Annu Rev Med 1995;46:57.

479 Bradley WG, Daroff RB, Fenichel GM, et al. (eds). Neurology in Clinical Practice (Vols I & II). Boston: Butterworth–Heinemann, 1991.

480. Adams RD, Victor M. Principles of Neurology (4th ed). New York: McGraw-Hill, 1989.

481. Rowland LP (ed). Merritt's Textbook of Neurology (8th ed). Philadelphia: Lea & Febiger, 1989.

482. Staedt J, Stoppe G, Kogler A, et al. Nocturnal myoclonus syndrome (periodic limb movements in sleep) related to central dopamine $D_2$ receptor alteration. Eur Arch Psychiatry Clin Neurosci 1995;245:8.

483. Staedt J, Stoppe G, Kogler A, et al. Dopamine $D_2$ receptor alteration in patients with periodic movements in sleep (nocturnal myoclonus). J Neurol Trans 1993; 93:71.

484. Staedt J, Stoppe G, Kogler A, et al. Single photon emission tomography (SPECT) imaging of dopamine $D_2$ receptor in the course of dopamine replacement therapy in patients with nocturnal myoclonus syndrome (NMS). J Neurol Trans 1995;99:187.

485. MacFarlane JG, List SJ, Moldofsky H, et al. Dopamine $D_2$ receptors quantified in vivo in human narcolepsy. Biol Psychiatry 1997;41:305.

486. Rinne JO, Hublin C, Partinen M, et al. Positron emission tomography study of human narcolepsy: no increase in striatal dopamine $D_2$ receptors. Neurology 1995;45:1735.

487. Staedt J, Stoppe G, Kogler A, et al. {$^{123}$1} IBZM SPET analysis of dopamine $D_2$ receptor occupancy in narcoleptic patients in the course of treatment. Biol Psychiatry 1996;39:107.

488. Bucher SF, Seelos KC, Oertel WH, et al. Cerebral generators involved in the pathogenesis of the restless legs syndrome. Ann Neurol 1997;41:639.

489. Saadeh A, Hauri PJ, Kripke DF, Lavie P. The role of actigraphy in the evaluation of sleep disorders. Sleep 1995;18:288.

490. Bates DV. Respiratory Function in Disease (3rd ed). Philadelphia: Saunders, 1989;106.

491. Black LF, Hyatt RE. Maximal static respiratory pressures in generalized neuromuscular disease. Am Rev Respir Dis 1971;103:641.

492. Guindi GM, Bannister R, Gibson W, et al. Laryngeal electromyography in multiple system atrophy with autonomic failure. J Neurol Neurosurg Psychiatry 1981;44:49.

493. Markand ON, Kincaid JC, Pourmand RA, et al. Electrophysiologic evaluation of diaphragm by transcutaneous phrenic nerve stimulation. Neurology 1984;34:604.

494. Chokroverty S, Deutsch A, Guha C, et al. Thoracic spinal nerve and root conduction: a magnetic stimulation study. Muscle Nerve 1995;18:987.

495. Sanders MH. The Management of Sleep Disordered Breathing. In RJ Martin (ed), Cardiorespiratory Disorders During Sleep. Mount Kisco, NY: Futura, 1990;141.

496. Issa FG, Sullivan CE. Upper airway closing pressures in snorers. J Appl Physiol 1984;57:528.

497. Krol RC, Knuth SL, Bartlett D Jr. Selective reduction of genioglossal muscle activity by alcohol in normal human subjects. Am Rev Respir Dis 1984;129:247.

498. Taasan VC, Block AJ, Boysen PG, et al. Alcohol increases sleep apnea and oxygen desaturation in asymptomatic men. Am J Med 1981;71:240.

499. Brownell LG, West P, Sweatman P, et al. Protriptyline in obstructive sleep apnea: a double-blind trial. N Engl J Med 1982;307:1037.

500. Hensley MJ, Saunders NA, Strohl KP. Medroxyprogesterone treatment of obstructive sleep apnea. Sleep 1980;3:441.

501. Rajagopal KR, Abbrecht P, Jabbari P. Effects of medroxyprogesterone acetate in obstructive sleep apnea. Chest 1986;90:815.

502. Skatrud JB, Dempsey JA, Kaiser DG. Ventilatory response to medroxyprogesterone acetate in normal subjects: time, course and mechanisms. J Appl Physiol 1978;44:939.

503. Strohl KP, Hensley M, Saunders NA, et al. Progesterone administration and progressive sleep apneas. JAMA 1981;245:1230.

504. Sutton FD, Zwillich CW, Creagh CE, et al. Progesterone for outpatient treatment of Pickwickian syndrome. Ann Intern Med 1975;83:476.

505. Lyons HA, Huang CT. Therapeutic use of progesterone in alveolar hypoventilation associated with obesity. Am J Med 1968;44:881.

506. McEvoy GK (ed). AHFS Drug Information 93. Bethesda, MD: American Society of Hospital Pharmacists, 1993; 44:2424.

507. Sharp J, Druz W, D'Souza V, et al. Effect of metabolic acidosis upon sleep apnea. Chest 1985;87:619.

508. Sutton JR, Gray GW, Houston CS, et al. Effects of duration at altitude and acetazolamide on ventilation and oxygenation during sleep. Sleep 1980;3:455.

509. Sutton JR, Houston CS, Mansell AC, et al. Effect of acetazolamide on hypoxia during sleep at high altitude. N Engl J Med 1979;301:1329.

510. White DP, Zwillich CW, Pickett CK, et al. Central sleep apnea: improvement with acetazolamide therapy. Arch Intern Med 1982;142:1816.

511. Guilleminault C, Kowall J. Central Sleep Apnea in Adults. In MJ Thorpy (ed), Handbook of Sleep Disorders. New York: Marcel Dekker, 1990;337.

512. Guilleminault C, Quera-Salva M, Nino-Murcia G, et al. Central sleep apnea and partial obstruction of the upper airway. Ann Neurol 1987;21:465.

513. Hoffstein V, Slutsky AS. Central apnea reversal by continuous positive airway pressure. Am Rev Respir Dis 1987;137:1210.

514. Issa FG, Sullivan CE. Reversal of central apnea using nasal CPAP. Chest 1986;90:165.

515. Martin TJ, Sanders MH. Chronic alveolar hypoventilation: a review for the clinician. Sleep 1995;18:617.

516. Tobin MJ. Mechanical ventilation. New Engl J Med 1994;330:1056.

517. Strumpf DA, Millman R, Hill NS. The management of chronic hypoventilation. Chest 1990;98:474.

518. Hill NS. Clinical application of body ventilators. Chest 1986;90:897.

519. Spalding JMK, Opie L. Artificial respiration with the Tunnicliffe breathing jacket. Lancet 1958;613.

520. Collier CR, Affeldt JE. Ventilatory efficiency of the cuirass respirator in totally paralyzed chronic poliomyelitis patients. J Appl Physiol 1954;6:531.

521. Levy RD, Bradley TD, Newman SL, et al. Negative pressure ventilation: effects on ventilation during sleep in normal subjects. Chest 1989;95:95.

522. Ellis ER, Bye PTP, Bruderer JW, Sullivan CE. Treatment of respiratory failure during sleep in patients with neuromuscular disease: positive-pressure ventilation through a nose mask. Am Rev Respir Dis 1987;135:148.

523. Bach JR, Alba AS, Bohatiuk G, et al. Mouth intermittent positive pressure ventilation in the management of postpolio respiratory insufficiency. Chest 1987;91:859.

524. Leger P, Bedicam JM, Cornett A, et al. Nasal intermittent positive pressure ventilation. Long-term follow-up in patients with severe chronic respiratory insufficiency. Chest 1994;105:100.

525. Gay PC, Patel AM, Viggiano RW, Hubmayr RD. Nocturnal nasal ventilation for treatment of patients with hypercapnic respiratory failure. Mayo Clin Proc 1991; 66:695.

526. Sanders MH, Kern NB, Stiller RA, et al. CPAP therapy via oronasal mask for obstructive sleep apnea. Chest 1994;106:774.

527. Prosise GL, Berry RB. Oral-nasal continuous positive airway pressure as a treatment for obstructive sleep apnea. Chest 1994;106:180.

528. Carroll N, Branthwaite MA. Control of nocturnal hypoventilation by nasal intermittent positive pressure ventilation. Thorax 1988;43:349.

529. Leger P, Jennequin J, Gerard M, Robert D. Home positive pressure ventilation via nasal mask for patients with neuromuscular weakness or restrictive lung or chest-wall disease. Resp Care 1989;34:73.

530. Segall D. Noninvasive nasal mask-assisted ventilation in respiratory failure of Duchenne muscular dystrophy. Chest 1988;93:1298.

531. Vianello A, Bevilacqua M, Salvador V, et al. Long-term nasal intermittent positive pressure ventilation in advanced Duchenne's muscular dystrophy. Chest 1994;105:445.

532. Heckmatt JZ, Loh L, Dubowitz V. Night-time nasal ventilation in neuromuscular disease. Lancet 1990;335:579.

533. Guilleminault C, Stoohs R, Schneider H, et al. Central alveolar hypoventilation and sleep: treatment by intermittent positive-pressure ventilation through nasal mask in an adult. Chest 1989;96:1210.

534. Bye PTB, Ellis ER, Donnelly PD, et al. Role of sleep in the development of respiratory failure in neuromuscular disease. Am Rev Respir Dis 1985;131:108.

535. Kerby DY, Meyer LS, Tingleton SK. Nocturnal positive pressure ventilation via nasal mask. Am Rev Respir Dis 1987;135:738.

536. Sanders MH, Black J, Stiller RA, Donahoe MP. Nocturnal ventilatory assistance with bi-level positive airway pressure. Operative Techniques in Otolaryngology. Head Neck Surg 1991;2:56.

537. Waldhorn RE. Nocturnal nasal intermittent positive pressure ventilation with bi-level positive airway pressure (BiPAP) in respiratory failure. Chest 1992;101:516.

538. Sanders MH, Kern NB. Nocturnal Bi-Level Positive Airway Pressure (BiPAP) in Patients with Chronic Ventilatory Failure: Long-term Experience, Clinical and Physiologic Implications. In K Togawa, S Katayama, Y Hishikawa, et al. (eds), Sleep Apnea and Rhonchopathy. Basel: Karger, 1993;23.

539. Martin RJ, Sanders MA, Gray BA, et al. Acute and long term ventilatory effects of hyperoxia in the adult sleep apnea syndrome. Am Rev Respir Dis 1982; 125:175.

540. Motta A, Guilleminault C. Effects of Oxygen Administration in Sleep-Induced Apneas. In C Guilleminault, WC Dement (eds), Sleep Apnea Syndrome. New York: Liss, 1978;137.

541. Chokroverty S, Barrocas M, Barron KD, et al. Hypoventilation syndrome and obesity: a polygraphic study. Trans Am Neurol Assoc 1969;94:240.

542. Gay PC, Edmonds LC. Severe hypercapnia after low-flow oxygen therapy in patients with neuromuscular disease and diaphragmatic dysfunction. Mayo Clin Proc 1995;70:327.

543. Sarnoff SJ, Whittenberger JL, Affeldt JA. Hypoventilation syndrome in bulbar poliomyelitis. JAMA 1951; 147:30.

544. Glenn WWL, Phelps M, Gersten LM. Diaphragm Pacing in the Management of Central Alveolar Hypoventilation. In C Guilleminault, WC Dement (eds), Sleep Apnea Syndromes. New York: Liss, 1978;333.

545. Chervin R, Guilleminault C. Diaphragm pacing: review and reassessment. Sleep 1990;17:176.

546. Kenan PD. Complications associated with tracheostomy: prevention and treatment. Otolaryngol Clin North Am 1979;12:807.

547. Satlin A, Volicer L, Ross V, et al. Bright light treatment of behavioral and sleep disturbance in Alzheimer's disease. Am J Psychiatry 1992;114:1028.

548. Okawa M, Hishikawa Y, Hozumi S, Hori H. Sleep-Wake Rhythm Disorder and Phototherapy in Elderly Patients with Dementia. In R Gracagri, et al. (eds), Biological Psychiatry (Vol 1). New York: Elsevier, 1991;837.

549. Okawa M, Mishima K, Shirakawa S, et al. Sleep Disorders in Elderly Patients with Dementia and Attempts of Bright Light Therapy: In Senile Dementia of Alzheimer's Type and Multi-Infarct Dementia. In T Hairoshige, K Honma (eds), Evolution of Circadian Clock. Sapporo, Japan: Hokkaido University Press, 1994;313.

550. Satlin A. Sleep disorders in dementia. Psychiatry Annu 1994;24:186.

551. Dement WC. A personal history of sleep disorders medicine. J Clin Neurophysiol 1990;7:17.

# Chapter 28
# Sleep in Psychiatric Disorders

## Virgil D. Wooten and Daniel J. Buysse

Numerous studies link psychopathology and poor sleep. Often, physicians who have exhausted all routine laboratory assessments and medical interventions in the effort to diagnose and treat a person with an undiscovered sleep problem refer the patient to a psychiatrist. Patients who present to sleep disorders centers frequently exhibit symptoms of psychopathology, which may or may not be due to psychiatric illness. According to the Epidemiological Catchment Area (ECA) study[1] of the National Institute of Mental Health (NIMH) consisting of 18,571 people aged 18 years and older, within 1 month of initial interview, 15.4% of the population had a mental disorder, 5.1% an affective disorder, 7.3% an anxiety disorder, and 3.8% a substance abuse disorder. The respective lifetime prevalence in these groups was estimated at 8.3%, 14.6%, and 16.4%. A survey of 7,954 people in scattered major U.S. cities between 1981 and 1985 as part of the NIMH/ECA study also revealed that 40% of those with insomnia and 46.5% of those with hypersomnia met the criteria for mental illness in the third edition of the American Psychiatric Association's *Diagnostic and Statistical Manual of Mental Disorders* (*DSM-III-R*).[2] Ten percent of the sample complained of insomnia and 3.2% of hypersomnia. Fourteen percent of the patients with insomnia met criteria for major depression, compared to 9.9% of those with hypersomnolence. The rate of new psychiatric disorders at 1-year follow-up was greater among respondents with persistent sleep complaints. The numbers in this study were thought to be low due to strict criteria for defining insomnia and the omission of generalized anxiety disorder and personality disorders from the survey. In a study by Mosko and colleagues,[3] 66.5% of 206 patients presenting to one sleep disorders center reported one episode of major depression in the previous 5 years and 25.7% described themselves as depressed on presentation. Additional studies have established substantial risk of developing major depression and generalized anxiety in patients with sleep disorders.[4–6] Mellinger and coworkers[4] reported that 21% of insomniacs had symptoms of major depression, and another 13% symptoms of generalized anxiety. Breslau et al.,[5] in a 3-year longitudinal study of 979 young adults, found a lifetime prevalence of 16% for insomnia and 8% for hypersomnolence. Patients with insomnia had a fourfold increase in risk for developing major depression compared to patients without insomnia; sleep disturbance was a stronger predictor of the subsequent development of depression than any other factor.

## SLEEP STUDIES OF PSYCHOPATHOLOGY

Studies of rapid eye movement (REM) sleep architecture in various psychopathologic states have been conducted since Dement first evaluated REM sleep in schizophrenic patients in 1955. More recently, REM sleep changes have most often been associated with affective disorders. Subsequently, numerous studies have attempted to use measures of REM sleep latency, REM density, and REM sleep distribution to link affective disorders to various other psychopathologic states such as schizophrenia, eating disorders, personality disorders, and substance abuse disorders. Others have attempted to use these same measures to distinguish various psychopathologic states from major depression. Unfortunately, a great deal of confusion has resulted from various methodologic issues and diagnostic uncertainties in psychiatric patients. Examples of methodologic differences in studies include the number of consecutive nights patients are studied, determination of the time between sleep onset and REM sleep onset (REM sleep latency), the definition of increased REM density, concurrent use of psychotropic drugs, period of withdrawal from psychotropic medications, sleep schedule, and the severity of the illness. Just as important is the overlap of symptoms among various disorders found in the Research Diagnostic Criteria, the fourth edition of the *DSM*, and other classifications for mental disorders. Although in theory psychiatric diagnoses are categorically distinct from one another, in clinical practice such distinctions are more difficult to make, and often patients have more than one psychiatric diagnosis.

## Affective Disorders

Major depression is the psychiatric disorder most studied by sleep researchers, and several theories of the mechanisms involved have been published.[7] Great efforts have been made to distinguish major depression from other psychopathologic states by use of sleep electroencephalography (EEG) and other biological markers. The primary well-documented changes in sleep architecture include shortened REM sleep–onset latency, increased REM density, reduced total sleep time, reduced sleep efficiency, increased awakenings, decreased slow-wave sleep (SWS), and a shift of SWS from the first non-REM (NREM) cycle to the second (Figure 28-1). More recently, high-amplitude fast-frequency EEG activity has been suggested as a marker for depression.[8] Sleep architecture changes found in depression may serve as a marker for the development of depression in those genetically predisposed to depression.[9,10] In comparison with major depressive disorder, dysthymia has not been extensively studied. Hypersomnolence,[11] reductions in K complexes, vertex

sharp waves, increased stage I sleep, decreased SWS, increased awakenings, spindles in REM sleep, theta bursts, and positive occipital sharp transients[12,13] have been cited in isolated studies.

Changes in sleep architecture, particularly in REM sleep and deep NREM sleep, are more pronounced with age in major depression. Prepubertal depressed children are less likely to show changes in sleep architecture than postpubertal depressives.[14,15] There has been some conflict in the literature about whether REM sleep latency in depressed children is normal or shortened.[16] Changes in sleep architecture in adolescents appear to depend on the severity of the illness. Inpatient, psychotic, or suicidal adolescents may exhibit the typical adult changes of major depression, whereas the sleep of adolescents who are not as severely depressed may show no changes.[17–19]

Aging has a marked shortening influence on REM sleep latency; elderly depressed patients often have a REM sleep onset of less than 10 minutes. Older patients with a history of suicide attempts have longer sleep-onset latency, reduced sleep efficiency, and increased REM density than "nonattempters."[20] Depressed men have less SWS than depressed women,[21] but women may have more and higher-amplitude beta activity.[22] Women with past depressive episodes appear to experience more sleep disruption and reduced REM sleep latency[23] in the immediate postpartum months.

In approximately 90% of cases, major depression results in insomnia. A smaller percentage of patients with major depression complain of excessive sleepiness; most are adolescents and young adults.[24] Whereas depressed adolescents and young adults may be more prone to be "long sleepers," studies of older depressed patients with the complaint of hypersomnolence have failed to show evidence of pathologic sleepiness.[25]

Studies of the effects of antidepressant medication on REM sleep measures in patients with major depression have suggested that when immediate and persistent antidepressant-induced prolongation of the REM sleep latency, reduction of total REM sleep time, and REM density are observed, clinical response is better.[26,27] The occurrence of sleep-onset REM sleep episodes and shorter REM sleep duration during maintenance treatment with antidepressants has been associated with increased risk of relapse during treatment.[28] Studies of the effects of electroconvulsive therapy (ECT) on REM sleep

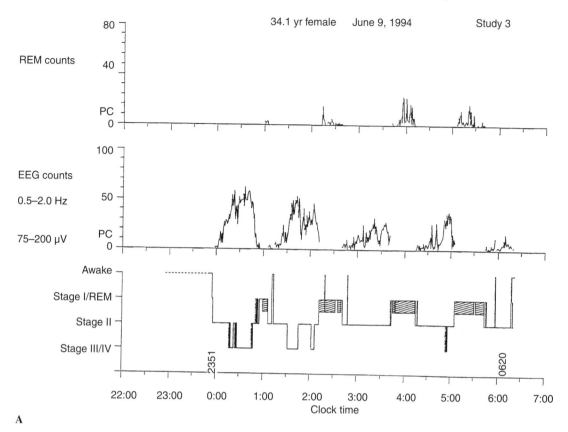

**Figure 28-1.** Representative sleep histograms for a healthy subject (**A**) and an age- and sex-matched patient with major depressive disorder (**B**). In each figure, the top panel shows the number and timing of REM counts identified by computer algorithm; the middle panel shows EEG delta activity during NREM sleep identified by computer algorithm; and the bottom panel shows the sleep histogram from visual sleep stage scoring. Relative to the control subject, the depressed patient has a longer sleep latency, more wakefulness during sleep, less visually scored stage III/IV and EEG delta activity, a larger percentage of REM sleep, more phasic REM activity, and shorter REM sleep latency.

architecture suggest that they are not as pronounced as those observed with most antidepressants.[29] As with pharmacotherapy, patients with post-ECT EEG signs of depression are more likely to have recurrence of the illness.[30]

Patients in the manic phase of bipolar disorder have been shown to have much reduced total sleep time, which gradually extends as the manic phase passes.[31] There is also a reduction in stage III and IV sleep. No consistent change in REM sleep has been found, probably due to excitability and subsequent reduction of total sleep in these patients, but most studies show the same changes as seen in major depression.[32,33] It has been suggested that the switch from euthymia or depression into the manic phase occurs during sleep.[34] Lithium, which is the primary drug used to treat the manic phase of bipolar disorder, has been found to increase SWS and reduce REM sleep.

### Anxiety Disorders

Patients with generalized anxiety disorder typically have prolonged sleep-onset latency, increased stage I and II sleep, less SWS, a smaller REM sleep percentage, and, with the exception of isolated reports, increased or normal REM sleep latency.[35,36] Compared to patients with major depression, patients with generalized anxiety disorder have fewer awakenings. No difference has been found between patients with generalized anxiety disorder alone and those with generalized anxiety disorder and

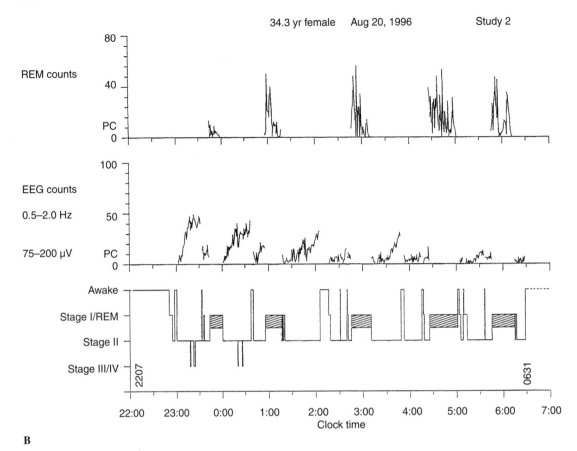

34.3 yr female    Aug 20, 1996          Study 2

**B**

**Figure 28-1.** *Continued*

depression.[37] Patients with social phobia show increased sleep-onset latency, awakening after sleep onset, and reduced total sleep time.[38]

Panic disorder has multiple somatic and emotional symptoms leading to diagnostic confusion. Similar presentations are seen in mitral valve prolapse syndrome, cardiovascular dysautonomia, and sleep choking syndrome. The diagnosis may depend on the presentation of psychiatric symptoms, as opposed to autonomic and respiratory symptoms. Controversy exists over the roles of increased brainstem carbon dioxide receptor sensitivity and dysautonomia in panic.[39–45]

Despite ample evidence for an autonomic component in panic disorder, the link to emotional status also appears to be important. Data from the ECA program indicated that the question "Are you a nervous person?" identified 60% of individuals who would experience panic within the following year.[46] It has been suggested that a number of substances and situations provoke panic attacks, such as caffeine, nicotine, over-the-counter cold remedies, cannabis, cocaine, sleep deprivation, excessive sugar intake, exercise, relaxation, hyperventilation, stress, and even fluorescent lighting.[47] As much as 70% of patients with panic disorder have difficulty with sleep-onset and maintenance insomnia.[48] Panic attacks can occur in any stage of sleep, but most occur during NREM sleep just before the onset of SWS. Nocturnal panic attacks may occur in as many as 69% of patients with panic disorder.[49] Nocturnal panic symptoms are typically more intense than those associated with daytime attacks. Patients with nocturnal panic attacks experience worse daytime panic attacks, more somatic symptoms,[50] and more comorbid psychiatric disorders[51] than daytime-only panic disorder patients. Symptoms similar to those associated with nocturnal panic attacks may be observed in patients with arrhythmias, gastroesophageal reflux, sleep apnea,[52] sleep terrors, REM sleep behavior disorder, and paroxysmal hypnogenic dystonia.[53] Patients with panic disorder often report sleep paralysis[54] and hypnagogic hallucinations.[55]

It has been suggested that patients with sleep-only panic attacks experience depression more frequently than panic disorder patients who do not experience sleep-related panic attacks.[56] Nondepressed patients with panic disorder have been reported to have normal sleep-onset latency and modestly reduced total sleep time and delta sleep.[57] Patients with major depression and panic, however, may have features typical of major depression, with substantially prolonged sleep-onset latency, reduced total sleep time, sleep disruption, reduced SWS, and early REM sleep onset.[58–61]

Patients with obsessive compulsive disorder show decreased total sleep time, increased number of awakenings, shortened REM sleep latency, reduced stage IV sleep, and reduced sleep efficiency.[62]

Post-traumatic stress disorder is caused by involvement in events not normally experienced, usually combat, torture, or other situations involving physical and psychological abuse. This disorder has been associated with increased sleep-onset latency, decreased sleep efficiency, increased wakefulness after sleep onset, decreased total sleep time, reduction in stage II sleep, and increased stage I sleep.[63] Frequent nightmares are a hallmark of post-traumatic stress disorder, involving both reliving of experiences and imaginary scenarios of gruesome or life-threatening content. There is controversy over the effects on REM sleep: Some authors report normal REM sleep parameters,[63] whereas others report reduced REM sleep latency and increased REM density.[64–66] Nightmares have been found to occur during both NREM and REM sleep.[67,68] REM sleep behavior disorder has also been associated with post-traumatic stress disorder.[69,70] Authors have speculated that post-traumatic stress disorder may be a disorder of REM sleep mechanisms.[71]

### Eating Disorders

Most studies of patients with bulimia show very little change in REM sleep measures compared with controls. REM sleep architecture studies of patients with anorexia nervosa have been more contradictory: Some report no change in REM sleep parameters,[72] whereas others suggest that there are changes similar to those seen in major depression.[73] These findings may be due to high rates of comorbidity with affective disorders and frequent family history of affective disorders in anorexia patients. Patients with severe untreated anorexia nervosa often show reduced total sleep time, decreased sleep efficiency, increased wakefulness after sleep onset, increased

stage I sleep, and decreased SWS. Sleep normalizes after weight is gained.[74,75] One study suggests that there is initial shortening of the REM sleep latency with severe weight loss but that with recovery of weight the REM sleep latency returns to normal.[76]

### Schizophrenia

Patients with schizophrenia often sleep worse than healthy individuals, with sleep continuity disturbance, reduced SWS, decreased REM latency, and increased REM sleep, although there are contrasting studies showing relatively little change in sleep. Variability in documented sleep architecture changes and sleep quality are most likely due to differences in the age of patients, medications, study techniques, and other variables. Sleep efficiency, stage II sleep, sleep continuity, total sleep time, and total REM sleep decrease on withdrawal of neuroleptics.[77–79] In one study,[77] patients with tardive dyskinesia had an earlier onset of REM suppression after withdrawal of medication. Mean REM sleep latency was shorter, and total REM sleep time was greater in patients with tardive dyskinesia than in those without tardive dyskinesia. NREM sleep parameters improved more on withdrawal of medication than REM sleep parameters. All had prolonged sleep-onset latencies. SWS was more abundant in patients without tardive dyskinesia. Studies have suggested an inverse relationship between SWS and sleep maintenance and brain ventricle size.[80–82] It has been suggested that reductions in SWS and increases in negative symptoms may be related to reduced anabolism and accelerated aging or atrophy of the brain.[83] SWS also does not rebound after sleep deprivation in patients with schizophrenia.[84]

The first attempt to establish a connection between REM sleep abnormalities and schizophrenia was reported by Dement in 1955.[85] This study, carried out before the advent of neuroleptics, found shortened REM sleep latency but no difference in eye movement activity in schizophrenics. Despite subsequent conflicts in the literature about whether there is shorter REM sleep latency in schizophrenia,[86–91] the similarity of the hallucinatory activity that normally occurs in REM sleep to the hallucinations of schizophrenics has continued to intrigue investigators.

Acute schizophrenics have no REM sleep rebound after REM sleep deprivation, whereas chronic schizophrenics without active symptoms have more rebound than normal.[86,92] A subsequent "hydraulic leakage" theory of schizophrenia was developed, positing that the hallucinatory activity of REM sleep leaks into wakefulness in schizophrenics.[93] This theory was developed because studies showed that there were reductions in intricate themes, clarity, and vividness in the dreams of these patients.[85,94]

Another theory later developed by Dement and coworkers[95] hypothesized that schizophrenics have hallucinations resulting from ponto-geniculo-occipital (PGO) discharges, or phasic events, in the waking state. Comparison of periorbital potentials (PIPs) and middle ear muscle activity (MEMA) before and after REM sleep showed no redistribution of MEMA or PIPs into other sleep stages in patients with schizophrenia that would suggest that PGO discharges are responsible.[96]

Models from artificial intelligence theory suggested that the central nervous system (CNS) malfunction in schizophrenia occurs because of ineffective REM sleep. REM sleep was theorized to be necessary to eliminate parasitic states in which too many neural connections interfere with information processing and memory.[97] One study that attempted to link REM sleep to schizophrenia was done by Weiler and colleagues.[98] Brain glucose metabolism was evaluated in 49 awake schizophrenics, 30 awake controls, and 12 controls during REM sleep by positron emission tomography. No relationship was found between glucose utilization for awake schizophrenics and controls in REM sleep, including patients with active hallucinations. The glucose utilization in awake schizophrenics most closely resembled that of awake controls.

A more accepted theory of schizophrenia suggests that it is due to an imbalance of dopamine and acetylcholine in key CNS structures. Dopaminergic activity has been shown to increase in the psychotic phase, and a compensatory increase of muscarinic acetylcholine activity in turn results in increased negative symptoms. A study of the effects of biperiden, an antimuscarinic $M_1$ agent, on REM sleep latency in schizophrenics and controls found that the psychotic patients had a smaller increase in REM sleep latency.[99] Biperiden also increased positive symptoms and decreased negative ones. It has also been reported that prolactin secretion is increased during sleep in schizophrenics.[100] This may reflect abnormalities in the dopaminergic system. One study linked decreased REM sleep latency and increased REM density with the negative symptoms of schizophrenia and attributed these changes to increased CNS muscarinic activity.[101] Alternatively,

there may be increased cholinergic sensitivity in patients with schizophrenia.[102]

Assuming that the dopaminergic-acetylcholinergic imbalance theory is correct, variations in REM sleep parameters that have been reported by numerous investigators could be explained by the phase of the illness, the degree of neurotransmitter imbalance, and the influence of short- and long-term use of medication.

Sleep apnea has also been reported to aggravate schizophrenia symptoms.[103]

### Borderline Personality Disorder

Borderline personality disorder as defined by the *DSM-IV* encompasses a number of symptoms of other psychiatric disorders, including major depression. In numerous studies of borderline personality disorder, it has been shown repeatedly that the sleep architecture changes are very similar to those observed in patients with major depression.[104–107] Borderline personality disorder patients have less total sleep time, less sleep efficiency, reduced SWS, increased stage II sleep, reduced REM sleep latency, and increased REM density. Subjects with borderline personality disorder frequently have symptoms of depression and have been shown to have abnormalities of other biological markers associated with depression.[108]

### Childhood Psychiatric Disorders

Attention-deficit hyperactivity disorder may be associated with childhood insomnia.[109] Most polysomnographic studies show relatively normal sleep parameters, however, in most patients.[110–112] Stimulants in the evenings can have beneficial effects on sleep and usually cause little or no sleep disturbance. Gilles de la Tourette's syndrome often results in sleep disruption. Motor tics may disturb sleep, and patients with comorbid attention deficit hyperactivity disorder experience the most sleep disturbance.[109,113]

### Medication Effects and Substance Abuse

The reader is referred to Table 28-1 for a review of the acute, chronic, and withdrawal effects on sleep parameters of various medications and substances of abuse.

**Table 28-1.** Drugs That Affect Sleep

| Drug | | Effects on Sleep | Comments |
|---|---|---|---|
| Barbiturates | Acute: | ↑TST | Rapid development of tolerance |
| | | ↓WASO | Withdrawal insomnia |
| | | ↓REM | Daytime sedation |
| | | ↑Stage II, ↑spindles | |
| | | ↑ or ↓Delta | |
| | Withdrawal: | ↓TST | |
| Benzodiazepines | Acute: | ↓SL (most agents) | Agents vary in onset and duration of action |
| | | ↑TST | Daytime sedation (with long-acting agents) |
| | | ↓WASO | Tolerance develops (with short-acting agents) |
| | | ↓REM | Withdrawal insomnia (with short-acting agents) |
| | | ↑Stage II, ↑spindles | |
| | | ↓Delta (most agents; some ↑delta) | |
| | Withdrawal: | ↓TST | |
| Benzodiazepine receptor agents (zolpidem) | Acute: | ↓SL | Sleep architecture not typically altered |
| | | ↑TST | Withdrawal effects inconsistently seen |
| | | →REM | |
| | | →Delta | |
| | Withdrawal: | → or ↑WASO | |
| Chloral hydrate | | ↑TST | Little information on tolerance or withdrawal |
| | | →REM | |
| | | →Stage II | |
| | | →Delta | |
| L-Tryptophan | | → or ↑TST | Effects are mild and inconsistent and may |
| | | → or ↑REM | be delayed |
| | | ↑Delta | |
| Alcohol | Acute: | ↑TST 1st half of night, ↓2nd half | Acute effects variable |
| | | ↓WASO 1st half of night, ↑2nd half | |
| | | ↓REM 1st half of night | |
| | | ↑Delta | |
| | Chronic: | →TST | |
| | | →REM | |
| | | ↓Delta | |
| | Withdrawal: | ↓TST | Degree of REM rebound may correlate with |
| | | ↑WASO | likelihood of withdrawal delirium |
| | | ↑REM | |
| | | ↓Delta | |
| Narcotics | Acute: | ↑WASO | Effects vary with specific agents |
| | | ↓REM | |
| | | ↓Delta (total), with ↑delta "bursts" | |
| | Chronic: | →WASO | |
| | | →Delta | Hypersomnolence may occur during withdrawal |
| | Withdrawal: | ↓WASO | |
| Aspirin | Acute: | ↓Delta | May act via prostaglandin inhibition and temperature effects |
| Amphetamines | Acute: | ↓TST | Sleep-wake cycle may be severely disrupted |
| | | ↑WASO, ↑movements | during acute use and withdrawal |
| | | ↓REM | |
| | | ↓Delta | |
| | Withdrawal: | ↑TST | |
| | | ↑REM | |
| Caffeine | | ↑SL | May have effects on sleep EEG even when no |
| | | ↓TST | subjective disturbance occurs |
| | | ↑WASO | |
| | | ↓REM | |
| | | ↓Delta (1st half of night) | |

**Table 28-1.** *Continued*

| Drug | | Effects on Sleep | Comments |
|---|---|---|---|
| Miscellaneous stim- ulants (e.g., nico- tine, cocaine, pemoline, methyl- phenidate) | | ↑SL ↓TST ↓REM | |
| Antidepressants (e.g., tricyclic and monoamine oxi- dase inhibitors, except trimipra- mine) | Acute: | ↓WASO ↓REM ↑Stage II ↑Delta | Sleep effects vary with sedative potential of specific agent; MAOIs may cause ↑WASO |
| | Withdrawal: | ↑WASO ↑REM | |
| Selective serotonin- reuptake inhibitors | Acute: | → or ↑WASO →TST ↓REM →Delta | May cause insomnia or hypersomnia May produce eye movements in non-REM sleep |
| Trazodone | Acute: | ↓WASO → or ↓REM → or ↑Delta | Less suppression of REM sleep than tricyclics and MAOIs |
| Lithium | | ↓REM ↑Delta | |
| Phenothiazine | | ↑TST ↑Delta | Effects mild and variable, according to specific agent REM effects inconsistent |
| Reserpine | | ↑WASO ↑REM ↑Delta | Can cause insomnia, nightmares |
| Yohimbine | | ↑REM ↓Delta | |
| Clonidine | | →TST ↑WASO ↑Stage shifts ↓REM | Can cause insomnia, daytime sedation |
| α-Methyldopa | | ↑REM (1st half of night) ↓Delta | Can cause nightmares |
| Diuretics | | ↑WASO | Probably acts via nocturia, hemodynamic effects |
| Cimetidine | | ↑Delta | Can cause daytime sedation |
| Baclofen | | ↑TST | |
| L-Dopa | | →TST → or ↑REM →Delta | In toxic doses, causes insomnia, delirium |
| Methysergide | | →TST → or ↑REM ↑Delta | |
| γ-Hydroxybutyrate | | ↑TST | |
| Steroids | | ↑WASO | |

SL = sleep latency; WASO = wakefulness after sleep onset; TST = total sleep time; MAOIs = monoamine oxidase inhibitors; ↑ = increased; ↓ = decreased; → = unchanged.

Source: Adapted from DJ Buysse, CF Reynolds. Insomnia. In MJ Thorpy (ed), Handbook of Sleep Disorders. New York: Marcel Dekker, 1990;18:373.

## APPROACH TO SLEEP DISORDERS PATIENTS WITH PSYCHIATRIC ILLNESS

Patients with sleep disorders frequently have symptoms of psychiatric illness. It is the task of the sleep disorders specialist to determine whether there is an underlying organic disorder such as sleep apnea, restless legs syndrome, or periodic limb movements that may cause or contribute to the symptoms. In addition, the sleep specialist can be especially helpful in assessing and correcting behaviors that contribute to sleep impairment. The sleep disorders specialist should have knowledge of the pharmacologic properties of sedatives and stimulants (i.e., onset of action, duration of action, relative toxicity, drug interactions, drug withdrawal effects, and relative effects on alertness and sleep parameters).

Because many sleep practitioners do not have extensive psychiatric training, it is often necessary to engage the assistance of a psychiatrist or psychologist to evaluate a patient with suspected or known psychiatric illness. Psychological tests such as the Minnesota Multiphasic Personality Inventory, Beck Depression Inventory, and State Trait Anxiety Inventory are useful for screening patients with sleep disorders for psychopathology. These tests alone, however, are somewhat limited. Many patients with untreated organic sleep disorders such as sleep apnea show changes in psychological tests that are suggestive of psychopathology, but the changes may resolve following effective treatment of the disorder.

There is mounting objective evidence to support the claim that behavioral techniques are useful in improving insomnia in patients with psychiatric illness. In addition, there are data to support the argument that patients with chronic insomnia have sustained benefit with and without adjunctive sedative administration.[114]

As should be evident from the earlier discussion on various psychopathologic states, the severity of the insomnia of a psychiatric patient often parallels the severity of the illness. Therefore, the aggressiveness of medication and behavioral management of insomnia in psychiatric patients should parallel the severity of psychiatric symptoms present. Patients with severe sleep disturbance due to schizophrenia or affective psychosis often require sedating neuroleptics as well as adjunctive sedative-hypnotics. Patients with schizophrenia and affective disorders

with nocturnal hallucinations may need additional neuroleptic medication for better control of their illness to reduce nighttime hallucinations. Chronic psychiatric illnesses with associated insomnia are much more difficult to manage and may require long-term administration of benzodiazepines, including sedatives of that class. Psychiatric illnesses that are intermittent (e.g., major depression) may require sedatives only during the active phase of the illness.

Insomnia in patients with affective disorders can be addressed in one of several ways: The patient can be given an antidepressant alone, a combination of two antidepressants, a benzodiazepine sedative alone, or a combination of a sedative and an antidepressant. Some antidepressants, such as most of the tricyclic antidepressants and trazodone, have the advantage of causing sedation without the addition of another drug but are limited by side effects, toxicity, and daytime cognitive and alertness impairment. Selective serotonin-reuptake inhibitors (SSRIs) are sometimes combined with other sedating antidepressants such as trazodone to improve sleep. The potential for drug interaction between some antidepressants[115] as well as developing the "serotonin syndrome" exists in this scenario. There is little evidence that sedative treatment of insomnia due to depression without other interventions such as psychotherapy, ECT, or antidepressant therapy relieves depression.[116] Combinations of antidepressants and sedatives can improve insomnia without interfering with the antidepressant effectiveness or onset of action.[117,118]

In some instances, medications used in psychiatric patients aggravate an existing organic sleep problem or insomnia. Antidepressants, antipsychotics, and antihistamines may aggravate restless legs syndrome. Sometimes, nocturnal akathisia, which has symptoms almost identical to restless legs syndrome, is caused by neuroleptic compounds. Medications such as the monoamine oxidase inhibitors, fluoxetine, sertraline, bupropion, protriptyline, and buspirone, which have stimulant properties, may aggravate insomnia. Despite studies showing sleep disruption with stimulating antidepressants, however, patients placed on these compounds often report subjective improvement in their sleep, particularly with the SSRIs.

It is not unusual for patients with psychiatric illness, particularly schizophrenia, to have pseudoinsomnia. The underlying cause for the inability to perceive sleep when it occurs is unknown and is often vexing to the patient, family, and physician. The problem is often identified when the patient complains of little or no sleep but exhibits no daytime fatigue or other impairment. Although the patient is rarely reassured by an overnight study that confirms adequate sleep, the family and health care providers are often relieved to have the information. When obsessive characteristics are identified, medications with specific antiobsessive effects, such as clomipramine and SSRIs, are sometimes helpful.

The appropriate selection of a sedative-hypnotic for patients with psychiatric illness is often more difficult than for the general population. There is greater potential for adverse drug interactions with multiple psychotropic medications than between most sedatives prescribed along with medications used for other conditions. Particular attention must be paid to the duration of action of sedatives in patients with anxiety. There may be a tendency for increased daytime anxiety in patients taking short- and intermediate-acting sedative hypnotics.[119] This problem might be circumvented by using longer-acting sedatives such as flurazepam or quazepam at bedtime, relying on the long-life (80 and 20 hours, respectively) to reduce anxiety during the day. Alternative approaches include using multiple doses of intermediate-acting benzodiazepines (e.g., lorazepam, alprazolam, oxazepam) during the day, and using the same medication at bedtime as a sedative. Another approach is to use a long-acting antianxiety agent such as diazepam, clonazepam, or chlordiazepoxide less frequently during the day and also as a sedative. As most of the intermediate- and long-acting benzodiazepine antianxiety agents have delayed onset, it is often best that they be given approximately an hour before bedtime for the sedative properties to have enough time to take effect. Patients with nocturnal panic attacks may benefit from benzodiazepines such as alprazolam, estazolam, or clonazepam. In addition, various antidepressants, β-blockers, calcium channel blockers, and α-agonists may be useful.

In relatively normal patients, DuPont[120] has suggested that there is a subset of individuals with chronic insomnia who develop performance anxiety specifically about sleep and can benefit from benzodiazepines. In addition, DuPont and Saylor[121] believed that the anxiolytic effects of the benzodi-azepines are sustained for months or years, and that individuals may be able to function well on small doses of benzodiazepines without tending to abuse the drug or increase the dose. As with all patients, those with chronic psychiatric illness with associated chronic insomnia require careful follow-up to ensure that no long-term adverse effects result from psychotropic drugs and, in cases where abusable medications are necessary, that the patients do not develop tolerance leading to excessive usage. When any patient presents to the sleep disorders center taking an excessive amount of a sedative with abuse potential, or taking a normal dose of a sedative for a prolonged period, it is very important to determine whether there is a psychiatric illness or any underlying tendency to abuse drugs. After treatment of underlying organic sleep disorders and training in sleep hygiene and relaxation skills, patients without psychiatric illness may be able to sleep without the help of habituating medication.

## REFERENCES

1. Regier DA, Burke JD, Christie KA. Comorbidity of Affective and Anxiety Disorders in Population Based Studies: The NIMH Epidemiological Catchment Area (ECA) Program. In JD Maser, CR Cloninger (eds), Comorbidity of Anxiety and Depressive Disorders. Washington, DC: American Psychiatric Press, 1990.
2. Ford DE, Kamerow DB. Epidemiological study of sleep disturbances and psychiatric disorders. JAMA 1989;262:1479.
3. Mosko S, Zetin M, Glen S, et al. Self-reported depressive symptomatology, mood ratings, and treatment outcome in sleep disorders patients. J Clin Psychol 1989;45:51.
4. Mellinger GD, Balter MB, Uhlenhuth EH. Insomnia and its treatment: prevalence and correlates. Arch Gen Psychiatry 1985;42:225.

5. Breslau N, Roth T, Rosenthal L, Andreski P. Sleep disturbance and psychiatric disorders: a longitudinal epidemiological study of young adults. Biol Psychiatry 1996;39:411.

6. Eaton WW, Badawi M, Melton B. Prodromes and precursors: epidemiologic data for primary prevention of disorders with slow onset. Am J Psychiatry 1995; 152:967.

7. Gillin JC. Sleep studies in affective illness. Diagnostic, therapeutic and pathophysiological implications. Psychiatr Annu 1983;13:367.

8. Armitage R. Microarchitectural findings in sleep EEG in depression: diagnostic implications. Biol Psychiatry 1995;37:72.

9. Giles DE, Roffwarg HP, Kupfer DF. Secular trend in unipolar depression: a hypothesis. J Affect Disord 1989;14:51.

10. Lauer CJ, Shreiber W, Holsboer F, Kreig JC. In quest of identifying vulnerability markers for psychiatric disorders by all night polysomnography. Arch Gen Psychiatry 1995;52:145.

11. Billiard M, Dolenc L, Aldaz C, et al. Hypersomnia associated with mood disorders: a new perspective. J Psychosom Res 1994;38:S41.

12. Paiva T, Arriaga F, Rosa A, Leitao JN. Sleep phasic events in dysthymic patients: a comparative study with normal controls. Physiol Behav 1993;54:819.

13. Arriaga F, Rosado P, Paiva T. The sleep of dysthymic patients: a comparison with normal controls. Biol Psychiatry 1990;27:649.

14. Puig-Antich J, Goetz R, Hanlon C, et al. Sleep architecture and REM sleep measures in prepubertal major depressives during an episode. Arch Gen Psychiatry 1982;39:932.

15. Young W, Knowles JB, MacLean AW. The sleep of childhood depressives: comparison with age-matched controls. Biol Psychiatry 1982;17:1163.

16. Emslie GH, Roffwarg HP, Rush AJ, et al. Children with major depression show reduced rapid eye movement latencies. Arch Gen Psychiatry 1990;47:119.

17. Dahl RE, Puig-Antich J, Ryan N, et al. EEG sleep in adolescents with major depression: the role of suicidality and inpatient status. J Affect Disord 1990;19:63.

18. Naylor MW, Shain BN, Shipley JE. REM latency in psychotically depressed adolescents. Biol Psychiatry 1990;28:161.

19. Emslie GJ, Rush AJ, Weinberg WA, et al. Sleep EEG features of adolescents with major depression. Biol Psychiatry 1994;36:573.

20. Sabo E, Reynolds DF, Kupfer DJ, et al. Sleep, depression and suicide. Psychiatry Res 1991;36:265.

21. Reynolds CF, Kupfer DF, Thase ME, et al. Sleep, gender and depression: an analysis of gender effects on the electroencephalographic sleep of 302 depressed outpatients. Biol Psychiatry 1990;28:673.

22. Armitage R, Hudson A, Trivedi M, Rush AJ. Sex differences in the distribution of EEG frequencies during sleep: unipolar depressed outpatients. J Affect Disord 1995;34:121.

23. Coble PA, Reynolds CF, Kupfer DJ, et al. Childbearing women with and without a history of affective disorder. II. Electroencephalographic sleep. Compr Psychiatry 1994;35:215.

24. Hawkins DR, Taub JM, van de Castle RL. Extended sleep (hypersomnia) in young, depressed patients. Am J Psychiatry 1985;142:905.

25. Nofzinger EA, Thase ME, Reynolds CF, et al. Hypersomnia in bipolar depression: a comparison with narcolepsy using the multiple sleep latency test. Am J Psychiatry 1991;148:1177.

26. Hoch CC, Buysse DJ, Reynolds DF. Sleep and depression in late life. Clin Geriatr Med 1989;5:259.

27. Reynolds CF. Sleep and affective disorders. A minireview. Psychiatr Clin North Am 1987;10:583.

28. Kupfer DJ, Ehlers CL, Frank E, et al. Persistent effects of antidepressants: EEG sleep studies in depressed patients during maintenance treatment. Biol Psychiatry 1994;35:781.

29. Dealy RS, Reynolds CF, Spiker DG, et al. Effect of ECT on EEG sleep measures in depression. Sleep Res 1982;11:119.

30. Grunhaus L, Shipley JE, Eiser A, et al. Shortened REM latency post ECT is associated with rapid recurrence of depressive symptomatology. Biol Psychiatry 1994; 36:214.

31. Hartman E. Longitudinal studies of sleep and dream patterns in manic-depressive patients. Arch Gen Psychiatry 1968;19:312.

32. Linkowski P, Kerkhofs M, Rielaert C, Mendlewicz J. Sleep during mania in manic-depressive males. Eur Arch Psychiatry Neurol Sci 1986;235:339.

33. Hudson JI, Lipinski JF, Frankenburg FR, et al. Electroencephalographic sleep in mania. Arch Gen Psychiatry 1988;45:267.

34. Bunny WE, Wehr RT, Gillin JC, et al. The switch process in manic-depressive psychosis. Ann Intern Med 1977;87:319.

35. Reynolds CF, Shaw DH, Newton TF, et al. EEG sleep in outpatients with generalized anxiety: a preliminary comparison with depressed outpatients. Psychiatry Res 1983;8:81.

36. Papadimitriou GN, Kerkhofs M, Kempenaers C, et al. EEG sleep studies in patients with generalized anxiety disorder. Psychiatry Res 1988;26:183.

37. Papadimitriou GN, Linkowski P, Kerkhofs M, et al. Sleep EEG recordings in generalized anxiety disorder with significant depression. J Affect Disord 1988;15:113.

38. Stein MB, Kroft CD, Walker JR. Sleep impairment in patients with social phobia. Psychiatry Res 1993;49:251.

39. Stein MB, Millar TW, Larsen DK, Kryger MH. Irregular breathing during sleep in patients with panic disorder. Am J Psychiatry 1995;152:1168.

40. Koenigsberg HW, Pollack CP, Fine J, Kakuma T. Cardiac and respiratory activity in panic disorder: effects

of sleep and sleep lactate infusions. Am J Psychiatry 1994;151:1148.

41. Styres KS. The phenomenon of dysautonomia and mitral valve prolapse. J Am Acad Nurse Pract 1994;6:11.

42. Benarroch EE. The central autonomic network: functional organization, dysfunction and perspective. Mayo Clin Proc 1993;68:988.

43. Pine DS, Weese-Mayer DE, Silvestri JM, et al. Anxiety and congenital central hypoventilation syndrome. Am J Psychiatry 1994;151:864.

44. Craske MG, Barlow DH. Nocturnal panic: response to hyperventilation and carbon dioxide challenge. J Abnorm Psychol 1990;99:302.

45. Ley R. The "suffocation alarm" theory of panic attacks: a critical commentary. J Behav Ther Exp Psychiatry 1994;25:269.

46. Eaton WW, Badawi M, Melton B. Prodromes and precursors: epidemiologic data for primary prevention of disorders with slow onset. Am J Psychiatry 1995;152:967.

47. Roy-Byrne PP, Uhde TW. Exogenous factors in panic disorder. Clinical and research implications. J Clin Psychiatry 1988;49:56.

48. Sheehan DV, Ballenger J, Jacobsen G. Treatment of endogenous anxiety with phobic, hysterical, and hypochondriacal symptoms. Arch Gen Psychiatry 1980;37:51.

49. Mellman TA, Uhde TW. Sleep in Panic and Generalized Anxiety Disorders. In JC Ballenger (ed), Neurobiological Aspects of Panic Disorder. New York: Liss, 1987;5:94.

50. Craske MG, Barlow DH. Nocturnal panic. J Nerv Ment Dis 1989;177:160.

51. Labbate LA, Pollack MH, Otto MW, et al. Sleep panic attacks: an association with childhood anxiety and adult psychopathology. Biol Psychiatry 1994;36:57.

52. Edlund MJ, McNamara EM, Millman RP. Sleep apnea and panic attacks. Compr Psychiatry 1991;32:130.

53. Stoudemire A, Ninan PT, Wooten V. Hypnogenic paroxysmal dystonia with panic attacks responsive to drug therapy. Psychosomatics 1987;28:280.

54. Patterson WM, Koplan AL, Shehi GM, et al. Clinical Correlates in Patients with Panic Disorder: Depression, Sleep Disturbances, Memory Recall and Rage Reactions. Presented to the 34th Annual Meeting of the Academy of Psychosomatic Medicine, November 12–15, 1988. Kalamazoo, MI: Upjohn, 1989.

55. Friedman S, Paradis CM, Hatch M. Characteristics of African-American and white patients with panic disorder and agoraphobia. Hosp Community Psychiatry 1994;45:798.

56. Mellman TA, Uhde TW. Sleep panic attacks: new clinical findings and theoretical implications. Am J Psychiatry 1989;146:1204.

57. Stein MB, Enns MW, Kryger MH. Sleep in nondepressed patients with panic disorder: II. Polysomnographic assessment of sleep architecture and sleep continuity. J Affect Disord 1993;28:1.

58. Mellman TA, Uhde TW. Electroencephalographic sleep in panic disorder. Arch Gen Psychiatry 1989;46:178.

59. Dube S, Jones DA, Bell J, et al. Interface of panic and depression: clinical-EEG correlates. Psychiatry Res 1986;19:119.

60. Uhde TW, Roy-Byrne P, Gillin JC, et al. The sleep of patients with panic disorder: a preliminary report. Psychiatry Res 1985;12:251.

61. Stein MB, Chartier M, Walker JR. Sleep in nondepressed patients with panic disorder: I. Systematic assessment of subjective sleep quality and sleep disturbance. Sleep 1993;16:724.

62. Insel TR, Gillin JC, Moore A, et al. The sleep of patients with obsessive compulsive disorders. Arch Gen Psychiatry 1982;39:1372.

63. van Kammen W, Christiansen C, van Kammen D, et al. Sleep and the POW experience. Sleep Res 1987;16:291.

64. Greenberg R, Pearlman CA, Gampel D. War neuroses and the adaptive function of REM sleep. Br J Med Psychol 1972;45:27.

65. Kauffman CD, Reist C, Djenderedjian A, et al. Biological markers of affective disorders and post traumatic stress disorder: a pilot study with desipramine. J Clin Psychiatry 1987;45:366.

66. Schlosberg A, Benjamin M. Sleep patterns in three acute combat fatigue cases. J Clin Psychiatry 1978;39:546.

67. van der Kolk B, Blitz R, Burr W, et al. Nightmares and trauma: a comparison of nightmares after combat with lifelong nightmares in veterans. Am J Psychiatry 1984;41:187.

68. Hefez A, Metz L, Lavie P. Long term effects of extreme situational stress on sleep and dreaming. Am J Psychiatry 1987;144:344.

69. Schenck CH, Hurwitz TD, Mahowal MW. REM sleep behavior disorder. Am J Psychiatry 1988;145:652.

70. Ross RJ, Ball WA, Sullivan KA, et al. Sleep disturbances as the hallmark of post traumatic stress disorder. Am J Psychiatry 1989;146:697.

71. Mellman TA, Kulick-Bell R, Ashlock LE, Nolan B. Sleep events among veterans with combat-related posttraumatic stress disorder. Am J Psychiatry 1995;152:110.

72. Lauer C, Zulley J, Krieg JC, et al. EEG sleep and the cholinergic induction test in anorexic and bulimic patients. Psychiatry Res 1988;26:171.

73. Katz JL, Kuperberg A, Pollack CP, et al. Is there a relationship between eating and affective disorders? New evidence from sleep recordings. Am J Psychiatry 1984;141:753.

74. Neil JF, Merikangas JR, Foster FG, et al. Waking and all-night sleep EEGs in anorexia nervosa. Clin Electroencephalogr 1980;11:9.

75. Lacey JH, Crips AH, Kalucey RS, et al. Weight gain and the sleeping electroencephalogram: study of ten patients with anorexia nervosa. BMJ 1975;4:556.

76. Bergiannaki JD, Soldatos CR, Sakkas PN, et al. Longitudinal studies of biologic markers for depression in male anorectics. Psychoneuroendocrinology 1987;12:237.

77. Thaker GK, Wagman AMI, Tamminga CA. Sleep polygraphy in schizophrenia: methodological issues. Biol Psychiatry 1990;28:240.

78. Neylan TC, van Kammen DP, Kelley ME, Peters JL. Sleep in schizophrenic patients on and off haloperidol therapy. Clinically stable vs relapsed patients. Arch Gen Psychiatry 1992;49:643.

79. Nofzinger EA, van Kammen DP, Gilbertson MW, et al. Electroencephalographic sleep in clinically stable schizophrenic patients: two-weeks versus six-weeks neuroleptic free. Biol Psychiatry 1993;33:829.

80. van Kammen DP, van Kammen WB, Peters J, et al. Decreased slow wave sleep and enlarged lateral ventricles in schizophrenia. Neuropsychopharmacology 1988;1:265.

81. Benson KL, Zarcone VP. Slow Wave Sleep and Brain Structural Imaging in Schizophrenia. Presented at the 6th Annual Meeting of the Association of Professional Sleep Societies, June 2, 1992. Rochester, MN: APSS Meeting Abstracts, 1992;128.

82. Keshavan MS, Reynolds CF, Ganguli R, et al. Encephalographic sleep and cerebral morphology in functional psychoses: a preliminary study with computed tomography. Psychiatry Res 1991;39:293.

83. Keshavan MS, Pettegrew JW, Reynolds CF, et al. Biological correlates of slow wave sleep deficits in functional psychoses: $^{31}$P-magnetic resonance spectroscopy. Psychiatry Res 1995;57:91.

84. Benson KL, Sullivan EV, Lim KO, Zarcone VP. The effect of total sleep deprivation on slow wave recovery in schizophrenia. Sleep Res 1993;22:143.

85. Dement WC. Dream recall and eye movements in schizophrenics and normals. J Nerv Ment Dis 1955;122:263.

86. Gulevich GD, Dement WC, Zarcone VP. All night sleep recordings of chronic schizophrenics in remission. Compr Psychiatry 1967;8:141.

87. Jus K, Bouchard M, Jus AK, et al. Sleep EEG variables in untreated long-term schizophrenic patients. Arch Gen Psychiatry 1973;29:386.

88. Hiatt JF, Floyd TC, Katz PH, et al. Further evidence of abnormal non-rapid-eye-movement sleep in schizophrenia. Arch Gen Psychiatry 1985;42:797.

89. Caldwell DF, Domino DF. Electroencephalographic and eye movement patterns during sleep in chronic schizophrenia. Electroencephalogr Clin Neurophysiol 1967;22:414.

90. Reich L, Weiss BL, Coble P, et al. Sleep disturbance in schizophrenia: a revisit. Arch Gen Psychiatry 1975;32:51.

91. Ganguli R, Reynold CF, Kupfer DJ. Electroencephalographic sleep in young never-medicated schizophrenics. Arch Gen Psychiatry 1987;44:36.

92. Azumi K. A polygraphic study of sleep in schizophrenics. Seishin Shinkeigaku Zasshi 1966;68:1222.

93. Wyatt R, Termini BA, Davis J. A review of the literature 1960–1970. Part II. Sleep studies. Schizophr Bull 1969;1:45.

94. Cartwright RD. Sleep fantasy in normal and schizophrenic persons. J Abnorm Psychol 1972;80:275.

95. Dement WC, Zarcone VP, Feruson J, et al. Some Parallel Findings in Schizophrenic Patients and Serotonin Depleted Cats. In S Sankar (ed), Schizophrenia: Current Concepts and Research. Hicksville, NY: PJD, 1969;1:775.

96. Benson KL, Zarcone VP. Testing the REM sleep phasic event intrusion hypothesis of schizophrenia. Psychiatry Res 1985;15:163.

97. Crick F, Michelson G. The function of dream sleep. Nature 1983;304:111.

98. Weiler MA, Buchsbaum MS, Gillin JC, et al. Explorations in the relationship of dream sleep to schizophrenia using positron emission tomography. Neuropsychobiology 1990;23:109.

99. Tandon R, Shipley JE, Greden JF, et al. Muscarinic cholinergic hyperactivity in schizophrenia. Relationship to positive and negative symptoms. Schizophr Res 1991;4:23.

100. Cauter EV, Linkowski P, Kerkhofs M, et al. Circadian and sleep-related endocrine rhythms in schizophrenia. Arch Gen Psychiatry 1991;48:348.

101. Tandon R, Shipley JE, Eiser AS, et al. Association between abnormal REM sleep and negative symptoms, in schizophrenia. Psychiatry Res 1988;27:359.

102. Riemann D. Cholinergic REM induction test: muscarinic supersensitivity underlies polysomnographic findings in both depression and schizophrenia. J Psychiatr Res 1994;49:185.

103. Berrettini WH. Paranoid psychosis and sleep apnea syndrome. Am J Psychiatry 1980;137:493.

104. Akiskal HS. Subaffective disorders. Dysthymic, cyclothymic and bipolar II disorders in the borderline realm. Psychiatr Clin North Am 1981;4:25.

105. Akiskal HS, Yerevanian BI, Davis GC, et al. The nosologic status of borderline personality: clinical and polysomnographic study. Am J Psychiatry 1985;142:192.

106. Reynolds CF, Soloff PH, Taska LS, et al. EEG sleep evaluation of depression in borderline patients: a prospective replication. Sleep Res 1984;13:124.

107. Bell J, Lycaki H, Jones D, et al. Effect of preexisting borderline personality disorder on clinical and EEG sleep correlates of depression. Psychiatry Res 1983;9:115.

108. Lahmeyer HW, Val E, Gaviria FM, et al. EEG sleep, lithium transport, dexamethasone suppression, and monoamine oxidase activity in borderline personality disorder. Psychiatry Res 1988;25:19.

109. Allen RP, Singer HS, Brown JE, Salam MM. Sleep disorders in Tourette syndrome: a primary or unrelated problem? Pediatr Neurol 1992;8:275.

110. Kent JD, Blader JC, Koplewicz HS, et al. Effects of late-afternoon methylphenidate administration on behavior and sleep in attention-deficit hyperactivity disorder. Pediatrics 1995;96:320.

111. Busby K, Firestone P, Pivik RT. Sleep patterns in hyperkinetic and normal children. Sleep 1981;4:366.

112. Greenhill L, Puig-Antich J, Goetz R, et al. Sleep architecture and REM sleep measures in prepubertal chil-

dren with attention deficit disorder with hyperactivity. Sleep 1983;6:91.

113. Drake ME, Hietter SA, Bogner JE, Andrews JM. Cassette EEG sleep recordings in Gilles de la Tourette syndrome. Clin Electroencephalogr 1992;23:142.

114. Morin CM, Wooten V. Psychological and pharmacological approaches to treating insomnia: critical issues in assessing their separate and combined effects. Clin Psychol Rev 1996;16:521.

115. Nemeroff CB, DeVane CL, Pollock BG. Newer antidepressants and the cytochrome P450 system. Am J Psychiatry 1996;153:311.

116. Dominguez RA, Jacobson AF, Goldstein BJ, Steinbook RM. Comparison of triazolam and placebo in the treatment of insomnia in depressed patients. Curr Ther Res 1984;36:856.

117. Scharf MB, Hirshkowitz J, Zemlan FP, et al. Comparative effects of limbitrol and amitriptyline on sleep efficiency and architecture. J Clin Psychiatry 1996;47:587.

118. Cohn JB. Triazolam treatment of insomnia in depressed patients taking tricyclics. J Clin Psychiatry 1983;44:401.

119. Buysse DJ, Reynolds CF, Houck PR, et al. Does adjunctive lorazepam impair the antidepressant response to nortriptyline in elderly depressed patients? Sleep Res 1996;25:153.

120. DuPont RL. Overcoming Sleep Disorders. A Guide for Insomniacs. Rockville, MD: Institute for Behavior and Health, 1990;1:1.

121. DuPont RL, Saylor KE. Sedatives/Hypnotics and Benzodiazepines. In RV Frances, SI Miller (eds), Clinical Textbook of Addictive Disorders. New York: Guilford, 1991;1:69.

# Chapter 29

# Sleep Disturbances
# in Other Medical Disorders

## Sudhansu Chokroverty

Sleep disturbances associated with seven medical disorders are listed under the category of other medical disorders in the *International Classification of Sleep Disorders (ICSD)*[1]: sleeping sickness, nocturnal cardiac ischemia, chronic obstructive pulmonary disease (COPD), sleep-related asthma, sleep-related gastroesophageal reflux, peptic ulcer disease, and fibromyalgia. A number of other medical disorders may cause severe disturbances of sleep and breathing that have important practical implications, in terms of diagnosis, prognosis, and treatment. These other medical disorders not listed in the *ICSD* are also briefly reviewed in this chapter to give an overview of sleep disturbances in the general medical disorders. They are included because sleep disturbance may adversely affect the course of the medical illness, and, of course, the medical disorders and drugs prescribed to treat them may have deleterious effects on sleep and breathing.

When a patient presents to a sleep specialist with sleep disturbance, either with the complaint of insomnia or hypersomnia, the first important step is to obtain a detailed medical history and other histories, followed by physical examination to uncover a cause for the sleep disturbance. Often, the patient presents to an internist or a family practice physician, who may then refer for a consultation to a sleep specialist if there are sleep complaints. Therefore, a comprehensive knowledge of major medical disorders that may present with sleep disturbance is essential, and in this section a brief outline of the salient clinical diagnostic points is offered, followed by some key laboratory investigations of some important medical disorders presenting with sleep disturbance.

Gislason and Almqvist[2] made an epidemiologic study in a random sample of 3,201 Swedish men aged 30–69 years. Difficulty initiating or maintaining sleep and too little sleep were the major complaints, followed by excessive daytime somnolence (EDS) or too much sleep. Sleep maintenance problems became more frequent with increasing age. The following conditions were associated with the sleep complaints: systemic hypertension, bronchitis and bronchial asthma, musculoskeletal disorders, obesity, and diabetes mellitus. The authors suggested that the reported increased mortality among patients with sleep complaints might be related to the intercurrent somatic diseases.

In a questionnaire of 100 adult male medical and surgical patients in a teaching hospital in Melbourne, Australia, Johns and coworkers[3] found sleep duration to be the same as that in the general population. The sleep duration decreased from 20 to 50 years of age, then increased again after age 60. Daytime sleep duration increased with age. These authors found that increasing age and ischemic heart disease were mostly associated with long-term sleep disturbances.

## MEDICAL DISORDERS THAT CAUSE SLEEP DISTURBANCES

A brief description of the clinical features of some of the medical disorders associated with sleep disturbances is given in this section, but for further details readers should consult general textbooks of internal medicine.

- Cardiovascular diseases: cardiac arrhythmia, congestive cardiac failure (CCF), ischemic heart disease, nocturnal angina
- Intrinsic respiratory disorders: COPD, asthma (including nocturnal asthma), restrictive lung disease
- Gastrointestinal diseases: peptic ulcer disease and reflux esophagitis
- Endocrine diseases: hyperthyroidism, hypothyroidism, diabetes mellitus, growth hormone (GH) deficiency and excess
- Renal disorders: chronic renal failure (CRF), sleep disturbances associated with renal dialysis
- Hematologic disorders
- Rheumatic disorders, including fibromyalgia syndrome (FMS)
- Miscellaneous disorders: acquired immunodeficiency syndrome (AIDS), Lyme disease, medical and surgical disorders of patients in medical and surgical intensive care units (ICU), chronic fatigue syndrome (CFS), sleeping sickness

## MECHANISM OF SLEEP DISTURBANCES IN MEDICAL DISORDERS

Sleep disturbance may have an adverse effect on the course of a medical illness. Thus, a vicious cycle may result from the effect of sleep disturbance on the medical disease and the effect of the medical illness on sleep architecture.

Sleep may be disturbed in medical disorders by a variety of mechanisms, including

- Indirect effects on the hypnogenic neurons in the diencephalon and brain stem, and respiratory neurons in the brain stem by metabolic disturbances (e.g., renal, hepatic, or respiratory failure; electrolyte disturbances; hypoglycemia or hyperglycemia; ketosis; toxic states)
- Adverse effects on sleep organization and sleep structure by drugs used to treat medical illness
- Disturbances of circadian rhythm (i.e., sleep-wake schedule)
- Effects on the peripheral respiratory mechanism (including respiratory muscles) causing respiratory sleep disorder

- Esophageal reflux, which may be due to prolongation of acid clearance of the lower esophagus, aspiration, and reflex mechanism (see Chapter 6)
- Adverse effect on sleep structure after prolonged immobilization resulting from medical disorders
- Dysfunction of the autonomic nervous system caused by medical disorder (e.g., diabetes mellitus, amyloidosis)

## GENERAL FEATURES OF SLEEP DISTURBANCES IN MEDICAL ILLNESS

Sleep architecture, sleep continuity, and sleep organization may be affected in a variety of medical illnesses. Patients may present with either insomnia or hypersomnolence, but most medical disorders present with insomnia. Some patients may have a mixture of insomnia and hypersomnolence (e.g., those with COPD or nocturnal asthma).

Patients with insomnia may complain of lack of initiation of sleep, inability to maintain sleep, repeated arousals at night, early morning awakening. Daytime symptoms of fatigue, inability to concentrate, irritability, anxiety, and sometimes depression[4] may be related to the sleep deprivation. Polysomnographic (PSG) findings include prolonged sleep latency, reduction of rapid eye movement (REM) and slow-wave sleep (SWS), more than 10 awakenings per night, frequent stage shifts, early morning awakening, increased waking after sleep onset (WASO), and increased percentage of wakefulness and stage I non-REM (NREM) sleep.[5]

Patients with hypersomnolence may present with repeated daytime somnolence, fatigue, depression, headache, and intellectual deterioration related to repeated sleep-related disordered breathing and hypoxemia.[6–9] PSG findings consist of sleep-disordered breathing (SDB), repeated arousals with oxygen desaturation at night, sleep fragmentation, sleep stage shifts, reduced SWS, shortened sleep-onset latency on the Multiple Sleep Latency Test (MSLT), and sometimes REM sleep abnormalities.[6–9]

Systemic medical disorders may cause neurologic disturbances, which in turn may cause sleep disturbances either directly by affecting sleep-wake systems in the central nervous system (CNS) or indirectly by affecting breathing. Sleep-related breathing dysfunction and neurologic illness are described in Chapter 27.

## SPECIFIC MEDICAL DISORDERS AND SLEEP DISTURBANCES

### Cardiovascular Disease

It is generally well-known that sleep disturbances may occur in cardiovascular diseases, particularly in patients with ischemic heart disease, myocardial infarction, or CCF. Cardiac arrhythmias and sudden cardiac death at night are also known to occur, although adequate objective tests, including PSG study to document such disturbances, are lacking.

### Ischemic Heart Disease

A careful inquiry into history is most important in making the diagnosis. The patient complains of a sense of tightness in the middle of the chest and a bandlike feeling around the chest. The pain is often induced by exertion and relieved by rest. Generally, it lasts only a few minutes. When the patient complains of pain on lying supine, it is known as *angina decubitus*, whereas pain that awakens the patient at night is known as *nocturnal angina*. Infrequently, the pain results from coronary artery spasm accompanied by transient ST elevation in the electrocardiogram (ECG), and the entity is then known as *Prinzmetal's* or *variant angina*. The condition is most common in middle-aged men but may affect postmenopausal women. Complications include cardiac arrhythmias; left ventricular failure; acute myocardial infarction; and sudden cardiac, often nocturnal, death.

Sleep disturbances are very common in patients with ischemic heart disease. Pain may awaken the patient, causing frequent awakenings and reduced sleep efficiency. Obstructive sleep apnea syndrome (OSAS) is associated sometimes with arterial hypoxemia causing cardiac ischemia. Simultaneous recording of ECG may show ST depression at least 1 mm below the horizontal, whereas ST elevation occurs in Prinzmetal's or variant angina. Often, the patient complains of discomfort in the arms during the retrosternal pain. Pain may sometimes radiate to the epigastrium or to the neck and the jaw. It may be accompanied by shortness of breath. ECG is essential for the diagnosis of ischemic heart disease or myocardial infarction. Coronary angiography provides information about the site of coronary artery occlusion.

Treatment consists of avoiding exertion for patients susceptible to angina attacks and administration of drugs such as nitrates, β-blockers, and calcium antagonists. Patients with severe symptoms that persist despite medical treatment may need surgical treatment in the form of coronary artery bypass grafting.

**Nocturnal Angina and Sleep Disturbance.** Nocturnal angina is known to occur during both REM and NREM sleep stages. Karacan and coworkers[10] found increased sleep-onset latency, reduced stage III and IV NREM sleep, decreased sleep efficiency, and very little change in REM sleep on PSG study in 10 patients with a history of nocturnal angina.

Nowlin and colleagues[11] noted an increased number of nocturnal anginal attacks (32 of 39 attacks associated with REM sleep) with ECG changes of ST segment depression in four patients with a history of angina. King and coworkers[12] described Prinzmetal's or variant angina during REM sleep. In contrast, Stern and Tzivoni[13] recorded ECG continuously for 24 hours in 140 patients with ischemic heart disease and could not ascribe ST segment changes to dreaming. It should be pointed out, however, that these authors did not record electroencephalography (EEG) or electrooculography (EOG) to document sleep stages objectively. Murao and colleagues,[14] after all-night polygraphic studies in 12 patients with nocturnal angina, found more episodes of ischemic ECG changes during REM sleep.

Epidemiologically, there is a clear relationship between increased cardiovascular morbidity and mortality and sleep disturbances associated with SDB. Patients with coronary artery disease (CAD) and OSA may have an increased cardiac risk due to nocturnal myocardial ischemia triggered by apnea-associated oxygen desaturation. Schafer et al.[15] studied 14 patients with OSA and coronary heart disease and seven patients with OSA but without coronary arterial disease using overnight PSG and ECG recordings. They found an increased number of apnea-related ischemic episodes associated with low oxygen desaturation. Nitrate administration did not reduce ischemic episodes. Sleep architecture showed reduction of SWS and REM sleep as well as increased and more severe arousals during periods with myocardial ischemia than during control episodes. They also noted that approximately 78% of ischemic episodes occurred during REM sleep. Andreas et al.[16] investigated the prevalence of OSA in 50 patients with CAD diagnosed by coronary angiography. They found a high apnea index in 25 patients and EDS in eight of these patients. In 19 of the patients who had an all-night PSG, the mean apnea-hypopnea index was 32.4, the mean oxygen saturation was 87.3, and the minimum oxygen saturation was 75.5. The authors concluded that CAD patients may have a high prevalence of OSA.

In an important study, Kripke and associates[17] noted increased mortality rates among patients with ischemic heart disease, stroke, and cancer who slept 4 hours or less, or more than 10 hours. Wingard and Berkman[18] in their study of approximately 7,000 adults over a period of 9 years also found excessive mortality from ischemic heart disease in short sleepers (less than 7 hours) and long sleepers (more than 9 hours). Poor sleep is thus associated with increased risk of future cardiovascular morbidity or mortality.[17–19]

**Sleep in Myocardial Infarction.**   In 12 patients who had experienced acute myocardial infarction studied in the ICU, Broughton and Baron[20] found decreased sleep efficiency, increased sleep stage shifts, increased awakenings, and decreased REM sleep. Sleep pattern became normal by the ninth day of the illness. Circadian susceptibility to myocardial infarction (attacks are most likely between midnight and 6:00 AM) has been noted.[21,22] Karacan and coworkers[23] studied four patients with myocardial infarction in the ICU continuously from the second to the sixth day and found increased wakefulness, reduced REM sleep, absent stage III and IV NREM sleep, and a partial breakdown in the circadian cycling.

**Sleep in Congestive Cardiac Failure.**   Sleep disturbances, periodic breathing, and hypoxemia at night have been described in patients with CCF.[24–28] The increased morbidity and mortality in CCF results from multiple factors, including associated SDB and nocturnal oxygen desaturation. Cheyne-

Stokes respiration, commonly associated with CCF, (approximately 40% of patients with a left ventricular ejection fraction of less than 40%)[28] may result in hypoxemia, hypercapnia, sleep disruption due to repeated arousals, EDS, and impaired cognitive function.[26,27,29–31] Thus, Cheyne-Stokes respiration in CCF may present as sleep apnea syndrome. The recognition of this syndrome as a distinct entity in CCF is important because of its impact on heart failure and of treatment implications. Javaheri and colleagues[26,32] studied 42 patients with stable heart failure without other comorbid factors. Nineteen of these patients (45%) had an apnea-hypopnea index higher than 20. All episodes were associated with increased arousals and arterial desaturation. After treatment with nocturnal oxygen administration, continuous positive airway pressure (CPAP) titration, and medications such as theophylline, the patient showed improvement. These authors[32] suggested that large-scale control studies are needed to further delineate the central sleep apnea-hypopnea syndrome and to understand its pathogenesis and effects of various treatment modalities. Previously, Hanly et al.[33] performed two consecutive overnight sleep studies in nine men from outpatients with severe but stable CCF to determine the effects of supplemental oxygen on Cheyne-Stokes respiration and sleep in these patients. They found that nocturnal oxygen therapy reduced Cheyne-Stokes breathing, controlled hypoxemia, and consolidated sleep by reducing arousals caused by the hyperapneic phase of Cheyne-Stokes respiration. Because of increased mortality associated with CCF,[26,34,35] various therapeutic modalities have been directed at alleviating Cheyne-Stokes respiration with central sleep apnea in these patients. CPAP has been used, but its role in central apnea of heart failure is not clear. Takasaki et al.[36] reported the first case-controlled trial of nocturnal CPAP for the treatment of Cheyne-Stokes respiration and central apnea in five patients with CCF. This treatment alleviated Cheyne-Stokes respiration and improved left ventricular ejection fraction. Bradley[37] and Granton and colleagues[38] later demonstrated that nasal CPAP, if applied nightly at high enough pressure (10.0–12.5 cm $H_2O$) over a period of at least 1–3 months, can alleviate Cheyne-Stokes respiration and central sleep apnea in patients with CCF as well as bring about hemodynamic improvement. Whether this intervention can provide long-term clinical benefit to these patients requires longer trials of CPAP. A single-night study[39] and a well-designed blinded protocol[40] failed to show any improvement in sleep quality, daytime sleepiness, or left ventricular ejection fraction as a result of CPAP therapy in CCF patients. Calverley[41] has cautioned that substantial questions remain to be answered before the role of CPAP in the maintenance treatment of CCF can be considered established.

*Sleep and Cardiac Arrhythmias*

An understanding of the interaction between the autonomic nervous system, cardiac innervation, and sleep is important to appreciating the effects of sleep on cardiac rhythms. Readers are referred to Chapters 6 and 27 for such review. A relationship between sleep and atrioventricular arrhythmias has been noted, but reports in the literature are somewhat contradictory. Atrial arrhythmias, such as atrial flutter, atrial fibrillation, paroxysmal atrial tachycardia,[42] and first- and second-degree atrioventricular block,[43] have been described in normal subjects during REM sleep, but no clear relationship between different sleep stages and atrial arrhythmias has emerged. A prominent sinus arrhythmia has been noted in several studies in normal subjects using Holter monitoring.[44] Brodsky and colleagues[45] monitored 24-hour continuous ECG in 50 male medical students with no apparent heart disease and observed sinus pauses of 1.8–2.0 seconds' duration in 30% of them, as well as episodes of second-degree heart block (Mobitz type I) in another 6%. Guilleminault and associates[46] noted 42 episodes of sinus arrest in four young, healthy adults that lasted 2–9 seconds during REM sleep. No associated apneas or significant oxygen desaturation was observed. The incidence of nocturnal bradyarrhythmias decreases with advancing age.[47]

Contradictory results have been noted in human studies of the effects of sleep on ventricular arrhythmia, but the majority show an antiarrhythmic effect of sleep on ventricular premature beats (VPB).[48] This seems to be due to enhanced parasympathetic tone during sleep, confirming protection against ventricular arrhythmia and sudden cardiac death. Pitzalis et al.[49] evaluated 45 patients with frequent premature ventricular contractions to find out whether the phenomenon of sleep suppression may be a sensitive and specific parameter for predicting

the anti-arrhythmic effect of β-blockers and premature ventricular contractions. Based on Holter recordings, these authors concluded that sleep suppression of the premature ventricular contractions was a sensitive characteristic for identifying those patients with premature ventricular contractions who are likely to benefit from administration of β-blockers. Ventricular arrhythmias are also noted to occur during arousal from sleep.[48] A classic example was provided by Wellens and colleagues,[50] who described a 14-year-old girl awakened from sleep by a loud auditory stimulus who had ventricular tachyarrhythmia. The authors postulated that increased sympathetic activity triggered these episodes, because they could be prevented by the (β-blocker propranolol).

Holter monitoring may reveal several ECG changes during sleep in patients with ischemic heart diseases, including ST segment depression and T wave inversion.[13] Cardiac ischemia associated with ST segment depression or elevation during sleep at night has been noted in some middle-aged men and postmenopausal women. In contrast, subjects with normal ECG findings showed no ST segment changes.[51]

Lown's group[52] noted reduction of VPB by at least 50% in 22 subjects and 25–35% in 13 others during sleep. De Silva[53] noted reduction in VPB in all stages except REM sleep, with stages III and IV NREM sleep showing the most effect. Pickering and colleagues[54] described 12 untreated patients with frequent ventricular extrasystoles who showed a significant decrease in both the heart rate and extrasystoles during sleep. Intravenous propranolol (a β-blocker), and to a lesser extent intravenous phenylephrine, produced similar decrease in the heart rate and ventricular arrhythmias during wakefulness. These changes appear to be mediated by the autonomic nervous system, the sympathetic system dominating the parasympathetic system. They found that the frequency of ventricular arrhythmias was similar in both REM and NREM sleep. Their findings are similar to those of Lown and colleagues.[52] In contrast, Rosenblatt's group[55] observed arrhythmias during stage III and IV NREM sleep. These authors noted VPB with similar frequency during wakefulness and REM sleep.

It is known that there is an imbalance between sympathetic and parasympathetic tone during REM and NREM sleep. Gillis and colleagues[56] observed no group difference in the frequency of ventricular premature depolarization (VPD) during REM and NREM sleep. After studying 14 patients with ventricular arrhythmias, they concluded that heart rate determined the diurnal variation of VPD. The reduction of VPD frequently correlated with the reduction in the heart rate and was independent of sleep state or wakefulness.

The observations of Pickering's group[54] also contrast with those of Smith and coworkers,[57] who studied 18 patients in a coronary care unit to document frequency of cardiac arrhythmias in wakefulness and sleep. They found no significant difference in the occurrence of ventricular or atrial premature contractions during sleep and wakefulness. Similarly, Richards et al.,[58] in a pilot overnight sleep study on nine patients with cardiovascular disease in the medical ICU, did not find any increase in incidence of dysrhythmia during any sleep stages or during sleep state in these critical care unit patients. Disturbed sleep in coronary care patients[20] may explain the discrepancies in these data.

*Sleep and Sudden Cardiac Death*

An analysis of the time of sudden cardiac death in 2,203 individuals by Muller and associates[21] revealed a low incidence during the night and a high incidence from 7:00 to 11:00 AM. Similarly, nonfatal myocardial infarction and myocardial ischemic episodes are more likely to occur in the morning. It is known that sympathetic activity increases in the morning, causing increased myocardial electrical instability; thus, sudden cardiac death may result from a primary fatal arrhythmia.

LaRovere and associates[59] correlated increased cardiovascular mortality among patients with a first myocardial infarction with reduced baroreflex sensitivity (BRS). *Reduced BRS* is defined as less slowing in heart rate for a given rise in arterial blood pressure, which indicates reduced vagal tone.

McWilliams[60] first suggested that ventricular fibrillation is the cause of sudden death and that sympathetic discharges play an important role in causing this fatal arrhythmia. During sleep, cardiovascular hemodynamic activity is decreased, as are heart rate and blood pressure, owing to withdrawal of sympathetic tone and increased vagal tone (see Chapter 6).

Reduced vagal tone, as measured by decreased heart rate variability in 24-hour Holter monitoring, was found by Kleiger and colleagues[61] to be a powerful predictor of increased mortality and sudden cardiac death after myocardial infarction. Autonomic imbalance (either sympathetic overactivity or parasympathetic underactivity) may trigger ventricular arrhythmias.[62]

Besides myocardial infarction, another clinical entity known as *congenital long QT syndrome* (CLQTS) may cause syncope or sudden death.[63] In CLQTS, ECG shows a prolonged QT interval with abnormal U waves and torsades de pointes (polymorphic ventricular tachycardia).

Tanchaiswad[64] concluded in his review that sudden unexplained nocturnal death syndrome during sleep in healthy, young men from the northeastern part of Thailand may be related to the instability of the physiologic systems, particularly respiration during the REM stage.

*Sleep and Hypertension*

There is a high prevalence (22–48%) of sleep apnea and related symptoms (e.g., EDS) in patients with systemic hypertension.[65–68] In contrast, studies by Escourrour and colleagues[69] found no significant difference between 21 hypertensive and 29 normotensive patients in sleep stage distribution and disorganization, apnea-hypopnea index and duration, and oxygen saturation. These 50 patients did not have airway obstruction as evidenced by forced expiratory volume in 1 second ($FEV_1$) value or daytime hypoxemia and were selected from 65 patients referred to the sleep clinic complaining of daytime hypersomnolence and snoring. The prevalence of hypertension in sleep apnea patients is approximately 50–90%.[6,70–81] In the Wisconsin Sleep Cohort study, a dose-response relationship between hypertension and the apnea-hypopnea index as well as snoring has been described.[82,83] Furthermore, the studies have confirmed that treatment of sleep apnea by nasal CPAP reduces blood pressure.[84,85]

Stradling and Davies[86] made a persuasive argument based on a critical analysis of the literature and taking into consideration the confounding variables (e.g., age, sex, smoking, obesity, and alcohol consumption) that there is no convincing evidence yet supporting the contention that OSA is a significant independent risk factor for sustained hypertension in humans. They suggested that a large randomized controlled trial by CPAP on blood pressure in patients with a range of OSA severity is needed before CPAP can be recommended for asymptomatic OSA patients. Several reports support this conclusion.[87-91] Silverberg and Oksenberg,[92,93] however, contend that even when the confounding factors are taken into consideration, OSA is an independent risk factor for hypertension and that treatment of OSA reduces daytime as well as nighttime blood pressure. Based on an analysis of the research data in the literature, Silverberg and Oksenberg[93] suggested a unifying hypothesis that essential hypertension is mainly due to increased upper airway resistance during sleep.

### Intrinsic Respiratory Disorders

#### Chronic Obstructive Pulmonary Disease

To understand sleep disturbances it is important to have some knowledge of gas exchange during sleep.[94] In COPD patients, $SaO_2$ and $PaO_2$ fall and $PaCO_2$ rises during sleep; these values worsen during REM sleep.[95-98] Some patients' SDB (e.g., apnea, hypopnea, or periodic breathing) is associated with reduced $SaO_2$ saturation, which is generally short-lived (less than 1 minute) and mild to moderate in intensity.[99-101] Episodes of $SaO_2$ desaturation during REM sleep last more than 5 minutes and are more severe than in NREM sleep.[99,102,103] Physiologic changes in respiration, respiratory muscles, and control of breathing (see Chapter 6) during sleep adversely affect breathing in these patients. In COPD patients, two basic mechanisms worsen hypoxemia during sleep: alveolar-hypoventilation, which is worse during REM sleep, and ventilation-perfusion mismatching.[104-107]

Other groups at risk for hypoxemia include the middle-aged and elderly (particularly men), postmenopausal women, and obese individuals.[94] Diminished ventilatory response to hypoxia and hypercapnia in some COPD patients contributes to increasing nocturnal oxygen desaturation.[94] Nocturnal hypoxemia causes repeated disruption and fragmentation of sleep architecture.[94]

COPD includes chronic bronchitis and emphysema. The salient clinical features include chronic cough, exertional dyspnea, tightness in the chest, and sometimes wheeze. Physical examination reveals inspiratory and expiratory rhonchi and crepitations. Patients with resting hypoxemia and hypercapnia may exhibit cyanosis. Investigations should include radiographic examination of the chest and pulmonary function tests. Complications include polycythemia, pulmonary hypertension, cor pulmonale, and cardiac arrhythmias.

COPD patients are traditionally divided into two groups, "pink puffers" and "blue bloaters."[108,109] Pink puffers generally have normal blood gases, hyperinflated lungs, no hypoxemia or hypercapnia, and no cardiomegaly or cor pulmonale.[94] On the other hand, blue bloaters are generally hypoxemic and hypercapnic and have cor pulmonale, polycythemia, enlarged heart, and reduced ventilatory response to hypoxemia and hypercapnia.[94] In general, blue bloaters have more severe hypoxemia of longer duration than pink puffers.[110,111] It should be noted that oxygen saturation for both groups is somewhat similar during wakefulness and in the upright position but is markedly different during sleep. The worse value is noted in blue bloaters. There are no absolute criteria for determining which groups of COPD patients have more severe nocturnal hypoxemia. Patients must be monitored at night, which is impractical considering the large number of patients who should be monitored. In some patients, COPD may coexist with OSAS—a condition called *overlap syndrome*, a term introduced by Flenley.[112] In a study[113] of 265 consecutive unselected OSAS patients, COPD was found to be present in 30 (11%) of these patients. Coexistence of COPD and OSAS results in a higher risk of pulmonary hypertension and CCF than in those with only OSAS.[104,105]

#### Changes in Sleep Architecture

Disturbances in sleep architecture in COPD patients have been reported by several authors.[96,114-119] These disturbances may be summarized as follows: a reduction of sleep efficiency, delayed sleep onset, increased WASO, frequent stage shifts, and frequent arousals. Arand and coworkers[114] correlated these findings with EDS.

A number of factors cause sleep disturbances in COPD patients, resulting in disturbed EEG sleep patterns, including the use of drugs that have a sleep-reducing effect, such as methylxanthines; increased nocturnal cough resulting from accumulated bronchial secretions; and associated hypoxemia and hypercapnia.[104,120] In a study by Calverley,[121] administration of supplemental oxygen at 2 liters per minute by nasal cannula during sleep improved both oxygen saturation at night and sleep architecture, in terms of decreasing sleep latency and increasing all stages of sleep including REM and SWS. Other reports did not note improved sleep quality, but the nocturnal hypoxemia did improve after oxygen administration.[114,115]

### Cardiac Arrhythmias in Chronic Obstructive Pulmonary Disease

There are several reports of increasing prevalence of cardiac arrhythmias, particularly during sleep, in COPD patients. According to Flick and Block,[122] the incidence of premature ventricular contractions peaks between 3:00 and 5:00 AM and between 6:00 and 7:00 AM. In a study by Shepard and colleagues,[123] a relationship between nocturnal oxygen desaturation and cardiac arrhythmias was established in 42 COPD patients. These authors found premature ventricular contractions in 64% of patients. In six patients with oxygen desaturation below 80% during REM sleep, there was a 150% increase in premature ventricular contractions. The authors concluded that factors such as hypoxemia, hypercapnia, elevation of systemic blood pressure with increased myocardial oxygen demands, and increased catecholamines contributed to increasing irritability.

### Treatment of Nocturnal Oxygen Desaturation

Investigators have become aware of severe nocturnal hypoxemia in many patients with COPD.[95–98] This nocturnal hypoxemia may or may not be accompanied by sleep-related apnea, hypopnea, or periodic breathing and impairment of gas exchange.[99–101] It is clear that repeated or prolonged oxygen desaturation at night may cause cardiac arrhythmias and may lead to pulmonary hypertension and cor pulmonale.[123] In addition, patients with COPD show changes in sleep[96,114–119] architecture that may be related to the poor quality of sleep or may be secondary to nocturnal hypoxemia causing disruption of nocturnal EEG sleep stages. Oxygen desaturation during sleep in COPD patients can be identified only if PSG, using sleep staging or continuous monitoring of oxygenation, is performed. Several studies show episodes of oxygen desaturation during sleep in COPD patients.

An important study by Wynne's group[99] showed that oxygen desaturation could be associated with two types of patients: those with SDB (apnea and hypopnea) and those without SDB. In patients with SDB, the desaturation typically lasts less than 1 minute and is mild. In the other group, the desaturation lasts 1–30 minutes and is associated with a profound decrease in oxygen saturation. The maximum episodes, lasting longer than 5 minutes, occur during REM sleep. Similar episodes of nocturnal oxygen desaturation have been described in patients with kyphoscoliosis,[124,125] in young patients with cystic fibrosis,[103,126,127] and in patients with interstitial lung disease.[128,129]

Modern treatment of nocturnal hypoxemia is administration of oxygen by nasal cannula at a slow flow rate, usually less than 2 liters per minute. The multiple-center study by the Nocturnal Oxygen Therapy Trial Group[130] and the Medical Research Council Working Party study[131] showed increased longevity for patients who used continuous supplemental oxygen at home.

Particular indications for supplemental oxygen can be summarized as follows: daytime $Pao_2$ below 55 mm Hg; and daytime $Pao_2$ between 55 and 60 mm Hg accompanied by signs of right-sided heart failure, unexplained polycythemia, pulmonary hypertension, and cor pulmonale.[120,132] Oxygen administration may also improve sleep architecture.[121]

The question of safety of oxygen administration has to be determined.[94] Some patients become more hypercapnic after oxygen administration.[96] Furthermore, Motta and Guilleminault[133] showed the worsening effects of administration of oxygen at night in patients with OSAS. Many patients with COPD may have OSA (overlap syndrome),[96,112,113] so physicians must be careful during administration of oxygen. Kearley and colleagues[134] have shown that administration of oxygen at 2 liters per minute reduces the episodic desaturation. Fleetham and associates[135] confirmed this finding, but Guilleminault and coworkers[101] contradicted these findings in five patients with excessive sleepiness associated with chronic obstructive airflow disease. The multiple-institution studies by the Nocturnal Oxygen Therapy Trial Group[130] showed the relative safety of oxygen therapy, however, including home oxygen. In COPD patients undergoing long-term oxygen therapy, it may be useful to monitor breathing and oxygen saturation by pulse finger oximetry during sleep at night.[136]

Some patients with COPD and nocturnal hypoxemia benefit from treatment with medroxyprogesterone acetate, a respiratory stimulant,[137,138] but the results have not been consistent. Similarly, acetazolamide, which improves sleep hypoxemia and periodic breathing in patients with acute mountain sickness,[139] has not been found effective in the majority of patients with COPD.

Almitrine[120,139–141] has been found to improve ventilation in COPD patients. Almitrine acts by stimulating peripheral chemoreceptors, thus improving hypoxic ventilatory drive. A dangerous side effect of almitrine noted both in animals and humans with COPD is acute rise of pulmonary artery pressure, as reported by MacNee and coworkers.[142] The long-term effect of the drug treatment, in terms of morbidity and mortality, as well as the natural history of COPD must be clearly assessed before recommending judicious use of these drugs.

### Bronchial Asthma, Including Nocturnal Asthma

The characteristic clinical triad of asthma is the paroxysm of dyspnea, wheezing, and cough. The paroxysmal attacks of wheezing and breathlessness may occur at any hour of the day or night, and the nocturnal attacks are distributed at random without any relationship to a particular sleep stage. Breathing is characterized by prolonged expiration accompanied by wheezing and unproductive cough. There may be tightness of the chest and palpitation. The attacks last for 1–2 hours. When the attacks last hours, the disorder is called *acute severe asthma* or *status asthmaticus*; this is a life-threatening condition because of extreme respiratory distress and arterial hypoxemia.

Pulmonary function tests and radiographic examination of the chest are important for confirming the diagnosis of bronchial asthma. Abnormalities of certain pulmonary function tests (i.e., $FEV_1$, vital capacity [VC], peak expiratory flow [PEF]) suggest airflow obstruction. Chest radiography may reveal hyperinflated lungs and emphysema.

### Sleep Disturbances in Bronchial Asthma

A variety of sleep disturbances have been noted in patients with asthma. Janson and associates,[143] using questionnaires and sleep diaries, studied the prevalence of sleep complaints and sleep disturbances prospectively in 98 consecutive adult asthma patients attending an outpatient clinic in Uppsala, Sweden. Compared with 226 age- and sex-matched controls, they found a high incidence of sleep disturbances in asthma patients, including early morning awakening, difficulty in maintaining sleep, and EDS. Sleep disturbances in general consist of a combination of insomnia and hypersomnia. PSG studies may reveal disruption of sleep architecture as well as sleep apnea in some patients.

Nocturnal exacerbation of symptoms during sleep is a frequent finding in asthma patients.[105] There is also evidence of progressive bronchoconstriction and hypoxemia during sleep in patients with asthma.[144] In an important study by Turner-Warwick,[145] 94% of 7,729 asthmatics surveyed woke up at least once a night with symptoms of asthma, 74% at least one night a week, 64% at least three nights a week, and 39% every night. Nocturnal asthma is a potentially serious problem, as there is a high incidence of respiratory arrests and sudden death in adult asthmatics between midnight and 8:00 AM.[146,147]

To understand the relationship between the attacks of asthma and sleep stage and time of night, Kales and colleagues[148] studied six men and six women aged 20–45 years with PSG, each for two to three consecutive nights. They observed a total of 93 asthma attacks in these patients, 73 during NREM sleep and 18 during REM. They did not find a relationship between asthma attacks and sleep stage or time of night. Sleep pattern showed less total sleep time, frequent WASOs, early final awakenings, and reduced stage IV sleep. Kales' group[149] observed similar findings in a PSG study of 10 asthmatic children. Montplaisir and colleagues[150] studied 12 asthmatics, eight of whom showed nocturnal attacks on sleep studies (six women and two men aged 20–51 years).

Two questionnaire surveys from the European community[151,152] found that bronchial asthma was associated with increased daytime sleepiness and impaired subjective quality of sleep (difficulty initiating sleep and early morning awakenings). One survey also noted increased prevalence of snoring and sleep-related apneas during sleep.[151] In the same survey, associated allergic rhinitis may have been a confounding variable. Twenty-six attacks were documented. No attacks occurred in stage III or IV NREM sleep, nor were attacks more frequent during REM than NREM sleep. Thus, stage III and IV sleep was "protective." Sleep efficiency was decreased. The number and duration of apneas were not significantly greater in asthmatics than in controls. Episodes of oxygen desaturation occurred only in the asthmatics. Sleep efficiency and waking time after sleep onset were altered in asthmatics. When there were no attacks, no difference in sleep architecture was noted between the controls and the patients, which suggested that sleep disturbances are characteristic of unstable asthma with nocturnal attacks.

A number of pathogenic mechanisms for sleep disturbances and nocturnal exacerbations of asthma have been suggested[105,143,153,154]:

- Sleep deprivation[155]
- Impaired ventilatory function in the supine posture[156]
- A decrease in circulating epinephrine at night, with an increase in histamine[157]
- Gastroesophageal reflux[158] (a study by Tan and associates[159] casts doubt on this)
- Marked fluctuation in airway tone during REM sleep[160]
- Theophylline, a commonly used asthma drug that may cause insomnia[161,162] and increase episodes of gastroesophageal reflux[163,164] (a study by Hubert's group[165] found no such increase in asthmatics taking theophylline)
- Prolonged administration of corticosteroids in some asthmatics, which may have adverse effects on sleep and daytime functioning because of increased incidence of OSA[166,167]
- Increased cellular inflammatory response in the bronchopulmonary region at night[153,168]
- Miscellaneous factors, including allergens (e.g., house dust); increased bronchial secretions combined with suppression of cough, especially during REM sleep; airway cooling at night; increased pulmonary resistance; altered bronchial reactivity; normal propensity for worsening of lung function during sleep; normally increased vagal tone during sleep; suppressed arousal response to bronchoconstriction in severe nocturnal asthma[153]
- Certain circadian factors[153,154]

Three pieces of evidence support the claim that circadian factors contribute to nocturnal exacerbation of asthma:

1. PEFR typically is highest at 4:00 PM and lowest at 4:00 AM.[153] The variation is ordinarily approximately 5–8%, but if it reaches 50%, as it can in some asthmatics, there is the danger of respiratory arrest.[153] This circadian variation in PEFR is related to sleep and not to recumbency or the hour.[153,154]

2. Airway resistance as measured breath by breath is not increased in normal individuals at night, but asthmatics show a circadian rhythm of increased airway resistance at night that is related to the duration of the sleep and not to sleep stages.[153,169]

3. As with OSAS and COPD, nocturnal asthma is associated with sleep-disturbed breathing[167,170] (hypopneas more than apneas, of mixed, obstructive, or central type) accompanied by awakening, which is worse during REM sleep.

*Treatment of Bronchial Asthma*

Treatment of bronchial asthma, including nocturnal asthma,[153] consists of judicious use of bronchodilators and corticosteroids, preferably inhaled in a compressor; oral theophylline, maximizing the serum concentration at around 4:00 AM when most nocturnal attacks occur; and, for a small subset of patients who show the lowest plasma cortisol levels accompanied by the lowest PEFR at night or early morning, nocturnal steroids.[171] Other measures include treating the reversible factors such as allergens, nasal congestion, or bronchopulmonary infections, and using a humidifier.[153]

In a double-blind, placebo-controlled crossover study, Kraft et al.[172] reported that salmeterol, an inhaled $\beta_2$-agonist with a prolonged duration of action, improved the number of nocturnal awakenings in 10 patients with nocturnal asthma without significant alteration in lung function test and airway inflammation. Previously, several studies showed efficacy of salmeterol in nocturnal asthma, primarily in combination with inhaled corticosteroids.[173–177]

### Sleep in Restrictive Lung Disease

Restrictive lung disease is characterized functionally by a reduction of total lung capacity, functional residual capacity, VC, expiratory reserve volume, and diffusion capacity but preservation of the normal ratio of $FEV_1$ to FVC.[129] This may be due to intrapulmonary restriction (e.g., interstitial lung disease) or extrapulmonary restriction resulting from diseases of the chest wall (e.g., kyphoscoliosis) or pleura; neuromuscular diseases; obesity; or pregnancy, which may abnormally elevate the diaphragm.

### Interstitial Lung Disease

**Etiopathogenesis.**    Interstitial lung disease may result from a variety of causes, including idiopathic pulmonary fibrosis, fibrosing alveolitis associated with connective tissue disorders, pulmonary sarcoidosis, occupational dust exposure, pulmonary damage resulting from drugs, or radiotherapy to the thorax.[178] The common features of all these conditions include alveolar thickening due to fibrosis, cellular exudates, or edema; increased stiffening of the lungs causing reduced compliance; and ventilation-perfusion mismatch giving rise to hypoxemia, hyperventilation, and hypocapnia.

**Clinical Features.**    Features of interstitial lung disease include progressive exertional dyspnea, a dry cough, clubbing of the fingers, and pulmonary crepitations on auscultation of the lungs. The diagnosis is based on a combination of characteristic clinical features, radiographic findings (e.g., diffuse pulmonary fibrosis), and pulmonary function test results.

**Sleep Abnormalities.**    Bye[128] and Perez-Padilla and their coworkers[179] reported on sleep studies in interstitial lung disease. Sleep abnormalities consist of repeated arousals with sleep fragmentation and multiple sleep stage shifts, increased stage I and reduced REM sleep accompanied by oxygen desaturation during REM and NREM sleep owing to episodic hypoventilation and ventilation-perfusion mismatch, and occasionally OSA.

**Treatment.**    For approximately 30% of cases of interstitial lung disease, corticosteroids are effective. George and Kryger[129] advocate symptomatic treatment with supplemental nocturnal oxygen therapy, according to the guidelines developed by the Nocturnal Oxygen Therapy Trial Group.[130]

### Kyphoscoliosis

Kyphoscoliosis is a thoracic cage deformity that causes extrapulmonary restriction of the lungs and gives rise to impairment of pulmonary functions, as described earlier for restrictive lung diseases. The condition may be primary (idiopathic) or secondary to neuromuscular disease, spondylitis, or Marfan syndrome.[129]

In severe cases of kyphoscoliosis, breathing disorders during sleep (e.g., central, obstructive, and mixed apneas associated with oxygen desaturation) and sleep disturbances (e.g., disrupted night sleep, reduced NREM stages II through IV and REM sleep, and EDS) have been described.[124,125,129]

CPAP or tracheostomy may benefit patients with moderate to severe obstructive apnea. Some patients may also require nighttime mechanical ventilation, including nasal intermittent positive pressure ventilation.[180,181] Patients with mild respiratory failure may benefit from medical treatment with acetazolamide, medroxyprogesterone, or almitrine, as discussed for COPD patients.

### Gastrointestinal Diseases

### Peptic Ulcer Disease

A peptic ulcer is an ulcer in the lower esophagus, stomach, or duodenum. The prevalence of peptic ulcer in the general population is fairly high—approximately 10% of the adult population—and men are most often affected. The commonest presentation of peptic ulcer is episodic pain localized to the epigastrium that is relieved by food, antacids, or other acid suppressant. The pain has a characteristic periodicity and extends over many years. The patient generally can localize the pain to the epigastrium. Occasionally, however, it is referred to the interscapular region at the lower chest and is usually described as burning or gnawing. Duodenal pain is often described as "hunger pain" and is relieved by eating. An important feature is that the pain awakens patients 2–3 hours after they retire to bed, disturbing sleep. An important physical sign is the so-called pointing sign and localized epigastric tenderness.

The natural history of the disease is episodic occurrence over a course of days or weeks, after which the pain disappears, to recur weeks or months later. Between attacks the patient feels well. Presentation may be secondary to complications of ulcer, such as an acute episode of bleeding or perforation, or even an episode of gastric obstruction.

The differential diagnosis of ulcer pain should include cholecystitis, angina, gastroesophageal reflux, and esophagitis or pancreatitis. Definitive diagnosis is established by barium examination of the gastroduodenal tract and, if necessary, by endoscopic examination and biopsy.

In the last decade, it has been clearly established that the commonest cause of peptic ulcer disease is *Helicobacter pylori* (HP) infection.[182–186] The second most common cause is ingestion of aspirin and other nonsteroidal anti-inflammatory drugs (NSAIDs).[182,186] HP infection is responsible for 90% of duodenal and more than 75% of gastric ulcers.[182,186]

*Sleep, Nocturnal Acid Secretion, and Duodenal Ulcer*

To understand the role of nocturnal gastric acid secretion in duodenal ulcer, Dragstedt[187] studied hourly collections of nocturnal gastric acid from patients with duodenal ulcer and from normal subjects. They found 3–20 times greater volumes of nocturnal acid secretion in patients than in normal controls. Vagotomy abolished this increased secretion and improved healing of ulcers. Studies by Orr and colleagues[188] have shown that patients with duodenal ulcer exhibit failure of inhibition of gastric acid secretion during the first 2 hours after onset of sleep. A study by Watanabe et al.[189] confirmed the findings of Orr et al.[188] and found that the intragastric pH values increased during NREM and REM sleep in healthy controls and gastric acid patients but the intragastric pH of duodenal patients did not change.

Sleep disturbances in duodenal ulcer patients characteristically result from episodes of nocturnal epigastric pain. These symptoms cause arousals and repeated awakenings, thus fragmenting and disturbing the sleep considerably in these patients.

*Treatment*

In light of the evidence about the role of HP infection and NSAIDs in the pathogenesis of gastroduodenal ulcers, the theory of hypersecretion of the acid in peptic ulcer patients has been relegated to a secondary role.[186] The first step is to find the causes of ulcer based on the history and laboratory tests such as serology; urea breath test; and endoscopic biopsy and histology, particularly in patients with gastric ulcer.[185,186] The purpose of treatment is to relieve symptoms; heal the ulcer; and either cure the disease, in case of HP ulcers, or prevent recurrences in NSAID ulcers.[186] To cure the ulcer, the best approach is triple combination therapy (e.g., tetracycline hydrochloride 500 mg qid, metronidazole 250 mg tid, and bismuth subsalicylate at two tablets qid for 2 weeks).[186,190] To accelerate healing, the triple combination is combined with antisecretory agents ($H_2$-receptor antagonists) such as 800 mg cimetidine (Tagamet), 300 mg of ranitidine (Zantac) or nizatidine (Axid), 20 mg of famotidine (Pepcid) for 6–8 weeks.[186,191–196] Acid-pump inhibitors (e.g., omeprazole) inhibit the $H^+$-$K^+$-ATPase responsible for acid secretion and are the most potent antisecretory agents.[186,190] Because of high cost and the marginal benefit obtained with 20 mg of omeprazole compared with $H_2$-receptor antagonists, however, omeprazole is not recommended as first-line therapy.[186] For treatment of NSAID ulcers, NSAID therapy should be stopped and treated with traditional antisecretory agents. Patients who require continued NSAID therapy, however, may be treated with misoprostol (200 µg two to four times a day).[186] General measures of treatment of peptic ulcer disease should consist of avoidance of tobacco and alcohol.

The importance of nocturnal acid suppression in the healing of duodenal ulcer and in preventing the reoccurrence of such ulcers in patients is well established.[197] It has been found that some patients treated with cimetidine remain symptomatic, and in these patients acid secretion remains high. When these patients are treated with ranitidine, a more potent acid suppressant, both the symptoms and the amount of acid secretion decrease considerably. Patients who show little improvement in response to medical treatment can opt for vagotomy, which suppresses the acid secretion, relieving symptoms and healing the ulcers.[198] In addition, maintenance of nocturnal acid suppression by ranitidine prevents the recurrence of duodenal ulcers.[199–201] These therapeutic measures clearly document the importance of the nocturnal acid suppression in the healing of duodenal ulcer.[197] Other factors, such as mucosal resistance, may also play a role.[197]

*Gastroesophageal Reflux Disease*

**Clinical Features.**   *Gastroesophageal reflux disease* (GERD) is preferable to the term *reflux esophagi-*

*tis.*[202] GERD frequently occurs in middle-aged and elderly women, and sometimes in younger women during pregnancy. Hiatal hernia is often associated with reflux esophagitis. The characteristic symptom is heartburn, described as retrosternal burning pain exacerbated by lifting or straining or when the patient lies down at night.[202–205] The burning pain causes difficulty in initiating sleep, frequent awakenings, and fragmentation of sleep. The nocturnal pain is characteristically relieved by sitting up or ingesting food or by acid-suppressant agents. An important differential diagnosis would be angina, particularly when the pain radiates to the neck, jaws, and arms, but an important point to remember is that the esophageal pain is usually not related to exertion. Other symptoms include transient or persistent dysphagia if the patient has developed stricture and regurgitation of gastric contents associated with coughing, wheezing, and shortness of breath due to the aspiration of the gastric contents into the bronchopulmonary region.[202–205] A serious complication of repeated episodes of gastroesophageal reflux and esophagitis is Barrett's esophagus, which may be a precursor to esophageal adenocarcinoma.[202,204–208] Another potential complication is exacerbation of nocturnal asthma.

**Differential Diagnosis, Pathogenesis, and Diagnostic Tests.** Peptic ulcer disease, ischemic heart disease, sleep apnea, abnormal swallowing, and sleep choking syndromes may be mistaken for gastroesophageal reflux.[197,202,204,205] It has been shown that the fundamental mechanism of GERD is the inappropriate, transient, and frequent relaxation of the lower esophageal sphincter causing episodes of acid reflux.[202,205,209] The esophagitis resulting from acid reflux in the esophagus reduces the sphincter pressure and impairs esophageal contractility.[209] An additional mechanism is the presence of a hiatal hernia. Other factors, such as the acid clearance time, frequency of swallowing, and secretion of saliva play an important role in the pathogenesis. The diagnosis of gastroesophageal reflux and prolonged acid secretion can be made by continuous monitoring of lower esophageal pH.[210] When the pH falls below 4, gastroesophageal reflux occurs.[211] Repeated prolonged episodes of gastroesophageal reflux during sleep at night can cause esophagitis.[212] Suppression of saliva, decreased swallowing frequency, and prolonged mucosal contact with the gastric acid all contribute to the development of esophagitis. After repeated prolonged episodes of gastroesophageal reflux at night for many years, patients may develop Barrett's esophagus, which results from replacement of the squamous epithelium of the lower esophagus by the columnar epithelium of the stomach.[202,204–208] Documentation of spontaneous gastroesophageal reflux and prolonged acid clearance is important for diagnosis and treatment of esophagitis resulting from repeated episodes of gastroesophageal reflux.

### Role of Gastroesophageal Reflux in Bronchopulmonary Disease

In some patients with asthma and chronic bronchitis or COPD, spontaneous gastroesophageal reflux at night plays a role in the pathogenesis of symptoms such as nocturnal wheeze, cough, or shortness of breath.[202,205,213–216] In such patients, intraesophageal pH monitoring has shown prolonged acid clearance.[214] This is important from a therapeutic point of view, because administration of acid suppressants to such patients improves pulmonary symptoms.[202,205] A study by Tan and coworkers,[217] however, casts doubt on the relevance of gastroesophageal reflux to asthma.

The mechanisms of pulmonary symptoms in gastroesophageal reflux associated with asthma and bronchitis may include[202,205,218,219] (1) aspiration of the gastric contents in the lungs causes pneumonitis and (2) acid contact with the lower esophagus initiates reflex stimulation of the vagus nerve, which causes bronchoconstriction. Actual aspiration of gastric contents into the lungs can be documented with the method used by Chernow and associates,[216] a scintigraphic technique. These authors instilled a radionuclide into the stomach before sleep. A lung scan the next morning showed the radioactive material in the lung, suggesting nocturnal pulmonary aspiration. It should be noted that children with asthma and bronchopulmonary disease may have sleep apnea, in addition to the other complications of gastroesophageal reflux.[220] Gastroesophageal reflux has been implicated in some cases of sudden infant death syndrome, possibly causing apnea and sudden death, but this has been found in only a small percentage of cases.[220,221]

**Diagnostic Tests.** No single test is diagnostic for GERD, but a combination of tests to assess the potential for reflux damage to the esophagus and actual presence of reflux is necessary to make the diagnosis. The diagnosis is confirmed by barium examination, and, if necessary, by endoscopic examination and biopsy. Measurement of lower esophageal sphincter pressure and a diagnosis of hiatal hernia may detect risk factors for reflux.[202,204] Damage to the esophagus may be assessed by Bernstein's test (acid perfusion test), esophagography, esophagoscopy, and mucosal biopsy.[204] The actual presence of reflux may be established with the following tests: esophagography, acid reflux test, prolonged esophageal pH monitoring, and gastroesophageal scintigraphy.[202,204] The importance of 24-hour ambulatory esophageal pH monitoring has been emphasized by Triadafilopoulos and Castillo.[222]

**Treatment.** Treatment[202,204,205,209] includes general measures such as avoidance of fatty foods and stooping, weight reduction, and elevation of the head end of the bed to reduce reflux at night. Smoking should also be avoided. These simple measures decrease the frequency and length of reflux episodes as demonstrated by 24-hour pH monitoring.[202] If the patients fail to improve as a result of these simple measures, $H_2$-receptor antagonists (cimetidine, ranitidine, famotidine, and nizatidine) in the usual dose range as used for peptic ulcer patients (see earlier) will improve the symptoms of GERD.[202,205,209] For patients who are resistant to $H_2$-receptor antagonists, a proton pump inhibitor (omeprazole, 20 mg once a day) may be used.[202,205,209] Other measures found to be useful are prokinetic agents (e.g., metoclopramide, 10 mg qid; cisapride, 10 mg qid; bethanechol, 10 mg qid).[202] For patients who fail to respond to medical treatment, antireflux surgery (e.g., fundoplication) is indicated.

In conclusion, an awareness of the role of sleep in the pathogenesis and treatment of peptic disease, particularly duodenal ulcer and esophageal reflux, is important for diagnosis and treatment. Facilities for all-night PSG study and 24-hour esophageal pH monitoring have contributed to an understanding of the association between sleep and these diseases. These disorders are good examples of diseases that benefit from a multidisciplinary approach to patient management by a gastroenterologist, a pulmonologist, and a sleep specialist. This review also shows that sleep adversely affects patients with GERD by increasing the episodes of reflux and prolonging the acid clearance time. Furthermore, repeated spontaneous reflux episodes adversely affect sleep by causing arousals, frequent awakenings, and sleep fragmentation.

### Sleep in Nonulcer Dyspepsia and Irritable Bowel Syndrome

Nonulcer dyspepsia (NUD) includes functional disorders of the upper gut and presents with upper abdominal pain or discomfort, nausea, gaseous distention, and early satiety.[223–226] A number of patients with NUD also have symptoms originating from the lower gut consistent with irritable bowel syndrome (IBS).[227] Many patients with NUD and IBS have a history of sleep complaints (e.g., frequent awakenings with or without pain and nonrestorative sleep).[228,229] Such functional disorders may be associated with FMS.[230–232] Patients with FMS complain of a variety of sleep problems (see later).

In a questionnaire and sleep diary survey of 65 NUD patients and 43 controls, David et al.[223] reported sleep disturbances (i.e., repeated awakenings and early morning awakenings) more commonly in NUD patients than in controls (67% vs. 23%). Nonrestorative sleep in IBS similar to that in FMS has also been reported by Moldofsky.[233]

### Endocrine Diseases

#### Thyroid Disorders

It is important to be aware of the association between thyroid disorders, disordered breathing, and sleep disturbances. History and physical examination may direct attention to a thyroid disorder, in which case thyroid function tests should be performed to confirm the clinical diagnosis.

#### Hypothyroidism

The salient diagnostic features suggestive of myxedema consist of presentation in a middle-aged or elderly individual of fatigue, weight gain, decrease of physical and mental faculties, dryness and coarsening of the skin, pretibial edema, hoarse voice, cold sensitivity (sometimes presenting with hypothermia), constipation, and bradycardia or evidence of ischemic heart disease in the ECG. Both upper airway obstructive[234] and central sleep apneas,[235] which disappeared after thyroxine treatment, have been described in patients with myxedema. Mechanisms include deposition of mucopolysaccharides in the upper airways as well as central respiratory dysfunction as evidenced by impaired hypercapnic and hypoxic ventilatory response.[236]

In an important paper by Rajagopal and coworkers,[237] OSA was reported in nine of 11 consecutive hypothyroid patients (apnea index, 17–176). These authors noted improvement of the OSA after thyroid replacement treatment. In a sleep EEG study of myxedema patients, Kales and colleagues[238] noted a reduction of SWS, which normalized after treatment. Grunstein and Sullivan[239] recommended nasal CPAP treatment in patients with hypothyroidism and concomitant OSA while the patient is receiving thyroxine treatment.

## Hyperthyroidism

Clinical features suggestive of thyrotoxicosis are presentation in a woman (female-to-male ratio, 8 to 1) of apparent increased energy, weight loss despite increased appetite, staring or bulging of the eyes, exophthalmos, tachycardia or atrial fibrillation, heat intolerance with excessive sweating, feelings of warmth, and a fine tremor of the outstretched fingers.

Few sleep studies have been made in patients with thyrotoxicosis. Dunleavy and colleagues[240] observed an increased amount of SWS, which returned to normal after treatment. In contrast, Passouant and colleagues[241] did not find any change in SWS but described an increase in sleep-onset latency in hyperthyroid patients. Johns and Rinsler[242] found no relationship between stages of sleep and alteration of thyroid function.

## Diabetes Mellitus

For sleep disturbance and sleep apnea in diabetes see the section on autonomic neuropathy in Chapter 27.

## Growth Hormone Deficiency and Sleep

In eight adults with isolated GH deficiency (aged 18–28 years), Astrom and Lindholm[243] found a reduction of stage IV sleep but increases in stage I and II NREM sleep, with a net result of an increase of total sleep time. In a later paper, Astrom and others[244] studied these patients after daily treatment with GH for 6 months and found a decrease in total sleep time that was due mainly to a reduction in stage II sleep, unchanged slow waves, and an increase in REM sleep time. In contrast to these findings in adults, Wu and Thorpy[245] found normal stage IV sleep but increased stage III NREM sleep in seven children with GH deficiency.

## Excessive Growth Hormone Release and Sleep

Sullivan and colleagues[246] reported sleep apnea in association with GH release from the pituitary in patients with acromegaly. The most common explanation for sleep apnea in these patients is enlargement of the tongue and pharyngeal wall, which causes narrowing of the upper airway. Sullivan's group[246] studied 40 patients with acromegaly and observed central sleep apnea in 30%. Increased respiratory drive with increased hypercapnic ventilatory response is present in these patients. Sandostatin, a somatostatin analog, cured central apnea and normalized the ventilatory response.

Grunstein and coworkers[247] studied 53 patients with acromegaly who were consecutively referred for consultation. Sleep apnea was a reason for referral of 33 patients, whereas 20 patients were referred without any suspicion of apnea. Thirty-one patients of the group of 33 referred for apnea had sleep apnea; 12 of the 20 patients referred without suspected apnea were found to have apnea. Central apnea was predominant in 33% of patients. The authors concluded that sleep apnea is common in individuals with acromegaly and central sleep apnea is associated with increased disease activity as reflected by biochemical measurement. They speculated that alteration of the respiratory control may be a mechanism for sleep apnea in these patients. In a later study of 54 patients with acromegaly, Grunstein and collaborators[248] found increased hypercapnic ventilatory responses in those patients with central sleep apnea but not in those with OSA or those without sleep apnea. These authors also found that acromegalic patients with central sleep apnea have increased GH and insulinlike growth factor–1 levels compared with their counterparts with OSA. The authors concluded that increased ventilatory responsiveness and elevated hormonal parameters of disease activity contribute to the pathogenesis of central sleep apnea and acromegaly.

In a retrospective cohort study, Rosenow et al.[249] found a relative frequency of sleep apnea in patients with treated acromegaly of at least 21%.

Octreotide, a long-acting somatostatin analog, has been found to be an effective noninvasive treatment for sleep apnea in acromegaly.[250,251] The relationship between sleep apnea and the GH level in active acromegaly remains unresolved.[247,252,253] Grunstein et al.[247] did not find a correlation between GH level and severity of sleep apnea in their patients. Similarly, Liebowitz et al.[250] found no correlation between GH hypersecretion and the severity of sleep apnea syndrome in two acromegalic patients. In contrast, Hart et al.[254] previously found a correlation between hormone levels and the presence of sleep apnea syndrome. Tsai et al.[255] reported an absence of the sleep-related GH peak in the acromegaly subjects.

### Renal Disorders

#### Sleep Disturbances and Chronic Renal Failure

Sleep disturbances are relatively common in patients with CRF with or without dialysis, particularly in those with end-stage renal disease (ESRD).[256–265] The sleep complaints in these patients include insomnia, EDS, and day-night reversal with disturbed nocturnal sleep. Several studies have used PSG to objectively document the sleep disturbances, which consist of reduced sleep efficiency, increased sleep fragmentation, frequent awakenings with difficulty in maintenance of sleep, decreased SWS, and disorganization of sleep cycle.[256,257,259–261,265] In the studies by Williams[256] and Karacan's group,[257] sleep disturbances remained unchanged in patients on dialysis, even in those who underwent renal transplantation, suggesting that an irreversible CNS deficit causes sleep dysfunction. In contrast, a more recent report[266] showed that the uremic form of restless legs syndrome (RLS) causing sleep disturbance can be cured after successful kidney transplantation. Daly and Hassall[258] reported that subjective sleep complaints were worse on dialysis nights. Passouant's group,[259] however, reported that dialysis improved nighttime sleep and sleep abnormalities.

#### Sleep Apnea in Patients Receiving Dialysis

Many CRF patients on and off dialysis suffer from sleep apnea syndrome, mainly obstructive in nature,[262,265,267–273] and may have periodic limb movements in sleep (PLMS).[267–269] It is important to diagnose sleep apnea in these patients, which may be difficult because of the similarity of uremic symptoms to those of sleep apnea syndrome.[265] Because CPAP titration has been found to be an effective form of treatment in hemodialysis patients with OSAS,[272] a PSG study to establish the diagnosis of OSAS should be performed in any patients with a history of EDS and disturbed night sleep. One study based on PSG recording suggested that 7–9% of the ESRD patients treated with hemodialysis have sleep apnea.[267]

Mendelson and colleagues[270] observed significant sleep apnea in six of 11 patients with CRF. Six of the 11 patients had diabetes mellitus, however, which is known to be associated with sleep apnea. These authors did not find any alteration after hemodialysis in the sleep architecture and the number of sleep-related disordered breathing events (both obstructive and central sleep apneas). They did find an increase in the percentage of obstructive apnea time on the night after hemodialysis, which may have been due to modulation of chemical control of ventilation.

Millman and colleagues[269] studied 29 men on long-term dialysis. In 12 (41%), symptoms (EDS, repeated arousals at night, and morning headache) suggested sleep apnea. According to PSG, six of these patients had OSA. These authors did not find any significant effect of testosterone, which is often given to CRF patients to stimulate erythropoiesis, on sleep apnea.

Kimmel and colleagues[267] performed a PSG study of 26 CRF patients treated with hemodialysis. Twenty-two had a history suggestive of sleep apnea, and 16 of these symptomatic (73%) patients had sleep apnea syndrome. In nine of 16 patients, the sleep apnea was of obstructive type. These authors concluded that EDS in some patients with CRF may be related to disturbed nocturnal sleep and sleep apnea.

The following mechanisms have been suggested for the pathogenesis of sleep apnea in CRF:

- Upper airway edema causing partial airway obstruction coupled with decreased muscle tone during sleep[273]
- CNS depression during sleep resulting from so-called uremic toxins causing excessive reduction of upper airway muscle tone[265,273] (persistence of sleep apnea after dialysis speaks against this suggestion)
- Disturbance of the ventilatory control of breathing in renal failure and hemodialysis[262,263,268,274–276] making the respiratory control unstable, causing an imbalance between diaphragmatic and upper airway muscle
- CCF, which may occur in association with CRF, itself causing SDB[277]
- Chronic metabolic acidosis, as noted in patients with CRF[278] (Kimmel's group,[267] however, did not find any relationship between disordered-breathing events and hydrogen ion concentrations or carbon dioxide tension in the symptomatic patients.)
- Alteration of the hydrogen ion set point for stimulation of respiration[274]
- Anatomic narrowing of the upper airway (not yet documented by computed tomography in CRF patients[267])
- Hypertension associated with CRF
- Metabolic derangement associated with uremia (Soreide et al.[279] reported that an infusion of branched-chain amino acids stimulated nocturnal respiration and resulted in a decreased number of obstructive apneas.)
- Alteration in cytokine metabolism in patients treated with hemodialysis causing abnormal somnolence (interleukin-1 is a sleep-promoting factor[268])

After doing a multidisciplinary case review, Kimmel et al.[265] suggested that despite the absence of adequate clinical data correlating the intensity of dialysis and SDB, it is plausible that adequate dialysis and reduced uremic toxicity may improve sleep problems in CRF patients.

*Restless Legs Syndrome*
*in Chronic Renal Failure Patients*

RLS has been described as a symptomatic or secondary form of RLS in many patients with CRF and the prevalence in hemodialyzed patients varies from 15–40%.[280–282] Symptomatic RLS is associated with CRF and not with the hemodialysis itself.[282–284] It should be noted that the uremic RLS and idiopathic RLS resemble each other and cannot be distinguished clinically.[284] As stated earlier, there has been a report of the cure of this form of RLS after successful kidney transplantation.[266]

### Rheumatic Diseases: Fibrositis or Fibromyalgia Syndrome

According to Goldenberg,[285] an estimated 3–6 million Americans are afflicted with FMS, a syndrome characterized by diffuse muscle aches and pains not related to diseases of the joints, bones, or connective tissues. Common sites of these aches and pains include the neck and shoulder joints, and the sacrospinal and gluteal regions. Yunus and colleagues[286] listed specific diagnostic criteria for FMS. An important item in the differential diagnosis is polymyalgia rheumatica, which is also characterized by diffuse muscle aches and pains but is often associated with accelerated erythrocyte sedimentation rate and evidence of temporal arteritis. Other differential diagnostic considerations include CFS (see later) and other myofacial pain syndrome. The etiology and pathogenesis of the condition remain undetermined.[285–290]

Sleep disturbance is very common in FMS.[285–292] The characteristic PSG finding is intermittent alpha activity during NREM sleep giving rise to the characteristic alpha-delta or alpha-NREM sleep pattern in the recording (Figure 29-1). Another important association is the presence of PLMS on PSG examination. It should be noted that although alpha-delta sleep is seen in this condition, this variant is not specific for the syndrome. Alpha-NREM sleep has also been reported in other rheumatic disorders,[293] febrile illness, postviral fatigue syndrome,[294] psychiatric patients,[295] and even normal individuals.[296,297] Nonrestorative sleep associated with nonspecific PSG abnormalities of sleep fragmentation, increased awakenings, decreased sleep efficiency, and alpha-NREM sleep is the most prominent complaint in these patients.

There is often an overlap between FMS and CFS (see later). This is particularly true in juvenile FMS.[297–299] Treatment of this condition remains unsatisfactory. Three lines of therapy have been rec-

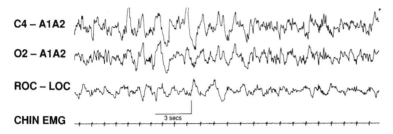

C4 – A1A2

O2 – A1A2

ROC – LOC

CHIN EMG

3 secs

**Figure 29-1.** Portion of a poly-somnographic recording. Note alpha intrusion into non-REM sleep (alpha-delta sleep) in the EEG channels.

ommended[290,291,300] for these patients: (1) pharmacologic treatment with tricyclic antidepressants and short-term treatment with zolpidem,[300] (2) an exercise program, and (3) education and reassurance.

### Hematologic Disorders

The hematologic disorders that may be adversely affected by sleep include paroxysmal nocturnal hemoglobinuria (PNH), sickle cell anemia, and hereditary hemorrhagic telangiectasis. Hansen[301] noted increased levels of plasma hemoglobin in five of seven patients with PNH and the maximum values were found at midnight or at 4:00 AM. However, the author did not record EEG or EOG to document any relationship with different sleep stages. Patients with sickle cell anemia occasionally show reduced arterial oxygen saturation during sleep.[302] OSA and sleep disturbances resulting from reduced arterial oxygen saturation can occur in patients with sickle cell anemia; when these diagnoses are suspected, therefore, they should be confirmed by overnight PSG recording so that appropriate treatment with CPAP titration can be instituted.[303] Progressive somnolence accompanied by confusion has been described in a patient with hereditary hemorrhagic telangiectasis.[304]

### Miscellaneous Disorders

#### Sleep of Intensive Care Unit Patients (Medical and Surgical)

Generally, patients are admitted to the medical ICU because of acute respiratory failure resulting from COPD, bronchial asthma, sleep apnea syndrome, restrictive lung disease, acute cardiovascular disor-

ders (e.g., ischemic heart disease with or without myocardial infarction, cardiac arrhythmias, CCF), acute neurologic disorders causing respiratory disturbances (e.g., brain stem lesion, status epilepticus, high cervical cord lesions, neuromuscular disorders), renal failure, or gastroesophageal reflux causing acute respiratory tract symptoms. All of these conditions can be associated with sleep disturbances (insomnia, hypersomnia, and sleep-related respiratory dysrhythmia), which become intense in severely ill patients admitted to the ICU who require life-saving cardiorespiratory support.[256,305–307]

Other factors (e.g., a variety of drugs used in the ICU) may aggravate sleep and sleep-related respiratory disturbances in the ICU. The ICU environment itself is deleterious to normal sleep and conducive to sleep deprivation with its attendant complications, such as ICU psychosis. In addition to sleep deprivation, physiologic and physical factors contribute to ICU psychosis. Noise, bright light, and constant activity on the part of the ICU personnel for monitoring and drug administration play significant roles in disturbing the sleep of ICU patients.

The ICU syndrome is a characteristic mental state defined as a reversible confusional state developing 3–7 days after ICU admission and is secondary to sleep deprivation.[306,307] The ICU psychosis is more common in surgical than in medical ICUs and the prevalence has been estimated to be between 12.5% and 38.0% of patients admitted to the ICU.[306–308] Sleep deprivation has been cited as the major cause of the ICU syndrome.[306,307] In a study by Helton et al.,[309] 10% of patients with moderate sleep deprivation and 33% with severe sleep deprivation develop the ICU syndrome.

An important cause of sleep disruption in the ICU is noise.[306,307,310–316] Technological advances in the ICU setting have been cited as the major culprits for contributing to the ICU noise. The role of the noise in contributing to sleep disruption has been documented objectively by continuous sleep monitoring and recording of the environmental peak sound levels.[313,315]

In the surgical ICU, patients are usually admitted in the postoperative period because they are recovering from anesthesia, are beginning to suffer from pain, are experiencing metabolic disturbances, or have an infection related to surgical care. All these factors may cause severe disturbance of sleep and breathing.

Another condition noted in many patients admitted to the ICU is REM behavior disorder. Schenck and Mahowald[317] reported REM behavior disorder in 17 of 20 patients admitted to the ICU over an 8-year period.

Several authors have studied ICU patients using PSG to document disruption of sleep structure.[318–322] These disturbances consist of marked diminution of stage III and IV NREM and REM sleep, frequent awakenings, sleep fragmentation, and reduced total sleep time. Because of night sleep disturbances, ICU patients often have EDS.[318,321] Adequate and controlled PSG studies to document the prevalence of sleep disruption and deprivation in ICU patients have not been conducted.

*Treatment*

The physicians and paramedical personnel who take care of ICU patients must be aware of these various ICU factors contributing to the problem of sleep disturbances, so that correct diagnosis and management of secondary complications (in addition to treatment of the primary disorders) can be effected promptly. The treatment for sleep disturbance in the ICU environment consists of nonpharmacologic and pharmacologic intervention. Nonpharmacologic treatment includes measures to decrease or eliminate many of the factors causing sleep deprivation in the ICU patients. Hypnotics are needed in some ICU patients, but benzodiazepine drugs should be used with caution because of adverse effects. Zolpidem, a nonbenzodiazepine hypnotic that binds selectively to one of the benzodiazepine receptors in the brain,[323] may be useful in patients admitted to the ICU because of its lesser side effects. Adequate control ICU studies

are needed, however, to determine the efficacy of zolpidem for these patients.

In addition to treating the primary disorder, it is important to treat secondary sleep-related respiratory problems. If a sleep disturbance persists after the patient leaves the ICU, a primary sleep disorder may be suspected and appropriate investigations, such as PSG study and MSLT, should be performed.

*Acquired Immunodeficiency Syndrome*

AIDS is a multisystem disorder caused by infection with human immunodeficiency virus (HIV). Its manifestations are protean. Neurologic manifestations include both CNS and peripheral neuromuscular dysfunction. Encephalitis, due to either opportunistic infection or direct invasion by the virus, may cause a variety of disorders such as memory impairment, seizures, and pyramidal or extrapyramidal manifestations. Some patients have sleep disturbances.

Norman and colleagues[324,325] studied groups of asymptomatic HIV-positive men and found an increase in SWS and a disruption of the NREM-REM cycle. A follow-up study[326] of 17 of the initial group of patients 19–63 months later showed a decrease in SWS, an increase of sleep fragmentation, and disruption of the NREM-REM cycle as the disease became symptomatic.

Moller and associates[327] obtained nocturnal PSG recordings for 14 patients with HIV infection. They found increased sleep-onset latency, short total sleep time, reduced sleep efficiency, increased time in wakefulness and stage I, and reduced stage II sleep. They found that asymptomatic patients had similar sleep abnormalities. The authors suggested that sleep study may be a sensitive method for detecting and monitoring CNS infection in HIV-positive patients.

White and colleagues[328] studied 23 HIV-positive and 13 seronegative men using nocturnal and daytime sleep recordings. They found that asymptomatic HIV-positive patients with CD4+ T cell counts higher than $400 \times 10^6$/liter demonstrated a statistically significant increase in SWS and decreased arousability during the later portion of the night. These authors further concluded that sleep structure distortion remained one of the earliest and most consistently replicable physiologic signs of HIV infection. The same group of investigators[329,330] suggested that there is evidence to support a role for the somnogenic immune peptides tumor necrosis factor–$\alpha$ and interleukin-1$\beta$ in the sleep changes and fatigue commonly seen in HIV infection. These authors[329] stated that these peptides were elevated in the blood of HIV-infected individuals and these are somnogenic in clinical use and animal models. Impaired sleep quality in HIV-infected individuals has also been documented by questionnaire surveys.[331,332]

HIV infection can cause SDB. Epstein et al.[333] identified three HIV patients with OSA due to adenotonsillar hypertrophy. They also surveyed 134 patients with asymptomatic HIV disease with a self-administered questionnaire designed to detect OSA and EDS. Those patients whose responses suggested possible OSA were studied by overnight PSG recording. Twelve HIV-positive patients with OSA were identified. The consistent risk factor in this young and nonobese population was the presence of adenotonsillar hypertrophy, which was found in 11 of 12 patients with OSA. In a previous paper, these authors[334] reported the first cases of severe OSA in HIV-infected men. Garrigo et al.[335] obtained PSG recording in asymptomatic HIV-positive men and reported an elevated apnea index in seven of 24 patients who did not have symptoms related to SDB.

Whether PSG can document significant and specific abnormalities in asymptomatic individuals or warn of the development of encephalopathy remains to be determined. A systematic study of a large number of cases needs to be done to answer these questions.

### Lyme Disease

Lyme disease[336–342] is a multisystem disease caused by the spirochete *Borrelia burgdorferi* and transmitted to humans by tick bite. The clinical manifestations may be divided into three stages: (1) Initially there is a characteristic skin lesion, erythema migrans, which is followed in the course of time by a febrile illness (acute or stage I). (2) In the subacute or stage II, which occurs in several weeks to months of the onset of the illness, approximately 15% of patients may develop neurologic manifestations and approximately 8% may have cardiac involvement (conduction disturbance or cardiomyopathy).[341] Neurologic manifestations may present as axonal polyneuropathy, radiculoneuropathy, cranial neuropathy (particularly affecting the facial nerve), lymphocytic meningitis, encephalitis, or encephalopathy. Encephalitis is rare. Patients with CNS manifestations may have sleep disturbances. (3) In the chronic or stage III, which occurs weeks to as long as 2 years after the onset of illness, approximately 60% of patients develop arthritis.[341]

Sleep complaints are common in Lyme disease,[336] but no large-scale study using PSG is available to characterize the sleep disturbances in this condition. Greenberg et al.[343] obtained two nights of PSG in 11 patients meeting Centers for Disease Control and Prevention criteria for late Lyme disease with serologic confirmation and 10 age-matched controls. In addition, the authors performed MSLT in the Lyme disease patients. All patients had complaints of difficulty initiating sleep, frequent nocturnal awakenings, and EDS; a small percentage had restless legs or nocturnal leg jerking. PSG findings included a decreased sleep efficiency, increased arousal index with sleep fragmentation, and alpha intrusion into NREM sleep. These authors concluded that these sleep abnormalities may have contributed to the sleep complaints and fatigue that are commonly present in this disease.

Because Lyme disease is treatable, every attempt should be made to diagnose it accurately. Diagnosis depends on the serologic detection of antibodies against *B. burgdorferi* in the serum (or in case of CNS infection, in cerebrospinal fluid samples).[342] The usual method of testing is the enzyme-linked immunosorbent assay,[342] but antibodies usually are not detectable until 4–6 weeks after the initial infection. Diagnosis may be complicated by false-positive results and lack of a standardized technique to assay for antibodies. Polymerase chain reaction has been shown to be useful in demonstrating *B. burgdorferi* DNA in clinical material.[341,342] The disease shows an excellent response to antibiotic therapy (amoxicillin, 500 mg tid for 21 days; doxycycline, 100 mg bid for 21 days; or ceftriaxone, 2 mg daily for 2–4 weeks).[341]

### Chronic Fatigue Syndrome

CFS is an ill-defined heterogeneous condition.[344–349] Certain diagnostic criteria, both major and minor, have been established for it.[345] Two major manifestations are (1) insidious onset of fatigue for at least 6 months and (2) no evident cause for the fatigue despite extensive laboratory investigation. The minor manifestations include arthralgias, myalgias, headache, and sleep disturbances. The cause is undetermined. Various psychological and psychiatric illnesses (e.g., major affective disorder) may present as CFS. In many cases of CFS, however, depression is one of the minor manifestations. A variety of viruses, particularly herpes simplex, enterovirus, retroviruses, and Epstein-Barr virus, have been incriminated without any firm evidence. Several patients with CFS had orthostatic hypotension on tilt table study, which was thought to be responsible for some of the symptoms.[350,351] However, further studies are needed to understand the significance and the prevalence of orthostatic hypotension in CFS. There have been some inconsistent abnormalities in the magnetic resonance imaging studies showing small, discreet, patchy brain stem and subcortical lesions in patients with CFS, and single photon emission computerized tomography revealed reduction of blood flow in many patients, particularly in the hind brain.[352] Increased brain serotonin levels have been postulated in CFS but no reliable data are available.[353] In a study comparing the effect of D-fenfluramine, a selective serotonin-releasing agent, in 10 men with CFS and 10 controls, prolactin levels 3–4 hours after administration of the drug were significantly higher in patients with CFS than in controls, indicating indirectly increased brain serotonin levels.[353] Whether this is simply an epiphenomenon or whether there was a real increase of serotonin level causing fatigue in CFS, however, cannot be determined at present.

Sleep disturbances (e.g., disturbed nighttime sleep, sleep disorganization, EDS) are important problems in some CFS patients, but in many cases these have not been adequately characterized by PSG studies. Sleep complaints and PSG abnormalities have been found in a few studies. Fischler et al.,[353] in a PSG study in 49 CFS patients and 20 healthy controls, found more sleep initiation and maintenance disturbances and significantly lower percentage of stage IV NREM sleep in the CFS patients than in the control group. However, they did not find any association between sleep disorders and the degree of functional impairment. In some studies,[354–356] PSG recordings in CFS patients have shown a high incidence of the associated or coexistent primary sleep disorders such as sleep apnea,

PLMS, or narcolepsy. In conclusion, the entity of CFS remains ill defined and the treatment, at present, should be nonpharmacologic in nature.[357]

## African Sleeping Sickness (Trypanosomiasis)

African sleeping sickness is caused by *Trypanosoma gambiense* or *Trypanosoma rhodesiense* and is transmitted to humans by the bite of tsetse flies. The clinical features are characterized by lymphadenopathy, fever, and later, after several months or years, excessive sleepiness due to encephalopathy or encephalitis. The clinical manifestations in the type caused by *T. rhodesiense* (Rhodesian sleeping sickness) is more rapidly progressive, resulting in cardiac failure and acute neurologic manifestations.[358] The Gambian sleeping sickness, caused by *T. gambiense*, is a more chronic illness with predominant neurologic manifestations.[358] Within 6 months to several years after the onset of the first symptoms, the Gambian type progresses into a late meningoencephalitic stage. CNS involvement is initially characterized by personality changes followed by delusions, hallucinations, and reversal of sleep-wake rhythm.[358] The patient remains somnolent in the daytime and progresses gradually into the stage of stupor and coma. The cerebrospinal fluid examination shows increased cells and protein.

Several PSG studies lasting for at least 24 hours and correlating with several plasma hormone levels have been conducted in patients with human African trypanosomiasis.[359–365] These studies documented disruption of the circadian sleep-wake rhythm, which is proportional to the severity of the illness. In less severely affected patients, the relationship between hormonal pulses (cortisol, prolactin, and plasma renin activity) and specific sleep stages persists.[359] Circadian disruption of plasma cortisol, prolactin, and sleep-wake rhythms is noted in the most advanced patients, but not in patients with less severe illness.[364,365] These findings of circadian disruption suggest selective changes in the suprachiasmatic nucleus (SCN), resulting in circadian rhythm changes in the advanced stage of the illness. The association between SWS and GH secretion persisted in the patients, even in the presence of disrupted circadian rhythms.[362] In one study, circadian periodicity of sleep-wake cycle was disturbed and proportional to the severity of the illness, but the patients' melatonin rhythm was similar to that in normal individuals, suggesting additional control for melatonin besides SCN.[363] In three advanced patients, the cytokine interferon-$\gamma$ levels were increased 7- to 12-fold.[364] In an experimental study, rats infected with the parasite *Trypanosoma brucei brucei* showed selective changes in c-*fos* expression in the SCN, supporting the hypothesis that in human trypanosomiasis, changes in SCN are responsible for circadian rhythm dysregulation and changes in sleep-wake pattern.[365]

The diagnosis of trypanosomiasis is based on history as well as confirmation that the organism is in the blood, bone marrow, CSF, lymph node aspirates, or a scraping from the chancre.[358] The treatment of choice for patients in the meningoencephalitic stage is arsenical melarsoprol.[358]

## REFERENCES

1. Diagnostic Classification Steering Committee. The International Classification of Sleep Disorders (revised): Diagnostic and Coding Manual. Rochester, MN: American Sleep Disorders Association, 1990;1997.
2. Gislason T, Almqvist M. Somatic diseases and sleep complaints. An epidemiological study of 3201 Swedish men. Acta Med Scand 1987;221:475.
3. Johns MWW, Egan P, Gay TJ, et al. Sleep habits and symptoms in male medical and surgical patients. BMJ 1970;2:509.
4. Aldrich MS. Cardinal Manifestations of Sleep Disorders. In Kryger MH, Roth T, Dement WC (eds), Principles and Practice of Sleep Medicine (2nd ed). Philadelphia: Saunders, 1994.
5. Wooten V. Medical Causes of Insomnia. In MH Kryger, T Roth, WC Dement (eds), Principles and Practice of Sleep Medicine. Philadelphia: Saunders, 1989;456.
6. Guilleminault C, Hoed JVD, Mitler MM. Clinical Overview of the Sleep Apnea Syndromes. In C Guilleminault, WC Dement (eds), Sleep Apnea Syndromes. New York: Liss, 1978;1.
7. Remmers JE, Anch AM, deGroot WJ. Respiratory disturbances during sleep. Clin Chest Med 1980;1:57.
8. Guilleminault C, Tilkian A, Dement WC. The sleep apnea syndromes. Annu Rev Med 1976;27:465.
9. Chokroverty S. Sleep and Breathing in Neurological Disorders. In NH Edelman, TV Santiago (eds), Breathing Disorders of Sleep. New York: Churchill Livingstone, 1986;225.
10. Karacan I, Williams RL, Taylor WJ. Sleep characteristics of patients with angina pectoris. Psychosomatics 1969;10:280.
11. Nowlin JB, Troyer WG, Collins WS, et al. The association of nocturnal angina pectoris with dreaming. Ann Intern Med 1965;63:1040.

12. King MJ, Zir LM, Kaltman AJ, et al. Variant angina associated with angiographically demonstrated coronary artery spasm and REM sleep. Am J Med Sci 1973;265:419.
13. Stern S, Tzivoni D. Dynamic changes in the ST-T segment during sleep in ischemic heart disease. Am J Cardiol 1973;32:16.
14. Murao S, Harumi K, Katayama S, et al. All-night polygraphic studies of nocturnal angina pectoris. Jpn Heart J 1972;13:295.
15. Schafer H, Koehler U, Ploch T, Peter JH. Sleep-related myocardial ischemia and sleep structure in patients with obstructive sleep apnea and coronary artery disease. Chest 1997;111:387.
16. Andreas S, Schulz R, Werner GS, Kreuzer H. Prevalence of obstructive sleep apnea in patients with coronary artery disease. Coron Artery Dis 1996;7:541.
17. Kripke D, Simons R, Garfinkel L, et al. Short and long sleep and sleeping pills. Arch Gen Psychiatry 1979;36:103.
18. Wingard DL, Berkman LF. Mortality risk associated with sleep pattern among adults. Sleep 1983;6:102.
19. Partinen M, Putkonen PTS, Kaprio J, et al. Sleep disorders in relation to coronary heart disease. Acta Med Scand (Suppl) 1982;660:69.
20. Broughton R, Baron R. Sleep of acute coronary patients in an open ward type intensive care unit. Sleep Res 1973;2:144.
21. Muller JE, Stone PH, Turi ZG, et al. Circadian variation in the frequency of onset of acute myocardial infarction. N Engl J Med 1985;313:1315.
22. Mitler MM, Kripke DF. Circadian variation in myocardial infarction. N Engl J Med 1986;314:1187.
23. Karacan I, Green JR, Taylor WJ, et al. Sleep characteristics of acute myocardial infarct patients in an ICU. Sleep Res 1973;2:159.
24. Dark DS, Pingleton SK, Kerby GR, et al. Breathing pattern abnormalities and arterial oxygen desaturation during sleep in the congestive heart failure syndrome. Chest 1987;91:833.
25. Baylor P, Tayloe D, Owen D, et al. Cardiac failure presenting as sleep apnea: elimination of apnea following medical management of cardiac failure. Chest 1988;94:1298.
26. Javaheri S, et al. Occult sleep-disordered breathing in stable congestive heart failure. Ann Intern Med 1995;122:487.
27. Dowdell WT, Javaheri S, McGinnis W. Cheyne-Stokes respiration presenting as sleep apnea syndrome. Am Rev Respir Dis 1990;141:871.
28. Quaranta AJ, D'Alonzo GE, Krachman SL. Cheyne-Stokes respiration during sleep in congestive heart failure. Chest 1997;111:467.
29. Yamashiro Y, Kryger MH. Review: sleep in heart failure. Sleep 1993;16:513.
30. Hanly P, Zuberi-Khokhar N. Daytime sleepiness in patients with congestive heart failure and Cheyne-Stokes respiration. Chest 1995;107:952.

31. Adreas S, Clemens C, Sandholzer H, et al. Improvement of exercise capacity with treatment of Cheyne-Stokes respiration in patients with congestive heart failure. J Am Clin Cardiol 1996;27:1486.

32. Javaheri S. Central sleep apnea-hypopnea syndrome in heart failure: prevalence, impact and treatment. Sleep 1996;19:S229.

33. Hanly P, Miller TW, Steljes DG, et al. The effect of oxygen on respiration and sleep in patients with congestive heart failure. Ann Intern Med 1989;111:777.

34. Naughton MT, Liu PP, Bernard DC, et al. Treatment of congestive heart failure and Cheyne-Stokes respiration during sleep by continous positive airway pressure. Am J Respir Crit Care Med 1995;151:92.

35. Hanly PJ, Zuberi-Khokhar N. Increased mortality associated with Cheyne-Stokes respiration in patients with congestive heart failure. Am J Respir Crit Care Med 1996;153:272.

36. Takasaki Y, Orr D, Popkin J, et al. Effect of nasal continuous positive airway pressure on sleep apnea in congestive heart failure. Am Rev Respir Dis 1989;140:1578.

37. Bradley TD. Hemodynamic and sympathoinhibitory effects of nasal CPAP in congestive heart failure. Sleep 1996;19:S232.

38. Granton GA, Naughton MT, Benard DC, et al. CPAP improves inspiratory muscle strength in patients with heart failure and central sleep apnea. Am J Respir Crit Care Med 1996;153:277.

39. Buckle P, Miller T, Kreger M. The effect of short-term nasal CPAP on Cheyne-Stokes respiration in congestive heart failure. Chest 1992;102:31.

40. Davies RJO, Harrington KJ, Oliver J, et al. Nasal continuous positive airway pressure in chronic heart failure with sleep-disordered breathing. Am Rev Respir Dis 1993;147:630.

41. Calverley PMA. Nasal CPAP in cardiac failure: case not proven. Sleep 1996;19:S236.

42. Otsuka K, Ichimaru Y, Yanaga T. Studies of arrhythmias by 24-hour polygraphic recordings: relationship between arterioventricular block and sleep states. Am Heart J 1983;105:934.

43. Nevins DB. First- and second-degree A-V heart block with rapid eye movement sleep. Ann Intern Med 1972;76:981.

44. Parish JM, Shepherd JW Jr. Cardiovascular effects of sleep disorders. Chest 1990;97:1220.

45. Brodksy M, Wu D, Denes P, et al. Arrhythmias documented by 24-hour continuous electrocardiographic monitoring in 50 male medical students without apparent heart disease. Am J Cardiol 1977;39:390.

46. Guilleminault C, Pool P, Motta J. Sinus arrest during REM sleep in young adults. N Engl J Med 1984;311:1006.

47. Fleg JC, Kennedy HL. Cardiac arrhythmias in a healthy elderly population. Chest 1982;81:302.

48. Verrier RL, Kirby DA. Sleep and cardiac arrhythmias. Ann N Y Acad Sci 1988;533:238.

49. Pitzalis MV, Mastropisqua F, Massari F, et al. Sleep suppression of ventricular arrhythmias: a predictor of β-blocker efficacy. Eur Heart J 1996;17:917.

50. Wellens HJJ, Vermeulen A, Durrer D. Ventricular fibrillation occurring on arousal from sleep by auditory stimuli. Circulation 1971;46:661.

51. Tzivoni D, Stern S. Electrocardiographic changes during sleep in normal individuals. Clin Res 1972;20:401.

52. Lown V, Tykocinski M, Gartein A, et al. Sleep and ventricular premature beats. Circulation 1973;48:691.

53. De Silva RA. Central nervous system risk factors for sudden coronary death. Ann N Y Acad Sci 1982;382:143.

54. Pickering TG, Johnston JM, Honour AJ. Comparison of the effects of sleep, exercise and autonomic drugs on ventricular extrasystoles, using ambulatory monitoring of electrocardiogram and electroencephalogram. Am J Med 1978;65:575.

55. Rosenblatt G, Zwillig G, Hartman E. Electrocardiographic changes during sleep in patients with cardiac abnormality [abstract]. Psychophysiology 1969;6:233.

56. Gillis AM, MacLean KE, Guilleminault C. The QT interval during wake and sleep in patients with ventricular arrhythmias. Sleep 1988;11:333.

57. Smith R, Johnson L, Rothfield D, et al. Sleep and cardiac arrhythmias. Arch Intern Med 1972;130:751.

58. Richards KC, Curry N, Lyons W, et al. Cardiac dysrhythmia during sleep in the critically ill: a pilot study. Am J Crit Care 1996;5:26.

59. LaRovere MT, Specchia G, Mortara A, et al. Baroreflex sensitivity, clinical correlates and cardiovascular mortality among patients with a first myocardial infarction: a prospective study. Circulation 1988;78:816.

60. McWilliams JA. Ventricular fibrillation and sudden death. BMJ 1923;2:215.

61. Kleiger RE, Miller JP, Bigger JWT, et al. Decreased heart rate variability and its association with increased mortality after acute myocardial infarction. Am J Cardiol 1987;59:256.

62. Verrier RL. Mechanisms of behaviorally induced arrhythmias. Circulation 1987;76:148.

63. Bhandari AK, Scheinman M. The long QT syndrome. Mod Concepts Cardiovasc Dis 1985;54:45.

64. Tanchaiswad W. Is sudden unexplained nocturnal death a breathing disorder? Psychiatry Clin Neurosci 1995;49:111.

65. Kales A, Bixler EO, Cadieux RJ, et al. Sleep apnoea in a hypertensive population. Lancet 1984;2:1005.

66. Lavie P, Ben-Yosef R, Rubin AE. Prevalence of sleep apnea syndrome among patients with essential hypertension. Am Heart J 1984;108:373.

67. Fletcher EC, DeBehnke RD, Lovoi MS, et al. Undiagnosed sleep apnea in patients with essential hypertension. Ann Intern Med 1985;103:190.

68. Williams AJ, Houston D, Finberg S, et al. Sleep apnea syndrome and essential hypertension. Am J Cardiol 1985;55:1019.

69. Escourrou P, Jirani A, Nedelcoux H, et al. Systemic hypertension in sleep apnea syndrome. Chest 1990; 98:1362.

70. Tilkian AG, Guilleminault C, Schroeder JS, et al. Hemodynamics in sleep-induced apnea studies during wakefulness and sleep. Ann Intern Med 1976;85:714.

71. Burach B, Pollack C, Borowiecki B, et al. The hypersomnia-sleep apnea syndrome: a reversible major cardiovascular hazard. Circulation 1977;56:177.

72. Guilleminault C, Simmons FB, Motta J, et al. Obstructive sleep apnea syndrome and tracheostomy: long term follow-up experience. Arch Intern Med 1981;141:985.

73. Lugaresi E, Coccagna G, Cirignotta F. Breathing during sleep in man in normal and pathological conditions. Adv Exp Med Biol 1978;99:33.

74. Lavie P, Yoffe N, Berger J, Peled R. The relationship between the severity of sleep apnea syndrome and 24-hour blood pressure values in patients with obstructive sleep apnea. Chest 1993;103:717.

75. Stoohs RA, Gingold J, Cohrs F, et al. Sleep-disordered breathing and systemic hypertension in the elderly. J Am Geriatr Soc 1996;44:1295.

76. Carlson JT, Hedner JA, Ejnell H, Peterson LE. High prevalence of hypertension in sleep apnea patients independent of obesity. Am J Respir Crit Care Med 1994;150:72.

77. Hoffstein V. Blood pressure, snoring obesity, and nocturnal hypoxaemia. Lancet 1994;344:643.

78. Guilleminault C, Stoohs R, Young-Do K, et al. Upper airway sleep-disordered breathing in women. Ann Intern Med 1995;122:493.

79. Pankow W, Nable B, Lies A, et al. Influence of obstructive sleep apnea on circadian blood pressure profile. Sleep Res 1995;19:410.

80. Coy TV, Dimsdale JE, Ancoli-Israel S, Clausen JL. The role of sleep-disordered breathing in essential hypertension. Chest 1996;108:890.

81. McGinty D, Beahn E, Stern N, et al. Nocturnal hypertension in older men with sleep-related breathing disorders. Chest 1988;94:305.

82. Hla K, Young T, Bidwell T, et al. Sleep apnea and hypertension: a population-based study. Ann Intern Med 1994;120:382.

83. Young T, Finn L, Hla KM, et al. Snoring as part of a dose-response relationship between sleep-disordered breathing and blood pressure. Sleep 1996;19:S202.

84. Mayer J, Weichler U, Becker H, et al. Sleep Apnea Induced Changes in Blood Pressure and Heart Rate. In Horn J (ed), Sleep 88. Stuttgart: Gustave Fischer Verlag, 1989;270.

85. Wilcox I, Hedner JA, Grenstein RR, et al. Non-pharmacological reduction of systemic blood pressure in patients with sleep apnea by treatment with continuous positive airway pressure. Circulation 1991;84:II-480.

86. Stradling J, Davies RJO. Sleep apnea and hypertension—what a mess! Sleep 1997;20:789.

87. Nabe B, Lies A, Pankow W, et al. Determinants of circadian blood pressure rhythm and blood pressure variability in obstructive sleep apnea. J Sleep Res 1995; 4:S97.

88. Olson LG, King MT, Kensley MJ, Saunders NA. A community study of snoring and sleep-disordered breathing. Am J Respir Crit Care Med 1995;152:717.

89. Davies RJO, Crosby J, Prothero O, Stradling JR. Ambulatory blood pressure and left ventricular hypertrophy in subjects with untreated obstructive sleep apnea and snoring compared with matched control subjects and their response to treatment. Clin Sci 1994;86:417.

90. Worsnop CJ, Pierce RJ, Naughton M. Systemic hypertension and obstructive sleep apnea. Sleep 1993;16:S148.

91. Rauscher H, Popp W, Zwich H. Systemic hypertension in snorers with and without sleep apnea. Chest 1992;102:67.

92. Silverberg DS, Oksenberg A. Essential and secondary hypertension and sleep-disordered breathing: a unifying hypothesis. J Hum Hypertens 1996;10:353.

93. Silverberg DS, Oksenberg A. Essential hypertension and abnormal upper airway resistance during sleep. Sleep 1997;20:794.

94. Wynne JW. Gas Exchange During Sleep in Patients with Chronic Airway Obstruction. In NA Saunders, CE Sullivan (eds), Sleep and Breathing. New York: Marcel Dekker, 1984;485.

95. Pierce AK, Jarret CE, Werkle G Jr, et al. Respiratory function during sleep in patients with chronic obstructive lung disease. J Clin Invest 1966;45:631.

96. Leitch AJ, Clancy LJ, Leggett RJ, et al. Arterial blood gas tensions, hydrogen ion, and electroencephalogram during sleep in patients with chronic ventilatory failure. Thorax 1976;31:730.

97. Coccagna G, Lugaresi E. Arterial blood gases and pulmonary and systemic arterial pressure during sleep in chronic obstructive pulmonary disease. Sleep 1978;1:117.

98. Koo KW, Sax DS, Snider GL. Arterial blood gases and pH during sleep in chronic obstructive pulmonary disease. Am J Med 1975;58:663.

99. Wynne JW, Block AJ, Hemenway J, et al. Disordered breathing and oxygen desaturation during sleep in patients with chronic obstructive lung disease (COLD). Am J Med 1979;66:573.

100. Littner MR, McGinty DJ, Arand DL. Determinants of oxygen desaturation in the course of ventilation during sleep in chronic obstructive pulmonary disease. Am Rev Respir Dis 1990;122:849.

101. Guilleminault C, Cummiskey J, Motta J. Chronic obstructive airflow disease and sleep studies. Am Rev Respir Dis 1980;122:397.

102. Douglas NJ, Calverley PM, Leggett RJ, et al. Transient hypoxemia during sleep in chronic bronchitis and emphysema. Lancet 1979;1:1.

103. Francis PW, Muller NL, Gurwitz D, et al. Hemoglobin desaturation: its occurrence during sleep in patients with cystic fibrosis. Am J Dis Child 1980;134:734.

104. Weitzenblum E, Chaouat A, Charpentier C, et al. Sleep-related hypoxemia in chronic obstructive pulmonary

disease: causes, consequences and treatment. Respiration 1997;64:187.

105. McNicholas WT. Impact of sleep in respiratory failure. Eur Respir J 1997;10:920.

106. Mulloy E, McNicholas WT. Ventilation and gas exchange during sleep and exercise in patients with severe COPD. Chest 1996;109:387.

107. Martin RJ. The sleep-related worsening of lower airways obstruction: understanding an intervention. Med Clin North Am 1990;74:701.

108. Fletcher CM, Hugh-Jones P, McNicol MW, et al. The diagnosis of pulmonary emphysema in the presence of chronic bronchitis. Q J Med 1963;123:33.

109. Filley GF, Beckwitt HJ, Reeves JT, et al. Chronic obstructive bronchopulmonary disease. II. Oxygen transport in two clinical types. Am J Med 1968;44:26.

110. Flenley DC, Claverly PM, Douglas NJ, et al. Nocturnal hypoxemia and long-term domiciliary oxygen therapy in "blue and bloated" bronchitics. Physiopathological correlations. Chest 1980;77:305.

111. DeMarco FJ, Wynne JW, Block AJ, et al. Oxygen desaturation during sleep as a determinant of the "blue and bloated" syndrome. Chest 1981;79:621.

112. Flenley DC. Sleep in chronic obstructive lung disease. Clin Chest Med 1985;6:51.

113. Chaouat ARI, Weitzenblum E, Krieger J, et al. Association of chronic obstructive pulmonary disease and sleep apnea syndrome. Am J Respir Crit Care Med 1995; 151:82.

114. Arand DL, McGinty DJ, Littner MR. Respiratory patterns associated with hemoglobin desaturation during sleep in chronic obstructive pulmonary disease. Chest 1981;80:183.

115. Fleetham JA, Bradley CA, Kryger MH, et al. The effect of low flow oxygen therapy in chemical control of ventilation in patients with hypoxemic COPD. Am Rev Respir Dis 1980;122:833.

116. Brezinova A, Catterall JR, Douglas NJ, et al. Night sleep of patients with chronic ventilatory failure and age matched controls: number and duration of the EEG episodes of intervening wakefulness and drowsiness. Sleep 1982;5:123.

117. Fletcher EC, Martin RJ, Monlux RD. Disturbed EEG sleep patterns in chronic obstructive pulmonary disease. Sleep Res 1982;11:186.

118. Fleetham J, Wes P, Mezon B, et al. Sleep, arousals and oxygen desaturation in chronic obstructive pulmonary disease: the effect of oxygen therapy. Am Rev Respir Dis 1982;126:429.

119. Calverly PMA, Brezinova V, Douglas NJ, et al. The effect of oxygenation on sleep quality in chronic bronchitis and emphysema. Am Rev Respir Dis 1982; 126:206.

120. Fletcher EC. Respiration During Sleep and Cardiopulmonary Hemodynamics in Patients with Chronic Lung Disease. In RJ Martin (ed), Cardiorespiratory Disorders During Sleep. Mt. Kisco, NY: Futura, 1990;215.

121. Calverly PMA, Brezinova V, Douglas NJ, et al. The effect of oxygenation on sleep quality in chronic bronchitis and emphysema. Am Rev Respir Dis 1982;126:206.

122. Flick MR, Block AJ. Nocturnal vs. diurnal cardiac arrhythmias in patients with chronic obstructive pulmonary disease. Chest 1979;75:8.

123. Shepard JW Jr, Garrison MW, Grither DA, et al. Relationship of ventricular ectopy to nocturnal oxygen desaturation in patients with chronic obstructive pulmonary disease. Am J Med 1985;78:28.

124. Mezon BL, West P, Israel J, et al. Sleep breathing abnormalities in kyphoscoliosis. Am Rev Respir Dis 1980;122:617.

125. Guilleminault C, Kurland G, Winkle R, et al. Severe kyphoscoliosis, breathing and sleep. Chest 1981;79:626.

126. Muller NL, Francis PW, Gurwitz D, et al. Mechanism of hemoglobin in desaturation during rapid-eye-movement sleep in normal subjects and in patients with cystic fibrosis. Am Rev Respir Dis 1980;121:463.

127. Stokes DC, McBride JT, Wall MA, et al. Sleep hypoxemia in young adults with cystic fibrosis. Am J Dis Child 1980;134:741.

128. Bye PT, Issa F, Berthan-Jones M, et al. Studies of oxygenation during sleep in patients with interstitial lung disease. Am Rev Respir Dis 1984;129:27.

129. George CF, Kryger MH. Sleep in restrictive lung disease. Sleep 1987;10:409.

130. Nocturnal Oxygen Therapy Trial Group. Continuous or nocturnal oxygen therapy in hypoxemic chronic obstructive lung disease. Ann Intern Med 1980;93:391.

131. Medical Research Council Working Party. Long-term domiciliary oxygen therapy in chronic hypoxic cor pulmonale complicating chronic bronchitis and emphysema. Lancet 1981;1:681.

132. Fulmer JD, Snider GL. ACCP-NHLBI national conference on oxygen therapy. Chest 1984;86:234.

133. Motta J, Guilleminault C. Effects of Oxygen Administration in Sleep-Induced Apneas. In C Guilleminault, WC Dement (eds), Sleep Apnea Syndrome. New York: Liss, 1978;137.

134. Kearley RW, Wynne JW, Block AJ, et al. Effects of low flow oxygen on sleep disordered breathing in patients with COPD. Chest 1980;78:682.

135. Fleetham JA, Conway W, West P, et al. The effect of oxygen therapy on sleep profile and arousal frequency in hypoxemic COPD patients. Am Rev Respir Dis 1981;123:S72.

136. Damato S, Frigo V, Dell'Oca M, et al. Utility of monitoring breathing during night hours in COPD patients undergoing long-term oxygen therapy. Monaldi Arch Chest Dis 1997;52:106.

137. Tyler JM. The effect of progesterone on the respiration of patients with emphysema and hypercapnia. J Clin Invest 1960;39:34.

138. Dolly R, Block AJ. Medroxyprogesterone and COPD: effect on breathing and oxygenation in sleep and awake patients. Chest 1983;84:394.

139. Sutton JR, Gray GW, Houston CS, et al. Effects of duration at altitude and acetazolamide in ventilation and oxygenation during sleep. Sleep 1980;3:445.

140. Prefaut C, Bourgouin-Karaouni D, Ramonatxo M, et al. Blood gases and pulmonary haemodynamic follow-up during a one-year double blind bismesylate almitrine therapy in COPD patients. Am Rev Respir Dis 1985;131:A71.

141. Connaughton JJ, Douglas NJ, Morgan AD, et al. Almitrine improves oxygenation when both awake and asleep, in patients with hypoxia and $CO_2$ retention due to chronic bronchitis and emphysema. Am Rev Respir Dis 1985;132:206.

142. MacNee W, Connaugton JJ, Hayhurst MD, et al. The effects of almitrine on pulmonary artery pressure and right ventricular performance in chronic bronchitis and emphysema. Respiration 1984;46:157.

143. Janson C, Gislason T, Boman G, et al. Sleep disturbances in patients with asthma. Respir Med 1990;84:37.

144. Deegan PC, McNicholas WT. Continuous non-invasive monitoring of evolving acute severe asthma during sleep. Thorax 1994;49:613.

145. Turner-Warwick M. Epidemiology of nocturnal asthma. Am J Med 1988;85:6.

146. Cochrane GM, Clark TJH. A survey of asthma mortality in patients between ages 35 and 65 in the greater London hospitals in 1971. Thorax 1975;30:300.

147. Hetzel MR, Clark TJH, Branthwaite MA. Asthma: analysis of sudden deaths and ventilatory arrests in hospital. BMJ 1977;1:808.

148. Kales A, Beall GN, Bajor GF, et al. Sleep studies in asthmatic adults: relationship of attacks to sleep stage and time of night. J Allergy 1968;41:164.

149. Kales J, Kales JD, Sly R, et al. Sleep patterns of asthmatic children: all night electroencephalographic studies. J Allergy 1970;46:300.

150. Montplaisir J, Walsh J, Malo JL. Nocturnal asthma: features of attacks, sleep and breathing patterns. Am Rev Respir Dis 1982;125:18.

151. Janson C, De Backer W, Gislason T, et al. Increased prevalence of sleep disturbances and daytime sleepiness in subjects with bronchial asthma: a population study of young adults in three European countries. Eur Respir J 1996;9:2132.

152. van Keimpema ARG, Ariaanz M, Nauta JJP, Postmus PE. Subjective sleep quality and mental fitness in asthmatic patients. J Asthma 1995;32:69.

153. Martin RJ. Nocturnal Asthma. In RJ Martin (ed), Cardiorespiratory Disorders During Sleep. Mt. Kisco, NY: Futura, 1990;189.

154. Clark TJH, Hetzel MR. Diurnal variation of asthma. Br J Dis Chest 1977;71:87.

155. Catterall JR, Rhind GB, Stewart IC, et al. Effect of sleep deprivation on overnight bronchoconstriction in nocturnal asthma. Thorax 1986;41:676.

156. Jonsson E, Mossberg B. Impairment of ventilatory function by supine posture in asthma. Eur J Respir Dis 1984;65:496.

157. Barnes PJ, Fitzgerald G, Brown M, et al. Nocturnal asthma and changes in circulating epinephrine, histamine and cortisol. N Engl J Med 1980;303:263.

158. Goodall RJR, Earis JE, Cooper DN, et al. Relationship between asthma and gastroesophageal reflux. Thorax 1981;36:116.

159. Tan WC, Ballard RD, Martin RJ, et al. The role of gastroesophageal reflux in nocturnal asthma. Am Rev Respir Dis 1988;137:55.

160. Sullivan CE, Zamel N, Kozar LF, et al. Regulation of airway smooth muscle tone in sleeping dogs. Am Rev Respir Dis 1979;119:87.

161. Rhind GB, Connaughton JJ, McFie J, et al. Sustained release choline theophyllinate in nocturnal asthma. BMJ 1985;291:1605.

162. Janson C, Gislason T, Almqvist M, et al. Theophylline disturbs sleep mainly in caffeine-sensitive persons. Pulm Pharmacol 1989;2:125.

163. Berquist WE, Rachelefsky GS, Kadden M, et al. Effect of theophylline on gastroesophageal reflux in normal adults. J Allergy Clin Immunol 1981;67:407.

164. Stein MR, Towner TG, Weber RW, et al. The effect of theophylline on the lower esophageal sphincter pressure. Ann Allergy 1980;45:238.

165. Hubert D, Gaudric M, Guerre J, et al. Effect of theophylline on gastroesophageal reflux in patients with asthma. J Allergy Clin Immunol 1988;81:1168.

166. Guilleminault C, Silvestri R. Aging, drugs and sleep. Neurobiol Aging 1982;3:379.

167. Chan CS, Woolcock AJ, Sullivan CE. Nocturnal asthma: role of snoring and obstructive sleep apnea. Am Rev Respir Dis 1988;137:1502.

168. Martin RJ, Cicutto LC, Smith HR, et al. Airway inflammation in nocturnal asthma. Am Rev Respir Dis 1991;143:351.

169. Ballard RD, Saathoff MC, Patel DK, et al. The effect of sleep on nocturnal bronchoconstriction and ventilatory patterns in asthmatics. J Appl Physiol 1989;67:243.

170. Catterall JR, Douglas NJ, Calverley PMA. Irregular breathing and hypoxemia during sleep in chronic stable asthma. Lancet 1982;1:301.

171. Soutar CA, Costello J, Ijuduola O, et al. Nocturnal and morning asthma. Thorax 1975;30:436.

172. Kraft M, Wenzel SE, Bettinger CM, Martin RJ. The effect of salmeterol on nocturnal symptoms, airway function and inflammation in asthma. Chest 1997;111:1249.

173. Greening AP, Ind PW, Northfield M, et al. Added salmeterol versus higher-dose cortical steroid in asthma patients with symptoms on existing inhaled cortical steroids. Lancet 1994;344:219.

174. Fitzpatrick NF, Mackay T, Driver H, et al. Salmeterol in nocturnal asthma: a double-blind placebo trial of a long acting inhaled $\beta_2$ agonist. BMJ 1990;301:1365.

175. Brambilla C, Chastang C, Georges D, et al. Salmeterol compared with slow-release terbutaline in nocturnal asthma. Allergy 1994;49:421.

176. Britton MG, Earnshaw JS, Palmer JBD. A 12-month comparison of salmeterol with salbutamol in asthmatic patients. Eur Respir J 1992;5:1062.

177. Lundbeck B, Rawlinson DW, Palmer JBD. A 12-month comparison of salmeterol and salbutamol as dry powder formulations in asthmatic patients. Thorax 1993;48:148.

178. Warren CPW. Lung Restriction. In M Kryger (ed), Pathophysiology of Respiration. New York: Wiley, 1981;43.

179. Perez-Padilla RR, West P, Lertzman M, et al. Breathing during sleep in patients with interstitial lung disease. Am Rev Respir Dis 1985;132:224.

180. Hoeppner VH, Cockcroft DW, Dosman JA, et al. Nighttime ventilation improves respiratory failure in secondary kyphoscoliosis. Am Rev Respir Dis 1984;129:240.

181. Bach JR, Robert D, Leger P, Langevin B. Sleep fragmentation in kyphoscoliotic individuals with alveolar hypoventilation treated by NIPPV. Chest 1995;107:1552.

182. Soll AH. Peptic Ulcer: Pathophysiology. In JC Bennett, F Plum (eds), Cecil Textbook of Medicine. Philadelphia: Saunders, 1996;662.

183. Cover TL, Blaser MJ. *Helicobacter pylori* and gastroduodenal disease. Annu Rev Med 1992;43:135.

184. Dooley CP, Cohen H. *Helicobacter pylori* infection. Gastroenterol Clin North Am 1993;22:1.

185. Isenberg JI, Soll AH. Peptic Ulcer, Epidemiology, Clinical Manifestations and Diagnosis. In JC Bennett, F Plum (eds), Cecil Textbook of Medicine. Philadelphia: Saunders, 1996;664.

186. Graham DY. Peptic Ulcer: Medical Therapy. In JC Bennett, F Plum (eds), Cecil Textbook of Medicine. Philadelphia: Saunders, 1996;667.

187. Dragstedt LR. A concept of the etiology of gastric and duodenal ulcers. Gastroenterology 1956;30:208.

188. Orr WC, Hall WH, Stahl ML, et al. Sleep patterns and gastric acid secretion in duodenal ulcer disease. Arch Intern Med 1976;136:655.

189. Watanabe M, Nakazawa S, Yoshino J, et al. A study of the relationship between nocturnal intragastric pH and sleep stages of peptic ulcer. Nippon Shokakibyo Gakkai Zasshi 1995;92:1241.

190. Graham DY. Treatment of peptic ulcers caused by *Helicobacter pylori*. N Engl J Med 1993;328:349.

191. Kildebo S, Aronsen O, Bernersen B, et al. Cimetidine 800 mg at night, in the treatment of duodenal ulcers. Scand J Gastroenterol 1985;20:1147.

192. Graham DY, Lew GM, Klein PD, et al. Effect of treatment of *Helicobactor pylori* infection on the long-term recurrence of gastric or duodenal ulcer. A randomized controlled study. Ann Intern Med 1992;116:705.

193. McGuigan JE. Peptic Ulcer and Gastritis. In JD Wilson, E Braunwald, KJ Isselbacher, et al. (eds), Harrison's Principles of Internal Medicine (2nd ed). New York: McGraw-Hill, 1991;1229.

194. Penstone JG, Wormsley KG. Review article: maintenance treatment with $H_2$-receptor antagonist for peptic ulcer disease. Aliment Pharmacol Ther 1992;6:3.

195. Howden CW, Jones DB, Hunl RH. Nocturnal doses of $H_2$ receptor antagonists for duodenal ulcer. Lancet 1985;1:647.

196. Van Deventer GM, Elashoff JD, Reedy TJ, et al. A randomized study of maintenance therapy with ranitidine to prevent the recurrence of duodenal ulcer. N Engl J Med 1989;30:1113.

197. Orr WC. Gastrointestinal Disorders. In MH Kryger, T Roth, WC Dement (eds), Principles and Practice of Sleep Medicine. Philadelphia: Saunders, 1989;622.

198. Gledhill T, Buck M, Paul A, et al. Comparison of the effects of proximal gastric vagotomy, cimetidine, and placebo on nocturnal intragastric acidity and acid secretion in patients with cimetidine resistance duodenal ulcer. Br J Surg 1983;70:704.

199. Gough KR, Bardhan KD, Crowe JP, et al. Ranitidine and cimetidine in prevention of duodenal ulcer relapse. Lancet 1984;2:659.

200. Silvis SE. Final report on the United States multicenter trial comparing ranitidine to cimetidine as maintenance therapy following healing of duodenal ulcer. J Clin Gastroenterol 1985;7:482.

201. Santana IA, Sharma BK, Pounder RE, et al. 24-hour intragastric acidity during maintenance treatment with ranitidine. BMJ 1984;289:1420.

202. Cohen S, Parkman HP. Diseases of the Esophagus. In JC Bennett, F Plum (eds), Cecil Textbook of Medicine. Philadelphia: Saunders, 1996;650.

203. Klauser AG, Schindlbeck NE, Muller-Lissner SA. Symptoms in gastroesophageal reflux disease. Gut 1988;29:886.

204. Richter JE, Castell DO. Gastroesophageal reflux. Ann Intern Med 1982;97:93.

205. Pope CE II. Acid-reflux disorders. N Engl J Med 1994;331:656.

206. Barrett NR. Chronic peptic ulcer of the oesophagus and "oesophagitis." Br J Surg 1950;38:175.

207. Allison PR, Johnstone AS. The oesophagus lined with gastric mucous membrane. Thorax 1953;8:87.

208. Bozymski EM, Herlihy KJ, Orlando RC. Barrett's esophagus. Ann Intern Med 1982;97:103.

209. Mittal RK, Balabin DH. The esophagogastric junction. N Engl J Med 1997;336:924.

210. Johnsson F, Joelsson B. Reproducibility of ambulatory oesophageal pH monitoring. Gut 1988;29:886.

211. Johnson LF, DeMeester TR. Twenty-four hour pH monitoring of the distal esophagus. Am J Gastroenterol 1974;62:325.

212. DeMeester R, Johnson LF, Guy JJ, et al. Patterns of gastroesophageal reflux in health and disease. Ann Surg 1976;184:459.

213. Allen CJ, Newhouse MT. Gastroesophageal reflux and chronic respiratory disease. Am Rev Respir Dis 1984;129:645.

214. David P, Denis P, Nouvet G, et al. Lung function and gastroesophageal reflux during chronic bronchitis. Bull Eur Physiopathol Respir 1982;18:81.

215. Orringer MB. Respiratory symptoms and esophageal reflux. Chest 1979;76:618.
216. Chernow B, Johnson LF, Janowitz WR, et al. Pulmonary aspiration as a consequence of gastroesophageal reflux: a diagnostic approach. Dig Dis Sci 1979;24:839.
217. Tan WC, Martin RJ, Pandey R, et al. Effects of spontaneous and simulated gastroesophageal reflux on sleeping asthmatics. Am Rev Respir Dis 1990;141:1394.
218. Mansfield LE. Gastroesophageal reflux and respiratory disorders: a review. Ann Allergy 1989;62:158.
219. Pack AI. Acid: a nocturnal bronchoconstrictor? Am Rev Respir Dis 1990;141:1391.
220. Herbst JJ, Minton SD, Book LS. Gastroesophageal reflux causing respiratory distress and apnea in newborn infants. J Pediatr 1979;95:763.
221. Herbst JJ, Book LS, Bray PF. Gastroesophageal reflux in the "near miss" sudden infant death syndrome. J Pediatr 1978;92:73.
222. Triadafilopoulos G, Castillo T. Nonpropulsive esophageal contractions and gastroesophageal reflux. Am J Gastroenterol 1991;86:153.
223. David D, Mertz H, Fefer L, et al. Sleep and duodenal motor activity in patients with severe non-ulcer dyspepsia. Gut 1994;35:916.
224. Talley NJ, Phillips SF. Non-ulcer dyspepsia: potential causes and pathophysiology. Ann Intern Med 1988; 108:8665.
225. Barbara L, Camilleri M, Corinaldesi R, et al. Definition and investigation of dyspepsia. Consensus of an international ad hoc working party. Dig Dis Sci 1989; 34:1272.
226. Talley NJ, Zinsmeister AR, Schleck CD, Melton LJ. Dyspepsia and dyspepsia subgroups: a population-based study. Gastroenterology 1992;102:1259.
227. Talley NJ. Spectrum of chronic dyspepsia in the presence of the irritable bowel syndrome. Scand J Gastroenterol 1991;182:7.
228. Whorwell PJ, McCallum M, Creed FH. Non-colonic features of irritable bowel syndrome. Gut 1986;27:37.
229. Maxton DG, Morris J, Whorwell PJ. More accurate diagnosis of irritable bowel syndrome by the use of "non-colonic" symptomatology. Gut 1991;32:784.
230. Veale D, Kavanch G, Fielding JF, Fitzgerald O. Primary fibromyalgia and irritable bowel syndrome: different expressions of a common pathogenetic process. Br J Rheumatol 1991;30:220.
231. Triadafilopoulos G, Simms RW, Goldenberg DL. Bowel Dysfunction in Fibromyalgia. In JR Friction, EA Awad (eds), Advances in Pain Research (Vol 17). New York: Raven, 1990;227.
232. Yunus M, Masi AT, Calabro JJ, et al. Primary fibromyalgia (fibrositis): clinical study of 50 patients with matched normal controls. Semin Arthritis Rheum 1981;11:151.
233. Moldofsky H. The Contribution of Sleep-Wake Physiology to Fibromyalgia. In JR Friction, EA Awad (eds), Advances in Pain Research (Vol 17). New York: Raven, 1990;227.
234. Skatrud J, Iber C, Ewart R, et al. Disordered breathing during sleep in hypothyroidism. Am Rev Respir Dis 1981;124:325.
235. Millman RP, Bevilacqua J, Peterson DD, et al. Central sleep apnea in hypothyroidism. Am Rev Respir Dis 1983;127:504.
236. Zwillich CW, Pierson DJ, Hofeldt FD, et al. Ventilatory control in myxedema and hypothyroidism. N Engl J Med 1975;292:662.
237. Rajagopal KR, Abbrecht PH, Derderian SS, et al. Obstructive sleep apnea in hypothyroidism. Ann Intern Med 1984;101:491.
238. Kales A, Heuser G, Jacobson A, et al. All-night sleep studies in hypothyroid patients before and after treatment. J Clin Endocrinol 1967;27:1593.
239. Grunstein RR, Sullivan CE. Sleep apnea and hypothyroidism: mechanisms and management. Am J Med 1988;85:775.
240. Dunleavy DLF, Oswald I, Brown P, et al. Hyperthyroidism, sleep and growth hormone. Electroencephalogr Clin Neurophysiol 1974;36:259.
241. Passouant P, Passouant-Fountaine T, Cadilhac J. L'influence de l'hyperthyrodie sur le sommeil. Étude clinique et experimentale. Rev Neurol (Paris) 1966;115:353.
242. Johns MW, Rinsler MG. Sleep and thyroid function. Further studies in healthy young men. J Psychosom Res 1977;21:161.
243. Astrom C, Lindholm J. Growth hormone–deficient young adults have decreased deep sleep. Neuroendocrinology 1990;51:82.
244. Astrom C, Pedersen SA, Lindholm J. The influence of growth hormone on sleep in adults with growth hormone deficiency. Clin Endocrinol 1990;33:495.
245. Wu RHK, Thorpy MJ. Effect of growth hormone treatment on sleep EEGs in growth hormone deficiency children. Sleep 1988;11:425.
246. Sullivan CE, Parker S, Grunstein RR, et al. Ventilatory Control in Sleep Apnea: A Search for Brain's Neurochemical Defects. In FG Issa, PM Suratt, JE Remmers (eds), Sleep and Respiration. New York: Wiley-Liss, 1990;325.
247. Grunstein RR, Ho KY, Sullivan CE. Sleep apnea in acromegaly. Ann Intern Med 1991;115:527.
248. Grunstein RR, Ho KY, Berthon-Jones M, et al. Central sleep apnea is associated with increased ventilatory response to carbon dioxide and hypersecretion of growth hormone in patients with acromegaly. Am J Respir Crit Care Med 1994;150:496.
249. Rosenow F, Reuter S, Deuss U, et al. Sleep apnea in treated acromegaly: relative frequency and predisposing factors. Clin Endocrinol 1996;45:563.
250. Leibowitz G, Shapiro MS, Salameh M, Glaser B. Improvement of sleep apnea due to acromegaly during short-term treatment with octreotide. J Intern Med 1994;236:231.
251. Buyse B, Michiels E, Bouillon R, et al. Relief of sleep apnea after treatment of acromegaly: report of three cases and review of the literature. Eur Respir J 1997;10:1401.

252. Rosenstock J, Doyle A, Joplin J, et al. Acromegaly with sleep disturbance relieved by yttrium-90 pituitary implantation. J Roy Soc Med 1982;75:209.

253. Pekkarinen T, Partinen M, Pelkonen R, Iivanainen M. Sleep apnea and daytime somnolence in acromegaly: relationship to endocrinological factors. Clin Endocrinol 1987;27:649.

254. Hart TB, Radow SK, Blackard WG, et al. Sleep apnea in active acromegaly. Arch Intern Med 1985;145:865.

255. Tsai JS, Zorilla LL, Jacob KK, et al. Nocturnal monitoring of growth hormone, insulin, C-peptide, and glucose in patients with acromegaly. Am J Med Sci 1996;311:281.

256. Williams RL. Sleep Disturbances in Various Medical and Surgical Conditions. In RL Williams, I Karacan, CA Moore (eds), Sleep Disorders. New York: Wiley, 1988;265.

257. Karacan I, Williams RL, Bose J, et al. Insomnia in hemodialytic and kidney transplant patients. Abstracts of papers presented to the eleventh annual meeting of the Association for the Psychophysiological Study of Sleep. Psychophysiology 1972;9:137.

258. Daly RJ, Hassall C. Reported sleep on maintenance haemodialysis. BMJ 1970;2:508.

259. Passouant P, Cadihac J, Baldy-Moulinier M, et al. Etude du sommeil nocturne chez des uremiques chroniques soumis a une epuration extrarenael. Electroencephalogr Clin Neurophysiol 1970;29:441.

260. Strub B, Schneider-Helmert D, Gnirss F, et al. Sleep disorders in patients with chronic renal insufficiency in long-term hemodialysis treatment. Schweiz Med Wochenschr 1982;112:824.

261. Fraser C, Arieff AI. Nervous system complications in uremia. Ann Intern Med 1988;109:143.

262. Kimmel PL. Sleep disorders in chronic renal disease. J Nephrol 1989;1:59.

263. Kimmel PL. Sleep Disorders in Hemodialysis Patients. In JP Bosch (ed), Hemodialysis: High Efficiency Treatment. Contemporary Issues in Nephrology (Vol 27). New York: Churchill Livingstone, 1993;95.

264. Walker S, Fine A, Kryger MH. Sleep complaints are common in a dialysis unit. Am J Kidney Dis 1995;26:751.

265. Kimmel PL, Gavin C, Miller G, et al. Disordered sleep and non-compliance in a patient with end-stage renal disease. Adv Ren Replace Ther 1997;4:55.

266. Yasuda T, Nishimura A, Katsuki Y, et al. Restless legs syndrome treated successfully by kidney transplantation: a case report. Clin Transplant 1986;138:138.

267. Kimmel PL, Miller G, Mendelson WB. Sleep apnea syndrome in chronic renal disease. Am J Med 1989;86:308.

268. Kimmel PL. Sleep apnea in end-stage renal disease. Semin Dialys 1991;4:52.

269. Millman RP, Kimmel PL, Shore ET, et al. Sleep apnea in hemodialysis patients: the lack of testosterone effect on its pathogenesis. Nephron 1985;40:407.

270. Mendelson WB, Wadhwa NK, Greenberg HE, et al. Effects of hemodialysis on sleep apnea syndrome in end-stage renal disease. Clin Nephrol 1990;33:247.

271. Pressman MR, Benz RL, Schleifer CR, et al. Sleep-disordered breathing in ESRD: acute beneficial effects of treatment with nasal continuous positive airway pressure. Kidney Int 1993;43:1134.

272. Hallet M, Barden S, Stewart D, et al. Sleep apnea in end-stage renal diseased patients on hemodialysis and continuous ambulatory peritoneal dialysis. ASAIO J 1995;41:M435.

273. Fein AM, Niederman MS, Imbriano L, et al. Reversal of sleep apnea in uremia by dialysis. Arch Intern Med 1987;147:1355.

274. Anderton J, Harris E, Robson J. The ventilatory response to carbon dioxide and hydrogen ion in renal failure. Clin Sci 1965;28:251.

275. Hamilton R, Epstein P, Henderson L, et al. Control of breathing in uremia: ventilatory response to $CO_2$ after hemodialysis. J Appl Physiol 1976;41:216.

276. Frasier C, Arieff AI. Nervous system complications in uremia. Ann Intern Med 1988;109:143.

277. Crabb JE, Pingleton SK, Gollub S, et al. Sleep-disordered breathing in decompensated congestive heart failure [abstract]. Am Rev Respir Dis 1985;105:68.

278. Ingbar DH, Gee BL. Pathophysiology and treatment of sleep apnea. Annu Rev Med 1985;36:365.

279. Soreide E, Skeie B, Kirvela O, et al. Branched-chain amino acid in chronic renal failure patients: respiratory and sleep effects. Kidney Int 1991;40:539.

280. Trenkwalder C, Walters AS, Hening W. Periodic limb movements and restless legs syndrome. Neurol Clin 1996;14:629.

281. Winkleman JW, Chertow GM, Lazarus JM. Restless legs syndrome in end-stage renal disease. Am J Kidney Dis 1996;28:372.

282. Roger SD, Harris DCH, Stewart JH. Possible relation between restless legs and anemia in renal dialysis patients. Lancet 1991;337:1551.

283. Callaghan N. Restless legs syndrome in uremic neuropathy. Neurology 1966;16:359.

284. Trenkwalder C, Stiasny K, Pollmaecher T, et al. L-Dopa therapy of uremic and idiopathic restless legs syndrome: a double-blind crossover trial. Sleep 1995;18:681.

285. Goldenberg DL. Fibromyalgia syndrome: an emerging but controversial condition. JAMA 1987;257:2782.

286. Yunus M, Masi AT, Calabro JJ, et al. Primary fibromyalgia (fibrositis): clinical study of 50 patients with matched normal controls. Semin Arthritis Rheum 1981;11:151.

287. Reiffenberger DH, Amundson LH. Fibromyalgia syndrome: a review. Am Fam Physician 1996;53:1698.

288. Neeck G, Riedel W. Neuromediator and hormonal perturbations in fibromyalgia syndrome: results of chronic stress? Baillieres Clin Rheumatol 1994;8:763.

289. Lorenzen I. Fibromyalgia: a clinical challenge. J Intern Med 1994;235:199.

290. Harvey CK, Cadena R, Dunlap L. Fibromyalgia. Part I. Review of the literature. J Am Podiatr Med Assoc 1993;83:412.

291. Schaver JL, Lentz M, Landis CA, et al. Sleep, psychologic distress, and stress arousal in women with fibromyalgia. Res Nurs Health 1997;20:247.

292. Tishler M, Barak Y, Parin D, Yaron M. Sleep distur- bances, fibromyalgia and primary Sjogeren's syndrome. Clin Exp Rheumatol 1997;15:71.

293. Moldofsky H, Lue FA, Smythe H. Alpha EEG sleep and morning symptoms of rheumatoid arthritis. J Rheumatol 1983;10:373.

294. Moldofsky H, Saskin P, Lue FA. Sleep and symptoms in fibrositis syndrome after a febrile illness. J Rheuma- tol 1988;15:1701.

295. Hauri P, Hawkins H. Alpha-delta sleep. Electroen- cephalogr Clin Neurophysiol 1973;34:233.

296. Scheuler W, Kubicki ST, Marquardt J, et al. The Alpha Sleep Pattern—Quantitative Analysis and Functional Aspects. In WP Koella, et al. (eds), Sleep 86. Stuttgart: Gustav Fischer, 1988;284.

297. Horne JA, Shackett BS. Alpha-like EEG activity in non- REM sleep and the fibromyalgia (fibrositis) syndrome. Electroencephalogr Clin Neurophysiol 1991;79:271.

298. Roizenblatt S, Tufik S, Goldenberg J, et al. Juvenile fibromyalgia: clinical and polysomnographic aspects. J Rheumatol 1997;24:579.

299. Buchwald D. Fibromyalgia and chronic fatigue syn- drome: similarities and differences. Rheum Dis Clin North Am 1996;22:219.

300. Moldofsky H, Lue FA, Mously C, et al. The effect of zolpidem in patients with fibromyalgia: a dose ranging, double-blind, placebo control, modified cross-over study. J Rheumatol 1996;23:529.

301. Hansen NE. Sleep related plasma haemoglobin levels in paroxysmal nocturnal haemoglobinuria. Acta Med Scand 1968;184:547.

302. Scharf MB, Lobel JS, Cadwell E, et al. Nocturnal oxy- gen desaturation in patients with sickle cell anemia. JAMA 1983;249:1753.

303. Brooks LJ, Koziol SM, Chiarucci AM, Berman BW. Does sleep-disordered breathing contribute to the clini- cal severity of sickle cell anemia? J Pediatr Hematol Oncol 1996;18:135.

304. Samandari T, Smith BD, Morgan HJ. Progressive som- nolence and confusion in a patient with hereditary hem- orrhagic telangiectasia. Tenn Med 1996;89:417.

305. Hara KS, Shepard JW Jr. Sleep and Critical Care Med- icine. In RJ Martin (ed), Cardiorespiratory Disorders During Sleep. Mt. Kisco, NY: Futura, 1990;323.

306. Krachman SL, D'Alonzo GE, Criner GJ. Sleep in the intensive care unit. Chest 1995;107:1713.

307. Schwab RJ. Disturbances of sleep in the intensive care unit. Crit Care Clin 1994;10:681.

308. Easton C, MacKenzie F. Sensory-perceptual alterations: delirium in the intensive care unit. Heart Lung 1988;17:229.

309. Helton MC, Gordon SH, Nunnery SL. The correlation between sleep deprivation and the intensive care unit syndrome. Heart Lung 1980;9:464.

310. Heller SS, Frank KA, Malm JR, et al. Psychiatric com- plications of open-heart surgery. N Engl J Med 1970;283:1015.

311. Weber RJ, Soak MA, Bolender BJ, et al. The intensive care unit syndrome: causes, treatment and prevention. Drug Intell Clin Pharm 1985;19:13.

312. Hansell HN. The behavioral effects of noise on man: the patient with intensive care unit psychosis. Heart Lung 1984;13:59.

313. Aaron JN, Carlisle CC, Carskadon MA, et al. Environ- mental noise as a cause of sleep disruption in an inter- mediate respiratory care unit. Sleep 1996;19:707.

314. Topf M, Bookman M, Arand D. Effects of critical care unit noise on the subjective quality of sleep. J Adv Nurs 1996;24:545.

315. Bentley S, Murphy F, Dudley H. Perceived noise in sur- gical wards and an intensive care area: an objective analysis. BMJ 1977;2:1503.

316. Meyers TJ, Eveloff SE, Bauer MS, et al. Adverse envi- ronmental conditions in the respiratory and medical ICU settings. Chest 1994;105:1211.

317. Schenck CH, Mahowald MW. Injurious sleep behavior disorders (parasomnias) affecting patients on intensive care units. Intensive Care Med 1991;17:219.

318. Richards KC, Bairnsfather L. A description of night sleep patterns in the critical care unit. Heart Lung 1988;17:35.

319. Orr WC, Stahl ML. Sleep disturbances after open heart surgery. Am J Cardiol 1977;39:196.

320. Karacan I, Green JR Jr, Taylor WJ, et al. Sleep in Post- myocardial Infarction Patients. In RS Eliot (ed), Stress and the Heart: Contemporary Problems in Cardiology. Mt. Kisco, NY: Futura, 1974;163.

321. Aurell J, Elmqvist D. Sleep in the surgical intensive care unit: continuous polygraphic recording of sleep in nine patients receiving postoperative care. BMJ 1985; 290:1029.

322. Buckle B, Pouliot Z, Miller T, et al. Polysomnography in acutely ill intensive care unit patients. Chest 1992;102:288.

323. Langtry HD, Benfield P. Zolpidem—a review of its pharmacodynamic and pharmacokinetic properties and therapeutic potentials. Drugs 1990;40:291.

324. Norman SE, Chediak AD, et al. Sleep disturbances in HIV-infected homosexual men. AIDS 1990;4:775.

325. Norman SE, Chediak AD, Freeman C, et al. Sleep dis- turbances in men with asymptomatic human immuno- deficiency (HIV) infection. Sleep 1992;15:150.

326. Norman SE, Chediak AD. Longitudinal analysis of sleep disturbances in HIV-infected men. Sleep Res 1992;21:304.

327. Moller WM, Schreiber W, Krieg J-C, et al. Alterations of nocturnal sleep in patients with HIV infection. Acta Neurol Scand 1991;83:141.

328. White JL, Darko DF, Brown SJ, et al. Early central ner- vous system response to HIV infection: sleep distortion and cognitive motor decrements. AIDS 1995;9:1043.

329. Darko DF, Mitler ML, Henricksen SJ. Lentiviral infec- tion, immune response peptides and sleep. Adv Neu- roimmunol 1995;5:57.

330. Darko DF, Miller JC, Gallen C, et al. Sleep electroencephalogram delta-frequency amplitude, night plasma levels of tumor necrosis factor alpha, and human immune deficiency virus infection. Proc Natl Acad Sci U S A 1995;92:12080.

331. Nokes KL, Kendrew J. Sleep quality in people with HIV disease. J Assoc Nurses AIDS Care 1996;7:43.

332. Cohen FL, Ferrans CE, Vizgirda V, et al. Sleep in men and women infected with human immunodeficiency virus. Holist Nurse Pract 1996;10:33.

333. Epstein LJ, Strollo PJ Jr, Donegan RB, et al. Obstructive sleep apnea in patients with human immunodeficiency virus (HIV) disease. Sleep 1995;18:368.

334. Epstein LJ, Strollo PJ, Westbrook PR. Severe obstructive sleep apnea in HIV infected men: a case series. Am Rev Respir Dis 1993;147:A234.

335. Garrigo J, Norman S, Chediak F. Occult obstructive sleep apnea in HIV infected asymptomatic homosexual men cannot be explained by alterations of waking upper airway compliance. Sleep Res 1992;21:292.

336. Logigian EL, Kaplan RF, Steere AC. Chronic neurologic manifestations of Lyme disease. N Engl J Med 1990;323:1438.

337. Halperin JJ. Neurological applications of Lyme disease. Neurol Chron 1992;1:1.

338. Dinerman H, Steere AC. Lyme disease associated with fibromyalgia. Ann Intern Med 1992;117:281.

339. Steere AC, Beraidi VP, Weeks KE, et al. Evaluation of the intrathecal antibody response to *Borrelia burgdorferi* as a diagnostic test for Lyme neuroborreliosis. J Infect Dis 1990;161:1203.

340. Rahn DW, Malawista SE. Lyme disease: recommendations for diagnosis and treatment. Ann Intern Med 1991;114:472.

341. Malawista SE. Lyme Disease. In JC Bennett, F Plum (eds), Cecil Textbook of Medicine. Philadelphia: Saunders, 1996;1715.

342. Tugwell P, Dennis DT, Weinstein A, et al. Guidelines for laboratory evaluation in the diagnosis of Lyme disease. Clinical guidelines part 1 and part 2. Ann Intern Med 1997;127:1106.

343. Greenberg HE, Ney G, Seharf SM, et al. Sleep quality in Lyme disease. Sleep 1995;18:912.

344. Krupp LB, Mendelson WB, Friedman R. An overview of chronic fatigue syndrome. J Clin Psychiatry 1991;52:403.

345. Holmes GP, Kaplan JE, Gantz NM, et al. Chronic fatigue syndrome: a working case definition. Ann Intern Med 1988;108:385.

346. Komaroff AL, Fagioli LR, Geiger AM, et al. An examination of the working case definition of chronic fatigue syndrome. Am J Med 1996;100:56.

347. Chester AC. Chronic fatigue syndrome criteria in patients with other forms of unexplained chronic fatigue. J Psychiatr Res 1997;31:45.

348. Schluederberg A, Straus SE, Peterson P. Chronic fatigue syndrome research. Definition and medical outcome assessment. Ann Intern Med 1992;117:325.

349. Wilson A, Hicki I, Lloyd A, et al. The treatment of chronic fatigue syndrome: science and speculation. Am J Med 1994;96:544.

350. Bou-Holaigah I. The relationship between neurally mediated hypotension and the chronic fatigue syndrome. JAMA 1995;274:961.

351. Dickinson CJ. Chronic fatigue syndrome—etiological aspects. Eur J Clin Invest 1997;27:257.

352. Sharpe M, et al. Increased brain serotonin function in men with chronic fatigue syndrome. BMJ 1997; 315:164.

353. Fischler B, Le Bon O, Hoffmann G, et al. Sleep anomalies in the chronic fatigue syndrome. A comorbidity study. Neuropsychobiology 1997;35:115.

354. Manu P, Lane TJ, Matthews DA, et al. Alpha-delta sleep in patients with a chief complaint of chronic fatigue. South Med J 1994;87:465.

355. Buchwald D, Pascualy R, Bombardier C, Kith P. Sleep disorders in patients with chronic fatigue. Clin Infect Dis 1994;18:S68.

356. Sharpe M, Chalder T, Palmer I, Wessely S. Chronic fatigue syndrome. A practical guide to assessment and management. Gen Hosp Psychiatry 1997;19:185.

357. Quinn TC. African Trypanosomiasis (Sleeping Sickness). In JC Bennett, F Plum (eds), Cecil Textbook of Medicine. Philadelphia: Saunders, 1996;1896.

358. Brandenberger G, Buguet A, Spiegel K, et al. Disruption of endocrine rhythms in sleeping sickness with preserved relationship between hormonal pulsatility and the REM-NREM sleep cycles. J Biol Rhythms 1996; 11:258.

359. Billiard M. Other Hypersomnias. In MJ Thorpy (ed), Handbook of Sleep Disorders. New York: Marcel Dekker, 1990;353.

360. Buguet A, Bert J, Tapie P, et al. The distribution of sleep and wakefulness in human African trypanosomiasis. Bull Soc Pathol Exot 1994;87:362.

361. Radomski MW, Buguet A, Doua F, et al. Relationship of plasma growth hormone to slow-wave sleep in African sleeping sickness. Neuroendocrinology 1996; 63:393.

362. Claustrat B, Buguet A, Geoffriau M, et al. The nyctohemeral rhythm of melatonin is preserved in human African trypanosomiasis. Bull Soc Pathol Exot 1994;87:380.

363. Radomski MW, Buguet A, Bogui P, et al. Disruptions in the secretion of cortisol, prolactin and certain cytokines in human African trypanosomiasis patients. Bull Soc Pathol Exot 1994;87:376.

364. Radomski MW, Buguet A, Montmayeur A, et al. Twenty-four hour plasma cortisol and prolactin in human African trypanosomiasis patients and healthy African controls. Am J Trop Med Hyg 1995;52:281.

365. Bentivoglio M, Grassi-Zucconi G, Peng ZC, et al. Trypanosomes cause dysregulation of c-fos expression in the rat suprachiasmatic nucleus. Neuroreport 1994; 5:712.

# Chapter 30
# Circadian Rhythm Disorders

## Mark W. Mahowald and Milton G. Ettinger

Chronobiology, the study of biological rhythms (normal and abnormal), is a field whose time has come. Although giant strides have been made, much remains to be learned. The staggering medical, social, and economic consequences of chronobiological dysfunction are imperatives for further advancement of this exciting field.

Disorders of biological rhythms are of more than academic interest. These disorders affect alertness, concentration, and performance, all of which may be crucial for safety in certain occupations, such as transportation and manufacturing. The *Report of the National Commission on Sleep Disorders Research* has underscored the startling, disastrous socioeconomic consequences of sleepiness in our society at a personal, national, and international level.[1] Sleep-wake schedules play a major role in these consequences. Job-related and social demands on the sleep-wake schedules of individuals may result in circadian rhythm disorders that can be life-threatening. Studies have shown a circadian pattern of motor vehicle accidents, with an approximately threefold higher incidence in early morning hours and another (lesser) peak in the afternoon.[2] Human deaths and births show circadian patterns, with a tendency for both to occur in the late night or early morning.[3,4] Many circadian rhythm disorders that do not have an obvious cause can result in significant impairment if affected individuals are required to perform when sleepy or fatigued as they attempt to adjust to the geophysical world.

Most living creatures follow a consistent and pervasive daily rhythm of activity and rest that is ultimately linked to the periodic energy flow from the sun to a spot on Earth as it rotates. Plants, animals, and even unicellular organisms show daily variations in metabolic activity, locomotion, feeding, and many other functions.[5–8] When isolated from time cues such as sunlight, many creatures show intrinsic rhythms of nearly, but rarely exactly, 24 hours. Certain mice, for example, will run on an exercise wheel for several hours approximately once every 23 hours, when kept in an environment with constant lighting.[7] Such a near–24-hour rhythm is called a *circadian rhythm*, a term coined by Franz Halberg from the Latin *circa*, "about," and *dies*, "day."[9]

In humans and other mammals, the suprachiasmatic nucleus (SCN) of the hypothalamus controls most circadian rhythms, such as the rest-activity rhythm[10,11] and drinking rhythm. There is good evidence that the circadian pacemaker promotes wakefulness.[12] The discovery of a retinohypothalamic tract in animals indicated that the biological clock may be directly influenced by environmental light.[13–16] This led to the application of bright light to reset rhythms of activity in animal studies and the sleep-wake cycle in humans.[17,18] The timing of exposure to bright light with respect to the animal's intrinsic rhythm controls the nature of the resetting. For example, in a diurnal or day-active animal, bright light administered just as activity is beginning, say at 6:00 AM, will typically advance the onset of the next activity onset, which might occur at 5:00 AM the next day. Bright light administered in the middle of the day, at 1:00 PM, for example, usually has no effect on the timing of the next day's activity. The time interval of little effect is called the *dead zone*. Bright light administered at the end of the day a few hours before sleep onset, say at 8:00 PM, often delays the activity rhythms. The animal experiences a delay in activity onset, which in this example, might not occur until 7:30 AM rather than the usual 6:00 AM.

Data obtained from research on bright light administration has led to the concept of the phase response curve (PRC), which indicates the various responses of advance, dead zone, and delay of the activity cycle.[19–21] The PRC is determined by exposing an individual or population to bright light or other stimulus at a variety of clock times in the free-running condition, and noting the effects on subsequent activity onsets. The same stimulus will have dramatically different effects on the underlying rhythm, depending on the timing of administration within the rhythm. The effect on the underlying rhythm is much greater when the light is administered during the subjective night, and may be negligible when the light is administered during the day. Light at the beginning of the "night" will delay the rhythm, whereas light administered toward the end of the night will advance the rhythm.[17,22,23] The PRC may differ substantially among individuals and differ systematically with the intensity of the light stimulus.

The importance of the light-dark cycle on the human biological clock is underscored by the fact that in totally blind humans, only one-third are entrained to the environment. One-third have a cycle that is 24 hours in length but out of phase with the environment, and the remaining one-third experience a free-running pattern longer than 24 hours.[24] In blind individuals, there is a striking relationship between the timing of daytime production of melatonin and the timing of daytime naps.[25]

The fact that some blind individuals become entrained to the light-dark cycle is explained by the persistence of a retinohypothalamic tract that is independent of the tracts for vision. This fact should be taken into account before undertaking bilateral enucleation in blind individuals with normal circadian entrainment.[26] Treatment of totally blind people with a variety of pharmacologic agents may be useful in demonstrating the effect of these drugs on biological rhythms.[27]

It is important to keep in mind that factors such as changes in activity, posture, meals, timed caloric restriction, and the environment may affect circadian rhythms.[28–31] Some evidence exists that age may affect circadian rhythms, as there appears to be a dampening or advancement of the rhythms in the elderly.[32,33]

In humans, many biological variables show circadian rhythms in isolation studies, including temperature, sleep, serum potassium, sodium, calcium, urination, white blood cell count, attention, short-term memory, ability to perform calculations, and performance. Such isolation studies have been carried out for decades and typically require a subject to live in a set of rooms sequestered from external time cues for weeks or longer. In these studies, there are no windows, clocks, radios, televisions, nor current newspapers or magazines. Instruments record activity, core temperature, and electroencephalographic sleep recordings. The laboratory may obtain a variety of other tests, such as serum electrolytes, cortisol, and melatonin.[5]

The human biological clock has two "sleepy" periods—the primary one occurs during the conventional "night" between midnight and 6:00 AM, with a secondary period at "siesta time" in early to midafternoon. The magnitude of this postlunch dip in performance and alertness is individually determined.[34]

Figure 30-1 is a schematic example of a sleep-wake pattern typical of a free-run study. The schematic is not from an actual recording, but is contrived to illustrate some conventions and terms used in the following discussion of circadian rhythm disorders. A free-running pattern like that illustrated in Figure 30-1 is observed briefly in the transition from the chaotic sleep-wake pattern of the newborn to the well-developed sleep-wake, day-night pattern in normal adults.[35]

In addition to overall circadian sleep-wake schedule abnormalities, there may be ultradian (less than 24-hour) dysrhythmias of state (wake, rapid eye movement [REM] sleep, and non-REM [NREM] sleep). These are beyond the scope of this review.[36]

A fascinating study suggests that in one seasonal mammal, longevity may depend on a fixed number of seasonal cycles rather than on a fixed biological age.[37] This finding warrants further study.

## MEDICAL CHRONOBIOLOGY

*Chronobiology* is the study of the timing and mechanisms of biological rhythms. *Medical chronobiology* is a developing field of medicine concerned with two important issues: (1) *chronopathology*, the effect of circadian rhythms on health and their relationship to disease, and (2) *chronopharmacology*, the circadian variability of efficacy and toxicity of various treatments for a wide variety of medical conditions.[38]

### *Chronopathology*

As more physiologic systems and disease states are studied, it has become apparent that many, if not all, have a predictable circadian variation in activity or severity. For instance, blood pressure is lowest at 3:00 AM and epidermal mitosis is maximal at midnight. The same holds true for disease states: Asthma is worst at 4:00 AM and cerebral hemorrhage peaks in the early evening.[39] Nocturnal asthma is probably one of the most studied medical conditions that exhibit marked chronobiological aspects.[40,41] As more is learned about the peaks of occurrence of physiologic variables and disease states, more effective treatment approaches can be developed.[39]

### *Chronopharmacology*

Not only may pharmacologic agents influence biological rhythms, conversely, the timing of administration of a wide variety (and, perhaps all) medications and other therapies such as irradiation may have profound effects on their efficacy and toxicity.[42–44] Substantial work demonstrates that the therapeutic benefits may be maximized and the toxic side effects minimized by administration of the drug at the appropriate time of day. Circadian rhythms in rates of metabolism and inactivation have been demonstrated,[45] along with variation in rates of excretion of drug products.[46] Circadian variations in blood volume and extracellular fluid volume, resulting in varying degrees of dilution of the drug; the susceptibility of the target organ or organs to the circulating drug; and other rhythms all contribute to the net effect of circadian variation in response to a specific med-

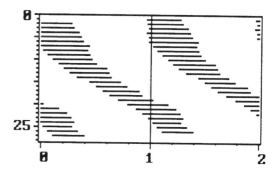

**Figure 30-1.** Schematic example of a free-run study. Black bars represent sleep, double-plotted to highlight patterns. Two 24-hour intervals extend to the right of each number, which represents a day of the study. The left end of the first bar represents the first sleep onset, which occurs at approximately 11:00 PM on day 1. The second sleep onset is represented to the right of the first and also below it. On day 2, sleep begins also at 11:00 PM. During the first 6 days of the study, the subject is "entrained," or synchronized with external time cues, or *zeitgebers*. The sleep onsets are almost all at 11:00 PM. On day 7, isolation begins. Sleep onset is delayed by approximately 30 minutes on day 8. From days 7 through 17, there is a fairly constant delay of approximately 1 hour per day. Sleep onsets occur throughout the hours of the day. The average time between sleep onsets, which is one measure of the "period" of the cycle, is approximately 25 hours, typical for humans in free-run conditions.

ication. There is compelling evidence of the importance of considering time of day in drug administration from clinical areas such as cancer chemotherapy, use of anesthetics and antiepileptic drugs, and steroid administration.[47] Some specific examples of circadian variability include the facts that evening administration of diltiazem is more effective than other dosage schedules[48] and continuous intravenous infusion of heparin has a maximum anticoagulant effect between 4:00 and 8:00 AM and a minimum effect at 12:00 PM, indicating that laboratory control should be performed at fixed times.[49]

To date, very little work has been done on the circadian considerations of drugs used to treat sleep disorders. Narcolepsy is a good example of a sleep disorder that requires life-long stimulant therapy. Data are not currently available to help plan timing of medication to maximize therapeutic effects and minimize toxic effects. This concept presents a challenging new opportunity for investigation of drug therapy in sleep disorders.

## CLINICAL EVALUATION

Sleep-wake schedule disorders fall into two categories: (1) primary, meaning that there has been a malfunction of the biological clock per se, and (2) secondary, indicating that the disorder is due to environmental effects on the underlying clock. The secondary disorders (e.g., jet lag and shift work) are usually immediately apparent on simple questioning of the patient. The primary disorders may be much more difficult to diagnose, as they typically masquerade as other disorders such as hypersomnia, insomnia, substance abuse, or psychiatric conditions.

Clinical evaluation must include a thorough medical and psychiatric history, physical examination, and a detailed analysis of the sleep-wake pattern. Careful attention must be given to drug use (prescription and otherwise). One crucial piece of information is whether sleep is uninterrupted and normal once it has begun. If sleep is uninterrupted and normal, it is not the sleep per se, but rather the *timing* of sleep that is the problem. The patient's report of his or her pattern in free-running conditions may be invaluable. Even if there has been no opportunity to obtain such a report, the patient may be amazingly accurate when asked to speculate what the pattern would likely be if he or she were to spend 2 weeks on a South Sea island with absolutely no environmental time constraints (e.g., work, school, meals, family obligations). When free-running, it is usually clear that the issue is the timing, not the duration or quality, of sleep.

A subjective log reflecting at least 2 weeks of the patient's sleep-wake pattern should be available for the initial interview. Often, analysis of such sleep diaries is sufficient to establish a tentative diagnosis. If not, objective data may be invaluable. Such data may be obtained by actigraphy, a technique that provides an objective record of activity that supplements the log. An actigraph is a small wrist-mounted device worn for 1–2 weeks while the device records the activity per time epoch—often 1 minute for a 1-week study. In one model of the actigraph, the recorded unit is the number of zero-crossings of a voltage that is affected by movements of a tiny beam within the actigraph. Like a seismometer, the beam moves with respect to the actigraph when the actigraph moves with the subject's wrist. There are different models of actigraphs, whose principles are reviewed elsewhere.[50] When data collection has been completed, the results are transferred into a personal computer, where software permits display of activity versus time. Figure 30-2 shows an actigraphic report and demonstrates how the pattern is apparent at a glance. There is high correlation between the rest and activity recorded by the actigraph and the sleep-wake pattern.[51]

## TREATMENT MODALITIES

For many years, the circadian rhythm disorders were only of academic interest, as no proven effective treatments existed. This has changed, however, and the majority of patients with these often incapacitating disorders will benefit from accurate diagnosis and appropriate treatment. The mainstays of treatment are chronotherapy and phototherapy.[52] In addition, promising new pharmacologic treatments are on the horizon.

### *Chronotherapy*

In chronotherapy, the desired total sleep time is determined by sleep logs during a free-running period. The patient then delays or advances sleep onset by a few hours every day, sleeping only the predetermined number of hours, until the sleep onset occurs at the desired time. The patient then attempts to maintain the sleep-onset time.[53–55] This method requires several days of free time, and can be derailed if sleeping quarters are not kept dark and quiet during the periods when the patient must sleep.[56]

### *Phototherapy*

As discussed earlier, it has been discovered that exposure to bright light at strategic times of the sleep-wake cycle results in a change in the underlying rhythm. This discovery has led to effective treatment of circadian dysrhythmias.[17,22,56] The timing and duration of the phototherapy depend on diagnosis and individual response. The patient sits at a prescribed distance from a bright light that provides an illumination of more than 2,500 lux at that distance. Fluorescent lights are commonly used. Commercially available light boxes for treatment of seasonal affective disorder typically provide

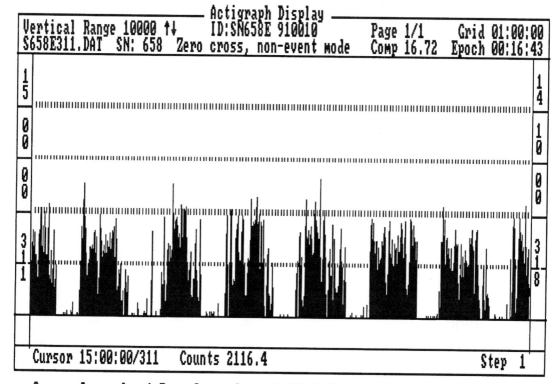

**Figure 30-2.** The vertical bars represent activity levels plotted over seven consecutive 24-hour periods, permitting rapid assessment of the objective rest/activity pattern, which correlates with the wake/sleep patern. The difference between that of a normal adult (**A**) and an adult male with a chaotic wake/sleep pattern (**B**) is immediately apparent.

5,000–10,000 lux, depending on the model. Distance from the light is critical in determining the degree of illumination, according to the inverse square law. Doubling the distance cuts the illumination by three-fourths. The effect of light on human rhythms varies with intensity, wavelength, timing, and duration of exposure. Much remains to be learned regarding these variables and the effectiveness of phototherapy in the clinical setting.[57,58]

To diminish eyestrain, the light should not be aimed directly at the patient's eyes. For patients with a history of eye disorders, the patient's ophthalmologist should be consulted before beginning treatment. Light units should be safety-tested and should include measures to screen ultraviolet rays.[59]

Adverse effects of this treatment include headache, eyestrain, and excessive advance of sleep onset. Possible remedies for these problems include analgesics, change in light position, and decrease in exposure time, respectively. Bright light exposure has been reported to precipitate mania in bipolar individuals.[60,61] In such cases, light therapy should be discontinued immediately, and appropriate measures instituted to control the mania, such as neuroleptics, other mood-stabilizing medication, and hospitalization. Candidates for light therapy should be questioned about both personal and family histories of psychiatric disorders and should be warned about the possible precipitation of mania.

Little information exists regarding the interaction of light and a variety of commonly used medications. Caution is urged in the use of light with medication said to cause photosensitization.[62,63]

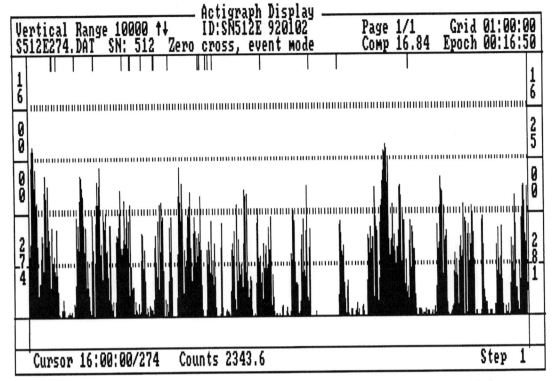

**Figure 30-2.** *Continued.*

### Pharmacologic Manipulation

Drugs that shift biological rhythms are called *chronobiotics*. Numerous neurotransmitters and peptides that affect the circadian clock have been identified[64] and are discussed in Chapter 5. A number of exciting therapeutic possibilities are in development. Although promising, pharmacologic manipulation of biological rhythms is still in its developmental phase. None of these treatments is of proven efficacy for any given clinical application, and a thorough review is beyond the scope of this chapter. Compelling data suggest that benzodiazepines are capable of affecting biological rhythms.[65–68] There have been scattered reports of the effect of vitamin $B_{12}$ in some circadian rhythm abnormalities.[69–72] Tricyclic antidepressants, monoamine oxidase inhibitors, and lithium may also influence biological rhythms.[73,74]

One of the most promising pharmacologic treatments under development is melatonin. Melatonin is secreted by the pineal gland. This secretion is suppressed by exposure to light, and is entrained by the light-dark cycle. It is coupled to the sleep-wake cycle and to the circadian cortisol rhythm and is a valuable marker of the underlying sleep-wake period. It is likely that melatonin plays an important role in biological rhythms, and evidence exists that administration of exogenous melatonin may alter biological rhythms.[24,75,76] The discovery of melatonin receptors in the SCN in humans suggests its importance in biological rhythms.[77] The timing of melatonin administration results in variable changes in the underlying rhythm, resulting in a PRC similar to that of light exposure but in the opposite direction (melatonin at the beginning of the "night" advances the sleep phase and vice versa).[76,78] The effects of melatonin on sleep and performance are complicated. Melatonin diminishes alertness (possibly by reducing body temperature), impairs performance, and may affect the circadian rhythm. The soporific and circadian effects may be independent effects of melatonin.[79–82] It should be remembered that melatonin is best thought of as a "dark" hormone, rather than a "sleep" hormone, as it is released during the dark phase of both light- and dark-active animals.

### Other Treatment Possibilities

#### Exercise

Preliminary evidence exists that appropriately timed exercise can phase shift circadian rhythms. Therefore, exercise might be used to promote circadian adaptation.[83] More work needs to be done in this area to determine the effect of exercise on human circadian timing. The necessary timing and amount of exercise as well as the nature of its interaction with nonphotic and photic *zeitgebers* are unknown.[84]

#### Light Exposure

Evidence exists that exposure to bright light may improve alertness and performance during nighttime waking hours, possibly due to light-induced suppression of melatonin and the attendant nocturnal decrease in temperature.[85] The combination of bright light and caffeine has been shown to enhance alertness and performance during periods of sleep deprivation.[86]

## RELATIONSHIP WITH MAJOR PSYCHIATRIC DISORDERS

Although beyond the scope of this chapter, the striking relationship between circadian rhythms and psychiatric disorders, particularly seasonal affective disorder, primary depression, and bipolar affective disorder, must be mentioned.[87] These disorders are often associated with abnormalities of the sleep-wake cycle and of the cycling of REM and NREM sleep within the sleep-wake cycle.[88–90] Many of the treatment modalities for these conditions (i.e., sleep deprivation; phototherapy; and many medications, such as tricyclic antidepressants, monoamine oxi-

dase inhibitors, and lithium) affect the sleep-wake cycle and the REM-NREM cycle.[73,91–93]

## PRIMARY CIRCADIAN DYSRHYTHMIAS

### Delayed Sleep Phase Syndrome

In delayed sleep phase syndrome (DSPS), the patient falls asleep late and rises late. The inability to fall asleep at an earlier, more desirable time is striking. For example, a college student is habitually unable to fall asleep until 2:00 AM, and has great difficulty getting up in time for her 8:00 AM classes Monday through Friday. She finds herself dozing off during morning classes. On Saturday and Sunday she sleeps in until approximately 10:00 AM and feels rested on arising, with no episodes of dozing during the day.

This disorder may represent 5–10% of cases with presenting complaints of insomnia at sleep disorders centers.[94] Onset is often during adolescence, but some patients report onset in childhood. A history of DSPS in family members has been noted clinically. DSPS may follow head trauma.[95]

Some individuals may experience disruption of school and work. The consequences depend partly on the tolerance of the patient's environment. A lenient employer and flexible schedule may allow a person to perform unimpaired, if permitted to begin and end work a few hours later than others. More demanding or rigid work or school schedules may not allow this, however, and the patient is forced to quit if treatment is not available. A disrupted family life may also result, if other family members do not have a similar schedule. The pervasive misperception that "sleeping in" is the result of an undesirable personality characteristic such as laziness or an example of avoidance behavior often leads to interpersonal stress and hostility. Attempts to adhere to a normal schedule result in sleep deprivation, making driving and operating machinery more dangerous. Individuals with DSPS may use alcohol or sedative-hypnotics in an attempt to induce sleep earlier, sometimes developing alcohol or drug dependence.[96]

Differential diagnosis includes irregular sleep-wake pattern; obstructive sleep apnea syndrome; narcolepsy (particularly during its development in adolescents)[97]; periodic limb movement disorder with or without restless legs syndrome; and psychiatric disorders associated with disturbed sleep, such as major depression, mania, dysthymia, obsessive-compulsive disorder, and schizophrenia. It may be very difficult to differentiate true, physiologic DSPS from sleep phase delay, which is a volitional sleep-wake schedule adopted by an individual to avoid contact with family, school, or work.[98]

As mentioned later, there appears to be an association between DSPS and depression.[99] The cause-and-effect relationship between DSPS and depression is unknown.[99] Some evidence exists that indicates a correlation between DSPS and personality disorders, and that the DSPS may predispose to the development of personality disorders.[100,101]

Exposure to bright light on awakening (toward the end of the PRC) has been shown to be effective in advancing sleep onset as well as in advancing temperature rhythm in a placebo-controlled study. The patient is asked to sit near a bright light, providing 5,000–10,000 lux, for approximately 1 hour on awakening every day. The response may not be evident for 2 weeks, and the treatment may have to be continuous.[56] There is some evidence that melatonin secretion may be suppressed by relatively low levels of illumination. Therefore, evening low-level light exposure could serve to maintain the DSPS.[102] A case report of a patient with non–24-hour sleep-wake syndrome whose sleep onset displayed intermittent changes attributed to exposure to light in the "delay" portion of the PRC supports this theory.[103]

Other treatment for DSPS includes chronotherapy and schedule change. For example, the patient goes to sleep at 2:00 AM the first night, then at 5:00 AM, 8:00 AM, and so on, until reaching 10:00 PM. The sleep onset of patients does not always stabilize at the desired time, but continues to be delayed, sometimes coming back to the time of sleep onset the patient started treatment with. There are case reports of individuals who developed non–24-hour cycle disorder on attempting chronotherapy for DSPS. Their sleep onsets never stopped changing once they were progressively delayed.[104]

Some individuals with DSPS report temporary resolution when in environments with strong time cues, such as staying with friends or relatives who set limits on staying up late and assist the patients in arising at the desired time. There are isolated reports of response to vitamin B$_{12}$,[69] benzodiazepines,[105] and melatonin.[106] The (often unconscious) secondary gain in the intentional sleep phase delay syndrome can make this condition very difficult to treat.

DSPS may be difficult to treat and tends to relapse if the treatment is suspended. A combination of approaches such as chronotherapy, phototherapy, and pharmacotherapy may produce better results.[67,99,107,108]

*Case Example*

Ms. K is a 36-year-old woman who referred herself to the sleep center to discuss treatment options for her nearly life-long pattern of an inability to fall asleep before 5:00 AM with a tendency to sleep until 3:00 PM. She has lost two jobs due to an inability to get to work on time, and her sleep-wake pattern played a role in her divorce. She currently works an afternoon shift, and has no sleep-wake complaints.

On her sleep center questionnaire, she wrote the following:

> Over the past many years I have been unable to wake up in the morning by an alarm or naturally—my body's sleep cycle seems "stuck" in a schedule where I sleep all day and am awake during the night and early morning hours. It has *totally* baffled most physicians and I have and still am being treated for depression, since this is the "diagnosis"—which I feel is not the case. If I indeed do have delayed sleep phase syndrome, and it can't be cured by techniques or medications, I will then fully accept this condition after learning more about it. This condition has totally disrupted my life and has created financial hardship, and seeing friends and family is difficult with my schedule.
>
> I would simply like to know if this condition is temporary or permanent. I would like to be awake during the day again! My life has changed drastically due to this condition, and I feel life is passing me by. Social activities and relationships are rare to nonexistent.

There is no history of true psychiatric or neurologic disease. Her father has a similar sleep-wake pattern. Ms. K brought sleep diaries to the appointment that confirmed the report of her sleep-wake pattern (Figure 30-3).

Treatment options discussed with Ms. K include (1) continuing to accommodate her sleep-wake pattern by working the afternoon-evening shift and (2) combinations of chronotherapy, phototherapy, and possibly the use of sedative/hypnotic agents and melatonin.

This patient's response on her questionnaire emphasizes the devastating nature of this condition.

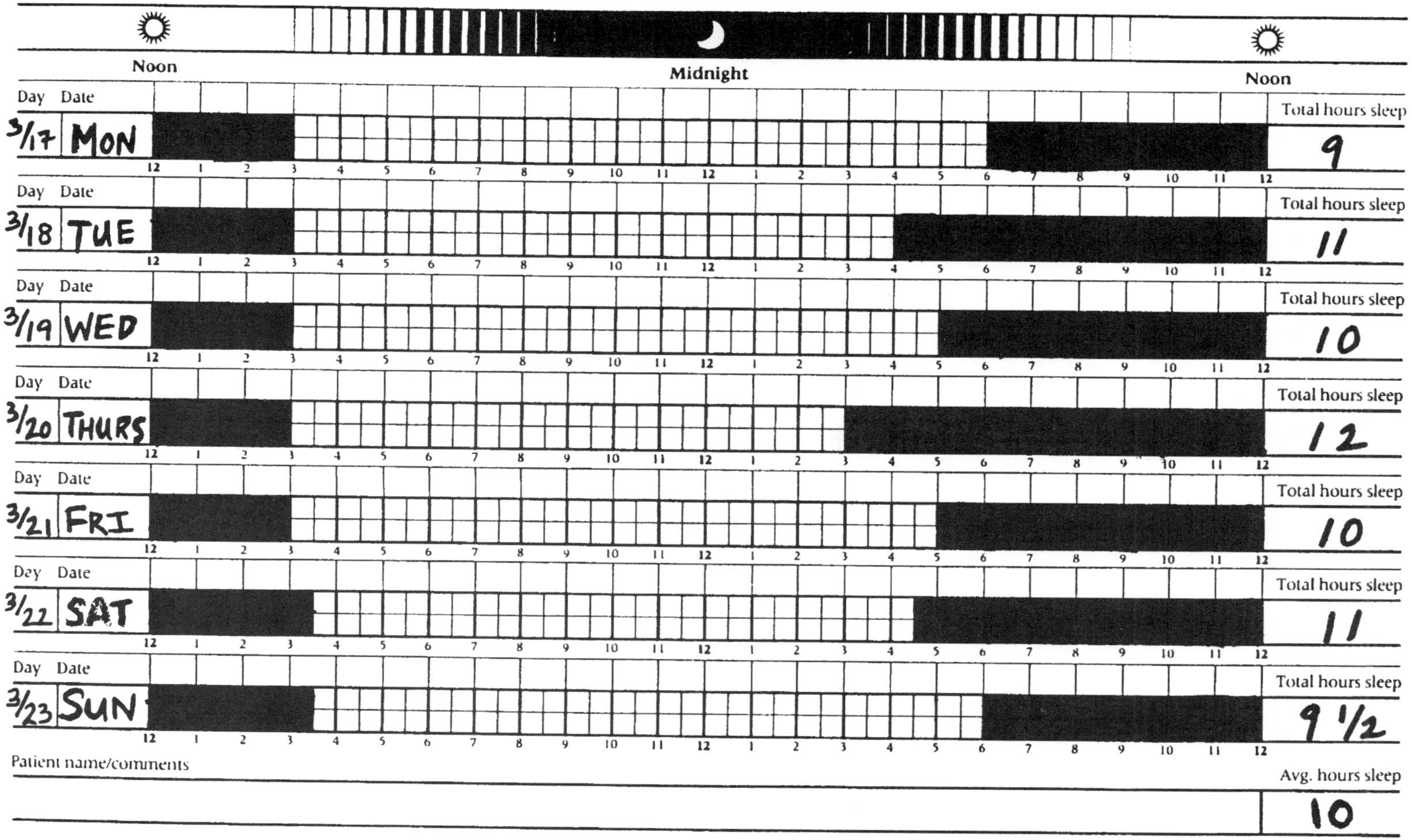

**Figure 30-3.** Sleep diary of a patient with delayed sleep phase syndrome. It is clear that this patient's problem is the timing, rather than the duration or continuity of sleep, as she is unable to fall asleep earlier than approximately 5:00 AM, and sleeps until approximately 3:00 PM.

This case underscores the value of sleep diaries. The history and sleep diaries speak for themselves, and indicate that DSPS is a clinical diagnosis. (She had undergone a totally unnecessary formal sleep study at another sleep center.)

### Advanced Sleep Phase Syndrome

Individuals with advanced sleep phase syndrome (ASPS) fall asleep early and awaken early. They are unable to remain awake until the desired time, falling asleep in the early evening and awakening in the very early hours of the morning.

No studies of the prevalence and incidence of this disorder exist, but clinical experience suggests that it may be less common than DSPS. The onset of the disorder occurs in later years, with most patients being older than 50 years. ASPS may be responsible for some of the deterioration in the sleep-wake pattern experienced by the elderly.

Patients complain of interruption of evening activities by their sleepiness. They may avoid evening social activities, fearing the intrusive sleepiness. They are also distressed by the very early awakenings. Driving and operating machinery in the evening can be dangerous for these patients.

The differential diagnosis includes psychiatric disorders with sleep disturbance. The early morning awakenings are often erroneously assumed to be a manifestation of depression. The early evening hypersomnia may be misinterpreted as a symptom of a primary sleep disorder such as obstructive sleep apnea syndrome or narcolepsy.

Bright light administered in the late afternoon or early evening (at the early portion of the PRC) has been reported effective in delaying both sleep onset and temperature rhythm.[8] The technique is the same as that for DSPS, except for the timing of exposure. Adverse effects are similar, but there is no advance of sleep onset. There may be excessive delay of sleep onset, however, until the early hours of the morning. Shorter light exposures may prevent this. Some flexibility may be needed in establishing the timing of the exposure, as the patient may have social activities in the early evening. Occasionally, an exposure just before supper is convenient and effective. Chronotherapy, with a 3-hour advance every other day until the desired sleep-onset time has been reached, may also be effective.[109]

Contributing to the growing body of evidence suggesting that in many cases of insomnia there are underlying organic factors,[110,111] one study has suggested that early morning awakening insomnia may arise from phase-advanced circadian rhythms.[112]

### Non–24-Hour Sleep-Wake Syndrome

Individuals with non–24-hour sleep-wake syndrome, also know as *hypernychthemeral syndrome*, cannot maintain a regular bedtime and find their sleep onsets wandering around the clock. Most patients experience a gradually increasing delay in sleep onset, often approximately 1 hour per sleep-wake cycle. A typical pattern of sleep onsets might be 9:00 PM the first cycle, then 10:00 PM, 11:30 PM, 12:00 AM, 1:30 AM, 3:00 AM, and so on, eventually progressing through daytime hours into the evening again. This likely reflects the fact that most humans have an intrinsic circadian rhythm of approximately 25 hours, slightly longer than the 24-hour geophysical day. Rarely, patients experience a gradually increasing advance in sleep-onset time. Individuals with non–24-hour sleep-wake syndrome lack the ability to be entrained or synchronized by the usual time cues such as sunlight and social activity.

Non–24-hour sleep-wake syndrome is apparently extremely uncommon. In each of our few cases, the patient has been diagnosed with a major psychiatric disorder, including recurrent major depression, panic disorder with agoraphobia, and post-traumatic stress disorder. Two had history consistent with DSPS before the onset of the non–24-hour sleep-wake syndrome. In one, the onset of the non–24-hour sleep-wake syndrome followed a period of shift work. The course of this syndrome is chronic, with many patients reporting years of the disturbance.

Structural lesions of the central nervous system, such as hypothalamic tumors, have been associated with this disorder. Magnetic resonance imaging studies of the head, with special attention to the hypothalamic and pituitary regions, are recommended in these patients.[94] Totally blind individuals, who have lost or experienced impairment of their retinohypothalamic pathway, frequently develop this disorder. Approximately one-third of blind subjects had this disorder in one series.[24]

Complications include severe disruption of work or studies and accidents when attempting to drive or operate machinery while sleepy. As with DSPS, the tolerance of the patient's environment plays an important role in determining the degree of disruption. Some individuals with a flexible work schedule may experience no disruption of work, which they accomplish when convenient. The lives of many patients are completely disrupted by this disorder, however, having been fired from work or expelled from school as a result of poor performance when sleepy, tardiness, or absences associated with inopportune episodes of sleep.

The differential diagnosis includes irregular sleep-wake pattern; DSPS; psychiatric disorders associated with changes in sleep-wake patterns; and primary sleep disorders, such as narcolepsy and obstructive sleep apnea.

Treatment attempts have included strengthening of time cues, with one individual reporting temporary resolution of symptoms when living with a relative who kept her to a strict schedule. Phototherapy,[113] benzodiazepines,[114] and vitamin $B_{12}$[69,115,116] have been successful in isolated cases, but controlled studies are not available. Melatonin was used to entrain a sighted man with non–24-hour sleep-wake syndrome.[117]

### Irregular Sleep-Wake Pattern

Individuals with irregular sleep-wake pattern show a disorganized sleep-wake pattern with variable sleep and wake lengths. Patients may complain of insomnia, excessive sleepiness, cognitive disturbance, and fatigue. Sleep onsets may occur at a variety of clock times. To meet the official criteria for this diagnosis, there must be at least three sleep episodes per 24-hour period.[94] The disturbance must be present for at least 3 months. The average total sleep time per 24 hours is normal for the patient's age. There must be objective evidence of disturbed rhythms by 24-hour polysomnographic monitoring or by 24-hour temperature monitoring. The patient has no medical or psychiatric disorder that could explain the symptoms and does not have another sleep disorder that would account for insomnia or excessive daytime sleepiness.

The incidence and prevalence of this disorder are unknown. Irregular sleep-wake pattern may occur in individuals with central nervous system disorders such as head injury,[118] hypothalamic lesions,[119] senile

dementia of the Alzheimer type,[120] or developmental disabilities. The uncontrollably irregular pattern of sleep may interfere with work and family activities. These disorders may result in a high cost to society by forcing the institutionalization of a demented or developmentally impaired individual previously living at home. One major reason for institutionalization of demented elderly individuals is the inability of caregivers at home to monitor the irregular, around-the-clock activity of their impaired relative.[120]

Many elderly individuals, including most nursing home residents, receive very little exposure to natural light, as they spend nearly all day inside.[121] Stronger social time cues help some patients resume a regular 24-hour pattern. In uncontrolled reports, exposure to bright light[122] and vitamin $B_{12}$ administration[123] have reportedly been effective. The relative lack of exposure to time cues may contribute to the development of this disorder. Some associated diagnoses in patients at our center include alcohol abuse in remission and major depression.

Profound abnormalities of the sleep-wake cycle appear to be common and disabling for patients with static encephalopathies and some individuals after traumatic brain injury. No systematic studies are available in these groups.[124]

Other sleep disorders such as obstructive sleep apnea syndrome, narcolepsy, periodic limb movement disorder, and restless legs syndrome could result in irregular patterns of sleep and wake, and should be ruled out. Medical disorders causing multiple awakening, such as those causing bladder or bowel dysfunction, could result in a similar pattern.

## SECONDARY CIRCADIAN DYSRHYTHMIAS

In contrast to the primary circadian dysrhythmias that represent malfunctioning of the biological clock within the conventional geophysical environment, the secondary circadian dysrhythmias occur *because* the biological clock is working properly but is functioning out of phase due to an imposed shift in the geophysical environment. Technological advances such as electric lights and jet planes have allowed us to override or ignore our physiologic biological rhythms. The numbers of people involved in transmeridian flight or shift work are startling (nearly one-fourth of all workers in industrialized countries work unconventional shifts). This fact coupled with the well-documented impairment of performance and judgment that comes with trying to "disobey" the biological clock has staggering implications at the personal, national, and international levels.[1] The changes associated with time-zone crossing are transient and self-limited; the changes associated with shift work persist as long as the shift work. The symptoms of secondary circadian dysrhythmias have been experienced by most of us, and are well reviewed elsewhere.[125,126] Schedule-induced decrements in alertness and performance have enormous implications for shuttle diplomats, traveling athletes, and shift workers. Effective treatment to reduce or minimize the consequences of the secondary circadian dysrhythmias is in the developmental stage and includes chronotherapy,[127] benzodiazepines,[128–130] phototherapy,[131] and melatonin.[132–135]

The primary consequence of shift work is impaired performance. In addition, some evidence links shift work to increased cardiovascular morbidity and mortality as well as gastrointestinal disease.[136,137] There is a high degree of variability in the short- and long-term adjustment to shift work.[138,139] This is in part due to the exposure to bright light on the drive home in the morning. This exposure can impair or prevent circadian adaptation.[140]

In the past, one approach to improving adjustment to shift work has been to use sedative-hypnotic agents to promote sleep. Inasmuch as the human circadian pacemaker promotes alertness, however, it has been suggested that emulation of the biological function of the circadian pacemaker by administering wake-promoting agents may be more effective in combating the sleepiness experienced by shift workers during working hours.[141] Shift work schedules should be individualized to accommodate the goals of the employer, the desires of the employee, and ergonomic recommendations for the design of shift systems.[142] Night shift workers rarely develop circadian adaptation to the night shift.

## CONCLUSION AND FUTURE DIRECTIONS

The study of chronobiology has taught us much about circadian rhythms. The negative consequences of all types of circadian dysrhythmias are starting to be appreciated. The biological clock is a powerful physiologic force and may cause disabling symptoms when out of synchrony with the environment. In primary circadian rhythm disorders, the clock is defective; in secondary disorders, there is difficulty or delay in the clock's adjustment to a shift in environmental time cues.

With the advent of effective treatment, the identification of these disorders is of the utmost importance. The primary circadian dysrhythmias are undoubtedly much more prevalent than previously thought, masquerading as psychiatric, substance abuse, or primary sleep disorders. Careful history taking and the use of sleep diaries and actigraphy usually lead to a proper diagnosis with practical therapeutic implications. Like any field in its infancy, chronobiology is exploding with excitement as new treatments emerge. Few fields have such important implications for so many people.

## REFERENCES

1. National Commission on Sleep Disorders Research. Report of the National Commission on Sleep Disorders Research. Research DHHS Pub. No. 92-XXXX. Washington, DC: U.S. Government Printing Office, 1992.
2. Mitler MM, Carskadon MA, Czeisler CA, et al. Catastrophes, sleep, and public policy. Sleep 1988;11:100.
3. Smolensky M, Halberg F, Sargent F. Chronobiology of the Life Sequence. In S Ito, K Ogata, H Yoshimura (eds), Advances in Climatic Physiology. Tokyo: Igaku Shoin, 1972;281.
4. Kaiser IH, Halberg F. Circadian periodic aspects of birth. Ann N Y Acad Sci 1962;98:1056.
5. Wever RA. The Circadian System of Man: Results of Experiments Under Temporal Isolation. New York: Springer, 1979.
6. Minors DS. Circadian Rhythms and the Human. Bristol: Wright, 1981.
7. Moore-Ede MC, Sulzman FM, Fuller CA. The Clocks That Time Us: Physiology of the Circadian Timing System. Cambridge, MA: Harvard University Press, 1982.
8. Murphy PJ, Campbell SS. Physiology of the circadian system in animals and humans. J Clin Neurophysiol 1996;13:2.
9. Halberg F. Physiologic 24-Hour Periodicity in Human Beings and Mice: The Lighting Regimen and Daily Routine. In RB Withrow (ed), Photoperiodism and Related Phenomena in Plants and Animals. Washington, DC: American Association for the Advancement of Science, 1959;803.
10. Ibuka N, Kawamura H. Loss of circadian rhythm in sleep-wakefulness cycle in the rat by suprachiasmatic nucleus lesions. Brain Res 1975;96:76.

11. Miller JD, Morin LP, Schwartz WJ, Moore RY. New insights into the mammalian circadian clock. Sleep 1996;19:641.

12. Edgar DM, Dement WC, Fuller CA. Effect of SCN lesions on sleep in squirrel monkeys: evidence for opponent processes in sleep-wake regulation. J Neurosci 1993;13:1065.

13. Moore R. Retinohypothalamic projections in mammals: a comparative study. Brain Res 1973;49:403.

14. Rawson KS. Homing Behavior and Endogenous Activity Rhythms (cited in Weaver, 1979[5]) [PhD]. Cambridge, MA: Harvard University, 1956.

15. Burchard JE. Re-setting a Biological Clock (cited in Weaver, 1979[5]) [PhD]. Princeton, NJ: Princeton University Press, 1958.

16. Pittendrigh CS, Bruce VG. An Oscillator Model for Biological Clocks. In D Rudnick (ed), Rhythmic and Synthetic Processes in Growth. Princeton, NJ: Princeton University Press, 1957;75.

17. Czeisler CA, Kronauer RE, Allen JS, et al. Bright light induction of strong (type 0) resetting of the human pacemaker. Science 1989;244:1328.

18. Lewy AJ, Wehr TA, Goodwin FK, et al. Light suppresses melatonin secretion in humans. Science 1980;210:1267.

19. DeCorsey PJ. Daily light sensitivity rhythm in the flying squirrel (cited in Wever, 1979) [PhD] Madison, WI: University of Wisconsin, 1959.

20. DeCorsey PJ. Daily light sensitivity rhythm in a rodent. Science 1960;131:33.

21. Pittendrigh CS. Circadian rhythms and the circadian organization of living systems. Cold Spring Harb Symp Quant Biol 1960;25:159.

22. Eastman CI. Squashing versus nudging circadian rhythms with artificial bright light: solutions for shift work? Perspect Biol Med 1991;34:181.

23. Moore-Ede MC, Czeisler CA, Richardson GS. Circadian timekeeping in health and disease. Part 1. Basic properties of circadian pacemakers. N Engl J Med 1983;3009:469.

24. Sack RL, Lewy AJ, Blood ML, et al. Circadian rhythm abnormalities in totally blind people; incidence and clinical significance. J Clin Endocrinol Metab 1992;75:127.

25. Lockley SW, Skene DJ, Tabandeh H, et al. Relationship between napping and melatonin in the blind. J Biol Rhythms 1997;12:16.

26. Czeisler CA, Shanahan TL, Klerman EB, et al. Suppression of melatonin secretion in some blind patients by exposure to bright light. N Engl J Med 1995;332:6.

27. Sack RL, Lewy AJ, Blood ML, et al. Melatonin administration to blind people: phase advances and entrainment. J Biol Rhythms 1991;6:249.

28. Rietveld WJ, Minors DS, Waterhouse JM. Circadian rhythms and masking: an overview. Chronobiol Int 1993;10:306.

29. Challet E, Pevet P, Vivien-Roels B, Malan A. Phase-advanced daily rhythms of melatonin, body temperature, and locomotor activity in food-restricted rats fed during the daytime. J Biol Rhythms 1997;12:65.

30. Edgar DM, Martin CE, Dement WC. Activity feedback to the mammalian circadian pacemaker: influence on observed measures of rhythm period length. J Biol Rhythms 1991;6:185.

31. Welch DK, Richardson GS, Dement WC. Effect of running wheel availability on the circadian pattern of sleep and wakefulness in the mouse. Sleep Res 1985;14:316.

32. Copinschi G, Van Cauter E. Effects of ageing on modulation of hormonal secretions by sleep and circadian rhythmicity. Hormone Res 1995;43:20.

33. Witting W, Mirmiran M, Bos NPA, Swaab DF. The effect of old age on the free-running period of circadian rhythms in rats. Chronobiol Int 1994;11:103.

34. Monk TH, Buysse DJ, Reynolds CFI, Kupfer DJ. Circadian determinants of postlunch dip in performance. Chronobiol Int 1966;13:123.

35. Kleitman N. Sleep and Wakefulness. Chicago: University of Chicago Press, 1963.

36. Mahowald MW, Schenck CH, O'Connor KA. Dynamics of sleep/wake determination—normal and abnormal. Chaos 1991;1:287.

37. Perret M. Change in photoperiodic cycle affects life span in a prosimian primate (Microcebus murinus). J Biol Rhythms 1997;12:136.

38. Smolensky MH, D'Alonzo GE. Medical Chronobiology: Concepts and Applications. In RJ Martin (ed), Nocturnal Asthma: Mechanisms and Treatment. Mt. Kisco, NY: Futura, 1993;1.

39. Pincus DJ, Beam WR, Martin RJ. Chronobiology and chronotherapy of asthma. Clin Chest Med 1995;16:699.

40. Martin RJ. Nocturnal Asthma: Mechanisms and Treatment. Mt. Kisco, NY: Futura, 1993.

41. Martin RJ. Chronotherapy of asthma: how to use standard medications for better results. Semin Respir Crit Care Med 1994;15:128.

42. Smolensky MH, D'Alonzo GE. Biological Rhythms and Medications: Chronopharmacology and Chronotherapeutics. In JR Martin (ed), Nocturnal Asthma: Mechanisms and Treatment. Mt. Kisco, NY: Futura, 1993;25.

43. Hallberg F. Chronobiology. Ann Rev Physiol 1969; 31:675.

44. Moore-Ede MC. Circadian rhythms of drug effectiveness and toxicity. Clin Pharmacol Ther 1973;14:925.

45. Radzialowski RM, Bousquet WF. Daily rhythmic variation in hepatic drug metabolism in the rat and mouse. J Pharmacol Exp Ther 1968;163:229.

46. Reinberg A. The hours of changing responsiveness or susceptibility. Perspect Biol Med 1967;11:111.

47. Koren G, Ferrazzini G, Sohl H, et al. Chronopharmacology of methotrexate pharmacokinetics in childhood leukemia. Chronobiol Int 1992;9:434.

48. Kohno I, Iwasaki H, Okutani M, et al. Administration-time-dependent effects of diltiazem on the 24-hour blood pressure profile of essential hypertension patients. Chronobiol Int 1997;14:71.

49. Krulder JWM, Van Den Besselaar AMHP, Van Der Meer FJM, et al. Diurnal changes in heparin effect during continuous constant-rate infusion. J Int Med 1994; 235:411.

50. Tryon WK. Activity Measurement in Psychology and Medicine. New York: Plenum, 1991.

51. Brown A, Smolensky M, D'Alonzo G, et al. Circadian Rhythm in Human Activity Objectively Quantified by Actigraphy. In DK Hays (ed), Chronobiology: Its Role in Clinical Medicine, General Biology, and Agriculture. New York: Wiley, 1990;A77.

52. Richardson GS, Malin HV. Circadian rhythm disorders: pathophysiology and treatment. J Clin Neurophysiol 1996;13:17.

53. Moore-Ede MC, Czeisler CA, Richardson GS. Circadian timekeeping in health and disease. Part 2. Clinical implications of circadian rhythmicity. N Engl J Med 1983;309:530.

54. Czeisler CA, Richardson GS, Coleman RM. Chronotherapy: resetting the circadian clocks of patients with delayed sleep phase insomnia. Sleep 1981;4:1.

55. Weitzman ED, Czeisler CA, Coleman RM, et al. Delayed sleep phase syndrome. A chronobiological disorder with sleep-onset insomnia. Arch Gen Psychiatry 1981;38:737.

56. Rosenthal NE, Joseph-Vanderpool JR, Levendosky AA, et al. Phase-shifting effects of bright morning light as treatment for delayed sleep phase syndrome. Sleep 1990;13:354.

57. Lewy AJ, Sack RL. Intensity, Wavelength, and Timing: Three Critical Parameters for Chronobiologically Active Light. In DJ Kupfer, TH Monk, JD Barchas (eds), Biological Rhythms and Mental Disorders. New York: Guilford, 1988;197.

58. Terman M. Light Therapy. In MH Kryger, T Roth, WC Dement (eds), Principles and Practice of Sleep Medicine. Philadelphia: Saunders, 1994;717.

59. Terman M, Williams JB, Terman JS. Light Therapy for Winter Depression: A Clinician's Guide. In PA Keller (ed), Innovations in Clinical Practice: A Source Book. Sarasota, FL: Professional Resource Exchange, 1991.

60. Kripke DF. Timing of phototherapy and occurrence of mania. Biol Psychiatry 1991;29:1156.

61. Schwitzer J, Neudorfer C, Blecha HG, Fleischhacker WW. Mania as a side effect of phototherapy. Biol Psychiatry 1990;28:523.

62. Roberts JE, Reme CE, Dillon J, Terman M. Exposure to bright light and the concurrent use of photosensitizing drugs. N Engl J Med 1992;326:1500.

63. Terman M, Reme CE, Rafferty B, et al. Bright light therapy for winter depression: potential ocular effects and theoretical implications. Photochem Photobiol 1990;51:781.

64. Dawson D, Armstrong SM. Chronobiotics—drugs that shift rhythms. Pharmacol Ther 1996;69:15.

65. Turek FW, Losee-Olson S. Entrainment of the circadian activity rhythm to the light-dark cycle can be altered by short-acting benzodiazepine, triazolam. J Biol Rhythms 1987;2:249.

66. Turek FW. Manipulation of a central circadian clock regulating behavioral and endocrine rhythms with a short-acting benzodiazepine used in the treatment of insomnia. Psychoneuroendocrinology 1988;13:217.

67. Alvarez B, Dahlitz MJ, Vignau J, Parkes JD. The delayed sleep phase syndrome: clinical and investigative findings in fourteen subjects. J Neurol Neurosurg Psychiatry 1992;55:665.

68. Ozaki N, Iwata T, Itoh A, et al. A treatment of delayed sleep phase syndrome with triazolam. Jpn J Psychiatry Neurol 1989;43:51.

69. Okawa M, Mishima K, Nanami T, et al. Vitamin $B_{12}$ treatment for sleep-wake rhythm disorders. Sleep 1990;13:15.

70. Tshjimaru S, Kideaki E, Honma G, et al. Effects of vitamin $B_{12}$ on the period of free-running rhythm in rats. Jpn J Psychiatry Neurol 1992;46:225.

71. Ohta T, Iwata T, Kayukawa Y. Daily activity and persistent sleep-wake schedule disorders. Prog Neuropsychopharmacol Biol Psychiatry 1991;16:529.

72. Ohta T, Ando K, Iwata T, et al. Treatment of persistent sleep-wake schedule disorders in adolescents with methylcobalamin (vitamin $B_{12}$). Sleep 1991;12:414.

73. Hallonquist JD, Goldberg MA, Brandes JS. Affective disorders and circadian rhythms. Can J Psychiatry 1986;31:259.

74. Nagayama H. Chronic administration of imipramine and lithium changes the phase-angle relationship between the activity and core body temperature circadian rhythms in rats. Chronobiol Int 1996;13:251.

75. Erlich SS, Apuzzo MLJ. The pineal gland: anatomy, physiology, and clinical significance. J Neurosurg 1985;63:321.

76. Lewy AJ, Sack RL, Singer CM. Melatonin, Light and Chronobiological Disorders. In Ciba Foundation Symposium 117: Photoperiodism, Melatonin, and the Pineal. London: Pitman, 1985;231.

77. Reppert SM, Weaver DR, Rivkees SA, Stopa EG. Putative melatonin receptors in a human biologic clock. Science 1988;242:78.

78. Lewy AJ, Ahmed S, Latham Jackson JM, Sack RL. Melatonin shifts human circadian rhythms according to a phase-response curve. Chronobiol Int 1992;9:380.

79. Deacon S, Arendt J. Melatonin-induced temperature suppression and its acute phase-shifting effects correlate in a dose-dependent manner in humans. Brain Res 1995;688:77.

80. Brzezinski A. Melatonin in humans. N Engl J Med 1997;336:186.

81. Reid K, Van Den Heuvel C, Dawson D. Day-time melatonin administration: effects on core temperature and sleep onset latency. J Sleep Res 1996;5:150.

82. Hughes RJ, Badia P. Sleep-promoting and hypothermic effects of daytime melatonin administration in humans. Sleep 1997;20:124.

83. Eastman CI, Hoese EK, Youngstedt SD, Liu L. Phase-shifting human circadian rhythms with exercise during the night shift. Physiol Behav 1995;58:1287.

84. Redlin U, Mrosovsky N. Exercise and human circadian rhythms: what we know and what we need to know. Chronobiol Int 1997;14:221.

85. Daurat A, Aguirre A, Foret J, et al. Bright light affects alertness and performance rhythms during a 24-h constant routine. Physiol Behav 1993;53:929.

86. Wright KP Jr, Badia P, Myers BL, Plenzler SC. Combination of bright light and caffeine as a countermeasure for impaired alertness and performance during extended sleep deprivation. J Sleep Res 1997;6:26.

87. Rosenthal NE, Blehar MC (eds). Seasonal Affective Disorders and Phototherapy. New York: Guilford, 1989.

88. Wehr TA. Effects of Wakefulness and Sleep on Depression and Mania. In J Montplaisir, R Godbout (eds), Sleep and Biological Rhythms. Basic Mechanisms and Applications to Psychiatry. New York: Oxford University Press, 1990;42.

89. Kupfer DJ, Monk TH, Barchas JD (eds). Biological Rhythms and Mental Disorders. New York: Guilford, 1988.

90. Benca R, Obermeyer WH, Thisted RA, Gillin JC. Sleep and psychiatric disorders. A meta-analysis. Arch Gen Psychiatry 1992;49:651.

91. Schigen B, Tolle R. Partial sleep deprivation as therapy for depression. Arch Gen Psychiatry 1980;37:267.

92. Rosenthal NE, Sack DA, Gillin JC, et al. Seasonal affective disorder. A description of the syndrome and preliminary findings with light therapy. Arch Gen Psychiatry 1984;41:72.

93. Wehr TA, Jacobsen FM, Sack DA, et al. Phototherapy of seasonal affective disorder. Arch Gen Psychiatry 1986;43:870.

94. Diagnostic Classification Steering Committee, MJ Thorpy, Chairman. International Classification of Sleep Disorders: Diagnostic and Coding Manual. Rochester, MN: American Sleep Disorders Association, 1990.

95. Patten SB, Lauderdale WM. Delayed sleep phase disorder after traumatic brain injury. J Am Acad Child Adolesc Psychiatry 1992;31:100.

96. Institute of Medicine National Academy of Sciences. Sleeping Pills, Insomnia and Medical Practice. Washington, DC: NAS Office of Publications, 1971.

97. Guilleminault C. Narcolepsy and Its Differential Diagnosis. In C Guilleminault (ed), Sleep and Its Disorders in Children. New York: Raven, 1987;181.

98. Ferber R, Boyle MP. Delayed sleep phase syndrome versus motivated sleep phase delay in adolescents. Sleep Res 1983;12:239.

99. Regestein QR, Monk TH. Delayed sleep phase syndrome: a review of its clinical aspects. Am J Psychiatry 1995;152:602.

100. Dagan Y, Sela H, Omer H, et al. High prevalence of personality disorders among circadian rhythm sleep disorders (CSRD) patients. J Psychosom Res 1996;41:357.

101. Dagan Y, Stein D, Steinbock M, et al. Frequency of delayed sleep phase syndrome (DSPS) among hospitalized psychiatric patients (in press).

102. Trinder J, Armstrong SM, O'Brien C, et al. Inhibition of melatonin secretion onset by low levels of illumination. J Sleep Res 1966;5:77.

103. Uchiyama M, Okawa M, Ozaki S, et al. Delayed phase jumps of sleep onset in a patient with non-24-hour sleep-wake syndrome. Sleep 1996;19:637.

104. Oren DA, Wehr TA. Hypernyctohemeral syndrome after chronotherapy for delayed sleep phase syndrome. N Engl J Med 1992;327:1762.

105. Uruha S, Mikami A, Teshima Y, et al. Effect of triazolam for delayed sleep phase syndrome. Sleep Res 1987;16:650.

106. Dahlitz M, Alvarez B, Vignau J, et al. Delayed sleep phase syndrome response to melatonin. Lancet 1991;337:1121.

107. Ito A, Ando K, Hayakawa T, et al. Long-term course of adult patients with delayed sleep phase syndrome. Jpn J Psychiatry Neurol 1993;47:563.

108. Regestein QR, Pavlova M. Treatment of delayed sleep phase syndrome. Gen Hosp Psychiatry 1995;17:335.

109. Moldofsky H, Musisi S, Phillipson EA. Treatment of a case of advanced sleep phase syndrome by phase advance chronotherapy. Sleep 1986;9:61.

110. Bonnet MH, Arand DL. 24-hour metabolic rate in insomniacs and matched normal sleepers. Sleep 1995;18:581.

111. Bonnet MH, Arand DL. The consequences of a week of insomnia. Sleep 1996;19:453.

112. Lack LC, Mercer JD, Wright H. Circadian rhythms of early morning awakening insomniacs. J Sleep Res 1996;5:211.

113. Hoban TM, Sack RL, Lewy AJ, et al. Entrainment of a free-running human with bright light. Chronobiol Int 1989;2:277.

114. Wollman M, Lavie P, Peled R. A hypernychthemeral sleep-wake syndrome: a treatment attempt. Chronobiol Int 1985;2:277.

115. Kamgar-Parsi B, Wehr TA, Gillin JC. Successful treatment of human non-24-hour sleep-wake syndrome. Sleep 1983;6:257.

116. Sugita Y, Ishikawa H, Mikami A, et al. Successful treatment of a patient with hypernychtohemeral syndrome. Sleep Res 1987;17:642.

117. McArthur AJ, Lewy AJ, Sack RL. Non-24-hour sleep-wake syndrome in a sighted man: circadian rhythm studies and efficacy of melatonin treatment. Sleep 1996;19:544.

118. Okawa M, Takahashi K, Sasaki H. Disturbance of circadian rhythms in severely brain-damaged patients correlated with CT findings. J Neurol 1986;233:274.

119. Cohen RA, Albers HE. Disruption of human circadian and cognitive regulation following a discrete hypothalamic lesion: a case study. Neurology 1991;41:726.

120. Bliwise DL. Sleep in normal aging and dementia. Sleep 1993;16:40.

121. Ancoli-Israel S, Kripke D, Williams-Jones D, et al. Light exposure and sleep in nursing home patients. Soc Light Treat Biol Rhythms Abs 1991;3:18.

122. Satlin A, Vilicer L, Ross V, et al. Bright light treatment of behavioral and sleep disturbances in patients with Alzheimer's disease. Am J Psychiatry 1992;149:1028.

123. Mishima K, Okawa M, Hishikawa Y. Effect of methyl-cobalamin ($VB_{12}$) injection on sleep-wake rhythm in demented patients. Jpn J Psychiatry Neurol 1992;46:227.

124. Mahowald MW, Mahowald ML. Sleep Disorders. In M Rizzo, D Trandel (eds), Head Injury and Postconcussive Syndrome. New York: Churchill Livingstone, 1996;285.

125. U.S. Congress, Office of Technology Assessment. Biological rhythms: implications for the worker. Washington, DC: U.S. Government Printing Office, 1991; OTA-BA-463.

126. Loat CER, Rhodes EC. Jet-lag and human performance. Sports Med 1989;8:226.

127. Czeisler CA, Moore-Ede MC, Coleman RM. Rotating shift work schedules that disrupt sleep are improved by applying circadian principles. Science 1982;217:460.

128. Cohen AS, Seidel WF, Yost D, et al. Triazolam used in the treatment of jet lag: effects on sleep and subsequent wakefulness. Sleep Res 1991;20:61.

129. Walsh JK, Sugerman JL, Muehlbach MJ, Schweitzer PK. Physiological sleep tendency on a simulated night shift: adaptation and effects of triazolam. Sleep 1988;11:251.

130. Bonnet MH, Dexter JR, Gillin JC, et al. The use of triazolam in phase-advanced sleep. Neuropsychopharmacology 1988;1:225.

131. Czeisler CA, Johnson MP, Duffy JF, et al. Exposure to bright light and darkness to treat physiologic maladaptation to night work. N Engl J Med 1990;322:1253.

132. Samel A, Wegmann H-M, Vejvoda M, et al. Influence of melatonin treatment on human circadian rhythmicity before and after a simulated 9-hr time shift. J Biol Rhythms 1991;6:235.

133. Petrie K, Dawson AG, Thompson L, Brook R. A double-blind trial of melatonin as a treatment for jet lag in international cabin crew. Biol Psychiatry 1993;33:526.

134. Redfern P, Minors D, Waterhouse J. Circadian rhythms, jet lag, and chronobiotics: an overview. Chronobiol Int 1994;11:253.

135. Arendt J, Deacon S. Treatment of circadian rhythm disorders—melatonin. Chronobiol Int 1997;14:185.

136. Harrington JM. Shift work and health—a critical review of the literature on working hours. Ann Acad Med Singapore 1994;23:699.

137. Kawachi I, Colditz GA, Stampfer MJ, et al. Prospective study of shift work and risk of coronary heart disease in women. Circulation 1995;92:3178.

138. Costa G. The problem: shiftwork. Chronobiol Int 1997; 14:89.

139. Quera-Salva MA, Defrance R, Claustrat B, et al. Rapid shift in sleep time and acrophase of melatonin secretion in short shift work schedule. Sleep 1996;19:539.

140. Mitchell PJ, Hoese EK, Liu L, et al. Conflicting bright light exposure during night shifts impedes circadian adaptation. J Biol Rhythms 1997;12:5.

141. Edgar DM. Circadian Control of Sleep/Wakefulness: Implications in Shiftwork and Therapeutic Strategies. In K Shiraki, S Sagawa, MK Yousef (eds), Physiological Basis of Occupational Health; Stressful Environments. Amsterdam: SPB Academic, 1996;253.

142. Knauth P. Changing schedules: shiftwork. Chronobiol Int 1997;14:159.

# Chapter 31
# Behavioral Parasomnias

## Roger J. Broughton

*Parasomnias* are events that occur intermittently or episodically during sleep, as opposed to other sleep disorders, which are characterized by an overall increase or decrease from the normal sleep amount or relate to abnormalities of circadian sleep-wake regulation. In one sense, all brief behavioral phenomena during sleep can be considered parasomnias, including sleep apnea, periodic leg movements, sleep-related choking, swallowing, laryngospasm, gastroesophageal reflux, asthmatic attacks, and epileptic seizures, all of which are discussed elsewhere in this volume. Although the most recent classification of sleep disorders[1] lists and describes 24 distinct parasomnias, a number of these are either exceedingly rare (e.g., sleep-related swallowing syndrome and congenital central hypoventilation syndrome) or are not disorders of behavior (e.g., rapid eye movement [REM]-related sinus arrest). This chapter restricts itself to the main behavioral parasomnias.

Parasomnias may be classified according to the sleep-wake state during which they preferentially or exclusively occur: sleep onset, deep slow-wave sleep (SWS), REM sleep (either in fully integrated or dissociated forms), light sleep stages, or all sleep stages indiscriminately. The 17 main parasomnias discussed in this chapter are organized according to sleep-wake state in Table 31-1.

## WAKE-TO-SLEEP TRANSITION DISORDERS

### Intensified Sleep Starts (Hypnic Jerks)

Sleep starts are variously referred to as *hypnagogic jerks, hypnic jerks,* or *predormital myoclonus.* They consist of bilateral and sometimes asymmetric brief body jerks, usually in isolation, but occasionally several in succession, that occur during the process of sleep onset. Sleep starts principally involve the legs but may also affect the arms and head. Asymmetry of the jerks may occur due to asymmetric body position in bed. Sleep starts may be spontaneous or evoked by stimuli. At times they are accompanied by sensory symptoms such as a flash of light, a feeling of falling, or more organized hypnagogic hallucinations. There is a wide variety of intensity of sleep starts in the general population. The intensity of the contraction may cause an abrupt expiratory cry. Rarely, mild injury such as bruises may occur.

One of the earliest careful descriptions of sleep starts was that of S. Weir Mitchell[2] in 1890, who also discussed the possibility that particularly intense and frequent jerks can lead to a form of sleep-onset insomnia with consequent sleep deprivation. The early French neurologist Roger[3] also fully recognized this latter clinical expression.

The cause of the intensification of this otherwise normal physiologic event to clinically significant

**Table 31-1.** Classification of Behavioral Parasomnias

Wake-sleep transition disorders
    Intensified sleep starts (hypnic jerks)
    Rhythmic movement disorder (jactatio capitis nocturna)
    Terrifying hypnagogic hallucinations
Non-REM sleep disorders
    Confusional arousals (nocturnal sleep drunkenness)
    Sleep terrors (pavor nocturnus, incubus attacks)
    Sleepwalking (somnambulism)
    Nocturnal paroxysmal dystonia
REM sleep disorders
    Nightmares (terrifying dreams, anxiety dreams)
    REM sleep behavior disorder
    Sleep paralysis, isolated form
    Painful erections
Light sleep disorders (stages I, II, and REM)
    Sleep talking
    Bruxism (tooth grinding)
    Sleep-related panic attacks
Diffuse sleep disorders (no stage preference)
    Enuresis nocturna (bed-wetting)
    Nocturnal leg cramps
    Violent behavior in sleep

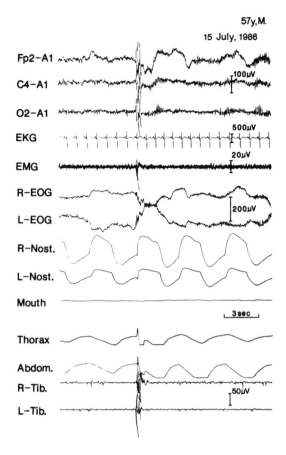

**Figure 31-1.** Hypnic jerk in stage I drowsiness. The jerk involved both legs and submental and facial muscles synchronously, and created a movement artifact on the respiratory and EEG channel. The EEG was initially that of stage I drowsiness succeeded by an arousal with return of alpha rhythm and tonic muscle artifact.

levels is often unknown. It has at times been related to intake of stimulants, including excessive nicotine or caffeine, intense evening exercise, and stress. Small doses of strychnine may produce it.[4] There are no known familial cases and both sexes appear to be equally affected.

Electroencephalographic (EEG) correlates in asymptomatic individuals were first described by Oswald,[5] who noted the presence of stage I drowsiness with at times a vertex sharp wave occurring at the time of the jerk. Superficial electromyographic (EMG) features were subsequently described by Gastaut and Broughton[6] and consist of brief 75- to 250-msec high-amplitude potentials occurring bilaterally and synchronously over homologous muscles in the affected regions (Figure 31-1). Broughton[7] has polygraphically confirmed the intensification of sleep starts to levels causing sleep-onset insomnia.

From a pathophysiologic point of view, clinically significant sleep starts appear to represent simple intensification of an otherwise normal physiologic event. It is important to recall that during sleep onset, hypnogenic brain structures actively inhibit those responsible for wakefulness, thereby temporarily creating an unstable state before sleep maintenance mechanisms become fully functional.

During this transitional state, synchronous volleys that are believed to be the mechanism of the jerks occur in the pyramidal tracts.[8]

The differential diagnosis includes a number of other motor phenomena that may occur at sleep onset. The fragmentary partial myoclonus described by De Lisi[9] and documented polygraphically by Loeb and coworkers,[10] and by Gastaut and Broughton,[6] involves contraction of local areas of musculature independently and asynchronously in various body regions. Startle disease or the so-called hyperekplexia syndrome[11] is characterized by pathologic responsiveness to sensory stimuli during wakefulness and during sleep, including deep non-REM (NREM) sleep.[4] Epileptic brief generalized myoclonus is associated with a coexisting polyspike-and-wave EEG discharge,[12] and the patient typically also has waking seizures. In so-called periodic movements in sleep,[13] the contractions last much longer, occur throughout various sleep stages, and show pseudoperiodic repetition every 20–60 seconds. This pattern also characterizes the pseudorhythmic myoclonus of subacute sclerosing panencephalitis.[14] Restless legs syndrome[15] consists of crampy dysesthesias in the lower legs during presleep and sleep onset that produce an almost irresistible urge to move the legs and that are improved by getting out of bed and walking around.

Treatment of intense hypnagogic jerks involves mainly avoidance of precipitating factors such as chemical stimulants or very irregular sleep-wake patterns. The condition is often self-limiting and disappears spontaneously. Rarely, patients require intermittent treatment with a benzodiazepine hypnotic, the most effective being clonazepam and diazepam in the usual hypnotic doses.

### *Rhythmic Movement Disorder (Jactatio Capitis Nocturna)*

Rhythmic movement disorder consists of repetitive stereotyped movements involving large body areas, usually of the head and neck (head banging) or the entire body (body rocking), that typically occur just before sleep onset and persist into light sleep. Early descriptions include those of Zappert[16] in 1905, who introduced the term *jactatio capitis nocturna*, and of Cruchet.[17] Several comprehensive reviews exist.[18–20] The phenomenon is much more common in children, although adult cases are well documented.

In the head-banging form, the patient often lies prone and repeatedly lifts the head or entire body, then bangs the head down onto the pillow or mattress. The head may also be struck rhythmically against the headboard. At times, a sitting posture is associated with backward banging of the occiput. In typical body rocking, the entire body is most usually rolled forward and backward from a sitting position, or side-to-side from a supine position. Such movements are repeated rhythmically with a frequency of 0.5–2.0 seconds in long clusters.

Rhythmic chanting or other vocalizations may occur during head banging or body rocking.

The condition is relatively common in infants and young children, the majority of affected children being otherwise normal.[18–20] The rare persistence into, or appearance during, later childhood or adulthood is more often associated with significant psychopathology including autism and mental retardation. At all ages, the condition has been found to predominate in males by a ratio of approximately 3 to 1.[21] Genetic factors are occasionally involved, and the condition has been described in twins. Older patients, in particular, may have organic brain disease.

When particularly persistent or intense, significant complications can arise. These include scalp and other body wounds, subdural hematoma, retinal petechiae, skull callus formation, and significant family and psychosocial problems.

First reported by Gastaut and Broughton[6] and confirmed by others,[22–25] polysomnography (PSG) has shown the presence of rhythmic movement artifacts, primarily in the immediate presleep period during light stages I and II sleep. Head rolling has been described as sometimes occurring mainly[26] or exclusively[27,28] during REM sleep. In very serious cases, persistence into deep SWS has been noted.[6] A remarkable typical feature is the absence of any EEG signs of arousal during, or immediately after, intense rocking movements (Figure 31-2).

Diagnosis seldom poses a problem, owing to the stereotyped nature of the movements. In infants and in very young children, it may have to be distinguished from bruxism (tooth grinding), thumb sucking, and other such disorders. Periodic limb movements in sleep are easily differentiated, as they appear only after sleep begins, involve mainly the legs, and, although "pseudorhythmic," show several seconds or dozens of seconds between individual contractions. Rhythmic epileptic behaviors, including infantile spasms, are distinguished by their usual associated EEG discharge.

Treatment in the majority of infants and children is not required and the parents should be reassured. Padding the bed area or a protective helmet is sometimes indicated. Restraining is generally ineffective. Behavior modification procedures[28,29] have been used with varying degrees of success. After early childhood, psychiatric and neurologic evaluation may be needed. Benzodiazepine and tricyclic medications have occasionally been helpful.[20]

**7 yrs.**

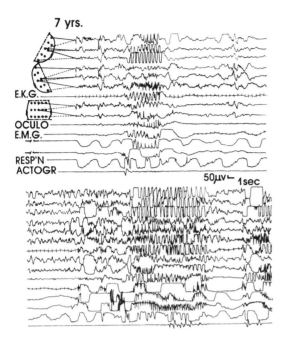

E.K.G.

OCULO
E.M.G.

RESP'N
ACTOGR

50μv — 1sec

**Figure 31-2.** Body rolling in sleep (jactatio capitis nocturna) all stages. This 7-year-old mentally handicapped girl rolled with a 1- to 3-second frequency in all stages of sleep. Rhythmic artifacts from total body movement are shown in both stage II sleep (above) and slow-wave sleep (below). They occur without significant arousal.

### Terrifying Hypnagogic Hallucinations (Sleep-Onset Nightmares)

Terrifying hypnagogic hallucinations are nightmares or bad dreams that occur at sleep onset and are otherwise indistinguishable clinically from the much more common nightmares that occur in later stages of sleep. Initially, the mental content is typically like that of normal sleep-onset reverie and mild hallucinations. The content increases in intensity and becomes threatening in its specifics, the dreamer often awakening in a state of anxiety. Before awakening there may be major body movements, gestures, apparent labored breathing, moaning, vocalizations, and even screaming. A characteristic feature is the detailed recall of the content of the bad dream on awakening.[30,31] Rarely, patients may exhibit a simultaneous awareness of both the environment and the disturbing dream mentation during the episodes, a situation that has been called "double consciousness."[32]

The prevalence of sleep-onset nightmares in the general population is unknown but appears to be low. Both sexes seem to be equally affected. The condition presents both in isolation and as one of the cardinal tetrad of symptoms of narcolepsy,[33] appearing as a symptom in approximately 10–30% of narcoleptics.[34] Facilitating factors are poorly defined for the isolated form but there is evidence that mental and physical stress, irregular sleep habits, and recovery from sleep deprivation or various central nervous system (CNS)-active drugs may play a role. The course is usually benign, although deterioration of waking levels of psychological functioning may lead to increase in frequency and chronicity. Recurrence of terrifying hypnagogic hallucinations may lead to a form of sleep-onset insomnia because of fear of the disturbing experiences at that time.

PSG shows that the sleep state consists of a sleep-onset REM period in both isolated form and when presented as part of the narcolepsy syndrome.[30] Before awakening there may be elevated amounts of movement artifact and REM and phasic EMG twitch potentials, at times associated with mild increases in heart and respiratory rate. Awakening is not associated with signs of intense autonomic activation.

The differential diagnosis includes several other parasomnias occurring at sleep onset or with similar symptoms. Normal hypnagogic reverie may consist variously of vague drifting thoughts; misperceptions and distortions of reality (illusions); simple sensations (e.g., flashes of light, sounds); or organized, dreamlike hallucinations that are not frightening and do not lead to awakening with feelings of anxiety. "Exploding head syndrome"[35,36] is a rare, bothersome but benign condition consisting of the experience of sudden loud noises in the head, sometimes associated with other sounds or flashes of light, that occurs either at sleep onset or after falling asleep. Studies have shown that the patients are almost always awake, although they believe they were asleep.[37] REM sleep nightmares occur during a later stage of sleep, usually in the last third of sleep, but otherwise are identical to the SOREMP (sleep-onset rapid eye movement period) form of terrifying hypnagogic hallucination. Sleep terrors also do not occur at sleep onset but during arousals from SWS, usually in the first third of the night, and are associated with marked autonomic activation (increased heart and respiratory rate and sweating) and little if any recall of associated mentation. Complex partial epileptic seizures with hallucinations in sleep are extremely rare and are associated with an EEG epileptic discharge and possibly a similar or other form of epileptic seizure in the daytime.

Treatment is sometimes unnecessary when the sleep-onset nightmares are rare or associated with avoidable precipitating factors such as specific stresses or sleep deprivation. When they are a bothersome chronic symptom, medication may be indicated. The usual treatment[31] is by tricyclic antidepressants, the most usual being clomipramine, 25–75 mg taken 1 hour before retiring, which appears effective both for episodes in NREM and in REM sleep onsets. Mild psychotherapy, desensitization from specific fears, hypnosis, and reassurance of the benign nature of the attacks may all be helpful in individual patients.

## NON–RAPID EYE MOVEMENT SLEEP DISORDERS (INCLUDING SLOW-WAVE SLEEP AROUSAL DISORDERS)

### Confusional Arousals (Nocturnal Sleep Drunkenness)

Episodes of marked confusion during and after arousal from sleep, but without sleepwalking or sleep terrors, have been referred to as *confusional arousals*, *nocturnal sleep drunkenness*, and *excessive sleep inertia*. Such episodes arise most typically from a deep sleep state in the first part of the night.

Early descriptions include those of Marc,[38] physician to the king of France, who called the phenomenon *l'ivresse du sommeil*, and von Gudden,[39] who used the equivalent term *Schlaftrunkenheit*. During episodes, the subject awakens only partially and exhibits marked confusion with slow mentation, disorientation in time and place, and perceptual impairment. Behavior is often inappropriate. Cognition is typically altered from full wakefulness with confused thinking, misunderstandings, and errors of logic. One personal medicolegal case involved an on-call physician, who, when called in the early morning hours approximately 1 hour after sleep onset to obtain medical advice, gave recommendations he would never give in normal wakefulness with consequent serious repercussions for the patient. Rarely, aggressive

behavior is observed, and there are several well-documented cases of homicide being committed immediately on sudden arousal from deep sleep.[40,41] The confusion lasts several minutes to dozens of minutes. Patients may make inappropriate decisions due to impaired cognition, a phenomenon not infrequently seen in (often sleep-deprived) medical residents and physicians when aroused from a deep sleep. Memory for any associated mental activity or for the episode itself is typically totally absent. Confusional arousals are more common in children[6] and may be universal before approximately 5 years of age.[6,42] In such cases, they are usually relatively benign and disappear with time. In adults, however, the condition can be more serious and is usually stable, varying only with the precipitating causes.

Predisposing factors include anything that deepens sleep or impairs ease of awakening. The major factors are young age, recovery from sleep deprivation, fever, and CNS-depressant medications, including hypnotics and tranquilizers. Confusional arousals can be associated with medical diseases characterized by deep or disturbed sleep, including metabolic, toxic, and other encephalopathies; idiopathic hypersomnia; symptomatic hypersomnias; and sleep apnea syndrome. In cases of confusional arousal of unknown mechanism, a family history of the episodes and deep sleep is common.

PSG has shown that the episodes typically have their onset during SWS.[6,43] They most commonly occur in the first third of nocturnal sleep but have also been described later at night during light NREM sleep and NREM/REM transitions and during afternoon naps. They rarely, if ever, accompany arousal from REM sleep, after which rapid return to clear mentation is usual. During confusional episodes, the EEG may show some residual slow-wave activity, stage I theta patterns, repeated microsleeps, or a diffuse and poorly reactive alpha rhythm,[6] all indicating incomplete awakening. Cerebral evoked potentials have also been described as altered during confusion accompanying experimental forced arousals from SWS.[43,44]

Pathophysiologically, confusional arousals represent incomplete awakenings from sleep, most commonly deep SWS, leading to intensification of the normal period of sleep inertia before full wakefulness is achieved.

The differential diagnosis of confusional awakenings includes four other parasomnias that occur during sleep and have amnesic qualities: (1) sleep-walking; (2) sleep terrors, in which there are signs of acute fear, usually including screams; (3) REM sleep behavior disorder, associated with explosive movements such as fighting or diving out of bed; and (4) nocturnal epileptic seizures of complex partial type associated with ictal EEG discharges, usually occurring in patients exhibiting similar attacks during the daytime and wakefulness.

Treatment is rarely necessary for the confusional arousals of children, who typically outgrow them. Parents may be reassured and should be told to let the episodes run their course rather than trying to cut them short. Facilitating causes (i.e., sleep deprivation, CNS depressants, stress) should be avoided. Treatment of the associated disease is indicated for rare symptomatic forms. Efforts to lighten the sleep of deep sleepers with a mild stimulant has proved useful in some cases.[31]

Confusional arousals, sleepwalking, and sleep terrors all primarily occur during abnormal arousals from SWS, and all can be experimentally induced in some patients by simple attempts at forced awakenings during SWS in the first third of the night. Arousal from SWS is therefore by itself sufficient to produce the attacks in predisposed individuals, demonstrating that the arousal mechanisms themselves are abnormal in such patients. This has led to the proposal that these parasomnias represent disorders of arousal.[43] Moreover, attacks with intermediate or combined features of the classic forms occur, and there is also a significant degree of genetic overlap. These findings indicate that the three prototypic clinical expressions are part of a continuum.

### Sleep Terrors (Incubus Attacks, Pavor Nocturnus)

Typically, a patient with sleep terrors sits up suddenly during sleep and emits a scream. The patient appears to be in a state of acute terror; shows tachypnea, tachycardia, mydriasis, and increased muscle tone; and is impossible to console.[1,6] The attacks appear to "run themselves out." Sleep terrors characteristically begin during the deep sleep of the first third of the night[6]; however, when episodes are very frequent, they may be diffusely distributed across the sleep period and occur in any NREM stage. The usual duration is from approximately 30 seconds to 3 minutes. As attacks may also occur during daytime naps, the term *sleep terror* is preferable to *night terror*. Once awake, the subject often remembers having difficulty breathing or marked palpitations, but recall of detailed mental activity is rare. If present, it consists almost always of a static scene like a single photograph,[6,44a] rather than the progressive succession of images that characterize a typical dream.

Attacks in children are sometimes referred to as *pavor nocturnus* (Latin for sleep terror) and in adults as *incubus* attacks. They have also been referred to as *nightmares*, but this creates confusion with the true terrifying dream or REM nightmare. The terrifying dream has been known at least since Ernest Jones[44a] to be a distinctly different parasomnia. The words *incubus* (Latin: *in*, upon; *cubare*, to press) and nightmare (Teutonic: *mar*, devil) reflect the medieval belief that sleep terrors are caused by a devil sitting or pressing on the chest of the sleeper, which leads to the breathing difficulties and acute terror.[43]

The attacks can occur from early childhood on. The prevalence of the condition is low, affecting approximately 3% of children and 1% of adults.[45] Sleep terrors are sometimes familial[46] and are associated with increased personal and family incidence of sleepwalking and confusional arousals. Males are more frequently affected than females. In children, psychopathology is very rare, and the attacks tend to disappear in adolescence. Psychopathology is common in adults. Adult attacks are most frequent in the 20- to 30-year range and less frequent in old age.

As reported by Gastaut and Broughton[6] and Broughton,[43] and confirmed by Fisher and colleagues,[47,48] PSG has shown that sleep terrors occur mainly during arousals from SWS (Figure 31-3). When many episodes occur during a single night, they may occasionally arise in stage II sleep as well. Marked tachycardia, polypnea, and reduced skin resistance are all present[6] and testify to an acute autonomic discharge. A correlation exists between the amount of prior SWS and the degree of autonomic activation as indexed by level of increase in heart rate,[47] which often doubles. In predisposed subjects, attacks may be elicited experimentally by forced arousals during monitored SWS.[6,43,47,48] PSGs often show a tendency for a more marked than usual increase in heart rate even outside of behavioral episodes, with arousals in NREM sleep and an increased frequency of SWS-to-wake arousals.[49]

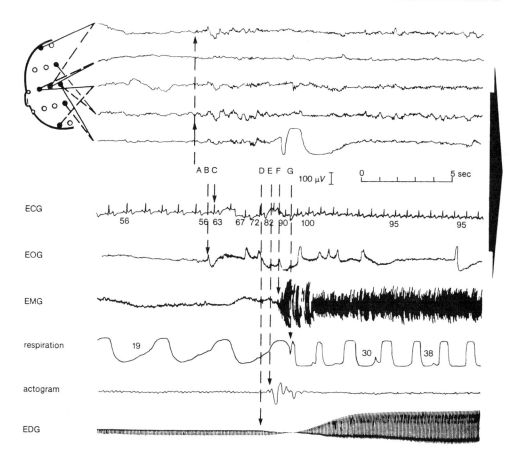

**Figure 31-3. (A)** Sleep terror beginning in stage II sleep (sleep spindles were recorded shortly before); was one of many experienced in a single night. Sequential onset of polysomnography changes is indicated by letters: A = a series of delta waves or K complexes; B = eye movements; C = tachycardia; D = reducing skin resistance in electrodermography (EDG); E = bed movement by actigraphy (actogram); F = increase in submental electromyographic (EMG) activity; G = tachypnea. (ECG = electrocardiography; EOG = electro-oculography.)

In the differential diagnosis, a distinction must be made between terrifying dreams and sleep terrors. The former typically occur in the last (rather than first) third of the night; do not have the same intensity of terror, autonomic arousal, or motor activity; and are not followed by such intense mental confusion. Moreover, the person typically recalls an organized dream that evolved in theme and became personally threatening. Nocturnal anxiety related to obstructive sleep apnea, nocturnal cardiac ischemia, sleep-related epileptic seizures, or other such events rarely pose problems for differential diagnosis.

Treatment is often unnecessary when episodes are rare. Parents of young patients may be reassured

that, even if the terror episodes are dramatic, they seldom cause injury and are almost always outgrown. Diazepam at bedtime in the usual hypnotic doses is effective in suppressing the attacks.[50] Although diazepam was first introduced because it reduces SWS, there is no correlation between the sleep architecture effect and the timing or degree of the clinical effect.[50] The latter appears more likely to be related to diazepam's suppressant effect on the autonomic or motor responsiveness to arousing stimuli.[51] Other benzodiazepines, especially clonazepam, may be effective, as are tricyclic antidepressants for adult patients.[52,53] Psychotherapy[54] and general stress reduction techniques are at times effective, particularly in adults.

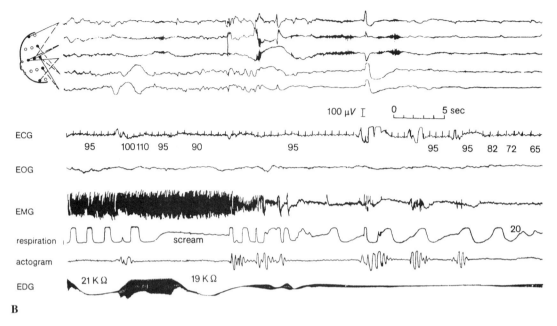

**B**

**Figure 31-3.** *Continued.* (**B**) Continuation of the recording. The EEG was desynchronized; heart rate doubled to 110 bpm; an intense, piercing scream was uttered during sustained expiration; and skin resistance continued to decrease (sweating). The attack was terminated by several body movements that are visible in the actigraphic and submental EMG channels. (ECG = electrocardiography; EOG = electro-oculography.)

## Sleepwalking (Somnambulism)

Sleepwalking consists of recurrent episodes in which the subject arises from a deep sleep, typically in the first third of the night, and, without awakening, exhibits complex automatic behaviors, which include leaving the bed and walking for some distance.[6,43] Communication with sleepwalkers is difficult or impossible and the behavior seems to have to play itself out. A pattern of repetitive behavior that has obvious symbolic meaning may occur, such as a child repeatedly crawling into his or her parents' bed or an adult trying to prepare meals. Rarely, eating may occur and the patient may present as having a sleep-related eating syndrome. Mumbling or even comprehensible speech may occur as well as, rarely, aggression, especially as a response to attempts to restrict the sleepwalker's mobility. Injury may arise from walking into dangerous situations or from cuts or burns.

The usual duration of an episode of sleepwalking is 1–5 minutes, but prolonged complex behaviors, including driving, have been documented as lasting more than 1 hour.[55] Rarely, a sleep terror immediately precedes and evolves into a sleepwalking episode as a combined or hybrid attack. The episodes may terminate either spontaneously or by forced awakening. The patient is usually very hard to awaken and, once aroused, shows mental confusion with amnesia for the event. Such amnesia varies in degree, however, and a small proportion of patients have recall of the events. One patient stated that she was aware of the environment and of her movements during a sleepwalking episode but simply could not change her behavior during it. Such recall, however, is very uncommon. Very rarely, violent or aggressive behaviors may occur and at least one well-documented case of apparent homicidal somnambulism has been reported.[56]

Sleepwalking can occur at any age after a person learns to walk. It is most common in children aged 4–6 years[43] and frequently disappears during adolescence. Adult cases, however, are not infrequent. A strong family history is common,[57,58] and there is often a family or personal history of other arousal disorders from SWS, specifically sleep terrors and confusional arousals.[59]

Facilitating and precipitating factors that increase the probability of an episode on a particular night have been identified. These are mainly factors that deepen

**20 yrs.**

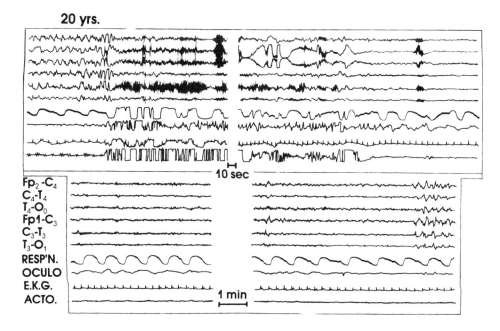

Fp₂-C₄
C₄-T₄
T₄-O₀
Fp1-C₃
C₃-T₃
T₃-O₁
RESP'N.
OCULO
E.K.G.
ACTO.

**Figure 31-4.** Sleepwalking in a 26-year-old man was recorded by cable electrodes. The upper left fragment shows onset in slow-wave sleep, followed by arousal and movement artifact as the sleeper got out of bed. Approximately 10 seconds of recording has been removed and is followed by a quiescent stage I pattern (continued below) after the patient went back to bed. One minute later the patient was in stage II sleep (lower right). (RESP'N = respiration; OCULO = electro-oculography; EKG = electrocardiography; ACTO = actigraphy.)

sleep, particularly sleep deprivation and CNS-depressant medication. The presence of factors that disrupt SWS, including stress, pain, sleep apnea, or distended bladder, can also trigger an attack. In chronic sleepwalkers, episodes can at times be "experimentally" precipitated by simple forced arousal during deep sleep in the early part of the night.[6]

PSGs first reported by Gastaut and coworkers[60] and Gastaut and Broughton[6] and confirmed by the University of California, Los Angeles, group[61,62] have shown that episodes arise in deep stage III or IV sleep (Figure 31-4), most often at the end of the first or second cycle of NREM sleep. EEG during sleepwalking has been recorded by both long cables[61] and telemetry.[6] It has typically shown lightening from SWS to stage I patterns or an abnormal diffuse and slow alpha rhythm that is unresponsive to bright light stimulation. The marked autonomic activation characteristic of sleep terrors is absent. Episodes occasionally occur in light stage II sleep or even during NREM-to-REM transitions,[43] especially when frequent throughout the night. On nights without episodes, PSG often shows three or more direct slow-wave–wakefulness transi-

tions,[49] an infrequent finding in normal subjects. There is also evidence of more frequent and higher-amplitude delta bursts during incomplete arousals from NREM sleep[61,63] and a higher frequency of brief microarousals.[64]

The pathophysiology includes strong sleep pressure due to genetic factors (familial deep sleepers), young age, recent sleep deprivation, head trauma, drugs or other factors causing difficulty in sleep-to-wake transitions, combined with causes of sleep fragmentation such as stress, noises, and pain. This combination appears to be at least part of the cause of the dissociative features in which behaviors that an observer might conclude are in wakefulness are in fact associated with some degree of cerebral sleep.

Diagnosis is seldom a problem, although "escape" behaviors during certain sleep terrors or REM sleep behavior disorder must be distinguished. If eating or drinking is a common behavior during sleepwalking, the disorder must be differentiated from the nocturnal eating (drinking) syndrome in which the consummatory behaviors consist of recurrent awakenings with inability to return to sleep without food or drink.

Sleep-related partial complex seizures with ambulatory automatisms are exceedingly rare[65]; they are associated with an ictal EEG discharge, and similar episodes usually occur in the daytime.

Treatment[66] of young children for sleepwalking is often unnecessary. Parents may be reassured that the child will most likely outgrow the episodes. When the behavior seriously distresses the patient or the family or risks injury, treatment should be instituted. Precipitating factors should be carefully avoided. Efforts should be made to minimize possible injury by locking doors and windows, removing sharp objects, and so forth. Hypnosis and psychotherapy have both been reported to have favorable effects in some patients. Drug treatment, especially benzodiazepines (diazepam, clonazepam, oxazepam) or tricyclic medication (imipramine, clomipramine), may be helpful for relatively short drug trials during periods of frequent attacks.[67] The tricyclic antidepressant amineptine has been described as being particularly effective.[68] Adult cases are typically more difficult to treat than childhood ones, and psychopathology is much more frequent.

### Nocturnal Paroxysmal Dystonia

Nocturnal paroxysmal dystonia consists of repeated dystonic or dyskinetic (ballistic, choreoathetoid) movement episodes that are repeated in stereotypical fashion during sleep.[69,70] Two varieties exist: (1) a short-lived form lasting 15–60 seconds and often repeated several times per night, and (2) a prolonged form that lasts up to 1 hour.[71] The nature of the movements is similar in both varieties. The attacks arise from tranquil sleep and consist of such dystonic movements as rotation of the head or trunk, often with abductor limb posturing, in either extension or flexion. The eyes are open but unresponsive. The sleeper may sit up and subsequently fall back, or may exhibit opisthotonus. Vocalization may occur; and the dystonic posturing is at times associated with wild ballistic or slower choreoathetoid movements. Subjects can remain asleep during episodes, or they may awaken, in which case they are usually coherent and have no difficulty going back to sleep.

The movements are intense and can cause severe sleep disruption with secondary daytime sleepiness. The sleeper or sleeping partner may be injured. Episodes typically occur most nights, and in the brief form several times per night. They can begin in childhood to late middle age and may persist into old age. Birth history, neurologic status, and psychological examination findings are typically all normal. Patients may have a history of daytime generalized tonic-clonic or other epileptic seizures, particularly those with the brief form, although ictal EEG discharges have not been recorded to date at the time of the dystonic episodes. The attacks typically persist for years without showing any tendency to spontaneous remission.

PSG[69–72] has shown that the attacks occur exclusively in NREM sleep, typically in stage II (Figure 31-5) but at times in stage III or IV. There is desynchronization of the EEG, indicating arousal without evident epileptic medial frontal discharge. Increased muscle tone rapidly obscures the brain wave patterns. Just before an episode, a central respiratory pause, slowing of heart rate, or change in electrodermal activity may occur.[69,70]

Differential diagnosis from other parasomnias is seldom difficult, given the unusual dystonic nature of the movements and the characteristic PSG. The nocturnal tonic spasms described by Lance[73] have similar PSG correlates[74] but occur in the context of demyelinating disease, especially multiple sclerosis. Epileptic seizures of frontal lobe origin most closely resemble nocturnal paroxysmal dystonia, but an ictal EEG discharge is usually recorded with the seizures and patients typically have similar episodes in the daytime.[71]

Treatment is usually required. Attacks do not respond to normal tranquilizers, sedatives, barbiturates, or diphenylhydantoin. Most patients with the short form of attacks are controlled by carbamazepine, in the usual clinical dose of approximately 15 mg/kg daily.[69,71] Serum drug levels should be monitored, as should hematologic status for possible side effects. There is evidence to support the suggestion that at least some episodes of the short form of attacks are occult epileptic seizures.[71] The longer attacks, however, appear to represent a form of dyskinesia of neurochemical origin.

## RAPID EYE MOVEMENT SLEEP DISORDERS

### Nightmares (Terrifying Dreams)

The term *nightmare* is best reserved for dreams with progressive content that becomes frightening

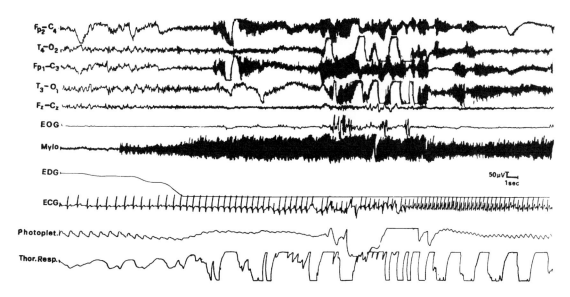

**Figure 31-5.** Paroxysmal nocturnal dystonia begins in stage II sleep. The EEG shows desynchronization with some alpha and then is obscured by sustained electromyography (EMG) artifact. A marked increase in muscle tone is visible in the submental EMG (mylohyoid muscle), associated with decreasing skin resistance, tachycardia, decreased pulsation (photo-plethysmography), and hyperpnea with tachypnea. (EOG = electro-oculography; EDG = electrodermography; ECG = electro-cardiography.) (Figure appears courtesy of Professor Elio Lugaresi.)

to the sleeper and leads to awakening.[75,76] The term has also been applied to the sleep terror, a condition that is a distinctly different form of parasomnia. Nightmares occur mainly in the second half of the night within REM sleep. Movements, mumbling, or vocalizations may occur during sleep before awakening. The awakening is seldom accompanied by the cry typical of an episode of sleep terror, and palpitations and labored breathing, if present, are much less marked. The sensorium is relatively intact, with little of the confusion and disorientation that are characteristic of sleep terrors. Most important for differentiating nightmares from sleep terrors, a patient with nightmares typically can report detailed recall of a succession of dream images whose content became threatening. Nightmares usually last approximately 4–15 minutes, although shorter and longer episodes do occur. Subjective perception of imminent injury or death is not infrequent. Nightmares never evolve into sleepwalking as can sleep terrors.

Nightmares are not uncommon in children and have been said to occur in 10–50% of 3- to 6-year-olds.[76] Nightmares may persist into, or initially appear in, adolescence or adulthood. Approximately 40–50% of adults report at least occasional nightmares. Certain personality characteristics appear to be associated with lifelong nightmares. Hartmann[76] and Kales and coworkers[77] have noticed an increased frequency of borderline personality disorder, schizoid personality disorder, and schizophrenia. Patients may feel that their childhood was unusually difficult, although often no specific major trauma occurred. Sufferers are often vulnerable with soft ego boundaries and strong artistic tendencies. In military personnel with combat shock, nightmares may be particularly intense and recurrent, and the relationship to life stresses is evident.[78,79] A common cause of nightmares is so-called REM rebound during a period of recuperation after REM sleep deprivation either from stress, drugs, or other causes. A number of drugs also predispose to nightmares, including β-adrenergic blockers, L-dopa, and related medications, as does withdrawal from REM-suppressant medications such as tricyclic antidepressants, monoamine oxidase (MAO) inhibitors, selective serotonin-reuptake inhibitors (SSRIs) alcohol, and certain stimulants and sedative-hypnotics. In 50% of adult sufferers, no psychiatric or other medical diagnosis can be made, and the nightmares appear to be related simply to daytime stress.

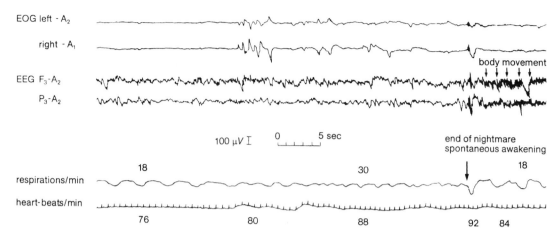

**Figure 31-6.** A REM nightmare in a chronic adult sufferer. Mild to moderate increases in heart and respiratory rate in REM sleep before arousal are followed by body movement and awakening. The patient subsequently described in detail a terrifying dream sequence in which he was viciously attacked by man-sized cats. The remarkable degree of dissociation between terrifying dream content and minimal autonomic or EEG activation is evident, a phenomenon referred to as "desomatization." (EOG = electro-oculography.) (Reprinted with permission from the late Dr. Charles Fisher.)

PSG[47,48,50] shows changes within REM sleep followed by awakening. During REM sleep, the amount of actual eye movement activity and brief EMG twitch potentials may be increased. There may be a mild increase in frequency or variability in heart or respiratory rate but the explosive tachycardia and tachypnea characteristic of sleep terror on awakening are absent (Figure 31-6). Nightmares may occur during NREM sleep, especially stage I or II, particularly after severe mental or physical trauma.

The principal item of differential diagnosis is sleep terror, the distinguishing features of which have already been detailed, including typical occurrence in the first third of the night, cry on awakening, marked tachycardia and tachypnea, and lack of recall of a detailed dream sequence. Occasionally, differentiation from REM sleep behavior disorder poses a problem. This condition is more common in the elderly, some of whom have CNS lesions. The explosive, violent movements; markedly increased muscle tone; frequent intense myoclonus; and typical PSG features of REM sleep behavior disorder help make the distinction.

Treatment of recurrent disturbing nightmares is often necessary.[80] Stresses that appear recurrently and are related to precipitation of nightmares should be avoided. Drugs known to promote nightmares should, whenever possible, be substituted. Psy-

chotherapy, including strengthening ego boundaries by assertiveness training, dream content analysis, and techniques to acquire some degree of dream content control (so-called lucid dreaming) have all been helpful in individual cases. In patients with irregular sleep-wake patterns, a simple sleep hygiene regimen may reduce the frequency of nightmares. Rarely, patients with severe recurrent nightmares require a REM-suppressant medication (tricyclics, MAO inhibitors). REM-suppressant medications should be withdrawn very slowly, to avoid recurrence during the REM-rebound period.

### Rapid Eye Movement Sleep Behavior Disorder

A condition recently documented independently by Hishikawa et al.[81] and by Schenck, Mahowald, and colleagues,[82–84] REM sleep behavior disorder is characterized by intermittent absence of the normal atonia of REM sleep associated with intense motor activity related to dream mentation. The movements are often explosive, including sudden jerking, leaping or diving from the bed, rapid ambulatory collisions with walls or furniture, and other behaviors that appear to be dream enactment. Injury to self or to the bed partner is common. Similar but less violent movements, such as hand and arm waving, reaching gestures, and punching or kicking may occur while the patient remains in bed. Episodes may repeat only a few times a week, but if several occur each night, they may reappear in cyclic fashion approximately every 90 minutes after sleep onset. On awakening, recall of an intense dream in which the patient must fend off or flee from an attacker is typical. The violent nocturnal behavior is typically discordant with the dreamer's daytime personality. Duration of attacks is typically 2–10 minutes.

In at least one-third of patients, a prodromal period of talking, yelling, or vigorous movements in sleep precedes the full-blown episodes by a number of years.[84] In a similar number of patients, there is a history of significant neuropathology that can include dementia, subarachnoid hemorrhage, stroke, Parkinson's disease, olivopontocerebellar degeneration, multiple sclerosis, or Guillain-Barré syndrome. The condition is common during, and was first identified in, chronic alcoholics.[81] Despite this variety of possible associations with pathology, at least 60% of cases are idiopathic. No consistently associated psychopathology has been documented.

It is believed that REM sleep behavior disorder is generally lesional and due to dysfunction of the brain stem mechanisms responsible for the normal suppression of muscle tone in REM sleep. An essentially identical behavior has long been described after experimental dorsal pontine lesions in cats.[85] The precise prevalence is unknown, but the condition is far more common in males, and, although it can occur at any age, it is most frequent after age 60 years.

PSG shows a number of characteristic features.[81–83] During REM sleep, there are recurrent periods of persistent muscle tone that is normally abolished. Marked increases of phasic motor activity are present during REM sleep, particularly during the episodes. These include eye movements, brief twitch potentials, and longer 0.5- to 2.0-second phasic EMG potentials. During the episodes, such phasic increases are superimposed on marked sustained tonic increases in background EMG tone (Figure 31-7).

The differential diagnosis is extensive and includes post-traumatic stress syndrome, classic REM nightmares, sleep terrors, nocturnal paroxysmal dystonia, sleep-related epileptic seizures, and nocturnal delirium. Although the history is often suggestive, definitive diagnosis is based on the characteristic PSG features.

Treatment of this parasomnia is mainly by drugs.[82,83] Most cases respond to the benzodiazepine clonazepam (1–2 mg at bedtime). The mechanisms of its effectiveness are not fully understood, but clonazepam suppresses both the violent behavior and the intense subjective dream recall. Desipramine (25–50 mg at bedtime) has also been successful in a smaller percentage of cases. Because the clinical attacks occasionally break through drug therapy, sharp objects should be removed from the sleeping environment and other precautions should be taken against injury. Cessation of medication inevitably leads to recurrence of the attacks.

### Sleep Paralysis (Isolated)

Sleep paralysis[86,87] consists of episodes of inability to perform voluntary movements, either at sleep onset (hypnagogic or predormital form) or on awakening (hypnopompic or postdormital form). Although sleep paralysis is one of the so-called symptom tetrad of the narcolepsy-cataplexy syndrome, it is much more common in its isolated form. Characteristically, limb, trunk, and head movements are impossible, but the patient can move the eyes and make some degree of respiratory effort. The sufferer is usually conscious of the environment and feels vulnerable and often frightened and anxious. Fragments of dream imagery may be recalled; when present, they are occasionally superimposed on the environment, leading to a form of "double consciousness."[32] Episodes typically last 1–3 minutes. The paralysis typically either disappears spontaneously or is aborted by someone else touching or moving part of the person's body.

Isolated sleep paralysis is not infrequently experienced by rotating shift workers experiencing irregular sleep-wake patterns,[88] individuals with recurrent exposure to jet lag,[89] and medical students and interns.[90,91] It has been suggested that sleep paralysis is experienced at least once during the lifetime of approximately 30–50% of normal subjects. Both sexes are equally affected. Isolated sleep paralysis occasionally occurs in a familial form[92] that tends to be more chronic, affects females more often than males, and has an X-linked dominant transmission. No autopsy reports have been published in cases of isolated sleep paralysis but as patients are neurologically intact on physical examination, any organic

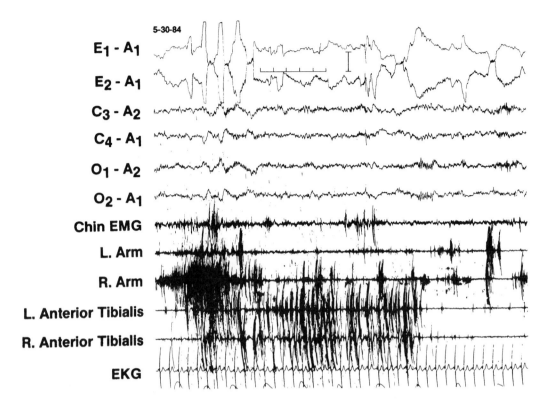

**Figure 31-7.** REM sleep behavior disorder in a 64-year-old man. The polygraph fragment is taken from the middle of a sequence that lasted several minutes. It shows REM sleep features, indicated by the stage I EEG pattern combined with REM. The chin electromyography (EMG), however, shows the characteristic sustained muscle tone of this disorder. The four limb EMGs show tonic increase in muscle tone with superimposed phasic increases. The phasic increases are associated with visible myoclonus ("twitching"). (EKG = electrocardiography.) (Courtesy of Drs. Carlos Schenck and Mark Mahowald.)

cause in chronic cases most likely is microstructural, neurochemical, or neuroimmunologic.

PSG recordings have been described in detail for sleep paralysis in association with the narcolepsy syndrome only.[87,93] They have shown the condition to occur during direct transitions into or out of REM sleep and to consist of absence of muscle tone in submental, other axial, and peripheral EMGs in association with an EEG of wakefulness plus waking ocular movements and blink patterns. Occasionally, drowsy stage I patterns with slow eye movements occur. H-reflex studies during episodes have shown total suppression of this monosynaptic reflex, indicating loss of anterior motoneuron excitability, which normally occurs during full-blown REM sleep. Sleep paralysis is thus considered a dissociated REM state in which the motor atonia of REM sleep is present in isolation. Patho-

physiologically, sleep paralysis may therefore be considered the inverse of REM sleep behavior disorder, in which sleep is preserved but the mechanisms of REM atonia are absent.

The differential diagnosis seldom poses a problem, as the episodes are so characteristic. Narcolepsy syndrome can be excluded by absence of its other features, including cataplectic attacks triggered in wakefulness by emotional stimuli; irresistible sleep attacks; multiple sleep-onset REM periods on the Multiple Sleep Latency Test; and positive histocompatibility testing in Caucasians and Japanese for HLA-DR15 (formerly -DR2) and -DQw1 antigens. Nocturnal nerve compression palsies must be considered but are usually self-evident and local. Hypokalemic paralysis must be distinguished. Hypokalemic paralysis usually occurs in wakefulness; is more common in adolescents; exhibits familial transmission; and, above all, shows characteristic low serum potassium levels during episodes, which can be reversed by taking potassium.

Successful treatment in isolated cases associated with irregular sleep-wake patterns may consist of improved sleep hygiene alone. In chronic cases, especially in the familial ones, medication may be necessary. The usual drug treatment is clomipramine hydrochloride, 25 mg at bedtime.[31] Desipramine is less effective, and imipramine has little if any effect. In exceptionally resistant cases, an MAO inhibitor such as phenelzine may be indicated, although the risk of serious side effects and the necessary dietary precautions with these drugs seriously limit their usefulness.

### *Painful Erections*

The occurrence of painful nocturnal erections is a rare parasomnia[1,94] often associated with recall of dreams. If recurrent, the patient may develop a form of sleep maintenance insomnia with subsequent daytime sleepiness, anxiety, and irritability. Concern over the symptom may become intense. Penile erections during wakefulness usually are not affected. In most cases, the cause is unknown. Painful nocturnal erections can be associated with Peyronie's disease or phimosis and can be seen intermittently during intense REM rebound after REM sleep deprivation resulting from stress, REM-suppressant medication, or other factors.

PSG confirms the presence of recurrent awakenings from REM sleep associated with penile erections monitored by strain gauge devices or observation.

Treatment in symptomatic cases (e.g., painful erections associated with Peyronie's disease) is by surgical correction of the underlying disease. In idiopathic cases, the symptom often disappears spontaneously. A small proportion of patients require REM-suppressant medication.[95]

## LIGHT SLEEP STAGE DISORDERS (STAGES I, II, AND REM)

### *Sleep Talking*

Sleep talking is usually a benign phenomenon and seldom represents a significant sleep disorder. It consists of speech or sound uttered during sleep without awareness of the behavior.[96] The duration varies from a few seconds to dozens of minutes. Sleep talking typically becomes a problem only when it is sufficiently frequent or loud to disturb the sleep of others. It is usually spontaneous (somniloquy); more rarely, however, it can be elicited, resulting in a dialogue with others.[97] The occurrence of two sleepers having a dialogue between them, none of which is recalled by either on awakening, has also been reported. Arkin and coworkers[98] have shown that recalled mental activity after awakening, when present, generally shows a reasonable degree of concordance with speech content. This supports the premise that such utterances reflect ongoing mental activity in sleep.

The course of sleep talking is typically benign. Sleep talking may occur only for short intermittent periods, then disappear completely. Chronic sleep talking may be related to significant psychopathology or to intercurrent sleep disturbances. The phenomenon shows no gender preference. Occasionally, it appears to be familial.

PSG has shown that sleep talking most commonly occurs in stages I, II, and REM sleep,[6,96] and only rarely in SWS. Speech utterances typically are associated[6] with increased muscle tone and a transient and incomplete EEG arousal (Figure 31-8). Autonomic activation during the EEG arousals is minimal. The phenomenon seldom requires treatment, and, in any event, no specific treatment is known.

### *Bruxism*

Bruxism is repeated grinding or crunching of the teeth during sleep,[99,100] often disturbing the bed partner. Bruxism is frequently associated with a pre-existing dental, mandibular, or maxillary condition such as dental disease, malocclusion, and others.[101] Repeated sleep-related bruxism may lead secondarily to excessive tooth wear and decay or periodontal tissue damage[102] and is often associated with jaw pain, including the temporomandibular variety.

Tooth grinding is often associated with stress and may be seen in otherwise normal individuals. However, it is particularly common in children who have some degree of mental deficiency.[103] Tooth grinding in wakefulness as a habit or tic is often associated. There is no gender preference. Rarely, apparent familial cases have been described.

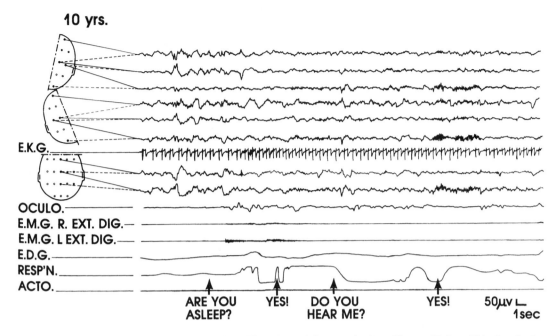

**Figure 31-8.** Sleep talking (dialogue) in NREM sleep. The polygraph fragment begins with stage II sleep. This chronic sleep talker, a 10-year-old boy, was asked "Are you asleep?" The question evoked a K complex. Transient arousal (return of alpha rhythm) was associated with the answer, "Yes." Subsequently (not shown) he was asked "Do you hear me?" (K complex) and answered "Yes" (alpha burst). The child heard, understood, and appropriately answered the two questions while remaining asleep, arousing only briefly during answers. A few seconds later he was awakened and recalled nothing. (EKG = electrocardiography; OCULO = electro-oculography; EMG = electromyography; EDG = electrodermography; RESP'N = respiration; ACTO = actigraphy.)

PSG shows repeated phasic increases of masseter muscle tone that cause rhythmic EMG artifacts in the EEG (Figure 31-9). These repeat at a frequency of approximately 0.5 to 1.5 per second in bursts lasting a few to several dozens of seconds and occur mainly in stages I, II, and REM sleep.[6,104,105] Some cases in which phasic increases occur exclusively in REM sleep have been described. [105]

Diagnosis seldom poses a problem. Rhythmic jaw movements in epileptic seizures associated with an ictal EEG discharge are rare but occasionally must be excluded.

Evaluation for treatment[106] includes a comprehensive dental examination and correction of any causal anatomic anomalies. Rare patients have treatable CNS lesions. In most cases, no evident jaw or brain abnormality is found. Stress may be reduced by appropriate counseling or psychotherapy. In some cases, relaxation techniques or biofeedback have been useful. A few patients require a rubber mouth guard over the teeth to prevent further dental and jaw damage.

### Sleep-Related Panic Attacks

Some or all of the attacks of panic characterizing sleep-related panic disorder occur with sudden awakenings from sleep.[107] The attacks consist of sudden acute fear, often of impending doom or death, associated with a variety of somatic symptoms. These symptoms may include dizziness, palpitations, trembling, chest discomfort, choking, sweating, and so on. After the attack, the patient remains in an excessively aroused condition for a significant period of time and has difficulty falling back to sleep.

Patients usually have daytime attacks as well and exhibit various phobias between attacks, the most common being agoraphobia, the fear of being in places (e.g., a car, a plane, a meeting room with the doors closed) and situations from which escape is difficult or impossible or embarrassment might ensue.

Etiology and precipitating factors are variable. The exact prevalence is unknown but the sleep-only form is rare. Most patients are young adults and

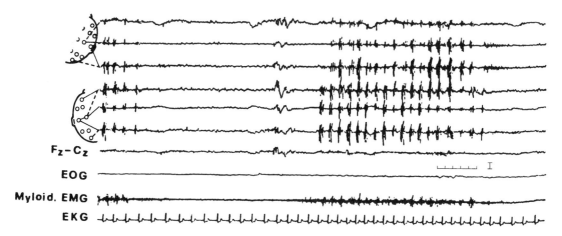

**Figure 31-9.** Teeth grinding (bruxism) in an 18-year-old woman. One series of four teeth grindings is followed by stage I patterns, stage II (K complex), and some degree of EEG arousal associated with return of rhythmic electromyography (EMG) artifacts with a frequency of approximately 0.5–1.0 Hz. (EOG = electro-oculography; EKG = electrocardiography.)

women are more commonly afflicted than men with a 3-to-1 ratio. There are no known genetic factors. Separation anxiety from parents in childhood is common in the patient history. Depression is seen in approximately one-half of patients.[108] Alcohol abuse is often associated. Triggering is usually by exposure to the particular objects feared during the daytime before attacks.

PSG shows the attacks to be most common during transitions from stage II to early stage III of SWS and, to a lesser degree, in light NREM stages I and II.[109,110] Occasionally, attacks are seen during sleep onset at the start of the night. There are usually some tachycardia and tachypnea during a nocturnal panic attack but their intensity is much less than one might expect and certainly less than during sleep terrors. Outside of the attacks, the overall sleep architecture tends to show some increase in sleep onset and increased wakefulness with corresponding reduced sleep efficiency and increased movement time. There is usually little daytime sleepiness, as patients tend to be hyper-aroused, and MSLT is typically normal.

The differential diagnosis is mainly that of sleep terror, which is characterized by a cry and the sense of respiratory oppression; occurrence in the first third of the night in SWS; and marked activation of the autonomic nervous system, expressed as increased heart and respiratory rate and increased sweating. The occurrence of daytime panic attacks

and the presence of specific phobias help clarify the diagnosis. Rarely, nocturnal choking syndrome may also be considered in the diagnosis, but its typical choking sensation and the lack of daytime panic attacks and agoraphobia make diagnosis straightforward.

Treatment is that of the underlying clinical panic disorder and agoraphobia, which can include psychotherapy, desensitization programs for specific phobias, relaxation therapies, and use of antianxiety medication.[111]

## DIFFUSE SLEEP DISORDERS (NO STAGE PREFERENCE)

### *Enuresis Nocturna*

Enuresis nocturna, or bed-wetting, consists of involuntary micturition during sleep. It is often classified into primary and secondary types. In primary enuresis, full urinary continence, which should occur by 5 years of age, has never been achieved. In secondary enuresis, after learning bladder control for at least 6 months, patients lose control and become enuretic.[112,113]

Bed-wetting is also often divided into idiopathic and symptomatic forms, the latter being associated with genitourinary pathology such as small bladder size, increased renal output, or other medical condi-

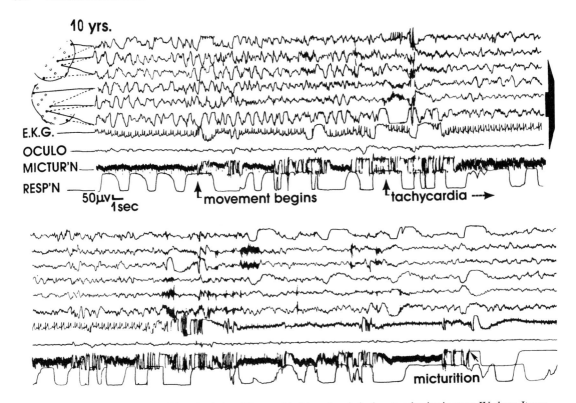

**Figure 31-10.** Enuresis nocturna. This episode in a 10-year-old girl, a chronic bed-wetter, begins in stage IV sleep. It consists of body movement, tachycardia, EEG desynchronization evolving eventually to stage I patterns, and, lower right, micturition indicated by loss of the dark 60-Hz main lines artifact in the micturition channel. (EKG = electrocardiography; OCULO = electro-oculography.)

tions. Idiopathic primary enuresis is by far the most common type. Bed-wetting tends to occur in the first third of the night during a partial or complete arousal. Dreaming may be recalled in association with the enuresis, but it has been shown that dreams about fluids represent postevent incorporation of the wet bed stimuli rather than being causal.[53] Bed-wetting often leads to embarrassment and secondary psychological trauma, especially in older children, adolescents, and adults. Bladder control during daytime wakefulness is typically normal.

The reasons for the perpetuation or reappearance of bed-wetting after age 5 years vary. In some children toilet training is not fully provided or acquired.[114] A small functional bladder[115] or an insensitive bladder[116,117] may be present without demonstrable organic disease. Idiopathic enuresis is more common in males, lower socioeconomic classes, and institutionalized children.[112] In adults, idiopathic enuresis is much more rare, and an organic cause, an associated metabolic or endocrine

disorder, or coexisting sleep apnea syndrome is more common. A hereditary factor appears to be present in primary enuresis[118,119] and in symptomatic cases with urogenital malformations.

PSG (Figure 31-10) has determined that enuresis episodes can occur in all stages of sleep, with or without concomitant arousal.[120,121] In NREM sleep episodes there is a tendency for increasing episode duration (from first signs of state change to micturition) associated with lighter sleep-wake patterns at the moment of bed-wetting.[6] Sleep cystometry[6,122] has shown increased bladder reactivity to environmental stimuli; increased detrusor contractions in sleep before onset of micturition; and waves of elevated bladder pressure during sleep at the onset of the enuretic event that later reach levels sufficient to trigger involuntary micturition, at least in wakefulness (Figures 31-11 and 31-12).

The diagnosis of idiopathic enuresis requires the exclusion of organic and metabolic causes. Urogenital disease, chronic urinary tract infection, diabetes

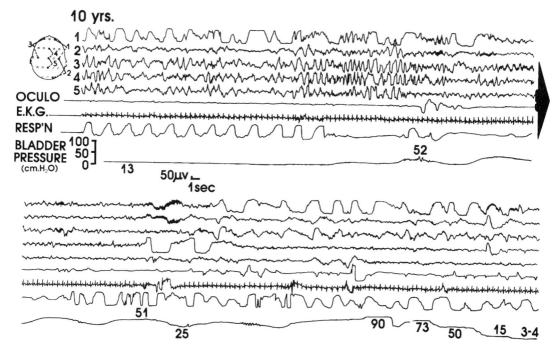

**Figure 31-11.** Bladder pressure changes during an enuretic episode. The recording comes from another night in the same patient as in Figure 31-10 and shows increasing pressure with waves reaching levels at which suppression of the micturition reflex is impossible (bottom right). Bed-wetting ensues with precipitous pressure decrease in the lower right. Polysomnography also shows transition from stage III/IV to stage I, then to wake, which closely parallels the episode without intravesicular pressure recording (Figure 31-10). Respiratory changes are also prominent. (Note that the baseline pressure is artificially elevated due to the location of the manometer head.) (EKG = electrocardiography; OCULO = electro-oculography.)

insipidus, diabetes mellitus, neurologic disease, sleep apnea syndrome, and nocturnal epileptic seizures must all be ruled out by appropriate tests.

Treatment of the symptomatic form is that of the underlying disease. This may include surgical correction of genitourinary pathology, treatment of diabetes insipidus, and so on. In the case of the much more common idiopathic primary enuresis, a number of approaches are helpful. Avoidance of fluids in late evening may be sufficient. Bladder training exercises during wakefulness, in which the patient is taught to hold increasingly larger amounts of urine in the bladder, may help,[123] as may sphincter training exercises in which the patient repeatedly interrupts the stream of urine while voiding.[124] Patients may respond positively to a conditioning device in which a bell or alarm triggered by the release of urine stimulates the patient, who becomes more aware of the enuresis over time.[125] This apparently leads eventually to learning to sense the detrusor contractions during sleep and, consequently,

awakening in time to void. Family support and avoidance of teasing may be crucial.

Medication may be necessary, particularly for children who are under much social stress and for adults. The most effective substance is imipramine hydrochloride, 10–75 mg at bedtime.[126] Its effect does not appear to relate to any change in sleep structure, but to a direct anticholinergic effect on the bladder myoneural junction. Various tricyclics and other drugs have also been found to be of help in individual cases.

### Nocturnal Leg Cramps

Nocturnal leg cramps are painful leg sensations of muscular tightness or cramping, typically in the calf but sometimes in the foot, that occur in sleep and frequently are the cause of awakening.[127] The acute discomfort is associated with objective cramping with muscle hardness or tightness in one or rarely both

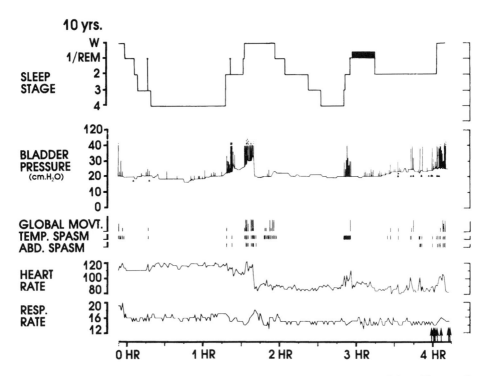

**Figure 31-12.** Detailed sleep histogram in a 10-year-old boy bed-wetter for the first 4 hours of sleep. The recording included intravesicular bladder pressure as measured by indwelling catheter. Enuresis occurred approximately 100 minutes after sleep onset. Up to that point, there was increasing baseline bladder pressure with superimposed vesicular contractions (vertical lines) and some degree of sustained tachycardia and tachypnea. These led to a crescendo during lightening of sleep, from NREM stages IV to II to I, followed by micturition around the catheter. Micturition was followed by an abrupt drop of baseline bladder pressure, heart rate, and, to a lesser extent, respiratory rate. With the bladder empty, there were no further bladder contractions for approximately 1.5 hours. This period was followed by increased bladder pressure and a return of contractions. (Note that the baseline pressure is artificially high owing to the location of the manometer head).

legs. Although often not considered a parasomnia, the condition occurs in episodic, unpredictable fashion and leads to awakening. It typically lasts a few seconds to several minutes, although it may persist for 30–45 minutes. The frequency of recurrence is variable but is generally of the order of once or twice a week to two per night. Frequent occurrence of leg cramps may lead to a form of sleep maintenance insomnia and possible consequent daytime sleepiness and fatigue. Similar leg cramps are occasionally experienced in daytime wakefulness. The condition is most common in the elderly but can be experienced at all ages from young childhood on. Males and females appear equally afflicted. The prevalence is not well known but some studies suggest that nocturnal leg cramps affect at least 15–20% of individuals at some time during their lifetime.[127,131]

Several facilitating and etiologic factors exist. Genetic factors are not well documented, although some familial cases have been reported.[128–130] Pregnancy; diabetes mellitus; excessive exercise; metabolic diseases; various neuromuscular disorders; peripheral vascular disease; and disorders associated with reduced mobility, such as arthritis involving leg joints and the rigidity of Parkinson's disease, are all predisposing factors.

On PSG, the condition is expressed as sustained tonic EMG patterns over the affected muscles (typically the gastrocnemius) associated with nocturnal leg cramps that have been documented to occur in all stages of sleep.[131] There are no characteristic EEG, autonomic, or other correlates.

The differential diagnosis seldom poses a problems as the cramp sensations and actual muscle

**Table 31-2.** Etiology of Violent Behavior in Sleep

**Parasomnias**
Disorders of arousal
    Confusional arousals (CA)
    Sleep terrors (ST)
    Sleepwalking (SW)
REM sleep behavior disorder
Nocturnal paroxysmal dystonia
Sleep-related epileptic seizures
    Frontal
    Inferomesial temporal
Nocturnal delirium
"Overlap" parasomnias (in single patient)
    CA/ST/SW
    Non-REM/REM
    Nonepileptic/epileptic

**Nonparasomnia disorders**
Obstructive sleep apnea
Idiopathic central nervous system hypersomnia with sleep
    drunkenness
Alcohol- and hypnotic-related hypersomnias
Cerebral degenerative disorders
Restless legs syndrome and periodic movements in sleep
Intensified sleep starts
Waking aggression
Malingering

Source: Adapted from R Broughton, T Shimizu. Dangerous
Behaviors by Night. In C Shapiro, A McCall (eds), Forensic
Aspects of Sleep. London: Wiley 1997;65.

**Table 31-3.** Pathophysiologic Factors Potentially
Involved in Violent Behaviors in Sleep

Immediate prior sleep stage
Circadian time of day
Degree of concurrent sleep pressure
    Prior total or partial sleep deprivation
    Microfragmentation of sleep
Rate of awakening from sleep
Physiologic level of central nervous system arousal
Microarousal presence after awakening
Dissociated or incomplete sleep-wake states
Overlapping sleep-wake states
Cognitive difficulties, including misperceptions, illusions,
    hallucinations, and dreams
Effects of drugs, alcohol, and other chemical substances
Hypoxemia during sleep
Brain lesion effects
Ictal and postictal epileptic confusional states
Environmental resistance against behaviors
Psychogenic dissociative states

Source: Adapted from R Broughton, T Shimizu. Dangerous
Behaviors by Night. In C Shapiro, A McCall (eds), Forensic
Aspects of Sleep. London: Wiley 1997;65.

tightening are characteristic. Restless legs syndrome, fasciculation syndromes, peripheral neuropathy, and disorders of calcium metabolism, however, should all be excluded.

Treatment often consists of slow stretching of the leg and muscle, massage, or application of heat, all of which may reverse the muscle spasm. Episodes may sometimes be avoided by taking either clonazepam (0.5–2.0 mg) or quinine sulfate before retiring.

### Violent Behaviors in Sleep

Aggressive and violent behaviors in sleep do not represent a single parasomnia but are included because of their personal, social, and forensic implications. The nature of the behaviors is highly variable (see references in Broughton and Shimizu[132]).

The etiology of aggressive and violent behavior is as variable as the kinds of behaviors exhibited. The primary causes are summarized in Table 31-2 and the common pathophysiologic factors are listed in Table 31-3. That the incidence is much higher in males than females for all parasomnias in which violent behaviors in sleep have been studied raises the strong possibility that the behavior may be related to endocrine differences between the genders. Testosterone is particularly implicated, as giving it experimentally to female animals markedly enhances their aggression.

There is nothing in PSGs that marks violent behaviors in sleep, the patterns being those of the causal parasomnia often with greater EMG and movement artifact than is usual. As with most parasomnias, documentation of episodes is best with videotelemetry or other means that permit full, unimpeded movement of the patient, such as ambulatory monitoring.

Treatment involves three approaches. The first consists of handling the violent behavior while it is happening. Physically impeding the behavior of a person with an asleep, or a partially asleep and con-

**Table 31-4.** Comparison of the Behavioral Parasomnias

| Clinical features | Sleep Starts | Rhythmic Movements | Hypnagogic Hallucinations | Confusion Episodes | Sleep Terrors | Nocturnal Sleep-walking | Paroxysmal Dystonia | REM Behavior Disorder | Sleep Talking | Bruxism | Nocturnal Enuresis |
|---|---|---|---|---|---|---|---|---|---|---|---|
| Motor | Repeated jerks | Body rocking, head rolling | None or minor twitching | May sit up | Sits, screams | Gets out of bed | Dystonia in bed | Explosive behaviors | Speech, vocalization | Tooth grinding | Bed-wetting |
| Subjective | Simple sensations | None | Dreams, nightmares | Confusion | Single image, if any | Little or none | None | Detailed dream | Unaware | Unaware | Unaware |
| ANS activation | Minimal | None or minimal | Minimal | Low | Extreme | Low | Low to moderate | Low to moderate | Absent | Absent | Bladder contractions |
| Memory | Vague recall | None | Detailed recall | None | Little or none | Little or none | None | Good | None to little | None to little | Absent |
| Violence | None | None, can self-injure | Extremely rare | Possible | Possible | Possible | None | Possible | Absent | Absent | Absent |
| Duration | 1 msec to 1 sec | 1–3/sec for 1 min | 2–25 mins | 1–3 mins | 30 secs to 5 mins | 2–145 mins, rarely longer | 10–60 secs (short form), 60 secs to 60 mins (long form) | 5–20 mins | Minutes to hours | Minutes to hours | 20 secs to 3 mins |
| Predisposing factors | Caffeine, nicotine | Cognitive impairment | Stress, fears, and phobias | Deep sleep arousals | Deep sleep arousals | Deep sleep arousals | None known | Pontine lesions, stress | Stress | Dental problems | Small bladder, deep sleeper |
| Sleep stage preferred | Sleep onset | Sleep onset and in sleep | Sleep onset | SWS arousal | SWS arousal | SWS arousal | NREM stages | Dissociated REM | Light SI, SII, REM | Light SI, SII, REM | All equally |
| Pathophysiology | Startle increase | Uncertain and variable | SOREMP | Arousal disorder | Arousal disorder | Arousal disorder | Epileptic (short form), neurochemical (long form) | Absent REM atonia | Mentation-induced? | Sleep tic, dental | Poor bladder sensation |
| Treatment (main) | Off stimulants, clonazepam | Variable | Stress reduction, clomipramine | Avoid predisposing factors | Clonazepam, diazepam | Clonazepam, tricyclics | Carbamazepine | Clonazepam | Unnecessary | Protective devices | Reduce fluid intake, imipramine, conditioning |

REM = rapid eye movement; ANS = autonomic nervous system; SOREMP = sleep-onset rapid eye movement period; SWS = slow-wave sleep; SI = stage I sleep; SII = stage II sleep.

fused brain usually enhances the level of aggression and should therefore be avoided. Typically, the best approach is to let the episode run itself out while attempting to awaken the person by talking to him or her or using other nonphysical methods. Efforts to protect the person from self-injury or injury may also be necessary. Most such behaviors stop after 1–3 minutes. The second approach is treatment of the underlying parasomnia, which, if successful, will prevent further aggressive episodes. Counseling and reassurance of the patient and family to help them understand the unconscious nature of the behaviors can be helpful. Medicolegal implications of the violent behavior determine the third treatment approach. If violent behaviors are chronic and not under medical control, the law generally (and in all constituencies based on British common law) considers the patient to be a risk to society and himself and therefore requires institutionalization while such behaviors persist.

## SUMMARY

The primary behavioral parasomnia disorders have been considered in detail in this chapter. The main features of the nonepileptic parasomnias are summarized in Table 31-4. Sleep-related epileptic seizures, an important group of parasomnias, are considered in Chapter 34.

## REFERENCES

1. Diagnostic Classification Steering Committee. International Classification of Sleep Disorders: Diagnostic and Coding Manual. Rochester, MN: American Sleep Disorders Association, 1990.
2. Mitchell SW. Some disorders of sleep. Int J Med Sci 1890;100:109.
3. Roger H. Les Troubles du Sommeil—Hypersomnies, Insomnies, Parasomnies. Paris: Masson, 1932.
4. Gastaut H, Broughton R. Epileptic Seizures: Clinical and Electrographic Features, Diagnosis and Treatment. Springfield, IL: Thomas, 1972.
5. Oswald I. Sudden body jerks on falling asleep. Brain 1959;82:92.
6. Gastaut H, Broughton R. A clinical and polygraphic study of episodic phenomena during sleep. Rec Adv Biol Psychiatry 1965;7:197.
7. Broughton R. Pathological Fragmentary Myoclonus, Intensified Hypnic Jerks and Hypnagogic Foot Tremors:

Three Unusual Sleep-Related Movement Disorders. In WP Koella, F Obal, H Schulz (eds), Sleep '86. Stuttgart: Gustav Fischer, 1988;240.
8. Creutzfeldt O, Jung R. Neuronal Discharge in Cat's Motor Cortex During Sleep and Arousal. In GEW Wolstenholme, M O'Connor (eds), The Nature of Sleep. London: Churchill Livingstone, 1961;131.
9. De Lisi L. Su un di fenomeno motorio costanti del sonno normale: le mioclonie ipniche fisiologiche. Riv Pat Nerv Ment 1932;110:481.
10. Loeb C, Massazza G, Sacco G, et al. Etude polygraphique de myoclonies hypniques chez l'homme. Rev Neurol (Paris) 1964;110:258.
11. Gastaut H, Villeneuve A. The startle disease or hyperexplexia: pathological surprise reaction. J Neurol Sci 1967;5:523.
12. Gastaut H. Semeiologie des myoclonies et nosologie analytique des syndromes myocloniques. Rev Neurol (Paris) 1968;119:1.
13. Coleman RM, Pollak CP, Weitzman ED. Periodic movements in sleep (nocturnal myoclonus): relation to sleep disorders. Ann Neurol 1980;8:416.
14. Petre-Quadrans O, Sfello Z, Bogaert L, van Moya G. Sleep study in subacute sclerosing panencephalitis. Neurology 1968;18:60.
15. Ekbom KA. Restless legs. Acta Med Scand Suppl 1944;158:1.
16. Zappert J. Uber nachtliche Kopfbewegungen bei Kindern (jactatio capitis nocturna). Jahrbuch Kinderheilk 1905;62:70.
17. Cruchet R. Tics et sommeil. Presse Med 1905;13:33.
18. De Lissovoy V. Headbanging in early childhood. Child Dev 1962;13:43.
19. Klackenburg G. Rhythmic movements in infancy and early childhood. Acta Paediatr Scand Suppl 1971;224:74.
20. Thorpy MJ, Glovinsky P. Jactatio Capitis Nocturnea. In M Kryger, T Roth, WC Dement (eds), Principles and Practice of Sleep Medicine. Philadelphia: Saunders, 1989;648.
21. Sallustro F, Atwell CW. Body rocking, head banging and head rolling in normal children. J Pediatr 1978;93:704.
22. Freidin MR, Jakowski JJ, Singer WD. Nocturnal head banging as a sleep disorder: a case report. Am J Psychiatry 1979;136:1469.
23. Baldy-Moulinier M, Levy M, Passouant P. Etude de la jactatio capitis au cours de sommeil de nuit. Rev Neurol (Paris) 1969;120:460.
24. Walsh JK, Kramer M, Skinner JE. A case of jactatio capitis nocturna. Am J Psychiatry 1981;138:524.
25. Oswald I. Rocking at night. Electroencephalogr Clin Neurophysiol 1964;16:577.
26. Regenstein RR, Hartman E, Reich P. A head movement disorder occurring in REM sleep. J Nerv Ment Dis 1977;164:432.
27. Gagnon P, de Koninck J. Repetitive head movements during REM sleep. Biol Psychiatry 1985;20:176.

28. Decatanzaro DA, Baldwin G. Effective treatment of self-injurious behavior through a forced arm exercise. Am J Ment Defic 1978;82:422.

29. Weiher RG, Harman RE. The use of omission training to reduce self-injurious behavior in a retarded child. Behav Res Ther 1975;6:261.

30. Hishikawa Y, Nan'no H, Tachibana M, et al. The nature of the sleep attack and other symptoms of narcolepsy. Electroencephalogr Clin Neurophysiol 1968;24:1.

31. Roth B. Narcolepsy and Hypersomnia. Basel: Karger, 1980.

32. Broughton R. Human consciousness and sleep/waking rhythm: a review and some neuropsychological considerations. J Clin Neuropsychol 1982;4:193.

33. Yoss RE, Daly DD. Criteria for the diagnosis of the narcolepsy syndrome. Proc Mayo Clin 1957;32:320.

34. Broughton R. Narcolepsy. In MJ Thorpy (ed), Handbook of Sleep Disorders. New York: Dekker, 1990;197.

35. Pierce JMS. Exploding head syndrome. Lancet 1988;2:270.

36. Pierce JMS. Clinical features of the exploding head syndrome. J Neurol Neurosurg Psychiatry 1989; 52:902.

37. Sachs C, Svanborg E. The exploding head syndrome: polysomnographic recordings and therapeutic suggestions. Sleep 1991;14:263.

38. Marc C. De la Folie. Paris: Bailliere, 1840.

39. von Gudden H. Die physiologische und pathologische Schlaftrunkenheit. Arch Psychiatr Nervenkrank 1905; 40:989.

40. Bonkalo A. Impulsive acts and confusional states during incomplete arousal from sleep: criminological and forensic implications. Psychiatr Q 1974;48:400.

41. Broughton RJ, Shimizu T. Sleep-related violence: a medical and forensic challenge. Sleep 1995;18:727.

42. Ferber RF. Sleepwalking, confusional arousals, and sleep terrors in the child. In M Kryger, T Roth, WC Dement (eds), Principles and Practice of Sleep Medicine. Philadelphia: Saunders, 1989;640.

43. Broughton R. Disorders of sleep: disorders of arousal? Science 1968;59:1070.

44. Saier J, Regis H, Mano T, et al. Potentiels Evoquees Visuels Pendant les Differents Phases de Sommeil Chez L'Homme: Etudes de la Reponse Visuelle Evoquee Apres le Reveil. In H Gastaut, E Lugaresi, G Berti Ceroni, et al. (eds), The Abnormalities of Sleep in Man. Bologna: Aulo Gaggi, 1968;55.

44a. Jones E. On the Nightmare. London: Hogarth, 1949.

45. Cirignotta F, Zucconi M, Mondini S, et al. Enuresis, Sleepwalking and Nightmares: An Epidemiological Survey in the Republic of San Marino. In C Guilleminault, E Lugaresi (eds), Sleep-Wake Disorders: Natural History, Epidemiology and Long-Term Evolution. New York: Raven, 1983;237.

46. Hallstrom T. Night terror in adults through three generations. Acta Psychiatr Scand 1972;48:350.

47. Fisher C, Byrne J, Edwards A, et al. A psychophysiological study of nightmares. J Am Psychoanal Assoc 1970;18:747.

48. Fisher C, Kahn E, Edwards A, et al. A psychophysiological study of nightmares and sleep terrors. J Nerv Ment Dis 1973;157:75.

49. Broughton R. Phasic and Dynamic Aspects of Sleep: A Symposium Review and Synthesis. In MG Terzano, P Halasz, AC Declerck (eds), Phasic Events and the Dynamic Organization of Sleep. New York: Raven, 1991;185.

50. Fisher C, Kahn E, Edwards A, et al. A psychological study of nightmares and sleep terrors: the suppression of stage 4 sleep terrors with diazepam. Arch Gen Psychiatry 1973;28:252.

51. Broughton R. Pathophysiology of Enuresis Nocturne, Sleep Terrors and Sleepwalking: Current Status and the Marseille Contribution. In RJ Broughton (ed), Henri Gastaut and the Marseille School's Contribution to the Neurosciences. Amsterdam: Elsevier, 1982;401.

52. Pesikoff RB, Davis PC. Treatment of pavor nocturnus and somnambulism in children. Am J Psychiatry 1971;128:778.

53. Marshall JR. The treatment of night terrors associated with the post-traumatic syndrome. Am J Psychiatry 1975;132:293.

54. Kales JD, Cadieux RJ, Soldatos C, et al. Psychotherapy with night-terror patients. Am J Psychother 1982;36:399.

55. Schneck CH, Mahowald MW. A polysomnographically documented case of adult somnambulism with long-distance automobile driving and frequent nocturnal violence: parasomnia with continuing danger as a non-insane automatism. Sleep 1995;11:765.

56. Broughton R, Billings R, Cartwright R, et al. Homicidal somnambulism: a case report. Sleep 1994;17:235.

57. Abe K, Shimakawa M. Predisposition to sleepwalking. Psychiatr Neurol 1966;152:306.

58. Bakwin H. Sleepwalking in twins. Lancet 1970;2:466.

59. Kales A, Soldatos CR, Bixler EO, et al. Hereditary factors in sleepwalking and sleep terrors. Br J Psychiatry 1980;137:111.

60. Gastaut H, Batini C, Broughton R, et al. Etude electroencephyalographique des manifestations paroxystique au cours du sommeil nocturne. Rev Neurol (Paris) 1964;110:309.

61. Jacobson A, Kales A, Lehmann D, et al. Somnambulism: all night electroencephalography studies. Science 1965;148:975.

62. Kales A, Jacobson A, Paulson M, et al. Somnambulism: psychophysiological correlates: I. All-night EEG studies. Arch Gen Psychiatry 1966;14:585.

63. Jacobson A, Kales A. Somnambulism: all-night EEG and related studies. Res Publ Assoc Res Nerv Ment Dis 1967;45:424.

64. Halasz P, Ujszaszi J, Gadorvo P. Are microarousals preceded by electroencephalographic slow-wave synchro-

nization precursors of confusional awakenings? Sleep 1985;8:231.

65. Pedley TA, Guilleminault C. Episodic nocturnal wanderings responsive to anticonvulsant drug therapy. Ann Neurol 1977;2:30.

66. Guilleminault C. Sleepwalking and Night Terrors. In MH Kryger, T Roth, WC Dement (eds), Principles and Practice of Sleep Medicine. Philadelphia: Saunders, 1989;379.

67. Cooper AJ. Treatment of coexistent night terrors and somnambulism in adults with imipramine and diazepam. J Clin Psychiatry 1987;48:209.

68. de Villard R, Dalery J, Mouret J. Le somnabulisme de l'enfant: etude clinique, polygraphique et therapeutique: a propos de 37 observations. Lyon Med 1978;240:65.

69. Lugaresi E, Cirignotta F. Hypnogenic paroxysmal dystonia: epileptic seizure or a new syndrome? Sleep 1981;4:129.

70. Cromwell JA, Anders TF. Hypnogenic paroxysmal dystonia. J Am Acad Child Psychiatry 1985;24:353.

71. Lugaresi E, Cirignotta F. Two Variants of Nocturnal Paroxysmal Dystonia with Attacks of Short and Long Duration. In R Degen, E Neidermeyer (eds), Epilepsy, Sleep and Sleep Deprivation. Amsterdam: Elsevier, 1984;169.

72. Godbout R, Montplaisir J, Rouleau J. Hypnogenic paroxysmal dystonia: epilepsy or sleep disorder? Electroencephalogr Clin Neurophysiol 1985;16:136.

73. Lance JW. Sporadic and familial varieties of tonic seizures. J Neurol Neurosurg Psychiatr 1963;26:51.

74. Tassinari CA, Broughton RJ, Poire R, et al. Sur l'Evolution des Mouvements Anormaux au Cours du Sommeil. In H Fischgold (ed), Le Sommeil de Nuit Normal et Pathologique. Paris: Masson, 1965;314.

75. Hartmann E. The Nightmare: The Psychology and Biology of Terrifying Dreams. New York: Basic Books, 1984.

76. Hartmann E. A preliminary study of the personality of the nightmare sufferer: relationship to schizophrenia and creativity. Am J Psychiatry 1981;136:794.

77. Kales A, Soldatos CR, Caldwell AB, et al. Nightmares: clinical characteristics and personality patterns. Am J Psychiatry 1980;137:1197.

78. Lavie P, Hefez A, Halpern G, et al. Long-term effects of traumatic war related events on sleep. Am J Psychiatry 1979;136:1175.

79. Kramer M, Schoen LS, Kinney L. Nightmares in Vietnam veterans. J Am Acad Psychoanal 1987;15:67.

80. Hartmann E. Normal and Abnormal Dreams. In MH Kryger, T Roth, WC Dement (eds), Principles and Practice of Sleep Medicine. Philadelphia: Saunders, 1989;191.

81. Hishikawa Y, Sugita Y, Teshima Y, et al. Sleep Disorders in Alcoholic Patients with Delirium Tremens. Reevaluation of the REM Rebound and Intrusion Theory. In I Karacan (ed), Psychophysiological Aspects of Sleep. Park Ridge, NJ: Noyes Medical, 1981;109.

82. Schenck CH, Bundlie SR, Ettinger MC, et al. Chronic behavior disorders of human REM sleep: a new category of parasomnia. Sleep 1986;9:293.

83. Schenck CH, Bundlie SR, Patterson AL, et al. Rapid eye movement sleep behavior disorder: a treatable parasomnia affecting older patients. JAMA 1987;257:1786.

84. Mahowald MW, Schenck CH. REM Sleep Behavior Disorder. In MH Kryger, T Roth, WC Dement (eds), Principles and Practice of Sleep Medicine. Philadelphia: Saunders, 1989;389.

85. Jouvet M, Delorme JF. Locus coeruleus et sommeil paradoxal. C R Soc Biol (Paris) 1965;159:895.

86. Goode GB. Sleep paralysis. Arch Neurol 1962;6:228.

87. Hishikawa Y. Sleep Paralysis. In C Guilleminault, WC Dement, P Passouant (eds), Narcolepsy. New York: Spectrum, 1976;97.

88. Folkard S, Condon R, Herbert M. Night sleep paralysis. Experientia 1984;40:510.

89. Snyder S. Isolated sleep paralysis after rapid time zone changes (jet-lag syndrome). Chronobiologica 1983;10:377.

90. Everett HC. Sleep paralysis in medical students. J Nerv Ment Dis 1963;136:283.

91. Penn NE, Kripke DF, Scharff J. Sleep paralysis among medical students. J Psychol 1981;107:247.

92. Roth B, Buhova S, Berkova L. Familial sleep paralysis. Schweiz Arch Neurol Neurochir Psychiatr 1968;102:321.

93. Nan'no H, Hishikawa Y, Koida H, et al. A neurophysiological study of sleep paralysis in narcoleptic patients. Electroencephalogr Clin Neurophysiol 1970;28:382.

94. Ware JC. Monitoring Erections During Sleep. In MH Kryger, T Roth, WC Dement (eds), Principles and Practice of Sleep Medicine. Philadelphia: Saunders, 1989;689.

95. Fisher C, Kahn E, Edwards A, et al. Total suppression of REM sleep with the MAO inhibitor Nardil in a subject with painful nocturnal REM erection. Psychophysiology 1972;9:91.

96. Arkin AM. Sleep talking: a review. J Nerv Ment Dis 1966;143:101.

97. Aarons L. Evoked sleep talking. Percept Mot Skills 1970;31:27.

98. Arkin AM, Toth MF, Baker J, et al. The degree of concordance between the content of sleep talking and mentation recalled in wakefulness. J Nerv Ment Dis 1970;151:375.

99. Glaros AG, Rao SM. Bruxism: a critical review. Psychol Bull 1977;84:767.

100. Ahmed R. Bruxism in children. J Pedol 1986;10:105.

101. Funch DP, Gale EN. Factors associated with nocturnal bruxism and its treatment. J Behav Med 1980;3:385.

102. Glaros AG, Rao SM. Effects of bruxism: a review of the literature. J Prosthet Dent 1977;38:149.

103. Richmond G, Rugh JD, Dolfi R, et al. Survey of bruxism in an institutionalized mentally retarded population. Am J Ment Defic 1984;88:418.

104. Reding GR, Zepelin H, Robinson JE, et al. Nocturnal tooth-grinding: all-night psychophysiological studies. J Dent Res 1968;47:786.

105. Ware JC, Rugh J. Destructive bruxism: sleep stage relationship. Sleep 1988;11:172.

106. Hartmann E. Bruxism. In MH Kryger, T Roth, WC Dement (eds), Principles and Practice of Sleep Medicine. Philadelphia: Saunders, 1989;385.

107. Sussman N. Anxiety disorders. Psychiatric Ann 1988;18:134.

108. Grunhaus L, Rabin D, Harel Y, et al. Simultaneous panic and depressive disorders. Psychiatry Res 1986;17:251.

109. Uhde TW, Roy Byrne P, Gillin JC, et al. The sleep of patients with panic disorder: a preliminary report. Psychiatry Res 1985;12:251.

110. Hauri PJ, Friedman M, Ravaris CL. Sleep in patients with spontaneous panic attacks. Sleep 1989;12:323.

111. Ballenger JC. Pharmacology of panic attacks. J Clin Psychiatry 1986;47(suppl 6):27.

112. Agarwal A. Enuresis. Amer Acad Fam Phys 1982;25:203.

113. Scharf MB. Waking Up Dry: How to End Bedwetting Forever. Cincinatti: Writer's Digest Books, 1986.

114. Ferber R. Sleep-Associated Enuresis in the Child. In MH Kryger, T Roth, WC Dement (eds), Principles and Practice of Sleep Medicine. Philadelphia: Saunders, 1989;643.

115. Muellner SR. Development of urinary control in children: a new concept in cause, prevention and treatment in primary enuresis. J Urol 1960;84:714.

116. Di Perri R, Meduri MA. A Polygraphic Approach to the Study of Enuresis Nocturna. In P Levin, WP Koella (eds), Sleep 1974. Basel: Karger, 1975;413.

117. Bradley WE. Electroencephalography and bladder innervation. J Urol 1977;118:412.

118. Hallgren B. Enuresis—a clinical and genetic study. Acta Psychiatr Neurol Scand 1957;32(suppl 114):1159.

119. Bakwin H. The Genetics of Enuresis. In I Kolvin, RC MacKeith, SR Meadow (eds), Bladder Control and Enuresis. Clin Dev Med 1973;48/49:73.

120. Kales A, Kales JD, Jacobson A, et al. Effects of imipramine on enuresis frequency and sleep states. Pediatrics 1977;60:431.

121. Mikkelsen EJ, Rapaport JL, Nee L, et al. Childhood enuresis. I. Sleep patterns and psychopathology. Arch Gen Psychiatry 1980;27:1139.

122. Broughton R, Gastaut H. Further polygraphic studies of enuresis nocturna (intra-vesicular pressure). Electroencephalogr Clin Neurophysiol 1964;16:626.

123. Marshall S, Marshall HH, Lyon RP. Enuresis: an analysis of various therapeutic approaches. Pediatrics 1973;52:813.

124. Starfield B, Mellits ED. Increase in functional bladder capacity and improvement of enuresis. J Pediatr 1968;72:483.

125. Goel KM, Thomson RB, Gibb EM, et al. Evaluation of nine different types of enuresis alarms. Arch Dis Child 1984;59:748.

126. Kardash S, Hellman E, Werry J. Efficacy of imipramine in childhood enuresis: a double-blind control study with placebo. Can Med Assoc J 1968;99:236.

127. Layzer RB, Rowland LP. Leg cramps. N Engl J Med 1971;283:31.

128. Jacobsen JH, Rosenberg RS, Huttenlocher PR, Spire JP. Familial nocturnal cramping. Sleep 1986;9:54.

129. Saskin P, Whelton C, Moldofsky H, Akin F. Sleep and nocturnal leg cramps. Sleep 1988;11:307.

130. Weiner IH, Weiner HL. Nocturnal leg muscle cramps. JAMA 1980;244:2332.

131. Norris FH, Gasteiger EL, Chatfield PO. An electromyographic study of induced and spontaneous muscle cramps. Electroencephalogr Clin Neurophysiol 1957;9:139.

132. Broughton R, Shimizu T. Dangerous Behaviors by Night. In C Shapiro, A McCall (eds), Forensic Aspects of Sleep. London: Wiley, 1997;65.

# Chapter 32
# Sleep Disorders in the Elderly

## Sudhansu Chokroverty

To understand the sleep disorders of the elderly it is important to know what changes in sleep structure and sleep cycle are normal in disease-free aged individuals. It is also important to understand the neurology of aging and, in particular, changes in central nervous system (CNS) physiology and morphology in normal healthy older individuals.

In 1900, 4% of the American population was older than age 65; according to the best current estimate, that figure will be 13% in the year 2000, and 21% by 2050.[1] It is life expectancy that has been increasing rather than the human life span, which is determined biologically and genetically and remains fixed.[2] We do not know what determines aging and the changes associated with aging. See Behnke et al.[3] and Comfort[4] for a review of this topic. Older individuals are at risk for sleep disturbances owing to a variety of factors, including social and psychosocial problems; increasing prevalence of concurrent medical, psychiatric, and neurologic illnesses; increasing use of medications (often sedative-hypnotics) and alcohol; and alterations in circadian rhythms.

## NEUROLOGY OF AGING

### Clinical Aspects of Central Nervous System Changes

Before discussing the neurology of aging it is important to define what is meant by *aging*. No standard definition is available, but for this discussion I arbitrarily define age 65 as the start of old age. A normal elderly person is one who is free of obvious diseases of the central and peripheral neurologic system as well as general systemic diseases (e.g., cardiovascular, respiratory, renal, metabolic, hematologic, skeletal, and muscular diseases). Accepting this definition, a variety of changes in mental functions and the general nervous system of healthy elderly individuals have been noted. At the outset I must point out certain difficulties in studying the neurology of aging. It is difficult to get a large number of elderly subjects who meet the criteria by being free of neurologic and other systemic disorders. Even if a number of such subjects can be recruited, without many years' subsequent longitudinal study, it often remains problematic to decide whether certain abnormal findings are related to a subclinical affliction of the nervous system that is expressed in overt manifestations later in life.[5] A large number of elderly individuals have general medical and neurologic disorders, particularly dementia of the Alzheimer's type. In addition, there could be subclinical cerebral infarction, as noted in large series of autopsy examinations,[6] in which half the individuals with cerebral infarction remained asymptomatic. The following discussion of the neurologic changes of normal aging was written with these limitations in mind.

On mental function examination, the most striking changes in old age are in learning new information and in central processing of information.[5] In the

Wechsler Adult Intelligence Scale,[7] the performance scale declines much more rapidly than the verbal tests.[5,8] This has been confirmed in several cross-sectional and longitudinal studies comparing young and old individuals.[7–11] The past and the immediate memory remain relatively intact until approximately the middle 70s, but recent memory is impaired. There is often forgetfulness and difficulty remembering names and remembering several objects at one time, which suggests impairment of central processing time. Speed of learning is retarded, as is speed of processing new information.[5] The reaction time to simple and complex stimuli is often delayed, and there is impairment of motor speed.[12–16] The cognitive impairment of the normal elderly is often termed *benign forgetfulness of senescence*[17] or *age-associated memory impairment.*[18]

In a classic paper in 1931, Critchley[19] first directed attention to certain changes in the nervous system of normal healthy elderly individuals. Since then, several studies have appeared in the literature documenting the presence of abnormal neurologic signs in a small number of such people,[20,21] but these signs may represent asymptomatic subclinical disease[5] (e.g., cerebrovascular disease or cervical spondylosis), and without longitudinal studies it is impossible to exclude these definitely. Despite this limitation, there is a general consensus about the presence of certain findings in normal elderly individuals. There are changes in both the somatic and autonomic nervous system (ANS).[5,22,23] In the somatic system an important finding is impairment of gait and stance.[5,24,25] It is difficult to stand on one leg with eyes closed.[20,21,25] The so-called senile gait is characterized by stooped posture with flexed attitude, accompanied by short steps, reduced arm swings, shortening of the stride, and impaired speed and balance.[2,5,24] The gait resembles that of patients in the early stage of Parkinson's disease, which may be due to the loss of dopaminergic neurons and striatal dopamine receptors.[5,24] Grip strength declines with age.[21] The ankle reflex may be diminished, which may be related to the loss of the large-diameter nerve fibers.[5] In the sensory examination, the striking abnormality is impairment of the vibration sense in the lower extremities.[21] Rowe and Troen[26] suggested that old age represents a hyperadrenergic state. If this is the case, sympathetic overactivity may explain some of the changes noted in the cardiovascular reflex, galvanic skin response, erection,

maturation, and pupillary response of elders. Over-activity of the sympathetic nervous system may also interfere with cognitive function.

## Physiologic Changes in Old Age

### Electroencephalographic Changes

**Awake Electroencephalography.** The question remains whether electroencephalography (EEG) changes in old age are maturational changes or are related to pathologic alterations of the CNS. Many elderly individuals are afflicted with a variety of dementing illnesses, cerebrovascular disease, or systemic medical disorders that may cause metabolic encephalopathy.[27] Thus it is important to select healthy elderly individuals who are free from any of these diseases for EEG study. Such a selection was made in the study of healthy septuagenarians by Katz and Horowitz.[28] The subjects were screened by careful neurologic, psychiatric, and neuropsychological examination and found to represent normative EEG data. The EEG was normal, with an average alpha frequency of 9.8 Hz, and was therefore similar to that of young and middle-aged adults. This study can be contrasted with the report by Torres and colleagues,[29] in which they found that 52% of a group of normal volunteers with a mean age of 69 years had mild to moderate EEG abnormalities. Obrist[30] summarized the EEG changes in old age as follows: slowing of the alpha rhythm and an increase of fast activities, diffuse slow activity, and focal slow waves. In an important longitudinal study by Obrist and colleagues,[31] alpha frequency fell from 9.4 Hz at age 79 to 8 Hz intermixed with 6- to 7-Hz theta waves at age 89. Spectral analysis by Matejcek[32] and Nakano and coworkers[33] supported the progressive slowing of the alpha rhythm with aging. Duffy and associates[34] found no significant change in the frequency of the posterior EEG rhythm in a study of 63 men between 30 and 80 years of age. Oken and Kaye[35] analyzed conventional EEG and computerized EEG frequency in 22 extremely healthy subjects between 84 and 98 years old. The posterior peak frequency was higher than 8 Hz in those younger than 84, but between 7 and 8 Hz in five of 22 subjects older than 84 years. Alpha slowing appears to be related to the decline in mental function, which may be an early stage of progressive dementia of old age.[36] Alpha blocking and photic driving response to intermittent photic stimulation are also diminished in old age.[37] These findings may be related to the structural CNS alterations in elderly individuals (see Pathologic Central Nervous System Changes of Normal Aging).

An increase of fast activity was noted by Busse and Obrist[38] in elderly volunteer community subjects, especially women. In an EEG spectral analysis, Brenner et al.[39] also found more beta activity in elderly women than men. Kugler[40] also reported an increase of fast activity with increasing age. The significance of this is uncertain, but Kugler[40] stated that the presence of fast activity in old age correlates with preserved mental functioning.

Intermittent focal slow waves in the temporal regions (particularly in the middle and anterior temporal regions and greater on the left side) are noted in 17–59% of healthy elderly individuals.[29,30,35,41–43] This temporal slow activity may be accompanied by sharp transients, which may be related to cerebral vascular disease causing asymptomatic small infarction of the temporal lobe,[36] ventricular enlargement with cerebral atrophy,[44] or white matter hyperintensities on magnetic resonance imaging (MRI).[35] Klass and Brenner listed[45] some of the characteristics of what they called *benign temporal delta transients of the elderly* as follows: Slow waves occur in patients older than 60 years and are maximally noted in the left temporal, particularly anterior temporal, region; the voltage is usually less than 70 μv and these waves do not disrupt background activity; these delta transients are attenuated by mental alerting and eye opening and are increased by drowsiness and hyperventilation; the transients generally occur as single waves or in pairs but not in rhythmic trains; and the transient waves are present for up to 1% of recording time. The elderly may also have an increased amount of theta activity.[41,46]

Transient bursts of anteriorly dominant rhythmic delta waves are often noted in elderly subjects in the early stage of sleep. Gibbs and Gibbs[47] used the term *anterior bradyrhythmia* for this finding. Katz and Horowitz[48] obtained sleep-onset frontal intermittent rhythmic delta activity in normal elderly subjects, which should be differentiated from that associated with a variety of neurologic disorders. These are highly stimulus-sensitive and disappear in deeper stages of sleep. In demented elders, however, one can see diffuse slow waves in the delta and theta frequencies.

There is no clear relationship between intellectual deterioration and EEG slowing.[30,35] Whether the EEG changes are correlated with cerebral blood flow (CBF) study remains controversial. There is no correlation, however, between areas that show the maximum blood flow reduction and those that show prominent EEG slowing, or between the blood flow changes and the alpha frequency changes in normal elderly subjects.[49,50] The other suggestion is that the alpha slowing is related to the loss of choline acetyltransferase, the enzyme for synthesis of acetylcholine.[5]

### Sleep Electroencephalography Changes, Including Changes in Sleep Architecture and Organization.

In addition to awake EEG changes, there are changes during sleep in the elderly.[51,52] It is interesting to note that Liberson[53] in 1945 described paroxysmal bursts of sleeplike EEG lasting 1–10 seconds in the eyes-resting state in elderly subjects, and the incidence of these bursts increased with the age of the subject. Liberson[53] termed these episodes *microsleeps*. Normal elders show normal sleep patterns with certain modifications. The delta waves during slow-wave sleep (SWS) are reduced in amplitude and incidence.[22,54,55] The amplitude of delta waves decreases, and, in the usual Rechtschaffen and Kales[56] scoring technique, therefore, stages III and IV decrease. Feinberg and colleagues[57] discussed this point and suggested that quantification of the amount of time spent in a specified frequency, rather than using an amplitude criterion, be used for scoring SWS in elderly individuals. This reduction of amplitude of delta waves could be related to three factors: (1) reduction of neuronal synchronization in the neocortex, (2) alterations in the skull, and (3) changes in the subarachnoid spaces.[22,57]

Sleep spindles may show a variety of changes in old age,[58,59] including decreased frequency, amount, and amplitude. The frequency may decrease from 16 to 14 Hz, and then from 14 to 12 Hz. The spindles are often poorly formed and poorly developed. Sleep spindle changes thus resemble those noted with alpha frequency in old age.

The cyclic pattern from rapid eye movement (REM) to non-REM (NREM) remains unchanged, but the first cycle may be reduced.[22,60–62] REM density (i.e., number of eye movement bursts per minute of REM sleep) and total REM sleep time are reduced, but the percentage of REM in relation to total sleep time (TST) remains unaltered.[22,51,63] Sleep fragmentation is due to frequent interruptions at night. In addition, there are frequent sleep stage shifts, and, thus, frequent awakenings.[22,51] Regarding nocturnal TST (lights out to lights on), there is discrepancy between subjective report and objective data based on the technician's schedule.[22]

Nighttime sleep of elders usually is reported to be decreased (e.g., 5.5–6.5 hours, in contrast to the usual 7.5-hour TST average of young adults).[64,65] This may not be an accurate observation, because elders often take daytime naps; 24-hour TST of elders probably is no different from the 24-hour TST of young adults.

Increased fragmentation of sleep and increased numbers of transient arousals accompanied by increased daytime sleepiness have been described in the studies by Carskadon and coworkers.[66,67] Kales et al.[68] and Feinberg et al.[55] demonstrated the following changes in sleep with advancing age: state changes; frequent stage shifts; reduction of SWS (NREM stages III and IV) and the EEG amplitude of delta waves; increased stage I owing to frequent arousals; decreased total nocturnal sleep; and reduction of total REM sleep time but normal REM percentage in relation to the TST.

Williams and colleagues[69] recruited 120 healthy seniors through advertisements, without mentioning sleep. They tried to carefully screen out sleep disorders by excluding those who had sleep complaints. These authors found that the seniors' sleep quality was poorer than that of young individuals. In particular, there was a decrease of stage III and IV sleep and an increase in nighttime wakefulness.[69,70] Prinz and Vitiello[71] considered these findings as a benchmark level of sleep change associated with aging per se. In another study involving the Veterans Administration Survey, Cashman and colleagues[72] found that nighttime hypoxemia, which correlated with sleep apnea, was worse in several medical disorders (i.e., diabetes, cardiovascular disease, history of alcoholism, and vascular headaches). Thus, the data suggest that the disease states may interact with sleep disorders.

Between the ages of 60 and 90 years there are differences in the sleep architecture of men and women.[59] Between 60 and 70 years, men have more frequent arousals and more decrements in stage III and IV sleep. Between 60 and 80 years, women spend 9% of TST in the slow-wave stage, whereas men spend only 2%. The percentages of REM and total REM sleep are not different for men and women between 60 and 90 years.

In a longitudinal polysomnographic (PSG) and diary-based study, Hoch et al.[73] found deterioration of measures of sleep quality, continuity, and depth but not other sleep measures over a 3-year follow-up period in a group of 27 healthy "old old" subjects (75–87 years) as contrasted with a group of 23 "young old" subjects (61–74 years). The decline in sleep measures was manifested by impaired sleep efficiency, prolonged sleep latency, increased wakefulness after sleep onset, and decreased SWS percentage. These changes were accompanied by increased napping in the "old old" group.

**Changes in the Circadian Rhythm.** Circadian rhythm changes[52] in the elderly result from fundamental changes in social, including family, interaction. Interaction is governed by alterations of daily routine and activities, health needs, and psychosocial factors (e.g., loneliness, divorce).[22] There may also be intrinsic changes in the circadian rhythm related to the pathologic changes noted in apparently normal individuals. Animal studies lend support to this conclusion.[74–78] In long-term care facilities, circadian rhythm disturbances may be related to alterations of *Zeitgebers* (external time cues), such as bedtime, medication time, mealtime, and special institutional regulations on lights out and lights on.[17] Wessler and colleagues[79] made an intensive study of 69- to 94-year-old institutionalized patients under strict environmentally controlled conditions and found a remarkable regularity in circadian synchronization. In a study involving 69- to 86-year-old subjects, however, Scheving et al.[80] did not find support for the other group's conclusion. In all of these studies involving institutionalized patients, the effect of chronic illnesses must be considered in explanations of circadian rhythm disturbances. Thus, these changes may not be related to "normal" old age.

A study of evolution of sleep shows that the strong monophasic circadian rhythm of youth gives way to a polyphasic ultradian rhythm in old age. Frequent awakenings at night, with reduction of wakefulness, are accompanied by increased daytime naps. These physiologic changes may be related to the structural alterations noted in the suprachiasmatic nucleus (SCN) and brain stem hypnogenic neurons in experimental studies in several species of animals.[81–84]

There is also phase advance in the elderly—that is, there is a tendency to go to sleep early and awaken early. These changes may be related to age-related changes in the core body temperature rhythm.[85,86] In elderly individuals the amplitude of the temperature rhythm is attenuated and phase advanced.[86]

*Autonomic Nervous System Changes with Age*

A number of changes occur in the ANS in sleep, and there are striking changes in ANS functions in elders.[22,23] Five important aspects of ANS changes are sympathetic nerve activity, thermoregulation, cardiovascular changes, respiration, and nocturnal penile tumescence.

**Sympathetic Nerve Activity.**    The most consistent abnormalities in old age are increased muscle sympathetic nerve activity and elevated plasma concentration of the sympathetic neurotransmitter norepinephrine.[87,88]

**Thermoregulation.**    Thermoregulation is impaired in old age.[23] In response to passive heating, the sweating response of elders is impaired.[89,90] They are susceptible to hypothermia (both postoperative and in response to low ambient temperature in the environment)[91–93] and hyperthermia.[94,95] There is a paucity of studies that show ANS changes during sleep in elders.

**Cardiovascular Changes.**    Blood pressure and pulse rate fall at sleep onset, rise on awakening, and fluctuate during the night.[96] The increased incidence of stroke in elders during sleep may be related to these factors.[22] Orthostatic hypotension is common in elders and may be due to impaired baroreflex responsiveness and neuroeffector function.[23]

**Respiration.**    Age-related changes in the respiratory system and pulmonary function include[22,97–99] a reduction of vital capacity, chest wall compliance, diffusion capacity, elastic recoil, arterial oxygen tension, mismatch of the ventilation-perfusion ratio, decreased respiratory muscle strength, and respiratory center sensitivity. There is a higher

incidence of periodic breathing, including Cheyne-Stokes breathing and snoring in elders at night.[96,100–102] Patients with chronic obstructive pulmonary disease, who are often elderly, are at special risk for periodic breathing during sleep (both at night and during the day) because of increasing oxygen desaturation, hypercapnia, and apnea during sleep.[103,104]

**Nocturnal Penile Tumescence.**    Penile erection occurs during REM sleep. This REM-related penile tumescence shows a linear decrease from youth to old age (from 88% at 20–26 years old to 64–74% at 60–90 years old).[105,106]

*Endocrine Changes with Age*

**Plasma Cortisol.**    The circadian rhythm for plasma cortisol concentration is normal, and the plasma concentration of cortisol does not change in 60- to 95-year-old subjects.[107–109] In depressed patients (both young and old), however, the plasma cortisol level remains high during sleep and wakefulness, and the dexamethasone suppression test does not block secretion of cortisol.[110,111]

**Growth Hormone.**    Sleep-related growth hormone release is diminished in old age,[112–114] but the response of the growth hormone secretion to insulin hypoglycemia is normal.[115] Whether the decreased release of growth hormone is related to reduction of stage IV sleep in the elderly is not known.[22]

**Prolactin Secretion.**    Prolactin secretion in old age shows a normal pattern of episodic secretion with a sharp rise just after sleep onset and a sharp fall during morning awakening.[22,116,117] Although older subjects wake up several times during the night and have daytime naps, these episodes are not correlated with the prolactin secretion pattern.[22]

**Gonadotropins (Follicle-Stimulating Hormone and Luteinizing Hormone).**    No good studies correlate sleep changes in the elderly with gonadotropin secretion.[22]

**Plasma Insulin and Glucose.**    Insulin secretion shows a clear circadian variation in healthy young adults, but there is no adequate study of aged individuals.[22]

**Thyroid-Stimulating Hormone.**    Plasma thyroid-stimulating hormone (TSH) shows a circadian periodicity in adults: peak levels occur just before sleep onset at night.[118,119] In subjects older than 50 years, there are progressive changes in thyroid function causing a modest decrease in serum triiodothyronine concentration and minimal changes in TSH and thyroxine concentrations.[120]

**Melatonin Secretion.**    Serum melatonin concentration shows an age-related decrease in old age.[121] Impaired melatonin secretion has been reported to be associated with sleep complaints in the elderly.[122,123]

*Changes in the Cerebral Blood Flow
and Cerebral Metabolism*

Despite some inconsistent early findings,[5] there is a direct relationship between normal aging, CBF, and cerebral metabolism. Kety,[124] using his own nitrous oxide method, showed a direct relationship between a decrease in CBF and cerebral metabolism and advancing age in normal individuals. Others, however, contended that the changes were secondary to associated diseases.[125] Later, introduction of noninvasive and improved technique of xenon-133 inhalation method[126] related a clear-cut decline in the regional blood flow exclusively to advancing age, without the compounding factors of associated diseases.[127–129] This decline with advancing age was noted more in the gray than in the white matter CBF values.[125] Maximal declines were seen in the prefrontal and parietal regions and minimal declines in the frontal and frontotemporal regions.[5,125] This decline in old age seems to be related to a progressive decrease in the cerebral metabolic rate,[130,131] and possibly also to the morphologic changes in the neurons in the brains of elderly individuals.[125] It should be noted, however, that the decrease of CBF during SWS and the increase during REM sleep are similar in normal subjects of all ages.[125] In elderly sleep apnea patients, however, this decrease during SWS becomes excessive, placing elderly individuals at increasing risk for sudden death and development of stroke during sleep when combined with hypoxemia related to apnea.[125]

*Pathologic Central Nervous System Changes
of Normal Aging*

Aging represents biologic maturation, which may be accompanied by a variety of pathologic changes in the CNS. The neuropathologic changes of old age can be summarized as follows[5,132]: shrinkage of the brain; alterations in the outline and loss of neurons in various locations; lipofuscin accumulation; collection of corpora amylacea; intraparenchymal vascular changes; loss of dendritic arbor and dendritic spines; and presence of senile plaques and amyloid deposits, neurofibrillary tangles and granulovacuolar degeneration, and Hirano bodies. The presence of senile plaques and amyloid deposits, neurofibrillary tangles and granulovacuolar degeneration, and Hirano bodies is correlated with dementia, but the other neuropathologic changes are considered nonspecific changes of aging.

From the standpoint of sleep disorders medicine, the cell loss in the locus coeruleus, pontine and midbrain reticular formation, selective hypothalamic regions, and the suprachiasmatic neurons, as well as accumulation of neurofibrillary tangles and abnormal pigment in the hypothalamus are important morphologic correlates for widespread sleep disturbances in the elderly. Animal experiments on suprachiasmatic nuclei show the relationship between destruction of these nuclei and alteration of circadian rhythmicity of adrenal cortical secretion, body temperature, activity-rest cycle, and sleep cycle loss.[22]

## SLEEP COMPLAINTS IN OLD AGE

In an epidemiologic study, Ford and Kamerow[133] interviewed 7,954 subjects and observed that 40% of patients with insomnia and 46.5% of those with hypersomnia had a psychiatric disorder, compared with 16% of those with no sleep complaints. Complaints of persistent insomnia are important late in life. There is a high incidence of depression with insomnia in the elderly. Among the 1,801 elderly respondents aged 65 and older, the prevalence of insomnia was 12% and the incidence of insomnia was 7.3%.[133] For hypersomnia, the figures for prevalence and incidence were 1.6% and 1.8%, respectively. There was a strong association between persistent insomnia (longer than 1 month) and the risk of major depression. Clayton and coworkers[134] noted that in late-life spousal bereavement there is also a persistent and debilitating complaint of insomnia.

Brabbins et al.[135] noted an overall prevalence of 35% for insomnia complaints (more in women) after an interview of 1,070 noninstitutionalized elderly individuals. In contrast, Henderson et al.[136] found a prevalence of approximately 12% in the institutionalized and approximately 16% amongst the community elderly at 70 years or older after interviewing 59 institutionalized and 874 community residents. Insomnia complaints are more prevalent amongst women; whites; and those with depression, pain, and poor health. In another study from Germany, Hohagen et al.[137] investigated the prevalence of insomnia in 330 patients older than 65 years attending the offices of five general practitioners. Using the *Diagnostic and Statistical Manual of Mental Disorders* (3rd revision) diagnostic criteria, they found severe insomnia in 23%, moderate insomnia in 17%, and mild insomnia in another 17% of the patients. There was a significant association between insomnia, depression, and dementia.

Foley et al.[138] conducted an important epidemiologic study limited to interviews in more than 9,000 elderly subjects aged 65 years and older from three communities in the United States in the National Institute on Aging's multicentered study entitled "Established Populations for Epidemiologic Studies of the Elderly." These authors observed at least one of the following complaints in over half the subjects: trouble falling asleep, multiple awakenings, early morning awakening, daytime naps, and tiredness. These complaints are more common in women than in men and are often associated with respiratory symptoms, depression, nonprescription and prescription medications, poor self-esteem, and physical disabilities. The authors observed 33% of men and 19% of women with snoring and 13% of men and 4% of women with observed apneas. In this cross-sectional study, the authors did not find a clear relationship of loud snoring, observed apneas, or daytime sleepiness to hypertension or cardiovascular disease in the elders.

Excessive daytime somnolence (EDS) is often associated with fragmentation of nocturnal sleep, which may have been due to sleep-disordered breathing and periodic leg movements in sleep (PLMS).[139] Other factors are changes in the circadian rhythms of temperature, alertness and sleepiness, and social time cues.

Vitiello and Prinz[140] found that CNS degenerative disorders (e.g., dementia of the Alzheimer's type) may cause polyphasic sleep-wake patterns, which constitute a significant problem among old nursing home residents. In demented elderly subjects, nocturnal agitation, night wandering, shouting, and incontinence contribute to a variety of sleep disturbances.[133] There are many factors in the pathogenesis of nocturnal agitation, including loss of social *Zeitgebers* and circadian timekeeping, sleep apnea, REM-related parasomnias, low ambient light, and cold sensitivity.[141]

An important behavioral disturbance during sleep late in life is snoring. According to Koskenvuo and associates,[142,143] habitual snoring was found in 9% of men and 3.6% of women aged 40–69 years in their study done in Finland. Hypertension, ischemic heart disease, and stroke are risk factors for snoring. In an epidemiologic survey, Lugaresi and colleagues[144] found that approximately 60% of men and 40% of women between the ages of 41 and 64 years were habitual snorers. Enright et al.[145] recruited 5,201 adults aged 65 and older who were participants in a cardiovascular health study that enrolled a random sample of Medicare subjects in four U.S. communities. The purpose of the study was to ascertain the prevalence of snoring, observed apneas, and daytime sleepiness in older men and women and to study the relationship of these sleep disturbances to cardiovascular disease.

Many other factors can disrupt sleep: nocturia, leg cramps, pain, coughing or difficulty breathing, temperature sensitivity, and dreams.[139]

What is the relationship between sleep duration and mortality in elders? In 1989, Ancoli-Israel[146] re-examined the 1979 data of Kripke and coworkers[147] and concluded that 86% of deaths associated with short (less than 7 hours) or long (more than 8 hours) sleep occurred among those older than 60 years. Thus, it could be concluded by extrapolation from these data that older individuals who sleep less than 5 hours or more than 9 hours may be at greater risk for death.[139]

The high frequency of sleep complaints in aged individuals may be related to the physiologic sleep changes of normal aging as well as to concomitant medical, psychiatric, neurologic, and other disorders that are prevalent in this group.[52] Subjective sleep complaints are common in older subjects, as many reports attest.[147–151] The subjective complaints were corroborated by objective laboratory data. In contrast to the increasing incidence of subjective complaints from women, however, elderly men had more sleep disturbances than elderly women by objective reports.[152]

## CLINICAL ASSESSMENT OF SLEEP DISORDERS

Clinical assessment consists of a sleep, medical, drug, and psychiatric history. A general approach for making a clinical assessment is described in Chapter 18; only the points relevant to elders are emphasized in this section.

### Sleep History

Kales and coworkers[153] developed excellent guidelines for taking an adequate sleep history, summarized as follows:

1. The specific sleep problem should first be defined from the history. It is important with elders to understand the significance of daytime fatigue, which may result either from insomnia at night or from EDS. The latter condition can be an indirect effect of repeated arousals at night owing to sleep-related respiratory disorders, with or without PLMS. The other important factor to note is that the sleep of elders becomes polyphasic, associated with frequent daytime naps and less sleep at night. Therefore, every daytime nap is not necessarily indicative of EDS.

2. The onset and the clinical course of the condition should be assessed from the history. The course of the illness in some sleep disorders (e.g., night terrors, nightmares, and sleepwalking) is different.[154] Nightmares have a chronic course, whereas night terrors may be of recent onset. It should be noted that the relatively sudden onset of sleepwalking or night terrors in an elderly person is indicative of an organic CNS disorder, and appropriate investigation should be directed toward that diagnosis.[154]

3. Inquiries should be made into a family history of a sleep disorder. Certain sleep disorders (e.g.,

narcolepsy, hypersomnia, sleep apnea, sleepwalking, night terrors, and restless legs syndrome) may have a family history.[153–156]

4. Various sleep disorders should be distinguished from one another, and any previous diagnosis should be reassessed.

5. It is important to obtain a complete 24-hour sleep-wakefulness pattern. This is important in elderly individuals, because in old age the sleep cycle becomes polycyclic, rather than monophasic as in young adults. In elders, because of the tendency to take frequent naps, the sleep-wake schedule becomes irregular and may cause circadian rhythm disorders.

6. It might be important to keep a sleep diary or sleep log, and it is very important to question the bed partner or other caregivers about sleep disturbances of elders. Keeping a sleep diary may help assess the 24-hour sleep-wake cycle pattern.

7. The bed partner or caregiver should be questioned carefully, as they may have clues to the diagnosis of sleep apnea syndrome (SAS). For example, excessively loud snoring, temporary cessation of breathing, or restless movements in the bed are important pointers to the diagnosis of SAS[155] or PLMS.

8. It is essential to evaluate the impact of the sleep disorder and to determine the presence of other sleep disorders. The history may suggest a diagnosis of sleepwalking, night terror, or REM behavior disorder. A careful sleep history may also suggest nocturnal epilepsy, which is sometimes mistaken for a sleep disorder.

### Medical History

It is vital that a complete medical history be obtained from the patient.[157] Elderly individuals often have a variety of medical disorders, including congestive cardiac failure, hypertension, ischemic heart disease, chronic bronchopulmonary disorders, gastrointestinal disorders, arthritis and musculoskeletal pain syndromes, cancer, chronic renal disorders, endocrinopathies, and a variety of neurologic disorders. All of these conditions may disrupt sleep by virtue of the uncomfortable symptoms or because of the medications prescribed for them. Therefore, patients often complain of insomnia, but sometimes also of hypersomnia.

### Drug History

It is important to obtain drug history[153] because many medications can cause insomnia, including[157] CNS stimulants; bronchodilators; β-blockers; antihypertensives; benzodiazepines, particularly the short-acting ones; steroids; and theophylline. Withdrawal from short- and intermediate-acting benzodiazepines and nonbenzodiazepine hypnotics causes rebound insomnia. Many CNS depressants, such as hypnotics, sedatives, and antidepressants, may cause EDS. Finally, drinking coffee or cola at night may cause difficulty initiating sleep. Alcohol consumption may cause difficulty maintaining sleep.

### Psychiatric History

Psychophysiologic and psychiatric problems are the most common causes of insomnia in elders.[157] Elderly insomniacs can have a variety of psychological and psychiatric problems, such as anxiety, depression, organic psychosis, and obsessive compulsive neurosis. A patient with depression complains of early morning awakenings, whereas a patient with obsessive compulsive neurosis has difficulty initiating sleep. Some drugs (e.g., thioridazine) may increase nightmares.[154] Marital and sexual problems may give rise to interpersonal problems that cause sleep disturbances, particularly insomnia.[157]

### SLEEP DISORDERS IN OLD AGE

It is well-known that the prevalence and intensity of sleep disturbances increase with age.[157–159] Factors that affect the prevalence of sleep disturbances in the elderly are (1) physiologic (e.g., age-related changes in sleep patterns), (2) medical, (3) psychiatric, (4) pharmacologic (e.g., use, misuse, and abuse of drugs), and (5) social (changing rest-activity schedules, and, therefore, sleep-wake patterns).[157–161]

The prevalence of sleep-related breathing disorders, PLMS, and snoring are all greater among elders. The prevalence of sleep apnea increases with age and is greater in men than in women, and in menopausal women than in premenopausal women.[146] There is controversy over the exact prevalence of sleep apnea in the older population. In a study in 1971, Webb and Swinburne[162] noted that 75% of healthy volunteer men had periodic apneas. The prevalence rates for sleep apnea defined as *repetitive episodes of upper airway obstruction* in elders in various studies have been estimated to range from 5.6% to 70%.[163–171] The prevalence is greater in the elderly than in younger adults,[172,173] and in men than in women.[174] There is a lack of consistency in study methods, so it is very difficult to generalize from these studies.[174] It should be noted, however, that the prevalence of SAS in the population aged 30–60 years has currently been estimated to be 2% in women and 4% in men.[175] Because of the high prevalence of SAS in elders, questions have been raised as to the significance of sleep-disordered breathing in the elderly. Prinz et al.[176] stated that because apneic episodes in the elderly may not have the same clinical symptoms as noted in younger people, it is more difficult to determine if further investigations are needed. Fleury[177] suggested that SAS in the elderly not be considered different from SAS in middle aged men, however, assuming that appropriate diagnostic apnea index (AI) or respiratory disturbance index (RDI) was taken into consideration. Ancoli-Israel and Coy[170] agreed that if SAS is severe enough to cause symptoms in the elderly, treatment should be similar to that in a younger patient.

Reasons for the variation in the prevalence of sleep apnea could be sampling of different populations without using a random sampling method, small sample size, or use of different criteria to define sleep apnea.[174] An important problem has been the definition of AI or RDI.[174] RDI is equivalent to apnea-hypopnea index. *Hypopnea* is defined as a 50% decrease in thoracoabdominal effort for at least 10 seconds.[178] Another problem has been the clinical significance of an AI or RDI of 5. According to Ancoli-Israel,[174] an AI of 5 or more may be epidemiologically important but may not be equivalent to the diagnosis of SAS. Some authors have suggested that an AI of 20 or more is related to increased risk of death.[179] In a survey by Ancoli-Israel and coworkers[163] among 427 randomly selected community-dwelling people aged 65 years and older in San Diego, California, the prevalence rate of sleep-disordered breathing was 24% for an AI higher than 5 and 62% for an RDI higher than 10. The prevalence rate was 10% for an AI higher than 10, 4% for an AI higher than 20, and 1% for an AI higher than 40.[163] Another problem has been night-to-night variation of sleep apnea.[163,180–183]

The question of the relationship between sleep apnea or sleep-disordered breathing and increased morbidity or mortality remains controversial. Several studies have found a positive relationship.[179,184,185] In a nearly 10–year follow-up of a randomly selected, population-based probability sample of 426 men and women (65–95 years old), however, Ancoli-Israel et al.[186] found that those with severe sleep-disordered breathing (RDI of 30 or more) had a significantly shorter survival but that the RDI was not an independent predictor of death. Similar results were reported from a sleep disorders clinic patient population study by Lavie et al.[187] Ancoli-Israel et al.[186] stated that other confounding variables such as age, hypertension, and cardiovascular or pulmonary disease might be responsible for the increased morbidity and mortality. Chronologic or biological age (determined by biological markers of physiologic aging) may be the single most important factor for increased morbidity and mortality in sleep-disordered breathing (i.e., sleep apnea may be an age-dependent condition). To address this controversy, well-designed controlled clinical studies are needed.

### Diagnosis of Sleep Disorders in Old Age

Recognition of a variety of sleep disorders in elders is important for treatment of sleep disturbances and the associated medical or psychiatric conditions. Some examples of sleep disorders that have been recognized in the aged population[152,176,188] are insomnia, sleep-related respiratory dysfunction with periods of apneas and hypopneas, PLMS, sleep disturbances secondary to a variety of medical or psychiatric illnesses (particularly depression in the elderly), sleep disturbances associated with dementia (particularly of the Alzheimer's type), sleep disturbances related to the abuse of alcohol and sedative-hypnotic drugs, narcolepsy, restless legs syndrome, parasomnias, and circadian rhythm sleep disorders.

Insomnia and EDS are the two most common symptoms noted in normal aged individuals.[176] There is a high incidence of insomnia in the elderly, particularly elderly women[139,157] (see Chapter 24 for further details about insomnia).

### Sleep Apnea Syndrome

For the diagnosis of SAS, questioning the bed partner is very important. A history of loud snoring with periods of cessation of breathing at night accompanied by EDS and daytime fatigue suggests SAS.[189] The diagnosis is strongly suspected if the patient is also obese and hypertensive. For a definitive diagnosis, and to quantify the severity, an all-night PSG study is essential. The usual type is upper airway obstructive sleep apnea, but often it is mixed with central apnea, giving rise to mixed apnea (see Chapter 22). It is important to diagnose the condition because of possible adverse consequences,[189] such as congestive cardiac failure, cardiac arrhythmias, hypertension, neuropsychological impairment,[170,190] increased risk of traffic accidents,[191,192] and increased mortality related to cardiovascular events.[193] Lugaresi and colleagues[144] reported a high prevalence of snoring in elderly individuals, and this can be the forerunner of full-blown SAS.

### Periodic Limb Movements in Sleep

PLMS is reported more often in older normal subjects than in younger ones.[166,194–196] According to Coleman and associates,[196] the occurrence of PLMS may be related to disturbance of circadian sleep-wake rhythm in the elderly. In the study by Kripke and coworkers,[195] 20–30% of subjects 65 years and older had PLMS, whereas Ancoli-Israel and colleagues[194] reported an incidence of 37% of PLMS in 24 older subjects. PLMS is often associated with SAS.

### Sleep Disturbances Secondary to Medical Illness

A variety of medical disorders may be associated with insomnia—congestive cardiac failure; ischemic heart disease; arthritis and musculoskeletal pain syndrome; chronic respiratory disorder associated with bronchospasm; and dyspnea, which is often worse at night (see Chapter 24). Diabetics with autonomic neuropathy may have SAS.[197] For medical disorders that cause sleep-disordered breathing, EDS, and other sleep disturbances, see Chapter 29. Treatment should be directed at the primary condition to alleviate secondary sleep disturbances.

### Sleep Disturbances Secondary to Psychiatric Illness

An important psychiatric illness that causes sleep disturbances in the elderly is depression,[136,139,188,198–202] which should be carefully evaluated through a thorough psychiatric history. The condition is treatable, and misdiagnosis and prescription of hypnotics for insomnia would lead to a vicious cycle of worsening sleep complaints. An important sleep complaint in these patients is early morning awakening, resembling advanced sleep phase syndrome.[198–200] Anxiety disorders also cause sleep disturbances,[202] and various psychotic disorders may cause both hypersomnolence and insomnia[202] (see Chapter 28).

### Sleep Disturbances Secondary to Organic Brain Syndrome

Alzheimer's disease and related dementias in the elderly may cause sleep disturbances, including nocturnal confusional episodes (sun-downing syndrome), which may require antipsychotic medication (see Chapter 27).

### Sleep Disturbances Associated with Drugs and Alcohol

A careful drug and alcohol history is important, as elderly individuals often take a variety of medications, including sedative-hypnotics for associated medical conditions, and over-the-counter drugs to promote sleep.[136,152,157,188] Sleeping medications produce secondary drug-related insomnia. Alcohol worsens sleep disturbances and may exacerbate existing SAS.

### Narcolepsy

Narcolepsy is a disease of earlier onset than old age, and the diagnosis will probably have been made much earlier, but it is a lifelong condition. The diagnosis rests on a history of sudden sleep attacks lasting a short time and associated with auxiliary symptoms such as cataplexy, hypnagogic hallucinations, and sleep paralysis. A history of narcoleptic sleep attacks and cataplexy may be sufficient for diagnosis, but an all-night PSG study, followed by the Multiple Sleep Latency Test (MSLT), which will show reduced sleep-onset latency and sleep-onset REM in two out of five recordings, is needed for confirmation.

### Restless Legs Syndrome

Restless legs syndrome (see Chapter 26) is primarily a lifelong condition, although it may be secondary to diabetic or uremic peripheral neuropathy. In addition to the characteristic restless movements during the daytime, nighttime sleep is severely disturbed. The prevalence increases with age, and the symptoms may occur initially in old age.

### Parasomnias

The important parasomnias in the elderly are REM sleep behavior disorder, sleepwalking, and night terrors. The latter two conditions usually present in childhood or adolescence, but if they have a relatively sudden onset in an elderly person an acute neurologic condition should be suspected and excluded by appropriate laboratory investigations.[203,204] REM sleep behavior disorder can be suspected from the history given by the bed partner and by simultaneous video polygraphic evaluation at night. See Chapter 31 for a general discussion of parasomnias.

### Disorders of Circadian Function

Morgan and associates[205] reported that occasional sleep complaints are noted by 40% of older individuals, and according to Garma and colleagues,[206] older individuals complain of frequent and prolonged awakenings during the night. It has been speculated by Czeisler and coworkers[207] that these disorders may be due to changes in the human circadian pacemaker with advancing age. Work with light by Czeisler and colleagues[208,209] showed that, with appropriately timed exposure to bright light, one can change the temperature cycle—that is, circadian phase—and may be able to correct the circadian sleep disorder. Further research is needed in this area.

In 1962, McGhie and Russell[149] reported that 15% of older individuals complained of early morning awakenings, and in 1988 Mant and Eyland[210] reported that 33% of elderly individuals woke up early in the morning several times a week. Sleep parameters thus show an advanced phase, which is also noted with other circadian rhythms such as activity rhythm, body temperature rhythm, and timing of REM sleep and the cortisol rhythm.[207] An advance in the circadian phase due to a reduction of the endogenous period of the circadian pacemaker with advancing age is suggested by animal experiments.[211,212] Human data for such studies are lacking, but a cross-sectional study by Weitzman's group[213] documented that the free-running period of the temperature rhythm was significantly shorter in six subjects aged 53–60 years than in six healthy young adults. Study by Czeisler and colleagues[208] suggested a strong relationship between period reduction and phase advance in the circadian rhythms of older people.

The pathophysiologic mechanism of these changes remains speculative. In 1972,[214,215] a cluster of neurons was discovered in the anterior tip of the hypothalamus on either side of the third ventricle, the SCN. This is the circadian pacemaker. With advancing age, the volume of SCN cells shrinks—that is, the number of neurons decreases,[216–218] which may result in functional impairment.

## LABORATORY ASSESSMENT

The diagnostic evaluation should begin with a thorough history of sleep disturbances, which may be EDS, difficulty initiating or maintaining sleep, and intrusions of unusual behavior during sleep. Physical examination may direct attention to systemic disease. Based on the history and findings of the physical examination, a decision should be made regarding referrals to specialized sleep centers for PSG and MSLT studies. Tests should be performed when clinical interview and examination cannot resolve the problems.

Most of the sleep disturbances of elders can be diagnosed by a careful history and physical examination. For some conditions, however, laboratory assessment is important. In SAS it is important to have an all-night PSG study to quantify and determine the severity of sleep-related respiratory disturbances. Sleep apnea is a treatable condition, so it is important to make this diagnosis correctly. In addition, MSLT and PSG studies are important for narcolepsy diagnosis, although in elderly people this diagnosis may have been made many years earlier. All-night video recordings are necessary to diagnose some conditions, such as REM behavior disorder, that require the examiner to differentiate from among a number of sleep disorders with similar symptoms. Appropriate tests should be performed if other medical or neurologic disorders are suspected.

## TREATMENT

The objective of treatment is to reduce the risk of mortality and morbidity and improve quality of life.[219] The first step is accurate assessment and diagnosis.

### Indications for Treatment of Obstructive Sleep Apnea

Indications for treatment of obstructive sleep apnea are reviewed briefly in this section. The reader is referred to Chapters 22 and 23 for details. Obstructive sleep apnea is a major cause of hypersomnia in elders, and it is often a reversible condition if appropriately diagnosed and treated. For moderate to severe obstructive sleep apnea, treatment is recommended. PSG and MSLT studies should be able to decide the severity of the apnea when findings are considered with the RDI, the degree of oxygen saturation, and abnormally short sleep latency. Before instituting any specific treatment, certain general measures, including weight loss; avoidance of alcohol, sedatives and hypnotics; avoidance of the supine sleep position; and management of nasopharyngeal disorders are recommended. The majority of patients respond to continuous positive airway pressure (CPAP) treatment. If all measures including CPAP fail, surgical procedures such as uvulopalatopharyngoplasty (UPP) may be appropriate, particularly if the site of obstruction is in the pharyngeal region. The success rate of UPP is variable. Tracheostomy, which is modified to keep the trachea closed during the day and open at night, has been an option in most severe cases. The primary criteria for recommending tracheostomy[220] include severe daytime symptoms that interfere with function, severe hypertension or dangerous cardiac arrhythmias, and an AI of 20 or greater or a decrease in oxygen saturation of more than 10% below average baseline values. Tracheostomy is now rarely used and only reserved for morbidly ill patients who cannot tolerate CPAP. In selected patients with a moderate degree of sleep apnea, oral appliances[221] have been tried with moderate success.

### Indications for Treatment of Insomnia

Multiple factors are responsible for insomnia in elders, and, therefore, evaluation and treatment of insomnia should be multidisciplinary.[154,157] Elimination or avoidance of factors that are causing insomnia is the first step in treatment. The next important general measure is paying attention to sleep hygiene. See Chapter 24 for more information on the treatment of insomnia.

Insomnia is a very common complaint in the elderly and may be the result of a variety of medical or psychiatric conditions. Insomnia may also result from PLMS, or occasionally from sleep apnea. An important cause is pharmacologic agents (i.e., drugs and alcohol), so a careful history and physical examination are important before any treatment is instituted.

PLMS is an important condition in elders, but its incidence and natural history are unknown. Even the relationship between PLMS and insomnia is not clear. Therefore, any pharmacologic treatment for PLMS is subject to controversy, and the long-term effect of drug treatment on patients is unknown. For selected cases in which PLMS clearly disrupts sleep, therapy may be indicated (see Chapter 26).

Circadian rhythm disorder, another important cause of insomnia, results from changes in the daily routine or sleep pattern, shift work, or transmeridian travel. Therefore, environmental control and adequate counseling should be the first line of treatment.

When a medical or psychiatric disorder causes insomnia, appropriate treatment should be directed toward the primary condition. In the case of depression, appropriate treatment with tricyclic antidepressants, often those with sedative effect (e.g., amitriptyline, doxepin, trazodone), could be used to advantage.

Medical conditions such as cardiac failure, hyperthyroidism, respiratory disorders, arthritis and other painful conditions, and esophageal reflux syndrome should be treated appropriately. It should be remembered, however, that medications (e.g., theophylline, steroids) themselves may cause sleep disturbance.

For transient or temporary disturbances of sleep, short-term intermittent use of hypnotics and sedative tricyclics may be useful. Long-term use of hypnotics is not recommended. The drug of choice for insomnia in the elderly is a benzodiazepine (see Chapter 24).

An intermediate-acting benzodiazepine (e.g., flurazepam, temazepam) in a dose of 15 mg at bedtime is as effective as a short-term treatment that produces minimal daytime sedation.[222,223] A short-acting benzodiazepine (e.g., triazolam) is used with success for short-term treatment.[222,223] Limiting side effects include behavior disturbances (e.g., confusion, delirium, amnesia), rebound insomnia, and rebound anxiety. These side effects have triggered controversy that necessitated suspension of the drug in the United Kingdom and restriction of its use by the U.S. Food and Drug Administration. The nonbenzodiazepine hypnotic zolpidem, an imidazopyridine,[223,224] in a dose of 5–10 mg at bedtime has been found to be as efficacious as benzodiazepine but with fewer side effects. Reynolds et al.[225] reviewed 1,082 patients in 23 randomized, double-blind trials in elderly patients with chronic insomnia and found scientific support for the short-term (after 3 weeks) efficacy of zolpidem and triazolam in the elderly, as well as temazepam, flurazepam, and quazepam.

Melatonin, an indoleamine secreted by the pineal gland at night, has received considerable attention as a hypnotic based mostly on anecdotal rather than scientific evidence. Garfinkel et al.[226] found melatonin to be superior to placebo in improving sleep efficiency in the elderly in a double-blind, placebo-controlled study. This finding needs to be confirmed, however, before accepting melatonin as a hypnotic in the elderly. In a subgroup of elderly insomniacs with a melatonin deficiency, Haimov et al.[227] found melatonin replacement therapy to be beneficial in the initiation and maintenance of sleep in these patients.

### Special Pharmacologic Considerations

Vestal and Dawson[228] directed attention to the important factors of alterations of drug metabolism, with its attendant changes in pharmacokinetics in the elderly. It is important to start with a dose smaller than younger subjects require and then gradually to increase the dose, depending on the response. It is also extremely important to obtain a drug history, to prevent drug-drug interactions and exacerbation of sleep disturbances by hypnotics or other agents.

### Situational and Lifestyle Considerations

Lifestyle factors are different for elders.[188] Retirement, with disturbance of the sleep-wake schedule (e.g., napping in the daytime and consequent inability to sleep at the scheduled night time); so-called "empty nest syndrome" that develops when children leave home; and bereavement over the death of a spouse or close friend may lead to loneliness and depression with attendant sleep disturbances. Other causes of sleep disturbances in the elderly include institutionalization, prolonged bed rest, poor sleep hygiene, unsatisfactory bed environment, poor diet habits, and caffeine and alcohol consumption.

### Treatment of Sleep Cycle Changes Related to Age

Treatment of sleep cycle changes related to age consists of educating the patient about sleep disruptions in old age, discouraging multiple naps, and urging participation in special interests and other activities and hobbies.[203]

Future research may determine the role of appropriately timed exposure to bright light in treating sleep maintenance insomnia and other circadian rhythm sleep disorders in elders.[208,209,229–231]

### Treatment of Situational Stress

Patients should be given supportive psychotherapy and behavior modification treatment, as well as clear explanations, to reduce stress and sleeplessness.[203]

### Treatment of Nocturnal Confusional Episodes

Nocturnal confusional episodes are characterized by disorientation, agitation, and wandering at night, and often result from acute or chronic organic neurologic dysfunction (see Chapter 27).[203,232] Relatively sudden onset of night terror or sleepwalking indicates an organic brain disorder, and an appropriate investigation should be made. Nocturnal confusional episodes can be precipitated by other associated medical illnesses. The treatment should be directed toward the precipitating or causal factors for these confusional episodes. Often episodes are precipitated when the patient is transferred from home to an institution. As much as possible, the home environment of such patients should be preserved. The darkness of night often precipitates episodes, so a night light is helpful. A careful drug history should be obtained, and medications that are not absolutely necessary should be gradually reduced and eliminated. The use of barbiturates or hypnotics may further aggravate the condition. The treatment of choice is high-potency antipsychotics, such as haloperidol and thiothixene, in small doses.[188,232]

### Treatment of Medication-Induced Sleep-Wakefulness Disturbances

Some medications cause insomnia, whereas others cause EDS.[203,223,233] Elderly individuals often take a variety of medications because of the increased prevalence of other illnesses. Furthermore, because of their altered metabolism, they are susceptible to the side effects of various medications. The patient should avoid alcohol, caffeine, and cigarettes, and should gradually eliminate drugs that are not essential.

### Special Environmental Considerations in Treatment

Treatment should be designed and tailored to different environmental situations (e.g., nursing home, hospital, home), as different types of sleep disturbances have been noted in different environments.[51]

### Exercise Program

Exercise, particularly 5–6 hours before sleep, is thought to have a beneficial effect on sleep quality.

However, there is a dearth of well-controlled studies.[234,235] Vitiello and colleagues[236] found beneficial effects of aerobic exercise on PSG-defined sleep in a group of elderly volunteers without sleep complaints. King et al.[237] found that older adults with moderate sleep complaints can improve self-rated sleep quality by initiating a regular, moderate-intensity, endurance exercise program.

### Nonpharmacologic Treatment

Time-limited and sleep-focused nonpharmacologic interventions have been found to improve sleep in many chronic insomniacs.[238,239] The most common nonpharmacologic interventions include stimulus control therapy, sleep restriction therapy, relaxation techniques, and sleep hygiene education. It remains an open question until further studies whether nonpharmacologic interventions could be combined with pharmacotherapy to improve the quality of sleep.[238]

## REFERENCES

1. Monjan AA. Sleep disorders of older people: report of a consensus conference. Hosp Community Psychiatry 1990;41:743.
2. Adams RD, Victor M. Principles of Neurology (5th ed). New York: McGraw-Hill, 1993.
3. Behnke JA, Finch CE, Momoent BG (eds). The Biology of Aging. New York: Plenum, 1978.
4. Comfort A. The Biology of Senescence (3rd ed). New York: Elsevier, 1979.
5. Katzman R, Terry R. Normal Aging of the Nervous System. In The Neurology of Aging. Philadelphia: Davis, 1983;15.
6. Jorgensen L, Torvik A. Ischaemic cerebrovascular diseases in an autopsy series. Part I. Prevalence, location, and predisposing factors in verified thromboembolic occlusions, and their significance in the pathogenesis of cerebral infarction. J Neurol Sci 1966;3:490.
7. Wechsler D (ed). Manual for the Wechsler Adult Intelligence Scale. New York: Psychological Corporation, 1955;75.
8. Wechsler D (ed). The Measurement and Appraisal of Adult Intelligence (4th ed). Baltimore: Williams & Wilkins, 1958;297.
9. Green RF. Age-intelligence relationship between ages sixteen and sixty-four: a rising trend. Dev Psychol 1969;1:618.
10. Schaie KW, Labouvie-Vief G. Generational versus ontogenetic components of change in adult cognitive behavior: a fourteen-year cross-sequential study. Dev Psychol 1974;10:305.
11. Schaie KW, Labouvie GV, Buech BU. Generational- and cohort-specific differences in adult cognitive functioning: a fourteen-year study of independent samples. Dev Psychol 1973;9:151.
12. Birren JE. Age Changes in Speed of Behavior: Its Central Nature and Physiological Correlates. In AT Welford, JE Birren (eds), Behavior, Aging and the Nervous System. Springfield, IL: Thomas, 1963;191.
13. Birren JE. Translations in gerontology—from lab to life. Psychophysiology and speed of response. Am Psychol 1974;29:808.
14. Birren JE, Woods AM, Williams MV. Speed of Behavior as an Indicator of Age Changes and the Integrity of the Nervous System. In F Hoffmeister, C Muller (eds), Brain Function in Old Age. Berlin: Springer, 1979;10.
15. Welford AT. Motor Performance. In JE Birren, KW Schaie (eds), Handbook of the Psychology of Aging. New York: Van Nostrand Reinhold, 1977;450.
16. Welford AT. Sensory, Perceptual, and Motor Processes in Older Adults. In JE Birren, RB Sloane (eds), Handbook of Mental Health and Aging. Englewood Cliffs, NJ: Prentice-Hall, 1980;192.
17. Krall VA. Senescent forgetfulness: benign and malignant. Can Med Assoc J 1962;86:257.
18. Crook T, Bartus RT, Ferris SH, et al. Age-associated memory impairment: proposed diagnostic criteria and measures of clinical change-report of a National Institute of Mental Health Work Group. Dev Neuropsychol 1986;2:261.
19. Critchley M. The neurology of old age. Lancet 1931;1:1119,1221,1331.
20. Potvin AR, Syndulko K, Tourtellotte WW, et al. Human neurologic function and the aging process. J Am Geriatr Soc 1980;28:1.
21. Potvin AR, Syndulko K, Tourtellotte W, et al. Quantitative Evaluation of Normal Age Related Changes in Neurologic Function. In FJ Pirozzolo, GJ Maletta (eds), Advances in Neurogerontology (Vol 2). New York: Praeger, 1981;13.
22. Weitzman ED. Sleep and Aging. In R Katzman, RD Terry (eds), The Neurology of Aging. Philadelphia: Davis, 1983;167.
23. Low PA. The Effect of Aging on the Autonomic Nervous System. In PA Low (ed), Clinical Autonomic Disorders (2nd ed). Philadelphia: Lippincott–Raven, 1997;161.
24. Hazzard WR, Bierman EL. Old Age. In D Smith, EL Bierman (eds), Biological Ages of Man from Conception Through Old Age (2nd ed). Philadelphia: Saunders, 1978;229.
25. Cowley M. The View from 80. New York: Viking, 1976;1.
26. Rowe JW, Troen BR. Sympathetic nervous system and aging in man. Endocr Rev 1980;1:167.

27. Blass JP, Plum F. Metabolic Encephalopathies in Older Adults. In R Katzman, RD Terry (eds), The Neurology of Aging. Philadelphia: Davis, 1983;189.

28. Katz RI, Horowitz GR. The septuagenarian EEG: normative EEG studies in a selected normal ambulatory geriatric population [abstract]. Electroencephalogr Clin Neurophysiol 1981;51:35.

29. Torres A, Faoro A, Loewenson R, et al. The electroencephalogram of elderly subjects revisited. Electroencephalogr Clin Neurophysiol 1983;56:391.

30. Obrist WD. Problems of Aging. In A Remond (ed), Handbook of Electroencephalography and Clinical Neurophysiology (Vol 6A). Amsterdam: Elsevier, 1976;275.

31. Obrist WD, Henry CE, Justiss WA. Longitudinal Changes in the Senescent EEG: A 15-Year Study. In Proceedings of the 7th International Congress of Gerontology. Vienna: International Association of Gerontology, 1966;35.

32. Matejcek M. The EEG of the aging brain. A spectral analytic study [abstract]. Electroencephalogr Clin Neurophysiol 1981;51:51.

33. Nakano T, Miyasaka M, Ohtaka T, et al. A follow up study of automatic EEG analysis and the mental deterioration in the age [abstract]. Electroencephalogr Clin Neurophysiol 1982;54:27.

34. Duffy FH, Albert MS, McAnulty TG, et al. Age-related differences in brain electrical activity of healthy subjects. Ann Neurol 1984;16:430.

35. Oken BS, Kaye JA. Electrophysiologic function in the healthy, extremely old. Neurology 1992;42:519.

36. Niedermeyer E. EEG and Old Age. In E Niedermeyer, F Lopes da Silva (eds), Electroencephalography. Baltimore: Urban & Schwarzenberg, 1987;301.

37. Kelley J, Reilly P, Bellar S. Photic driving and psychogeriatric diagnosis. Clin Electroencephalogr 1983;14:78.

38. Busse EW, Obrist WD. Pre-senescent electroencephalographic changes in normal subjects. J Gerontol 1965;20:315.

39. Brenner RP, Ulrich RF, Reynolds CF. EEG spectral findings in healthy, elderly men and women—sex differences. Electroencephalogr Clin Neurophysiol 1995; 94:1.

40. Kugler J. Fast EEG activity in normal people of advanced age [abstract]. Electroencephalogr Clin Neurophysiol 1983;56:67.

41. Arenas AM, Brennar RP, Reynolds CF III. Temporal slowing in the elderly revisited. Am J EEG Technol 1986;26:105.

42. Katz RI, Horowitz GR. Electroencephalogram in the septuagenarian: studies in a normal geriatric population. J Am Geriatr Soc 1982;3:273.

43. Hughes JR, Cayafa JJ. The EEG in patients at different ages without organic cerebral disease. Electroencephalogr Clin Neurophysiol 1977;42:776.

44. Visser SL, Hooijer C, Jonker C, et al. Anterior temporal focal abnormalities in EEG in normal aged subjects: correlations with psychopathological and CT brain scan findings. Electroencephalogr Clin Neurophysiol 1987;66:1.

45. Klass DW, Brenner RP. Electroencephalography of the elderly. J Clin Neurophysiol 1995;12:116.

46. Pedley TA, Miller JA. Clinical neurophysiology of aging and dementia. Adv Neurol 1983;38:31.

47. Gibbs FA, Gibbs EL. Atlas of Electroencephalography (2nd ed). Reading, MA: Addison, 1964;3.

48. Katz RI, Horowitz GR. Sleep-onset frontal rhythmic slowing in a normal geriatric population [abstract]. Electroencephalogr Clin Neurophysiol 1983;56:27.

49. Libow LS, Obrist WD, Sokoloff L. Cerebral Circulatory and Electroencephalographic Changes in Elderly Men. In S Granick, RD Patterson (eds), Human Aging, II. HSM 71-9037. Rockville, MD: U.S. Department of Health, Education and Welfare, 1971.

50. Obrist WD, Sokoloff L, Lassen NA, et al. Relation of EEG to cerebral blood flow and metabolism in old age. Electroencephalogr Clin Neurophysiol 1963; 15:610.

51. Miles LE, Dement WC. Sleep and aging. Sleep 1980;3:119.

52. Bliwise DL. Sleep in normal aging and dementia: review. Sleep 1993;16:40.

53. Liberson WT. Functional electroencephalography in mental disorders. Dis Nerv Syst 1945;5:357.

54. Feinberg I. Functional Implications of Changes in Sleep Physiology with Age. In RD Terry, S Gershon (eds), Neurology of Aging. New York: Raven, 1976;23.

55. Feinberg I, Koresko R, Heller N. EEG sleep patterns as a function of normal and pathological aging in man. J Psychiatr Res 1967;5:107.

56. Rechtschaffen A, Kales A. A Manual of Standardized Terminology: Techniques and Scoring Stages of Human Subjects. Los Angeles: UCLA Brain Information Service/Brain Research Institute, 1968.

57. Feinberg I, Hibi S, Carlson V. Changes in EEG Amplitude During Sleep with Age. In K Nandy, I Sherwin (eds), The Aging Brain and Senile Dementia (Vol 23). New York: Plenum, 1977;85.

58. Feinberg I. Effects of Age on Human Sleep Patterns. In A Kales (ed), Sleep Physiology and Pathology: A Symposium. Philadelphia: JB Lippincott, 1969;39.

59. Williams R, Karacan I, Hursch C (eds). Electroencephalography of Human Sleep: Clinical Applications. New York: Wiley, 1977;49.

60. Kahn E, Fisher C. The sleep characteristics of the normal aged male. J Nerv Ment Dis 1969;148:477.

61. Feinberg I. Changes in sleep cycle patterns with age. J Psychiatr Res 1974;10:283.

62. Brezinova V. Sleep cycle content and sleep cycle durations. Electroencephalogr Clin Neurophysiol 1974; 36:275.

63. Kales A, Wilson T, Kales J. Measurements of all night sleep in normal elderly persons. J Am Geriatr Soc 1967;15:405.

64. Tune GS. Sleep and wakefulness in 509 normal human adults. Br J Med Psychol 1969;42:75.

65. Tune GS. The influence of age and temperament on the adult human sleep-wakefulness pattern. Br J Psychol 1969;60:431.

66. Carskadon M, Brown E, Dement W. Sleep fragmentation in the elderly: relationship to daytime sleep tendency. Neurobiol Aging 1982;3:321.

67. Carskadon MA, Dement WC. Sleep loss in elderly volunteers. Sleep 1985;8:207.

68. Kales A, Kales J, Jacobson A, et al. All night EEG studies: children and elderly. Electroencephalogr Clin Neurophysiol 1966;21:415.

69. Williams DE, Vitiello MV, Ries RK, et al. Successful recruitment of elderly, community dwelling subjects for Alzheimer's disease research: cognitively impaired, major depressive disorder, and normal control groups. J Gerontol 1988;43:69.

70. Prinz P, Halter J. Sleep Disturbances in the Elderly: Neurohormonal Correlates. In M Chase, E Weitzman (eds), Sleep Disorders: Basic and Clinical Research, Advances in Sleep Research (Vol 8). New York: SP Medical & Scientific, 1983;463.

71. Prinz PN, Vitiello M. Sleep in Alzheimer's Dementia and in Healthy Not-Complaining Seniors. In Program and Abstracts of NIH Consensus Development Conference on the Treatment of Sleep Disorders in Older People. Bethesda, MD: National Institutes of Health, 1990;41.

72. Cashman MA, Prinz PN, Personius J, et al. Nighttime hypoxemia events in patient groups and in controls. Sleep Res 1989;18:329.

73. Hoch CC, Dew MA, Reynolds CF, et al. Longitudinal changes in diary- and laboratory-based sleep measures in healthy "old age" and "young old" subjects: a three-year follow-up. Sleep 1997;20:192.

74. Pittendrigh CS, Daan S. Circadian oscillations in rodents: a systematic increase of their frequency with age. Science 1974;186:548.

75. Wax T. Effects of age, strain, and illumination intensity on activity and self-selection of light-dark schedules in mice. J Comp Physiol Psychol 1977;91:51.

76. Wax T. Runwheel activity patterns of mature-young and senescent mice: the effect of constant lighting conditions. J Gerontol 1975;30:22.

77. Samis H. 24-H rhythmic variations in white blood cell counts of the rat with advancing age. Chronobiologia 1977;4:147.

78. Witting W, Mirmiran M, Bos NPA, Swaab DF. The effect of old age on the free-running period of circadian rhythms in rat. Chronobiol Int 1994;11:103.

79. Wessler R, Rubin M, Sollberger A. Circadian rhythm of activity and sleep-wakefulness in elderly institutionalized persons. J Interdiscipl Cycle Res 1976;7:333.

80. Scheving L, Roig C, Halberg F, et al. Circadian Variations in Residents of a "Senior Citizens" Home. In L Scheving, F Halberg, J Pauly (eds), Chronobiology. Proceedings of the International Society for the Study of Biological Rhythms, Little Rock, Arkansas. Tokyo: Igaku Shoin, 1974;353.

81. Ibuka N, Kawamura H. Loss of circadian rhythm in sleep-wakefulness cycle in the rat by suprachiasmatic nucleus lesions. Brain Res 1975;96:76.

82. Moore RY, Eichler VB. Loss of a circadian adrenal corticosterone rhythm following suprachiasmatic lesions in the rat. Brain Res 1972;42:201.

83. Mouret J, Coindet J, Debilly G, et al. Suprachiasmatic nuclei lesions in the rat: alterations in sleep circadian rhythms. Electroencephalogr Clin Neurophysiol 1978;45:402.

84. Nagai K, Nishio T, Nakagawa H, et al. Effect of bilateral lesions of the suprachiasmatic nuclei on the circadian rhythm of food intake. Brain Res 1978;142:384.

85. Vitiello MV, Smallwood RG, Avery DH, et al. Circadian temperature rhythms in young and aged men. Neurobiol Aging 1986;72:97.

86. Weitzman ED, Moline ML, Czeisler CA, et al. Chronobiology of aging: temperature, sleep-wake rhythms and entrainment. Neurobiol Aging 1982;3:299.

87. Esler MD, Turner AG, Kaye DM, et al. Aging effects on human sympathetic neuronal function. Am J Physiol 1995;268:R278.

88. Ng AV, Callister R, Johnson DG, Seals DR. Age and gender influence muscle sympathetic nerve activity at rest in healthy humans. Hypertension 1993;21:498.

89. Fennell W, Moore R. Responses of aged men to passive heating [abstract]. J Appl Physiol 1973;231:118.

90. Foster K, Ellis F, Dore C, et al. Sweat responses in the aged. Age Aging 1976;91:91.

91. For R, Woodward P, Fry A, et al. Diagnosis of accidental hypothermia of the elderly. Lancet 1971;1:424.

92. Taylor G. The problem of hypothermia in the elderly. Practitioner 1964;193:761.

93. Wollner L, Spalding J. The Autonomic Nervous System. In J Brockelhurst (ed), Textbook of Geriatric Medicine and Gerontology. Edinburgh: Churchill Livingstone, 1973;235.

94. Friedfield L. Heat reaction states in the aged. Geriatrics 1949;4:211.

95. Oechsli F, Buechley R. Excess mortality associated with three Los Angeles September hot spells. Environ Res 1970;3:277.

96. Snyder F, Hobson J, Morrison D, et al. Changes in respiration, heart rate and systolic blood pressure in human sleep. J Appl Physiol 1964;19:417.

97. Crapo RO. The Aging Lung. In DA Mahler (ed), Pulmonary Disease in the Elderly Patient. New York: Dekker, 1993;1.

98. Peterson DD, Pack AI, Silage DA, et al. Effects of aging on ventilatory and occlusion pressure responses to hypoxia and hypercapnia. Am Rev Respir Dis 1981;124:387.

99. Rossi A, Ganassini A, Tantucci C, Grassi V. Aging and the respiratory system. Aging Clin Exp Res 1996;8:143.

100. Lugaresi E, Coccagna C, Parneti P, et al. Snoring. Electroencephalogr Clin Neurophysiol 1975;39:59.

101. Orem J. Breathing During Sleep. In DG Davies, CD Barnes (eds), Regulation of Ventilation and Gas Exchange. New York: Academic, 1978;131.

102. Webb P. Periodic breathing during sleep. J Appl Physiol 1974;37:899.

103. Coccagna G, Lugaresi E. Arterial blood gases and pulmonary and systemic arterial pressure during sleep in chronic obstructive pulmonary disease. Sleep 1978;1:117.

104. Wynne J, Block A, Flick M. Disordered breathing and oxygen desaturation during daytime naps. Johns Hopkins Med J 1978;143:3.

105. Karacan I, Hursch C, Williams R. Some characteristics of nocturnal penile tumescence in elderly males. J Gerontol 1972;27:39.

106. Kahn E, Fisher C. REM sleep and sexuality in the aged. J Geriatr Psychiatry 1969;2:181.

107. Copinschi G, Van Cauter E. Effects of aging on modulation of hormonal secretions by sleep and circadian rhythmicity. Horm Res 1995;43:20.

108. Colucci CF, D'Alessandro B, Bellastella A, et al. Circadian rhythm of plasma cortisol in the aged (Cosinor method). Gerontol Clin (Basel) 1976;17:89.

109. Silverberg A, Rizzo F, Krieger DT, et al. Nycterohemeral periodicity of plasma 17: OHCS levels in elderly subject. J Clin Endocrinol Metab 1968;28:1661.

110. Carroll B, Curtis G, Mendels J. Neuroendocrine regulation in depression. Arch Gen Psychiatry 1976;33:1039,1051.

111. Sachar E. Twenty-Four Hour Cortisol Secretory Patterns in Depressed and Manic Patients. In W Gispen, B van Wimersma Greidanus, B Bohus, et al. (eds), Progress in Brain Research—Hormones, Homeostasis and the Brain (Vol 42). Amsterdam: Elsevier, 1975;81.

112. Vidalon C, Khurana C, Chae S, et al. Age related changes in growth hormone in non-diabetic women. J Am Geriatr Soc 1973;21:253.

113. Bazzarre T, Johanson A, Huseman C, et al. Human growth hormone changes with age. Excerpta Med ICS 1976;381:261.

114. Veldhuis JD, Iranmanesh A. Physiological regulation of the human growth hormone (GHS)—insulin-like growth factor type I (IGF-I) axis: predominant impact of age, obesity, gonadal function and sleep. Sleep 1996;19(Suppl 10):221.

115. Calderon L, Ryan N, Kovacs K. Human pituitary growth hormone cells in old age. Gerontology 1978;24:441.

116. Sassin J, Frantz A, Kapen S, et al. The Nocturnal Rise of Human Prolactin Is Dependent on Sleep. In MH Chase, WC Stern, PL Walter (eds), Sleep Research (Vol 2). Los Angeles: Brain Research Institute, 1973;199.

117. Sassin J, Frantz A, Weitzman E, et al. Human prolactin: 24-hour pattern with increased release during sleep. Science 1972;177:1205.

118. Van Cauter, Turek FW. Endocrine and Other Biological Rhythms. In LJ DeGroot, M Besser, HG Burger, et al. (eds), Endocrinology (3rd ed). Philadelphia: Saunders, 1995;2487.

119. Weitzman ED. Circadian rhythms and episodic hormone secretion in man. Ann Rev Med 1976;27:225.

120. Fisher DA. Physiological variations in thyroid hormones: physiological and pathophysiological considerations. Clin Chem 1996;42:135.

121. Waldhouser F, Weiszenbacher G, Tatzer E, et al. Alterations in nocturnal serum melatonin levels in humans with growth and aging. J Clin Endocrinol Metab 1988;66:648.

122. Haimov I, Laudon M, Zisapel N, et al. Impaired 6-sulfatoxymelatonin rhythms in the elderly: coincidence with sleep disorders. BMJ 1994;309:167.

123. Garfinkel D, Laudon M, Nof D, Zisapel N. Improvement of sleep quality in elderly people by controlled-release melatonin. Lancet 1995;346:541.

124. Kety SS. Human cerebral blood flow and oxygen consumption as related to aging. J Chron Dis 1956;8:478.

125. Meyer JS. Cerebral Blood Flow in Aging. AAN Course #142. Minneapolis: American Academy of Neurology, 1992;65.

126. Meyer JS. Improved method for non-invasive measurement for regional cerebral blood flow by 133xenon inhalation. Part II: Measurements in health and disease. Stroke 1978;9:205.

127. Naritomi H, Meyer JS, Sakai F, et al. Effects of advancing age on regional cerebral blood flow. Studies in normal subjects and subjects with risk factors for atherothrombotic stroke. Arch Neurol 1979;36:410.

128. Malamed E, Lavy S, Bentin S, et al. Reduction in regional cerebral blood flow during normal aging in man. Stroke 1980;11:31.

129. Imai A, Meyer JS, Kobari M, et al. LCBF values decline while Lk values increase during normal human aging measured by stable xenon enhanced computed tomography. Neuroradiology 1988;30:463.

130. Pantano P, Baron JC, Lebrun-Grandie P, et al. Regional cerebral blood flow and oxygen consumption in human aging. Stroke 1984;15:635.

131. Sokoloff L. Effects of Normal Aging on Cerebral Circulation and Energy Metabolism. In F Hoffmeister, C Muller (eds), Brain Function in Old Age. New York: Springer, 1979;367.

132. Foncin JF. Classical and ultrastructural neuropathology of aging processes in the human: a critical review [abstract]. Electroencephalogr Clin Neurophysiol 1981;52:30.

133. Ford DE, Kamerow DB. Epidemiological studies of sleep disturbances and psychiatric disorders: an opportunity for prevention. JAMA 1979;262:1479.

134. Clayton PJ, Halikas JA, Mauria WL. The depression of widowhood. Br J Psychiatry 1972;120:71.

135. Brabbins CJ, Dewey ME, Copeland JRM, et al. Insomnia in the elderly: prevalence, gender differences and

relationships with morbidity and mortality. Int J Geriatr Psychiatry 1993;8:473.

136. Henderson S, Jorm AF, Scott LR, et al. Insomnia in the elderly: its prevalence and correlates in the general population. Med J Aust 1995;162:22.

137. Hohagan F, Kappler C, Schramm E, et al. Prevalence of insomnia in elderly general practiced attendars and the current treatment modalities. Acta Psychiatr Scand 1994;90:102.

138. Foley DJ, Mongan AA, Brown SL, et al. Sleep complaints among elderly persons: an epidemiologic study of three communities. Sleep 1995;18:425.

139. Reynolds CF III. Subjective and Objective Sleep Complaints in Late Life. In Program and Abstracts of NIH Consensus Development Conference on the Treatment of Sleep Disorders of Older People. Bethesda, MD: National Institutes of Health, 1990;21.

140. Vitiello MV, Prinz PN. Alzheimer's disease: sleep and sleep/wake patterns. Clin Geriatr Med 1989;5:289.

141. Reynolds CF III, Hoch CC, Monk TH. Sleep and Chronobiologic Disturbances in Late Life. In EW Busse, DG Blazer (eds), Geriatric Psychiatry. Washington, DC: American Psychiatric, 1989;475.

142. Koskenvuo M, Kaprio J, Partinen M, et al. Snoring as a risk factor for hypertension and angina pectoris. Lancet 1985;1:893.

143. Koskenvuo M, Kaprio J, Telaviki T, et al. Snoring as a risk factor for ischemic heart disease and stroke in men. BMJ 1987;294:16.

144. Lugaresi E, Cirignotta F, Coccagna G, et al. Some epidemiological data on snoring and cardiocirculatory disturbances. Sleep 1980;3:221.

145. Enright PL, Newman AB, Wahl PW, et al. Prevalence and correlates of snoring and observed apneas in 5,201 older adults. Sleep 1996;19:531.

146. Ancoli-Israel S. Epidemiology of sleep disorders. Clin Geriatr Med 1989;5:347.

147. Kripke DF, Simons RN, Garfinkel L, et al. Short and long sleep and sleeping pills: is increased mortality associated? Arch Gen Psychiatry 1979;36:103.

148. Karacan I, Thornby J, Anch M, et al. Prevalence of sleep disturbance in a primarily urban Florida county. Soc Sci Med 1976;10:239.

149. McGhie A, Russell S. The subjective assessment of normal sleep patterns. J Ment Sci 1962;108:642.

150. Thornby J, Karacan I, Searle R, et al. Subjective Reports of Sleep Disturbance in a Houston Metropolitan Health Survey. In MH Chase, MM Mitler, PL Walter (eds), Sleep Research (Vol 6). Los Angeles: BIS/BRI, 1977;181.

151. Ganguly M, Reynolds CF III, Gilby JE. Prevalence and persistence of sleep complaints in a rural older community sample: the movies project. J Am Geriatr Soc 1996;44:778.

152. Vitiello MV, Prinz PN. Aging and Sleep Disorders. In RL Williams, I Karacan, CA Moore (eds), Sleep Disorders: Diagnosis and Treatment (2nd ed). New York: Wiley, 1988;293.

153. Kales A, Soldatos CR, Kales JD. Taking a sleep history. Am Fam Physician 1980;22:101.

154. Kales A, Soldatos CR, Kales JD. Sleep disorders: insomnia, sleep-walking, night terrors, nightmares, and enuresis. Ann Intern Med 1987;106:582.

155. Kales A, Vela-Bueno A, Kales JD. Sleep disorders: sleep apnea and narcolepsy. Ann Intern Med 1987;106:434.

156. Walters A, Picchietti D, Hening W, Lazzarini A. Variable expressivity in familial restless legs syndrome. Arch Neurol 1990;47:1219.

157. Kales A, Kales JD. Evaluation and Treatment of Insomnia. New York: Oxford University Press, 1984.

158. Bixler EO, Kales A, Soldatos CR, et al. Prevalence of sleep disorders in the Los Angeles metropolitan area. Am J Psychiatry 1979;136:1257.

159. Dement WC, Miles LE, Carskadon MA. "White paper" on sleep and aging. J Am Geriatr Soc 1982;30:25.

160. Cadieux RJ, Woolley D, Kales JD. Sleep Disorders in the Elderly. In RM Berlin, CR Soldatos (eds), Psychiatric Medicine. Sleep Disorders in Psychiatric Practice, 1986. Longwood, FL: Ryandic, 1987;165.

161. Prinz PN. Sleep patterns in the healthy aged: relationship with intellectual function. J Gerontol 1977;32:179.

162. Webb W, Swinburne H. An observational study of sleep in the aged. Percept Mot Skills 1971;32:895.

163. Ancoli-Israel S, Kripke DF, Klauber MR, et al. Sleep-disordered breathing in community-dwelling elderly. Sleep 1991;14:486.

164. Coleman RM, Miles LE, Guilleminault CC, et al. Sleep-wake disorders in the elderly: a polysomnographic analysis. J Am Geriatr Soc 1981;29:289.

165. Hoch CC, Reynolds CF III, Kupfer DJ, et al. Sleep-disordered breathing in normal and pathologic aging. J Clin Psychiatry 1986;47:499.

166. Prinz PN. Sleep and sleep disorders in older adults. J Clin Neurophysioi 1995;12:139.

167. McGinty DJ, Littner M, Beahm E, et al. Sleep-related breathing disorders in older men: a search for underlying mechanisms. Neurobiol Aging 1982;3:337.

168. Roehrs T, Zorick F, Sicklesteel J, et al. Age-related sleep-wake disorders at a sleep disorder center. J Am Geriatr Soc 1983;31:364.

169. Smallwood RG, Vitiello MV, Giblin EC, et al. Sleep apnea: relationship to age, sex, and Alzheimer's dementia. Sleep 1983;6:16.

170. Ancoli-Israel, Coy T. Are breathing disturbances in elderly equivalent to sleep apnea syndrome? Sleep 1994;17:77.

171. Ancoli-Israel S. Epidemiology of sleep disorders. Clin Geriatr Med 1989;5:347.

172. Block AJ, Boysen PG, Wynne JW, et al. Sleep apnea, hypopnea and oxygen desaturation in normal subjects. A strong male predominance. N Engl J Med 1979;300:513.

173. Bixler EO, Kales A, Soldatos CR, et al. Sleep apneic activity in a normal population. Res Commun Chem Pathol Pharmacol 1982;36:141.

174. Ancoli-Israel S. Critical Review of Epidemiological Studies on Sleep Apnea. Program and Abstracts of NIH Consensus Development Conference on the Treatment of Sleep Disorders of Older People. Bethesda, MD: National Institutes of Health, 1990;47.

175. Young T, Palta M, Dempsey J, et al. Occurrence of sleep-disordered breathing among middle-aged adults. N Engl J Med 1993;328:1230.

176. Prinz PN, Vitiello MV, Raskind MA, et al. Geriatrics: sleep disorders and aging. N Engl J Med 1990;323:520.

177. Fleury B. Sleep apnea syndrome in the elderly. Sleep 1992;15:S39.

178. Gould GA, Whyte KF, Rhind GB, et al. The sleep hypopnea syndrome. Am Rev Respir Dis 1988; 137:895.

179. He J, Kryger MH, Zorick FJ, et al. Mortality and apnea index in obstructive sleep apnea: experience in 385 male patients. Chest 1988;94:9.

180. Bliwise DL, Benkert RE, Ingham RH. Factors associated with nightly variability in sleep-disordered breathing in the elderly. Chest 1991;100:973.

181. Mason WJ, Ancoli-Israel S, Kripke DF. Apnea revisited: a longitudinal follow-up. Sleep 1989;12:423.

182. Mosko SS, Dickel MJ, Ashurst J. Night-to-night variability in sleep apnea and sleep in sleep-related periodic leg movements in the elderly. Sleep 1988;11:340.

183. Wittig RM, Romaker A, Zorick E, et al. Night to night consistency of apneas during sleep. Am Rev Respir Dis 1984;129:244.

184. Pertinen M, Jamieson A, Guilleminault C. Long-term outcome for obstructive sleep apnea syndrome patients—mortality. Chest 1988;94:1200.

185. Guilleminault C, Simmons FB, Motta J, et al. Obstructive sleep apnea syndrome and tracheostomy: long-term follow-up experience. Arch Intern Med 1981;141:985.

186. Ancoli-Israel S, Kripke DF, Klauber MR, et al. Morbidity, mortality and sleep-disordered breathing in community dwelling elderly. Sleep 1996;19:277.

187. Lavie P, Herer P, Peled R, et al. Mortality in sleep apnea patients: a multivariant analysis of risk factors. Sleep 1995;18:149.

188. Vitiello MV, Prinz PN. Sleep and Sleep Disorders in Normal Aging. In MJ Thorpy (ed), Handbook of Sleep Disorders. New York: Dekker, 1990;139.

189. Chervin RD, Guilleminault C. Obstructive sleep apnea and related disorders. Neurol Clin 1996;14:583.

190. Bliwise DL. Neuropsychological function and sleep. Clin Geriatr Med 1989;5:381.

191. Aldrich MS. Automobile accidents in patients with sleep disorders. Sleep 1989;12:487.

192. Findley LJ, Fabrizio M, Thommi G, et al. Severity of sleep apnea and automobile crashes. N Engl J Med 1989;320:868.

193. Ancoli-Israel S, Klauber MR, Kripke DF, et al. Sleep apnea in female patients in a nursing home: increased risk of mortality. Chest 1989;96:1054.

194. Ancoli-Israel S, Kripke DR, Mason W, et al. Sleep apnea and nocturnal myoclonus in a senior population. Sleep 1981;4:349.

195. Kripke DF, Ancoli-Israel S, Okudaira N. Sleep apnea and nocturnal myoclonus in the elderly. Neurobiol Aging 1982;3:329.

196. Coleman RM, Pollak CP, Weitzman ED. Periodic movements in sleep (nocturnal myoclonus): relation to sleep-wake disorders. Ann Neurol 1980;8:416.

197. Rees PJ, Cochrane GM, Prior JG, et al. Sleep apnoea in diabetic patients with autonomic neuropathy. J R Soc Med 1981;74:192.

198. Rodin J, McAvay G, Timko C. Depressed mood and sleep disturbance in the elderly: a longitudinal study. J Gerontol 1988;43:45.

199. Reynolds CF, Kupfer DJ, Taska LS, et al. EEG sleep in elderly depressed, demented, and healthy subjects. Biol Psychiatry 1985;20:431.

200. Reynolds CF, Kupfer DJ, Houck PR, et al. Reliable discrimination of elderly depressed and demented patients by EEG sleep data. Arch Gen Psychiatry 1987;44:982.

201. Ulrich RF, Shaw DH, Kupfer DJ. Effects of aging on sleep in depression. Sleep 1980;3:31.

202. Benca RM. Sleep in psychiatric disorders. Neurol Clin 1996;14:739.

203. Cadieux RJ, Woolley D, Kales JD. Sleep Disorders in the Elderly. In RM Berlin, CR Soldatos (eds), Psychiatric Medicine. Sleep Disorders in Psychiatric Practice, 1986. Longwood, FL: Ryandic, 1987;165.

204. Culebras A, Magana R. Neurologic disorders and sleep disturbances. Semin Neurol 1987;7:277.

205. Morgan K, Dalloso H, Ebrahim S, et al. Characteristics of subjective insomnia in the elderly living at home. Age Ageing 1988;17:1.

206. Garma L, Bouard G, Benoit O. Age and Intervening Wakefulness in Chronic Insomnia. In WP Koella (ed), Sleep 1980. Basel: Karger, 1981;391.

207. Czeisler CA, Dumont M, Richardson GS, et al. Disorders of Circadian Function: Clinical Consequences and Treatment. Program and Abstracts of NIH Consensus Development Conference on the Treatment of Sleep Disorders of Older People. Bethesda, MD: National Institutes of Health, 1990;95.

208. Czeisler CA, Allan JS, Strogatz SH, et al. Bright light resets the human circadian pacemaker independent of the timing of the sleep-wake cycle. Science 1986; 233:667.

209. Czeisler CA, Kronhauer RE, Allan JS, et al. Bright light induction of strong (type O) resetting of the human circadian pacemaker. Science 1989;244:1328.

210. Mant A, Eyland EA. Sleep patterns and problems in elderly general practice attenders: an Australian survey. Community Health Study 1988;12:192.

211. Pittendrigh CS, Daan S. Circadian oscillations in rodents: a systematic increase of their frequency with age. Science 1974;186:548.

212. Morin LP. Age-related changes in hamster circadian period, entrainment, and rhythm splitting. J Biol Rhythms 1988;3:237.

213. Weitzman ED, Moline ML, Czeisler CA, et al. Chronobiology of aging: temperature, sleep-wake rhythms and entrainment. Neurobiol Aging 1982;3:299.

214. Moore RY, Eichler VB. Loss of circadian adrenal corticosterone rhythm following suprachiasmatic lesions in the rat. Brain Res 1972;42:201.

215. Stephan FK, Zucker I. Circadian rhythms in drinking behavior and locomotor activity of rats are eliminated by hypothalamic lesions. Proc Natl Acad Sci U S A 1972;69:1583.

216. Hofman MA, Fliers E, Goudsmit E, et al. Morphometric analysis of the suprachiasmatic and paraventricular nuclei in the human brain: sex differences and age-dependent changes. J Anat 1988;160:127.

217. Swaab DF, Fliers E, Partiman TS. The suprachiasmatic nucleus of the human brain in relation to sex, age, and senile dementia. Brain Res 1985;342:37.

218. Swaab DF, Fisser B, Kempherst W, Troost D. The human suprachiasmatic nucleus: neuropeptide changes in serium and Alzheimer's disease. Basic Appl Histochem 1988;2:43.

219. Remmers JE, Issa FG. Indications and Rationale for Treatment of Sleep-Disordered Breathing in Older People. Program and Abstracts of NIH Consensus Development Conference on the Treatment of Sleep Disorders of Older People. Bethesda, MD: National Institutes of Health, 1990;55.

220. Kales A, Vela-Bueno A, Kales JD. Sleep disorders: sleep apnea and narcolepsy. Ann Intern Med 1987;106:434.

221. Schmidt-Nowara W, Lowle A, Wiegand L, et al. Oral appliances for the treatment of snoring and obstructive sleep apnea: a review. Sleep 1995;18:501.

222. Gottlieb GL. Sleep disorders and their management: special considerations in the elderly. Am J Med 1990;88(Suppl 3A):29.

223. Kupfer DJ, Reynolds CF III. Management of insomnia. N Engl J Med 1997;336:341.

224. Scharf MB, Roth T, Vogel JW, Walsh JK. A multi-center placebo-controlled study evaluating zolpedam in the treatment of chronic insomnia. J Clin Psychiatry 1994;55:192.

225. Reynolds CF III, Regestein Q, Nowell PD, Neylan TC. Diagnosis and Treatment of Insomnia in the Elderly. In C Salzman (ed), Clinical Geriatric Psychopharmacology (3rd ed). Baltimore: Williams & Wilkins, 1997.

226. Garfinkel D, Laudon M, Nof D, Zisapel M. Improvement of sleep quality in elderly people by controlled-release melatonin. Lancet 1995;346:541.

227 Haimov I, Lavie P, Laudon M, et al. Melatonin replacement therapy of elderly insomniacs. Sleep 1995;18:591.

228. Vestal R, Dawson G. Pharmacology and Aging. In CE Finch, EL Schneider (eds), Handbook of the Biology of Aging (2nd ed). New York: Van Nostrand Reinhold, 1985;744.

229. Campbell SS, Dawson D, Anderson FW. Alleviation of sleep maintenance insomnia with time exposure to bright light. J Am Geriatr Soc 1993;41:829.

230. Murphy PJ, Campbell SS. Enhanced performance in elderly subjects following bright light treatment of sleep maintenance insomnia. J Sleep Res 1996;5:165.

231. Campbell SS. Bright Light Treatment of Sleep Maintenance Insomnia and Behavioral Disturbance. In RW Lam (ed), Beyond Seasonal Affective Disorder: Light Therapy for Non-SAD Conditions. Washington, DC: American Psychiatric, 1996.

232. Kales JD, Carvell M, Kales A. Sleep and Sleep Disorders. In CK Cassell, DE Riesenberg, LB Sorensen, et al. (eds), Geriatric Medicine. New York: Springer, 1990;562.

233. Lacy C, Armstrong LL, Ingrim N, Lance LL (eds). Drug Information Handbook. Hudson, OH: Lexa-Comp, 1995.

234. O'Connor PJ, Youngstedt SD. Influence of exercise on human sleep. Exerc Sport Sci Rev 1995;23:105.

235. Vitiello MV, Prinz PN, Schwartz RS. The subjective sleep quality of healthy older men and women is enhanced by participation in two fitness training programs: a non-specific effect [abstract]. Sleep Res 1994;23:148.

236. Vitiello MV, Prinz PN, Schwartz RS. Slow wave sleep but no overall sleep quality of healthy older men and women is improved by increased aerobic fitness [abstract]. Sleep Res 1994;23:149.

237. King AC, Oman RF, Brassington JS, et al. Moderate-intensity exercise and self-rated quality of sleep in older adults. A randomized controlled trial. JAMA 1997;277:32.

238. Hohagan F. Non-pharmacological treatment of insomnia. Sleep 1996;19:S50.

239. Morin CM, Culbert GP, Schwartz SM. Non-pharmacological interventions for insomnia: a meta-analysis of treatment efficacy. Am J Psychiatry 1994;151:1172.

# Chapter 33
# Sleep Disorders of Childhood

## Richard Ferber

The same sleep disorders that occur in adults also occur in children: sleep apnea, narcolepsy, parasomnias, circadian rhythm disorders, and insomnias.[1] All have presentations that are peculiar to children, however, a fact that greatly affects proper evaluation and treatment. For example, narcolepsy in children may present initially as a form of hypersomnolence with a single prolonged sleep period, and only later evolve into the adult pattern of daytime sleepiness with short, refreshing naps and cataplexy.[2–4] Sleep apnea in children often looks more like an upper airway resistance syndrome than the typical pattern of clear-cut apneas and desaturations.[5] Bedwetting at age 3 years reflects normal function, not the disorder of enuresis. Confusional arousals are much more frequent in children than sleepwalking or sleep terrors.[6] The sleep disorders whose childhood presentations are most different from those seen in the adult are insomnias, particularly the forms of sleeplessness seen in young children (this is especially true if one is willing to include relevant circadian problems).[7–10] Thus, this chapter focuses primarily on a discussion of factors that need to be considered when dealing with a young child who has difficulty falling asleep or remaining asleep.

Newborns enter the world already able to sleep. They have rapid eye movement (REM) and non-REM (NREM) sleep. At birth, however, NREM sleep is not fully developed and is not yet divisible into four substages.[11–16] The pattern of sleep cycling itself is also immature, not yet fully organized into a circadian pattern.[14,17–20] Periods of sleeping and waking are spread almost randomly across the 24-hour day.

Changes occur rapidly, both in the electrophysiologic aspects of sleep and in its circadian control. The tracé alternant electroencephalographic pattern of NREM sleep in the newborn (2- to 6-second bursts of high-amplitude slow waves separated by 4–8 seconds of low-voltage mixed activity) disappears within a few weeks and is replaced by a more continuous pattern.[11,14,16] Division of NREM into four stages is clear by age 6 months. Sleep spindles appear by age 4–6 weeks and are prominent by 2 months.[13] Vertex waves suggestive of K complexes are usually seen by approximately 4 months, and are clearly defined by 6 months.[12]

Evidence exists that the circadian clock is already functioning at birth but that it does not become linked to the sleep rhythm it controls until age 6–12 weeks.[20,21] By 3 months there is consolidation of the major sleep period into the night and beginning organization of daytime sleep into a pattern of regularly recurring naps.[14–19] These changes progress rapidly, along with the decrease in the need for nighttime feedings, after 5–6 months. By the second half of the first year of life, sleep should be well-organized, with good nighttime sleep and approximately two daytime naps. The morning nap is typically dropped around the first birthday, and the afternoon nap is usually given up in the third year of life.

A child should not be expected to sleep through the night before the age of 3 months. It is reasonable to expect (and surveys confirm) that full-term, normally developing and growing infants should be sleeping through the night, or very nearly through the night, by age 5–6 months.[22,23] If bedtime problems or nighttime awakening continues to be a significant problem after this time, reasons can usually be identified and corrected, most often by behavioral means.[7,8,10,24–27]

## PROBLEM VERSUS DISORDER AND PROBLEM VERSUS NO PROBLEM

Youngsters are very adaptable in terms of their ability to vary their sleep patterns, change habits associated with sleep, sleep at different times, and divide their sleep into different numbers of segments. These variations are especially common during the early years of life, when sleep is normally still polyphasic (i.e., divided into day and nighttime segments).[1] Certain patterns may present significant problems for family members, although technically these patterns represent variations of normal function, not disorders. The bulk of the complaints of sleeplessness in young children seen in practice fall into this category.

For a problem of sleeplessness to truly represent a disorder, (1) the child should have difficulty falling asleep even at the correct circadian phase, and (2) regardless of environmental setting, the sleep of the child should be interrupted inappropriately (i.e., awakenings should be more than just those reflecting normal sleep cycling), total sleep time should be below the sleep requirements of the child, or daytime functioning should be affected. The last symptom is often difficult to assess. A 1-year-old child who sleeps only 7 hours a night but naps 5 hours during the day could be viewed as getting a normal amount of sleep, but in a manner that is difficult for the family to accommodate. This child could also be viewed as a youngster who gets insufficient sleep at night, however, and is therefore excessively sleepy during the day. The former interpretation is usually the correct one, as the cause of such a presentation generally is not related to any underlying disorder and is easily corrected. It is also difficult to evaluate the consequences of insufficient sleep in a child, because children frequently do not show obvious signs of mild sleepiness. Behavioral symptoms such as irritability and decreased attention are more common than yawning or dozing,[4] but even behavioral consequences may not be recognized if they are mild or long-standing. The existence of symptoms is often inferred only when behavior improves after adjustment of the sleep pattern.

Unlike adults, children generally do not deal with their sleep problems by themselves. There are interactions between child and parent (or caregiver), and it is often the specifics of these interactions that determine whether a sleep pattern is a problem.[7,8,25,26,28,29] If parents must get up at night to help a youngster return to sleep after awakening (even if the child sleeps in the parents' room), they may consider this a problem. What is a problem for one family, however, may not be for the next. Often what determines the existence or severity of a complaint is the ability of the parent who gets up at night to go back to sleep after intervening. Even a brief intervention required only once a night (perhaps covering the child) may represent a major problem to a parent who cannot go back to sleep for 2 hours.

Nighttime awakenings occur as part of the normal pattern of sleep cycling from the day a child is born. Many problems develop because parents, misinterpreting these awakenings as abnormal, establish patterns of intervention that disrupt normal sleep patterns.

What works for one family or child may not work at all for another, a fact that reflects individual differences and varied temperaments.[30,31] Although that observation may seem simplistic, it is actually quite important and frequently overlooked. Although two children may be managed exactly the same way at bedtime and at nighttime awakenings (if they occur), one child may go to sleep quickly and sleep through the night (i.e., return to sleep after normal nighttime awakenings without awakening the parents) and the other may protest loudly at bedtime and be up three times a night, unable (or unwilling) to go back to sleep without parental intervention. Management of the first child is appropriate; management of the second child requires modification. The decision for parents to change their approach should be dictated by their child's actual sleep pattern.

### *General Considerations*

A major advance in the treatment of insomnia in adults came with the realization that many factors are involved in causing the problem, various diagnoses are possible, and specific treatments can be designed to fit the specific causes of patients' complaints.[32,33] No longer is it appropriate to treat insomnia as a single diagnosis with a single treatment (e.g., barbiturates). The same considerations must be applied to children. By assuming that all sleepless youngsters have the same diagnosis and need the same treatment, a practitioner is sure to treat many children inappropriately and unsuccessfully.

When dealing with an insomniac adult, one must take the history directly from the patient. For children, this history is usually obtained from the parent or caregiver. In the adult, it is the degree of unhappiness of the patient with his or her sleep pattern that determines the severity of the complaint. For a child, it is the impact on the family that determines severity. It is uncommon for a young sleepless child to act like an insomniac adult, frustrated by an inability to sleep despite a desire to do so. It is much more common to see a youngster who does not want to sleep at the time the parents have established.

In most cases, a very careful history from the family provides enough information to diagnose the causes of a child's sleep problems and to decide on therapy.[9,34,35] A physical examination should not be neglected, but it only rarely provides the answers. The history itself cannot be rushed, and it should be extensive and wide ranging, as multiple factors often contribute to a child's sleep difficulties.

It is helpful to obtain the history in a circadian format, finding out what happens and at what time, around the clock.[9,34,35] Of course, there must be emphasis on the times of sleep (bedtime, actual time of falling asleep, naptimes) and awakenings, and the exact circumstances under which all sleep transitions take place (even after nighttime awakening). If variations exist from night to night, the relative incidence of each pattern should be determined (often requiring great effort on the part of the examiner). Weekend versus weekday schedules (even differences at the homes of a child's divorced parents) should be clarified. Parents often forget to mention short periods of sleep (e.g., in the car or stroller) that may have much impact on the rest of the sleep pattern. The timing and pattern of daytime events are also important: day care, other structured activities, peer interactions, and television viewing. A careful description of the sleeping environment may be crucial, including the organization of the house,

where the bedrooms are located, who sleeps where, whether there is a night-light (and how bright it is), if the child's bedroom door is open or closed, if there is a transitional object, if other children share the room, if the child sleeps with the parents, and if the parents are on the same floor of the house at bedtime and during the night. External stimulation, such as a parent coming home just as a youngster is about to go to sleep or a parent getting up and showering very early in the morning, may also be relevant.

A complete social history should be obtained.[9,34,35] The makeup of the family should be known, marital discord should be probed, alcohol or drug abuse should be ascertained, and any other factors that could lead to stress in the home should be investigated.

## SPECIFIC DISORDERS

Although intrinsic and extrinsic sleep disorders[36] are both possible in young children, the vast majority of disorders encountered are classified as extrinsic.[37]

### *Sleep-Onset Association Disorder*

When sleep-onset association disorder is the only problem, the child's ability to fall asleep at the desired time and to sleep the desired number of hours is not affected.[7,26,38] The child has come to associate falling asleep with some behavioral pattern that is partially outside his or her control.[7,8,24–27,29,36,39–45] It is generally necessary for the parents to establish this routine at bedtime and then to re-establish it at times of (normal) nighttime awakening.

Although the associated routine at bedtime may be the same as at nighttime awakenings, the routine might not be considered a problem at bedtime, as interventions at that hour are not usually disruptive to the family (who are still awake) and because interactive bedtime rituals are desirable. When the child is allowed to go to sleep in the location and under the conditions desired by the parents, the process of sleep transition must be extended (e.g., 45 minutes of rocking before a child can be transferred to the crib) to be considered a problem. Even if bedtime is not a problem, the nighttime may be; a youngster may go to sleep quickly by himself or herself but need help returning to sleep after awakenings several times during the night.

A pattern of specific associations with sleep transitions is common at all ages, but after a certain age, most individuals are able to take on the responsibility for generating these patterns by themselves (i.e., sleeping on the back or side; under a heavy or light blanket; with or without music, a light, or a transitional object; and with a fat or thin pillow). Whether by necessity or choice, parents of young children often become entangled in these associations. Such parent-assisted patterns may truly be necessary to help a very young infant smoothly negotiate the transition from wakefulness to sleep at bedtimes and after spontaneous interruptions of sleep (particularly from the unstable state of REM sleep). A youngster who is colicky in the early months may also need special help.[46,47]

By the age of 3–4 months, most youngsters have passed the age of colic and, in any case, have matured sufficiently to be able to handle these transitions by themselves if desired or required. As discussed earlier, sleep-onset associations that require parental intervention are not inherently problematic. Some youngsters are rocked to sleep quickly at bedtime, then transferred to the crib easily without awakening and sleep through the night. Although they continue to associate rocking with the initial sleep transition, they do not have to have it repeated at nighttime awakenings. For these children and their families, no problem exists and no changes need be made.

Bedtime routines may lead to major problems in children if the routines have to be repeated during the night. Rocking and back patting or rubbing are perhaps the most common routines for infants. Youngsters may require a bottle or cup of water, juice, or milk. They may be handed a pacifier, walked about, or driven in the car. They may fall asleep quickly and transfer easily to the crib, or they may fall asleep slowly and be difficult to move from arms to mattress until they reach stage IV sleep. Once asleep, children generally do well for several hours (the initial delta sleep epochs). Although awakenings may begin earlier, they typically start 3–4 hours after the child first falls asleep (at, or shortly after, the time the parents go to bed themselves). This middle third of the night is when sleep is lightest, as youngsters change back and forth between stages II and REM sleep and brief periods

of waking. If they wake sufficiently to sense that the patterns associated with sleep transitions are no longer present, they are aroused more completely and let the parents know of their dissatisfaction by crying or calling. This situation is commonly seen in children but only rarely seen in adults: falling asleep under one set of conditions but awakening during the night to find things completely changed. (Perhaps a version of this problem does occur in an adult who falls asleep with the television on but awakens during the night in a totally silent environment.) Often, a child falls asleep in a parent's arms in the living room with the lights and television on, only to awaken during the night alone, in a crib, in a dark, quiet room. It is not surprising that a youngster in such a situation has difficulty returning to sleep. (Perhaps it is only surprising that some do not.)

The key diagnostic feature comes from the description of the nighttime awakenings.[7,9,25,26,34,35,39] The youngster goes back to sleep promptly when the parents respond by quickly reinstituting conditions that have become associated with sleep transitions. If simply rocking a child at this point causes him or her to go back to sleep quickly, most other causes of sleeplessness, including pain and schedule disorders, can be ruled out. There certainly can be no problem with the child's inherent ability to sleep if he or she returns to sleep with such minimal intervention. A truly frightened child may behave similarly, but usually parents can make this distinction. When associations are at fault, a youngster may seem angry at the parents if they do not do what he or she wants, but the child does not appear frightened.

Parents of children with sleep-onset association disorder are usually aware of one to three awakenings per night. Often the last several hours of the night are quiet again, reflecting the tendency of young children to return to delta sleep toward morning.

Once sleep-onset associations have been identified as the cause of a child's problem (i.e., interfering with return to sleep after normal nighttime awakenings), and if the parents want to take steps to improve matters, an appropriate pattern of intervention can be designed. Typically, this involves giving the youngster a chance to learn to make the transition from wake to sleep under the conditions that will be present at the time of spontaneous nighttime awakenings.[1,7,25,26,29,45,48–53] If these conditions mean being in the crib alone, in a relatively dark and quiet room, then they should be the ones in which the youngster learns to go to sleep. Although some workers begin the training at nap-time,[48] it seems reasonable to start at bedtime, when the drive to sleep is greater. If there is any question about when the child is ready to fall asleep, the chosen time should be somewhat on the late side, to be sure. The youngster simply needs to be put down awake after an appropriate bedtime ritual and given increasing amounts of time to fall asleep, interrupted by brief parental visits for reassurance. The same patterns should be used at times of nighttime awakenings, increasing the waiting times as needed on successive nights.

Although some recommendations suggest starting before 2 months of age,[48] it seems appropriate to wait until it is clear that the youngster has the neurologic capability to manage these transitions smoothly. Because most children sleep through the night by the age of 5 or 6 months, this seems a reasonable time to start. Starting the training process from the beginning (i.e., always putting a youngster down awake) in an effort to avoid problems later on makes little sense, as it is unclear why trying to teach a neonate to negotiate the transitions to sleep alone is of any particular value. Parental closeness is very more important for neonates, and, if necessary, new patterns can be learned later on without much difficulty. The learning process generally takes only one to three nights.

Another approach is scheduled awakenings.[54–57] The child is awakened during the night before the expected time of natural awakening. The assumption is that the child is quite sleepy at that point (as opposed to being in a lighter sleep), can go to sleep more quickly with less parental intervention, will learn new habits at that time, and will sleep through subsequent times of usual awakenings.

In some situations it is best to have the parents sleep in the child's room for 1–2 weeks, so as to be present at times of awakening but not to reinstitute rocking or other learned associations. This is particularly useful for a child with separation (or other) anxiety. In this case, the reassurance of having a parent in the room is enough to let the child return to sleep. This differs from the situation of a youngster for whom the habitual nighttime interventions themselves, not parental reassurance, is desired. In fact, such a child often finds it more frustrating to have a parent nearby if the parent refuses to rock or pat him.

### Nocturnal Eating Disorder

A youngster with nocturnal eating disorder is fed at times of nighttime awakening (and usually also at bedtime).[1,7,22,28,36,44,45,58–61] To some degree, this is analogous to the problem just discussed, sleep-onset associations, if the youngster falls asleep at the breast or while taking a bottle. The difference is that when there are excessive feedings, the child has more awakenings at night than when the problem is just one of sleep-onset associations.

To make this diagnosis, one must be sure that the number of nighttime awakenings is more than is required for nutritional purposes. Although many children continue to be fed at night beyond age 5 or 6 months, this is generally the result of habit, not need. Continued nighttime feeding after 6 months does not define the existence of a problem; this depends on the frequency of awakenings at night and the effect they have on family members who have to deal with them. An 8-month-old child who is fed six times a night has his or her sleep disrupted to a degree that is unlikely to be in the child's best interests, however, regardless of whether the parents see the awakenings as a problem for themselves.

Beside the factor of associations, the feedings themselves have a major impact. The amount of milk or juice taken during the night is frequently extraordinary, up to a quart (four bottles) or more. It is easy to understand how such intake can disrupt sleep. With intake of food there is stimulation of digestive processes, increased body temperature and other disruptions of circadian cycling, and increased urine output—all factors that may lead to increased awakenings. In addition, a youngster who learns to expect feeding during the night learns to get hungry at those times.[1,7,8,23,24,39,45,62] The associated gastric contractions and central signals can also stimulate arousal. The effect on the circadian system should not be underestimated. A youngster who continues to feed multiple times during the night remains on a pattern typical of early infancy, when sleeping, waking, and feeding are all distributed across the 24-hour day.[24,39]

If the nighttime feedings take place through nursing, this must be carefully explored with the mother before changes are made. It must be clear what her desires are regarding nighttime nursing, when she plans or desires to wean, and what she would consider ideal. Although most nursing is done for appropriate reasons (i.e., the mother's desire to care for and nurture her child), some psychosocial settings have pathologic overtones (e.g., marital discord with parents looking for excuses to be apart during the night, self-image difficulties with the mother needing to be nurtured herself, nonparticipation of the father, depression). A youngster who is fed at night by bottle often does not even require the presence of a parent during the process of returning to sleep; the child just needs someone to hand him or her another bottle (in this case it is obvious that neither separation nor social nurturance issues are key).

If the family decides to decrease or eliminate the nighttime feedings, there are different ways it can be accomplished[7,45,62] and these should be discussed with the family so that they can choose the one they feel best suits them. Perhaps the easiest is simply to progressively lengthen the interval between feedings (e.g., increasing it by 30 minutes each night), eliminating the nighttime feedings over approximately 1 week. Decreasing the amount of milk or juice per bottle may also help. Some families prefer to water down the formula or juice progressively; once only water is given, the nutritional aspects of nighttime feedings are eliminated, and then the water may be stopped. The association problems that may be part of the difficulty can be dealt with at the same time or after the feedings stop.

It is not always necessary to eliminate the bedtime feeding. If bedtime feeding is kept, the youngster should be fed and put into the crib. He or she should not be allowed back to the breast or given another bottle after that (even if he or she wakes at time of transition), to prevent an extended problem of association from developing. Occasionally, a parent wants to decrease nighttime feedings from several to one. This can be attempted by spacing out the minimum time between feedings and then stopping at a preselected time (such as 5 hours). This is often, but not always, successful.

### Limit-Setting Sleep Disorders

Limit-setting sleep disorder is usually seen in youngsters aged 3–6 years (i.e., somewhat older than those discussed in the previous section). Problems often start the day a child learns how to climb out of a crib or is moved to a bed for other reasons. With the loss of the control previously represented by the bars of the crib, the locus of nocturnal control is shifted from the parents to the youngster. The child is now expected to control his or her own urges, including the desire to put off bedtime, make endless requests, and leave the bed and room. The same thing may occur even if the youngster sleeps in the parents' bed. If parents are unable to enforce control by setting appropriate limits, the youngster becomes increasingly anxious,[63–65] limits are further tested, tension increases, and the night becomes more difficult.

A typical scenario is that of a child stalling at bedtime with multiple requests for an extra story, another glass of water, to watch more television, or to make additional trips to the bathroom. The more the parents give in to these requests, the more the child continues to make them (often searching for the point at which a limit will be set). If the parents are not nearby, the child may get out of bed and search for them.

Many factors have to be considered in these situations. A parent may not understand the importance of setting limits or that it is actually part of appropriate nurturing and not punishment. This point must be made clear. The tension that exists in the home when parents are distraught at the child's continued demands is certainly not in the youngster's best interest. A little boy who climbs into his parents' bed and kicks his father until his father goes to another room to sleep is made to feel inappropriately powerful and may be frightened by that power rather than happy at getting what he wanted. Moreover, parents may have no idea how to set limits.

Another consideration is secondary gain. Although parents may not like their daughter getting up in the middle of the night, they may enjoy cuddling with her in front of the television in the late evening. This sends the child mixed messages.

The issue of guilt is a complicated one. It is very difficult to set limits for a youngster who has, or had, significant medical problems (e.g., prematurity, chronic illness, deafness). It may be impossible (and often is contraindicated) to set firm limits in a home where there is ongoing psychosocial stress owing to marital discord, depression, alcoholism, financial difficulties, or a recent move. A child in such circumstances who is not being appropriately nurtured during the day may use the struggles at night as a way of ensuring interaction with the parents, even though the tone of the interaction is negative.

Finally, to make the diagnosis of a limit-setting disorder, one assumes that the youngster is ready to fall asleep at the designated bedtime. If circadian factors are taken into consideration, what at first appears to be a limit-setting disorder may be a schedule disorder.[66,67] A careful history is usually sufficient to make this distinction.

Management must take into account why this disorder exists. If the need is clearly to replace limits that have been lost (or were never present), then considerable time must be spent working with the family. First is the process of education, helping the parents understand that setting limits is important to a youngster's development. Then a concrete plan for setting limits that the family can follow must be devised.[45,58,68,69] Often this can be done quite easily, such as replacing the bars of the crib with gates at the doorway. Parents can respond in a progressive manner, coming back to the gates (as outlined for an association problem). A youngster who can knock gates over or climb over even a double gate may have to be kept in the room with the door closed,[7,10] although it is never reasonable to leave a child behind a locked door. The closed door serves as a passive limit setter, to avoid major confrontation between parents and child while enforcing the parents' rules. This should be done with the parent by the door and starting with very short closure time (approximately 30 seconds). The objective is not to frighten the youngster, only to set and enforce rules.

Older children (at least age 3 years) may be motivated with a star chart or some other reward system.[7,26,45] If the child is motivated and is willing to follow through with such a program, that is preferred; a positive reinforcement system is always better than a negative one.

Often, to the parents' surprise, once limits are firmly set, anxiety decreases markedly[8,64] and the youngster becomes much happier in the evening as nighttime tensions disappear. In fact, such children frequently remind their parents to close the gate before they leave, to be sure the parents remain in control.

In situations involving guilt, secondary gain, or psychosocial difficulties, there must be careful evaluation and discussion before proceeding.[8,9,24,35] Parents who feel guilty may need to have more gradual limit-setting measures outlined for them; those who

get secondary gain from the nighttime experience may have to understand it and be willing to give it up; and families with psychosocial difficulties may require very individualized care. In this last setting, a child may actually need more access to the parents at night (as well as during the day), and it may be best to hold off on a strict limit-setting program until the psychosocial issues themselves can be better addressed. Counseling is often indicated.[8,9]

### *Food Allergy Insomnia*

Kahn and associates[70–72] have described a condition of food allergy insomnia in which young children with documented allergy to cow's milk protein have severely disrupted sleep. Typically, they have delayed sleep initiation and frequent and prolonged nighttime awakenings. Symptoms begin whenever cow's milk is introduced into the diet. Total sleep time is often significantly reduced. In addition, more typical systemic signs of milk allergy, such as eczema, wheezing, or gastrointestinal disturbances, may be minimal or absent. Regardless of treatment, there is generally spontaneous resolution by age 2–4 years.

Radioallergosorbent testing in children with this allergy to cow's milk shows elevated immunoglobulin E (IgE) against β-lactoglobulin. Eosinophil count, IgE titer, and skin reactivity may be normal, especially before the first birthday. There may be some cross-reactivity with soy-based products.

Switching to a hypoallergenic hydrolyzed formula is followed by resolution of symptoms within days to weeks. A challenge with even small amounts of cow's milk protein causes a return of symptoms until the apparent allergy is outgrown.

For some reason, this disorder has not frequently been described in the United States. Perhaps this is because of the tendency of U.S. pediatricians to switch formulas empirically when things are not going well. Sensitivity of children's sleep to other dietary agents has also been described.[73]

### *Circadian Rhythm Sleep Disorders*

#### *Delayed or Advanced Sleep Phase*

Circadian rhythm disorders have been well-described in adults (see Chapter 30).[21,74] The syndromes are conceptually the same in young children, except that it is the parents' dissatisfaction with the schedule that generates the complaint. Strictly speaking, these are situations in which a youngster gets (or is capable of getting) a normal amount of sleep at night but it does not occur during the desired hours (neither the start nor end of the spontaneous sleep period is at an appropriate time.[21,66,74,75]

A child with an advanced sleep phase may fall asleep by 7:00 PM but awaken at 4:00 or 5:00 AM. The complaint is one of early morning awakenings. The parents of a youngster with a delayed sleep phase may complain that it takes him several hours to fall asleep (perhaps not until 10:00 PM or later) but that the time of spontaneous morning awakening is at or later than the desired hour (perhaps anywhere from 7:00 to 10:00 AM).

A careful history of a child with an advanced sleep phase usually shows advance of other aspects of the daytime schedule, including meals and naptimes.[7,66,67] The child who awakens at 5:00 AM may be fed shortly after that and nap as early as 7:00 AM. Both the early feeding and early nap may contribute to persistence of this syndrome.[7,67] The bedtime behavior of a child with a delayed sleep phase may resemble that of a youngster with limit-setting difficulties, but there is one major difference. In the situation of a phase delay, the youngster is completely unable to fall asleep, even if the parents set very firm limits. Instead of calling and coming out of bed, some youngsters try to "be good" and lie in bed each night for hours, waiting for sleepiness (and sleep) to arrive. During that time they are generally not allowed to read, listen to the radio, or watch television. They must lie in the dark room, and they have nothing to do but think. Thinking in a dark room may lead to fantasy, and fantasy may lead to scary thoughts. Some of these youngsters end up scaring themselves, and nighttime fears may be the presenting complaint.

The diagnosis should come from a careful history.[9,34,35] The child with an advanced sleep phase falls asleep easily and sleeps normally. Although the child awakens early, it is after a normal amount of sleep (the amount of daytime sleep must be taken into account).

The youngster with a delayed sleep phase must be distinguished from one with a limit-setting disorder or true nighttime fears. Typically, the time of

sleep onset is fairly independent of the bedtime. A youngster who falls asleep at 10:00 PM usually does so regardless of what hour he or she is put to bed; only the sleep latency changes. If a history of occasional late bedtimes can be obtained, much shorter sleep latencies will usually be reported. On a night when the family does not get home until after the child's usual hour of sleep onset, the child likely falls asleep in the car. Weekend and vacation schedules may be similarly helpful in recognizing this syndrome. Also, a child who scares himself or herself because of long sleep latency will not experience nighttime fears on nights that he or she goes to bed late.

Often these children are allowed (or want) to sleep late in the morning. If they are attending school or day care, late morning sleep may be limited to weekends. Awakening them earlier during the week may be accomplished only with great difficulty. Although later sleep is expected on weekends, this is not always the case with children old enough to watch television by themselves. A 5-year-old boy may get up early on the weekends (despite having to be awakened at that hour during the week) only to creep into a dark room to watch television for several hours. He probably dozes by the television; he certainly is not fully awake. To determine the true end of the sleep phase, it is more important to find out when the youngster climbs out from under the blanket on the sofa, asks for breakfast, and appears to be wide awake.

In young children, a delayed sleep phase can usually be corrected easily by controlling morning awakening.[7,66,67] It is best to start with a late bedtime, at the time the youngster actually has been falling asleep, to remove the stresses that have been present during the presleep hours and to help the youngster become accustomed to falling asleep quickly. If she is awakened for school or day care 5 days a week, this schedule should be enforced on weekends as well. If she usually sleeps late, the time of awakening can be advanced gradually, perhaps by 15 minutes a day. Once awakening is better controlled, bedtime can be slowly advanced in a similar manner.

It is best to ensure that the youngster is up, fed, and moving about in the morning, preferably exposed to as much light as possible. Formal use of light boxes[76] or around-the-clock progressive phase delay[77] is not usually necessary at this age.

For a child with an advanced sleep phase, ensuring plenty of light in the evening, progressively delaying bedtime, and progressively delaying the early morning meal and naptimes should lead to resolution. Control of early morning light exposure may also be helpful.

### Regular but Inappropriate Schedule

**Inappropriately Timed Meal or Nap.**    It is well-known that a regular nap in the late afternoon may delay the onset of sleep in the evening. What is less well-known is that a very early meal or naptime may reinforce early morning awakening.[7,66,67] Youngsters who nap very early, perhaps at 6:00 or 7:00 PM, may awaken at 5:00 AM only to return to sleep after 1–2 hours. The youngster acts as if the last sleep cycle was broken off from the night and moved 1–2 hours later. An early feeding, such as 5:00 AM (usually given because the youngster has awakened at that hour), may only reinforce continued early awakening, because the youngster learns to get hungry at that hour and hunger may trigger arousal. In these cases, nap and feeding times may need adjustment. The morning nap may be delayed to an appropriate time, such as 10:00 AM, it may be moved into the afternoon as a single nap (if the child is older than 1 year), or it may be eliminated altogether (depending on the age of the child). Similarly, the first feeding in the morning may be delayed gradually to an appropriate breakfast time (perhaps 6:00 or 7:00 AM). Such interventions allow for later sleep in the morning.

**Time in Bed Is More Than Sleep Requirement.** The syndrome of spending too much time in bed is similar to one sometimes seen in elderly individuals, but again, it is not the child's own decision to do so but that of the parents. It is not at all uncommon for parents to incorrectly estimate the amount of sleep their youngster needs.[78] Their estimate is often based on desire rather than reason. Thus, parents may decide that their 18-month-old child should get 11 hours of sleep at night, and they keep him in the crib from 7:00 PM to 6:00 AM. In fact, this child may need and get 11 hours of sleep, but it is 11 hours per 24 hours. He may get 2 hours as part of a regular afternoon nap, leaving only 9 hours to sleep at night. These hours of nighttime sleep might run from 7:00 PM to 4:00 AM or, more commonly, from 9:00 PM to 6:00 AM. In both cases, the parents leave an unhappy, wakeful child in the crib for 2 hours. In the first case, these hours are from 7:00 (when the parents insist on putting the child to bed) until 9:00 PM (when the child finally is able to fall asleep). In the second case, it is from 4:00 (when the child finished sleeping) until 6:00 AM (when the parents are willing to take the child out of the crib). Older children may be forced to spend too much time in bed as well, but at least sometimes they are allowed to read or play (if they can do so quietly).

Some youngsters split their sleep time into two segments, separated by an extended period of nighttime wakefulness. A child might sleep from 7:00 PM to 1:00 AM and from 3:00 to 6:00 AM, and still get the same 9 hours at night. In this case, no type of parental intervention during the period of nighttime wakefulness will get the youngster back to sleep. He or she is wide awake, just wants to play, and is usually allowed to do so (although young children are sometimes simply left crying in the crib).

The solution to all of these problems is the same: The time in bed should be limited to the sleep requirement.[7,66,67,78,79] In the cases described earlier, bedtime and awakening should be 9 hours apart, whichever 9 hours the parents find most workable (perhaps 9:00 PM to 6:00 AM or even 10:00 PM to 7:00 AM). The child should not be allowed to play in the middle of the night. Daytime naps should continue but should not be extended. Problems generally resolve quickly.

Sometimes the total sleep time is inappropriately divided into nighttime sleep that is too short and daytime sleep that is too long. A 15-month-old may be taking a 3- or 4-hour nap (or two 2-hour naps), leaving time for only 7–8 hours to sleep at night. In this case, of course, part of the treatment involves limiting the naptime to that appropriate for age.

### Medical and Psychiatric Sleep Disorders

#### Sleep Disorders Associated with Mental Disorders

In young children, the most common "psychiatric" disorder affecting sleep is anxiety. Fears and worries of various kinds are common in young childhood, and many are considered normal, especially if they are transient. In some cases the fears are more pronounced, passing beyond the bounds of what might be considered a normal developmental stage.[52,63,80]

It is common for children to pass through a period of separation anxiety toward the end of the first year. In addition, as they go through other developmental hurdles, such as toilet training, the start of school, and accepting a new sibling into the home, transient regression is common with a return of anxiety. Other problems may reflect more general psychosocial issues in the home, such as marital strife, divorce, alcoholism, depression, parental fighting, abuse, drug use, and lack of appropriate nurturance. A child who has handicaps or undergoes frequent medical or surgical procedures may have good reason for increased needs or worries.

In terms of sleep, anxiety usually causes a child to be unwilling to separate from parents at night. If this is the only problem, the child is able to fall asleep without difficulty as long as parents are close by, either in the child's room or with the child in theirs. The fact that such a youngster falls asleep quickly when sleeping with or close to the parents helps rule out many other causes of sleeplessness, such as the circadian issues described earlier. Even a child who is using a complaint of fears as an excuse to be back in the living room watching television usually can be differentiated from one who is truly afraid. A manipulative youngster is not happy simply having a parent nearby, even in the child's room; such a child is happy only to get his or her own way, perhaps by going back to the living room (and there, the parents may not even have to be present).

Children who are truly frightened appear so, and most often the parents are able to recognize this and describe it in a convincing manner (they similarly can identify a youngster who is just demanding). Anxious youngsters may become quite panicky as bedtime approaches. They usually do not enjoy the bedtime routines because they are fearful of the separation that will follow, and they become progressively more upset. Some children are sufficiently frightened that they are willing to accept any punishment simply to be allowed to be near the parents.

The main challenge in making diagnostic and treatment decisions is to identify the severity (and source) of the anxiety. If it is very mild, firm reassurance is often all that is necessary. Because part of the anxiety can stem from a lack of limit setting,

setting limits or making existing limits more strict can be beneficial. However, a child who is truly frightened at night will not be helped by increased limits. In fact, increased limits (and separation) may only increase fears. Whatever is necessary to make such a child feel safe and comfortable at night should be provided. This may require that a parent sleep in the child's room temporarily, or that the child sleep in the parents' room or bed. If the child is old enough, a sleeping bag on the floor of the parents' bedroom is often sufficient.

A child who is sufficiently verbal can discuss his or her concerns with the examiner, allowing for appropriate planning of treatment. Sometimes the youngster only needs the reassurance of having a parent on the same floor of the house when he goes to sleep (being on the second floor of a house alone at bedtime may be frightening, even to a child without other major fears). A child may also indicate that having a parent upstairs to look into the room every 5 minutes until the child goes to sleep is sufficient to allay his or her fears. However, the child may make it clear that even that degree of separation cannot be tolerated.

If the anxiety is relatively mild, it can be dealt with often by providing the supports necessary, developing a reward system, and gradually, with the youngster's approval, decreasing the degree of support. Each time the youngster is successful, he feels more confident, is able to take the next step, and is reassured. When the fears are long-standing and significant, however, professional counseling (family or individual) is usually required.

*Sleep Disorders Associated with Neurologic Disorders*

The list of sleep disorders associated with neurologic disorders is large, including neonatal insults, abnormalities in the development of the nervous system, and epilepsy and associated drug therapy.[81] Children with central nervous system dysfunction are subject to the same type of sleep disorders as other youngsters, perhaps more so because of parents' guilt feelings, which affect the pattern of nighttime intervention. When the disorders are severe and psychomotor retardation is marked, normal interaction with family members may not be possible, sleep may become inappropriately distributed across the day, and nighttime sleep may be severely disrupted.[82] Much more careful control of the timing and regularity of sleep may be an important consideration.

Certain children have severe sleep disorders that do not fit into other categories. These sleep abnormalities appear to be due to dysfunction of the central systems that control sleep. This is seen with considerable frequency in youngsters with pervasive developmental delay (autism) and in those with severe malformations or injury of the central nervous system. In these cases, total (day plus night) sleep time may be severely limited.[2] Although the electrophysiologic aspects of sleep in an autistic child are generally normal, this is not necessarily the case when more clear-cut structural abnormalities are present.

Behavioral intervention may not be sufficient to manage these children. One must keep in mind that managing such a child at home may be extremely difficult for even the most caring of families. Such a child may require a great deal of attention throughout the day. If the child gets only 5 hours of sleep, the parents do not have sufficient time to recuperate. Because of this (and because of the central dysfunction), pharmacologic intervention may have to be considered. There are few formal studies of such drug interventions in young children, and it is difficult to generalize from studies in any case because many of these youngsters differ significantly in their structural abnormalities. Anecdotally, we can report from work in our center that the types of medication generally used for adult insomnia (such as benzodiazepines) usually are not effective in these youngsters.[2] (It is probably correct to assume that if such a mild sedative could induce sleep in one of these children, behavioral methods would work as well.)

The drug with which we have had the best and most consistent results is chloral hydrate, a drug that has been useful in pediatrics for many years.[2] However, the physician must be prepared to give sedative doses. Small doses that only make the child drowsy can actually worsen behavior and not improve sleep. We have found that doses of 500–2,500 mg (i.e., up to about 50 mg/kg) sometimes are necessary. The aim is to increase nighttime sleep and improve, or at least not worsen, daytime function. The smallest effective doses should be used, and periodically the dose should be tapered to see if it is still needed. Often a satisfac-tory dose can be found and maintained for months to years, increasing only to adjust for growth of the child. It is reasonable to obtain periodic blood screens, although hematopoietic or hepatic side effects are not common. One problem with chloral hydrate is its taste, however, which is very bitter and cannot be hidden in chocolate, sugar, or honey. It comes in a gelcap form for children who can take pills. It is preferable to avoid nightly use of suppositories, as they often are expelled. Alternative medications include clonidine and promethazine, which are sometimes successful in these settings. Clonidine is particularly useful in children who are being treated for attention-deficit hyperactivity disorder.[83] There have been reports of improvement in neurologically impaired children treated with melatonin.[84,85] Melatonin is a relatively nontoxic agent and may be a good choice if subsequent research documents efficacy and clarifies indications.

Although one should approach use of high levels of medication in children with great hesitancy, physicians must be willing to treat when indicated. Helping such a youngster increase sleep from 5 to 8 hours can have a tremendous impact on the family and may be the deciding factor that allows the family to keep the child at home rather than placing him or her in an institution. Parents often report some improvement in the child's daytime function with more sleep, a clear additional benefit.

### Sleep Disorders Associated with Other Medical Disorders

Almost any medical problem may be associated with a sleep disorder because of direct effects on the sleep system, associated fever, pain, medication, or parental concern. These are obvious in short-term situations and usually do not demand intervention.

Certain medical problems may be more chronic and problematic. Asthma, with nighttime wheezing (and associated fear), may be disruptive and is usually treated by medication and, if necessary, counseling.[86,87] The stimulant medications used to treat asthma (such as theophylline), however, may be directly responsible for sleep disruption. Changing the dosage or switching to an inhaled preparation is sometimes helpful.

Gastroesophageal reflux, chronic middle ear disease, or atopic dermatitis may be associated with poor sleep.[45,88] Often there are nighttime awakenings associated with these conditions, when the child seems to be in discomfort. Parental interventions are slow to aid return to sleep after such awakenings. Treating the underlying condition, medically or surgically, is usually curative.

Colic is the most common cause of sleep difficulties in an infant's early months. Typical symptoms include irritability and inconsolable crying, especially in the late afternoon and evening.[46,47,89–91] Colic usually resolves by 3 months of age, and because nighttime sleep is not expected to consolidate before then, it is actually the consequences of patterns developed during the colicky period that are most relevant. These youngsters often are held, walked, rocked, placed in a swing, or patted in an effort to calm them and help them fall asleep. The patterns may persist after the colic has disappeared, creating a routine that the child associates with sleep. If the child cannot fall asleep without this attention, the habits need to be modified.

Finally, every medication must be considered a potential sleep disrupter in a given child. Probably even certain additives in liquid preparations affect youngsters in undesirable ways. In addition, the underlying medical problem that requires a child to take medication routinely, as well as associated psychosocial effects, must be considered. For example, a young leukemia patient on chemotherapy has many reasons for sleeping poorly: the effects of the illness itself, the medication, concerns about the illness, family concerns about the illness, and altered patterns of parent-child interaction. Separating these variables and designing appropriate therapy are the greatest challenges to the sleep clinician.

## REFERENCES

1. Ferber R. Childhood sleep disorders. Neurol Clin 1996;14:493.
2. Ferber R. Unpublished data. 1997.
3. Dahl RE, Holttum J, Trubnick L. A clinical picture of child and adolescent narcolepsy. J Am Acad Child Adolesc Psychiatry 1994;33:834.
4. Brown LW, Billiard M. Narcolepsy, Kleine-Levin Syndrome, and Other Causes of Sleepiness in Children. In R Ferber, M Kryger (eds), Principles and Practice of Sleep Medicine in the Child. Philadelphia: Saunders, 1995;125.
5. Carroll JL, Loughlin GM. Obstructive Sleep Apnea Syndrome in Infants and Children: Clinical Features and Pathophysiology. In R Ferber, M Kryger (eds), Principles and Practice of Sleep Medicine in the Child. Philadelphia: Saunders, 1995;163.
6. Rosen G, Mahowald MW, Ferber R. Sleepwalking, Confusional Arousals, and Sleep Terrors in the Child. In R Ferber, M Kryger (eds), Principles and Practice of Sleep Medicine in the Child. Philadelphia: Saunders, 1995;99.
7. Ferber RA. Solve Your Child's Sleep Problem. New York: Simon & Schuster, 1985.
8. Ferber RA. Behavioral "insomnia" in the child. Psychiatr Clin North Am 1988;10:641.
9. Ferber RA. Assessment Procedures for Diagnosis of Sleep Disorders in Children. In JD Noshpitz (ed), Basic Handbook of Child Psychiatry (Vol V). New York: Basic Books, 1987;185.
10. Ferber R. Sleeplessness in the Child. In MH Kryger, T Roth, WC Dement (eds), Principles and Practice of Sleep Medicine. Philadelphia: Saunders, 1989;633.
11. Ellingson RJ. Ontogenesis of Sleep in the Human. In GC Lairy, R Salzarulo (eds), Experimental Study of Human Sleep: Methodological Problems. Amsterdam: Elsevier, 1975;120.
12. Metcalf D, Mondale J, Butler F. Ontogenesis of spontaneous K complexes. Psychophysiology 1971;8:340.
13. Metcalf D. Sleep Spindle Ontogenesis in Normal Children. In W Smith (ed), Drugs, Development, and Cerebral Function. Springfield, IL: Thomas, 1972;12.
14. Parmelee AH. Ontogeny of Sleep Patterns and Associated Periodicities in Infants. In E Faulkner, N Kretchmer, E Ross (eds), Pre- and Postnatal Development of the Human Brain. Basel: Karger, 1974;298.
15. Lenard HG. Sleep studies in infancy. Acta Paediatr Scand 1970;59:572.
16. Anders TF, Sadeh A, Appareddy V. Normal Sleep in Neonates and Children. In R Ferber, M Kryger (eds), Principles and Practice of Sleep Medicine in the Child. Philadelphia: Saunders, 1995;7.
17. Stern E, Parmelee AH, Harris MA. Sleep state periodicity in prematures and young infants. Dev Psychobiol 1973;6:357.
18. Stern E, Parmelee AH, Akiyama Y, et al. Sleep cycle characteristics in infants. Pediatrics 1969,43:65.
19. Coons S, Guilleminault C. Development of consolidated sleep and wakeful periods in relation to the day/night cycle in infancy. Dev Med Child Neurol 1984;26:169.
20. Glotzbach SF, Edgar DM, Boeddiker M, Ariagno RL. Biological rhythmicity in normal infants during the first 3 months of life. Pediatrics 1994;94:482.
21. Moore-Ede MC, Sulzman FM, Fuller CA. The Clocks That Time Us. Cambridge, MA: Harvard University Press, 1982.
22. Moore T, Ucko LE. Nightwaking in early infancy: Part 1. Arch Dis Child 1957;32:333.
23. Ragins N, Schachter S. A study of sleep behavior in two-year-old children. J Am Acad Child Psychiatry 1971;10:464.

24. Ferber R. The Sleepless Child. In C Guilleminault (ed), Sleep and Its Disorders in Children. New York: Raven, 1987;141.

25. Douglas J, Richman N. My Child Won't Sleep: A Handbook of Management for Parents. London: Penguin, 1984.

26. Douglas J, Richman N. Sleep Management Manual. London: Department of Psychological Medicine, Hospital for Sick Children, 1982.

27. Ferber R. Sleep, sleeplessness, and sleep disruptions in infants and young children. Ann Clin Res 1985;17:227.

28. Richman N. A community survey of characteristics of one- to two-year-olds with sleep disruptions. J Am Acad Child Psychiatry 1981;20:281.

29. Richman N. Sleep problems in young children. Arch Dis Child 1984;56:491.

30. Carey W. Night waking and temperament in infancy. J Pediatr 1974;84:756.

31. Atkinson E, Vetere A, Grayson K. Sleep disruption in young children. The influence of temperament on the sleep patterns of pre-school children. Child Care Health Dev 1995;21:233.

32. Zorick FJ, Roth T, Hartse K, et al. Evaluation and diagnosis of persistent insomnia. Am J Psychiatry 1981;138:769.

33. Kripke DF, Simons RN, Garfinkle L, et al. Short and long sleep and sleeping pills: is increased mortality associated? Arch Gen Psychiatry 1970;36:103.

34. Ferber R. Clinical assessment of child and adolescent sleep disorders. Child Adolesc Psychiatry Clin North Am 1996;5:569.

35. Ferber R. Assessment of Sleep Disorders in the Child. In R Ferber, M Kryger (eds), Principles and Practice of Sleep Medicine in the Child. Philadelphia: Saunders, 1995;45.

36. Diagnostic Classification Steering Committee. International Classification of Sleep Disorders: Diagnostic and Coding Manual. Rochester, MN: American Sleep Disorders Association, 1990.

37. Adair RH, Bauchner H. Sleep problems in childhood. Curr Probl Pediatr 1993;23:147.

38. Ferber R, Boyle MP. Sleeplessness in infants and toddlers: sleep initiation difficulty masquerading as a sleep maintenance insomnia. Sleep Res 1983;12:240.

39. Ferber R. Sleeplessness, night awakening, and night crying in the infant and toddler. Pediatr Rev 1987;9:1.

40. Illingworth R. The child who won't sleep and whose parents won't let him. Mims Mag 1976;71.

41. Illingworth RS. Sleep problems in the first three years. BMJ 1951;1:722.

42. Bax MCO. Sleep disturbance in the young child. BMJ 1980;280:1177.

43. Bax M. Sleep (Editorial). Dev Med Child Neurol 1983;25:281.

44. Ferber R. Childhood Insomnia. In M Thorpy (ed), Handbook of Sleep Disorders. New York: Marcel Dekker, 1990;435.

45. Ferber R. Sleeplessness in Children. In R Ferber, M Kryger (eds), Principles and Practice of Sleep Medicine in the Child. Philadelphia: Saunders, 1995;79.

46. Weissbluth M. Crybabies: Coping with Colic: What To Do When Baby Won't Stop Crying. New York: Arbor House, 1984.

47. Weissbluth M. Colic. In R Ferber, M Kryger (eds), Principles and Practice of Sleep Medicine in the Child. Philadelphia: Saunders, 1995;75.

48. Cutherbertson J, Schevill S. Helping Your Child Sleep Through the Night. Garden City, NY: Doubleday, 1985.

49. Jones DPH, Verduyn CM. Behavioral management of sleep problems. Arch Dis Child 1983;58:442.

50. Younger JB. The management of night waking in older infants. Pediatr Nurs 1982;8:155.

51. Largo RH, Hunziker UA. A developmental approach to the management of children with sleep disturbances in the first three years of life. Eur J Pediatr 1984;142:170.

52. Leach P. Babyhood. New York: Knopf, 1976.

53. Valman HB. Sleep problems. BMJ 1981;283:422.

54. Johnson CM, Bradley-Johnson S, Stack JM. Decreasing the frequency of infants' nocturnal crying with the use of scheduled awakenings. Fam Pract Res J 1981;1:98.

55. Johnson CM, Lerner M. Amelioration of infant sleep disturbances: II. Effects of scheduled awakenings by compliant parents. Infant Ment Health J 1985;6:21.

56. McGarr RJ, Hovell MF. In search of the sand man: shaping an infant to sleep. Treatment Child 1980;3:173.

57. Rickert VI, Johnson CM. Reducing nocturnal awakening and crying episodes in infants and young children: a comparison between scheduled awakenings and systematic ignoring. Pediatrics 1988;81:203.

58. Ferber R, Boyle MP. Nocturnal fluid intake: a cause of, not treatment for, sleep disruption in infants and toddlers. Sleep Res 1983;12:243.

59. Osterholm P, Lindeke LL, Amidon D. Sleep disturbance in infants aged 6 to 12 months. Pediatr Nurs 1983;9:269.

60. Van Tassel EB. The relative influence of child and environmental characteristics on sleep disturbances in the first and second years of life. J Dev Behav Pediatr 1985;6:81.

61. Wright P, MacLeod HA, Cooper MJ. Waking at night: the effect of early feeding experience. Child Care Health Dev 1983;9:309.

62. Panilla T, Birch LL. Help me make it through the night: behavioral entrainment of breast-fed infants' sleep patterns. Pediatrics 1993;91:436.

63. Fraiberg SH. The Magic Years. New York: Scribner's, 1959.

64. Leach P. Your Baby and Child, from Birth to Age Five. New York: Knopf, 1978.

65. Blampied NM, France KG. A behavioral model of infant sleep disturbance. J Appl Behav Anal 1993; 26:477.

66. Ferber R. Circadian and Schedule Disturbances. In C Guilleminault (ed), Sleep and Its Disorders in Children. New York: Raven, 1987;165.

67. Ferber R. Circadian Rhythm Sleep Disorders in Childhood. In R Ferber, M Kryger (eds), Principles and Prac-

tice of Sleep Medicine in the Child. Philadelphia: Saunders, 1995;91.

68. Jackson H, Rawlins MD. The sleepless child. BMJ 1979;2:509.

69. Kleitman N. Sleep and Wakefulness. Chicago: University of Chicago Press, 1939.

70. Kahn A, Mozin MJ, Casimir G, et al. Insomnia and cow's milk allergy in infants. Pediatrics 1985;76:880.

71. Kahn A, Rebuffat E, Blum D, et al. Difficulty in initiating and maintaining sleep associated with cow's milk allergy in infants. Sleep 1987;10:116.

72. Kahn A, Francois G, Sottiaux M, et al. Sleep characteristics in milk-intolerant infants. Sleep 1988;11:291.

73. Rowe KS, Rowe KJ. Synthetic food coloring and behavior: a dose response effect in a double-blind, placebo-controlled, repeated-measures study. J Pediatr 1994;125:691.

74. Weitzman ED, Czeisler CA, Coleman RM, et al. Delayed sleep phase syndrome: a chronobiologic disorder with sleep onset insomnia. Arch Gen Psychiatry 1981;38:737.

75. Ferber R, Boyle MP. Phase shift dyssomnia in early childhood. Sleep Res 1983;12:242.

76. Lewy AJ, Sack RL. Light therapy and psychiatry. Proc Soc Exp Biol Med 1986;183:11.

77. Czeisler CA, Richardson GS, Coleman RM, et al. Chronotherapy: resetting the circadian clocks of patients with delayed sleep phase insomnia. Sleep 1981;4:1.

78. Galofre I, Santacana P, Ferber R. The "TIB>TST" syndrome. A cause of wakefulness in children. Sleep Res 1992;21:199.

79. Hauri P. Behavioral treatment of insomnia. Med Times 1979;107:36.

80. Dahl RE. Sleep in Behavioral and Emotional Disorders. In R Ferber, M Kryger (eds), Principles and Practice of Sleep Medicine in the Child. Philadelphia: Saunders, 1995;147.

81. Brown LW, Maistros P, Guilleminault C. Sleep in Children with Neurologic Problems. In R Ferber, M Kryger (eds), Principles and Practice of Sleep Medicine in the Child. Philadelphia: Saunders, 1995;135.

82. Okawa M, Sasaki H. Sleep Disorders in Mentally Retarded and Brain-Impaired Children. In C Guilleminault (ed), Sleep and Its Disorders in Children. New York: Raven, 1987;269.

83. Prince JB, Wilens TE, Biederman J, et al. Clonidine for sleep disturbances associated with attention-deficit hyperactivity disorder: a systematic chart review of 62 cases. J Am Acad Child Adolesc Psychiatry 1996; 35:599.

84. Jan JE, O'Donnell ME. Use of melatonin in the treatment of paediatric sleep disorders. J Pineal Res 1996;21:193.

85. Lapierre O, Dumont M. Melatonin treatment of a non–24-hour sleep-wake cycle in a blind retarded child. Biol Psychiatry 1995;38:119.

86. Gaultier C. Respiration During Sleep in Children with Chronic Obstructive Pulmonary Disease and Asthma. In C Guilleminault (ed), Sleep and Its Disorders in Children. New York: Raven, 1987;225.

87. Kales A, Kales JD, Sly RM, et al. Sleep pattern of asthmatic children: all-night electro-encephalographic studies. J Allergy 1970;46:301.

88. Dahl RE, Bernhisel-Broadbent J, Scanlon-Holdford S, et al. Sleep disturbances in children with atopic dermatitis. Arch Pediatr Adolesc Med 1995;149:856.

89. Weissbluth M. Sleep and the Colicky Infant. In C Guilleminault (ed), Sleep and Its Disorders in Children. New York: Raven, 1987;129.

90. Illingworth RS. "Three months" colic. Arch Dis Child 1954;29:167.

91. Wiessbluth M. Infant Colic. In SS Gellis, BM Kagan (eds), Current Pediatric Therapy (12th ed). Philadelphia: Saunders, 1986.

# Chapter 34
# Sleep and Epilepsy

## Sudhansu Chokroverty and Christine Quinto

The relationship between sleep and epilepsy has intrigued researchers and thinkers since antiquity. Passouant[1] mentioned Hippocrates' description of "fears, rages, deliria, leaps out of bed, and seizures during the night." Aristotle observed that in many cases epilepsy began during sleep. Despite these early observations, the intriguing relationship between seizure and sleep was neglected by the medical profession until the end of the last century. Echeverria,[2] Fere,[3] and Gowers[4] gave clear descriptions of the relationship of epilepsy to the sleep-wake cycle. In a study of hospitalized epileptics, Fere[3] noted that in more than two-thirds of 1,985 patients the attacks occurred between 8:00 PM and 8:00 AM. It is interesting to note that even in those days, Fere mentioned the effect of epilepsy on sleep—he noted apparently associated difficulties with falling asleep and impairment of sleep efficiency, suggesting the facilitation of seizures by sleep deprivation.

In the beginning of this century, Turner,[5] Gallus,[6] and Amann[7] emphasized that many seizures were nocturnal and occurred at certain times of the night. These reports were followed by those of Langdon-Down and Brain,[8] Patry,[9] Busciano,[10] and Magnussen.[11]

All of these early observations were made on the basis of clinical features alone and without the benefit of electroencephalography (EEG), which was not described until 1929. The observation of Gibbs and Gibbs[12] in 1947 of the occurrence of paroxysmal discharges in the EEG twice as often during sleep as during the waking state marks the begin-

ning of the modern era in the study of the relationship between epilepsy and sleep. Combining clinical and EEG observations showed that indeed a distinct relationship between epilepsy and sleep exists. This report was followed by many original observations, notably those of Janz,[13] Passouant,[14] Gastaut et al.,[15] Cadilhac,[16] Niedermeyer,[17] Montplaisir,[18] Broughton,[19] Billiard,[20] Kellaway and coworkers,[21] and other researchers.

This chapter provides an overview of the effect of sleep on epilepsy as well as the effect of epilepsy on sleep. The usefulness of sleep in the diagnosis of epilepsy and the practical relevance to understanding the relationship between sleep and epilepsy are also discussed.

## INTERRELATIONSHIP BETWEEN SLEEP AND EPILEPSY: PHYSIOLOGIC MECHANISMS

There is a reciprocal relationship between sleep and epilepsy: Sleep affects epilepsy, and epilepsy in turn affects sleep. To understand this relationship, it is important to review briefly the mechanism that generates paroxysmal EEG discharges and clinical seizures as well as the mechanism of initiation of sleep.

### Basic Mechanism of Epilepsy

An understanding of the basic mechanism of epilepsy is derived primarily from studies of animal models and human clinical epilepsy.[22] Experimental animal models of epilepsy are produced by topical application of agents or focal electrical stimulation to the neocortex and limbic cortex to provoke partial seizures, whereas electric shock or systemic injection of convulsants and penicillin have been used for generalized epilepsy models.[22] Neuronal synchronization and neuronal hyperexcitability are fundamental physiologic factors that may transform an interictal to an ictal state.[22] Factors enhancing synchronization are conducive to active ictal precipitation in susceptible individuals. These factors include nonspecific influences, such as sleep, sleep deprivation, and so on. In addition, seizure itself may produce sleep disturbance. A fundamental mechanism in the epileptic neurons is a paroxysmal depolarization shift in the epileptic neurons, originally described by Matsumoto and Ajmone-Marsan,[23] followed by after-hyperpolarization.[24]

Nonspecific thalamic reticular nuclei are responsible for recruiting, and specific thalamic nuclei are responsible for augmenting responses; both are also responsible for triggering generalized seizures by synchronizing afferent inputs to the cortex from these nuclei.[25,26] This thalamocortical interaction is responsible for changing the name of centrencephalic epilepsy to corticoreticular epilepsy for petit mal absence seizure.[27] The generalized tonic-clonic seizure is initiated in the cortex but the pontine reticular formation participates in the tonic phase.[22]

Epileptogenesis of the neurons is dependent on factors, both genetic and acquired, that maintain increased neuronal hyperexcitability and increased neuronal synchronization.[22] Examples of some of these factors are decreased dendritic spines and branches, cortical sprouting of surviving axons to cause increased synchronization, altered ionic microenvironment in and around the epileptic neurons, attenuation of inhibitory influences causing enhanced synchronization, and alteration of calcium and chloride ion channel distribution.[22]

It is important to understand the interictal state and precipitation of ictus as well as the mechanism of ictal termination and postictal state. The hallmark of an interictal state from the physiologic point of view is the focal or diffuse interictal EEG spike and wave discharge.[22] The epileptic neuronal aggregates show increased synchronization but with a decrease in firing rates, which may explain hypometabolism of the interictal focus as noted on

positron emission tomography (PET) using $^{18}$F-fluorodeoxyglucose scans.[22] Prevention of ictal spread and maintenance of interictal state are determined by strong inhibitory influences that also keep the neurons in an excessively synchronous state.[22]

The ictal onset is determined by a combination of a failure of inhibitory interictal mechanisms and enhancement of excitatory synaptic activities, which may be initiated by an excess of subcortical synchronizing afferent input as in generalized seizures or focal hypersynchronous discharge.[22] The true ictus in a generalized seizure is initiated in the cortex and may depend on a failure of inhibitory mechanism coupled with synchronizing thalamocortical input, as well as the influence of the reticular formation of the brain stem, particularly in the pontine region for the tonic phase.[22] A combination of diminution of synaptic inhibition, nonspecific excitation, propagation along the efferent projection pathways, and trans-synaptic alteration in excitation determines the appearance of partial ictus.[22] For the ictal termination, the two most important mechanisms are active inhibition and the failure of synchronization.[22] If these mechanisms fail, the patient may develop status epilepticus. Postictal phenomena (neuronal depression, neuronal deficit, EEG slowing, etc.) are sequela to events that cause termination of the ictus.

### Mechanism of Sleep

In humans there are two sleep states: desynchronized or rapid eye movement (REM) sleep and synchronized or non-REM (NREM) sleep. These sleep states are determined by two different mechanisms.[28]

NREM or synchronized sleep seems to act as a convulsant because this state is characterized physiologically by an excessive diffuse cortical synchronization mediated by the thalamocortical input.[29] This predisposes to activation of seizure in an already hyperexcitable cortex.

In REM or desynchronized sleep there is inhibition of thalamocortical synchronizing influence as evidenced by depression of recruiting rhythms generated by low-frequency electrical stimulation of the nonspecific thalamic nuclei.[29] Thus, there is attenuation of bilaterally synchronous epileptiform discharges at this stage of sleep. During REM sleep there is also a tonic reduction in the interhemispheric impulse traffic through the corpus callosum.[30] This also contributes to the limitation of propagation of the generalized epileptiform discharges.

Cortical excitability for epileptogenesis is higher during sleep than during wakefulness.[29] This factor coupled with the fact that the inhibitory mechanism (e.g., postspike hyperpolarization and afferent inhibition) may be less effective during sleep favors activation of focal cortical epileptiform discharge.

According to Steriade,[31] *physiologic synchronization* can be defined as a state during which there is appearance of the same frequency in two or more oscillators due to coactivation of a large number of neurons. In NREM sleep, spindles and slow waves result from synchronization. The nonspecific thalamic reticular nucleus is the synchronizing pacemaker of EEG spindle rhythmicity.[31] In athalamic animals, spindles disappear but slow waves persist, suggesting extrathalamic origin for sleep slow waves.[32] It has been suggested that subcortical white matter participates in the production of EEG slow waves[33] (see also Chapter 4).

Lesions and stimulation experiments have shown the existence of structures responsible for cortical synchrony in the forebrain as well as in the hindbrain.[31,34] Fifty years ago, Morison and Dempsey[35] observed recruiting synchronizing cortical responses after low-frequency electrical stimulation of the midline thalamic nuclei, evidence of an intimate thalamocortical relationship. In 1944, Hess[36] even suggested the existence of a thalamic sleep center. Later studies, however, have shown that the thalamus is responsible for the genesis of spindles and not for sleep slow waves or the behavioral aspect of sleep.[34]

The theory about REM or desynchronized sleep suggests that there are anatomically distributed and neurochemically interpenetrated "REM-on" and "REM-off" cells in the brain stem[28,37] (see also Chapter 3). REM sleep is dependent on an interaction between REM-on cells and REM-off cells in the brain stem. During REM sleep there is maximum cholinergic hyperactivity and aminergic hypoactivity.[28,37] Thus the interaction and oscillation between the cholinergic REM promoting and aminergic REM inhibiting neurons generate the REM-NREM cycle. The various chemical mechanisms participating in NREM and REM sleep may also be responsible for activation or inhibition of epileptiform discharges during sleep.

An understanding of the basic mechanism of epilepsy and sleep helps us understand the mechanism of activation and suppression of seizure discharges during sleep and in particular during different stages of sleep. The activation of ictal and interictal seizures during NREM sleep seems to be related to the existence of a thalamocortical synchronizing mechanism, whereas suppression during REM sleep is due to depression of the thalamic synchronizing mechanism and a tonic reduction of interhemispheric transmission during REM sleep.[29,30]

### Interrelationship between Epilepsy and Sleep

The activation of 3-Hz spike and wave discharges during NREM sleep is supported by the hypothesis of corticoreticular epilepsy of Kostopoulos and Gloor[38] and Gloor.[27] Kostopoulos and Gloor[38] presented evidence that the 3-Hz spike and wave discharges of primary generalized corticoreticular ("centrencephalic") or petit mal epilepsy resulted from an excessive response of cortical neurons to those thalamocortical volleys that are responsible for production of normal sleep spindles. In 1942, Morison and Dempsey[35] produced recruiting responses after intralaminar thalamic stimulation. In 1947, Jasper and Droogleever-Fortuyn[39] succeeded in producing 3-Hz spike and wave discharges after similar stimulation in the presence of cortical hyperexcitability. Spencer and Brookhart[40] and Spencer and Kandel[41] showed similarities between recruiting responses and cortical sleep spindles in the cat. Both of these waves resulted from summated postsynaptic potentials of cortical neurons due to low-frequency thalamocortical volleys. Gloor[42] confirmed and extended these observations with the feline model of generalized epilepsy induced by intramuscular penicillin and concluded that spike and wave discharges resulted from summated postsynaptic potentials of the cortical neurons as a result of the thalamocortical volleys that would normally produce sleep spindles and recruiting responses. Penicillin obviously caused cortical hyperexcitability. In this connection it is important to note that Niedermeyer[43] was the first to suggest that generalized synchronous spike and wave discharges originated from the physiologic K complex.

Wyler[44] studied epileptic neurons during sleep and wakefulness in 14 normal and 17 abnormal neurons recorded from alumina gel–induced chronic neocortical epileptic foci in four male *Macaca mulatta* monkeys during transition between sleep and wakefulness. During sleep, the neurons that were mildly epileptic during wakefulness changed their firing pattern drastically and behaved like neurons that were grossly epileptic during wakefulness; normal neurons and those neurons that were grossly epileptic during wakefulness did not change the firing pattern significantly. The author concluded that the neurons may represent the "critical mass" for initiation of seizure activity during synchronized sleep, which is characterized by burst-synchronizing events such as sleep spindles.

Shouse et al.[45] studied the mechanism of seizure suppression during REM sleep in cats. They created two seizure models in 20 cats, systemic penicillin epilepsy and electroconvulsive shock, and produced two types of lesions: bilateral electrolytic lesions in the mediolateral pontine tegmentum producing a syndrome of REM sleep without atonia and systemic atropine injection producing REM sleep without thalamocortical EEG desynchronization. These authors made the following conclusions based on these experiments: (1) REM sleep retarded the spread of epileptiform discharges in the EEG. (2) The descending brain stem pathways responsible for lower motor neuron inhibition during REM sleep also protected against generalized motor seizure during REM sleep. (3) The mechanism to prevent spread of seizure discharge used a separate pathway in the ascending brain stem structures that caused thalamocortical EEG desynchronization during REM sleep. (4) Their data thus suggested a cholinergic mechanism for thalamocortical EEG desynchronization and for retardation of EEG discharges during wakefulness and REM sleep. They further concluded that for generalized epilepsy, REM sleep was the most potent antiepileptic state in the sleep-wake cycle. It is important to note that Cohen et al.[46] found lowered convulsive threshold during REM deprivation in cats. REM deprivation thus may exacerbate epilepsy.

## EFFECT OF SLEEP ON EPILEPSY

Because of the awareness of an intimate relationship between sleep and epilepsy, various authors have classified seizures according to the time of occurrence of the seizures (clinical and electrical) during certain times in the sleep-wake cycle. Thus, seizures have been classified as waking, sleep, diffuse (both diurnal and nocturnal), circadian, ultradian and infradian epilepsies.

As early as 1885, Gowers[4] analyzed 840 institutionalized patients with a variety of seizure disorders and observed that 21% of seizures occurred exclusively at night; 42% exclusively in the daytime; and 37% at random, both during the day and night. According to Gowers,[4] the two most susceptible periods were the onset of sleep and the end of sleep. Langdon-Down and Brain[8] and Patry[9] made similar observations. In all three series, the analysis was based on institutionalized patients. Langdon-Down and Brain[8] observed that in a series of 66 patients, 24% had sleep, 43% had diurnal, and 33% had diffuse epilepsies. In a sample size of 31, Patry[9] found 19% sleep, 45% diurnal, and 36% diffuse epilepsies. Using the average of these three groups of institutionalized epileptics, the incidence of each of these three types of seizures in relation to the sleep-wake cycle is 22% sleep, 44% diurnal, and 34% diffuse epilepsies. Thus, the incidence is similar in these three series. Langdon-Down and Brain[8] found the peak incidence of waking epilepsies 1–2 hours after awakening, approximately 7:00–8:00 AM; smaller peaks were found at approximately 3:00 PM and 6:00–8:00 PM. Sleep epilepsies had two peaks, 10:00–11:00 PM and 4:00–5:00 AM (i.e., early and late at night, similar to that noted by Gowers[4]).

Amongst the contemporary epileptologists, Janz[13,47] has contributed most towards classification of seizure based on sleep-wake cycle. Janz[13,47] analyzed two large series of outpatients with tonic-clonic generalized seizures. In the first series of 2,110 patients,[13] he found 45% sleep, 34% diurnal, and 21% diffuse epilepsies. In the second series of 2,825 similar patients,[47] the incidence was 44% sleep, 33% diurnal, and 23% diffuse epilepsies. Therefore, the two series were similar. Janz[13] called diurnal seizure *awakening epilepsies* because of the high prevalence of seizure during awakening from sleep. In a sample size of 314 outpatient seizure patients, Billiard[20] found 15% sleep, 53% diurnal, and 32% diffuse epilepsies. It should be noted that Billiard[20] included a variety of types of epilepsies in his analysis. Earlier, Hopkins[48] analyzed a series of outpatient tonic-clonic generalized seizures and found 51% sleep, 30% diurnal, and 19% diffuse epilepsies. Janz[13,47] also noted increased frequency at the beginning and end of the night in sleep epilepsies similar to that observed by Gowers[4] in the last century. It is important to note that the earlier classification was based only on clinical studies and no night-time EEGs were obtained. The contemporary epileptologists and neurologists had the benefit of obtaining the EEG and all-night polysomnographic (PSG) studies using standard sleep scoring criteria. As regards stability of type, Janz[13] reported that 10% of awakening epilepsies later became sleep epilepsies, whereas only 6% became diffuse epilepsies. According to Janz[13,47] and Hopkins,[48] sleep and diffuse epilepsies lasting for 2 years rarely become awakening epilepsies.

The differences in the incidence of the three types of seizures may be due to the selection of patients (i.e., outpatient, institutionalized, generalized or partial seizures). The importance of classification based on sleep-wake cycle is that this classification may shed light on the prognosis and etiology. Patients with diffuse epilepsies often have intractable seizures and structural neurologic deficits with poor prognosis as compared to patients with awakening or sleep epilepsies.[49] Analyzing the various data, Shouse[49] stated that idiopathic type is generally awakening type, those associated with organic structural lesions are of the diffuse type, and the sleep epilepsies are intermediate in terms of organicity. D'Alessandro et al.[50] analyzed 1,200 patients visiting the epilepsy center during a 5-year period (1974–1979). They found that 90 of 1,200 (7.5%) had sleep epilepsy (i.e., had one or more seizures exclusively during sleep). This frequency is lower than that found by Janz[13] and Kajtor[51] but similar to that noted by Gibberd and Bateson.[52] The authors concluded that pure sleep epilepsies have a good prognosis. They rarely have waking seizures during the first few years after the onset of epilepsy.

A number of investigators have studied the question of whether epilepsy manifests biorhythmicity—specifically, whether there are circadian, ultradian, or infradian epilepsies. Kellaway et al.[21,53] cited the specific relationship of epileptic phenomenon to the sleep-wake cycle as an example of a circadian rhythm. It should be noted, however, that Autret et al.[54] noted an increase in the focal discharges during NREM stages I and II and of generalized discharges during NREM stages III and IV and a reduction or disappearance of the discharges in REM sleep during any time of the day and night. This evidence argues against a circadian rhythmicity. Kellaway and coworkers[21,53,55] suggested that epileptiform activity is linked to two rhythms: circadian and ultradian, related to NREM-REM cycle at 90–100 minutes. Stevens et al.[56] suggested that focal EEG discharges in adults may at times show an ultradian 90–100 minute periodicity in phase with prior NREM-REM sleep cycles throughout the day and night. Binnie[57] and Martins da Silva and Binnie[58] also noted periodicities of interictal discharges, both during diurnal waking and nocturnal sleep EEG recordings. In most of their patients, periodicities were longer or shorter than the typical 90- to 100-minute REM-NREM cycle. However, Kellaway et al.[53] failed to document waking ultradian rhythmicity in petit mal spike and wave discharges. In one case of petit mal absence, Broughton et al.[59] provided strong evidence for ultradian daytime variations of spike-wave discharges, mainly at the REM cycle rate. However, these observations have been made based only on one case study.

There are clear methodological problems in studying biorhythmicity in epilepsy.[57] The classic methods include temporal isolation to observe the free running rhythms (entrainment) and shifting the time zone. Such studies in epilepsy, however, have not been performed in detail.[57]

Finally, the question of infradian rhythmicity in epilepsy as exemplified by the catamenial epilepsy (i.e., menstrual-related epilepsy) remains controversial. Almqvist[60] found a periodicity in 47 out of 146 long-stay patients with epilepsy. The author noted that in some of the patients the interval of the attack was equal to the period of the menstrual cycle. As mentioned by Newmark and Penry,[61] however, the concept of catamenial epilepsy, although generally accepted, remains questionable as far as published evidence is concerned.

In conclusion, epilepsy in some patients may show a circadian temporal periodicity and an association with sleep periodicity, but it is not known if this periodicity is "state"-linked (sleep vs. wakefulness) or "time"-linked (nocturnal vs. diurnal).[62] Epileptic events are thought to be "state-dependent" by Webb[62] but "time-dependent" by Martins da Silva and Binnie.[58] Thus, little is known why a seizure occurs at a particular time of the day or night. This understanding may be important for effective control of epilepsy by optimization of the drug regimen. Binnie[57] raised the question without an answer: Can we improve patient care if we learn about biorhythms in epilepsy? Because of inconsistencies and contradictions in terms of classification related to biorhythms, the modern epileptologists use the International Classification of Epilepsy.[63]

## EFFECT OF SLEEP ON SPECIFIC SEIZURE TYPES

In this section we briefly describe the effect of sleep on clinical seizures as well as on the interictal EEG epileptiform discharges in both generalized and partial seizures.

### Clinical Seizures

#### Generalized Epilepsies

Generalized epilepsies commonly include generalized tonic-clonic (grand mal) epilepsy, petit mal (absence epilepsy), juvenile myoclonic epilepsy, infantile spasms (West's syndrome), and Lennox-Gastaut syndrome. Diurnal or *awakening epilepsy*, a term introduced by Janz[64] to differentiate from sleep and diffuse epilepsies, also belongs to the category of generalized epilepsies, which include generalized tonic-clonic, absence, and benign juvenile myoclonic seizure. Some varieties of diffuse epilepsies (e.g., Lennox-Gastaut and West's syndrome, progressive myoclonic epilepsies) also belong to generalized seizures.

**Primary Generalized Grand Mal Seizure.**   Primary generalized grand mal seizure occurs almost exclusively in NREM sleep[65] and is most frequently seen 1–2 hours after sleep onset and at 5:00–6:00 AM, as noted originally in 1985 by Gowers[4] and later by others.[8,9,13] Grand mal seizure may occur only during sleep, only during the daytime, or be randomly distributed. In a study of 171 patients, Billiard et al.[66] found exclusively nocturnal seizures in only 8%. This study also confirmed the observations of Passouant et al.[67] and Bessett[65] that primary generalized seizure occurs exclusively in NREM sleep. Passouant et al.[68] called the seizure occurring exclusively during sleep *l'epilepsie morpheique*; this is considered a benign form of epilepsy. These patients

rarely go on to develop waking epilepsies, and when they do it is after the first 2 years of onset.[50]

**Petit Mal (Absence) Epilepsy.**   Absence seizures occurring during sleep are difficult to diagnose and clinical absence seizures are observed in the waking state. According to Niedermeyer[17] there may be fluttering of the eyelids during the spike and wave discharges in sleep. Gastaut and colleagues,[69] Gastaut and Broughton,[70] and Patry et al.[71] described occasional cases of petit mal status in REM sleep.

**Juvenile Myoclonic Epilepsy.**   Meier-Ewert and Broughton[72] noted increased myoclonic seizures shortly after awakening in the morning and the duration of the attack is longer on awakening from NREM than from REM sleep. Occasionally, these attacks occur on awakening in the middle of the night or later in the afternoon.[9,13,73]

**Lennox-Gastaut Syndrome.**   In Lennox-Gastaut syndrome, the clinical seizures consist of tonic, myoclonic, generalized tonic-clonic, atonic and atypical absence.[74] Information regarding the effect of sleep on the clinical seizures in this syndrome is lacking in the literature.[75] Tonic seizures, however, are typically activated by sleep,[76] are much more frequent during NREM sleep than during wakefulness, and are never seen during REM sleep.[77]

**West's Syndrome (Infantile Spasms).**   Maximum clinical seizures, often spasms in series, are seen on arousal from sleep or before going to sleep.[21,78] Less than 3% of spasms are obtained in sleep.

### Partial Epilepsies

Clinical seizures in simple partial seizures and complex partial seizures (CPS) are more frequent during the day.[20,50] In Billiard's[20] study of 156 patients, 61.5% had daytime and 11.5% had nocturnal seizures only. According to Montplaisir and coworkers,[79–81] Laverdiere and Montplaisir,[82] and Rossi et al.,[83] REM sleep did not facilitate temporal lobe seizure. However, other authors[67,84–86] observed ictal phenomena during both stages of sleep. In fact, Epstein and Hill[86] described a case of temporal lobe seizure with unpleasant dreams during REM sleep associated with increased

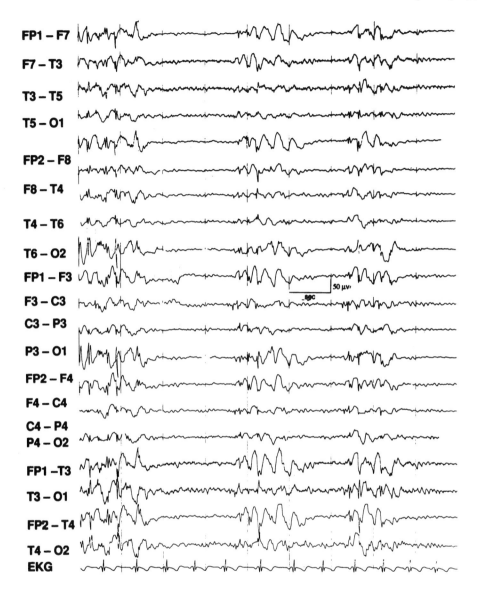

**Figure 34-1.** Interictal, primarily generalized epileptiform discharges (4- to 5-Hz spike and wave and multiple spike and wave discharges) seen synchronously and symmetrically with frontal dominance of amplitude in a patient with generalized tonic-clonic seizures. (EKG = electrocardiography.)

epileptiform activities in the EEG in the temporal region.

Pure sleep epilepsies mostly present as focal seizures with or without secondary generalization.[13,20] Benign rolandic epilepsy and electrical status epilepticus during sleep (ESES) are also typical examples of sleep epilepsies and are described in the next sections.

### Interictal Epileptiform Discharges

#### Primary Generalized Grand Mal Tonic-Clonic Seizures

Interictal EEG discharges (Figure 34-1) generally increase in NREM sleep and disappear in REM sleep.[18,20,54,70,87–89] Mostly the discharges are promi-

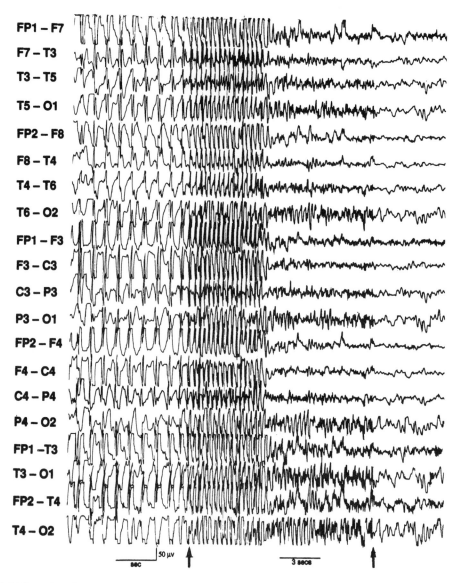

**Figure 34-2.** Three-Hz spike and wave discharges noted synchronously and symmetrically with dominance of the amplitude anteriorly in a patient with absence spells (petit mal). Note the paper speed on the panel to the left at 30 mm/sec (sec), and to the right at 10 mm/sec (3 secs; between the arrows).

nent at sleep onset and during the first part of the night. Sometimes the discharges are activated during NREM sleep in the late part of the night, possibly resulting from reduced serum levels of antiepileptic medications.[18] Interictal discharges may be fragmented or may appear as polyspikes or focal spikes during NREM sleep. According to Billiard,[20] interictal discharges are more frequent during NREM than during REM sleep (41% versus 9%) in pure sleep epilepsy but in waking or random epilepsy, interictal discharges are seen throughout the day and night. With nocturnal epilepsies, daytime EEG remains normal in a high percentage of patients.[90]

*Petit Mal (Absence Epilepsy)*

According to Sato et al.,[91] Tassinari et al.,[92] and Billiard et al.,[66] interictal EEG discharges (Figure 34-2)

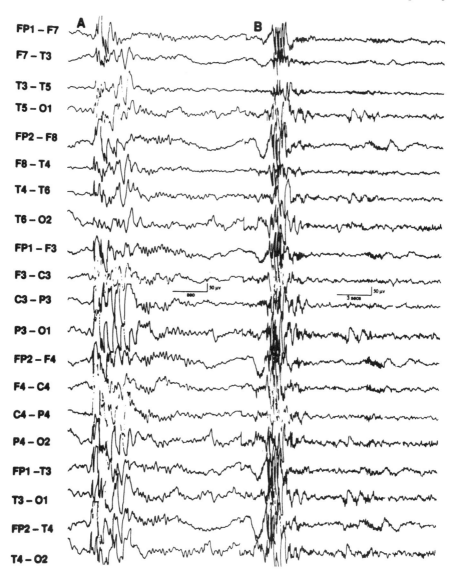

**Figure 34-3.** Interictal generalized multiple spike and wave discharges in the EEG of a patient with myoclonic epilepsy. Note the recording at 30 mm/sec (sec) on the left (**A**) and at 10 mm/sec (3 secs) on the right (**B**).

in absence attacks are present during all stages of NREM sleep. These are more marked during the first sleep cycle[91] but generally absent in REM sleep. The pattern during REM sleep is similar to that during wakefulness with reduced duration.[91,92] Sato et al.[91] described alterations of spike and wave discharge morphology during different sleep stages: regular or irregular spike and wave discharges in NREM stages I and II, and irregular polyspikes and slow waves during NREM stages III and IV. In addition, fragmentation or focalization of spikes can be seen over the frontal regions during NREM sleep.

*Juvenile Myoclonic Epilepsy*

Interictal discharges (Figure 34-3) in these patients are prominent at sleep onset and on awakening but are virtually nonexistent during the rest of the sleep

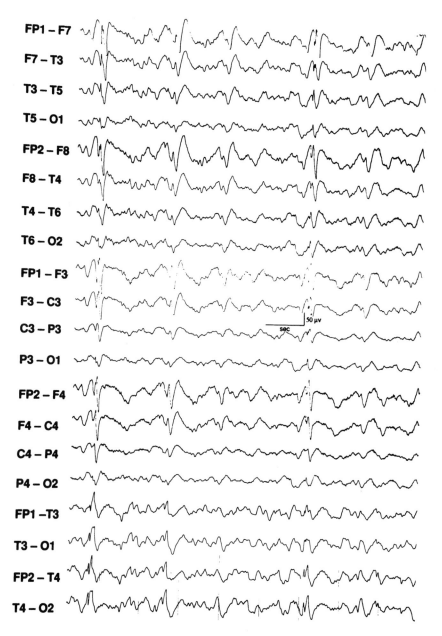

**Figure 34-4.** Generalized slow spike and wave (2.0–2.5 Hz) bursts in a patient with Lennox-Gastaut syndrome.

cycle.[18] According to Touchon,[73] induced awakening is a better facilitator than spontaneous awakening in these patients.

*Lennox-Gastaut Syndrome*

The typical EEG (Figure 34-4) finding in Lennox-Gastaut syndrome is slow spike and wave (1.5–2.5 Hz). In sleep, this may be intermixed with trains of fast spikes of 10–25 Hz lasting 2–10 seconds (so-called grand mal discharges) as interictal abnormalities. The spike and waves characteristically increase in NREM sleep.[75] Sometimes bursts of electrodecremental activity alternate with bursts of polyspikes, giving rise to a burst-suppression–like pattern.[75] According to Markand,[93] prognosis is better in those

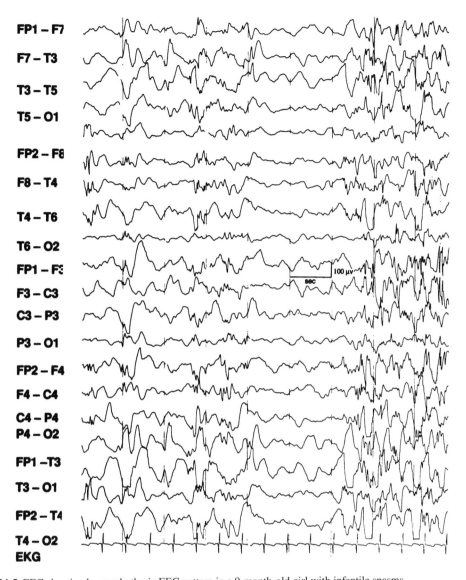

**Figure 34-5.** EEG showing hypsarrhythmic EEG pattern in a 9-month-old girl with infantile spasms.

patients with significant increase of interictal EEG abnormalities during sleep.

*West's Syndrome (Infantile Spasm)*

The characteristic EEG finding of West's syndrome (Figure 34-5) is hypsarrhythmia (high-amplitude slow waves and spike or sharp waves occurring irregularly), which may show progressive changes during sleep. The characteristic pattern seen during wakefulness may increase in NREM sleep. The hypsarrhythmic EEG of wakefulness may change

during NREM sleep into a periodic bilaterally synchronous diffuse pattern interspersed with flattening, resembling "burst suppression,"[67] and may even normalize during REM sleep. Occasionally waking EEG may be normal but NREM sleep EEG may show the irregular high-voltage slow waves and spikes.[94]

*Partial Epilepsies*

An increase of interictal EEG discharges (Figure 34-6) during NREM and diminution or disappear-

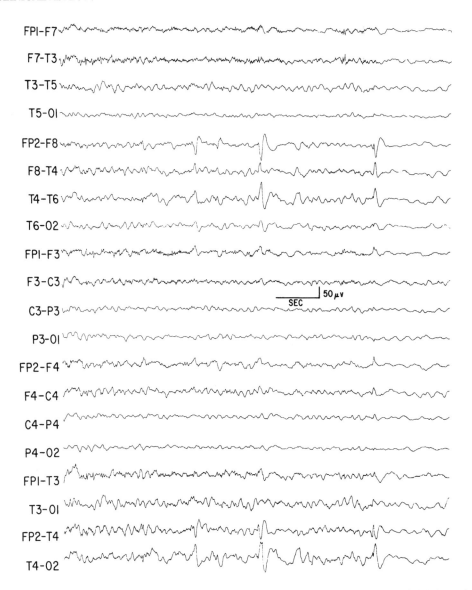

**Figure 34-6.** Focal right anterior and midtemporal sharp and slow waves showing phase reversal at F8-T4 electrodes in a patient with partial complex seizure.

ance during REM sleep have been found both in surface and depth electrode studies as well as in animal studies.[85,95–97] However, Touchon,[73] Passouant et al.,[98] Mayersdorf and Wilder,[99] and Epstein and Hill[86] found an increase of focal temporal discharges during REM sleep. An important point to note is that during NREM sleep the discharges spread ipsilaterally and contralaterally from the primary focus, whereas during REM sleep the discharges seem to focalize maximally.[80,88,100]

Activation of discharges during REM sleep were also found by Frank and Pegram[101] in alumina cream monkey models of temporal lobe epilepsies. However, Mayanagi[102] did not confirm these findings in a similar monkey model.

Depth electrode studies in humans by Montplaisir et al.[82] and Lieb et al.[100] showed increased spike discharges during NREM sleep and a reduction of the discharges during REM sleep. Depth electrode studies also showed that during REM sleep the spike discharges became maximally focalized.[82,83,100]

Autret et al.[89] reviewed 236 adult epileptics attending outpatient clinics and classified the seizures in two ways: (1) according to the time of onset of seizures by history (e.g., diurnal, nocturnal, and diffuse epilepsies); and (2) according to the interictal activation during all-night PSG study. They found more frequent myoclonic attacks and increased seizure frequency in patients with diurnal epilepsy. Patients with increased incidence of interictal activities during sleep have less generalized motor seizure, more frequent CPS, a higher seizure frequency, and the appearance of new interictal activities during sleep. These authors did not find a significant relationship between the two classifications. It should be noted that these data are at variance with the results of Janz.[13,47]

Lieb et al.[100] performed all-night depth electrode recordings in 10 patients with medically refractory CPS and used computer spike recognition technique for depth spike activities arising from medial temporal lobe sites. They found most frequent depth spike activity during deep sleep in six patients, during light sleep in three patients, and an equal number during deep and light sleep in one patient. They did not find a strong relationship between temporal lobe epilepsy and sleep pattern. Their findings that the discharge rates are greatest during NREM sleep and are suppressed during REM sleep are in agreement with the previous reports of temporal lobe epileptics. Similar depth electrode findings in temporal lobe epilepsies have been reported by Montplaisir and coworkers[79–82,103] and Passouant.[104] In some previous studies, however,[85,105] maximal spike activity was seen during light sleep. In the study by Lieb et al.,[100] the side showing maximal spike activity did not necessarily correspond to the site chosen for temporal lobectomy. This suggests that the interictal spikes and seizure generating capacity may not bear a close relationship to underlying pathology.

Malow et al.[106] studied the relationship of spikes to absolute delta log power (LDP), a continuous measure of sleep depth, in eight patients with partial epilepsy and found that within NREM sleep, spikes were most likely to occur at higher levels of LDP (i.e., deep sleep), on the ascending limb of LDP, and with more rapid rises in LDP (i.e., deepening sleep). They suggested that processes underlying the deepening of NREM sleep may contribute to spike activation in partial epilepsy.

Rossi et al.[83] obtained direct cerebral recordings (stereo EEG) by stereotactic implantation of stainless steel electrodes on preselected brain sites in 19 patients with medically refractory partial epilepsy and were potential candidates for surgery. They found that interictal spiking increased at the onset of sleep, reaching a maximum level during deep NREM sleep and returning to a lower level during REM sleep. The level in REM sleep was slightly lower as compared with that during wakefulness. They further noted that the spike rate was not influenced by spike location but was affected by the local level of epileptogenicity (i.e., the higher the epileptogenicity, the lower the variation), and that the interictal spiking across sleep and wakefulness showed wide variation in different patients and in the different regions of the same patients.

In conclusion, NREM sleep is the stage of augmentation of interictal focal and generalized EEG discharges. In REM sleep, generalized discharges are usually suppressed but focal discharges may persist.

To explain the variation in spiking during sleep and wakefulness, three factors may be cited[83]: (1) subcortical-cortical interplay of the mechanisms for sleep and wakefulness as well as EEG synchronization, (2) alteration in the cortical excitability during sleep and wakefulness, and (3) location of the epileptic lesion. The first factor may play a role in the generalized seizures and the second and the third factors may play a role in the genesis of the partial seizures.

### Status Epilepticus

The information regarding effect of sleep on status epilepticus is limited, as this is a neurologic emergency and the first priority is treatment of the patient rather than spending time on prolonged recording. Therefore, limited information is available in certain types of status epilepticus. Gastaut[107] defined *status epilepticus* as a condition in which seizure persists for a sufficient length of time or is repeated frequently enough to produce a fixed and enduring epileptic condition. An arbitrary time of 30–60 minutes has been accepted as a time to justify the term. Gastaut[107] classified status into three types: (1) generalized status epilepticus consisting of convulsive and nonconvulsive types, (2) simple and complex partial status epilepticus, and (3) unilateral status epilepticus.

Generalized tonic-clonic (grand mal) status epilepticus occurs during the early part of the night.[108] Tonic status as may be seen in patients with Lennox-Gastaut syndrome occurs almost exclusively during sleep and is seen mostly during NREM sleep.[109] Myoclonic status epilepticus can arise in two forms[107]: (1) as part of the primary generalized status epilepticus and (2) the type associated with acute or subacute encephalopathies. In both these conditions the myoclonic status epilepticus is markedly attenuated during sleep.[109] Petit mal status or absence status epilepticus may be terminated during sleep.[109] Gastaut and Tassinari[110] demonstrated that NREM sleep disrupts the EEG discharges, which are replaced by polyspikes or polyspike-wave complexes or even isolated bursts of spikes. According to several authors,[111–113] there may be recurrence of absence status on awakening during the night or in the morning. Occasionally the spike and wave discharges of petit mal status epilepticus may persist during NREM and REM sleep throughout the night.[111] In simple partial status epilepticus both improvement and activation during sleep have been noted.[109] According to Froscher,[109] the role of nocturnal sleep in complex partial status epilepticus has remained unknown. ESES is discussed in the next section.

## SPECIAL SEIZURE TYPES RELATED TO SLEEP-WAKE CYCLE

Certain varieties of epilepsy are seen during specific periods of the human sleep-wake cycle: (1) benign focal epilepsy of childhood with rolandic spikes (BERS), (2) juvenile myoclonic epilepsy of Janz, (3) epileptic syndrome with generalized tonic-clonic seizure on awakening, and (4) ESES.

### Benign Focal Epilepsy of Childhood with Rolandic Spikes

A clear description of BERS was given by Nayrac and Beaussart in 1958.[114] Later, Beaussart[115] drew attention to the benign nature of the condition. This is a childhood seizure seen mostly during drowsiness

and sleep. The clinical seizures are characterized by focal clonic facial seizures often preceded by perioral numbness. In many cases the patients have generalized tonic-clonic seizures that appear to be secondary generalization. On occasion, there is speech arrest. Consciousness is preserved. The EEG shows centrotemporal or rolandic spikes or sharp waves (Figure 34-7). These discharges are present throughout the night in all stages of sleep. The prognosis is excellent with cessation of seizures by the age of 15–20 years, without any neurologic sequelae. The patients respond to anticonvulsants satisfactorily.

### Juvenile Myoclonic Epilepsy of Janz

Juvenile myoclonic epilepsy, an electroclinical syndrome, was described by Janz and Mathes[116] and later published in detail by Janz and Christian.[117] The onset of the syndrome is usually between 13 and 19 years and is manifested by massive bilaterally synchronous myoclonic jerks, which are most commonly seen in the morning shortly after awakening.[117,118] The EEG is characterized by generalized spike and wave and typically polyspike and wave discharges (see Figure 34-3), seen in a synchronous and symmetric manner. The excellent response to anticonvulsants makes this condition benign and easily distinguishable from the malignant syndrome of progressive myoclonus epilepsies.

### Epileptic Syndrome with Generalized Tonic-Clonic Seizure on Awakening

Epileptic syndrome with generalized tonic-clonic seizure on awakening[118,119] is manifested by the occurrence in the second decade of generalized tonic-clonic seizures on awakening from sleep. This is a rare syndrome and clinically there may be occasional absence or myoclonic manifestations and photosensitivity resembling juvenile myoclonic epilepsy.

### Electrical Status Epilepticus during Sleep or Continuous Spike and Waves during Sleep

ESES is a disease of childhood characterized by generalized continuous spike and wave EEG discharges

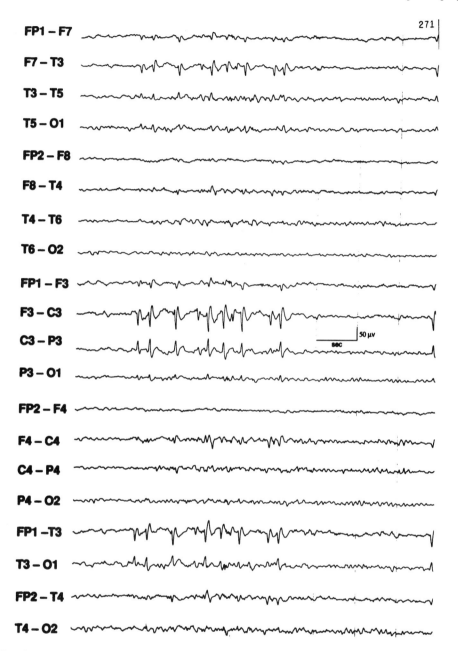

**Figure 34-7.** Left centrotemporal spikes and sharp waves in patient with benign focal epilepsy of childhood with rolandic spikes.

during slow-wave sleep. All-night PSG study is necessary for diagnosis. The patients display progressive behavioral disturbances, although the seizures disappear within months or years. This entity is rare and found in children between 5 and 15 years old. ESES was first described by Patry et al.[71] in 1971 in six children; later, Tassinari et al.[120] reviewed the litera-

ture and described 19 cases of their own. Most of the patients had a prior history of epilepsy. The characteristic EEG finding consists of 2.0–2.5 cycles per second generalized spike and wave discharges seen during at least 85% of NREM sleep and suppressed during REM sleep. Occasional bursts of spike and waves or focal frontal spikes were noted during REM sleep. There were a few bursts of generalized spike and wave discharges seen in the EEG during wakefulness. These EEG discharges disrupted the stages of NREM sleep. In particular, the vertex sharp waves, K complexes, and spindles could not be well-recognized. However, the cyclic pattern of REM-NREM persisted normally. Generally, there were no sleep disturbances but some children had difficulty awakening in the morning. However, Ortega et al.[121] reported a case of a 7-year-old girl with ESES hypersomnia, documented with an abnormal Multiple Sleep Latency Test (MSLT), and secondary nocturnal enuresis. These authors suggested that ESES is an intrinsic sleep disorder and not merely an EEG pattern.

*Nocturnal Paroxysmal Dystonia*

Initially described by Lugaresi and Cirignotta[122] and Lugaresi et al.,[123] this entity, particularly the short-lasting (15 seconds to 2 minutes) variety consisting of dystonic motor phenomena occurring during sleep, is now increasingly recognized as a form of frontal lobe epilepsy.[124,125,126]

*Autosomal Dominant Nocturnal*
*Frontal Lobe Epilepsy*

Scheffer et al.[127] described an autosomal dominant form of frontal lobe epilepsy in six families. Brief motor seizures usually occurred in clusters during sleep. The disorder usually started in childhood and persisted through adult life. Patients were of normal intellect and had normal neurologic examination and neuroimaging. Response to carbamazepine was excellent. In most cases, interictal EEGs were normal, although one family with daytime attacks had epileptiform discharges. Video-telemetry during the attacks confirmed their epileptic nature. Oldani et al.[128] studied 33 patients and found similar results.

## EFFECT OF SLEEP DEPRIVATION ON EPILEPSY

The diagnostic value of sleep-deprived EEG has been well-documented.[95,129–132] What is the mechanism of activation during sleep deprivation? This is probably not a sampling effect and not related to sleep alone.[129,130,132] Sleep deprivation increases the

epileptiform discharges mostly in the transition period between waking and light sleep and also has a localizing value.[130,132] Although the original study by Rodin et al.[133] in 1962 found epileptiform discharges in healthy subjects after sleep deprivation, later studies[132,134] failed to confirm these observations.

Rowan et al.[130] studied 43 consecutive patients using two types of activation: sleep deprivation (24 hours in adults and partial deprivation in children) and sedated sleep (after oral secobarbital). They obtained useful information in 44% of sleep-deprived as opposed to 14% of sedated sleep records. The patients were referred because of doubtful diagnosis of epilepsy or because seizure types could not be determined. They also found sleep deprivation superior to sedated sleep for differentiating those with a final diagnosis of seizure. It should be noted that sleep alone does not explain the activating effect of sleep deprivation. The mechanism remains largely unknown. Rowan et al.[130] suggested increased cerebral excitability after sleep deprivation in normal individuals.

Degen[131] studied 127 waking and sleep EEGs after sleep deprivation in 120 epileptic patients on anticonvulsant medication. He found seizure activity in 63% of the patients, although in the previous EEG records of these patients only 19% had shown seizure activity; thus, sleep deprivation increased the incidence of seizure activity. Approximately 48% of discharges occurred during slow-wave and 25% during REM sleep.

It is interesting to note that in 1896 Patrick and Gilbert[135] apparently performed sleep deprivation studies in human beings. The studies by Bennett[136] in 1963 and Mattson et al.[137] in 1965 established the value of sleep deprivation as a diagnostic tool in patients with seizure disorders. Rodin[138] computed the incidence of activation after sleep deprivation from an analysis of the literature and came up with a figure of approximately 45%.

## PHENOMENA DURING SLEEP THAT CAN BE MISTAKEN FOR EPILEPSY (NONEPILEPTIFORM DISORDERS)

Certain paroxysmal arousal disorders in NREM sleep may be mistaken for seizures, particularly for CPS. Some examples of these disorders are the following: night terror (pavor nocturnus), somnambu-

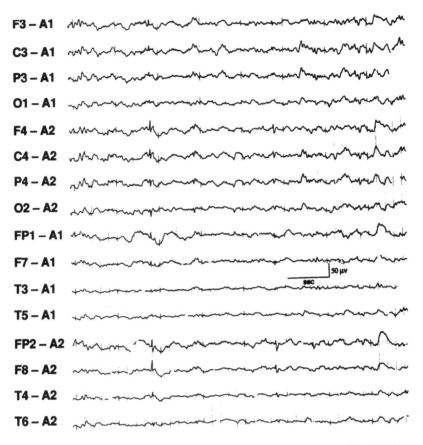

**Figure 34-8.** Small sharp spikes (benign epileptiform transients of sleep) seen in channels 5–8 and 13–16 from the top.

lism (sleepwalking), somniloquy (sleep talking), tooth grinding (bruxism), head banging (jactatio capitis nocturnas), and nocturnal enuresis. There are two other parasomnias usually associated with REM sleep, REM behavior disorder and nightmares (dream-anxiety attacks). These conditions are described in Chapter 31.

Paroxysmal nocturnal dystonia and periodic limb movements in sleep are two other nocturnal events that may be mistaken for seizures and these are described in Chapter 26.

Episodic nocturnal wanderings as described by Pedley and Guilleminault[139] may represent a special type of nocturnal seizure. Whether these are true nocturnal seizures or a type of parasomnias cannot be definitely ascertained, however, although the patients showed interictal EEG epileptiform abnormalities and responded to anticonvulsants. Finally, small sharp spikes or benign epileptiform transients

of sleep as noted in the EEG (Figure 34-8) in stages I and II NREM sleep may resemble true epileptiform spikes but the distribution, morphology, and occurrence during particular stages of sleep without any clinical accompaniments differentiate these from the true epileptiform spikes.[140]

The nocturnal events (clinical and electrographic) of nonepileptiform significance discussed earlier must be differentiated from true epileptic attacks. Otherwise, unnecessary medications and tests will be used. Characteristic clinical features combined with EEG and PSG recordings are important to differentiate these conditions. It should be noted that presence of EEG epileptiform discharges independent of nocturnal attacks may not be proof sine qua non that the attacks are of epileptic nature.[19] However, video-EEG recordings to correlate behavior with EEG manifestations may establish or exclude the diagnosis. Sometimes the two conditions (epileptic and nonepileptic attacks) may coexist. Finally, an improvement after empiric treatment with the anticonvulsant medication does not necessarily prove the epileptic nature of the condition.[19]

## EFFECT OF EPILEPSY ON SLEEP

An objective evaluation of the states of sleep in epileptic patients reveals that they are altered in a large percentage of patients studied. Although the utility of sleep in the diagnosis of epilepsy is well-established, the altered sleep characteristics in epileptics are not well-known. One of the difficulties has been that most of the studies have been conducted in patients who have been on anticonvulsants, thus adding the confounding factors of the effect of anticonvulsants on sleep architecture. Furthermore, there have not been good longitudinal studies to determine the effect of epilepsy on sleep in the early versus late stage of the illness. Despite these limitations, there have been several studies from which a general consensus has been reached regarding the effect of epilepsy on sleep and sleep structure. A variety of sleep disturbances have been observed in epileptics and can be summarized as follows[85,87,98,141,142]: a reduction in REM sleep; an increase in wake after sleep onset (WASO); increased instability of sleep states, such as unclassifiable sleep epochs; an increase in NREM stages I and II; a decrease in NREM sleep stages III and IV; a reduction in the density of sleep spindles; and an increase of sleep onset latency.

Three questions may be asked regarding the effect of epilepsy on sleep: (1) Is sleep quality related to the duration and type of seizures? (2) Is sleep quality related to repeated episodes of seizures or poorly controlled seizures? (3) Can epilepsy lead to a sleep disorder? These questions are discussed in the next section.

### Relationship between Seizure Type and Sleep

WASO, sleep stage shifts, and sleep fragmentation are found in all seizure types.[65,141,143–146] Reduction of REM sleep and an increase in NREM stages I and II are in part dependent on the type of epilepsy. Declerck et al.[141] found an increase of NREM stages I and II and a reduction of REM sleep in 258 patients with primary generalized or partial seizure with sec-ondary generalization as compared with 223 nonepileptic subjects. Similar findings were obtained by Bessett.[65] Baldy-Moulinier[143] noted a decrease of REM sleep in patients with CPS occurring during sleep. It is interesting to note that Bessett[65] in human epileptics and Baldy-Moulinier[143] in temporal lobe epilepsy models found no rebound REM sleep in subsequent recordings after REM sleep loss, which is contrary to the usual findings of REM rebound after REM deprivation. In summary, WASO and sleep fragmentation are found in all types of epilepsy, and generalized seizures are associated with reduction of NREM stages I and II and REM sleep. In CPS there is often REM reduction only.

Hoeppner et al.[147] studied self-reported sleep disorder symptoms in epilepsy. They gave a questionnaire relating to six aspects of sleep: delayed sleep onset, night awakenings, dreams, night terrors, sleepwalking, and fatigue on awakening. They evaluated four groups of subjects: (1) four patients with simple partial seizures, (2) 18 patients with CPS, (3) eight patients with generalized seizures, and (4) 23 controls (14 women and nine men aged 16–53 years). They found significantly more sleep disorder symptoms (particularly frequent awakenings at night) in patients with simple partial seizures and CPS. The generalized group behaved like the control group. Patients with most frequent seizures, irrespective of the type, had the most sleep disturbances.

Roder-Wanner et al.[148] obtained polygraphic sleep recordings in 43 patients with different types of epilepsies. They found that patients with generalized epilepsy had a higher percentage of deeper stages of sleep (NREM III and IV) than patients with focal epilepsy. These observations are correlated with the factor of photosensitivity, which was noted in a subgroup of these patients. The authors concluded that there was no real relationship between sleep structure and the type of epilepsy. Thus, there is some controversy regarding the relationship between seizure type and sleep. In previous studies, sleep structure abnormalities may have been related to clinical or subclinical seizure activity preceding the PSG investigation or to the medication received during the study.

There are contradictory reports regarding REM sleep disturbance.[87] On seizure-free nights, REM sleep is usually normal, but REM decrement is noted when there are primary or secondary generalized seizures during the night. There is no REM suppression during partial seizure without secondary generalization.[65,143] Bowersox and Drucker-Colin[149] stated that increased cortical neuronal excitability and reduced seizure threshold may result from chronic REM sleep deprivation secondary to repeated and frequent nocturnal generalized seizures.

In a series of 15 patients with temporal lobe seizure disorders, Touchon et al.[150] found increased WASO, shifting of the sleep stages, and increases in NREM sleep stages I and II. In a study of 23 patients with temporal lobe epilepsy, Kohsaka[151] found significantly decreased sleep efficiency and increased awakenings in both treated and untreated patients. He also noted increased NREM stage IV in untreated patients compared to healthy controls. The site of the primary focus may determine the type of the sleep disturbances.[18] Foci in the amygdalohippocampal region may lead to increased WASO and decreased sleep efficiency. Frontal lobe epileptics, however, may show a specific reduction in stages III and IV NREM sleep.

Bazil and Walczak[152] retrospectively studied video-EEG recordings of 1,116 seizures in 188 patients and found the following: (1) Thirty-five percent of CPS starting during sleep underwent secondary generalization, as compared with 18% in wakefulness. (2) Frontal lobe CPS secondarily generalized at equal rates during sleep and wakefulness, whereas temporal lobe CPS generalized more frequently during sleep. (3) Frontal lobe seizures were more likely to occur during sleep than were temporal lobe seizures. (4) CPS were more frequent in NREM stages I and II and rarely occurred in REM. (5) Seizures starting during slow-wave sleep lasted longer than those starting during wakefulness and stage II NREM sleep. In addition, they noted that psychogenic nonepileptic seizures rarely occurred between midnight and 6:00 AM and never during sleep.

In a questionnaire-based study of 40 children with tuberous sclerosis (TS), Hunt and Stores[153] found that concurrent epilepsy was significantly associated with sleep disturbances in these children. This observation was corroborated by Bruni and coworkers,[154] who found a more disrupted sleep architecture in patients with TS and epilepsy compared with seizure-free children.

### Severity of Seizure and Extent of Sleep Deficits

Seizure occurrence during sleep accentuates sleep deficits, which are more marked in primary gener-

alized and partial seizures with secondary generalization than in other types. In 25% of epileptics, Declerck et al.[141] could not evaluate PSG recordings because of severe encephalopathies associated with seizures. Bessett[65] could not discriminate NREM stages in the EEG or REM sleep because of disrupted sleep architecture due to the seizures (ictal and interictal). However, Baldy-Moulinier[143] found markedly reduced REM sleep in patients having only one attack of secondary generalized seizure during the night. It can be concluded, however, that the severity of sleep deficits is in part correlated with severity of the seizure disorder. Animal studies support such a conclusion.[155,156]

### Can Epilepsy Lead to a Sleep Disorder?

It is generally thought that sleep deficits in seizure disorders are secondary to the severity of the seizure disorder and are a direct result of seizures during sleep. However, studies by Tanaka and Naquet[157] demonstrated progressive sleep deficits in amygdala kindling models. In addition, the sleep deficits persisted 1 month after discontinuation of kindling procedures.

Shouse and Sterman[155] produced amygdala kindling in 10 adult cats and studied their sleep and waking patterns chronically. They found a progressive sleep disturbance and retention of the deficit over a prolonged period after termination of amygdala stimulation. These findings suggest the "kindling" of a sleep disorder in addition to a seizure disturbance. The authors further stated that sleep abnormalities cannot be viewed as a simple or temporary side effect of epileptiform activity. It appears that a permanent change in sleep physiology occurs in epilepsy. These observations of Shouse and Sterman[155] partially answer the question posed by Passouant[1]: "Can epilepsy lead to a sleep disorder?" Effective treatment of epilepsy with anticonvulsant medications or surgical methods normalizes sleep disturbances in human epilepsy.[145]

### Can a Sleep Disorder Lead to Epilepsy?

In 1995, Silvestri et al.[158] reported six patients who were diagnosed in childhood as having disorders of arousal and later developed epileptic seizures. The sleep disorders consisted of sleepwalking and night terrors, all confirmed by PSG studies. The seizures noted were complex partial in five and generalized tonic-clonic in one. Nocturnal monitoring confirmed the epileptic nature of these events. The authors hypothesized that because both disorders of arousal and epilepsy are related to sleep and share other common factors such as age of onset and precipitating factors, these disorders share common functional substrates and it is possible that disorders of arousal may later turn into epileptic seizures. It should be noted, however, that sleepwalking and sleep terrors are frequently noted in children and seizures may simply coexist with these NREM parasomnias. Most sleep specialists and epileptologists simply do not believe that such parasomnias can later turn into epileptic seizures. It should also be remembered that cases of typical disorders of arousal not associated with epileptic discharges in epileptic children have been described.[70,159,160]

## EFFECT OF ANTICONVULSANTS ON SLEEP IN EPILEPTICS

There is a dearth of well-controlled, careful studies documenting the effects of anticonvulsant medications on sleep architecture that properly take into account the effects of seizures on sleep. Only limited data are available. Johnson[145] reviewed the literature on acute and chronic exposure to anticonvulsant drugs in relation to the sleep pattern. Acute exposure to anticonvulsants may reduce REM and NREM stages III and IV and increase stage II NREM sleep. Acute and chronic drug trials in epileptics suggest that the main effects of anticonvulsants consist of sleep stabilization, however, which includes a reduction in WASO and an increase in NREM stages II, III, and IV, along with sleep spindle density. These improvements are concomitant with the reduction of seizures. The bulk of the evidence in the literature points to the fact that effective anticonvulsant treatment and seizure control result in reduction of sleep disturbance. Thus, the effects are due to the reduction of seizures and not to any specific effect of the anticonvulsants on sleep architecture.

In a survey of experimental epilepsy in animals, Wauquier et al.[161] observed that sleep fragmentation as obtained in epileptic animals as well as in humans may be the consequence of microarousals. Anticonvulsants may suppress microarousals because of their sedative properties and hence lead to stabilization of sleep fragmentation and normalization of sleep. Anticonvulsants may normalize sleep, however, because of a specific action on particular abnormal EEG patterns. Thus, despite the suggestion that anticonvulsants themselves may be responsible in part for the fragmentation and disruption of sleep architecture, the general consensus is that anticonvulsant medications normalize sleep architecture, most probably by reduction of the seizures.

Touchon et al.[162] studied sleep architecture in epileptic patients with CPS before and after treatment with carbamazepine. Initially, they studied 80 patients with CPS and found an increase in WASO and awakenings. These effects were not related to the seizure itself but may be related to the seizure duration or to the anticonvulsants. They also found a decrement of sleep efficiency. In a later study, these authors prospectively studied 10 patients with CPS and compared them with a group of normal, age-matched subjects. Seizure patients were on 800 mg carbamazepine daily. PSG studies were made on two consecutive nights, two nights before and two nights after the patient had been on carbamazepine treatment for 1 month. Before instituting carbamazepine, the authors found that the percentages of stage I NREM sleep, number of awakenings, and WASO were increased. After carbamazepine treatment, these sleep characteristics were partially modified and controlled by the treatment. They concluded that the length of seizure and drug treatment were not responsible for abnormal sleep architecture, the abnormal sleep structure may be related to the seizures, and carbamazepine treatment improves sleep architecture within limits.

Wolf et al.[163] reviewed the literature to assess the effect of barbiturates, phenytoin, carbamazepine, and valproic acid treatment on sleep. They noted significant reduction of REM sleep, a reduction in total awake time, and an increase in NREM stage II sleep as the short-term effects of barbiturates. The long-term effects of barbiturates are similar in general, but in some cases the sleep pattern returned to the premedication level.

Wolf et al.[163] performed a prospective polygraphic study of sleep in epileptic patients before and after medications using a cross-over design. They studied phenobarbital, phenytoin, ethosuximide, valproic acid, and carbamazepine. The authors included 40 unmedicated patients to study the effect of phenobarbital and phenytoin. The short-term effects of phenobarbital included reduction of WASO and REM sleep and increase of stage II NREM sleep. There was no relationship with the serum drug levels. The short-term effects of phenytoin included no change in the percentage of WASO, a decrease in NREM sleep stages I and II, and an increase in sleep stages III and IV; there was no change in REM sleep and no relationship with the serum drug levels.

Wolf et al.[163] studied the long-term effects of phenytoin in 12 patients. The long-term effects were in general a reversal of the short-term effects and consisted of an increase of NREM sleep stages I and II with a decrease of stages III and IV. REM sleep, however, remained unaltered. The effects of ethosuximide included an increase in stage I sleep, a decrease in stages III and IV sleep, and increased awakenings.[163] Valproic acid similarly increased stage I but did not decrease stages III and IV NREM sleep.[163]

Long-term phenytoin treatment by Hartmann[164] revealed a shortened sleep onset and an increase of light sleep in some subjects. Roder-Wanner et al.[165] noted a temporary increase of slow-wave sleep after phenytoin treatment.

Baldy-Moulinier[166] reported normalization of disturbed sleep pattern in temporal lobe epileptics after carbamazepine treatment. After acute carbamazepine administration in cats, Gigli et al.[167] reported an increase of NREM stage I sleep and total sleep time, a decrease of REM sleep, and reduced duration of awakenings.

Findji and Catani[168] reported an improvement of sleep organization and an increase of deep NREM sleep in epileptic children after treatment with valproic acid. At high dosage, however, Harding et al.[169] observed a decrease of delta and REM sleep.

Manni et al.[170] performed an objective and subjective assessment of daytime sleepiness using MSLT, clinical, and psychometric data on 10 patients with generalized epilepsy treated chronically with phenobarbital, 10 patients with cryptogenic partial epilepsy treated with carbamazepine, and 10 healthy controls. These authors found that patients on phenobarbital had a greater daytime sleep tendency and performed worse on the digit symbol substitution test compared to the other two

groups. In a similarly designed study,[171] they noted a shorter mean sleep latency in patients on phenobarbital compared with patients on sodium valproate and controls. Psychomotor functioning was also poor in patients on phenobarbital compared to controls, whereas patients on valproate had some attentional impairment and a tendency toward longer motor movement time. However, they did not find a correlation between the assessed parameters and serum drug concentrations.

A survey of the literature thus reveals that we need more studies to understand the interactions of the anticonvulsants, sleep, and epilepsy. Based on the literature and their own investigations, Declerck and Wauquier[172] emphasized the importance of the use and development of automatic methods to assess antiepileptic-induced sleep changes in patients with epilepsy. It may be that the anticonvulsants disrupt the circadian distribution of interictal discharges during the night and this may have practical relevance in terms of treatment.

## SLEEP, EPILEPSY, AND AUTONOMIC DYSFUNCTION

There are a number of autonomic nervous system (ANS) changes, particularly involving the respiratory and cardiovascular systems, during sleep[173] (see also Chapter 6). Furthermore, epilepsy itself may cause changes in the ANS and thus there is a close interrelationship between sleep, epilepsy, and the ANS.

ANS changes involving the cardiovascular system during sleep consist of reduction of the blood pressure and heart rate during NREM sleep and wide fluctuation of these during REM sleep.[173] Respiration shows considerable changes during NREM and in particular during REM sleep.[28] Sleep adversely affects breathing, even in normal individuals, and often triggers seizures in epileptic patients. Knowledge of the central autonomic network makes it easy to understand why this relationship between ANS, sleep, circulation, and respiration exists.[174] The nucleus tractus solitarius, a structure in the region of the medulla important for sleep, cardiovascular, and respiratory regulation, is reciprocally connected with the limbic-hypothalamic and other forebrain structures[174] (see Chapter 6). This connection explains why epileptic seizures triggered by the limbic-hypothalamic or other forebrain structures may interact with the cardiovascular and respiratory regulation during sleep. Respiratory dysrhythmia during generalized seizures, after seizure discharges in the limbic system, and after experimental stimulation of the limbic areas is documented.[175] The coexistence of sleep apnea and epilepsy, once thought to be rare, is increasingly recognized. There have been several reports[176–180] of upper airway obstructive, mixed, and central sleep apneas in patients with epilepsy (Figure 34-9) and of improvement in seizure control with treatment of the apneas.

It is well-known that in generalized tonic-clonic and CPS, transient abnormalities of ANS functions may occur and may consist of alterations in cardiac rhythm, blood pressure, and respiration.[181] In addition, it is well-known that epileptiform discharges without any clinical accompaniments may produce a variety of autonomic abnormalities. In patients after electroconvulsive[182] treatment and in animal models after pentylenetetrazol[183] injection, there are intense changes in blood pressure and cardiac rhythms. Similar changes have been observed in patients with focal temporal lobe discharges. Furthermore, the phenomenon of unexpected sudden death in patients with epilepsy,[184] which may account for up to 15%, may be the result of some unexplained autonomic dysfunction affecting the cardiac rhythm.

### Utility of Sleep in the Diagnosis of Epilepsy

Utility of sleep in the diagnosis of epilepsy was well-established after the landmark paper by Gibbs and Gibbs[12] in 1947 showing activation of epileptiform discharges in the sleep EEG. For the diagnosis of epilepsy, six sleep recordings are recommended: (1) standard sleep EEG recording, (2) EEG recording after sleep deprivation, (3) all-night PSG study, (4) video-PSG study, (5) MSLT, and (6) 24-hour ambulatory EEG and sleep recording. Table 34-1 outlines a suggested protocol for EEG recording in patients suspected to have epilepsy.

### Sleep Electroencephalography Recording and Sleep Deprivation Study

The usefulness of sleep EEG recording and sleep deprivation is discussed in detail in the previous para-graphs. For such recordings, a full complement of electrodes should be; various montages have been suggested (see Chapter 9). Broughton[19] listed some of the main indications and objectives of the daytime sleep EEG recording as follows: (1) normal EEGs in patients suspected of epilepsy to establish the diagnosis of true epilepsy; (2) normal waking EEGs in patients with known epilepsy to clarify the type of epilepsy; (3) patients with febrile convulsions showing normal waking EEGs; (4) assessment of the familial predisposition to epilepsy in family members; and (5) assessment of the degree of drug control, for example, in patients with hypsarrhythmia.

### All-Night Polysomnographic Recording

Broughton[19] listed the following important indications to perform all-night PSG study: (1) to differentiate between epileptic and nonepileptic nocturnal events (e.g., pseudoseizures, syncope due to cardiac arrhythmias, parasomnias); (2) to clarify the classification in patients with known sleep epilepsies; (3) to diagnose ESES; (4) to diagnose benign epilepsy of childhood with rolandic spikes; (5) to lateralize or localize the principal focus during REM sleep by use of stereo-EEG (this may be important before surgical treatment is considered); (6) to unmask the primary focus in a patient with secondary bilateral synchrony during REM sleep by causing suppression of the generalized discharges; (7) to reveal abnormalities in patients with hypsarrhythmia for whom waking EEGs rarely may be normal but sleep EEG may, and to clarify focal abnormalities in such patients; (8) to diagnose tonic seizures in patients with Lennox-Gastaut syndrome; (9) to diagnose sleep apnea or other primary sleep disorders, which may be mistaken for or associated with epilepsy; and (10) to investigate patients complaining of excessive daytime somnolence that cannot be explained by the anticonvulsant medication. Two additional indications are (1) to document cardiac arrhythmias that may arise during sleep and may be confused with, or even give rise to, seizures and (2) to document sleep disturbances and sleep architecture in epileptics so that these disturbances may be treated to prevent chronic sleep deprivation, which may in turn have deleterious effects on epilepsy itself. In suspected seizure disorders, all-night PSG recording should include multiple EEG leads and special montages (see Chapter 9).

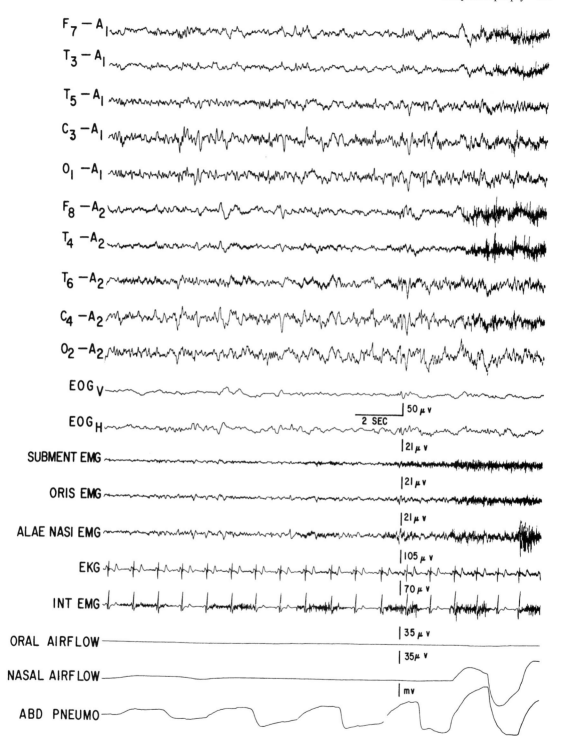

**Figure 34-9.** Polysomnographic recording in a patient with partial complex seizure and sleep apnea showing EEG (top 10 channels); vertical (EOG$_V$) and horizontal (EOG$_H$) electro-oculograms; submental (SUBMENT), orbicularis oris (ORIS), alae nasi, and intercostal (INT) electromyograms (EMG); electrocardiogram (EKG); oral and nasal airflow; and abdominal pneumogram (ABD PNEUMO). Note upper airway obstructive apnea during non-REM stage II sleep. No epileptiform discharges are seen in the EEG during the episodes. Paper speed is 15 mm/sec.

**Table 34-1.** Suggested Protocol for Electroencephalography Recording in Patients Suspected of Epilepsy

1. Routine EEG recording with hyperventilation and photic stimulation.
2. If negative for interictal epileptiform activity (IEA), EEG with sleep (natural or induced) recording.
3. If negative for IEA, EEG study with partial (at least 4 hours) or total (24 hours) sleep deprivation.
4. If negative for IEA after three to four EEGs, prolonged (4–6 hours) daytime EEG with sleep recording.
5. If negative for IEA, overnight polysomnographic (PSG) study, preferably video-PSG study for electroclinical correlation. If computer facilities exist for reformatting, change the paper speed to 30 mm/sec instead of the usual sleep recording speed of 10 mm/sec during interpretation of the recording. If computer facilities do not exist, use paper speed of 30 mm/sec as used during standard EEG recording, particularly during suspicious behavioral episodes. Use appropriately devised seizure montage with full complement of electrodes (see Chapter 9) or special electrode placements (e.g., T1 and T2 electrodes).
6. If still negative for IEA, cassette ambulatory 24-hour EEG recording.
7. If still negative for IEA, long-term video-EEG monitoring for 24–72 hours or longer if necessary.
8. Finally, in some patients, invasive intracranial EEG monitoring using subdural grids, strips, or depth electrodes may be necessary for localizing and lateralizing a focus.

### Video-Polysomnographic Study

The value of video-PSG for the diagnosis of parasomnias and seizure disorders has been well-documented by Aldrich and Jahnke[185] (see Chapter 18). Figure 34-10 is a PSG showing the onset of a partial seizure recorded at 10 mm per second and 30 mm per second paper speed.

### Multiple Sleep Latency Test

The MSLT[186] is indicated in patients complaining of excessive daytime somnolence that is not explained on the basis of anticonvulsant medication. Seizure during sleep may lead to repeated arousals, causing excessive daytime somnolence with further increase of seizure frequency, thus creating a vicious cycle. Sometimes narcolepsy may be mistaken for epilepsy, and an important diagnostic test for narcolepsy is MSLT. Finally, as discussed earlier, patients with epilepsy may have sleep apnea, which can be diagnosed by showing reduced sleep onset latency on MSLT, that is causing excessive daytime somnolence.

### Ambulatory 24-Hour Encephalographic Recording and Sleep Scoring

Ambulatory 24-hour encephalographic recording and sleep scoring allow for recording of the EEG discharges throughout the day to understand the circa-

dian and ultradian rhythmicity and the effects of sleep on the interictal discharges. The question of whether epilepsy manifests biorhythmicity was discussed earlier. Technical problems associated with unattended recordings, however, are serious limitations.

### Long-Term Video-Encephalography Monitoring

In some patients, simultaneous video and EEG monitoring in the inpatient unit for several days is necessary to document an ictal epileptiform discharge and its characteristic behavioral correlate, thus providing indisputable evidence of a true seizure episode.

### Intracranial Recordings

When both long-term monitoring and neuroimaging are unable to identify a seizure focus with certainty, intracranial recordings in a specialized epilepsy center are indicated. This usually entails the use of stereotactically implanted depth electrodes and subdural strips or grids.

### Other Investigations

Neuroimaging studies are indispensable in investigating the presence of structural lesions that may serve as epileptogenic foci. Anatomic studies (computed tomography and magnetic resonance imag-

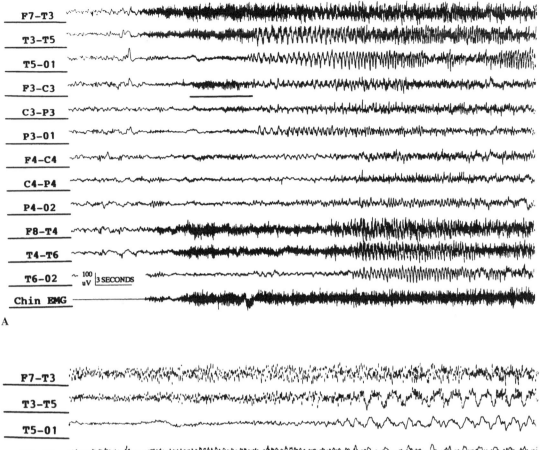

A

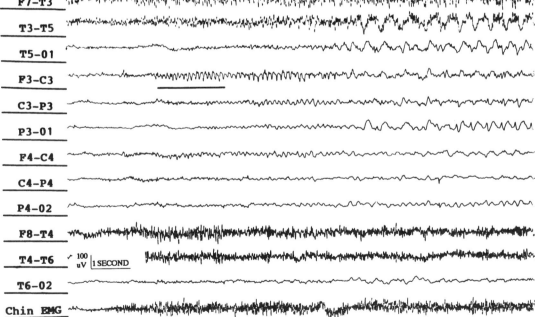

B

**Figure 34-10.** A portion of a polysomnographic recording using 12 channels of EEG showing the onset of a partial seizure recorded at 10 mm/sec paper speed. The underlined activity represents rhythmic ictal discharges beginning over the left hemisphere (F3-C3) and spreading rapidly to the right hemisphere, and is accompanied by clinical seizure. Although at 10 mm/sec paper speed (**A**) the underlined activity superficially resembles muscle artifacts, at 30 mm/sec paper speed (**B**) it becomes obvious that this activity is the beginning of the rhythmic epileptiform discharges in the EEG. (Reprinted with permission from M Aldrich, B Jahnke. Diagnostic value of video-EEG polysomnography. Neurology 1991;41:1060.)

ing) are usually performed in all adults with new onset seizures and in children without any characteristic epileptic syndromes. Functional or physiologic studies (single-photon emission computed tomography and PET) may be able to identify seizure foci by revealing areas of cerebral hypermetabolism or hyperperfusion during an ictal episode and areas of hypometabolism during the interictal period.

### Practical Relevance to Understanding the Relationship between Sleep and Epilepsy

An understanding of the relationship between sleep and epilepsy is important for three main purposes:

1. Such an understanding can aid in the diagnosis of seizure and in differential diagnosis between epileptic and nonepileptic events and among different types of seizures.

2. An understanding of this relationship can increase the understanding of the pathogenesis of triggering mechanisms of seizures during sleep and the mechanism and nature of sleep disturbances induced by epilepsy.

3. Therapeutic manipulation can be guided by the knowledge obtained through an understanding of the relationship between epilepsy and sleep. It may be possible to adjust the timing of the drug dose but this really has not been useful from a practical point of view. An understanding of the biorhythmicity and the relationship between sleep and epilepsy may be important to choose the type of anticonvulsant so that one may avoid those with marked hypnotic effects in nocturnal seizure patients and use drugs with less sedative effects (e.g., carbamazepine, valproic acid, felbamate). Finally, one may manipulate sleep stages—that is, give anticonvulsants that may increase REM or NREM stages III and IV to reduce the ictal or interictal discharges.

Finally, as Broughton[19] stated, it may be necessary to put some patients on a strict program of sleep hygiene (see Table 24-3) or to treat the sleep disorders with pharmacologic agents because of the deleterious effects the epilepsy has on sleep and sleep on epilepsy. Such patients may be advised to avoid sleep deprivation, alcohol in the evening, and late evening exercise, and to maintain regular sleep and waking hours. Broughton[19] suggested that the improvement of nocturnal sleep after such a regime may be associated with definite reduction of seizure frequency and overall improvement in general well-being.

---

## REFERENCES

1. Passouant P. Historical Aspects of Sleep and Epilepsy. In R Degen, E Niedermeyer (eds), Epilepsy, Sleep Deprivation. Amsterdam: Elsevier, 1984;67.
2. Echeverria MC. De l'epilepsie nocturne. Ann Med Psychol (Paris) 1879;5:177.
3. Fere L. Les Epilepsies et les Epileptiques. Paris: Alcan, 1890.
4. Gowers WR. Epilepsy and Other Chronic Convulsive Diseases (Vol 1). London: Williams Wood, 1885.
5. Turner WA. Epilepsy: A Study of the Idiopathic Disease. London: MacMillan, 1907.
6. Gallus R. Die allgemeinen Ursachen der Anfallshaufungen innerhalb grobgerer Gruppen von Kranken. Epilepsi (Leipzig) 1911;3:46.
7. Amann R. Untersuchungen uber die Veranderungen in der Haufigkiet der epileptischen Anfalle und deren Ursachen. Z Ges Neurol Psychiatry 1914;24:5.
8. Langdon-Down M, Brain WR. Time of day in relation to convulsions in epilepsy. Lancet 1929;2:1029.
9. Patry FL. The relation of time of day, sleep and other factors to the incidence of epileptic seizures. Am J Psychiatry 1931;87:789.
10. Busciano VM. Etiologia dell'accesso epilettica. Osped Psychiatry 1936;4:33.
11. Magnussen G. Eighteen cases of epilepsy with fits in relation to sleep. Acta Psychol (Amst) 1936;11:289.
12. Gibbs EL, Gibbs FA. Diagnostic and localizing value of electroencephalographic studies in sleep. Res Publ Assoc Res Nerv Ment Dis 1947;26:366.
13. Janz D. The grand mal epilepsies and the sleep-waking cycle. Epilepsia 1962;3:69.
14. Passouant P. Influence des Etats de Vigilance sur les Epilepsies. In WP Koella (ed), Sleep (Vol 3). Basel: Karger, 1977;57.
15. Gastaut H, Batini C, Fressy J, et al. Etude Electrocephalographique des Phenomenes Episodiques Course du Sommeil. In H Fischgold (ed), Le Sommeil de Nuit Normal et Pathologique. Paris: Masson, 1965;239.
16. Cadilhac JC. Le Sommeil Nocturne des Epileptiques. Étude Polygraphique. These de Medecine, Monsieur, 1967;150.
17. Niedermeyer E. Sleep electroencephalograms in petit mal. Arch Neurol 1965;12:625.
18. Montplaisir J. Epilepsy and Sleep: Reciprocal Interactions and Diagnostic Procedures Involving Sleep. In MJ Thorpy (ed), Handbook of Sleep Disorders. New York: Marcel Dekker, 1990;643.

19. Broughton RJ. Epilepsy and Sleep: A Synopsis and Prospectus. In R Degin, E Niedermeyer (eds), Epilepsy, Sleep and Sleep Deprivation. Amsterdam: Elsevier, 1984;317.

20. Billiard M. Epilepsy and the Sleep-Wake Cycle. In MB Sterman, MN Shouse, P Passouant (eds), Sleep and Epilepsy. New York: Academic, 1982;269.

21. Kellaway P. Sleep and epilepsy. Epilepsia 1985;26:S15.

22. Engel J Jr. Seizures and Epilepsy. Philadelphia: Davis, 1989;71.

23. Matsumoto H, Ajmone-Marsan C. Cortical cellular phenomena in experimental epilepsy: interictal manifestations. Exp Neurol 1964;9:286.

24. Margerison JH, Corsellis JA. Epilepsy and the temporal lobes: a clinical, electroencephalographic and neuropathological study of the brain in epilepsy, with particular reference to the temporal lobes. Brain 1966;69:499.

25. Gloor P, Quesney LF, Zumstein H. Pathophysiology of generalized penicillin epilepsy in the cat: the role of cortical and subcortical structures. II. Topical applications of penicillin to the cerebral cortex and to subcortical structures. Electroencephalogr Clin Neurophysiol 1977;43:79.

26. Quesney LF, Gloor P, Kratzenberg E, et al. Pathophysiology of generalized penicillin epilepsy in the cat: the role of cortical and subcortical structures. I. Systematic application of penicillin. Electroencephalogr Clin Neurophysiol 1977;42:640.

27. Gloor P. Generalized cortico-reticular epilepsy: some considerations on the pathophysiology of generalized bilaterally synchronous spike and wave discharge. Epilepsia 1968;9:249.

28. Chokroverty S. The Assessment of Sleep Disturbances in Autonomic Failure. In R Bannister, CJ Mathias (eds), Autonomic Failure. Oxford: Oxford University Press, 1992;422.

29. Pompeiano O. Sleep Mechanism. In HH Jasper, AA Ward Jr, A Pope (eds), Basic Mechanisms of the Epilepsies. Boston: Little, Brown, 1969;453.

30. Berlucchi G. Callosal activity in unrestrained, unanesthetized cats. Arch Ital Biol 1965;103:623.

31. Steriade M. Brain Electrical Activity and Sensory Processing During Waking and Sleep States. In MH Kryger, T Roth, WC Dement (eds), Principles and Practice of Sleep Medicine. Philadelphia: Saunders, 1989;86.

32. Villablanca J. Role of the Thalamus in Sleep Control: Sleep-Wakefulness Studies in Chronic Diencephalic and Athalamic Cats. In O Petre-Quadens, J Schlag (eds), Basic Sleep Mechanisms. New York: Academic, 1974;51.

33. Ball GJ, Gloor P, Schaul N. The cortical electromicrophysiology of pathological delta waves in the electroencephalogram of cats. Electroencephalogr Clin Neurophysiol 1977;43:346.

34. Jones BE. Basic Mechanisms of Sleep-Wake States. In MH Kryger, T Roth, WC Dement (eds), Principles and Practice of Sleep Medicine. Philadelphia: Saunders, 1989;121.

35. Morison RS, Dempsey EW. A study of thalamocortical relations. Am J Physiol 1942;135:281.

36. Hess WR. Das Schlafsyndrom als folge diencephaler Reizung. Healv Physiol Pharmacol Acta 1944;2:305.

37. Hobson JA, Lydic R, Baghdoyan HA. Evolving concepts of sleep cycle generation: from brain centers to neuronal populations. Behav Brain Sci 1986;9:371.

38. Kostopoulos G, Gloor P. A Mechanism for Spike-Wave Discharge in Feline Penicillin Epilepsy and Its Relationship to Spindle Generation. In MB Sterman, MM Shouse, P Passouant (eds), Sleep and Epilepsy. New York: Academic, 1982;11.

39. Jasper H, Droogleever-Fortuyn J. Experimental studies on the functional anatomy of petit mal epilepsy. Res Publ Assoc Res Nerv Ment Dis 1947;26:272.

40. Spencer WA, Brookhart JM. A study of spontaneous spindle waves in sensorimotor cortex of cats. J Neurophysiol 1961;24:50.

41. Spencer WA, Kandel ER. Synaptic Inhibition in Seizures. In HH Jasper, AA Ward Jr, A Pope (eds), Basic Mechanisms of the Epilepsies. Boston: Little, Brown, 1969;575.

42. Gloor P. Evolution of the Concept of the Mechanism of Generalized Epilepsy with Bilateral Spike and Wave Discharge. In JA Wada (ed), Modern Perspectives in Epilepsy. Montreal: Eden, 1978;99.

43. Niedermeyer E. The Generalized Epilepsies. Springfield: Thomas, 1972.

44. Wyler AR. Epileptic neurons during sleep and wakefulness. Exp Neurol 1974;42:593.

45. Shouse MN, Siegel JM, Wu MF, et al. Mechanism of seizure suppression during rapid-eye movement (REM) sleep in cats. Brain Res 1989;505:271.

46. Cohen HB, Thomas J, Dement WC. Sleep stages, REM deprivation and electroconvulsive threshold in the cat. Brain Res 1970;19:317.

47. Janz D. Epilepsy and the Sleeping-Waking Cycle. In PJ Vinken, GW Bruyn (eds), Handbook of Clinical Neurology: The Epilepsies. Amsterdam: North-Holland, 1974;457.

48. Hopkins H. The time of appearance of epileptic seizures in relation to age, duration and type of syndrome. J Nerv Ment Dis 1933;77:153.

49. Shouse MN. Epilepsy and Seizures During Sleep. In MH Kryger, T Roth, WC Dement (eds), Principles and Practices of Sleep Medicine. Philadelphia: Saunders, 1989;364.

50. D'Alesandro R, Santini M, Pazzagli P, et al. Pure Sleep Epilepsies: Prognostic Features. In G Nistico, R Di Perri, H Meinardi (eds), Epilepsy: An Update on Research and Therapy. New York: Liss, 1983;235.

51. Kajtor F. The influence of sleep and the waking state on the epileptic activity of different cerebral structures. Epilepsia 1962;3:274.

52. Gibberd FB, Bateson HC. Sleep epilepsy: its pattern and prognosis. BMJ 1974;2:403.

53. Kellaway P, Frost JD Jr, Crawley JM. Time modulation of spike-and-wave activity in generalized epilepsy. Ann Neurol 1980;8:491.

54. Autret A, Laffon F, Roux S. Influence of waking and sleep stages on the interictal paroxysmal activity in partial epilepsy with complex seizures. Electroencephalogr Clin Neurophysiol 1983;55:406.

55. Kellaway P, Frost JD Jr. Biorhythmic Modulation of Epileptic Events. In TA Pedley, Meldrum BS (eds), Recent Advances in Epilepsy. London: Churchill Livingstone, 1983;139.

56. Stevens JR, Lonsbury BL, Goel SL. Seizure occurrence and interspike interval. Arch Neurol 1972;26:409.

57. Binnie CD. Are Biological Rhythms of Importance in Epilepsy? In A Martins da Silva, CD Binnie, H Meinardi (eds), Biorhythms and Epilepsy. New York: Raven, 1985;1.

58. Martins da Silva A, Binnie CD. Ultradian Variations of Epileptiform EEG Activity. In A Martins da Silva, CD Binnie, H Meinardi (eds), Biorhythms and Epilepsy. New York: Raven, 1985;69.

59. Broughton R, Stampi C, Romano S, et al. Do Waking Ultradian Rhythms Exist for Petit Mal Absences? A Case Report. In A Martins da Silva, CD Binnie, H Meinardi (eds), Biorhythms and Epilepsy. New York: Raven, 1985;95.

60. Almqvist R. The Rhythm of Epileptic Attacks and Its Relationship to the Menstrual Cycle. Jonkoping: Tryckeriaktiebolaget Smaland, 1955.

61. Newmark ME, Penry JK. Catamenial epilepsy: a review. Epilepsia 1980;21:281.

62. Webb WB. Circadian Biological Rhythm Aspects of Sleep and Epilepsy. In A Martins da Silva, CD Binnie, H Meinardi (eds), Biorhythms and Epilepsy. New York: Raven, 1985;13.

63. Commission on Classification and Terminology of the International League Against Epilepsy. Proposal for classification of epilepsies and epileptic syndromes. Epilepsia 1985;26:268.

64. Janz D. "Aufwach-Epilepsien." Arch Psychiatr Nervenkr 1953;191:73.

65. Besset A. Influence of Generalized Seizures on Sleep Organization. In MB Sterman, MN Shouse, P Passouant (eds), Sleep and Epilepsy. New York: Academic, 1982;339.

66. Billiard M, Besset A, Zachariev Z, et al. Relation of Seizures and Seizure Discharged to Sleep Stages. In P Wolf, M Dam, F Janz, et al. (eds), Advances in Epileptology. New York: Raven, 1987;665.

67. Passouant P, Besset A, Carrier A, et al. Night Sleep and Generalized Epilepsies. In WP Koella, P Levin (eds), Sleep 1974. Basel: Karger, 1975;185.

68. Passouant P, Latour H, Cadilhac J. L'epilepsie morphepeique. Ann Med Psychol 1951;109:526.

69. Gastaut H, Batini C, Broughton R, et al. An electroencephalographic study of nocturnal sleep in epileptic patients [abstract]. Electroencephalogr Clin Neurophysiol 1965;18:96.

70. Gastaut H, Broughton R. A Clinical and Polygraphic Study of Episodic Phenomenon During Sleep. In J Wortis (ed), Recent Advances in Biological Psychiatry (Vol 7). New York: Plenum, 1965;197.

71. Patry G, Lyagoubi S, Tassinari CA. Subclinical electrical status epilepticus induced by sleep in children. Ann Neurol 1971;24:242.

72. Meier-Ewert K, Broughton R. Photomyoclonic response of epileptic subjects during wakefulness, sleep and arousal. Electroencephalogr Clin Neurophysiol 1967;23:142.

73. Touchon J. Effect of Awakening on Epileptic Activity in Primary Generalized Myoclonic Epilepsy. In MB Sterman, MN Shouse, P Passouant (eds), Sleep and Epilepsy. New York: Academic, 1982;239.

74. Gastaut H, Roger J, Soulayrol R, et al. Childhood epileptic encephalopathy with diffuse slow spike-waves (otherwise known as petit mal variant) or Lennox syndrome. Epilepsia 1966;7:139.

75. Dinner DS. Sleep and pediatric epilepsy. Cleve Clin J Med 1989;56:S234.

76. Gastaut H, Broughton R, Roger J, et al. Generalized Convulsive Seizures without Local Onset. In PJ Vinken, GW Bruyn (eds), Handbook of Clinical Neurology (Vol 15), The Epilepsies. Amsterdam: Elsevier, 1974;107.

77. Erba G, Moschen R, Ferber R. Sleep-related changes in EEG discharge activity and seizure risk in patients with Lennox-Gastaut syndrome. Sleep Res 1981;10:247.

78. Gomez MR, Klass DW. Epilepsies of infancy and childhood. Ann Neurol 1983;13:113.

79. Montplaisir J, Laverdiere M, Saint-Hilaire JM, et al. Sleep and temporal lobe epilepsy: a case study with depth electrodes. Neurology 1981;31:1352.

80. Montplaisir J, Laverdiere M, Saint-Hilaire JM. Sleep and Focal Epilepsy: Contribution of Depth Recording. In MB Sterman, MN Shouse, P Passouant (eds), Sleep and Epilepsy. New York: Academic, 1982;301.

81. Montplaisir J, Laverdiere M, Rouleau I, et al. Nocturnal sleep recording in partial epilepsy: a study with depth electrodes. J Clin Neurophysiol 1987;4:383.

82. Laverdiere M, Montplaisir J. Frequency of epileptic spike activity and sleep disturbances in temporal lobe epilepsy. Sleep Res 1984;13:177.

83. Rossi GF, Colicchio G, Polla P. Interictal epileptic activity during sleep: a stereo-EEG study in patients with partial epilepsy. Electroencephalogr Clin Neurophysiol 1983;58:97.

84. Cadilhac J. Complex Partial Seizures and REM Sleep. In MB Sterman, MN Shouse, P Passouant (eds), Sleep and Epilepsy. New York: Academic, 1982;315.

85. Kikuchi S. An electroencephalographic study of nocturnal sleep in temporal lobe epilepsy. Foli Psychiatr Neurol Jpn 1969;23:59.

86. Epstein AW, Hill W. Ictal phenomena during REM sleep of a temporal lobe epileptic. Ann Neurol 1966;15:367.

87. Montplaisir J, Laverdiere M, Saint-Hiliare JM. Sleep and Epilepsy. In J Gotman, JR Ives, P Gloor (eds), Long-Term Monitoring in Epilepsy (EEG Suppl No 37). Amsterdam: Elsevier, 1985;215.

88. Ross JJ, Johnson LC, Walter RD. Spike and wave discharges during stages of sleep. Ann Neurol 1966; 14:399.

89. Autret A, Lucas B, Laffont F, et al. Two distinct classifications of adult epilepsies: by time of seizures and by sensitivity of the interictal paroxysmal activities to sleep and waking. Electroencephalogr Clin Neurophysiol 1987;66:211.

90. Bittner-Manicka M. Investigations on the mechanism of nocturnal epilepsy. J Neurol 1976;211:169.

91. Sato S, Dreifuss F, Penry JK. The effect of sleep on spike-wave discharges in absence seizures. Neurology 1973;23:1335.

92. Tassinari CA, Bureau-Paillas M, Dalla-Bernardina B, et al. Generalized Epilepsies and Seizures During Sleep. A Polygraphic Study. In HM Van Praag, H Meinardi (eds), Brain and Sleep. Amsterdam: De Erven Bohn, 1974;154.

93. Markand ON. Slow spike-wave activity in EEG and associated clinical features: often called "Lennox" or "Lennox-Gastaut" syndrome. Neurology 1977;27:746.

94. Jeavons PM, Bower BD. The natural history of infantile spasms. Arch Dis Child 1961;36:17.

95. Niedermeyer E, Rocca U. The diagnostic significance of sleep electroencephalographs in temporal lobe epilepsy. A comparison of scalp and depth tracings. Eur Neurol 1972;7:119.

96. Frank G. Epileptiform discharges during various stages of sleep. Electroencephalogr Clin Neurophysiol 1970;28:95.

97. Angelieri F. Partial Epilepsies and Nocturnal Sleep. In P Levin, WP Koella (eds), Sleep 1974. Basel: Karger, 1975;196.

98. Passouant P, Cadilhac J, Delange M. Indications apportees par l'etude du dommeil du nuit sur la physiopathologie des epilepsies. Int J Neurol 1965;5:207.

99. Mayersdorf A, Wilder BJ. Focal epileptic discharges during all night sleep studies. Clin Electroencephalogr 1974;5:73.

100. Lieb J, Joseph JP, Engel J, et al. Sleep state and seizure foci related to depth spike activity in patients with temporal lobe epilepsy. Electroencephalogr Clin Neurophysiol 1980;49:538.

101. Frank GS, Pegram GV. Interrelations of sleep and focal epileptiform discharge in monkeys with alumina cream lesions. Aeromed Res Lab Publ 1974;27.

102. Mayanagi Y. The influence of natural sleep on focal spiking in experimental temporal lobe epilepsy in the monkey. Electroencephalogr Clin Neurophysiol 1977;43:813.

103. Montplaisir J, Laverdiere M, Walsh J, et al. Influence of nocturnal sleep on the epileptic spike activity recorded with multiple depth electrodes [abstract]. Electroencephalogr Clin Neurophysiol 1980;49:P85.

104. Passouant P. Epilepsie temporale et sommeil. Rev Roum Neurol 1967;4:151.

105. Giaquinto S. Sleep recordings from limbic structures in man. Confin Neurol (Basel) 1973;35:285.

106. Malow BA, Kushwaha R, Lin X, et al. Relationship of interictal epileptiform discharges to sleep depth in partial epilepsy. Electroencephalogr Clin Neurophysiol 1997;102:20.

107. Gastaut H. Classification of Status Epilepticus. In A Delgado-Escueta (ed), Status Epilepticus. New York: Raven, 1982.

108. Janz D. Die Epilepsien. Stuttgart: Thieme, 1969.

109. Froscher W. Sleep and Prolonged Epileptic Activity (Status Epilepticus). In R Degen, EA Rodin (eds), Epilepsy, Sleep and Sleep Deprivation (2nd ed). Amsterdam: Elsevier, 1991;165.

110. Gastaut H, Tassinari C. Status Epilepticus. In Remond A (ed), Handbook of Electroencephalography and Clinical Neurophysiology (Vol 13A). Amsterdam: Elsevier, 1975.

111. Passouant P. Influence des Etats de Vigilance sur les Epilepsies. In WP Koella, Levin P (eds), Sleep 1976. Basel: Karger, 1977;57.

112. Roger J, Lob H, Tassinari CA. Status Epilepticus. In PJ Vinken, GW Bruyn (eds), Handbook of Clinical Neurology (Vol 15). Amsterdam: Elsevier, 1974.

113. Tassinari CA, Terzano G, Capocchi G, et al. Epileptic Seizures During Sleep in Children. In JK Penry (ed), Epilepsy. The Eighth International Symposium. New York: Raven, 1977.

114. Nayrac P, Beaussart M. Les pointes-ondes pre-rolandiques: expression EEG tres particuliere. Etude electroclinique de 21 cas. Rev Neurol 1958;99:201.

115. Beaussart M. Benign epilepsy of children with rolandic (centrotemporal) paroxysmal foci. A clinical entity. Study of 221 cases. Epilepsia 1973;13:795.

116. Janz D, Mathes A. Die Propulsiv-Petit-Mal-Epilepsie. In Blitz-, Nick-, Salaamkrampfe (eds), Klinik and Verlauf der Sog. Basel: Karger, 1955.

117. Janz D, Christian W. Impulsive petit mal. Dtsch Z Nervenheilkd 1957;176:346.

118. Janz D. Epilepsy with impulsive petit mal (juvenile myoclinic epilepsy). Acta Neurol Scand 1985;72:449.

119. Wolf P. Epilepsy with Grand Mal on Awakening. In Roger J, Dravet C, Bureau M, et al. (eds), Epileptic Syndromes in Infancy, Childhood, and Adolescence. London: Libbey, 1985;259:270.

120. Tassinari CA, Bureau M, Dravet C, et al. Electrical Status Epilepticus During Sleep in Children (ESES). In MB Sterman, MN Shouse, P Passouant (eds), Sleep and Epilepsy. New York: Academic, 1982;465.

121. Ortega JJ, Belda VJ, Tripiana JL, et al. Electrical status epilepticus during sleep. Rev Neurol 1996;24(136):1551.

122. Lugaresi E, Cirignotta F. Hypnogenic paroxysmal dystonia: epileptic seizure or a new syndrome? Sleep 1981;4:129.

123. Lugaresi E, Cirignotta F, Montagna P. Nocturnal paroxysmal dystonia. J Neurol Neurosurg Psychiatry 1986;49:375.

124. Sellal F, Hirsch E, Maquet P. Postures et mouvements anormaux paroxystiques lors du sommeil: dystonie paroxystique hypnogenique ou epilepsie partielle? Rev Neurol (Paris) 1991;147:121.

125. Meierkord H, Fish DR, Smith JM, et al. Is nocturnal paroxysmal dystonia a form of frontal lobe epilepsy? Mov Disord 1992;7:38.

126. Oguni M, Oguni H, Kozam M, Fukuyama Y. A case with nocturnal paroxysmal unilateral dystonia and interictal right frontal epileptic EEG focus: a lateralized variant of nocturnal paroxysmal dystonia? Brain Dev 1992;14:412.

127. Scheffer IE, Bhatia KP, Lopes-Cendes I, et al. Autosomal dominant frontal epilepsy misdiagnosed as sleep disorder. Lancet 1994;343:515.

128. Oldani A, Zucconi M, Ferini-Strambi L, et al. Autosomal dominant nocturnal frontal lobe epilepsy: electroclinical picture. Epilepsia 1996;37:964.

129. Pratt KL, Mattson RH, Weikers NJ, et al. EEG activation of epileptics following sleep deprivation: a prospective study of 114 cases. Electroencephalogr Clin Neurophysiol 1968;24:11.

130. Rowan AJ, Veldhuisen RJ, Negelkerke NJD. Comparative evaluation of sleep deprivation and sedated sleep EEGs as diagnostic aids in epilepsy. Electroencephalogr Clin Neurophysiol 1982;54:357.

131. Degen R. A study of the diagnostic value of waking and sleep EEGs after sleep deprivation in epileptic patients on anticonvulsive therapy. Electroencephalogr Clin Neurophysiol 1980;49:577.

132. Arne-Bes MC, Calvet U, Thiberge M, et al. Effects of Sleep Deprivation in an EEG Study of Epileptics. In MB Sterman, P Passouant (eds), Sleep and Epilepsy. New York: Academic, 1982;339.

133. Rodin ES, Luby ED, Gottlieb JS. The electroencephalogram during prolonged experimental sleep deprivation. Electroencephalogr Clin Neurophysiol 1962;14:544.

134. Declerck AC. Interaction of Epilepsy, Sleep and Antiepileptics. Lisse: Swets & Zeitlinger, 1983.

135. Patrick GTW, Gilbert JA. On the effects of loss of sleep. Psychol Rev 1896;3:469. Cited in Kleitman N. Sleep and Wakefulness. Chicago: University of Chicago Press, 1963;219.

136. Bennett DR. Sleep deprivation and major motor convulsions. Neurology 1963;13:983.

137. Mattson RH, Pratt KL, Calverley JR. Electroencephalograms of epileptics following sleep deprivation. Ann Neurol 1965;13:310.

138. Rodin E. Sleep Deprivation and Epileptological Implications. In R Degen, EA Rodin (eds), Epilepsy, Sleep and Sleep Deprivation (2nd ed). Amsterdam: Elsevier, 1991;265.

139. Pedley TA, Guilleminault C. Episodic nocturnal wanderings responsive to anticonvulsant drug therapy. Ann Neurol 1977;2:30.

140. Niedermeyer E, Lopes da Silva F. Electroencephalography: Basic Principles, Clinical Applications and Related Fields. Baltimore: Urban & Schwarzenberg, 1987.

141. Declerck AC, Wauquier A, Sijben-Kiggen R, et al. A Normative Study of Sleep in Different Forms of Epilepsy. In MB Sterman, MN Shouse, P Passouant (eds), Sleep and Epilepsy. New York: Academic, 1982;329.

142. Delange D, Castan P, Cadilhac J, et al. Study of night sleep during centrencephalic and temporal epilepsides [abstract]. Electroencephalogr Clin Neurophysiol 1962;14:777.

143. Baldy-Moulinier M. Temporal Lobe Epilepsy and Sleep Organization. In MB Sterman, P Passouant (eds), Sleep and Epilepsy. New York: Academic, 1982;347.

144. Hamel AR, Sterman MB. Sleep and Epileptic Abnormalities During Sleep. In MB Sterman, MN Shouse, P Passouant (eds), Sleep and Epilepsy. New York: Academic, 1982;361.

145. Johnson LC. Effects of Anticonvulsant Medication on Sleep Patterns. In MB Sterman, MN Shouse, P Passouant (eds), Sleep and Epilepsy. New York: Academic, 1982;381.

146. Landau-Ferey J. A Contribution to the Study of Nocturnal Sleep in Patients Suspected of Having Epilepsy. In MB Sterman, MN Shouse, P Passouant (eds), Sleep and Epilepsy. New York: Academic, 1982;421.

147. Hoeppner J, Garron DC, Cartwright RD. Self-reported sleep disorder symptoms in epilepsy. Epilepsia 1984;25:434.

148. Roder-Wanner U, Wolf P, Danninger T. Are Sleep Patterns in Epileptic Patients Correlated with Their Type of Epilepsy? In A Martins da Silva, CD Binnie, H Meinardi (eds), Biorhythms and Epilepsy. New York: Raven, 1985;109.

149. Bowersox SS, Drucker-Colin R. Seizure Modification by Sleep Deprivation: A Possible Protein Synthesis Mechanism. In MB Sterman, MN Shouse, P Passouant (eds), Sleep and Epilepsy. New York: Academic, 1982;91.

150. Touchon J, Baldy-Moulinier M, Billiard M, et al. Organization du sommeil dans l'epilepsie recente du lobe temporal avant et apres traitement par carbamazepine. Rev Neurol (Paris) 1987;5:462.

151. Kohsaka M. Changes in epileptiform activities during sleep and sleep structures in temporal lobe epilepsy. Hokkaido J Med Sci 1993;68:630.

152. Bazil CW, Walczak TS. Effects of sleep and sleep stage on epileptic and nonepileptic seizures. Epilepsia 1997;38:56.

153. Hunt A, Stores G. Sleep disorder and epilepsy in children with tuberous sclerosis: a questionnaire-based study. Dev Med Child Neurol 1994;36:108.

154. Bruni O, Cortesi F, Gianotti F, Curatolo P. Sleep disorders in tuberous sclerosis: a polysomnographic study. Brain Dev 1995;17:52.

155. Shouse MN, Sterman MP. Sleep Pathology in Experimental Epilepsy: Amygdala Kindling. In MB Sterman, MN Shouse, P Passouant (eds), Sleep and Epilepsy. New York: Academic, 1982;151.

156. Cepeda C, Tanaka T. Limbic Status Epilepticus and Sleep in Baboons. In MB Sterman, MN Shouse, P Pas-

souant (eds), Sleep and Epilepsy. New York: Academic, 1982;165.

157. Tanaka T, Naquet R. Kindling effect and sleep organization in cats. Electroencephalogr Clin Neurophysiol 1975;39:449.

158. Silvestri R, de Domenico P, Mento G, et al. Epileptic seizures in subjects previously affected by disorders of arousal. Neurophysiol Clin 1995;25:19.

159. Tassinari CA, Mancia D, Della Bernadina B, Gastaut H. Pavor nocturnus of nonepileptic nature in epileptic children. Electroencephalogr Clin Neurophysiol 1972; 33:603.

160. Passouant P. Influence des Etats de Vigilance sur les Epilepsies. In WP Koella, Lenin P (eds), Sleep 1976. Basel: Karger, 1977;57.

161. Wauquier A, Clincake GHC, Declerck AC. Sleep Alterations by Seizures and Anticonvulsants. In A Martins da Silva, CD Binnie, H Meinardi (eds), Biorhythms and Epilepsy. New York: Raven, 1985;123.

162. Touchon J, Baldy-Moulinier M, Billiard M, et al. Sleep architecture in epileptic patients with complex partial seizures before and after treatment by carbamazepine [abstract]. Epilepsia 1986;27:640.

163. Wolf DP, Roder-Wanner UU, Brede M, et al. Influences of Antiepileptic Drugs on Sleep. In A Martins da Silva, CD Binnie, H Meinardi (eds), Biorhythms and Epilepsy. New York: Raven, 1985;137.

164. Hartmann E. The effects of diphenylhydantoin (DPH) on sleep in man. Psychophysiology 1970;7:316.

165. Roder-Wanner VV, Noachtar S, Wolf P. Response of polygraphic sleep to phenytoin treatment of epilepsy. A longitudinal study of immediate, short- and long-term effects. Acta Neurol Scand 1987;76:157.

166. Baldy-Moulinier M. Temporal lobe epilepsy and sleep organization. In MB Sterman, MN Shouse, P Passouant (eds), Sleep and Epilepsy. New York: Academic, 1982;347.

167. Gigli GL, Gotman J, Thomas ST. Sleep alterations after acute administration of carbamazepine in cats. Epilepsia 1988;29:748.

168. Findji F, Catani P. Readjustment des therapeutiques anticonvulsives chez l'enfant. L'Encephale 1982;8:595.

169. Harding GFA, Alford CA, Powell TE. The effect of sodium valproate on sleep, reaction times and visual evoked potential in normal subjects. Epilepsia 1985; 26:597.

170. Manni R, Ratti MT, Galimberti CA, et al. Daytime sleepiness in epileptic patients on long-term monotherapy: MSLT, clinical and psychometric assessment. Neurophysiol Clin 1993;23:71.

171. Manni R, Ratti MT, Perucca E, et al. A multiparametric investigation of daytime sleepiness and psychomotor functions in epileptic patients treated with phenobarbital and sodium valproate: a comparative controlled study. Electroencephalogr Clin Neurophysiol 1993; 86:322.

172. Declerck AC, Wauquier A. Influence of Antiepileptic Drugs on Sleep Patterns. In R Degen, EA Rodin (eds), Epilepsy, Sleep and Sleep Deprivation. Amsterdam: Elsevier, 1991;153.

173. Parmeggiani PL, Morrison AR. Alterations in Autonomic Functions During Sleep. In AD Loewy, KM Spyer (eds), Central Regulation of Autonomic Functions. Oxford, UK: Oxford University Press, 1990;366.

174. Chokroverty S. Functional anatomy of the autonomic nervous system: correlated with symptomatology of neurological disease. AAN Course No. 246, San Diego, 1992.

175. Nelson DA, Ray CD. Respiratory arrest from seizure discharges in limbic system. Arch Neurol 1968;19:199.

176. Wyler AR, Weymuller EA. Epilepsy complicated by sleep apnea. Ann Neurol 1981;9:403.

177. Chokroverty S, Sachdeo R, Goldhammer T, et al. Epilepsy and sleep apnea [abstract]. Electroencephalogr Clin Neurophysiol 1985;61:P26.

178. Vashista S, Ehrenberg B. Benefits of treating sleep-apnea in complex partial epilepsy [abstract]. Electroencephalogr Clin Neurophysiol 1988;70:P41.

179. Devinsky O, Ehrenberg B, Barthlen GM, et al. Epilepsy and sleep apnea syndrome. Neurology 1994;44:2060.

180. Vaughn BV, D'Cruz OF, Beach R, Messenheimer JA. Improvement of epileptic seizure control with treatment of obstructive sleep apnea. Seizure 1996;5:73.

181. Van Buren JM. Some autonomic concomitants of ictal automatisms. Brain 1958;81:505.

182. Brown ML. Cardiovascular changes associated with electroconvulsant therapy in man. Arch Neurol Psychiatry 1953;69:601.

183. Lathers CM, Schrader PL. Autonomic dysfunction in epilepsy. Characterization of cardiac neural discharge associated with pentylenetetrazol-induced seizures. Epilepsia 1982;23:633.

184. Jay GW, Leestma JE. Sudden death in epilepsy. Acta Neurol Scand Suppl 1981;82:1.

185. Aldrich M, Jahnke B. Diagnostic value of video-EEG polysomnography. Neurology 1991;41:1060.

186. Carskadon MA, Dement WC, Mitler MM, et al. Guidelines for the multiple sleep latency test (MSLT): a standard measure of sleepiness. Sleep 1986;9:519.

# Chapter 35

# Sleep-Related Violence and Forensic Medicine Issues

Mark W. Mahowald and Carlos H. Schenck

In all of us, even in good men, there is a lawless, wild-beast nature which peers out in sleep.
—Plato, *The Republic*

Acts done by a person asleep cannot be criminal, there being no consciousness.[1]

Increasingly, practitioners are asked to render legal opinions pertaining to violent or injurious behaviors arising from the sleep period. Automatic behaviors (automatisms) resulting in illegal behaviors have been described in many different conditions. Those automatisms arising from wakefulness are reasonably well-understood. Advances in sleep medicine have made it apparent that some complex behaviors, occasionally resulting in forensic science implications, are exclusively state-dependent (i.e., occur during the sleep period).

## Case Example

You are asked to see a 24-year-old single white male who enjoyed a stellar college academic and athletic record and has no history of psychiatric disease, drug or substance abuse, sleep disorders, or interpersonal violence. In December 1993, he was living in Japan, working as a teacher. He was very sleep deprived before returning to the United States. He estimates that he had received no more than 15 hours of sleep in the preceding 4 days. When he returned to the United States, he went to a friend's house, where he drank 1.5 beers and took one hit of marijuana. He was noticed to be acting "peculiar."

After leaving his friend's house, he got out of the car, saw a police officer approaching the car. He told his friends it was "okay," as he knew the officer (which was not true).

He sat down in the police car. The officer drove him to where his friends were waiting. Each got out of the car and met behind the car. He viciously attacked the officer, fracturing his jaw, knocking him unconscious. Another officer arrived. The patient was finally subdued by a number of people. According to his friends, his behavior was extremely inappropriate, irrational, and completely out of character.

He had no recollection of any of the event from riding in the car until he "came to" in a hospital. He does remember "dreamlike" images. He stated: "I thought I was in hell." He remembers being held down by a number of arms but could not identify bodies or faces. He thinks he thought he was in hell because of the burning sensation on his face. In retrospect, he thought this may have been fragmentary imagery of being held down by the policemen, and having been sprayed in the face with Mace. Extensive psychiatric and chemical dependency evaluations performed after the incident were unrevealing. He was charged with a felony. A conviction would destroy his developing business in Japan. Based on reports from his friends and the police, and on his fragmentary memories, he never denied having committed the violent act. He wanted to have his behavior declared a "noninsane automatism," which would have very different legal implications.

# NEUROPHYSIOLOGY OF SLEEP-RELATED VIOLENCE

## The State-Dependent Nature of Violence

The concept that sleep is simply the passive absence of wakefulness is no longer tenable. Not only is sleep an active, rather than passive, process, it is clear that sleep comprises two completely different states: rapid eye movement (REM) sleep, and non-REM (NREM) sleep. Therefore, our lives are spent in three entirely different states of being: wakefulness, REM sleep, and NREM sleep. Research has indicated that bizarre behavioral syndromes can occur as a result of the incomplete declaration or rapid oscillation of these states.[2,3] Although the automatic behaviors of some "mixed states" are relatively benign (i.e., shoplifting in narcolepsy),[4] others may be associated with violent behaviors.

The fact that violent or injurious behaviors may arise in the absence of conscious wakefulness and without conscious awareness raises the crucial question of how such complex behavior can occur. Examination of extensive animal experimental studies provides preliminary answers. The widely held concept that the brain stem and other more "primitive" neural structures primarily participate in elemental or vegetative rather than behavioral activities is inaccurate. Overwhelming data document that extremely complex emotional and motor behaviors can originate from these more primitive structures without involvement of "higher" neural structures such as the cortex.[5–11]

## Sleep-Related Disorders Associated with Violence

Violent sleep-related behaviors have been reviewed in the context of automated behavior in general. There are well-documented cases of (1) somnambulistic homicide, attempted homicide, and suicide; (2) murders and other crimes with sleep drunkenness (confusional arousals); and (3) sleep terrors or sleepwalking with potential violence or injury. A wide variety of disorders may result in sleep-related violence.[2] Conditions associated with sleep-period–related violence are listed in Table 35-1. These conveniently fall into two major categories: neurologic and psychiatric (see also Chapter 31).

**Table 35-1.** Conditions Associated with Sleep-Related Violent Behavior

**Neurologic sleep disorders**
Disorders of arousal (confusional arousals [sleep drunkenness], sleepwalking, sleep terrors)*
REM sleep behavior disorder*
Nocturnal seizures*
Automatic behavior
    Narcolepsy and idiopathic central nervous system
      hypersomnia
    Sleep apnea
    Sleep deprivation (including jet lag)

**Psychogenic sleep disorders**
Dissociative states (may arise exclusively from sleep)
    Fugues
    Multiple personality disorder
    Psychogenic amnesia
Malingering
Munchausen by proxy

*Obstructive sleep apnea may mimic or trigger these parasomnias.

# NEUROLOGIC CONDITIONS ASSOCIATED WITH VIOLENT BEHAVIORS

Extrapolating from animal data to the human condition, it has been shown that structural lesions at multiple levels of the nervous system may result in wakeful violence.[12–15] The animal studies provide insights into violent behaviors in the disorders of arousal, REM sleep behavior disorder (RBD), and sleep-related seizures.

## Disorders of Arousal

The disorders of arousal comprise a spectrum ranging from confusional arousals to sleepwalking to sleep terrors.[16,17] Although there is usually amnesia for the event,[18,19] vivid dreamlike mentation may be experienced and reported.[20] Contrary to popular opinion, these disorders may actually begin in adulthood, and are most often not associated with psychopathology.[20,21] The commonly held belief that sleepwalking and sleep terrors are always benign is erroneous: The accompanying behaviors may be violent, resulting in considerable injury to the individual, others, or damage to the environment.[2,20]

Febrile illness, alcohol, sleep deprivation, and emotional stress may serve to trigger disorders of arousal in susceptible individuals.[22–24] Sleep deprivation is well-known to result in confusion, disorientation, and hallucinatory phenomena.[25–30] Medications such as sedative-hypnotics, neuroleptics, minor tranquilizers, stimulants, and antihistamines, often in combination with each other or with alcohol, may also play a role.[31–33]

Confusional arousals (also called *sleep drunkenness*) occur during the transition between sleep and wakefulness and represent a disturbance of cognition and attention despite the motor behavior of wakefulness, resulting in complex behavior without conscious awareness.[34–36] These arousals may be potentiated by sleep deprivation or the ingestion of alcohol or sedative-hypnotics before sleep onset.[37] Episodes of "automatic behavior" occur in the setting of chronic sleep deprivation or other conditions associated with state admixture (shoplifting has been reported during a period of automatic behavior in a narcoleptic).[4,38,39]

Numerous associations exist between obstructive sleep apnea (OSA) and confusional arousals. Patients with OSA may experience frequent arousals that may serve to trigger arousal-induced precipitous motor activity.[40] Therefore, the observed clinical behavior, a confusional arousal, is actually the result of another underlying primary sleep disorder—OSA. Guilleminault and Silvestri[40] have made the following observations:

> It is well known that adult patients with OSA syndrome present nocturnal wandering during sleep. These patients frequently demonstrate yelling and screaming during sleep, as well as confusion, disorientation, and sleepwalking. . . . The nocturnal hypoxia and the repetitive sleep disruptions secondary to the OSA syndrome readily explain these symptoms.

This is another example of why overnight polysomnography (PSG) studies with extensive physiologic monitoring are mandatory in the evaluation of problematic motor parasomnias. Disorders of arousal may also be precipitated by adequate or incomplete treatment of sleep apnea with nasal continuous positive airway pressure.[41,42]

Apparently criminal acts performed without conscious awareness during sleep drunkenness (formerly termed *somnolentia*) are not recently observed phenomena; a classic book on sleep written well over a century ago contains dramatic descriptions of

cases. The author concluded that sleep drunkenness "is a natural phenomenon, to which all are liable."[43] Treatment of the disorders of arousal include both pharmacologic (benzodiazepine and tricyclic antidepressant) and behavioral (hypnosis) approaches.[44]

Some very dramatic cases have been tried using the confusional arousal defense. In one, the "Parks" case in Canada, the defendant drove 23 km, killed his mother-in-law, and attempted to kill his father-in-law. Somnambulism was the legal defense, and he was acquitted.[45] In another, the "Butler, PA" case, a confusional arousal attributed to underlying OSA was offered as a criminal defense for a man who fatally shot his wife during his usual sleeping hours. He was found guilty.[46]

Inappropriate sexual behaviors during the sleep state, presumably the results of an admixture of wakefulness and sleep, have been well-described.[47–51] Conversely, recurrent sexually oriented hypnagogic hallucinations experienced by patients with narcolepsy may be so vivid and convincing that they may lead to false accusations.[52]

Sleep talking has also been addressed by the legal system regarding the issue of whether utterances made during sleep are admissible in court.[53]

Specific incidents of sleep-related violence include

- Somnambulistic homicide and attempted homicide[31,54–68]
- Murders and other crimes with sleep drunkenness,[23] sleep apnea,[24] and narcolepsy[4]
- Suicide[69,70]
- Sleep terrors and sleepwalking with potential violence or injury[71–74]; episodes may be drug induced[31,75]

The behavioral similarities between documented sleepwalking and sleep terror violence in humans and "sham rage" as seen in the "hypothalamic savage" syndrome are striking.[76] Although it has been assumed that the sham rage animal preparations are awake, there is some suggestion that similar preparations are behaviorally awake but (partially) physiologically asleep, with apparent hallucinatory behavior possibly representing REM sleep dreaming occurring during wakefulness, dissociated from other REM state markers.[77]

The neural bases of aggression and rage in the cat have been reviewed, indicating that there is clearly an anatomic basis for some forms of violent behavior.[78] The prosencephalic system may serve to control and elaborate, rather than initiate, behaviors originating from deeper structures.[10] In humans with confusional arousals or sleep drunkenness, which can result in confusion or aggression, there is clear electroencephalographic (EEG) evidence of rapid oscillations between wakefulness and sleep.[35,36] It may be that such behaviors occurring in states other than wakefulness are the expression of motor or affective activity generated by lower structures unmonitored and unmodified by the cortex. Keeping in mind that not only is sleep a very active process, but that the generators or effectors of many components of both REM and NREM sleep reside in the brain stem and other "lower" centers, it is not surprising that prominent motoric and affective behaviors do occur during sleep.

Other, very important factors beyond the scope of this chapter include (1) the known effect of genetics on violence, and (2) the well-demonstrated effects of environmental and social factors on the structure and function of the nervous system.[79] In one study of 31 individuals awaiting trial or sentencing for murder, none was neurologically or psychiatrically normal.[13] Central nervous system plasticity may play a role in the environmental or social factors involved in violence.[80,81] These factors are undoubtedly operant in both waking and sleep-related violence.

### REM Sleep Behavior Disorder

RBD represents an experiment of nature predicted in 1965 by animal experiments[82] and identified in humans in 1986.[38] During REM sleep in normal individuals, there is active paralysis of all somatic muscles (excluding the diaphragm and eye movement muscles). In RBD, there is the absence of REM sleep atonia, which permits the "acting out" of dreams, often with dramatic and violent or injurious behaviors. The oneiric (dream) behavior demonstrated by cats with bilateral peri–locus coeruleus lesions and by humans with spontaneously occurring RBD clearly arises from and continues to occur during REM sleep.[38,82,83] These oneiric behaviors displayed by patients with RBD are often misdiagnosed as manifestations of a seizure or psychiatric

disorder. RBD is usually idiopathic, but may be associated with underlying neurologic disorders, particularly Parkinson's disease and related conditions.[38,84] The overwhelming male predominance (90%) of RBD[85] raises questions about the relationship of sexual hormones to aggression and violence.[86,87] The violent and injurious nature of RBD behaviors has been extensively reviewed elsewhere.[85,88] Treatment with clonazepam is highly effective.[85]

As with the disorders of arousal, underlying sleep apnea may simulate RBD, again underscoring the necessity for thorough formal PSG evaluation of these cases.[89]

### Seizures

The association between seizures and violence has been long debated. It is plain that, on occasion, seizures may result in violent, injurious, or even homicidal behavior.[2,90] Of particular note is the frantic and elaborate nocturnal motor activity that may result from seizures originating in the orbital, mesial, or prefrontal region.[91–96] "Episodic nocturnal wanderings," a condition clinically indistinguishable from other forms of sleep-related motor activity such as complex sleepwalking, but which is responsive to anticonvulsant therapy, has also been described.[97–99] Aggression and violence may be preictal, ictal, and postictal. The postictal violence is often induced or perpetuated by the good intentions of bystanders trying to calm the patient after a seizure.[100] Again, underlying sleep apnea may masquerade as nocturnal seizures.[101–103]

### PSYCHIATRIC CONDITIONS ASSOCIATED WITH VIOLENT BEHAVIORS

#### Psychogenic Dissociative States

Waking dissociative states may result in violence.[104] It is now apparent that dissociative disorders may arise exclusively or predominately from the sleep period.[2,105] Virtually all patients with nocturnal dissociative disorders evaluated at our center were victims of repeated physical or sexual abuse beginning in childhood.[106]

## Malingering

Although uncommon, malingering must also be considered in cases of apparent sleep-related violence. Our center has seen a young man who developed progressively violent behaviors, directed exclusively at his wife, apparently arising from sleep. This behavior included beating her and chasing her with a hammer. After extensive neurologic, psychiatric, and PSG evaluation, it was determined that this behavior represented malingering.

## Munchausen Syndrome by Proxy

In Munchausen syndrome by proxy, a child is reported to have medically serious symptoms, which, in fact, are induced by an adult—usually a caregiver, often a parent. The use of surreptitious video monitoring in sleep disorder centers during sleep (with the parent present) has documented the true etiology for reported sleep apnea and other unusual nocturnal spells.[107–109]

## MEDICOLEGAL EVALUATION

### Clinical and Laboratory Evaluation of Waking and Sleep Violence

The history of complex, violent, or potentially injurious motor behavior arising from the sleep period should suggest the possibility of one of the conditions discussed earlier. Our experience with more than 200 adult cases of sleep-related injury or violence has repeatedly indicated that clinical differentiation among RBD, disorders of arousal, sleep apnea, sleep-related psychogenic dissociative states, and other psychiatric conditions may be impossible without PSG study.[110] It is likely that violence arising from the sleep period is more frequent than previously assumed.[111]

The legal implications of automatic behavior have been discussed and debated in both the medical and legal literature.[1,112–116] As with nonsleep automatisms, the identification of a specific underlying organic or psychiatric condition does not establish causality for any given deed.

These conditions are diagnosable and most are treatable. Clinical evaluation should include a complete review of sleep-wake complaints from both the victim and bed partner (if available). This should be followed by a thorough general physical, neurologic, and psychiatric examination. The diagnosis may only be suspected clinically. Extensive polygraphic study using an extensive scalp EEG at a paper speed of 15 mm per second, electromyographic monitoring of all four extremities, and continuous audiovisual recording are mandatory for correct diagnosis in atypical cases.[16,40,98,117–122] Clinical and laboratory evaluations are best performed by experienced clinicians.[110]

Establishing the diagnosis of nocturnal seizures may be extremely difficult, as the motor activity associated with the spell often obscures the EEG pattern. Further, there may be no scalp-EEG manifestation of the seizure activity. Numerous well-documented cases of scalp electrode EEG–negative but depth electrode EEG–positive electrical seizure activity[123,124] or video-documented clinical seizure activity[125] have been reported. Another possible explanation for scalp electrode EEG–negative seizures is that some seizures are manifested electrically with only generalized low-voltage fast activity, not followed by postictal slowing.[126] Such activity arising from EEG-recorded sleep may be misinterpreted as an "arousal," rather than as electrical seizure activity. Seizure activity arising in the limbic system may spread to other more "primitive" structures, with resultant clinical behaviors, without EEG involvement of the neocortex.[9] The treatment of nocturnal seizures is similar to that of diurnal seizures. The difficulties in evaluating nocturnal seizures discussed earlier (obscuring of the record by movement artifact, absence of surface EEG abnormality or electrical seizure activity, lack of postictal slowing, misinterpretation of electrical seizure activity as an "arousal") emphasize the necessity of extensive, inperson laboratory monitoring. Scantily channeled "ambulatory" EEG monitoring has led to the misdiagnosis of functional psychiatric disease in a number of our patients subsequently demonstrated to have bona fide nocturnal seizures. If the history or physical examination suggests underlying neurologic disease, further studies such as magnetic resonance imaging or computed tomographic scanning of the brain, multimodal (visual, auditory, and somatosensory) evoked potentials, and formal neuropsychometric evaluation are indicated.

It is often possible to state that a given violent act may have arisen from the sleep period or from a mixed state of wakefulness and sleep; it is usually impossible to prove that a given incident did, in fact, represent a sleep-related automatism. To assist in the determination of the putative role of an underlying sleep disorder in a specific violent act, we have proposed guidelines, modified from Bonkalo (sleepwalking),[23] Walker (epilepsy),[127] and Glasgow (automatism in general)[128] and formulated from our clinical experience[2]:

1. There should be reason (by history or formal sleep laboratory evaluation) to suspect a sleep disorder. Similar episodes, with benign or morbid outcome, should have occurred previously.

2. The duration of the action is usually brief (minutes).

3. The behavior is usually abrupt, immediate, impulsive, and without apparent motivation. Although ostensibly purposeful, it is inappropriate to the situation, out of (waking) character for the individual, and without evidence of premeditation.

4. The victim is someone who merely happened to be present, and who may have been the stimulus for the arousal.

5. Immediately after return of consciousness, there is perplexity or horror, without attempt to escape, conceal, or cover up the action. There is evidence of lack of awareness on the part of the individual during the event.

6. There is usually some degree of amnesia for the event; however, this amnesia need not be complete.

7. In the case of night terrors, sleepwalking, or sleep drunkenness, the act may (a) occur on awakening after at least 1 hour of sleep or, rarely, immediately on falling asleep; (b) occur on attempts to awaken the subject; (c) have been potentiated by alcohol ingestion, sedative-hypnotic administration, or prior sleep deprivation.

The proposition that the presence of a sleep disorder may be a legitimate defense in cases of violence arising from the sleep period has been met with much skepticism.[129] For credibility, evaluations of such complex cases are best performed in experienced sleep disorders centers with interpretation by a veteran clinical polysomnographer. Due to the complex nature of many of these disorders, a multidisciplinary approach is highly recommended.

### Legal and Forensic Medicine Evaluation

With the identification of ever increasing causes, manifestations, and consequences of sleep-related violence comes the responsibility of neurologists and sleep medicine practitioners to educate the general public and practicing clinicians as to the occurrence and nature of such behaviors, and as to their successful treatment. More importantly, the onus is on the sleep medicine professional to educate and assist the legal profession in cases of sleep-related violence that result in forensic medicine issues. This often presents difficult ethical problems, as most "expert witnesses" are retained by either the defense or the prosecution, leading to the tendency for an expert witness to become an advocate or partisan for one side. Historically, this has been fertile ground for the appearance of "junk science" in the courtroom[130]—from Bendectin to triazolam to breast implants. Junk science leads to junk justice and altered standards of care.[131] Much attention has been paid to the existence and prevalence of junk science in the courtroom, with recommendations to minimize its occurrence. Before accepting a case, the sleep professional should become familiar with this most important issue. A good starting point is the highly informative book *Galileo's Revenge: Junk Science in the Courtroom.*[130] There is some hope that the judicial system is paying more attention to the process of authentic science and may move to accept only valid scientific evidence.[132,133] To address the problem of junk science in the courtroom, many professional societies are calling for guidelines and some have developed guidelines for expert witness qualifications and testimony.[134–136] The American Sleep Disorders Association and the American Academy of Neurology have adopted their own guidelines, which include the following qualifications for expert witnesses[137,138]: (1) a current, valid, unrestricted license; (2) a diploma from the American Board of Sleep Medicine; (3) familiarity with the clinical practice of sleep medicine; and (4) active involvement in clinical practice at the time of the event. Guidelines for expert testimony include the following:

1. The witness must be impartial. The ultimate test for accuracy and impartiality is the willingness of the witness to prepare testimony that can be presented unchanged for use by either the plaintiff or the defendant.

2. Fees should relate to time and effort and should not be contingent on the outcome of the claim. Fees should not exceed 20% of the practitioner's annual income.

3. The practitioner should be willing to submit his or her testimony for peer review.

4. To establish consistency, the expert witness should make records of previous expert witness testimony available to the attorneys and expert witnesses of both parties.

5. The expert witness must not become a partisan or advocate in the legal proceeding.

Familiarizing oneself with these guidelines may be helpful in a given case, as the expert witness from each side should be held to the same standards.[139]

The current legal system unfortunately must consider a parasomnia case strictly in terms of choosing between insane or noninsane automatism. Such a choice results in two very different consequences for the accused: if found insane, the individual is committed to a mental hospital for an indefinite period of time; if found sane, the individual is acquitted without any mandated medical consultation or follow-up or any stipulated deterrent concerning a recurrence of sleepwalking with criminal charges induced by high-risk behavior.

One fortunate but unexplained fact is that nocturnal sleep-related violence is rarely a recurrent phenomenon.[140] Recurrence is reported occasionally, and possibly should be termed a *noninsane automatism*. Thorough evaluation and effective treatment are mandatory before the patient can be regarded as no longer a menace to society.[141] In other cases, clear precipitating events can be identified, and must be avoided to be exonerated from legal culpability. This concept has led to the proposal of two new forensic categories: *parasomnia with continuing danger as a noninsane automatism* and *intermittent state-dependent continuing danger*.[141]

One reasonable approach to dealing with the automatisms mentioned earlier from a legal stand-point would be to add a category of acquittal that allowed for innocence based on lack of guilt consequent to certain diagnoses—specific disorders that could be categorized by a group of subspecialty clinicians in consultation with the legal profession.[142]

Another suggestion has been to hold a two-stage trial that would first establish who committed the act and then deal separately with the issue of culpability. The first part would be held before a jury; the second in front of a judge with medical advisors present.[143]

### Forensic Sleep Medicine Experts As Impartial Friends of the Court (**Amicus Curae**)

One infrequently used tactic to improve scientific testimony is to use a court-appointed "impartial expert."[130] If potential witnesses volunteer to serve as a court-appointed expert rather than one appointed by either the prosecution or defense, this practice may be encouraged. Other proposed measures include the development of a specific section in scientific journals dedicated to expert witness testimony extracted from public documents with request for opinions and consensus statements from appropriate specialists and the development of a library of circulating expert testimony that could be used to discredit irresponsible, professional, witnesses.[130] Good science is not determined by the credentials of the expert witness, but by scientific consensus.[131]

## SUMMARY AND DIRECTIONS FOR THE FUTURE

It is abundantly clear that violence may occur during any one of the three states of being. That which occurs during REM or NREM sleep may have occurred without conscious awareness and is due to one of a number of completely different disorders. Violent behavior during sleep may result in events that have forensic science implications. The apparent suicide, assault, or murder may be the unintentional, nonculpable, but catastrophic result of disorders of arousal, sleep-related seizures, RBD, or psychogenic dissociative states. The majority of these conditions are diagnosable and, more importantly, treatable. The social and legal implications are obvious.

The fields of neurology and sleep medicine must pursue further productive study and discourse, and request adequate funding to objectively study the following important questions: What is the prevalence of these disorders? How are they best and most accurately diagnosed? How can the usually present prodromes be taken seriously? Why is there a male predominance in many of these conditions? How can these disorders best be treated or, better yet, prevented? Are "social stressors" more prevalent in this population? What is the best way to deal with forensic science issues? What should be done with the offender? What is the likelihood of recurrence? Is such behavior a sane or an insane automatism?[68] How can the potential victim of the violence be protected?

More research, both basic science and clinical, is urgently needed to further identify and elaborate on the components of both waking and sleep-related violence, with particular emphasis on neurobiologic, neuroplastic, genetic, and socioenvironmental factors.[13–15] The study of violence and aggression will be greatly enhanced by close cooperation among clinicians, basic science researchers, and social scientists.

## REFERENCES

1. Fitzgerald PJ. Voluntary and Involuntary Acts. In AG Guest (ed), Oxford Essays in Jurisprudence. Oxford, UK: Oxford University Press, 1961;1.
2. Mahowald MW, Bundlie SR, Hurwitz TD, Schenck CH. Sleep violence—forensic science implications: polygraphic and video documentation. J Forensic Sci 1990;35:413.
3. Mahowald MW, Schenck CH. Dissociated states of wakefulness and sleep. Neurology 1992;42:44.
4. Zorick FJ, Salis PJ, Roth T, Kramer M. Narcolepsy and automatic behavior: a case report. J Clin Psychiatry 1979;40:194.
5. Grillner S, Dubic R. Control of locomotion in vertebrates: spinal and supraspinal mechanisms. Adv Neurol 1988;47:425.
6. Cohen AH. Evolution of the Vertebrate Central Pattern Generator for Locomotion. In AH Cohen, S Rossignol, S Grillner (eds), Neural Control of Rhythmic Movements in Vertebrates. New York: Wiley, 1988;129.
7. Corner MA. Brainstem Control of Behavior: Ontogenetic Aspects. In R Klemm, RP Vertes (eds), Brainstem Mechanisms of Behavior. New York: Wiley, 1990;239.
8. Siegel A, Pott CB. Neural substrates of aggression and flight in the cat. Prog Neurobiol 1988;31:261.
9. LeDoux JE. Emotion. In VB Montcastle, F Plum, SR Geiger (eds), Handbook of Physiology: The Nervous System: Higher Functions of the Brain, Part I. Baltimore: Williams & Wilkins, 1987;419.
10. Berntson GG, Micco DJ. Organization of brainstem behavioral systems. Brain Res Bull 1976;1:471.
11. Bandler R. Brain mechanisms of aggression as revealed by electrical and chemical stimulation: suggestion of a central role for the midbrain periaqueductal region. Prog Psychobiol Physiol Psychol 1988;13:67.
12. Weiger WA, Bear DM. An approach to the neurology of aggression. J Psychiatr Res 1988;22:85.
13. Blake PY, Pincus JH, Buckner C. Neurologic abnormalities in murderers. Neurology 1995;45:1641.
14. Elliott FA. Violence. The neurologic contribution: an overview. Arch Neurol 1992;49:595.
15. Greene AF, Lynch TF, Decker B, Coles CJ. A psychological theoretical characterization of interpersonal violence offenders. Aggress Violent Behav 1997;2:273.
16. Mahowald MW, Schenck CH. Parasomnia Purgatory—the Epileptic/Non-Epileptic Interface. In AJ Rowan, JR Gates (eds), Non-Epileptic Seizures. Boston: Butterworth–Heinemann, 1993;123.
17. Mahowald MW, Rosen GM. Parasomnias in children. Pediatrician 1990;17:21.
18. Fisher C, Kahn E, Edwards A, et al. A psychophysiological study of nightmares and night terrors. III. Mental content and recall of stage 4 night terrors. J Nerv Ment Dis 1974;158:174.
19. Thorpy MJ, Diagnostic Classification Steering Committee. ICSD—International Classification of Sleep Disorders: Diagnostic and Coding Manual. Rochester, MN: American Sleep Disorders Association, 1990.
20. Schenck CH, Hurwitz TD, Bundlie SR, Mahowald MW. Sleep-related injury in 100 adult patients: a polysomnographic and clinical report. Am J Psychiatry 1989;146:1166.
21. Hartmann E, Greenwald D, Brune P. Night-terrors—sleep walking. Sleep Res 1982;11:121.
22. Vela Bueno A, Blanco BD, Cajal FV. Episodic sleep disorder triggered by fever—a case presentation. Waking Sleeping 1980;4:243.
23. Bonkalo A. Impulsive acts and confusional states during incomplete arousal from sleep: criminological and forensic implications. Psychiatr Q 1974;48:400.
24. Raschka LB. Sleep and violence. Can J Psychiatry 1984;29:132.
25. Nielsen TA, Dumont M, Montplaisir J. A 20-h recovery sleep after prolonged sleep restriction: some effects of competing in a world record-setting cinemarathon. J Sleep Res 1995;4:78.
26. Williams HL, Morris GO, Lubin A. Illusions, Hallucinations and Sleep Loss. In L West (ed), Hallucinations. New York: Grune & Stratton, 1962;158.
27. Shurley JT. Hallucinations in Sensory Deprivation and Sleep Loss. In L West (ed), Hallucinations. New York: Grune & Stratton, 1962;87.
28. Babkoff H, Sing HC, Thorne DR, et al. Perceptual distortions and hallucinations reported during the course of sleep deprivation. Percept Mot Skills 1989; 68:787.

29. Brauchi JT, West LJ. Sleep deprivation. JAMA 1959;171:1.

30. Belenky GL. Unusual visual experiences reported by subjects in the British army study of sustained operations, exercise early call. Mil Med 1979;144:695.

31. Luchins DJ, Sherwood PM, Gillin JC, et al. Filicide during psychotropic-induced somnambulism: a case report. Am J Psychiatry 1978;135:1404.

32. Huapaya LVM. Seven cases of somnambulism induced by drugs. Am J Psychiatry 1979;136:985.

33. Charney DS, Kales A, Soldatos CR, Nelson JC. Somnambulistic-like episodes secondary to combined lithium-neuroleptic treatment. Br J Psychiatry 1979;135:418.

34. Lipowski ZJ. Delirium (acute confusional state). Am Med Assoc J 1987;258:1789.

35. Guilleminault C, Phillips R, Dement WC. A syndrome of hypersomnia with automatic behavior. Electroencephalogr Clin Neurophysiol 1975;38:403.

36. Roth B, Nevsimalova S, Sagova V, et al. Neurological, psychological and polygraphic findings in sleep drunkenness. Arch Suisses Neurol Neurochir Psychiatry 1981;129:209.

37. Roth B, Nevsimalova S, Rechtschaffen A. Hypersomnia with "sleep drunkenness." Arch Gen Psychiatry 1972;26:456.

38. Mahowald MW, Schenck CH. REM Sleep Behavior Disorder. In MH Kryger, WC Dement, T Roth (eds), Principles and Practice of Sleep Medicine (2nd ed), Philadelphia: Saunders, 1994;574.

39. Parkes JD. Sleep and Its Disorders. London: Saunders, 1985.

40. Guilleminault C, Silvestri R. Disorders of Arousal and Epilepsy During Sleep. In Sterman MB, Shouse MN, Passouant P (eds), Sleep and Epilepsy. New York: Academic, 1982;513.

41. Millman RP, Kipp GR, Carskadon MA. Sleepwalking precipitated by treatment of sleep apnea with nasal CPAP. Chest 1991;99:750.

42. Pressman MR, Meyer TJ, Kendrick-Mohamed J, et al. Night terrors in an adult precipitated by sleep apnea. Sleep 1995;18:773.

43. Hammond WA. Sleep and Its Derangements. Philadelphia: Lippincott, 1869.

44. Mahowald MW, Schenck CH. NREM parasomnias. Neurol Clin 1996;14:675.

45. Broughton R, Billings R, Cartwright R, et al. Homicidal somnambulism: a case report. Sleep 1994;17:253.

46. Nofzinger EA, Wettstein RM. Homicidal behavior and sleep apnea: a case report and medicolegal discussion. Sleep 1995;18:776.

47. Wong KE. Masturbation during sleep—a somnambulistic variant? Singapore Med J 1986;27:542.

48. Shapiro CM, Fedoroff JP, Trajanovic NN. Sexual behavior in sleep: a newly described parasomnia. Sleep Res 1996;25:367.

49. Hurwitz TD, Mahowald MW, Schenck CH, Schluter JL. Sleep-related sexual abuse of children. Sleep Res 1989;18:246.

50. Buchanan A. Sleepwalking and indecent exposure. Med Sci Law 1991;31:38.

51. Rosenfeld DS, Elhajjar AJ. Sleepsex: a variant of sleepwalking. Arch Sex Behav 1998;27:269.

52. Hays P. False but sincere accusations of sexual assault made by narcoleptic patients. Medico-Legal Bull 1992; 60:265.

53. Regina v. Warner. Ontario Reports 1995;136.

54. Hopwood JS, Snell HK. Amnesia in relation to crime. J Ment Sci 1933;79:27.

55. Tarsh MJ. On serious violence during sleep-walking [letter]. Br J Psychiatry 1986;148:476.

56. Bartholomew AA. On serious violence during sleep-walking [letter]. Br J Psychiatry 1986;148:476.

57. Sleepwalking and guilt [editorial]. BMJ 1970;2:186.

58. Oswald I, Evans J. On serious violence during sleep-walking. Br J Psychiatry 1985;147:688.

59. Morris N. Somnambulistic homicide: ghosts, spiders, and North Koreans. Res Judicatae 1951;5:29.

60. Fenwick P. Murdering while asleep. BMJ 1986; 293:574.

61. Podolsky E. Somnambulistic homicide. Dis Nerv Syst 1959;20:534.

62. Podolsky E. Somnambulistic homicide. Med Sci Law 1961;1:260.

63. Yellowlees D. Homicide by a somnambulist. J Ment Sci 1878;24:451.

64. Howard C, D'Orban PT. Violence in sleep: medico-legal issues and two case reports. Psychol Med 1987;17:915.

65. Schatzman M. To sleep, perchance to kill. New Scientist 1986;26:60.

66. Lochel M. Sleepwalking in children and adolescents— medical history, child psychiatric and electro-encephalographic aspects. Acta Paedopsychiatr 1989;52:112.

67. Ovuga EBL. Murder during sleepwalking. East Afr Med J 1992;69:533.

68. Brooks AD. Law, Psychiatry, and the Mental Health System. Boston: Little, Brown, 1974.

69. Kleitman N. Sleep and Wakefulness. Chicago: University of Chicago Press, 1963.

70. Chuaqui C. Suicide and abnormalities of consciousness. Can Psychiatr Assoc J 1975;20:25.

71. Hartmann E. Two case reports: night terrors with sleepwalking—a potentially lethal disorder. J Nerv Ment Dis 1983;171:503.

72. Rauch PK, Stern TA. Life-threatening injuries resulting from sleepwalking and night terrors. Psychosomatics 1986;27:62.

73. Ferber R, Boyle MP. Injury associated with sleepwalking and sleep terrors in children. Sleep Res 1984;13:141.

74. Chin CN. Sleep walking in adults: two case reports. Med J Malaysia 1987;42:132.

75. Scott AIF. Attempted strangulation during phenothiazine-induced sleep-walking and night terrors. Br J Psychiatry 1988;153:692.

76. Glusman M. The hypothalamic 'savage' syndrome. Assoc Res Nerv Ment Dis 1974;52:52.

77. Kitsikis A, Steriade M. Immediate behavioral effects of kainic acid injections into the midbrain reticular core. Behav Brain Res 1981;3:361.

78. Siegel A, Shaikh MB. The neural bases of aggression and rage in the cat. Aggression Violent Behav 1997;2:241.

79. Valzelli L. Psychobiology of Aggression and Violence. New York: Raven, 1981.

80. Pons TP, Garraghty PE, Ommaya K, et al. Massive cortical reorganization after sensory deafferentation in adult Macaques. Science 1991;252:1857.

81. Edelman GM. Neural Darwinism. New York: Basic Books, 1987.

82. Jouvet M, Delorme F. Locus coeruleus et sommeil paradoxal. C R Soc Biol 1965;159:895.

83. Hendricks JC, Morrison AR, Mann GL. Different behaviors during paradoxical sleep without atonia depend upon lesion site. Brain Res 1982;239:81.

84. Schenck CH, Bundlie SR, Mahowald MW. Delayed emergence of a parkinsonian disorder in 38% of 29 older men initially diagnosed with idiopathic rapid eye movement sleep behavior disorder. Neurology 1996;46:388.

85. Schenck CH, Hurwitz TD, Mahowald MW. REM sleep behavior disorder: a report on a series of 96 consecutive cases and a review of the literature. J Sleep Res 1993;2:224.

86. Goldstein M. Brain research and violent behavior. Arch Neurol 1974;30:1.

87. Moyer KE. Kinds of aggression and their physiological basis. Comm Behav Biol 1968;2:A65.

88. Dyken ME, Lin-Dyken DC, Seaba P, Yamada T. Violent sleep-related behavior leading to subdural hemorrhage. Arch Neurol 1995;52:318.

89. Nalamalapu U, Goldberg R, DePhillipo M, Fry JM. Behaviors simulating REM behavior disorder in patients with severe obstructive sleep apnea. Sleep Res 1996;1996:311.

90. Hindler CG. Epilepsy and violence. Br J Psychiatry 1989;155:246.

91. Collins RC, Carnes KM, Price JL. Prefrontal-limbic epilepsy: experimental functional anatomy. J Clin Neurophysiol 1988;5:105.

92. Quesney LF, Krieger C, Leitner C, et al. Frontal Lobe Epilepsy: Clinical and Electrographic Presentation. In RJ Porter, et al. (eds), Advances in Epileptology: XVth Epilepsy International Symposium. New York: Raven, 1984;503.

93. Ludwig B, Ajmone Marsan B, Strauss E, Wada JA. Cerebral seizures of probable orbitofrontal origin. Epilepsia 1987;16:141.

94. Waterman K, Purves SJ, Strauss E, Wada JA. An epileptic syndrome caused by mesial frontal lobe seizure foci. Neurology 1987;37:577.

95. Tharp B. Orbital frontal seizures. An unique electroencephalographic and clinical syndrome. Epilepsia 1972;13:627.

96. Williamson PD, Spencer SS. Clinical and EEG features of complex partial seizures of extratemporal origin. Epilepsia 1986;27(Suppl 2):46.

97. Maselli RA, Rosenberg RS, Spire JP. Episodic nocturnal wanderings in non-epileptic young patients. Sleep 1988;11:156.

98. Pedley TA, Guilleminault C. Episodic nocturnal wanderings responsive to anticonvulsant drug therapy. Ann Neurol 1977;2:30.

99. Plazzi G, Tinuper P, Montagna P, et al. Epileptic nocturnal wanderings. Sleep 1995;18:749.

100. Fenwick P. The nature and management of aggression in epilepsy. J Neuropsychiatry 1989;1:418.

101. Houdart R, Mamo H, Tomkiewicz H. La forme epileptogene du syndrome de Pickwick. Rev Neurol 1960;103:466.

102. Kryger M, Quesney LF, Holder D, et al. The sleep deprivation syndrome of the obese patient. Am J Med 1974;56:531.

103. Guilleminault C. Natural History, Cardiac Impact and Long-term Follow-up of Sleep Apnea Syndrome. In C Guilleminault, E Lugaresi (eds), Sleep/Wake Disorders: Natural History, Epidemiology, and Long-term Evolution. New York: Raven, 1983;107.

104. McCaldon RJ. Automatism. Can Med Assoc J 1964; 91:914.

105. Fleming J. Dissociative episodes presenting as somnambulism: a case report. Sleep Res 1987;16:263.

106. Schenck CH, Milner D, Hurwitz TD, et al. Dissociative disorders presenting as somnambulism: polysomnographic, video and clinical documentation (8 cases). Dissociation 1989;2:194.

107. Rosenberg DA. Web of deceit: a literature review of Munchausen syndrome by proxy. Child Abuse Negl 1987;11:547.

108. Light MJ, Sheridan MS. Munchausen syndrome by proxy and sleep apnea. Clin Pediatr 1990;29:162.

109. Griffith JC, Slovik LS. Munchausen by proxy and sleep disorders medicine. Sleep 1989;12:178.

110. Mahowald MW, Schenck CH, Rosen GR, Hurwitz TD. The role of a sleep disorders center in evaluating sleep violence. Arch Neurol 1992;49:604.

111. Broughton RJ, Shimizu T. Sleep-related violence: a medical and forensic challenge. Sleep 1995;18:727.

112. Whitlock FA. Criminal Responsibility and Mental Illness. London: Butterworths, 1963.

113. Prevezer S. Automatism and involuntary conduct. Criminal Law Rev 1958;440.

114. Prevezer S. Automatism and involuntary conduct. Criminal Law Rev 1958;361.

115. Williams G. Criminal Law. London: Stevens, 1961.

116. Forensic Psychiatry. In FE Camps (ed), Gradwohl's Legal Medicine (3rd ed). Chicago: Wright, 1976;505.

117. Soldatos CR, Vela-Bueno A, Bixler EO, et al. Sleepwalking and night terrors in adulthood, clinical and EEG findings. Clin Electroencephalogr 1980; 11:136.

118. Halbreich U, Assael M. Electroencephalogram with spheniodal needles in sleepwalkers. Psychiatr Clin 1978;11:213.

119. Popoviciu L, Szabo L, Corfariu O, et al. A Study of the Relationships of Certain Pavor Nocturnus (PN) Attacks with Nocturnal Epilepsy. In L Popoviciu, B Asgian, G Badiu (eds), Sleep 1978. Fourth European Congress on Sleep Research. Tirgu-Mures. Basel: Karger, 1980;599.

120. Dervent A, Karacan I, Ware JC, Williams RL. Somnambulism: a case report. Sleep Res 1978;7:220.

121. Amir N, Navon P, Silverberg-Shalev R. Interictal electroencephalography in night terrors and somnambulism. Isr J Med Sci 1985;21:22.

122. Broughton R. Childhood Sleepwalking, Sleep Terrors, and Enuresis Nocturna: Their Pathophysiology and Differentiation from Nocturnal Epileptic Seizures. In L Popoviciu, B Ashian, G Badiu (eds), Sleep 1978. Fourth European Congress on Sleep Research. Tirgu-Mures. Basel: Karger, 1980;103.

123. Ajmone Marsan C, Abraham K. Considerations on the use of chronically implanted electrodes in seizure disorders. Confin Neurol 1966;27:95.

124. Morris IHH, Dinner DS, Luders H, et al. Supplementary motor seizures: clinical and electroencephalographic findings. Neurology 1988;38:1075.

125. Devinsky O, Kelley K, Porter RJ, Theodore WH. Clinical and electroencephalographic features of simple partial seizures. Neurology 1988;38:1347.

126. Gastaut H, Roger J, Ouahchi S, et al. An electro-clinical study of generalized epileptic seizures of tonic expression. Epilepsia 1963;4:15.

127. Walker EA. Murder or epilepsy? J Nerv Ment Dis 1961;133:430.

128. Glasgow GL. The anatomy of automatism. N Z Med J 1965;64:491.

129. Guilleminault C, Kushida C, Leger D. Forensic sleep medicine and nocturnal wanderings. Sleep 1995;18:721.

130. Huber PW. Galileo's Revenge: Junk Science in the Courtroom. New York: Basic Books, 1991.

131. Weintraub MI. Expert witness testimony: a time for self-regulation? Neurology 1995;45:855.

132. Loevinger L. Science as evidence. Jurimetrics J 1995;153:153.

133. Foster KR, Bernstein DE, Huber PW. Phantom Risk: Scientific Inference and the Law. Cambridge, MA: MIT Press, 1993.

134. Committee on Medical Liability. Guidelines for expert witness testimony. Pediatrics 1989;83:312.

135. Anonymous. Guidelines for the physician expert witness. American College of Physicians. Ann Intern Med 1990;113:789.

136. Bone R, Rosenow E. ACCP guidelines for an expert witness. Chest 1990;98:1006.

137. American Sleep Disorders Association. ASDA guidelines for expert witness qualifications and testimony. APSS Newslett 1993;8:23.

138. American Academy of Neurology. Qualifications and guidelines for the physician expert witness (Newsletter). Neurology 1989;39:A9.

139. Mahowald MW, Schenck CH. Complex motor behavior arising during the sleep period: forensic science implications. Sleep 1995;18:724.

140. Guilleminault C, Moscovitch A, Leger D. Forensic sleep medicine: nocturnal wandering and violence. Sleep 1995;18:740.

141. Schenck CH, Mahowald MW. A polysomnographically documented case of adult somnambulism with long-distance automobile driving with frequent nocturnal violence: parasomnia with continuing danger as a noninsane automatism. Sleep 1995;18:765.

142. Beran RG. Automatisms—the current legal position related to clinical practice and medicolegal interpretation. Clin Exp Neurol 1992;29:81.

143. Fenwick P. Automatism, medicine, and the law. Psychol Med Monogr Suppl 1990;17:1.

# Glossary of Terms*

**Actigraph**  A biomedical instrument for the measurement of body movement.

**Active sleep**  A term used in the phylogenetic and ontogenetic literature for the stage of sleep that is considered to be equivalent to REM sleep (see *REM sleep*).

**Alpha activity**  An alpha EEG wave or sequence of waves with a frequency of 8–13 Hz.

**Alpha-delta sleep**  Sleep in which alpha activity occurs during slow-wave sleep. Because alpha-delta sleep is rarely seen without alpha occurring in other sleep stages, the term *alpha sleep* is preferred.

**Alpha intrusion (-infiltration, -insertion, -interruption)**  A brief superimposition of EEG alpha activity on sleep activities during a stage of sleep.

**Alpha rhythm**  An EEG rhythm with a frequency of 8–13 Hz in human adults that is most prominent over the parieto-occipital cortex when the eyes are closed. The rhythm is blocked by eye opening or other arousing stimuli. It is indicative of the awake state in most normal individuals and is most consistent and predominant during relaxed wakefulness, particularly with reduction of visual input. The amplitude is variable but typically is below 50 μV in adults. The alpha rhythm of an individual usually slows by 0.5–1.5 Hz and becomes more diffuse during drowsiness. The frequency range also varies with age; it is slower in children and older age groups than in young to middle-age adults.

**Alpha sleep**  Sleep in which alpha activity occurs during most, if not all, sleep stages.

**Apnea**  Cessation of airflow at the nostrils and mouth lasting at least 10 seconds. There are three types of apnea: obstructive, central, and mixed. Obstructive apnea is secondary to upper airway obstruction; central apnea is associated with a cessation of all respiratory movements; mixed apnea has both central and obstructive components.

**Apnea-hypopnea index**  The number of apneic episodes (obstructive, central, and mixed) plus hypopneas per hour of sleep as determined by all-night polysomnography. Synonymous with *respiratory disturbance index*.

**Apnea index**  The number of apneic episodes (obstructive, central, and mixed) per hour of sleep as determined with all-night polysomnography. Sometimes a separate obstructive apnea index or central apnea index is used.

**Arise time**  The clock time that an individual gets out of bed after the final awakening of the major sleep episode (distinguished from final wake up).

**Arousal**  An abrupt change from a deeper stage of non-REM sleep to a lighter stage, or from REM sleep to wakefulness, with the possibility of awakening as the final outcome. Arousal may be accompanied by increased tonic electromyographic activity and heart rate as well as body movements.

---

*Adapted with the permission of the American Sleep Disorders Association, Rochester, Minnesota.

**741**

**Arousal disorder** A parasomnia disorder presumed to be due to an abnormal arousal mechanism. Forced arousal from sleep can induce episodes. The classic arousal disorders are sleepwalking, sleep terrors, and confusional arousals.

**Awakening** The return to the polysomnographically defined awake state from any non-REM or REM sleep stage. It is characterized by alpha and beta EEG activity, a rise in tonic electromyography, voluntary REMs, and eye blinks. This definition of awakenings is valid only insofar as the polysomnogram is paralleled by a resumption of a reasonably alert state of awareness of the environment.

**Axial system** A means of presenting different types of information in a systematic manner using several "axes" to ensure that important information is not overlooked in light of a single major diagnosis. The International Classification of Sleep Disorders uses a three-axis system: axes A, B, and C.

**Axis A** The first level of the axial system devised by the International Classification of Sleep Disorders. Axis A includes the sleep disorder diagnoses, modifiers, and associated code numbers.

**Axis B** The second level of the axial system devised by the International Classification of Sleep Disorders. Axis B includes the sleep-related procedures, procedure features, and associated code numbers.

**Axis C** The third level of the axial system devised by the International Classification of Sleep Disorders. Axis C includes nonsleep diagnoses and associated code numbers.

**Baseline** The typical or normal state of an individual or of an investigative variable before an experimental manipulation.

**Bedtime** The clock time at which one attempts to fall asleep, as differentiated from the clock time when one gets into bed.

**Beta activity** A beta EEG wave or sequence of waves with frequency greater than 13 Hz.

**Beta rhythm** An EEG rhythm in the range of 13–35 Hz, when the predominant frequency, beta rhythm, is usually associated with alert wakefulness or vigilance and is accompanied by a high tonic EMG. The amplitude of beta rhythm is variable but usually is below 30 μV. This rhythm may be drug induced.

**Brain wave** Use of this term is discouraged. The preferred term is *EEG wave*.

**Cataplexy** A sudden decrement in muscle tone and loss of deep tendon reflexes leading to muscle weakness, paralysis, or postural collapse. Cataplexy usually is precipitated by an outburst of emotional expression, notably laughter, anger, or startle. One of the symptom tetrad of narcolepsy. During cataplexy, respiration and voluntary eye movements are not compromised.

**Cheyne-Stokes respiration** A breathing pattern characterized by regular "crescendo-decrescendo" fluctuations in respiratory rate and tidal volume.

**Chronobiology** The science of temporal, primarily rhythmic, processes in biology.

**Circadian rhythm** An innate, daily fluctuation of physiologic or behavioral functions, including sleep-wake states generally tied to the 24-hour daily dark-light cycle. Sometimes occurs at a measurably different periodicity (e.g., 23 or 25 hours) when light-dark and other time cues are removed.

**Circasemidian rhythm** A biological rhythm that has a period length of about half a day.

**Conditional insomnia** Insomnia produced by the development, during an earlier experience of sleeplessness, of conditioned arousal. Causes of the conditioned stimulus can include the customary sleep environment or thoughts of disturbed sleep. A conditioned insomnia is one component of psychophysiologic insomnia.

**Constant routine** A chronobiological test of the endogenous pacemaker that involves a 36-hour baseline monitoring period followed by a 40-hour waking episode of monitoring with the individual on a constant routine of food intake, position, activity, and light exposure.

**Cycle** Characteristic of an event exhibiting rhythmic fluctuations. One cycle is defined as the activity from one maximum or minimum to the next.

**Deep sleep** Common term for combined non-REM stage III and IV sleep. In some sleep literature, deep sleep is applied to REM sleep because of its high awakening threshold to nonsignificant stimuli (see *"Intermediary" sleep stage*; *Light sleep*).

**Delayed sleep phase** A condition that occurs when the clock hour at which sleep normally occurs is moved ahead in time within a given 24-hour sleep-wake cycle. This results in a temporarily displaced—that is, delayed—occurrence of sleep within the 24-hour cycle. The same term denotes a circadian rhythm sleep disturbance called *delayed sleep phase syndrome*.

**Delta activity**    EEG activity with a frequency of less than 4 Hz (usually 0.1–3.5 Hz). In human sleep scoring, the minimum characteristics for scoring delta waves are conventionally 75 μV amplitude (peak-to-peak) and 0.5 seconds' duration (2 Hz) or less.

**Delta sleep stage**    The stage of sleep in which EEG delta waves are prevalent or predominant—sleep stages III and IV, respectively (see *Slow-wave sleep*).

**Diagnostic criteria**    Specific criteria established in the International Classification of Sleep Disorders to aid in determining the unequivocal presence of a particular sleep disorder.

**Diurnal**    Pertaining to daytime.

**Drowsiness**    A stage of quiet wakefulness that typically occurs before sleep onset. If the eyes are closed, diffuse slowed alpha activity usually is present, which then gives way to early features of stage I sleep.

**Duration criteria**    Criteria (acute, subacute, chronic) established in the *International Classification of Sleep Disorders* for determining the duration of a particular disorder.

**Dyssomnia**    A primary disorder of initiating and maintaining sleep or of excessive sleepiness. The dyssomnias are disorders of sleep or wakefulness per se; not a parasomnia.

**Early morning arousal (early AM arousal)**    Premature morning awakening.

**Electroencephalogram (EEG)**    A recording of the electrical activity of the brain by means of electrodes placed on the surface of the head. With the electromyogram and electro-oculogram, the EEG is one of the three basic variables used to score sleep stages and waking. Sleep recording in humans uses surface electrodes to record potential differences between brain regions and a neutral reference point, or simply between brain regions. Either the C3 or C4 placement (central region, according to the International 10-20 System) is referentially (referred to an earlobe) recorded as the standard electrode derivation from which state scoring is done.

**Electromyogram (EMG)**    A recording of electrical activity from the muscular system; in sleep recording, same as muscle activity or potential. The chin EMG, along with EEG and electro-oculography, is one of the three basic variables used to score sleep stages and waking. Sleep recording in humans typically uses surface electrodes to measure activity from the submental muscles. These reflect maximally the changes in resting activity of axial body muscles. The submental muscle EMG is tonically inhibited during REM sleep.

**Electro-oculogram (EOG)**    A recording of voltage changes resulting from shifts in position of the ocular gloves, as each glove is a positive (anterior) and negative (posterior) dipole; along with the EEG and electromyogram, one of the three basic variables used to score sleep stages and waking. Sleep recording in humans uses surface electrodes placed near the eyes to record the movement (incidence, direction, and velocity) of the eyeballs. REMs in sleep form one part of the characteristics of the REM sleep state.

**End-tidal carbon dioxide**    Carbon dioxide value usually determined at the nares by an infrared carbon dioxide gas analyzer. The value reflects the alveolar or pulmonary arterial blood carbon dioxide level.

**Entrainment**    Synchronization of a biological rhythm by a forcing stimulus such as an environmental time cue (see *Zeitgeber*). During entrainment, the frequencies of the two cycles are the same or are integral multiples of each other.

**Epoch**    A measure of duration of the sleep recording, typically 20–30 seconds in duration, depending on the paper speed of the polysomnograph. An epoch corresponds to one page of the polysomnogram.

**Excessive sleepiness (-somnolence, -hypersomnia, excessive daytime sleepiness)**    A subjective report of difficulty in maintaining the alert awake state, usually accompanied by a rapid entrance into sleep when the person is sedentary. May be due to an excessively deep or prolonged major sleep episode. Can be quantitatively measured by use of subjectively defined rating scales of sleepiness, or physiologically measured by electrophysiologic tests such as the Multiple Sleep Latency Test (see *Multiple Sleep Latency Test*). Most commonly occurs during the daytime; however, excessive sleepiness may be present at night in a person whose major sleep episode occurs during the daytime, such as a shift worker.

**Extrinsic sleep disorders**   Disorders that originate, develop, or arise from causes outside of the body. The extrinsic sleep disorders are a subgroup of the dyssomnias.

**Final awakening**   The duration of wakefulness after the final wake-up time until the arise time (lights on).

**Final wake-up**   The clock time at which an individual awakens for the last time before the arise time.

**First-night effect**   The effect of the environment and polysomnographic recording apparatus on the quality of the subject's sleep during the first night of recording. Sleep is usually of reduced quality compared to what would be expected in the subject's usual sleeping environment without electrodes and other recording procedure stimuli. The subject usually is habituated to the laboratory by the time of the second night of recording.

**Fragmentation (of sleep architecture)**   The interruption of any stage of sleep owing to the appearance of another stage or wakefulness, leading to disrupted non-REM–REM sleep cycles; often used to refer to the interruption of REM sleep by movement arousals or stage II activity. Sleep fragmentation connotes repetitive interruptions of sleep by arousals and awakenings.

**Free-running**   A chronobiological term that refers to the natural endogenous period of a rhythm when *Zeitgebers* are removed. In humans, it most commonly is seen in the tendency to delay some circadian rhythms, such as the sleep-wake cycle, by approximately 1 hour every day, when a person has an impaired ability to entrain or is without time cues.

**Hertz**   A unit of frequency; preferred to the synonymous expression *cycles per second.*

**Hypercapnia**   Elevated level of carbon dioxide in blood.

**Hypersomnia**   Excessively deep or prolonged major sleep period. May be associated with difficulty in awakening. Hypersomnia is primarily a diagnostic term (e.g., idiopathic hypersomnia); *excessive sleepiness* is preferred to describe the symptom.

**Hypnagogic**   Descriptor for events that occur during the transition from wakefulness to sleep.

**Hypnagogic imagery (-hallucinations)**   Vivid sensory images occurring at sleep onset, but particularly vivid with sleep-onset REM periods. A feature of narcoleptic naps, when the onset occurs with REM sleep.

**Hypnagogic startle**   A "sleep start" or sudden body jerk (hypnic jerk), observed normally just at sleep onset and usually resulting, at least momentarily, in awakening.

**Hypnopompic (hypnopomic)**   Descriptor of an occurrence during the transition from sleep to wakefulness at the termination of a sleep episode.

**Hypopnea**   An episode of shallow breathing (airflow reduced by at least 50%) during sleep lasting 10 seconds or longer, usually associated with a fall in blood oxygen saturation.

***International Classification of Sleep Disorders* sleep code**   A code number of the *International Classification of the Sleep Disorders* that refers to modifying information of a diagnosis, such as associated symptom, severity, or duration of a sleep disorder.

**Insomnia**   Difficulty initiating or maintaining sleep. A term that is employed ubiquitously to indicate any and all gradations and types of sleep loss.

**"Intermediary" sleep stage**   A term sometimes used for non-REM stage II sleep (see *Deep sleep*; *Light sleep*). Often used, especially in the French literature, for stages combining elements of stage II and REM sleep.

**Into-bed time**   The clock time at which a person gets into bed. The into-bed time is synonymous with bedtime for many people, but not for those who spend time in wakeful activities in bed, such as reading, before attempting to sleep.

**Intrinsic sleep disorders**   Disorders that originate, develop, or arise from causes within the body. The intrinsic sleep disorders are a subgroup of the dyssomnias.

**K-alpha**   A K complex followed by several seconds of alpha rhythm; a type of microarousal.

**K complex**   A sharp, negative EEG wave followed by a high-voltage slow wave. The complex duration is at least 0.5 second, and may be accompanied by a sleep spindle. K complexes occur spontaneously during non-REM sleep, and begin and define stage II sleep. They are thought to be evoked responses to internal stimuli. They can also be elicited during sleep by external (particularly auditory) stimuli.

**Light-dark cycle**    The periodic pattern of light (artificial or natural) alternating with darkness.

**Light sleep**    A common term for non-REM sleep stage I and sometimes stage II.

**Maintenance of Wakefulness Test**    A series of measurements of the interval from lights out to sleep onset that is used in the assessment of the ability to remain awake. Subjects are instructed to try to remain awake in a darkened room when in a semireclined position. Long latencies to sleep are indicative of the ability to remain awake. This test is most useful for assessing the effects of medication on the ability to remain awake.

**Major sleep episode**    The longest sleep episode that occurs on a daily basis. Typically the sleep episode dictated by the circadian rhythm of sleep and wakefulness; the conventional or habitual time for sleeping.

**Microsleep**    An episode that lasts up to 30 seconds, during which external stimuli are not perceived. The polysomnogram suddenly shifts from waking characteristics to sleep. Microsleeps are associated with excessive sleepiness and automatic behavior.

**Minimal criteria**    Criteria of the *International Classification of Sleep Disorders* derived from the diagnostic criteria that provide the minimum features necessary for making a particular sleep disorder diagnosis.

**Montage**    The particular arrangement by which a number of derivations are displayed simultaneously in a polysomnogram.

**Movement arousal**    A body movement associated with an EEG pattern of arousal or a full awakening; a sleep-scoring variable.

**Movement time**    The term used in sleep record scoring to denote when EEG and electrooculography tracings are obscured for more than half the scoring epoch because of movement. It is scored only when the preceding and subsequent epochs are in sleep.

**Multiple Sleep Latency Test**    A series of measurements of the interval from lights out to sleep onset that is used in the assessment of excessive sleepiness. Subjects are allowed a fixed number of opportunities to fall asleep during their customary awake period. Excessive sleepiness is characterized by short latencies. Long latencies are helpful in distinguishing physical tiredness or fatigue from true sleepiness.

**Muscle tone**    A term sometimes used for resting muscle potential or resting muscle activity (see *Electromyogram*).

**Myoclonus**    Muscle contractions in the form of abrupt jerks or twitches generally lasting less than 100 msec. The term should not be applied to the periodic leg movements of sleep that characteristically have a duration of 0.5–5.0 seconds.

**Nap**    A short sleep episode that may be intentionally or unintentionally taken during the period of habitual wakefulness.

**Nightmare**    An unpleasant and frightening dream that usually occurs in REM sleep. Occasionally called a dream anxiety attack, it is not a sleep (night) terror. Nightmare in the past has been used to indicate both sleep terror and dream anxiety attacks.

**Nocturnal confusion**    Episodes of delirium and disorientation close to or during nighttime sleep; often seen in the elderly and indicative of organic central nervous system deterioration.

**Nocturnal dyspnea**    Respiratory distress that may be minimal during the day but becomes quite pronounced during sleep.

**Nocturnal penile tumescence**    The natural periodic cycle of penile erections that occur during sleep, typically associated with REM sleep. The preferred term is *sleep-related erections*.

**Nocturnal sleep**    The typical "nighttime" or major sleep episode related to the circadian rhythm of sleep and wakefulness; the conventional or habitual time for sleeping.

**Non-REM sleep**    See *Sleep stages*.

**Non-REM–REM sleep cycle (sleep cycle)**    A period during sleep composed of a non-REM sleep episode and the subsequent REM sleep episode; each non-REM–REM sleep couplet is equal to one cycle. Any non-REM sleep stage suffices as the non-REM sleep portion of a cycle. An adult sleep period of 6.5–8.5 hours generally consists of four to six cycles. The cycle duration increases from infancy to young adulthood.

**Non-REM sleep intrusion**    An interposition of non-REM sleep, or a component of non-REM sleep physiology (e.g., elevated EMG, K complex, sleep spindle, delta waves) in REM sleep; a portion of non-REM sleep not appearing in its usual sleep cycle position.

**Non-REM sleep period**    The non-REM sleep portion of non-REM–REM sleep cycle; such an episode consists primarily of sleep stages III and IV early in the night and of sleep stage II later (see *Sleep cycle*; *Sleep stages*).

**Obesity-hypoventilation syndrome** A condition of obese individuals who hypoventilate during wakefulness. Because the term can apply to several different disorders, its use is discouraged.

**Paradoxical sleep** Synonymous with *REM sleep*, which is the preferred term.

**Parasomnia** Disorder of arousal, partial arousal, or sleep stage transition, not a dyssomnia. It represents an episodic disorder in sleep (such as sleepwalking) rather than a disorder of sleep or wakefulness per se. May be induced or exacerbated by sleep.

**Paroxysm** Phenomenon of abrupt onset that rapidly attains maximum intensity and terminates suddenly; distinguished from background activity. Commonly refers to an epileptiform discharge on the EEG.

**Paroxysmal nocturnal dyspnea** Respiratory distress and shortness of breath due to pulmonary edema, which appears suddenly and often awakens the sleeper.

**Penile buckling pressure** The amount of force applied to the glans of the penis sufficient to produce at least a 30-degree bend in the shaft.

**Penile rigidity** The firmness of the penis as measured by the penile buckling pressure. Normally, the fully erect penis has maximum rigidity.

**Period** The interval between the recurrence of a defined phase or moment of a rhythmic or regularly recurring event—that is, the interval between one peak or trough and the next.

**Periodic leg movement** Rapid partial dorsiflexion of the foot at the ankle, extension of the big toe, and partial flexion of the knee and hip that occurs during sleep. The movements occur with a periodicity of 20–60 seconds in a stereotyped pattern lasting 0.5–5.0 seconds and are a characteristic feature of periodic limb movements in sleep disorder.

**Periodic limb movements in sleep** See *Periodic leg movement*.

**Phase advance** The shift of an episode of sleep or wake to an earlier position in the 24-hour sleep-wake cycle. A sleep period of 11 PM to 7 AM shifted to 8 PM to 4 AM represents a 3-hour phase advance (see *Phase delay*).

**Phase delay** A shift of an episode of sleep or wake to a later time of the 24-hour sleep-wake cycle. It is the exact opposite of *phase advance*. These terms differ from common concepts of change in clock time; to effect a phase delay, the clock is moved ahead or advanced. In contrast, to effect a phase advance, the clock moves backward (see *Phase advance*).

**Phase transition** One of the two junctures of the major sleep and wake phases in the 24-hour sleep-wake cycle.

**Phasic event (-activity)** Brain, muscle, or autonomic event of a brief and episodic nature occurring in sleep; characteristic of REM sleep, such as eye movements or muscle twitches. Usually the duration is milliseconds to 2 seconds.

**Photoperiod** The period of light in a light-dark cycle.

**Pickwickian** Descriptor for an obese person who snores, is sleepy, and has alveolar hypoventilation. The term has been applied to many different disorders and therefore its use is discouraged.

**PLM-arousal index** The number of sleep-related periodic leg movements per hour of sleep that are associated with an EEG arousal (see *Periodic leg movement*).

**PLM index** The number of periodic leg movements per hour of total sleep time as determined by all-night polysomnography. Sometimes expressed as the number of movements per hour of non-REM sleep because the movements are usually inhibited during REM sleep (see *Periodic leg movement*).

**PLM percentage** The percentage of total sleep time occupied with recurrent episodes of periodic leg movements.

**Polysomnogram** The continuous and simultaneous recording of multiple physiologic variables during sleep (i.e., EEG, electro-oculography, electromyography—the three basic stage-scoring parameters—electrocardiogram, respiratory airflow, respiratory movements, leg movements, and other electrophysiologic variables.

**Polysomnograph** A biomedical instrument for the measurement of physiologic variables of sleep.

**Polysomnographic (-recording, -monitoring, -registration, -tracings)** Describes a recording on paper, computer disc, or tape of a polysomnogram.

**Premature morning awakening** Early termination of the sleep episode, with inability to return to sleep, sometimes after the last of several awakenings. It reflects interference at the end, rather than at the commencement, of the sleep episode. A characteristic sleep disturbance of some people with depression.

**Proposed sleep disorder**   A disorder in which insufficient information is available in the medical literature to confirm the unequivocal existence of the disorder. A category of the International Classification of Sleep Disorders.

**Quiet sleep**   A term used to describe non-REM sleep in infants and animals when specific non-REM sleep stages I–IV cannot be determined.

**REM sleep**   Rapid eye movement sleep (see *Sleep stages*).

**Record**   The end product of the polysomnographic recording process.

**Recording**   The process of obtaining a polysomnographic record. The term is also applied to the end product of the polysomnographic recording process.

**REM density (-intensity)**   A function that expresses the frequency of eye movements per unit time during sleep stage REM.

**REM sleep episode**   The REM sleep portion of a non-REM–REM sleep cycle. Early in the night it may be as short as a half minute, in later cycles longer than an hour (see *Sleep stage REM*).

**REM sleep intrusion**   A brief interval of REM sleep appearing out of its usual position in the non-REM–REM sleep cycle; an interposition of REM sleep in non-REM sleep; sometimes appearance of a single, dissociated component of REM sleep (e.g., eye movements, "drop out" of muscle tone) rather than all REM sleep parameters.

**REM sleep latency**   The interval from sleep onset to the first appearance of stage REM sleep in the sleep episode.

**REM sleep onset**   The designation for commencement of a REM sleep episode. Sometimes also used as a shorthand term for a sleep-onset REM sleep episode (see *Sleep onset*; *Sleep-onset REM period*).

**REM sleep percent**   The proportion of total sleep time constituted by REM stage of sleep.

**REM sleep rebound (recovery)**   Lengthening and increase in frequency and density of REM sleep episodes, which results in an increase in REM sleep percent above baseline. REM sleep rebound follows REM sleep deprivation once the depriving influence is removed.

**Respiratory disturbance index**   The number of apneas (obstructive, central, or mixed) plus hypopneas per hour of total sleep time as determined by all-night polysomnography. Synonymous with *apnea-hypopnea index*.

**Restlessness**   Referring to quality of sleep, persistent or recurrent body movements, arousals, and brief awakenings in the course of sleep.

**Rhythm**   An event occurring with approximately constant periodicity.

**Sawtooth waves**   A form of theta rhythm that occurs during REM sleep and is characterized by a notched waveform. Occurs in bursts lasting up to 10 seconds.

**Severity criteria**   Criteria for establishing the severity of a particular sleep disorder according to three categories: mild, moderate, or severe.

**Sleep architecture**   The non-REM–REM sleep stage and cycle infrastructure of sleep understood from the vantage point of the quantitative relationship of these components to each other. Often plotted in the form of a histogram.

**Sleep cycle**   Synonymous with the non-REM–REM sleep cycle.

**Sleep efficiency (sleep efficiency index)**   The proportion of sleep in the episode potentially filled by sleep (i.e., the ratio of total sleep time to time in bed).

**Sleep episode**   An interval of sleep that may be voluntary or involuntary. In the sleep laboratory, the sleep episode occurs from the time of lights out to the time of lights on. The major sleep episode is usually the longest one.

**Sleep hygiene**   Conditions and practices that promote continuous and effective sleep. These include regularity of bedtime and arise time; conformity of time spent in bed to the time necessary for sustained and individually adequate sleep (i.e., the total sleep time sufficient to avoid sleepiness when awake); restriction of alcohol and caffeine before bedtime; and using exercise, nutrition, and environmental factors as strategies to enhance, rather than disturb, restful sleep.

**Sleepiness (somnolence, drowsiness)**   Difficulty maintaining alert wakefulness so that a person falls asleep if not actively aroused. This is not simply a feeling of physical tiredness or listlessness. When sleepiness occurs in inappropriate circumstances, it is considered excessive sleepiness.

**Sleep interruption**    Breaks in sleep resulting in arousal and wakefulness (see *Fragmentation*; *Restlessness*).

**Sleep latency**    The duration of time from lights out to the onset of sleep.

**Sleep log (-diary)**    A daily, written record of a person's sleep-wake pattern, containing information such as time of retiring and arising, time in bed, estimated total sleep time, number and duration of sleep interruptions, quality of sleep, daytime naps, use of medication or consumption of caffeine, nature of waking activities.

**Sleep-maintenance disorder (insomnia)**    Difficulty maintaining sleep, once achieved; persistently interrupted sleep without difficulty falling asleep. Synonymous with *sleep continuity disturbance*.

**Sleep mentation**    The imagery and thinking experienced during sleep. Sleep mentation usually consists of combinations of images and thoughts during REM sleep. Imagery is vividly expressed in dreams involving all the senses in approximate proportion to their waking representations. Mentation is experienced generally less distinctly in non-REM sleep, but it may be quite vivid in stage II sleep, especially toward the end of the sleep episode. Mentation at sleep onset (hypnagogic reverie) can be as vivid as in REM sleep.

**Sleep onset**    The transition from waking to sleep, normally into non-REM stage I sleep but in certain conditions such as infancy and narcolepsy into stage REM sleep. Most polysomnographers accept EEG slowing; reduction and eventual disappearance of alpha activity; presence of EEG vertex sharp transients; and slow, rolling eye movements (the components of non-REM stage I) as sufficient criteria for sleep onset; others require appearance of stage II patterns (see *Sleep latency*; *Sleep stages*).

**Sleep-onset REM period**    The beginning of sleep by entrance directly into stage REM sleep. The onset of REM occurs within 10 minutes of sleep onset.

**Sleep paralysis**    Immobility of the body that occurs in the transition from sleep to wakefulness; a partial manifestation of REM sleep.

**Sleep pattern (24-hour sleep-wake pattern)**    A person's clock-hour schedule of bedtime and arise time as well as nap behavior; may include time and duration of sleep interruptions (see *Sleep-wake cycle*; *Circadian rhythm*; *Sleep log*).

**Sleep-related erections**    The natural periodic cycle of penile erections that occur during sleep, typically associated with REM sleep. Sleep-related erectile activity can be characterized as four phases: T-up (ascending tumescence), T-max (plateau maximal tumescence), T-down (detumescence), and T-zero (no tumescence). Polysomnographic assessment of sleep-related erections is useful for differentiating organic from nonorganic erectile dysfunction.

**Sleep spindle**    Spindle-shaped bursts of 11.5- to 15.0-Hz waves lasting 0.5–1.5 seconds. Generally diffuse, but of highest voltage over the central regions of the head. The amplitude is typically less than 50 μV in the adult. One of the identifying EEG features of non-REM stage II sleep, it may persist into non-REM stages III and IV but is generally not seen in REM sleep.

**Sleep stage demarcation**    The significant polysomnographic characteristics that distinguish the boundaries of the sleep stages. In certain conditions and with drugs, sleep stage demarcations may be blurred or lost, making it difficult to identify certain stages with certainty or to distinguish the temporal limits of sleep stage lengths.

**Sleep stage episode**    A sleep stage interval that represents the stage in a non-REM–REM sleep cycle; easiest to comprehend in relation to REM sleep, which is a homogeneous stage (i.e., the fourth REM sleep episode is in the fourth sleep cycle unless a previous REM episode was skipped). If one interval of REM sleep is separated from another by more than 20 minutes, they constitute separate REM sleep episodes (and are in separate sleep cycles); a sleep stage episode may be of any duration.

**Sleep stage non-REM**    The other major sleep state apart from REM sleep; comprises sleep stages I–IV, which constitute levels in the spectrum of non-REM sleep "depth" or physiologic intensity.

**Sleep stage REM**    The stage of sleep with highest brain activity, characterized by enhanced brain metabolism and vivid hallucinatory imagery or dreaming. There are spontaneous rapid eye movements, resting muscle activity is suppressed, and awakening threshold to nonsignificant stimuli is high. The EEG is a low-voltage, mixed-frequency, non-alpha record. REM sleep is usually 20–25% of total sleep time. It is also called *paradoxical sleep.*

**Sleep stages**    Distinctive stages of sleep best demonstrated by polysomnographic recordings of the EEG, EOG, and EMG.

**Sleep stage I (non-REM stage I)**    A stage of non-REM sleep that occurs at sleep onset or that follows arousal from sleep stages II, III, IV, or REM. It consists of a relatively low-voltage EEG with mixed frequency, mainly theta and alpha activity of less than 50% of the scoring epoch. It contains EEG vertex waves; slow, rolling eye movements; and no sleep spindles, K complexes, or REMs. Stage I normally represents 4–5% of the major sleep episode.

**Sleep stage II (non-REM stage II)**    A stage of non-REM sleep characterized by the presence of sleep spindles and K complexes present in a relatively low-voltage, mixed-frequency EEG background. High-voltage delta waves may comprise less than 20% of stage II epochs. Stage II usually accounts for 45–55% of the major sleep episode.

**Sleep stage III (non-REM stage III)**    A stage of non-REM sleep defined by at least 20%, and not more than 50%, of the episode consisting of EEG waves less than 2 Hz and more than 75 μV (high-amplitude delta waves). Stage III is a delta sleep stage. "Deep" non-REM sleep, so-called slow-wave sleep, is made up of stages III and IV. Stage III is often combined with stage IV into non-REM sleep stage III/IV because of the lack of documented physiologic differences between the two. Stage III appears usually only in the first third of the sleep episode and typically comprises 4–6% of total sleep time.

**Sleep stage IV (non-REM stage IV)**    All statements concerning non-REM sleep stage III apply to stage IV except that high-voltage, EEG slow waves persist during 50% or more of the epoch. Non-REM sleep stage IV usually represents 12–15% of total sleep time. Sleepwalking, night terrors, and confusional arousal episodes generally start in stage IV or during arousals from this stage (see *Sleep stage III*).

**Sleep structure**    Similar to sleep architecture, sleep structure, in addition to encompassing sleep stages and sleep cycle relationships,

assesses the within-stage qualities of the EEG and other physiologic attributes.

**Sleep talking**    Talking in sleep that usually occurs in the course of transitory arousals from non-REM sleep. It can occur during stage REM sleep, at which time it represents a motor breakthrough of dream speech. Full consciousness is not achieved and no memory of the event remains.

**Sleep-wake cycle**    The clock-hour relationships of the major sleep and wake episodes in the 24-hour cycle (see *Phase transition*; *Circadian rhythm*).

**Sleep-wake shift (-change, -reversal)**    Displacement of sleep, entirely or in part, to a time of customary waking activity, and of waking activity to the time of the major sleep episode. Common in jet lag and shift work.

**Sleep-wake transition disorder**    A disorder that occurs during the transition from wakefulness to sleep or from one sleep stage to another. A parasomnia, not a dyssomnia.

**Slow-wave sleep**    Sleep characterized by EEG waves of duration slower than 4 Hz. Synonymous with sleep stages III and IV combined (see *Delta sleep stage*).

**Snoring**    A noise produced primarily with inspiratory respiration during sleep owing to vibration of the soft palate and the pillars of the oropharyngeal inlet. All snorers have incomplete obstruction of the upper airway, and many habitual snorers have complete episodes of upper airway obstruction.

**Spindle REM sleep**    A condition in which sleep spindles persist atypically during REM sleep, occasionally in the first REM period; seen in chronic insomnia conditions.

**Synchronized**    A chronobiological term used to indicate that two or more rhythms recur with the same phase relationship. In EEG it is used to indicate increased amplitude—and usually decreased frequency—of the dominant activities.

**Theta activity**    EEG activity with a frequency of 4–<8 Hz, generally maximal over the central and temporal cortex.

**Total recording time**    The interval from sleep onset to final awakening. In addition to total sleep time, it is comprised of the time taken up by wake periods and movement time until wake-up (see *Sleep efficiency*).

**Total sleep episode**    The total time available for sleep during an attempt to sleep. It comprises non-REM and REM sleep as well as wakefulness. Synonymous with (and preferred to) *total sleep period*.

**Total sleep time**    The amount of actual sleep time in a sleep episode; equal to total sleep episode minus awake time. Total sleep time is the total of all REM and non-REM sleep in a sleep episode.

**Tracé alternant**    EEG pattern of sleeping newborns, characterized by bursts of slow waves, at times intermixed with sharp waves, and intervening periods of relative quiescence with extreme low-amplitude activity.

**Tumescence (penile)**    Hardening and expansion of the penis (penile erection). When associated with REM sleep, it is referred to as a *sleep-related erection*.

**Twitch (body twitch)**    A very small body movement, such as a local foot or finger jerk; not usually associated with arousal.

**Vertex sharp transient**    Sharp negative potential, maximal at the vertex, occurring spontaneously during sleep or in response to a sensory stimulus during sleep or wakefulness. Amplitude varies but rarely exceeds 250 μV. Use of the term *vertex sharp wave* is discouraged.

**Wake time**    The total time scored as wakefulness in a polysomnogram occurring between sleep onset and final wake-up.

**Waxing and waning**    A crescendo-decrescendo pattern of activity, usually EEG activity.

*Zeitgeber*    German term for an environmental time cue that usually helps entrainment to the 24-hour day, such as sunlight, noise, social interaction, alarm clock.

# List of Abbreviations

| | | | |
|---|---|---|---|
| AHI | apnea-hypopnea index | MSLT | Multiple Sleep Latency Test |
| AI | apnea index | MWT | Maintenance of Wakefulness Test |
| ASDA | American Sleep Disorders Association | NPT | nocturnal penile tumescence |
| CNS | central nervous system | NREM | non–rapid eye movement (sleep) |
| CPS | cycles per second (hertz is preferred) | | |
| DIMS | disorder of initiating and maintaining sleep | PLM | periodic leg movement |
| | | PND | paroxysmal nocturnal dystonia |
| DOES | disorder of excessive somnolence | PSG | polysomnogram |
| DSM | *Diagnostic and Statistical Manual* | RDI | respiratory disturbance index |
| EEG | electroencephalogram | REM | rapid eye movement (sleep) |
| EMG | electromyogram | REMs | rapid eye movements |
| EOG | electro-oculogram | RLS | restless legs syndrome |
| Hz | hertz (cycles per second) | SDB | sleep-disordered breathing |
| ICD | International Classification of Diseases | SOREMP | sleep-onset REM period |
| ICSD | International Classification of Sleep Disorders | SWS | slow-wave sleep |
| | | TST | total sleep time |

# Index

Note: Page numbers followed by *f* indicate figures; page numbers followed by *t* indicate tables.